DATE DUE

MAY 29 1985			
MAY 29 REC'D			
MAY 19 1988			
MAY 19 REC'D			
NOV 9 1989			
OCT 31 REC'D			
DEC - 6 1998			
REC'D DEC 2 - 1998			

GAYLORD PRINTED IN U.S.A.

Ophthalmic Surgery

Fourth Edition

Ophthalmic Surgery is a volume from

Rob & Smith's

Operative Surgery

General Editors

Hugh Dudley ChM, FRCS(Ed), FRACS, FRCS
Professor of Surgery, St Mary's Hospital, London, UK

David C. Carter MD, FRCS(Ed.), FRCS(Glas.)
St Mungo Professor of Surgery, University of Glasgow;
Honorary Consultant Surgeon, Royal Infirmary, Glasgow, UK

Other volumes in this series

Ophthalmic Surgery

Fourth Edition

Edited by

Thomas A. Rice MD
Assistant Clinical Professor of Ophthalmology,
Case Western Reserve University School of Medicine,
Cleveland, Ohio, USA; formerly of The Wilmer Ophthalmological Institute

Ronald G. Michels MD
Professor of Ophthalmology, The Wilmer Ophthalmological Institute,
The Johns Hopkins University School of Medicine,
Baltimore, Maryland, USA

Walter J. Stark MD
Professor of Ophthalmology, The Wilmer Ophthalmological Institute,
The Johns Hopkins University School of Medicine,
Baltimore, Maryland, USA

The C V Mosby Company St Louis Toronto

Butterworths London Boston Durban Singapore Sydney Toronto Wellington

ISBN 0-407-00657-5

First edition published in eight volumes 1956–1958
Second edition published in fourteen volumes 1968–1971
Third edition published in nineteen volumes 1976–1981
Fourth edition published 1984

Library of Congress Cataloging in Publication Data

Main entry under title:
Rob & Smith's operative surgery.
Rev. ed. of: Operative surgery / under the general editorship of Charles Rob and Rodney Smith; associate editor, Hugh Dudley. 3rd ed. 1976–
Includes bibliographies and indexes.
Contents: [1] Alimentary tract and abdominal wall / edited by Hugh Dudley--[2] The hand / edited by Rolfe Birch, Donal Brooks--[3] Ophthalmic surgery / edited by Thomas A. Rice, Ronald G. Michels, Walter J. Stark.
1. Surgery, Operative, I. Dudley, Hugh Arnold Freeman. II. Pories, Walter J. III. Carter, David C. (David Craig) IV. Rob, Charles. V. Smith of Marlow, Rodney Smith, Baron, 1914–
VI. Operative surgery. [DNLM: 1. Hand--Surgery. W0 500 061 1982 v.7]
RD32.R6 1983 617'.91 83-14465
ISBN 0-407-00651-6 (v. 1)

Photoset by Butterworths Litho Preparation Department
Printed by Blantyre Printing & Binding Co, Ltd, Glasgow, Scotland

Contributors

Anthony J. Bron BSc, MB, FRCS
Margaret Ogilvie's Reader in Ophthalmology, University of Oxford, Oxford, UK

William E. Bruner MD
Assistant Professor of Ophthalmology, Case Western Reserve University School of Medicine, Cleveland, Ohio, USA; formerly of The Wilmer Ophthalmological Institute

David L. Guyton MD
Associate Professor of Ophthalmology, The Wilmer Ophthalmological Institute, The Johns Hopkins University School of Medicine, Baltimore, Maryland, USA

Lawrence W. Hirst MD
Associate Professor of Ophthalmology, St Louis University School of Medicine, St Louis, Missouri, USA; formerly of The Wilmer Ophthalmological Institute

Nicholas T. Iliff MD
Assistant Professor of Ophthalmology, The Wilmer Ophthalmological Institute, The Johns Hopkins University School of Medicine, Baltimore, Maryland, USA

W. Jackson Iliff MD
Assistant Professor of Ophthalmology, The Wilmer Ophthalmological Institute, The Johns Hopkins University School of Medicine, Baltimore, Maryland, USA

Peter J. McKenzie MB ChB, FARCS
Consultant Anaesthetist, Nuffield Department of Anaesthetics, Radcliffe Infirmary, Oxford, UK

A. Edward Maumenee MD
Professor of Ophthalmology and Director Emeritus, The Wilmer Ophthalmological Institute, The Johns Hopkins University School of Medicine, Baltimore, Maryland, USA

Ronald G. Michels MD
Professor of Ophthalmology, The Wilmer Ophthalmological Institute, The Johns Hopkins University School of Medicine, Baltimore, Maryland, USA

Neil R. Miller MD
Associate Professor of Ophthalmology, The Wilmer Ophthalmological Institute, The Johns Hopkins University School of Medicine, Baltimore, Maryland, USA

L. Harrell Pierce MD
Associate Professor of Ophthalmology, The Wilmer Ophthalmological Institute, The Johns Hopkins University School of Medicine, Baltimore, Maryland, USA

Harry A. Quigley MD
Associate Professor of Ophthalmology, The Wilmer Ophthalmological Institute, The Johns Hopkins University School of Medicine, Baltimore, Maryland, USA

Thomas A. Rice MD
Assistant Clinical Professor of Ophthalmology, Case Western Reserve University School of Medicine, Cleveland, Ohio, USA; formerly of The Wilmer Ophthalmological Institute

John D. Scott MA, FRCS, DO
Director, Retina Service, Addenbrooke's Hospital, University of Cambridge, Cambridge, UK

Jerry A. Shields MD
Director, Oncology Service, Wills Eye Hospital; Professor of Ophthalmology, Jefferson Medical College, Thomas Jefferson University, Philadelphia, Pennsylvania, USA

Walter J. Stark MD
Professor of Ophthalmology, The Wilmer Ophthalmological Institute, The Johns Hopkins University School of Medicine, Baltimore, Maryland, USA

Robert B. Welch MD
Associate Professor of Ophthalmology, The Wilmer Ophthalmological Institute, The Johns Hopkins University School of Medicine, Baltimore, Maryland, USA

Contributing Medical Artists

Nadine B. Sokol MA
Ophthalmic Illustrator, EyeSAT, St Louis, Missouri; formerly of Department of Art as Applied to Medicine, The Johns Hopkins University School of Medicine, Baltimore, Maryland, USA

Timothy C. Hengst MA
Assistant Professor, Department of Art as Applied to Medicine, The Johns Hopkins University School of Medicine, Baltimore, Maryland, USA

Contents

Preface

Ophthalmic surgery is one of the most interesting and technically demanding surgical disciplines, and there have been important advances during the past two decades because of expanding scientific knowledge, new operative techniques and improved instrumentation. Surgical methods have grown from a limited number of operations for conditions such as cataract, glaucoma and strabismus to a variety of refined techniques for improved treatment of these conditions and also effective management of other disorders for which no treatment methods were available before.

The purpose of this text is to describe current surgical methods and their role in treatment of various ocular disorders. We present the general principles of ophthalmic surgery and also the details of technique. In addition, each subject is organized to include information on the preoperative evaluation, indications for surgery, results, complications and postoperative management.

Each chapter deals with a different type of ophthalmic surgery and is written by a surgeon or surgeons specializing in that area. Although little of the material is original, the techniques described do reflect recent advances and the personal preferences of the authors, and they are illustrated with detailed drawings. Space limitations often prevent thorough presentation of alternative techniques, although these are frequently mentioned.

At a time when subspecialization in ophthalmology has resulted in a fragmentation of the ophthalmic literature, our intent is to provide a single, reasonably comprehensive source reflecting the current philosophies and methods of ophthalmic surgery. We believe now is an opportune time to compile this work because, in many areas, the rapid advances in surgical techniques of the past two decades have become more established. Some of the new procedures require expensive, specialized equipment or advanced surgical training, but often there are no equally effective, simpler alternatives.

We realize that some of the current methods presented will become outmoded. Even so, we present those approaches we now believe must have merit, and we hope that awareness of our present limitations in ophthalmic surgery will stimulate development of more effective methods to investigate and treat ocular diseases.

The editors gratefully acknowledge: (*1*) the capable and steadfast assistance of David Andrews of the Wilmer Institute in editing each of the chapters; (*2*) the exceptional skill and dedicated cooperation of the artists Timothy Hengst and Nadine Sokol in the preparation of the beautiful illustrations; and (*3*) the special assistance of Isabel Deleon, MD, Assistant Professor of Anesthesia, The Johns Hopkins University School of Medicine, for her scholarly review of the chapter dealing with anesthesia.

Thomas A. Rice

Ronald G. Michels

Walter J. Stark

1

Ocular anesthesia

Anthony J. Bron BSc, MB, FRCS
Peter J. McKenzie MBChB, FARCS

Introduction

The special needs of intraocular surgery are naturally the major consideration in any discussion of ocular anesthesia. This is because the eye is particularly vulnerable to damage, and the outcome of surgery may be influenced by anesthetic events. This chapter discusses general and local anesthesia for eye surgery, and the special requirements for intraocular and some extraocular procedures. The requirements for intraocular procedures are best understood by a consideration of the anatomy and physiology of the eye.

General anatomy and physiology

The eye may be considered as a fluid-filled semirigid sphere created by the corneoscleral envelope. Internally it is divided into two major compartments. The anterior chamber, containing aqueous humor, lies between the cornea anteriorly and the iris posteriorly. The iris and lens form a diaphragm between the anterior chamber and the vitreous, the largest compartment of the eye. The iris together with the ciliary body and choroid make up the uveal tract, the major vascular compartment of the globe. Choroidal thickness has been estimated to be 500–1000 μm[1,2]. Internal to the choroid lies the retina, whose axons leave the globe as the optic nerve.

Blood supply of the globe

Arterial supply

The blood supply to the globe is entirely from the ophthalmic artery, which supplies the central retinal artery and the long and short posterior ciliary arteries of the uveal tract (*Figure 1.1*). Ninety per cent of the blood flow of the eye passes through the uveal tract[3]. Blood flow through the choroid is very rapid; and despite the fact that the

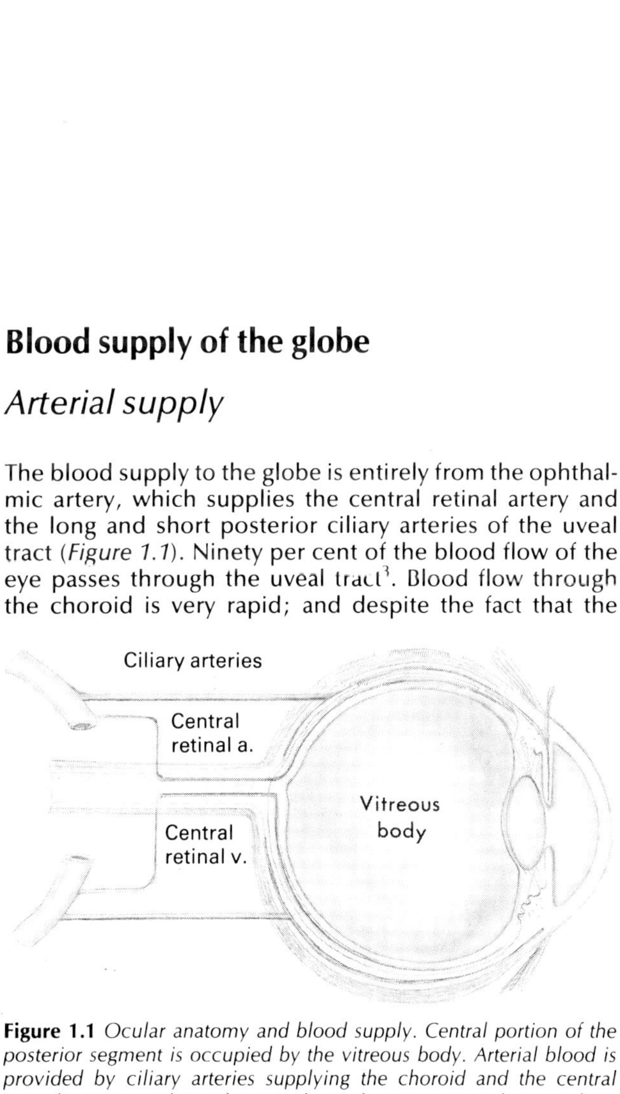

Figure 1.1 *Ocular anatomy and blood supply. Central portion of the posterior segment is occupied by the vitreous body. Arterial blood is provided by ciliary arteries supplying the choroid and the central retinal artery supplying the retinal circulation. Venous drainage from the retina is through the central retinal vein and choroidal drainage is through the vortex veins*

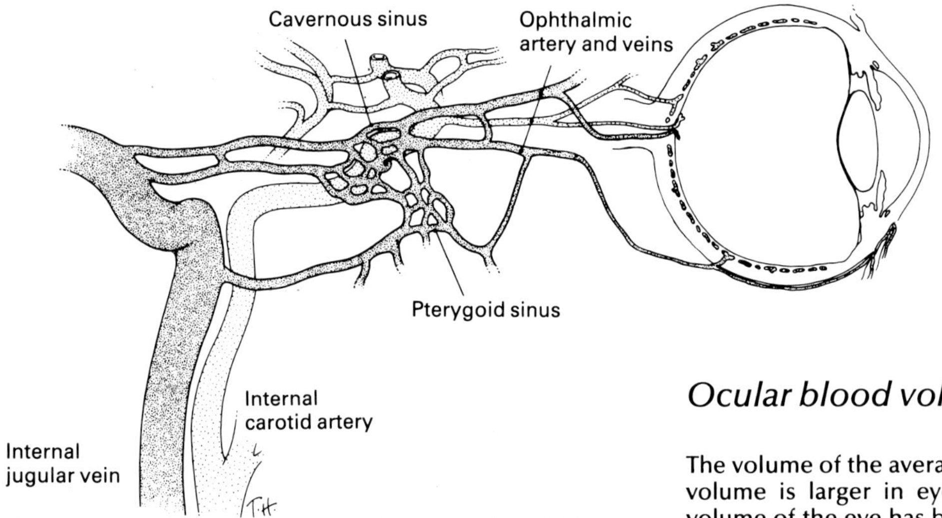

Figure 1.2 *Venous drainage from the eye joins the superior and inferior ophthalmic veins and then flows into the cavernous sinus and the pterygoid plexus. Blood leaving the eye and orbit drains into the valveless jugular veins so that pressure changes in the right side of the heart are transmitted directly to the eye*

choroid supplies the outer 60 per cent of the retina[4], the choroidal venous blood maintains a high level of oxygen saturation[5]. The responsiveness of the choroidal and retinal vasculatures to physiological changes in arterial oxygen tension (PaO_2) are different. Hypoxia leads to vasodilatation in the retinal vessels[6] but not the choroid[7]. Elevated PaO_2 leads to slight retinal arteriolar vasoconstriction with reduced blood flow[8], but has little effect on the choroidal circulation[7].

Venous drainage

Venous drainage of the retina and choroid is ultimately into the ophthalmic veins of the orbit, but within the eye the venous drainage is separate. The retinal tributary veins combine to form the central retinal vein, which crosses the subarachnoid space within the sheath of the optic nerve before exiting into the orbit. Choroidal venous blood is collected into four or five vortex veins, which exit through scleral channels to join the superior and inferior ophthalmic veins in the orbit. These drain mainly into the cavernous sinus, but they also connect with the pterygoid plexus of veins. The ophthalmic veins also connect anteriorly with the facial vein and other veins of the face (*Figure 1.2*).

Blood leaving the eye and orbit drains ultimately into the valveless internal and external jugular veins, and hence into the right side of the heart. Because of the lack of valves, pressure changes on the right side of the heart may be transmitted directly to the orbital venous system and can influence blood flow from the eye.

The lids and the conjunctiva receive their arterial supply from the branches of the internal and the external carotid artery. Venous drainage is mainly into the veins of the face, although the perilimbal bulbar veins drain partly into the episcleral venous plexus and then posteriorly into the ophthalmic veins of the orbit. This plexus also receives the aqueous humor outflow from the eye.

Ocular blood volume and flow

The volume of the average adult eye is about 6 ml, and the volume is larger in eyes with axial myopia. The blood volume of the eye has been estimated at between 200 and 300 μl[9]. Total ocular blood flow in man has not been measured, but in the dog a value of 680 μl/min has been found[10]. This represents a high blood flow perfusing the retina, equivalent to that perfusing the brain[5,11]. Because the uveal and retinal vascular systems are contained within the corneoscleral envelope, acute fluctuations in blood flow rapidly influence vascular volume and indirectly affect the intraocular pressure. However, the long-term homeostasis of intraocular pressure is determined by another fluid system, concerned with production and drainage of aqueous humor.

Ocular pressure and aqueous humor dynamics

Aqueous humor is formed by the ciliary body and circulates from the posterior chamber through the pupil into the anterior chamber. It leaves the anterior chamber through the filtering meshwork of the trabeculum and then Schlemm's canal, passing thence into the episcleral venous system. These veins connect with the ophthalmic veins of the orbit (*Figure 1.3*).

The aqueous humor volume is about 200 μl. Aqueous flow in man is about 1 per cent of the aqueous volume per minute, and thus about 2 μl/min[12]. By comparison, the blood flow of the eye is probably 400 times as great. This

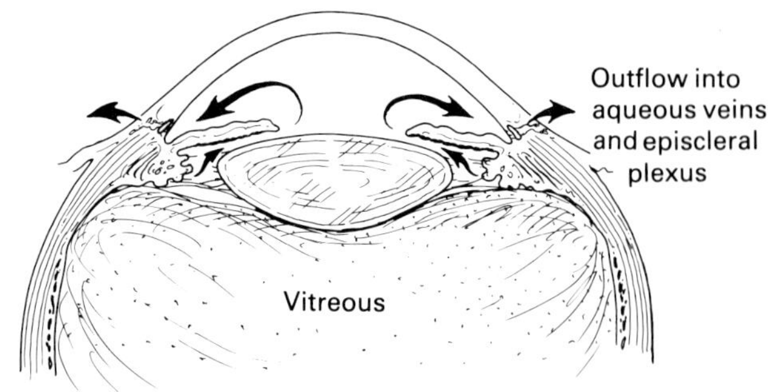

Figure 1.3 *Formation and drainage of aqueous humor. Aqueous humor is produced by the non-pigmented epithelium of the ciliary processes and passes from the posterior chamber, through the pupillary space, into the anterior chamber. It then drains out through the trabecular meshwork and canal of Schlemm into the episcleral venous plexus*

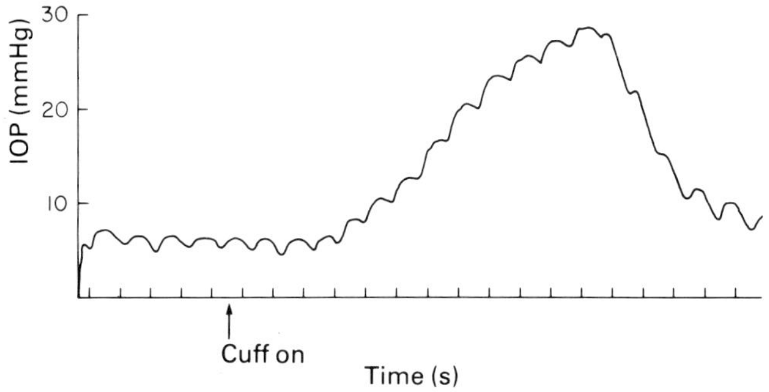

Figure 1.4 *Rapid rise in intraocular pressure following obstruction of venous drainage by inflation of a cuff around the neck*

difference in flow of the two systems results in part from the very different perfusion pressures acting in the aqueous and the vascular compartments; and it implies that obstruction of flow – for example, by totally obstructing either the aqueous or venous drainage – will produce very different effects. Obstruction of aqueous outflow will produce a comparatively slow rise in intraocular pressure, and obstruction of venous return will produce a rapid rise (*Figure 1.4*).

Perfusion pressures in the eye

Ocular fluid flow is determined by pressure gradients. In the case of aqueous flow, the 'upstream' pressure is the mean ocular pressure (e.g. 15 mmHg), and the 'downstream' pressure is that in the episcleral veins into which the aqueous drains (e.g. 9 mmHg). The usual pressure gradient for aqueous flow is therefore about 15 minus 9 = 6 mmHg (*Figure 1.5*).

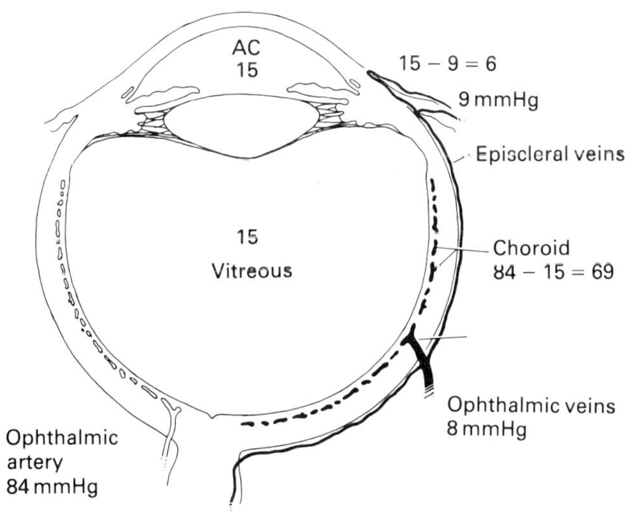

Figure 1.5 *Pressure gradients for aqueous outflow and perfusion pressure of the vascular compartment. Pressure gradient for aqueous outflow is low and is the difference between the intraocular pressure (15 mmHg) and the episcleral venous pressure (9 mmHg). The perfusion pressure of the vascular compartment is high and is the difference between the mean arterial pressure (84 mmHg) and the intraocular pressure (15 mmHg)*

The upstream pressure for vascular flow in the eye is probably the mean arterial pressure in the ophthalmic artery. This varies with posture, but it is about 84 mmHg in the supine posture in the awake subject[13,14]. The downstream pressure is mainly determined by the intraocular pressure, since the intraocular venous pressure (whether retinal or uveal) must be higher than the intraocular pressure to maintain patency of the veins. Therefore, the downstream pressure is about 15 mmHg, and the perfusion pressure in the vascular compartment is about 84 minus 15 = 69 mmHg.

The difference in perfusion pressure is the major factor determining the flow difference between the aqueous and vascular compartments. Changes in aqueous production or drainage are likely to involve such small changes in intraocular pressure, in a short period of time, that they would not be expected to cause significant clinical effects during anesthesia. However, vascular changes may produce rapid and wide fluctuations in intraocular pressure because of changes in ocular vascular volume within the corneoscleral envelope.

Another result of the difference in arterial and venous pressures is that changes in arterial and venous vascular volume do not affect the intraocular pressure in the same way. The systemic arterial pulse pressure is directly related to the ocular pulse pressure (*Figure 1.6*), but there is no relationship between mean systemic arterial pressure and the mean intraocular pressure. Although sudden changes in ocular arterial pressure will lead to changes in intraocular pressure of the same sign, a rise in arterial vascular volume, such as that due to fluctuations in arterial pressure during anesthesia, will be buffered acutely by expression of venous blood from the vascular compartment of the eye. Therefore, the ocular pressure fluctuation will be minimized. A rise in venous vascular volume of the eye, however, will not be buffered significantly by compression of the arterial compartment. Although the rise in intraocular pressure will be buffered eventually by increased aqueous drainage from the normal eye, this will

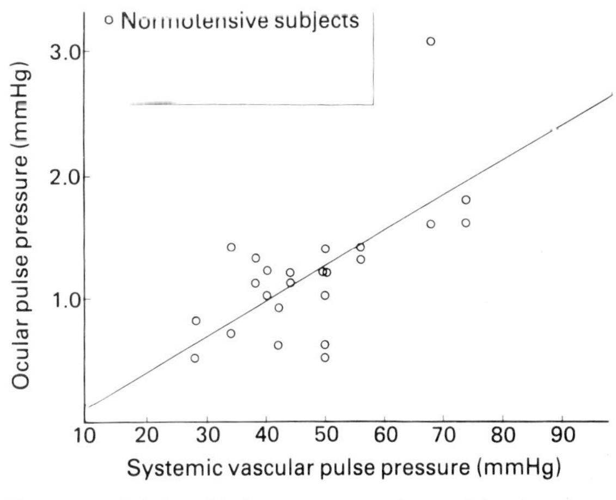

Figure 1.6 *Relationship between systemic arterial pulse pressure and the ocular pulse pressure. In normotensive patients, as the systemic vascular pulse pressure rises there is a linear rise of ocular pulse pressure*

be reduced if there is also a rise in episcleral venous pressure, thereby reducing the pressure gradient driving aqueous humor from the eye. Thus, a sustained rise in the central venous pressure would be expected to produce a sustained rise in intraocular pressure.

In the same way, compression of the globe will raise intraocular pressure, and the rise in pressure will be buffered acutely by expression of blood from the ocular vascular compartments and more slowly by expression of aqueous humor from the eye. With sustained external compression, further fluid is lost from the eye, so that when compression is released the intraocular pressure and volume will be below its usual level. Compression of the eye is of extreme importance in achieving low preoperative intraocular pressure and volume prior to cataract extraction, especially if intraocular lens (IOL) implantation is planned.

The closed eye and the open eye

The physiological relations discussed previously relate to the intact, or 'closed' eye. Once the eye is entered during surgery – as in cataract, corneal graft or glaucoma surgery – or after a penetrating injury, the intraocular pressure falls toward atmospheric pressure. With the eye thus opened, compression of the globe or a rise in the vascular volume will cause only a small rise in intraocular pressure, but it will result in displacement of the ocular contents toward the opening in the eye. This will also occur with expansion of the vascular compartment associated with a rise in the arterial and/or venous pressure within the eye and may be caused by a rise in the systemic arterial or central venous pressure. In still another situation, such as in pars plana vitrectomy, surgery may be performed in a 'closed-eye' system in which nearly watertight closure of the scleral incision(s) is maintained and there is an infusion system under hydrostatic control maintaining intraocular volume and pressure. The intraocular pressure is likely to be elevated during such surgery, thereby reducing the vascular perfusion pressure and counteracting the normal process of both aqueous humor production and outflow. In this special situation the physiological relations of the eye are dominated and altered by the more severe features of the infusion pressure and suction force that are inherent in the surgical method.

Pressure-volume relationship of the globe

When fluid is injected into the eye the intraocular pressure rises. The pressure-volume relationship of the globe is also affected by the ocular rigidity. It depends partly on the degree of distensibility of the ocular coats and partly on the compressibility of the vascular system. The corneoscleral envelope becomes increasingly more rigid and less elastic with age, so that a given change in volume causes a greater change in intraocular pressure. Another result of increased ocular rigidity with advancing age is a reduced tendency toward collapse of the globe when the eye is opened. Collapse of the globe is another factor tending to express ocular contents when the eye is opened.

Anesthetic factors in ocular surgery

Alterations in the physiology of the eye caused by anesthetic agents and other medications and procedures can have an important effect on the intraocular pressure and other features of the eye, thus affecting the safety and effectiveness of surgery. Of special importance is the relation between the eye and: (*1*) the central venous pressure (CVP); (*2*) changes in posture; (*3*) the Valsalva response; (*4*) blood-gas concentrations; and (*5*) direct ocular effects from anesthetic agents.

Central venous pressure

Recent studies suggest that, in the anesthetized supine subject, the CVP is about 5 mmHg lower than the intraocular pressure[15]. This implies that the pressure in veins immediately outside the eye (e.g. the episcleral venous plexus and ophthalmic veins of the orbit) are at a similar level, or slightly higher. If there is no major drop between the venous pressure within the eye and that outside the eye, then a rise in central venous pressure should retard venous outflow from the eye and raise intraocular vascular volume and intraocular pressure[15,16]. It would also be expected that a rise in venous pressure outside the globe would be associated with congestion of the conjunctival vasculature and perhaps increased bleeding in the operative field.

Hvidberg, Kessing and Fernandes[15] have shown that intraocular pressure closely follows changes in central venous pressure. This probably reflects the direct effect of elevated ophthalmic vein pressure on outflow from the vortex veins, rather than compression of the globe by expanded orbital vasculature. Comberg and Pilz[17] compared the effect of venous congestion produced by a neck cuff with that of injecting saline into the orbit. They found that saline injection produced a smaller rise in ocular pressure. Intraocular pressure rise induced by a neck cuff is also greatly diminished in man in the presence of diffuse choroidal sclerosis. These observations suggest that the elevated intraocular pressure is due to expanded intraocular vascular volume rather than a compressive effect by distended orbital veins.

Posture

In the non-anesthetized subject the intraocular pressure rises 1–2 mmHg in changing from the erect to the supine posture. In the anesthetized subject, adjustment of posture from the 15° head-up to the 15° head-down position is accompanied by an abrupt, square-wave rise of CVP of 5–10 mmHg[15]. This change in CVP is accompanied by a corresponding rise in intraocular pressure in the same range (*Figure 1.7*). The exact relationship between the CVP and intraocular pressure rise varies from subject to subject.

The smaller change in pressure with postural change in the awake subject may reflect a greater differential be-

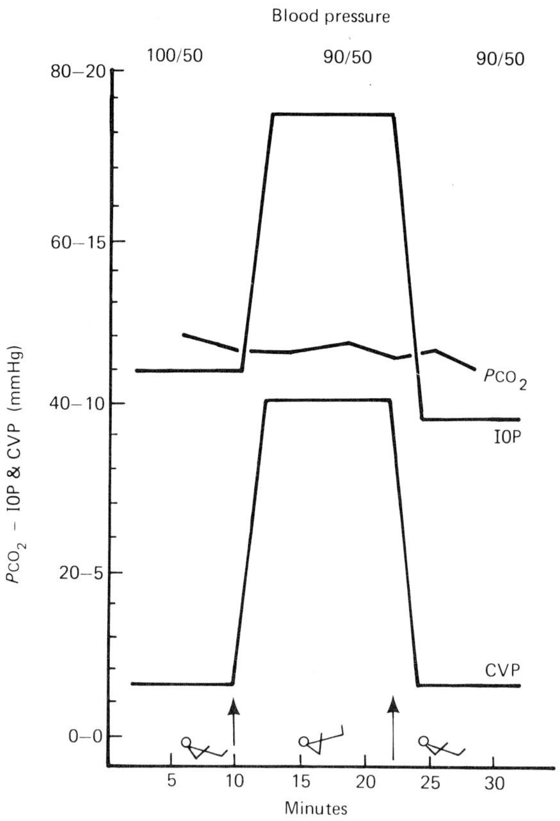

Figure 1.7 *Relationship between central venous pressure (CVP) and intraocular pressure (IOP). A rise in the CVP is accompanied by a corresponding rise in intraocular pressure in the same range (after Hvidberg, Kessing and Fernandes[15])*

tween the intraocular pressure and the ophthalmic vein pressure in the awake, erect subject. If there is a large drop in pressure between the intrascleral vortex veins and the ophthalmic veins in the orbit, then a moderate rise in CVP may not bring the ophthalmic vein pressure sufficiently close to the vortex vein pressure to retard outflow, expand the uveal vascular volume, and raise intraocular pressure. Langham and To'mey[14] suggested that cephalic venous pressure in the awake subject is about −25 mmHg in the erect posture.

Valsalva response

Such effects as laryngeal stimulation, airway obstruction, coughing, and 'straining' are all capable of stimulating a Valsalva response, involving a rise in intrathoracic pressure. This is transmitted to the cephalic arterial and venous systems, producing a square-wave rise in vascular pressures[18,19]. This vascular pressure rise is reflected precisely in the ocular vasculature, and it is associated with a rise in ocular pressure in the intact eye (*Figure 1.8*)[20,21]. A sustained Valsalva response is followed by further changes in cephalic arterial blood pressure and pulse, which are also reflected in the intraocular pressure response.

In the open eye, elevated intrathoracic pressure can be a major factor leading to prolapse of ocular contents. During cataract surgery this may lead to premature expulsion of the lens or prolapse of vitreous. In less severe cases there may be shallowing of the anterior chamber with iris prolapse and other conditions that prevent insertion of a lens implant. Elevated venous pressure might also increase the likelihood of choroidal hemorrhage.

Blood gases

Hypoxia results in vasodilation in the retinal circulation but not the uveal tract. A rise in arterial carbon dioxide tension ($Pa\text{CO}_2$) is a powerful stimulus to uveal vascular dilation[22] and a lesser stimulus to retinal vascular dilation[23,24]. Vasodilation will increase the volume of the vascular compartment of the eye and will result in a rise in intraocular pressure in the intact eye, as discussed before[25]. Conversely, positive pressure ventilation while maintaining a low $Pa\text{CO}_2$ is effective in constricting the choroidal vessels, reducing choroidal volume, and maintaining a low intraocular pressure[26–28].

Another mechanism may also account for elevated intraocular pressure with increased arterial carbon dioxide

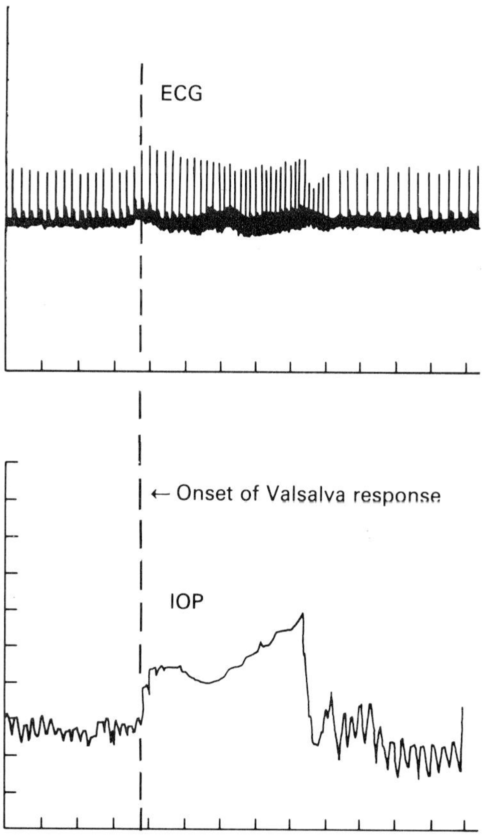

Figure 1.8 *Bottom graph: Valsalva response showing the pressure rise in IOP. The IOP shows a square-wave rise, with a later rise associated with tachycardia. Top record: ECG*

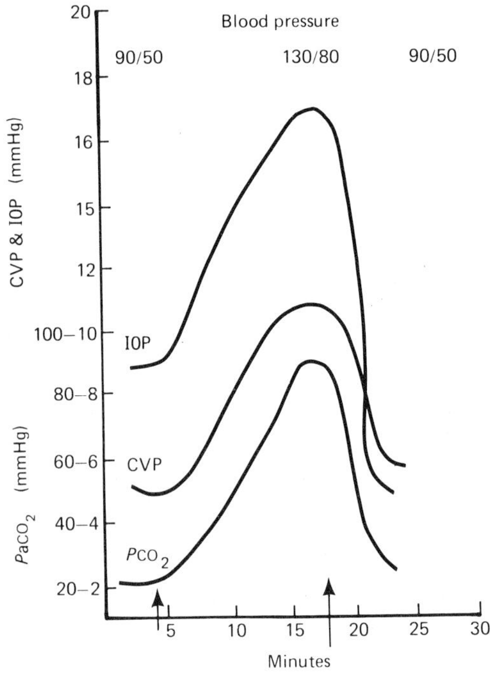

Figure 1.9 *Relationship between increased arterial carbon dioxide tension and the central venous pressure (CVP) and intraocular pressure (IOP). A rise in the* $PaCO_2$ *is accompanied by a corresponding rise in the CVP and IOP (after Hvidberg, Kessing and Fernandes[15])*

tension. In anesthetized supine patients, a rise in $PaCO_2$, whether induced by hypoventilation or by administration of a gas mixture containing 5 per cent CO_2, is accompanied by a rise in both intraocular pressure (a rise ranging from 5 to 9 mmHg) and in central venous pressure of a similar amount (*Figure 1.9*)[15].

Anesthetic agents

The uveal tract in man receives autonomic innervation, and it is assumed that this vasculature is responsive to effects of anesthetic agents that act on the sympathetic and parasympathetic nervous systems[29–31]. Although many anesthetic agents are known to have peripheral autonomic effects, their direct actions on the eye are unknown.

Preoperative considerations

The cardiovascular, respiratory, hepatic, renal, endocrine, and central nervous system (CNS) status must be assessed preoperatively by history and physical examination. Hemoglobin and/or hematocrit measurement is done on all patients, including children. Chest X-ray, electrocardiogram (ECG) and electrolyte determination should be performed routinely on patients over 50 years of age and on younger patients if there is a specific indication. All patients on diuretic therapy, diabetics, and those on long-term steroid therapy should have serum urea and electrolyte determinations. Liver function tests, pulmonary function tests and arterial blood gas determinations are performed if there are specific indications[32].

Based on experience in general surgery, general anesthesia is contraindicated after myocardial infarction within the previous 6 months except for urgent and essential procedures, because of an increased risk of another myocardial infarction. The reinfarction rate in the first 3 months is 37 per cent, decreasing to 16 per cent between 3 and 6 months, and 4 per cent thereafter. However, the risk of myocardial reinfarction associated with local anesthesia for ophthalmic surgery is not thought to be high, but information is limited[33–35].

Uncontrolled systemic hypertension is a contraindication to general anesthesia, because of cardiovascular instability and an increased risk of cardiovascular accidents[36]. The operation should be postponed, if possible, until blood pressure control is achieved. Anesthetic problems associated with dystrophia myotonica are prolonged contracture following use of succinylcholine, sensitivity to respiratory depressants, and regurgitation and aspiration due to smooth-muscle involvement[37]. Use of succinylcholine must be avoided in these cases[38].

Current upper respiratory tract infections, especially in children, are an indication to postpone surgery for a week or two. Patients with chronic bronchitis should have elective surgery when they are at their fittest, generally in the summer months. Prior respiratory physiotherapy is sometimes advisable, and smoking should be stopped.

Anticonvulsant and antihypertensive therapy, and in particular β-blockers, should be continued through the perioperative period. Monoamine oxidase inhibitors should be stopped 10–14 days before elective surgery under general anesthesia, because of possible interactions with drugs used in anesthesia, as mentioned below. Tricyclic antidepressants potentiate catecholamines, and use of epinephrine (adrenaline) and norepinephrine (noradrenaline) should be avoided in patients on these medications[39,40].

Any adverse reaction to previous anesthetic agents or other medications, and other allergies, should be noted. Repeated use of general anesthesia with the inhalation anesthetic halothane should be avoided because of possible liver damage[41].

Some commonly used drugs have perianesthetic side-effects that are especially important. Knowledge of these side-effects and their underlying mechanisms make the anesthetic management easier and safer.

The following discussion of these drugs and their side-effects has been provided by the Editors.

Methyldopa (Aldomet)

The problems encountered with methyldopa are postural hypotension and sedation. Its metabolite, α-methylnorepinephrine, replaces norepinephrine both centrally and peripherally, leading to decreased adrenergic compensatory activity. Inhibition of dopa-decarboxylase resulting in decreased synthesis of norepinephrine is another mechanism causing hypotension. Decreased norepinephrine, dopamine and serotonin in the central nervous system account for the sedative effect[42].

Propranolol (Inderal)

Problems associated with use of propranolol are acute cardiac failure and bronchoconstriction. Cardiac failure is due to decreased inotropic and chronotropic responses to adrenergic cardiac stimulation. Bronchoconstriction is caused by blockade of β_2 receptors of smooth muscles in the bronchi and bronchioli[42].

Hydrochlorothiazide (Esidrex)

Hydrochlorothiazide causes an increased exchange of potassium for sodium in the distal tubules of the kidney. This causes chronic potassium loss that affects myocardial and peripheral nerve conduction and increases sensitivity to non-depolarizing muscle relaxants[43]. Loss of potassium also exaggerates the activity of digitalis, leading to brady-arrhythmias and other disturbances of cardiac conduction[42].

Quinidine sulfate (quinidine sulphate)

Quinidine sulfate is an antiarrhythmic drug that increases the refractory period and decreases response to repetitive stimulation in skeletal muscle, probably by interfering with transmembrane sodium-potassium movement. Prolongation and increased depression of respiration have been reported with use of depolarizing and non-depolarizing muscle relaxants[42].

Anticonvulsants

Anticonvulsants can cause anesthetic-related problems because of increased biotransformation. This is due to an increase in the activity of drug-metabolizing enzymes and increased tolerance to CNS drugs[42]. Also anticonvulsants are CNS depressants that potentiate the CNS depressant effect of anesthetic agents.

Monoamine oxidase inhibitors

Monoamine oxidase inhibitors can cause orthostatic hypotension secondary to decreased release of norepinephrine (noradrenaline) from the cytoplasmic storage pool and formation of a false weak transmitter, octopamine. Hypertension, hypotension, hypothermia, convulsion and coma may occur with use of meperidine (pethidine; Demerol). Drug-metabolizing enzymes are inhibited by monoamine oxidase inhibitors, leading to the production of different metabolites or toxic metabolites of opioids[42].

Tricyclic antidepressants

Tricyclic antidepressants can cause hypotension due to blockage of norepinephrine reuptake at adrenergic nerve endings. Urinary retention, tachycardia and increased intraocular pressure may occur secondary to its marked anticholinergic effects. The combination of tricyclic antidepressants and monoamine oxidase inhibitors can lead to hypertensive crisis[42].

Echothiophate iodide (echothiopate iodide; Phospholine Iodide)

Echothiophate iodide is a pseudocholinesterase inhibitor which may cause prolonged apnea after administration of succinylcholine. Pseudocholinesterase activity begins to decrease after several days of application, and 3–6 weeks may be required for pseudocholinesterase to return to normal activity after discontinuing echothiophate[44].

Phenylephrine (neosynephrine)

Phenylephrine is used topically in ophthalmic practice to produce capillary decongestion and pupillary dilation. Systemic effects include severe hypertension and possible subarachnoid hemorrhage.

Timolol (Timoptic; Timoptol)

Timolol is an ophthalmic solution used for treatment of glaucoma. It is a β-adrenergic blocker and may cause bradycardia and bronchospasm.

General anesthesia

Patients undergoing eye surgery are often in the extreme age groups, i.e. young children for strabismus surgery or examination under anesthesia, and elderly patients for cataract extraction and other intraocular procedures. There is also an increasing frequency of chronically ill patients, such as diabetics, undergoing vitreous surgery. Factors to be considered relating to general anesthesia include: (*1*) premedication; (*2*) induction; (*3*) intubation; (*4*) maintenance of anesthesia; (*5*) extubation; and (*6*) recovery from anesthesia.

Premedication

The objective of premedication is to produce relief of anxiety and sedation, with appropriate drying of secretions. Opiates are avoided because they are unnecessary and increase the incidence of nausea and vomiting. Opiate-induced respiratory depression may also be troublesome if an anesthetic technique involving spontaneous respiration is chosen.

In some circumstances oral premedication is satisfactory, although in some hospitals premedication is routinely given by injection. An antisialogogue is not essential in elderly patients and may be unpleasant for the patient. It is, however, desirable in children, where secretions may provoke laryngeal spasm. If ketamine is to be used, an antisialogogue is probably essential. The antiemetic, sedative and antisialogogue actions of scopolamine (hyoscine) are useful. Scopolamine should not be used in elderly patients, because it may cause confusion and restlessness.

A satisfactory regimen is as follows. In adults under 65 years old, diazepam (Valium) 7.5–15 mg is given orally 2 hours before the operation, together with atropine 0.4–0.6 mg or scopolamine 0.4–0.6 mg intramuscularly. In adults over 65, diazepam 5–10 mg is given orally 2 hours before the operation, and this may be combined with atropine 0.4–0.6 mg intramuscularly. In the very frail or elderly patients, atropine 0.6 mg intramuscularly or no premedication whatsoever may be safer. Diazepam is a tranquilizing, centrally acting muscle relaxant and amnesic agent. Oral absorption is rapid and complete. Intramuscular injection is best avoided because it is painful and absorption is erratic.

In the United States, children over 2 years of age would commonly be given a combination selected from pentobarbital (pentobarbitone; Nembutal) 2–4 mg/kg intramuscularly 1 hour preoperatively; meperidine (pethidine; Demerol) 0.5–1 mg/kg intramuscularly; promethazine (Phenergan) 0.5 mg/kg intramuscularly; atropine 0.02 mg/kg intramuscularly. The usual combinations are meperidine-pentobarbital-atropine and meperidine-promethazine-atropine. If the exact time of surgery cannot be anticipated, it is recommended that intramuscular premedications be given 'on call'. In Great Britain a common approach would be trimeprazine syrup (Vallergan forte) 3–4 mg/kg body weight orally (to a maximum of 90 mg) and atropine 0.3–0.6 mg orally, both given 2 hours preoperatively. If desired, the atropine may be given 0.3–0.6 mg intramuscularly, 1 hour preoperatively. Infants less than 18 months of age are not given narcotics or sedatives because of the danger of respiratory depression and airway obstruction while they are unattended. Premedication is limited to atropine alone.

In patients undergoing outpatient surgery, premedication is omitted in most cases. Atropine is desirable for children, especially if ketamine is to be used or if intubation is planned.

Induction of anesthesia

Adults

Any of the currently available intravenous induction agents are satisfactory for use in adults, with the exception of ketamine, which often produces psychological disturbances in adults on awakening and cannot be used in 'open-eye' cases because it raises intraocular pressure. Thiopental sodium (thiopentone sodium; pentothal) produces reliably smooth induction, but it has a tendency to depress the cardiovascular system, especially in the debilitated patient. It produces a transient fall in intraocular pressure[45]. The long physiological half-life of thiopental causes a noticeable 'hangover' effect in the elderly but is now probably the most commonly used induction agent.

Etomidate, a new induction agent widely used outside the United States, is a derivative of imidazole, and it is now related to other agents used. It may have specific advantages in ophthalmic surgery. Etomidate produces an immediate and sustained fall in intraocular pressure of about 40 per cent lasting for at least 20 min[46]. Cardiovascular stability is excellent with etomidate, and no adverse allergic reactions have yet been reported. It is rapidly metabolized, and thus recovery is free from 'hangover'. However, troublesome side-effects include: (*1*) pain on injection, which can be reduced by use of a larger vein and mixing it with a local anesthetic agent; (*2*) myoclonic movements, which can be lessened by premedication. Furthermore etomidate abolishes the stress response after intravenous infusion and for this reason its more widespread use must await a fuller appraisal.

Children

Induction in children may be by inhalation or by the intravenous route. The preferences of the child and the anesthetist may be taken into account. If intubation is not required and where access is adequate with a mask, such as during probing of the nasolacrimal duct or examination under anesthesia, inhalational induction with halothane in nitrous oxide and oxygen is satisfactory.

If endotracheal intubation is planned, the intravenous route allows rapid induction and injection of a muscle relaxant to facilitate intubation. Alternatively, deep inhalational anesthesia with halothane, enflurane or isoflurane (Forane) will allow intubation.

Endotracheal intubation

Endotracheal intubation is necessary for intraocular surgery under general anesthesia to allow access to the eye and to ensure a clear airway. It also allows controlled ventilation, if desired, by using a cuffed endotracheal tube.

Spraying the trachea and larynx with 4 per cent lidocaine (lignocaine; Xylocaine) just before intubation reduces the likelihood of coughing or straining because of irritation caused by the tube and helps ensure smooth extubation. If local anesthetic spray is used, the patient should have nothing by mouth for about 3 hours after induction to avoid aspiration or thermal damage to the oropharynx. If intubation is used in young children, careful observation is needed after surgery because of the possibility of stridor from postintubation edema of the glottis or subglottic area.

Muscle relaxants are used to facilitate intubation without coughing or straining and to allow controlled intermittent positive pressure ventilation (IPPV) when necessary. Succinylcholine (suxamethonium; Scoline) is commonly used as the muscle relaxant. It is a short-acting 'depolarizing' drug that rapidly produces profound relaxation, and the effect lasts only about 5 minutes.

Succinylcholine causes a transient rise in intraocular pressure lasting less than 5 minutes[47]. The mechanism of this effect is probably a tonic contraction of the extraocular muscles[48–50]. However, it has also been suggested that the rise in intraocular pressure caused by succinylcholine is due to choroidal vasodilation[51], and pretreatment with a depolarizing muscle relaxant to abolish fasciculation does not reliably prevent the intraocular pressure rise[52].

Whatever the mechanism of action of succinylcholine that causes a rise in intraocular pressure, if this drug is used in cases with an 'open' eye, such as from a penetrating injury, contraction of the extraocular muscles and/or choroidal vasodilation could cause prolapse of the intraocular contents. Instead, a non-depolarizing relaxant such as pancuronium bromide (Pavulon) or curare can be used where it is safe to do so. Use of non-depolarizing relaxants may be hazardous in such cases if intubation proves difficult.

Succinylcholine is broken down by plasma pseudocholinesterase[53]. The topical antiglaucoma agent, echothiophate iodide (echothiopate; Phospholine Iodide), is a potent anticholinesterase agent and may cause prolongation of action of succinylcholine, leading to prolonged apnea. This event must be treated with IPPV until reversal occurs. Succinylcholine is avoided, therefore, in patients being treated with echothiophate, and echothiophate is discontinued preoperatively when possible.

Muscle relaxants of the non-depolarizing (curare-like) type tend to cause a fall in intraocular pressure by relaxing the extraocular muscles and by lowering the arterial pressure[54]. Alcuronium chloride (not yet available in the United States) can be used effectively, although it causes a small lowering of arterial blood pressure[55]. Pancuronium is an alternative if hypotension is undesirable[56].

Maintenance of anesthesia

The major choice in technique is between spontaneous or controlled ventilation. In both cases a volatile agent such as halothane (Fluothane), enflurane (Ethrane) or isoflurane (Forane) in nitrous oxide and oxygen is used to maintain anesthesia. The former agents lower intraocular pressure, perhaps by depression of midbrain and hypothalamic centers[57,58]. If an intraocular bubble will be injected during retinal or vitreous surgery, nitrous oxide is stopped at least 10 minutes before the bubble is injected and is withheld during the rest of the operation. This is done to permit clearing of the nitrous oxide through the lungs before intraocular gas injection, and thereby to avoid an equilibration between the soluble nitrous oxide and the injected gas that would cause rapid temporary expansion of the bubble size and possible marked elevation of the intraocular pressure.

Spontaneous ventilation

Spontaneous ventilation has the advantage of simplicity and ease of extubation without the need for reversal of muscle relaxation. Mean intrathoracic pressure is also negative, leading to low central venous pressure. However, the patient must be kept at a deep level of anesthesia to avoid coughing and straining due to irritation by the endotracheal tube. This causes respiratory depression and a raised $Paco_2$.

The deep anesthesia will help to counteract the rise in intraocular pressure produced by the raised $Paco_2$, but it is also desirable to position the patient in a 10–15° head-up tilt to lower venous pressure in the orbit. Problems of hypotension caused by these maneuvers may be troublesome, especially in the elderly. Deep anesthesia is also associated with a prolonged recovery time. The anesthetic system used to administer the gases must offer minimal expiratory resistance to prevent rises in intrathoracic pressure, and should not result in rises in $Paco_2$.

Controlled ventilation

Controlled ventilation with N_2O and a small (0.5–1 per cent) concentration of halothane has certain advantages for intraocular surgery. $Paco_2$ may be maintained at a normal level or lowered, if desired, to reduce intraocular pressure. Non-depolarizing muscle relaxants relax the extraocular muscles and reduce the risk of coughing or straining during the procedure, without the need for deep anesthesia. The synthetic opiate, fentanyl (phenoperidine; Sublimaze) (50–100 μg), may be given before induction to reduce the dose needed of induction and maintenance agents, and may reduce coughing on extubation.

It has been suggested that positive pressure ventilation may increase intraocular pressure because of increased intrathoracic pressure. However, this effect appears to be small and easily counteracted by control of $Paco_2$. Positive pressure ventilation with low $Paco_2$ causes choroidal vasoconstriction and therefore may discourage forward displacement of ocular contents when the eye is opened.

Controlled ventilation, therefore, may be of special value in certain cases in which: (*1*) spontaneous ventilation is likely to be inadequate or depressed; (*2*) deep anesthesia may not be well tolerated, as in elderly patients or those with cardiac disease; (*3*) there is an increased risk of vitreous loss as in cases of high myopia, young patients, and aphakic corneal grafts; and (*4*) forward displacement of the vitreous would cause special problems, as in intraocular lens implant surgery. Lowering of intraocular pressure may also be helpful in intraocular retinal detachment surgery, to allow easier indentation of sclera during examination and during placement of a scleral buckle.

Antiemetic

Administration of an antiemetic before the end of the operation reduces the incidence of vomiting and retching in the postoperative period. Perphenazine (Trilafon; Fentazin) 2–3 mg or prochlorperazine (Compazine; Stemetil) 5–12.5 mg intramuscularly about 15–20 minutes before the end of surgery is suitable for most adults. It also has a sedative effect. Care is taken in patients with cardiovascular disease, because both drugs can cause hypotension. Metoclopramide (not available in the United States) 10 mg intramuscularly may be preferable in these cases. A small dose of droperidol (Inapsine; Droleptan) 2.5 mg intravenously is also extremely effective and does not interfere with emergence from anesthesia. For children a small dose of cyclizine (Marezine; Valoid) intramuscularly is suitable. However, trimeprazine (Temaril; Vallergan), which is often used in premedication of children, is also an effective antiemetic.

Extubation

The airway is cleared of secretions by gentle pharyngeal suction prior to extubation, but endotracheal suction is avoided because it may cause coughing. If ventilation has been controlled using muscle relaxation, this is reversed with neostigmine and atropine. Administration of CO_2 may be necessary to resume spontaneous ventilation. Extubation is done as soon as respiration is adequate. Some coughing may occur, but this should be mild if the trachea and larynx were sprayed with a local anesthetic before intubation. Coughing after extubation cannot always be prevented, and therefore secure watertight closure of the ocular incision is important.

Recovery

The patient is turned onto his side with the operated eye uppermost to avoid accidental compression of the eye, unless an intraocular bubble was purposely left in the anterior chamber or vitreous cavity, in which case special posturing may be requested by the surgeon. The airway is supported until the patient is awake. Oxygen is given to all patients until they are awake and is continued for a variable period in the elderly and those with cardiovascular and respiratory disease.

Special situations and adjunctive techniques

Epinephrine and inhalational anesthesia

Halothane sensitizes the myocardium to catecholamines, especially in the presence of a raised $P\text{CO}_2$. Therefore, simultaneous use of epinephrine (adrenaline) and halothane is avoided. Where it is necessary to use topical or intraocular epinephrine, enflurane is preferable as the inhalation anesthetic agent, since the degree of myocardial sensitization is less[59].

Examination under anesthesia (EUA)

Examination under anesthesia is chiefly performed in infants and children, and involves limited manipulations of the globe. Ketamine anesthesia is ideal for this purpose, although inhalational anesthesia can also be used.

Ketamine is a dissociative and analgesic agent and provides anesthesia as the sole agent for minor procedures. It can be given in a dosage of 1–2 mg/kg intravenously or 5–10 mg/kg intramuscularly. The airway is maintained without intervention, and intubation is not necessary. Ketamine is particularly useful in the small child having EUA as an outpatient. Ketamine maintains intraocular pressure at normal or slightly high levels, and falsely low readings are avoided[60–62]. This must be considered in children being evaluated for control of congenital or juvenile glaucoma.

Strabismus and retinal detachment surgery

Pulling on a rectus muscle can induce the oculocardiac reflex, resulting in bradycardia[63–65], arrhythmia, or even cardiac arrest[66]. Atropine, given intravenously during induction, will inhibit this response, but a retrobulbar anesthetic block is ineffective[67]. Careful ECG monitoring is important, since atropine itself may occasionally give rise to cardiac arrhythmias.

Adjunctive techniques

Hyperosmotic agents given intravenously draw water from the eye, mainly from the vitreous space. They are used either to lower the intraocular pressure in eyes with severe glaucoma or to decrease the vitreous volume before cataract or aphakic corneal-graft surgery or during retinal reattachment procedures. During cataract surgery this reduction decreases the possibility of vitreous prolapse. The presence of a deeper anterior chamber after removal of the cataract greatly facilitates lens implantation.

Mannitol (Osmitrol) is the preferred hyperosmotic agent, and a 20 per cent solution can be given rapidly over 20–45 minutes in a dose of 1–2 g/kg. Refrigerated bottles should be gently warmed prior to infusion to remove crystals. The ocular hypotensive effect occurs in 30–60 minutes[68]. Marked diuresis follows and may require catheterization of the bladder if a prolonged operation is performed under general anesthesia. Also an acute expansion of extracellular volume may cause circulatory overload in a patient with cardiac decompensation.

In glaucoma cases it may be possible to lower the intraocular pressure preoperatively with an intravenous injection of acetazolamide (Diamox), a carbonic anhydrase inhibitor. This drug is a powerful inhibitor of aqueous secretion. Acetazolamide 500 mg may be given intravenously ½–1 hour before the operation[69]. It is contraindicated in renal acidosis, dehydration and low sodium and potassium states.

Local anesthesia

Most intraocular or extraocular procedures can be performed under local anesthesia. Local anesthesia permits surgery on patients who are otherwise unfit for general anesthesia. Some patients and many surgeons prefer local anesthesia because the risk of serious systemic complications may be lower. Also, the patient usually recovers from the anesthetic faster and is less likely to experience prolonged nausea or major metabolic disequilibrium. This is especially important in elderly patients and those with systemic illnesses such as diabetes. Elderly patients and those with significant medical problems having surgery under local anesthesia should be monitored by an anesthesiologist who will administer any intravenous sedatives or other medications.

It is not possible to control $PaCO_2$ and PaO_2 as readily as with general anesthesia, and effort should be made to avoid respiratory or cardiac depression. Inspired air may be enriched with a flow of oxygen under the drapes, but this is not safe if cautery or diathermy is used during the procedure. Instead, a forced flow of room air may be helpful.

To achieve adequate anesthesia of the globe and akinesia of the lids and globe, a retrobulbar injection is required in addition to a facial nerve block. A topical anesthetic is necessary to anesthetize the cornea and conjunctiva properly.

Premedication

Sedation is required without respiratory depression. Meperidine (pethidine; Demerol) in combination with promethazine (Phenergan) or hydroxyzine (Vistaril) intramuscularly may be used; alternatively diazepam 5 mg orally 2 hours preoperatively is effective. The premedication may sometimes be given intravenously just before the local anesthetic injections. Fentanyl 25–100 μg is given slowly, followed by diazepam in 2.5 mg increments at about 5 minute intervals until the desired level of sedation is obtained. Droperidol (Inapsine; Droleptan), which is an effective antiemetic, may be given in combination with fentanyl, and its sedative effect may last as long as 12 hours.

Topical anesthesia of the conjunctiva

The conjunctiva and cornea are anesthetized with topical medications before the facial nerve block and retrobulbar injection are given. This may be done with 0.5 per cent proparacaine (proxymetacaine; Ophthane), 1 per cent tetracaine (amethocaine), 0.4 per cent benoxinate hydrochloride (Oxybuprocaine hydrochloride), or occasionally 4 per cent cocaine. The patient is instructed to keep the eye closed after application of the drops, because these medications may cause severe corneal drying changes and other epithelial irregularities if exposed to the air. The lid is taped closed after the facial nerve is anesthetized, because voluntary control of lid closure is lost.

Choice of anesthetic for regional block

The choice of anesthetic agent(s) depends partly on the type and length of the operation. Lidocaine (lignocaine; Xylocaine), 2 per cent or 4 per cent, is satisfactory for most procedures lasting 1 hour or less. However, many surgeons routinely combine equal parts of 2 or 4 per cent lidocaine and 0.75 per cent bupivacaine (Marcaine) in the same syringe. Bupivacaine has a slower rate of onset of effect, but it lasts 2–12 hours. In short operations this prolonged anesthesia minimizes early postoperative discomfort.

Facial nerve block

Van-Lint technique

Five milliliters of a 1:1 mixture of 2 or 4 per cent lidocaine (lignocaine; Xylocaine) with 0.75 per cent bupivacaine (Marcaine; Marcain) are injected subcutaneously in three directions at the lateral margin of the orbit. A sharp 25 gauge 1½ inch (38 mm) needle is used. The first injection is directed nasally along the lower margin of the orbit. The second injection is directed upward along the superotemporal margin, and the third passes directly backward toward the ear. In an obese patient a larger volume (8 ml) may be required, delivered in two distinct planes (*Figure 1.10*).

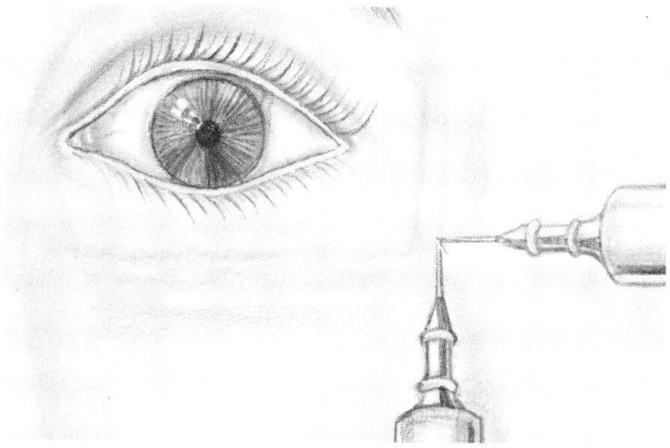

Figure 1.10 *Van-Lint technique for facial nerve block. Needle is introduced inferotemporal to lateral canthus and injections are made along the lower margin of the orbit, upward along the superotemporal orbital margin, and then directly backward toward the ear*

O'Brien technique

With the O'Brien technique the facial nerve trunk is injected where it leaves the stylomastoid canal and where its branches are directed forward through the parotid gland. The needle enters the skin 2 cm in front of and 1 cm below the external auditory canal (*Figure 1.11*). This point can be located (while the jaw is closed) as a palpable

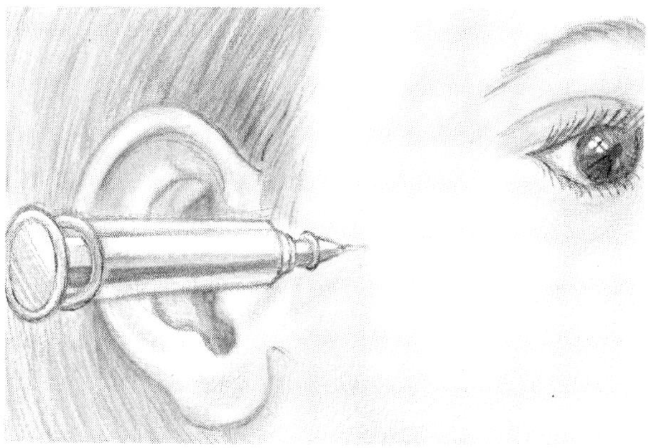

Figure 1.11 *O'Brien technique for facial nerve block. Injection is made 2 cm in front of and 1 cm below the external auditory canal to anesthetize the facial nerve trunk where it leaves the stylomastoid channel*

depression below the zygoma, which fills with the anterior condyle of the mandible when the jaw is opened. During injection the patient is instructed to keep the mouth closed.

About 5 ml of a mixture of 2 or 4 per cent lidocaine (lignocaine; Xylocaine) with 0.75 per cent bupivacaine are injected using a sharp 25 gauge, ⅝ inch (16 mm) needle, passed to its full depth. An alternative method, preferred by some, is to inject the facial nerve trunk by entering the skin just behind the earlobe and penetrating to the full extent of the ⅝ inch (16 mm) needle while directing it toward the deeper structures.

When a facial nerve block is used, 0.5 ml of anesthetic is injected separately to infiltrate the region of the lateral canthus to provide local anesthesia if a canthotomy is planned. This is often uncomfortable because the tissue is rather non-distensible. For those using lid sutures infiltration of the lid skin is also indicated.

Retrobulbar injection

The patient is asked to look upward and inward. The injection is made using a sharp 1½ inch (38 mm) 25 gauge needle introduced through the lower lid at the inferolateral third of the orbital rim (*Figure 1.12*). The needle is directed posteriorly, upward and medially toward the apex of the orbit, and gentle injection of anesthetic agent is given as the needle is advanced. Care must be exercised to avoid penetration of the globe, especially in myopic eyes because of the large size of the globe. Some surgeons prefer to inject with a blunt or tapered-tip 23 gauge needle which they feel is less likely to penetrate the globe inadvertently than a sharp, smaller-diameter needle.

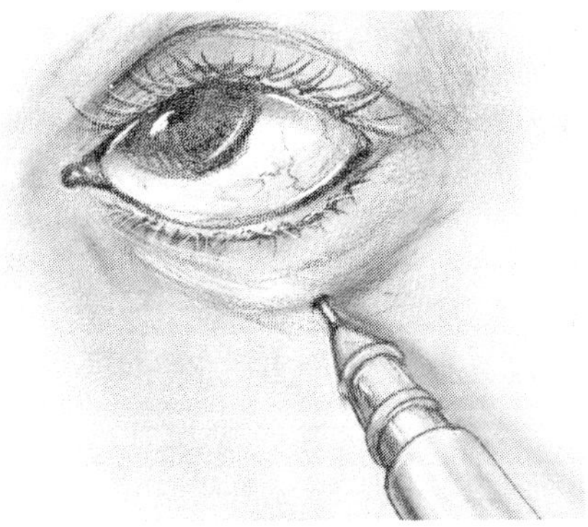

Figure 1.12 *Retrobulbar injection technique. Patient looks upward and inward and injection is made with sharp 1½ inch (38 mm) 25 gauge needle introduced through inferotemporal portion of lower lid and directed toward apex of the orbit behind the globe*

Penetration to a depth of 3.5 cm will give complete anesthesia of the globe, but little akinesia. Penetration to 5.0 cm gives akinesia also, but increases the risk of retrobulbar hemorrhage. Some surgeons believe that the risk of hemorrhage can be reduced by maintaining a steady slow injection of anesthetic while advancing the needle. Akinesia of the superior rectus can be augmented by a subconjunctival injection along the belly of the muscle itself (*Figure 1.13*).

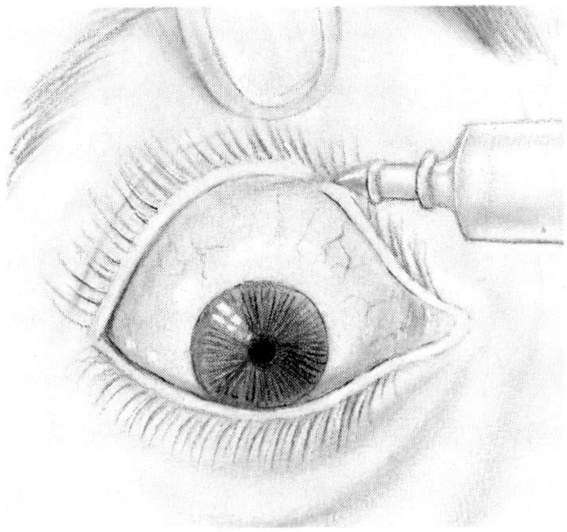

Figure 1.13 *Supplemental injection to ensure akinesia of the superior rectus muscle following retrobulbar injection. Subconjunctival injection is made along the superior rectus muscle belly*

Two to 4 ml of the lidocaine-bupivacaine mixture are injected, and complete anesthesia and akinesia are obtained in about 10 minutes. The injection can be repeated after 20–30 minutes if the effect is incomplete. During long retinal reattachment or vitrectomy operations, it may be necessary to supplement the injection during the operation. This is usually done with 2 or 4 per cent lidocaine.

Other medications may be added to the anesthetic agents, i.e. epinephrine (adrenaline) 0.3 ml of 1:1000 solution to prolong the action of the anesthetic. However, the cardiovascular status and overall degree of frailty of the patient should be considered. Hyaluronidase (4–8 u/ml) is routinely added to the anesthetic solution to encourage diffusion of the anesthetic to the ciliary ganglion and orbital nerves.

Retrobulbar hemorrhage may occur as a complication of retrobulbar injection. This is identified by the immediate onset of proptosis, with or without chemosis and subconjunctival or lid hematoma. Intermittent compression of the orbit through the closed lids may help to stop the bleeding. The fundus should be examined by indirect ophthalmoscopy. If there is no blood flow in the central retinal artery, then immediate lateral canthotomy and/or anterior chamber paracentesis is performed. The operation must be postponed for at least 2 weeks[70], except in the case of vitreous surgery. Here the operation can be performed, although the globe will be much less mobile.

Regional anesthesia

Periorbital region

Regional anesthesia in the periorbital area is achieved either by local infiltration subjacent to a small lesion or by regional nerve block at the level of the neurovascular plane of the nerve[71]. The points of exit of the trigeminal nerve on the face can be injected (*Figure 1.14*). Operations on the lower lid and cheek can be performed by blocking the infraorbital nerve at its exit from the infraorbital foramen. There is a palpable depression over this site, and

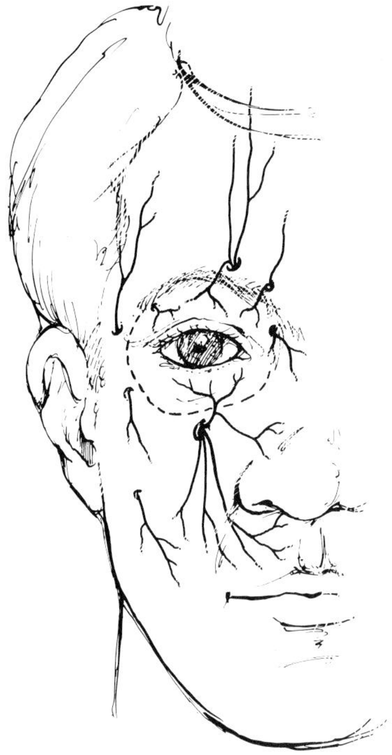

Figure 1.14 *Points of exit of the trigeminal nerve on the face. These locations can be injected to provide regional periorbital anesthesia*

it lies directly in line with the supraorbital notch. The lateral portion of the upper and lower lids is supplied by the lacrimal nerve, which can be infiltrated close to the lateral orbital margin. The major portion of the upper lid is supplied by the supraorbital and supratrochlear nerves, which can be blocked at their exit points. The most medial portion of both lids is supplied by the infratrochlear nerve, as discussed below.

Lacrimal surgery

Lacrimal surgery requires anesthesia of the tissues surrounding the lacrimal drainage system and of the mucous membrane of the nose. The anesthetic is injected 1 cm above the caruncle, at the level of the upper inner angle of the orbit (*Figure 1.15*). The needle is directed backward and medially to the level of the orbicularis fascia, to anesthetize the infratrochlear nerve. The needle is withdrawn and redirected toward the nose. It is inserted down to bone, and 0.5 ml is injected. The tissue is then firmly compressed. This anesthetizes the skin for the final injection. The needle is then inserted 1 cm below the caruncle and is directed to the bone of the nose. One ml is injected, and the tissue is firmly compressed[70].

To anesthetize the nasal mucous membrane, the middle fossa of the nasal cavity is packed with ribbon gauze or a pledget of cotton soaked in 4 per cent lidocaine (lignocaine; Xylocaine) with epinephrine (adrenaline) (1:100 000) (*Figure 1.16*). Alternatively, cocaine solution 4–10 per cent with or without epinephrine may be used. Mixtures of cocaine and epinephrine may be dangerous because of the potentiating interaction between these two drugs. A posterior nasal pack is used to prevent aspiration of blood.

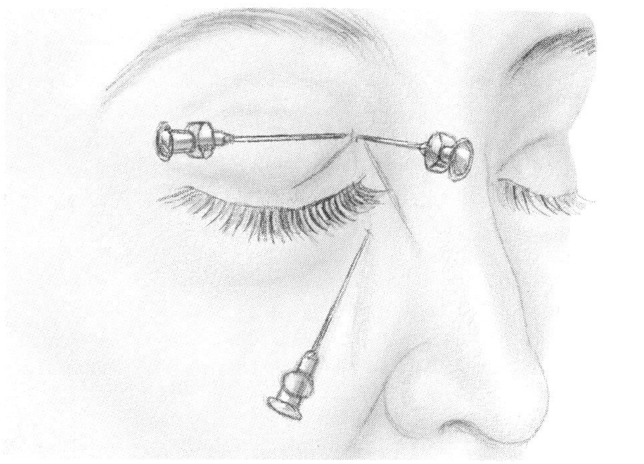

Figure 1.15 *Local anesthetic technique for lacrimal surgery. Injection is made 1 cm above the caruncle at the upper inner margin of the bony orbit and a second injection is made 1 cm below the caruncle directed toward the bone of the nose*

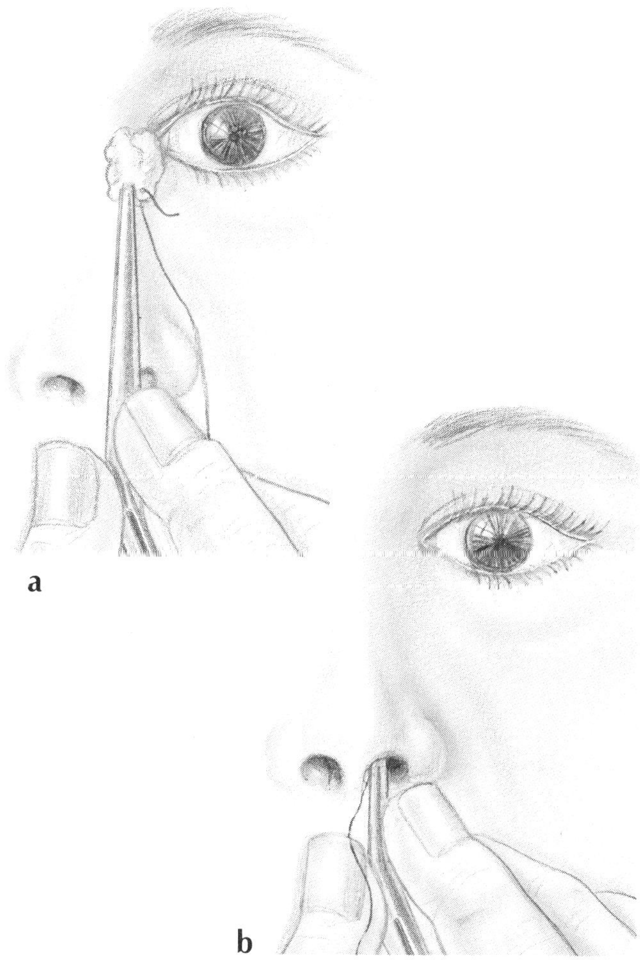

a

b

Figure 1.16 *Anesthesia of the nasal mucous membrane is provided by application of cotton pledget soaked in 4 per cent lidocaine and epinephrine.* **(a)** *Approximate location of the middle fossa of the nasal cavity is judged by measuring the distance from the external nares to the medial canthus before* **(b)** *introducing the cotton pledget*

Neuroleptanalgesia

For some patients with respiratory or cardiac disease, it is desirable to combine routine local anesthetic procedure with neuroleptanalgesia. This produces a quiet catatonic state with profound analgesia. Blood pressure, heart and respiratory rate are monitored throughout because there is some risk of respiratory depression. One standard regimen uses droperidol, which is also a strong antiemetic, and fentanyl (Sublimaze), a powerful narcotic analgesic.

The patient is premedicated with diazepam or droperidol, (Inapsine; Droleptan). During surgery fentanyl or a droperidol-fentanyl combination (Innovar) is given from time to time. Use of forced air under the drapes is advised. Respiratory depression may be combatted with naloxone 0.1–0.4 mg; and bradycardia is treated with atropine 0.4 mg intravenously.

References

1. Coleman, D. J., Abramson, D. H., Jack, R. L., Franzen, L. A. Ultrasonic diagnosis of tumours of the choroid. Archives of Ophthalmology 1974; 91:344–354
2. Coleman, D. J., Lizzi, F. *In vivo* choroidal thickness measurement. American Journal of Ophthalmology 1979; 88:369–375
3. Alm, A., Bill, A., Young, F. A. The effects of pilocarpine and neostigmine on the blood flow through the anterior uvea in monkeys. A study with radioactively labelled microspheres. Experimental Eye Research 1973; 15:31–36
4. Bill, A. Ocular circulation. In: Moses, R. A. ed. Adler's physiology of the eye: clinical application, 6th ed. St. Louis: C. V. Mosby, 1975:210
5. Wise, G. N., Dollery, C. T., Henkind, P. The retinal circulation. New York: Harper and Row, 1971:105
6. Sieker, H. O., Hickam, J. B. Normal and impaired retinal vascular reactivity. Circulation 1953; 7:79–83
7. Bill, A. A method for quantitative determination of the blood through the cat uvea. Archives of Ophthalmology 1962; 67:156–162
8. Hickam, J. B., Frayser, R., Ross, J. C. Study of retinal venous blood oxygen saturation in human subjects by a photographic means. Circulation 1963; 27:375–385
9. Duke-Elder, S., ed. System of Ophthalmology, Vol 4. The physiology of the eye and of vision. London: Kimpton, 1968:41–44
10. Pilkerton, R., Bulle, B., O'Rourke, J. Uveal blood flow determined by the nitrous oxide method. Investigative Ophthalmology 1964; 3:227–236
11. Cohan, B. E., Cohan, S. B. Flow and oxygen saturation of blood in the anterior ciliary vein of the dog eye. American Journal of Physiology 1963; 205:60–66
12. Moses, R. A. Intraocular pressure. In: Moses, R. A., ed. Adler's physiology of the eye: clinical application, 6th ed. St Louis: C. V. Mosby, 1975:179–209
13. Langham, M. E. Vascular pathophysiology of the ocular postural response. A pneumatonometric study. Transactions of the Ophthalmological Society of the United Kingdom 1975; 95:281–287
14. Langham, M. E., To'Mey, K. F. A clinical procedure for the measurement of the ocular pulse-pressure relationship and the ophthalmic arterial pressure. Experimental Eye Research 1978; 27:17–25
15. Hvidberg, A., Kessing, S. V., Fernandes, A. Effect of changes in PCO_2 and body positions on intraocular pressure during general anaesthesia. Acta Ophthalmologica 1981; 59:465–475
16. Le May, M. Aspects of measurement in ophthalmology. British Journal of Anaesthesia 1980; 52:655–662
17. Comberg, D., Pilz, A. Augeninnendruck und Rigiditätsverhalten bei experimenteller Venendruckerhöhung. Albrecht von Graefe's Archive für Ophthalmologie 1961; 163:189–202
18. Sharpey-Shafer, E. P. Effects of Valsalva's manoeuvre on the normal and failing circulation. British Medical Journal 1955; 1:693–695
19. Campbell, E. J. M., Dickinson, C. J., Slater, J. D. H. Clinical physiology, 2nd ed. 1963:80 Oxford: Blackwell Scientific
20. Rosen, D. A., Johnson, V. C. Ocular pressure patterns in the Valsalva manoeuvre. Archives of Ophthalmology 1959; 62:810–816
21. Bain, W. E. S., Maurice, D. M. Physiological variations in the intraocular pressure. Transactions of the Opthalmological Society of the United Kingdom 1959; 79:249–260
22. Alm, A., Bill, A. The oxygen supply to the retina. II. Effects of high intraocular pressure and of increased arterial carbon dioxide tension on uveal and retinal blood flow in cats. Acta Physiologica Scandinavica 1972; 84:306–319
23. Friedman, E., Chandra, S. R. Choroidal blood flow. III. Effects of oxygen and carbon dioxide. Archives of Ophthalmology 1972; 87:70–71
24. Frayser, R., Hickam, J. B. Retinal vascular response to breathing increased carbon dioxide and oxygen concentrations. Investigative Ophthalmology 1964; 3:427–431
25. Holloway, K. B. Control of the eye during general anaesthesia for intraocular surgery. British Journal of Anaesthesia 1980; 52:671–679
26. Duncalf, D., Weitzner, S. W. The influence of ventilation and hypercapnea on intraocular pressure during anaesthesia. Anaesthesia and Analgesia 1963; 43:232–237
27. Samuel, J. R., Beaugie, A. Effect of carbon dioxide on the intraocular pressure in man during general anaesthesia. British Journal of Ophthalmology 1974; 58:62–67
28. MacDiarmid, I. R., Holloway, K. B. Factors affecting intraocular pressure. Proceedings of the Royal Society of Medicine 1976; 69:601–602
29. Bill, A. Autonomic nervous control of uveal blood flow. Acta Physiologica Scandinavica 1962; 56:70–81
30. Chandra, S. R., Friedman, E. Choroidal blood flow. II. The effects of autonomic agents. Archives of Ophthalmology 1972; 87:67–69
31. Alm, A., Bill, A. The effect of stimulation of the cervical sympathetic chain on retinal oxygen tension and on uveal, retinal and cerebral blood flow in cats. Acta Physiologica Scandinavica 1973; 88:84–94
32. Tarhan, S., Moffitt, E. A., Taylor, W. F., Giulian, E. R. Myocardial infarction after general anesthesia. Journal of the American Medical Association 1972; 220:1451–1454
33. Breslin, P. P. Mortality in ophthalmic surgery. International Ophthalmology Clinics 1973; 13:215–226
34. Wolf, G., Lynch, S., Berlin, I. Intraocular surgery with general anesthesia. Archives of Ophthalmology 1975; 93:323–326
35. Backer, C. L., Tinker, J. H., Robertson, D. M., Vlietstra, R. E. Myocardial reinfarction following local anaesthesia for ophthalmic surgery. Anaesthesia and Analgesia 1980; 59:257–262
36. Foex, P., Prys-Roberts, C. Anaesthesia and the hypertensive patient. British Journal of Anaesthesia 1974; 46:575–588
37. Rosenberg, H. Neuromuscular diseases, myopathies and anesthesia. Annual Refresher Course Lectures 1980; 132:3
38. Adams, A. K., Jones, R. M. Anaesthesia for eye surgery: general considerations. British Journal of Anaesthesia 1980; 52:663–669
39. Boakes, A. J., Laurence, D. R., Teoh, P. C., Barar, F. S. K., Benedikter, L. T., Prichard, B. N. C. Interactions between sympathomimetic amines and antidepressant agents in man. British Medical Journal 1973; i:311–315
40. Perks, E. T. Monoamine oxidase inhibitors. Anaesthesia 1964; 19:376–386
41. Dundee, J. W. Problems of multiple inhalation anaesthetics. British Journal of Anaesthesia 1981; 53:63S–67S

42. Cascorbi, H. F. Perianesthetic problems with non-anesthetic drugs. Refresher Courses in Anesthesiology 1978; 6:15–30
43. Dripps, R. D., Eckenhoff, J. E., Vandam, L. D. Introduction to anaesthesia; the principles of safe practice. 5th ed. Philadelphia: W. B. Saunders, 1977
44. McCammon, R. L. Anesthetic considerations in the presence of ocular disease. Refresher Courses in Anesthesiology 1980; 8:127–137
45. Kornblueth, W., Aladjemoff, L., Magora, F., Gabbay, A. Influence of general anesthesia on intraocular pressure in man; the effect of diethyl ether, cyclopropane, vinyl ether, and thiopental sodium. Archives of Ophthalmology 1959; 61:84–87
46. Oji, E. O., Holdcroft, A. The ocular effects of etomidate. Anaesthesia 1979; 34:245–249
47. LIncoff, H. A., Ellis, C. H., DeVoe, A. G., *et al.* The effect of succinylcholine on intraocular pressure. American Journal of Ophthalmology 1955; 40:501–510
48. Kornblueth, W., Jampolsky, A., Tamler, E., Marge, E. Contraction of the oculorotary muscles and intraocular pressure: a tonographic and electromyographic study of the effect of edrophonium chloride (tensilon) and succinylcholine (anectine) on the intraocular pressure. American Journal of Ophthalmology 1960; 49:1381–1387
49. Eakins, K. E., Katz, R. L. The action of succinylcholine on the tension of extraocular muscle. British Journal of Pharmacology 1966; 26:205–211
50. Lincoff, H. A., Breinin, G. M., DeVoe, A. G. The effect of succinylcholine on the extraocular muscles. American Journal of Ophthalmology 1957; 43:440–444
51. Adams, A. K., Barnett, K. C. Anaesthesia and intraocular pressure. Anaesthesia 1966; 21:202–210
52. Bowen, D. J., McGrand, J. C., Hamilton, A. G. Intraocular pressures after suxamethonium and endotracheal intubation. The effect of pre-treatment with tubocurarine gallamine. Anaesthesia 1978; 33:518–522
53. Havener, W. H. Ocular pharmacology, 4th ed. St Louis: C. V. Mosby, 1978:103–105
54. Al-Abrak, M. H., Samuel, J. R. Effects of general anaesthesia on the intraocular pressure in man: comparison of tubocurarine and pancuronium in nitrous oxide and oxygen. British Journal of Ophthalmology 1974; 58:806–810
55. George, R., Nursingh, A., Downing, J. W., Welsh, N. H. Non-depolarizing neuromuscular blockers and the eye: a study of intraocular pressure. Pancuronium versus alcuronium. British Journal of Anaesthesia 1979; 51:789–792
56. Coleman, A. J., Downing, J., Leary, W. P., Moyes, D. G., Styles, M. The immediate cardiovascular effects of pancuronium, alcuronium, and tubocurarine in man. Anaesthesia 1972; 27:415–422
57. Runciman, J. C., Bowen-Wright, R. M., Welsh, N. H., Downing, J. W. Intraocular pressure changes during halothane and enflurane anaesthesia. British Journal of Anaesthesia 1978; 50:371–374
58. von Sallman, L., Macri, F. J., Wanko, T., Grimes, P. A. Some mechanisms of centrally induced eye pressure responses. American Journal of Ophthalmology 1956; 42:130–147
59. Reisner, L. S., Lippman, M. Ventricular arrhythmias after epinephrine injection in enflurane and in halothane anaesthesia. Anaesthesia and Analgesia 1975; 54:468–470
60. Yoshikawa, K., Murai, Y. The effect of ketamine on intraocular pressure in children. Anaesthesia and Analgesia 1971; 50:199–202
61. Peuler, M., Glass, D. D., Arens, J. F. Ketamine and intraocular pressure. Anesthesiology 1975; 43:575–578
62. Ausinch, B., Rayborn, R. L., Munson, E. S., Levy, N. S. Ketamine and intraocular pressure in children. Anaesthesia and Analgesia 1976; 55:773–775
63. Welhaf, W. R., Johnson, D. C. The oculo-cardiac reflex during extraocular muscle surgery. Archives of Ophthalmology 1965; 73:43–45
64. Apt, L., Isenberg, S., Gaffney, W. L. The oculocardiac reflex in strabismus surgery. American Journal of Ophthalmology 1973; 76:533–536
65. Dewar, K. M. S., Wishart, H. Y. The oculo-cardiac reflex. Proceedings of the Royal Society of Medicine 1976; 69:373–374
66. Alexander, J. P. Reflex disturbances of cardiac rhythm during ophthalmic surgery. British Journal of Ophthalmology 1975; 59:518–524
67. Bosomworth, P. B., Ziegler, C. H., Jacoby, J. The oculo-cardiac reflex in eye muscle surgery. Anesthesiology 1958; 19:7–10
68. Havener, W. H. Ocular Pharmacology, 4th ed. St Louis: C. V. Mosby, 1978:452
69. Aboul-Eish, E. Physiology of the eye pertinent to anaesthesia. International Ophthalmology Clinics 1972; 13(2):1–20
70. Arruga, H.: Ocular surgery, 4th ed. New York: McGraw-Hill, 1962
71. Allen, E. D., Elkington, A. R. Local anaesthesia and the eye. British Journal of Anaesthesia 1980; 52:689–694

2

Surgery of the eyelids and lacrimal drainage apparatus

Nicholas T. Iliff MD

Introduction

Ophthalmic plastic and reconstructive surgery is a rather new subspecialty dealing with cosmetic, functional and neoplastic abnormalities of the lids, orbit and lacrimal apparatus. Surgery on these adnexal structures presents unique challenges to the oculoplastic surgeon, and numerous alternatives have been described for each condition. Many of the clinical problems cannot be treated by a single standard approach, and they tax the ingenuity of the most experienced surgeon. Thus, a new surgical approach is often reported with enthusiasm, suggesting the discovery of a panacea, only to be followed by reports of alternative methods indicating that an optimum treatment still has not been found. Every case is different, as is each surgeon, and it is impossible to select one procedure that will always work. In this chapter, guidelines and procedures are presented that allow successful management of the majority of the oculoplastic problems, and which, in our opinion, have the highest chance for a satisfactory surgical result.

Basic principles

The unique properties of the skin of the lids necessitate special techniques for handling skin flaps and grafts. Lid skin is softer, thinner and more pliable than skin in any other part of the body. In addition, it is highly vascular, thereby minimizing the chance of necrosis. Free grafts 'take' readily, and infection is rarely a problem. Handling of the thin edges requires the finest instrumentation and care to prevent tearing, maceration and misalignment. Fine skin hooks and forceps with 0.12 or 0.3 mm teeth aid in tissue handling and prevent disruptive crushing.

The value of a constantly dry field cannot be overstressed. Identification of structures is facilitated, postoperative reaction and scarring are minimized, and overall results are better. Hemorrhage can be meticulously controlled with bipolar cautery.

Suturing technique

Interrupted and running suturing techniques each have advantages. Interrupted suturing prevents distortion caused by bunching of tissue, especially when closing curvilinear incisions. Individual stitch tension can be controlled, and adjacent edges can be shifted for flatter closure to help eliminate asymmetry. If one suture breaks or is cut, the suture line is not disrupted. Running sutures provide a flat suture line with only one or two knots, which can be buried. This is especially important if knots are on the conjunctival surface and could cause corneal abrasion.

When closing lid skin margins that are not under tension, interrupted 8/0 silk sutures using small tissue bites give the best closure. Control of suture tension can be achieved more readily with silk than with nylon. Use of small suture bites minimizes inturning of thin skin edges and bunching or distortion of tissue near the suture. These tiny sutures often fall out in 4–5 days; and even if left in longer, suture tracks are not a problem. These factors ensure an optimum cosmetic result. The disadvantage of interrupted 8/0 silk sutures is that they are tedious to insert and remove.

Heavier skin of the nose, cheek, temple or brow should be closed with 5/0 or 6/0 silk or nylon. Skin in these locations is less prone to distortion or inversion of the wound edges because the dermis is thicker. Running or subcuticular sutures work well. Vertical mattress sutures are only rarely needed for added strength. When used they should be taken out in 4 or 5 days to minimize the chance of suture tracks. Horizontal mattress sutures are helpful to evert the skin edges, and these are used when closing a tarsorrhaphy.

Choice of suture type and size is partly a personal preference. With the exception of levator resection procedures, we close deep tissues with absorbable sutures, usually 6/0 or 7/0 chromic catgut or polyglactin (Vicryl). Collagen sutures of 8/0 size are used in some cases of tarsal-conjunctival grafts. Absorbable sutures can be used on the skin in children, and we prefer 7/0 chromic catgut. There is slightly more postoperative inflammation, but elimination of the need for suture removal is often important. For lid skin 8/0 silk is used and for skin elsewhere 5/0 or 6/0 silk or nylon is used as mentioned before.

Scars

Scars cannot be avoided but should be minimized. Suture and tissue handling techniques are important, and correct location and orientation of incisions can also minimize scarring. Suture lines should be made in naturally occurring wrinkles or creases if possible. Careful handling of skin edges, avoidance of hemorrhage or infection, prevention of inversion of skin edges, and decreasing tension in suture lines by undermining and separate closure of deep tissue all minimize scarring.

All scars contract, and clinically this seems to occur more along the long axis of the scar, although percentage contraction is the same in all directions. It is contraction of scars that causes the serious postoperative and post-traumatic defects of hooding (*Figure 2.1*) and webbing of skin around the eyes, and notching and retraction of the lids. Therefore, orientation of incisions and revision of traumatic or surgical scars are aimed at minimizing these complications. The thin skin of the lid will scar much less than the surrounding thicker skin of the nose, forehead, temple and cheek. Whenever possible, surgical incisions should be confined to the lid skin.

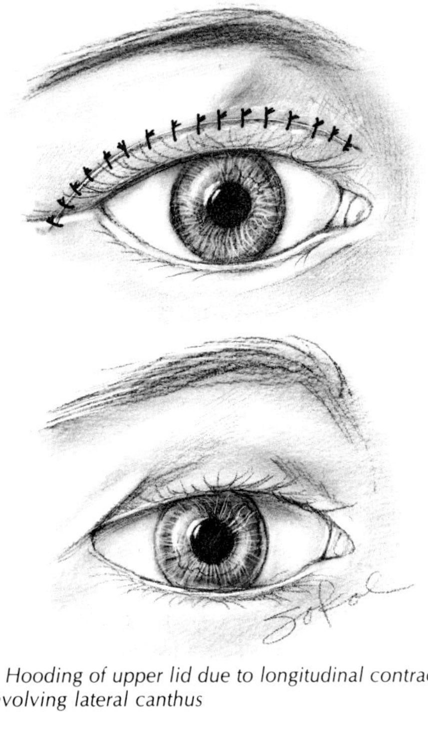

Figure 2.1 *Hooding of upper lid due to longitudinal contraction of an incision involving lateral canthus*

Postoperative application of steroid ointment may help decrease scar formation, but it should not be used at the time of surgery because it tends to enter the wound and delay primary closure. Hypertrophic scars may be treated with intrascar injection of steroid such as triamcinolone acetonide (Kenalog). A great improvement in scar contraction can be achieved by massage over several months with a lubricating ointment such as cocoa butter.

Skin grafts

Skin grafts to the lids must be thinner and more pliable than grafts to any other part of the body. Skin grafts rarely fail to 'take' on the lid because of the excellent blood supply. However, adequate functional and cosmetic results are harder to achieve. The best donor skin for full-thickness grafts is from the upper lid of the same or the fellow eye. Next best donor skin is from the postauricular area (*Figure 2.2*), followed by the supraclavicular area and medial aspect of the upper arm. Skin from the postauricular area is thicker than lid skin, but it is satisfactory for grafts to the upper lid and is excellent for the lower lid. Supraclavicular skin and that from the arm is considerably thicker than lid skin, and in Caucasians it tends to be yellower in color.

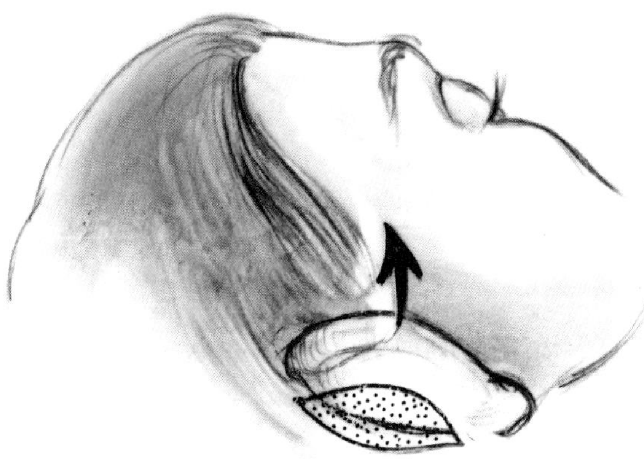

Figure 2.2 *Skin from the postauricular area used as free graft for upper or lower lid defect*

Full-thickness skin grafts contain sweat glands, sebaceous glands and hair follicles (*Figure 2.3*). They are preferred to split-thickness grafts for most lid reconstructions because (*1*) the dermal glands help improve the texture of the graft; (*2*) secondary shrinkage is less; and (*3*) the color tends to change less.

Split-thickness skin grafts are preferred when large areas must be covered and inadequate full-thickness material is available. Split-thickness skin works well for the lining of the orbit following exenteration, where texture and color match are not important and shrinkage is minimized by contact of the graft with the bone.

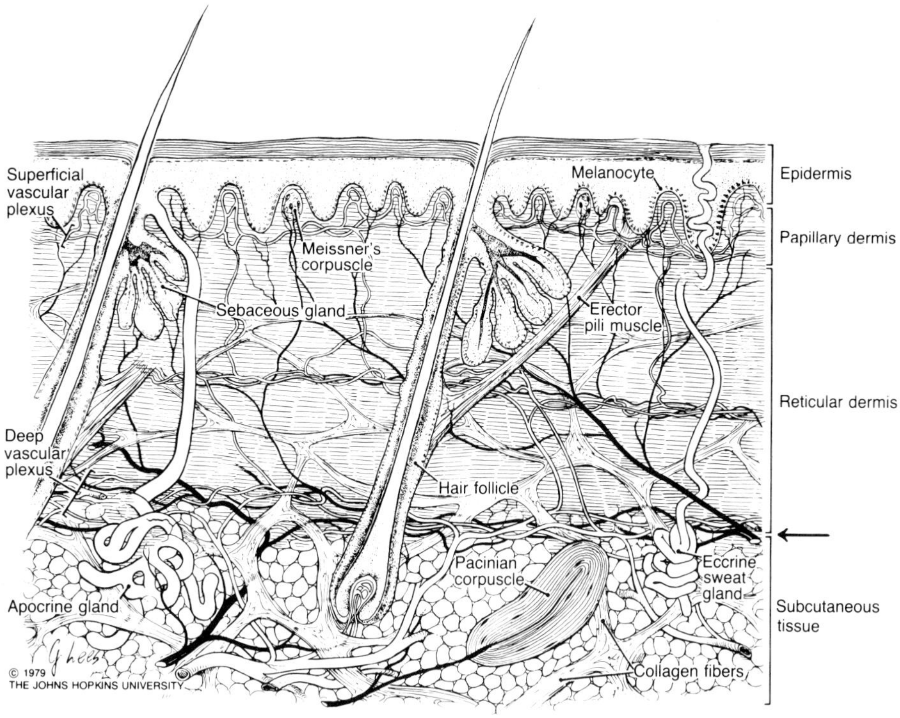

Figure 2.3 *Cross-section of skin with intradermal appendages. Full-thickness grafts are taken at level of lower reticular dermis (arrow) and include most glands and follicles*

Complete hemostasis in the recipient bed is essential, but avoiding excessive cauterization is also important to prevent charring and devascularization. Heavily irradiated tissue makes a poor recipient bed because of reduced blood supply, and the thinnest possible free graft should be used in such cases if a skin flap is not applicable. Fat is a poor bed for grafting, and it is helpful to cover fat with muscle to improve the chance of survival of the graft.

Skin for full-thickness grafts is usually excised as an ellipse to aid the closure of the donor site. The graft is then pinned on a small board, and the fat and connective tissue are excised from the undersurface with sharp iris scissors. The graft is made as thin as possible. After the graft has been partially sutured in place, it is cut to the final size.

Split-thickness grafts can be taken from the supraclavicular area (after injecting the skin with saline to facilitate use of the dermatome), from the abdomen or from a relatively hair-free portion of the thigh. Stryker adhesive strip is applied to the area, and the Stryker dermatome is set at 0.010–0.015 inch. Firm even pressure is maintained as the cut is made. Diffuse fine punctate bleeding indicates that the cut is of proper depth. Large areas of bleeding indicate that the cut is too deep. The adhesive tape stabilizes the very thin graft, keeps it from rolling in the dermatome and generally aids in its handling. The donor site is dressed with petroleum gauze and a firm dressing.

Good contact between the graft and recipient bed is essential for graft survival. During the initial 48 hours after grafting, a plasma-like transudate nourishes the graft. However, during this time only the deep graft layers are nourished, thereby emphasizing the importance of thin grafts, whether they be split- or full-thickness. Later, vascular circulation in the graft is re-established[2]. This occurs initially by anastomotic vessels between the graft and the recipient bed[3] followed by ingrowth of new capillaries and re-establishment of lymphatic drainage[4].

Any hemorrhage under the graft or bridging of the graft over a concavity in the underlying recipient bed prevents the nutrient plasmoid substance from being absorbed, which inhibits early anastomosis of vascular channels. Bridging is caused by too much tension on the graft. Conversely, an excessively large graft also presents problems because folding and gathering of the graft tissue prevents contact of parts of the graft with the vascularized bed, resulting in focal necrosis of the graft tissue and subsequent scarring. A moderate pressure dressing aids in promoting contact between the graft and the vascular bed, but it should not be so tight as to interfere with circulation in the bed. Drainage holes in the graft help prevent accumulation of serous or bloody fluid under the graft, but if fluid does accumulate, it should be evacuated.

Mucous membrane grafts

The preferred donor sites for mucous membrane grafts are the lower lip and the cheek. Adequate donor material can be obtained from these sites for most lid or cul-de-sac reconstruction problems. Nasal mucous membrane has been used; but, in our opinion, it is harder to harvest pieces of adequate size. We do not use mucous membrane-cartilage composite grafts, which can be obtained from the nose, for lid reconstruction.

We prefer full-thickness mucous membrane grafts removed by free-hand dissection. The donor site is injected with lidocaine (lignocaine) and 1:100 000 epinephrine (adrenaline) to expand and distend the tissue. The lower lip is then everted and stretched over a large lip clamp.

Dissection beneath the graft is done with Westcott scissors and then the graft margins are incised. The donor site is not sutured as it heals readily in a few days and causes surprisingly little discomfort. The graft is handled, thinned and placed in the recipient bed as has been described for skin grafts. It is attached with absorbable 7/0 or 8/0 sutures.

Skin flaps

Various types of skin flaps are useful for lid reconstruction. Flaps that have a tenuous blood supply and would not survive elsewhere can do well on the lid because of the excellent vascularity. Skin flaps are more difficult than free skin grafts to fashion so as to achieve the optimum result but when cartilage, scleral or composite grafts are needed, or when the recipient bed is of poor vascularity, skin flaps, conjunctival flaps or myocutaneous flaps are necessary. The most frequently used flaps are: pedicle (advancement and rotation), V–Y, and Z-plasty.

Pedicle flaps

A horizontal or vertical advancement flap is used most frequently in lid reconstruction (*Figure 2.4*). The flap can consist of skin alone or skin and muscle, depending on the depth of the defect to be filled. It takes advantage of skin elasticity, making use of excess skin at a site relatively distant from the defect. Excision of triangles of tissue (Burow's triangles) on either side of the base of the flap aids in advancement and facilitates closure of the defect.

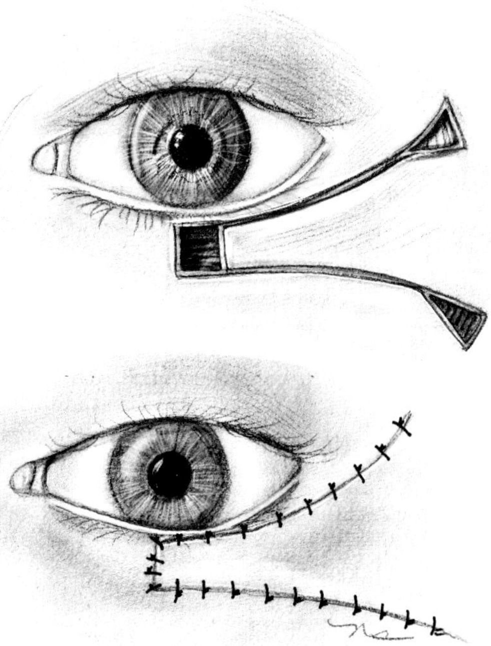

Figure 2.4 *Horizontal advancement flap used to fill lower lid defect. Skin is relatively elastic and can be advanced from lateral location. Excision of skin triangles near base of advancement flap aids closure of incisions*

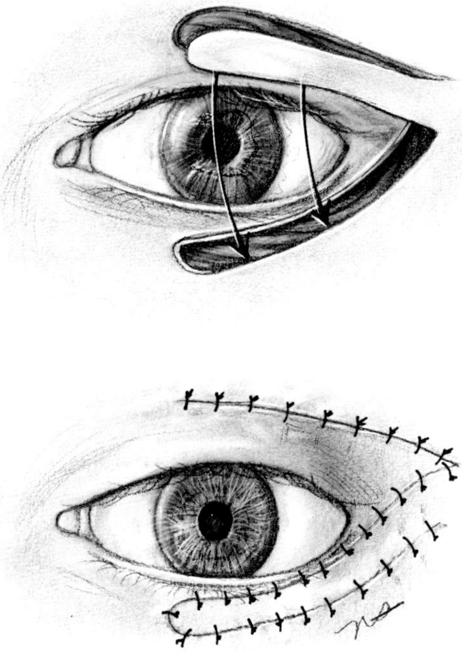

Figure 2.5 *Rotational pedicle flap using upper lid skin to fill lower lid defect. Pedicle remains attached temporally. Upper lid skin defect is easily closed because of excess skin in this area*

A rotational pedicle flap is used for transposing tissue from the upper lid to the medial canthus or to the lower lid (*Figure 2.5*). A rotational flap from the midforehead to the medial canthal area may be needed for closure of a defect which penetrates the bone into the nose. In general, pedicle flaps cannot be more than two to three times as long as they are wide or the vascular supply of the tip will not be adequate. However, a flap of lid skin of any shape will survive if there is a good recipient bed because it is thin and acts as a free graft. Myocutaneous flaps from the lid are more uncertain but they do quite well if the width-to-length ratio is about 1:3.

V–Y flaps

V–Y and Y–V flaps are advancement flap techniques that provide an increase in tissue dimensions in one direction and a decrease in another direction while making optimum use of adjacent tissues. A V-shaped incision can be converted to a Y to increase the amount of skin in the long axis of the Y while decreasing the skin perpendicular to that axis (*Figure 2.6*). Closing a Y-shaped incision as a V has the reverse effect.

Z-plasty

To perform a Z-plasty two triangular flaps are transposed with the effect that skin is added along the axis of the central arm of the Z and removed from the axis perpendicular to that central arm (*Figure 2.7*). The arms of the Z must be equal in length to the central member. The angle between the arms and center axis can be from 30 to 90°, but 60° is optimal in most cases. The greater the angle the greater the gain in length along the central axis. Zs with configurations greater than 60° are not very useful and are technically difficult. Z-plasties can be used to: (*1*) realign scar tissue in a more favorable position or make a scar less apparent by breaking its continuity; (*2*) lengthen tissue along the axis of a contracted scar – this may be combined with excision of the scar (*Figure 2.8*); and (*3*) move the position of structures such as the canthus or the brow when contained in the flaps of the Z (*Figure 2.9*).

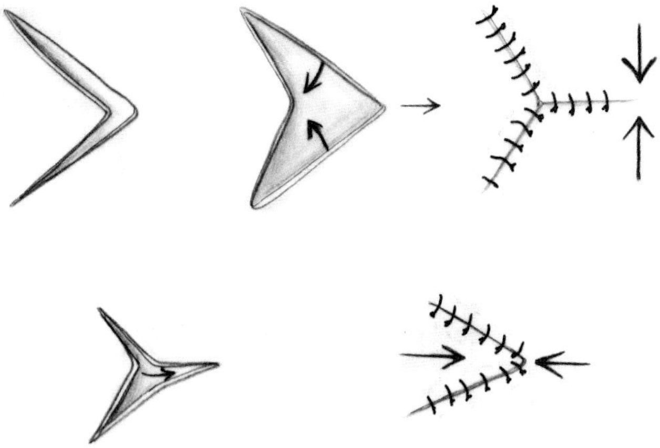

Figure 2.6 *V-Y and Y-V advancement flaps to increase tissue dimensions in one direction while decreasing dimensions in perpendicular direction. When V-shaped incision is closed as Y (top), length of incision along axis of V is increased while decreasing length in perpendicular direction. When Y-shaped incision is closed as V (bottom), length along axis of Y is decreased, and length in perpendicular direction is increased.*

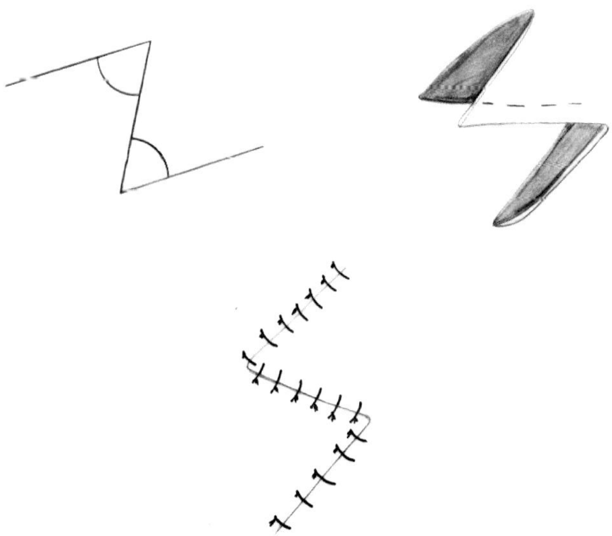

Figure 2.7 *Z-plasty to increase length along central arm of Z. Three incisions of equal length are made and transposed to give lengthening effect*

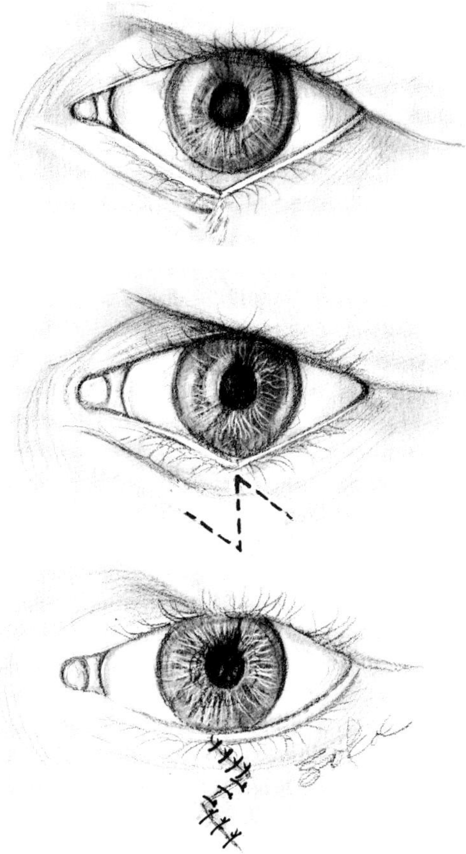

Figure 2.8 *Z-plasty used to treat contracted scar causing distortion of lower lid. Scar tissue is excised, and Z-plasty used to lengthen area of contracted tissue below lid margin*

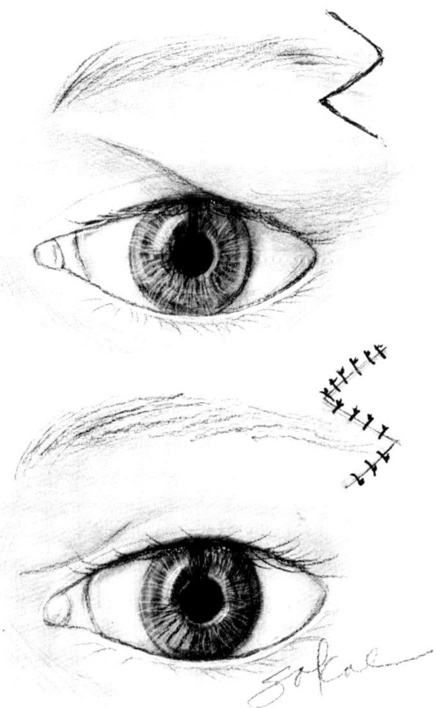

Figure 2.9 *Z-plasty used to lower updrawn brow. Brow included in upper portion of incision is moved inferiorly as the flaps of the Z are transposed*

Surgical anatomy of the lids

Skin

The upper lid skin is extremely thin, averaging 0.6 mm in depth and quite pliable. Upper lid skin is loose and moveable over the orbicularis muscle, becoming more fixed to the underlying tissues as it blends with the thicker surrounding skin of the nose, forehead and temple at the orbital rim. The skin of the lower lid is slightly thicker and also becomes less mobile where it joins the thicker cheek

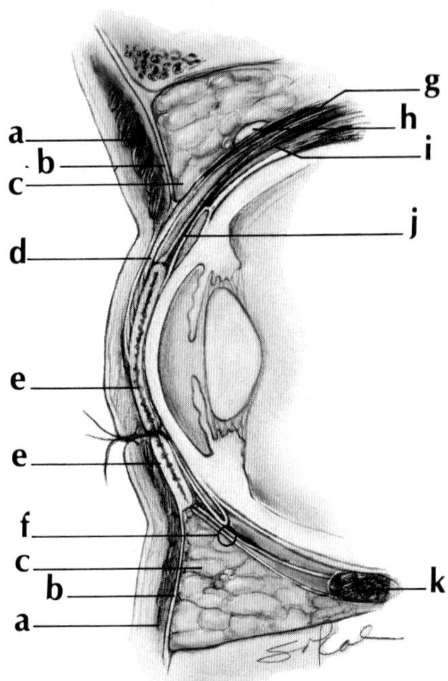

Figure 2.10 *Anatomy of the lids including:* **(a)** *orbicularis muscle;* **(b)** *orbital septum;* **(c)** *orbital fat;* **(d)** *levator tendon;* **(e)** *tarsi;* **(f)** *lower lid retractors;* **(g)** *levator muscle;* **(h)** *Whitnall's ligament;* **(i)** *Mueller's muscle;* **(j)** *conjunctiva;* **(k)** *inferior oblique muscle*

skin at the inferior orbital rim. At the lid margins the skin and the mucous membrane meet, forming a 'grey line' just anterior to the tarsus. This grey line is an important surgical landmark, separating the anterior skin-muscle layer from the posterior tarsus-conjunctiva layer. With aging the dermis thins and loses the normal elasticity of youth so that it becomes redundant.

The cilia (eyelashes) are arranged in two or three irregular rows at the anterior edge of the lid margin. The ducts of the eccrine sweat glands empty onto the skin. The glands of Zeis (holocrine sebaceous glands) and of Moll (apocrine sweat glands) empty into the lash follicles.

Orbicularis muscle

The orbicularis muscle fibers are oriented around the palpebral fissure in a horizontal ellipse and lie under a very thin layer of subcutaneous connective tissue (*Figure 2.10a*). The muscle, which extends from the lid margins to the oribital rim is divided into tarsal and preseptal segments and is innervated by the 7th cranial nerve. It is quite strong and serves to close the eye.

Frontalis muscle

The frontalis muscle is also innervated by the 7th cranial nerve. It is important in oculoplastic surgery because it controls the position and motion of the brow, and can be used to elevate a ptotic (drooping) lid. The origin of the frontalis is in the galea aponeurotica above the hairline, and the insertion is in the deep connective tissue and skin at the brow. It is a secondary elevator of the lid, its traction being transmitted through the skin, subcutaneous tissue and orbital septum.

Orbital septum

The orbital septum is a fibrous extension from the periosteum of the orbital rim (*Figure 2.10b*). It passes posterior to the orbicularis muscle and extends to a level just proximal to the retrotarsal margin where it joins the levator aponeurosis in the upper lid and fibers from the capsulo-palpebral fascia in the lower lid. The septum spreads nasally to the posterior lacrimal crest, temporally to the fascia of the lacrimal gland and attaches at the posterior aspect of the orbital rim around the remainder of the orbit.

Orbital fat

Orbital fat has a characteristic loose lobulated appearance. It is yellowish or whitish-yellow and contains many nerves, vessels and fibrous septa. In the upper lid it lies between the orbital septum anteriorly and the levator tendon posteriorly (*Figure 2.10c*). Thus it is an important surgical landmark because it aids in the identification of these structures. In the lower lid the orbital fat lies between the orbital septum and the fascial retractors (*Figure 2.10f*). The latter correspond to the levator tendon in the upper lid.

Levator muscle

The levator muscle (*Figure 2.10g*), the primary elevator of the upper lid, is innervated by the 3rd cranial nerve. It originates from the periorbita just above the annulus of Zinn and extends forward above the superior rectus muscle and under the frontal nerve. Soon after passing Whitnall's ligament, under the posterior aspect of the orbital rim, the muscle becomes a tendon (*Figure 2.10d*) which fans out into an aponeurosis. Just above the retrotarsal margin it fuses with the orbital septum, and it inserts on the anterior inferior one-third of the tarsus. Fibers from the aponeurosis pass into the orbicularis muscle near the level of the retrotarsal margin to form the lid crease.

A nasal extension of the aponeurosis inserts at the medial canthal tendon and sends a band to the area of the trochlea. Temporally the aponeurosis joins the lateral canthal tendon and sends a band to insert between the lobes of the lacrimal gland. These extensions to the trochlea and lacrimal areas (the so-called horns) can be tight in congenital ptosis and act as check ligaments.

Whitnall's ligament

Whitnall's ligament (the superior transverse ligament) (*Figure 2.10h*) extends from the fascia of the trochlea to the orbital lobe of the lacrimal gland. It usually lies anterior to the levator muscle, but sometimes surrounds the levator muscle and may act as a check ligament restricting its motion.

Mueller's muscle

Mueller's muscle, a sympathetically innervated smooth muscle, originates at the undersurface of the levator muscle just behind the level of Whitnall's ligament (*Figure 2.10i*). It is adherent to the underlying conjunctiva and inserts at the retrotarsal margin. The muscle is friable and slightly darker in appearance than the levator. There is a plexus of vessels on its anterior surface at the retrotarsal margin.

Capsulopalpebral fascia

The capsulopalpebral fascia, analogous to the levator aponeurosis of the upper lid, is an extension of the fascia surrounding the inferior oblique (*Figure 2.10k*) and inferior rectus muscles and Tenon's capsule. It extends forward, joining with the orbital septum and retrotarsal margin and sends strands to the inferior conjunctival fornix and the inferior tarsal muscle (which is analogous to Mueller's muscle).

Lacrimal gland

The lacrimal gland is divided into two lobes, the anterior palpebral lobe and the posterior orbital lobe. The gland lies in the lacrimal fossa in the superotemporal portion of the orbit. The upper extension of the lateral horn of the levator aponeurosis passes between the lobes. The ducts from both lobes pass around the edge of the aponeurotic extension and empty into the lateral superior conjunctival fornix.

Tarsus

The tarsus is the 'skeleton' of the lids. It is a fibrous plate about 1 mm thick and 22–25 mm in length (*Figure 2.10e*). In the upper lid it is 8–9 mm in its vertical dimension, and in the lower lid about 5 mm. The meibomian glands are located in the center of the tarsus and involve its entire height. Their openings are at the lid margins.

Conjunctiva

The conjunctiva is firmly attached to the posterior surface of the tarsus; it extends from the lid margin to the fornices of the cul-de-sacs and then anteriorly to the limbus of the globe (*Figure 2.10j*). It is suspended in the fornices by fine fibrous attachments from the levator muscle and fascia surrounding the rectus muscles. It contains the accessory lacrimal glands of Wolfring and Krause and numerous mucin-secreting goblet cells concentrated in the fornices.

Vascular supply

The abundant vascular supply to the lids promotes healing and helps prevent infection. The marginal vascular arcade runs anterior to the tarsus near the lid margin, while the peripheral arcade passes across the lid at the retrotarsal margin. These two plexi of vessels are fed by the medial superior palpebral artery, which is formed by a branch from the angular artery nasally and the zygomatico-orbital artery temporally. There are numerous veins in the lids. Those from the conjunctiva drain to the ophthalmic veins. Those from the anterior lamellae proceed to the angular vein medially and the superficial temporal vein laterally.

Lid malpositions

Senile or spastic entropion

Senile or spastic lower lid entropion is caused by a combination of factors. The skin and superficial fascia become atonic, redundant and less adherent to the orbicularis. The preseptal orbicularis is lax, decreasing pressure on the posterior part of the septum and the retrotarsal margin.

Aging also causes laxity of the capsulopalpebral fascia and absorption of orbital fat. This allows the globe to move posteriorly, thereby decreasing pressure on the lid margin, while the fascial laxness allows the retrotarsal margin and orbital septum to move forward. The preseptal orbicularis muscle rides up over the pretarsal orbicularis muscle, aggravating the situation. Entropion of 90–180° may occur (*Figure 2.11a*). Irritative factors such as ocular surgery, conjunctivitis or corneal abrasion from lashes cause orbicularis spasm that exacerbates the problem.

Numerous procedures have been devised for correction of entropion. They can be categorized as: (*1*) resections or transpositions of pieces of skin or tarsus; (*2*) cautery; (*3*) orbicularis tightening procedure; and (*4*) lid suturing procedures.

A rational and anatomical approach to the problem would tighten the capsulopalpebral fascia, stabilize the preseptal orbicularis and increase pressure of the lid against the globe, with tightening of the retrotarsal margin more than the lid margin further to stabilize the tarsus.

Correction of entropion by strategically placed sutures dates back to Hippocrates[5]. Recently, Feldstein[6] and Quickert and Rathbun[7] have described suture procedures; the latter's procedure has gained some popularity. However, recurrent entropion remains a problem, and we have developed a modification of these procedures to tighten the retractors and stabilize the tarsus and orbicularis by use of oblique scarring of the lids, which we believe gives more reliable results.

If there is also horizontal laxity of the lid from atonic tissues or orbital fat absorption, we combine the stitch procedure described below with a pentagonal full-thickness lid resection similar to that described by Hecht[8]. The combination of these measures tightens the retractors, stabilizes the orbicularis, firms contact between the lid and the globe and preferentially tightens the retrotarsal area.

Stitch operation for entropion

For anesthesia, local subcutaneous and subconjunctival injections of lidocaine (lignocaine) are used. The lid margin is grasped in its center with heavy (Adson) forceps and everted. The needle of a double-armed 4/0 chromic catgut suture (Ethicon No. 751-G provides a large, strong needle, which is essential) is passed directly down in the inferior fornix and through the retractors, which cause some resistance to its passage (*Figure 2.11b*). The needle is then angled up and outward so that it passes between orbicularis and tarsus to emerge from the skin 2 mm inferior to the cilia (*Figure 2.11c*). The second arm is passed 2 mm from the first to complete the mattress effect (*Figure 2.11d*). An additional suture is passed 3 or 4 mm on either side of the first. The three sutures are then tied to produce about a 30° overcorrection (*Figure 2.11e,f*).

Initial overcorrection of the entropion is extremely important to ensure the proper position and tightness of the stabilizing scar (*Figure 2.11g*). It is this aspect of the procedure that makes the operation highly successful. The sutures are left in place, and the external portions slough off in about 3–4 weeks. The lid remains overcorrected for 2–3 weeks and then returns to normal position.

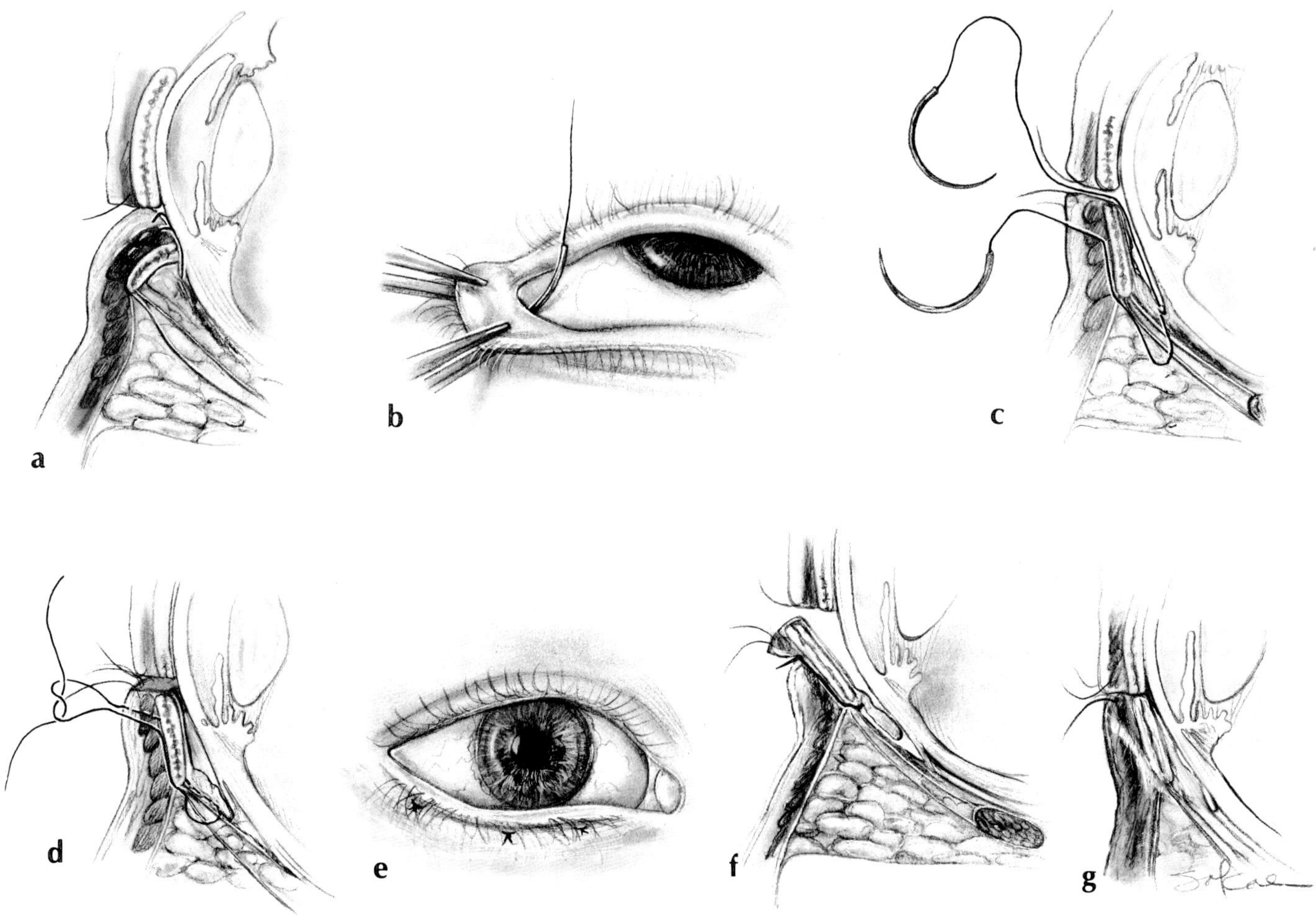

Figure 2.11 *Modified three-stitch procedure for treatment of senile or spastic entropion.* **(a)** *Lower lid is turned inward due to combination of factors including laxness of capsulopalpebral fascia and contracture of the pretarsal orbicularis muscle.* **(b,c)** *Double-armed 4/0 chromic catgut suture passed through conjunctiva near the fornix, through lower lid retractors and anteriorly in pretarsal plane to exit through skin below lash line.* **(d–f)** *Second arm of suture passed in same plane and two additional double-arm sutures used and tied to create 30° overcorrection.* **(g)** *Stabilizing scar maintains proper orientation of lid margin and overcorrection disappears*

Modified stitch operation for a very lax lid

A very lax lid is unstable and placement of the sutures described above can cause eversion of the lid by 90° or more. In these cases two mattress sutures are placed in the medial two-thirds of the lid. A pentagon of tissue is then removed from the lateral third of the lid. The incisions are shaped so that the widest part of the pentagon is at the retrotarsal margin (*Figure 2.12*)[8]. Usually a

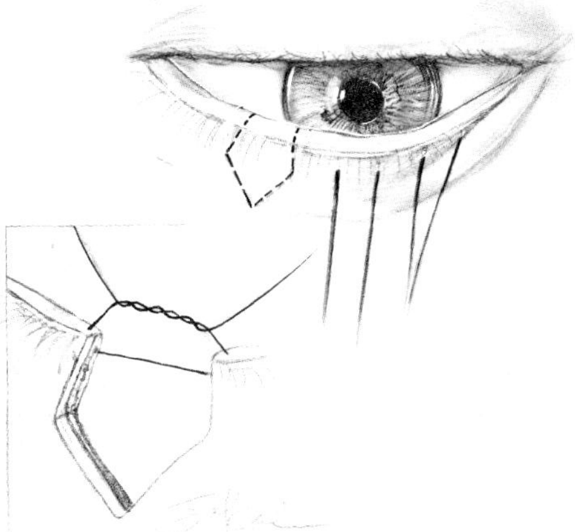

Figure 2.12 *Combination of stitch procedure with pentagonal excision of full-thickness portion of lateral lid margin to treat entropion and lax lid. Two sutures are used in nasal part of lid, and a portion of full-thickness lid margin is excised temporally to tighten lid*

total width of 5–7 mm is excised. The incision is closed first with 6/0 silk, taking a large bite through the tarsus to realign the lid margin. Absorbable 6/0 sutures are then used to reapproximate the cut tarsal edges, and the skin is closed with 8/0 black silk. A second 6/0 black silk suture is placed at the lash line. The preplaced 4/0 chromic mattress sutures are then tied so as to produce a 15–30° eversion of the lid margin.

Our overall success rate with these procedures has been about 95 per cent in more than 60 cases with a follow-up of 1–8 years. Two failures occurred in patients who had had previous entropion procedures. When failure occurs the suture procedure can be repeated with an increase in the initial overcorrection and horizontal lid tightening if needed.

Senile or spastic entropion of the upper lid is rare because the tarsal plate and firm traction from the levator and Mueller's muscle stabilize the lid margin.

Cicatricial entropion

Trachoma, recurrent chalazions, trauma and tumor surgery can cause scarring that distorts the lids. Scarring in the tarsus causes an inward curving of the lid margin, bringing the lashes into contact with the cornea. Contour abnormalities and trichiasis can further complicate the situation. Patients with trichiasis often pluck the lashes, breaking many and leaving stubs that do more corneal damage and may result in corneal ulceration and scarring.

Localized trichiasis can be treated by epilation with a diathermy unit. A long sharp diathermy needle is passed along the hair shaft to the level of the follicle. As current is applied a whitening occurs around the lash, and as the needle is withdrawn the hair comes with it.

More extensive trichiasis is best treated with cryotherapy. The cryotherapy probe is placed on the lashes, and the freezing effect is applied until a temperature of −20 °C is reached as measured by a thermocouple placed at the base of the lashes. If a thermocouple is not available, a freeze of 30–45 seconds is used. Two freezes are used in each location, with time allowed for a thaw between applications.

Effectiveness of freeze can be greatly enhanced by splitting the lid just posterior to the lashes and applying the freeze directly on the follicles. A retinal detachment probe can be used effectively when the lid is split, but a broad-tipped trichiasis unit (Cryomedics) is needed if the lid is not split. Cryotherapy causes depigmentation, and therefore in blacks the skin anterior to the follicles is dissected away and the freeze is applied to the posterior lamella of the lid.

Cicatricial entropion of either lid is extremely difficult to manage. Tarsectomy can be used if the tarsus is thickened, as occurs with trachoma[9]. Marginal rotations have also been used[10], but these may increase problems with contour deformity or retraction. We have found that a tarsal-conjunctival graft at the posterior edge of the lid margin gives the best results and can be used for either lid.

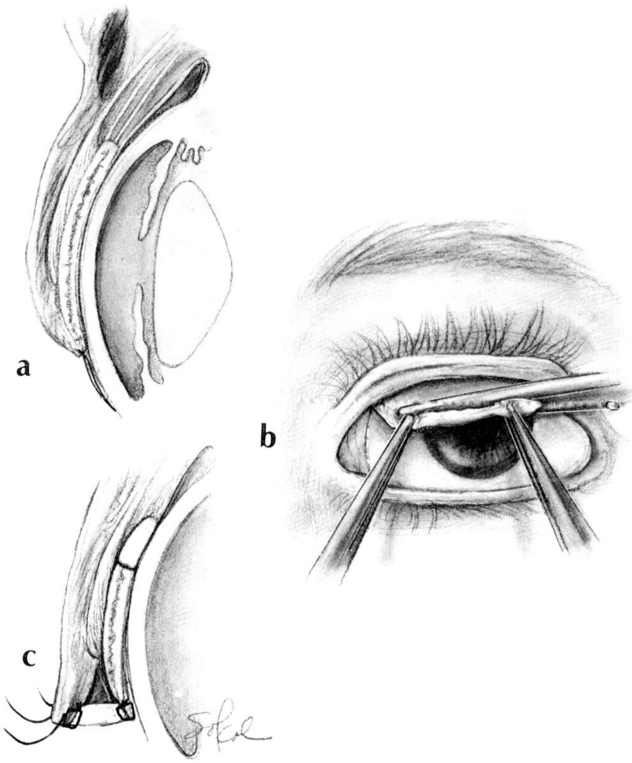

Figure 2.13 *Tarsal strip procedure for cicatricial entropion.* **(a)** *Cicatricial entropion causing contact between lid margin and lashes and globe.* **(b)** *After splitting eyelid along lid margin, lid is everted and 2 mm strip of superior tarsal edge and attached conjunctiva is excised.* **(c)** *Graft is then sutured between split edges of lid margin to rotate anterior part of lid and lashes away from globe*

The lid is split just posterior to the lashes or the keratinized epithelium. This is usually at the posterior edge of the lid. The skin flap containing the lashes is reflected forward with a traction suture, and dissection is performed anterior to the tarsus for about 2–3 mm. If there is severe trichiasis, the anterior flap can be treated with cryotherapy. The retrotarsal margin is then grasped with forceps, and scissors are used to excise 2 mm of the tarsal edge with the attached conjunctiva (*Figure 2.13a,b*). The graft is then sutured in the split lid with 8/0 absorbable sutures, carefully burying the knots (*Figure 2.13c*). The procedure creates a new lid margin that is free of lashes and keratinized epithelium. The preoperative lid contour, as determined by the lower portion of the tarsal plate, is unchanged. The donor site is not sutured.

For severe entropion of the upper lid, excision of the distorted tarsus is necessary. The lid is everted with a Desmarres retractor, and an incision is made at the retrotarsal edge through the conjunctiva and Mueller's muscle. The free edge of the tarsus is grasped, the retractor removed and blunt dissection used to separate the tarsus from the levator aponeurosis as far anterior as the insertion of the levator on the inferior anterior tarsus. The tarsus is excised proximal to this insertion. The conjunctiva and Mueller's muscle are sutured to the levator tendon at its insertion, using a running absorbable suture. The knots are buried to avoid contact with the cornea. The pull of the aponeurosis and Mueller's muscle on the anterior surface of this small remaining tarsal strip tends to rotate it and the lashes outwards. The bare cut edge of tarsus is in contact with the cornea, and it epithelializes quickly. A suture elevating the lower lid is used for 24 hours to hold the lower lid firmly against the upper lid margin, which also helps rotate the lashes outward.

Ectropion

Ectropion, like entropion, can have a cicatricial or non-cicatricial cause. Non-cicatricial ectropion of the upper lid is unusual but does occur and has been seen in both infants and adults[11,12]. It occurs mainly during sleep but can occur during tight lid closure. It is caused by excessive horizontal length of the tarsal plate. Correction is obtained by full-thickness lid resection.

Senile (non-cicatricial) ectropion of the lower lid is common. A persistent blepharoconjunctivitis often results. The conjunctiva along the lid margin dries, with resulting cornification and subepithelial inflammatory cell infiltration. Horizontal shortening of the lid is required with preferential tightening of the lid margin.

Senile ectropion of the lower lid

Byron Smith's modification of the original Kuhnt–Szymanowski procedure[13] in repairing senile ectropion of the lower lid (*Figure 2.14a*) provides excellent results. An incision is made just below the cilia through skin and muscle. The incision extends from just temporal to the punctum to the lateral canthus and is then angled upward and extended 1 cm further (*Figure 2.14b*). A skin-muscle flap is dissected along the length of the incision for about 15 mm inferiorly (*Figure 2.14c*). The posterior half of the lid – consisting of the lid margin, tarsus and conjunctiva – is shortened by removing a base-up triangle from its temporal third (*Figure 2.14d*). The lateral arm of the triangle is cut first with scissors. The two cut edges are then grasped with forceps and overlapped to estimate the amount of tissue removal needed to give a suitably tight lid. Usually about 1 cm of tissue is excised. The lid margin (*Figure 2.14e*) and tarsus (*Figure 2.15a*) are then reapproximated as has been described for entropion repair.

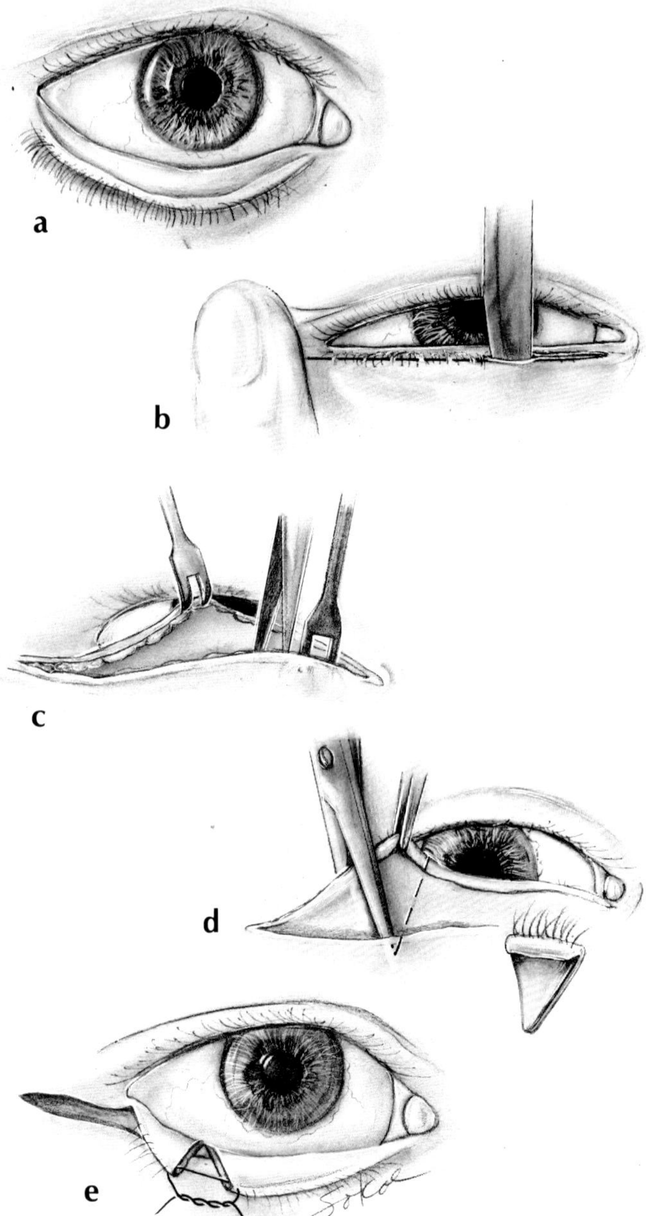

Figure 2.14 *Modified Kuhnt-Szymanowski procedure for correction of senile entropion of lower lid.* **(a)** *Senile ectropion of lower lid.* **(b)** *An incision is made just below the lid margin extending from nasal punctum to just beyond and superior to lateral canthus.* **(c)** *Skin-muscle flap is dissected throughout length of incision.* **(d)** *Base-up triangle of lid margin tissue is excised laterally.* **(e)** *Cut edges of lid margin are reapproximated*

The skin-muscle flap is then pulled temporally with a skin hook so that a fold of skin forms overlying the inferior crow's-foot crease. The fold of skin is excised with scissors angled so that when the incision is closed the suture line falls in the crow's-foot crease (*Figure 2.15b*). The skin at the temporal edge of the flap is then dissected away from the muscle for 2–3 mm to allow placement of two deep mattress sutures (*Figure 2.15c,d*). Two 5/0 absorbable sutures are passed through the muscle and tied. They are brought superotemporally and are passed through the firm fascia and muscle so that when tied there is an upward and outward sling effect on the muscle. The skin is then closed with multiple interrupted 8/0 silk suture (*Figure 2.15d, e*).

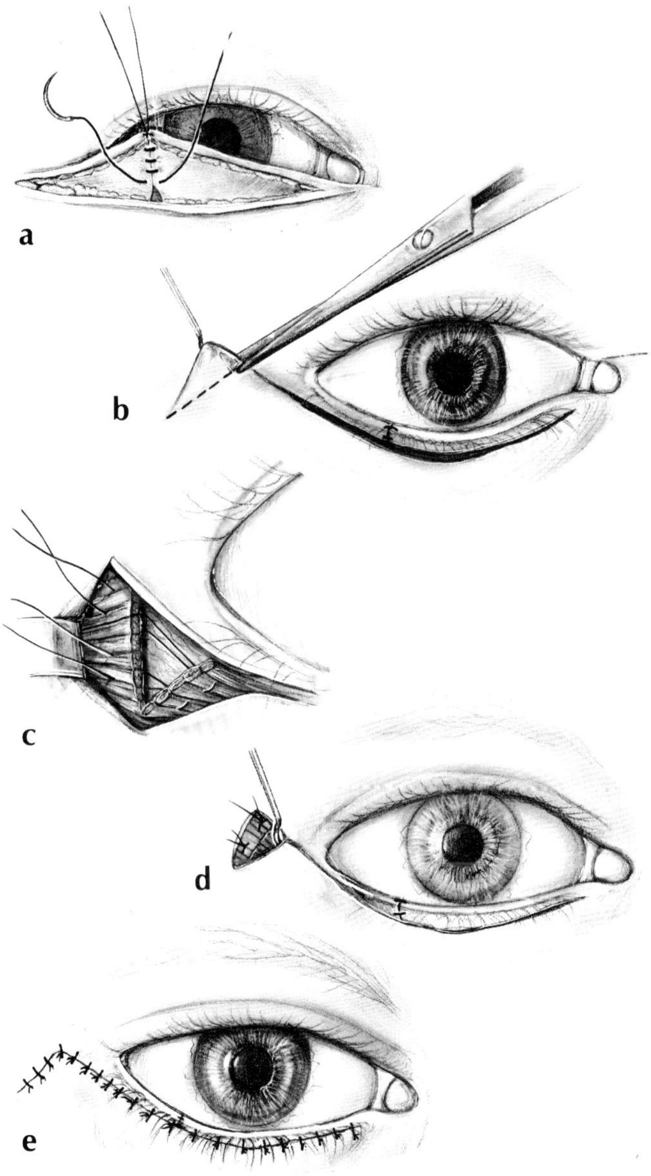

Figure 2.15 *Further steps in repair of senile ectropion of lower lid.* **(a)** *Cut tarsus is repaired with multiple sutures.* **(b)** *Skin-muscle flap is then pulled temporally and excess skin excised.* **(c,d)** *Two deep absorbable sutures are used to close the muscle layer.* **(e)** *Skin incision is closed with multiple fine sutures*

If the thickened roll of conjunctiva near the lid margin does not invert readily, it must be removed with scissors or cautery. No suturing is necessary; the denuded area rapidly epithelializes.

Ectropion of the punctum

Mild ectropion of the medial aspect of the lid may not be readily apparent, but it may cause the punctum to be everted away from the lacrimal lake, resulting in epiphora. The 'Lazy T' procedure, described by Byron Smith[14], works well for this problem (*Figure 2.16a–e*).

A lacrimal probe is placed in the canaliculus and a 1 cm horizontal incision is made 3 mm below the canaliculus through conjunctiva and tarsus parallel to the lid margin (*Figure 2.16b*). The area inferior to the incision is undermined for 3 mm, and a small triangle 3 mm wide and 1 cm long is excised (*Figure 2.16c*). A vertical, full-thickness lid incision extending to the lid margin is made 3 mm temporal to the punctum, corresponding to the temporal end of the horizontal incision. The temporal portion of lid is pulled nasally over the incision to estimate the amount of horizontal shortening needed. A base-up triangle is excised. The horizontal incision is closed with interrupted 7/0 absorbable sutures (*Figure 2.16d*), and the vertical incision is closed as has been described (*Figure 2.16e*).

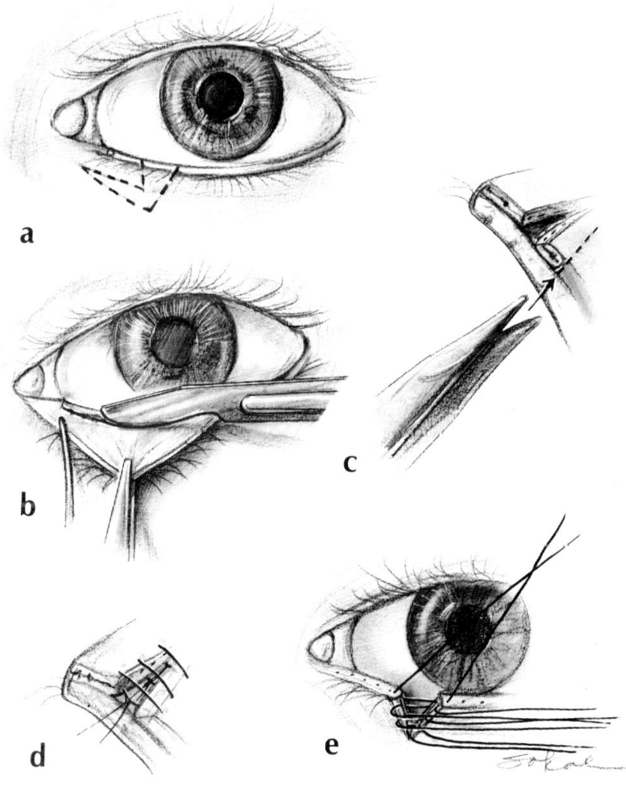

Figure 2.16 *'Lazy T' operation for ectropion of punctum.* **(a)** *Wedge-shaped portions of lid margin and deep tarsal-conjunctival surface will be removed.* **(b)** *Horizontal incision is made through conjunctiva and tarsus below canaliculus.* **(c)** *Wedge-shaped tissue strip 3 mm wide and vertical wedge-shaped section of lid margin are excised.* **(d,e)** *The two incisions are closed separately*

Cicatricial ectropion

Scarring from trauma, infection, irradiation, tumor or surgery can cause tightening of the lid skin with secondary ectropion. Removal of the abnormal scarred tissue and skin grafting are needed. Deep scarring must be completely released prior to grafting, and the lid is kept stretched for several days after grafting to minimize recurrence of deep scarring. Skin grafting techniques are discussed in the section on 'Basic principles'.

Ptosis

Blepharoptosis is one of the most challenging and commonly encountered oculoplastic problems. Especially in congenital ptosis, compromises among various factors have to be made to get the best result, and these compromises have to be discussed preoperatively with the patient or the parents. A defective levator muscle cannot be made to function properly, but the lid level can be changed. The dynamic limitations that persist postoperatively lead to lid lag and lagophthalmos. Often the best that can be hoped for is normal lid level and contour when the eyes are in the primary position.

The knowledge of lid anatomy gained from a textbook is inadequate for the ptosis surgeon. Only experience gained with a skilled surgeon will suffice. Photographs and drawings cannot depict the subtle shifting of tissue planes that occur and distort the operative picture. The levator tendon and orbital septum may be quite thin, tending to shred when held. Any description of ptosis surgery can only be taken as a starting point for treatment of this condition.

Types of ptosis

Congenital ptosis

Ptosis is considered congenital if it is present from birth, although it may not have a hereditary basis. Birth injury is often suggested (especially by parents) as a possible cause, although there is no good evidence to support this suggestion.

Berke and Wadsworth[15] found that striated muscle fibers were decreased in the levator in cases with mild congenital ptosis, and in cases with moderate ptosis muscle fibers could be identified in only 54 per cent. No striated muscle fibers were found in severe ptosis. Isaksson[16] confirmed Berke and Wadsworth's findings. It is unlikely that birth trauma is a cause of these findings. However, levator tendon dehiscence sometimes occurs in congenital ptosis[17], and this could be related to trauma. Ptosis can occur as a familial disorder, and the blepharophimosis-ptosis syndrome is a hereditary disease which follows an autosomal dominant pattern.

Blepharophimosis ptosis

Patients with this syndrome have bilateral severe ptosis, epicanthus and small palpebral fissures. Telecanthus and ectropion and ptosis of the lateral aspects of the lower lids are associated defects. The aponeurotic horns are very tight, often making the lids difficult to evert. The lids appear thickened and do not have creases.

Unilateral and bilateral ptosis

Any degree of ptosis can occur and, although usually sporadic, can be familial. Mild unilateral ptosis is only a cosmetic defect. Severe ptosis that covers the visual axis can cause amblyopia[18], even though previously it was felt that amblyopia would not occur unless ptosis was associated with strabismus, lid tumor or anisometropia. Therefore, young patients with severe ptosis should be carefully evaluated prior to corrective surgery. Children with severe bilateral ptosis may tilt the head back to see straight ahead. This abnormal head position tends to unbalance the body and can interfere with the baby's learning to walk. In such cases surgery is done at 9 months to a year of age.

Ptosis with superior rectus muscle weakness

Unilateral or bilateral ptosis can be associated with weakness of the superior rectus muscle, which is probably caused by a loss of muscle fibers as is the weakness of the levator muscle. The eye will not elevate in abduction. Passive ('forced') ductions show no resistance to motion. Fusion is possible in all lower fields. Occasionally, secondary contraction of the inferior rectus muscle occurs and makes strabismus surgery necessary.

Double elevator palsy

Children with unilateral or bilateral ptosis can have a double elevator palsy. There is decreased superior rectus and inferior oblique function. The eye will not elevate above the midline. The etiology is unknown, but preservation of the Bell's phenomenon in these cases suggests a supranuclear lesion.

Strabismus

Orthoptic evaluation should be done on all children with ptosis. When ptosis is associated with strabismus that requires corrective surgery, the strabismus procedure can be done at the same time as the ptosis surgery. If diplopia is present, corrective strabismus surgery should be done prior to ptosis surgery to rule out a 'protective' cause for the ptosis in which the lid is closed to avoid diplopia.

Jaw-winking (Marcus–Gunn phenomenon)

Jaw-winking is usually unilateral, but bilateral cases also occur. With the eyes in the primary position there is a variable amount of ptosis. (We have seen one case in which the wink occurred but no ptosis was present.) When the jaw is moved there is rapid elevation of the lid to a level that may be higher than the normal lid position, followed by a rapid return to the ptotic state. The wink may be induced by sucking, swallowing, chewing or lateral motion of the jaw.

The cause of jaw-winking is a congenital misdirection of 5th cranial nerve fibers into the branch of the 3rd cranial nerve supplying the levator muscle. The levator muscle in these cases is rather poorly innervated, accounting for the ptosis, and when stimulation of the muscles supplied by the 5th nerve occurs, impulses also go the levator muscle on the affected side. Although it has been thought that jaw-winking improves with age, Beard[19] believes that this is not the case. We agree that the Marcus–Gunn phenomenon can be seen in adults, and there are no documented cases of spontaneous disappearance of the symptoms. However, we have observed patients in whom the intensity of the reflex decreased with advancing age[20].

3rd nerve palsy

Congenital 3rd nerve palsy with ptosis usually does not improve with time. Amblyopia occurs unless vigorous orthoptic therapy is given. If the ptosis is severe enough to interfere with vision while the fellow eye is patched, ptosis surgery should be done at an early age.

Horner's syndrome

Congenital Horner's syndrome can be caused by trauma to the sympathetic fibers at the level of the brachial plexus at birth. The levator muscle is normal. Therefore, the amount of levator resection needed is less than for the same amount of congenital ptosis which is due solely to a levator abnormality.

Senile ptosis

Although loss of levator and Mueller's muscle tone undoubtedly occurs with age and can account for some decrease in upper lid height, it is now believed that the primary cause of 'senile' ptosis is thinning with stretching or dehiscence of the levator aponeurosis[21]. Despite the term 'senile', this condition can occur at any age and has been documented in children[17]. Inflammation, surgery and trauma can cause or hasten ptosis because of levator aponeurosis stretching or dehiscence. The usual site of dehiscence is just above the retrotarsal margin. The levator muscle is normal, and surgery must take this into account or overcorrection will result.

Myogenic ptosis

Progressive external ophthalmoplegia is a chronic, slowly progressive disorder with increasing interference with extraocular and levator muscle function. The disease begins in childhood or adolescence. Bell's phenomenon is absent, but the orbicularis muscle often is not affected until late in the course of the disease. A very conservative frontalis sling procedure to elevate the lid barely above the visual axis can be done.

Late hereditary ptosis is accompanied by difficulty in swallowing, as a result of oculopharyngeal dystrophy. Many patients with this disorder are members of a French Canadian family that was originally from Quebec[22].

Neurogenic ptosis

Vascular, traumatic, inflammatory or neoplastic lesions can damage the 3rd cranial nerve and cause exotropia, hypotropia, ptosis and pupillary dilatation. There is loss of accommodation, and diplopia occurs. The causes of 3rd nerve palsy are often of more serious concern than treatment of the ocular effects. After treatment of the underlying disorder, surgery can be done to correct the ptosis. The diplopia usually cannot be eliminated, and therefore elevation of the lid must be followed by occlusion of vision in the affected eye with an opaque contact lens. Usually a frontalis sling procedure is required.

Horner's syndrome is a frequent cause of neurogenic ptosis, and it is caused by interference with the sympathetic innervation to Mueller's muscle[23]. The ptosis is associated with miosis and slight elevation of the lower lid. Tumors, inflammatory disorders, injuries and aneurysms can be the cause. Failure of the pupil to dilate when cocaine drops are instilled is typical of a 3rd nerve type of Horner's syndrome. However, the pupil will dilate and the lid will elevate when phenylephrine is instilled. If there is a preganglionic lesion, hydroxyamphetamine (Paredrine) drops will dilate the pupil, indicating that norepinephrine (noradrenaline) is present at the myoneural junction. The pupil fails to dilate if the lesion is postganglionic, because no norepinephrine is present. A small levator resection can be done to repair the ptosis.

Myasthenia gravis

Patients with undiagnosed myasthenia gravis may be seen initially by the opthalmologist because of diplopia and/or ptosis. The condition is caused by a defect at the myoneural junction[24]. It is not known why the extraocular muscles, especially the levator muscle, are often affected first.

Ptosis may be unilateral or bilateral. The disease can begin in childhood, and it should be tested for in cases of acquired and variable ptosis in children. Testing is done by intramuscular injection of neostigmine (Prostigmin) or intravenous injection of edrophonium (Tensilon), which causes rapid temporary relief of symptoms. If involvement by the disease is confined to the ocular symptoms and the patient does not tolerate the medical therapy, ptosis surgery can be done.

Traumatic ptosis

Trauma to the lid can cause ptosis by damaging the levator muscle or tendon, or by subsequent scarring that restricts lid movement. Damage to the 3rd cranial nerve can also result in ptosis, as has been mentioned. Blunt trauma may cause an intramuscular hematoma or local neurological damage. The ptosis may resolve after several months, and a waiting period of at least 6 months is advised before operating.

Lacerations can produce localized or complete ptosis by dividing the levator aponeurosis. Often, associated swelling and damage to other tissues initially masks evidence of the levator tendon injury. If the levator damage is not repaired primarily, residual ptosis occurs and is difficult to correct with later surgery because of the associated scarring. Reattachment of a severed levator tendon must often be accompanied by a small levator resection because of scarring and fibrosis in the levator muscle.

Mechanical ptosis

Mechanical ptosis can be caused by added eyelid weight from severe edema, neurofibromas, hemangiomas or large basal cell carcinomas. Scarring of the conjunctiva, lid skin or deeper structures can restrict lid movement.

Pseudoptosis

The term 'pseudoptosis' is used to describe a drooping of the upper lid not caused by an abnormality of the levator apparatus, such as with enophthalmos or a poorly fitting prosthesis. In these cases there is decreased support to the back of the eyelid. The term pseudoptosis is then perhaps inappropriate because ptosis of the eyelid is present, for whatever reason.

The term pseudoptosis should be reserved for a lid that looks ptotic but actually isn't, as might occur with asymmetrical lid creases or severely redundant lid skin that hangs over the lid margin.

Preoperative evaluation

Proper preoperative evaluation is essential to determine accurately the type and degree of ptosis and to plan the appropriate surgical procedure.

History

Past medical history is recorded, with special attention to history of allergic reactions, bleeding tendency, use of medications and anesthesia problems in the patient or family members. Malignant hyperthermia during surgery is slightly more common in ptosis patients. It occurs as a rapid rise in body temperature caused by an abnormal response to anesthetic agents and/or neuromuscular blockers. Often there is a family history of anesthesia problems, and serum creatine phosphokinase (CPK) is elevated in susceptible patients. This can be tested for preoperatively in children who will be undergoing surgery for congenital ptosis, but this test has not been done routinely.

In children, features of the prenatal and perinatal history may be helpful in determining whether a 'congenital' ptosis is of developmental or traumatic origin. In adults, history of heart, lung, liver or kidney problems could have important bearing on the risks of anesthetic agents or antibiotics. A history of muscle weakness or difficulty in swallowing suggests muscular dystrophy or possibly myasthenia gravis.

Ophthalmic history of diplopia, variability of lid level, injury, infection or previous ophthalmic surgery may help in determining the cause of an acquired ptosis. Time of onset, duration and progression (if any) of the ptosis are noted. Many children with congenital ptosis have lagophthalmos, and often the parents give a history that the child sleeps with the affected eye slightly open. In such cases the lagophthalmos may be made more severe by surgery, and this possibility is discussed with the parents.

In adults it is important to record any history of asthenopic symptoms. Surgery for ptosis in patients with a history of dry eye problems should be approached with caution.

Examination

Ophthalmic examination of ptosis patients begins with a measure of visual function. In young children the fixation pattern and whether he or she objects to a bright light or to covering of each eye may be all that can be measured. A carefully done confrontation test of visual field is usually adequate to determine whether there is a disturbance of peripheral vision attributable to the ptosis. The presence of abnormal extraocular motility, muscle paresis or diplopia is noted. In children, cycloplegic retinoscopy is done. Amblyopia, when it occurs in patients with ptosis, is usually related to strabismus or anisometropia and only rarely is caused by ptosis alone. Bell's phenomenon is tested for. Slit-lamp, fundus examination and measurement of intraocular pressure are done. Schirmer testing is done in adults.

The lid contour, lashes and skin are evaluated. In adults, redundant skin or ptosis of the brow may require excision or repair. Palpation may reveal small masses not evident by observation. To test orbicularis function, the patient is asked to close his or her eyes. Children are asked to move their jaw or chew and infants are allowed to nurse as a test for jaw-winking.

Ptosis evaluation begins with observation of the level of the lids relative to the globe and to each other. The normal upper eyelid crosses the cornea 1.5–2 mm below the limbus. The cornea is about 11 mm in height; therefore, a 3.5 mm ptosis would cause the lid margin to split the visual axis. In an uncooperative child exact measurement may be impossible. However, the amount of ptosis can be estimated by the position of the lid and pupil. For example, if the lid margin is about 1.5 mm above the visual axis (perhaps at the edge of the pupil in a moderately lighted room), there is 2 mm of ptosis.

The position of the lids is measured if possible. If the lower lids are normal and equal, and if there is no strabismus, an accurate assessment of ptosis can be made by measuring the opening of the palpebral fissure. The use of Beard's classification[25] aids in grouping the degrees of ptosis that cannot be precisely measured. A mild ptosis is 1–2 mm; moderate, 3 mm; and severe, 4 mm or more (*Figure 2.17*).

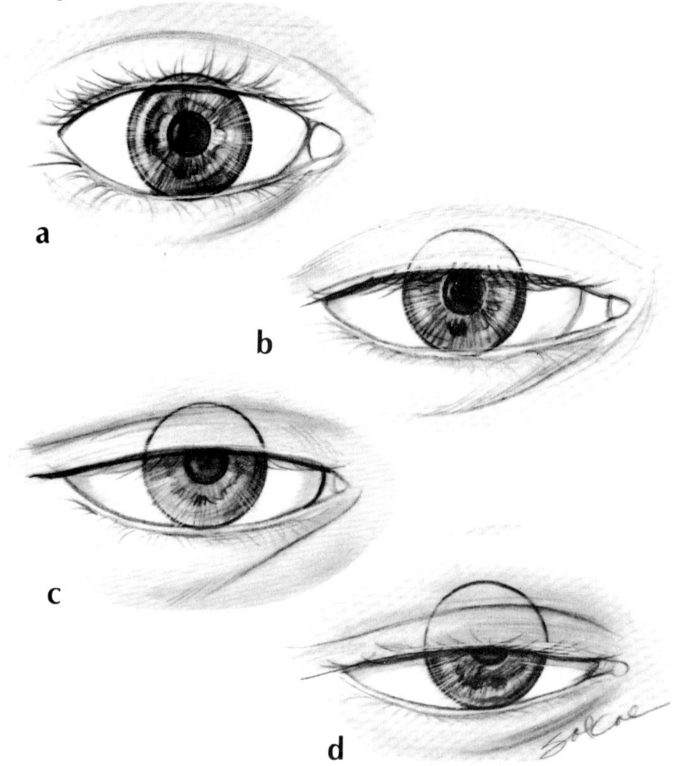

Figure 2.17 *Classification of degrees of ptosis.* **(a)** *Upper lid normally crosses cornea 1.5–2 mm below limbus.* **(b)** *Drooping of lid 1–2 mm is judged mild ptosis.* **(c)** *3 mm is moderate ptosis.* **(d)** *4 mm or more is severe ptosis*

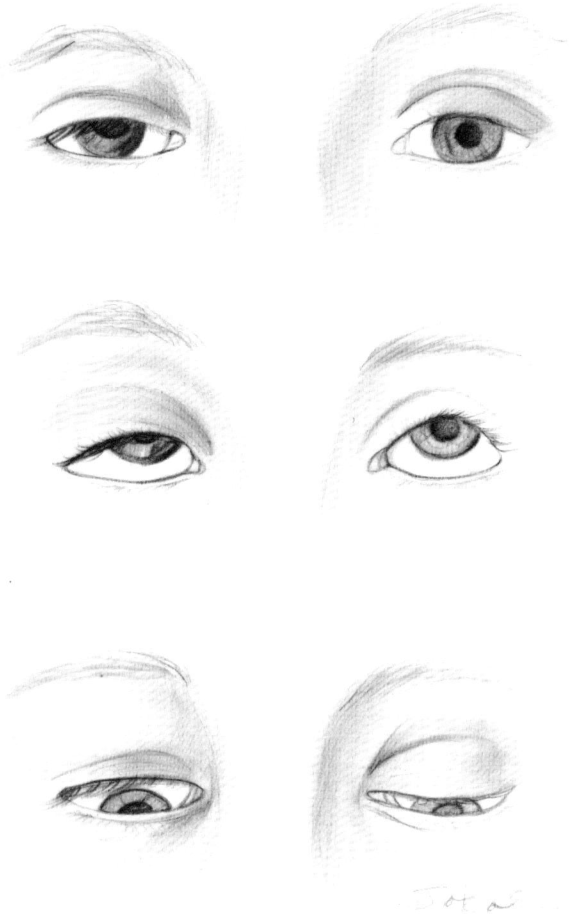

Figure 2.18 *Lid lag in ptotic right eye. Right lid droops in primary position and fails to follow globe downward during downgaze, suggesting fibrotic levator muscle*

Evaluation of levator function is extremely important and begins with observation of the lid creases. The presence of a lid crease suggests the existence of levator function, even if the lid moves poorly. In acquired ptosis due to aponeurosis dehiscence the crease often moves superiorly. An asymmetrical lid crease can be a significant cosmetic blemish requiring surgical correction, even in cases with very mild ptosis. The patient's ability to reduce an everted lid by looking up also indicates some levator function.

Exact measurement of the position of the lid margin in upgaze and downgaze gives the most accurate evaluation of ptosis. In severe congenital ptosis, the levator muscle is fibrotic (deficient of muscle fibers). Therefore, the amplitude of its action is diminished and the lid will fail to depress normally, producing a lid lag on downgaze (*Figure 2.18*). Lid lag is increased by surgery for congenital ptosis, and this situation must be discussed with the parents. Fibrosis of the levator, with lagophthalmos, causes the affected eye to be *less* ptotic when the patient is under anesthesia. We know of one case in which the wrong eye was operated on because of this change.

The levator muscle is normal in ptosis caused by dehiscence of the aponeurosis, and the levator is not fibrotic in neurogenic or myogenic ptosis. Therefore, the amount of ptosis stays the same in upgaze and downgaze (*Figure 2.19*). Movement of 4 mm or less is considered a sign of poor levator function; 5–7 mm indicates fair levator function; and 8 mm or more indicates good levator function.

Photographs

Preoperative photographs are an important part of the medical record, and they may be helpful in revealing aspects of the ptosis that are not obvious during examination. Photographs should be taken in the primary gaze position and in upgaze and downgaze. If the Marcus–Gunn phenomenon is present, the photographs should include the mouth and demonstrate the change in position of the lid as the jaw is moved.

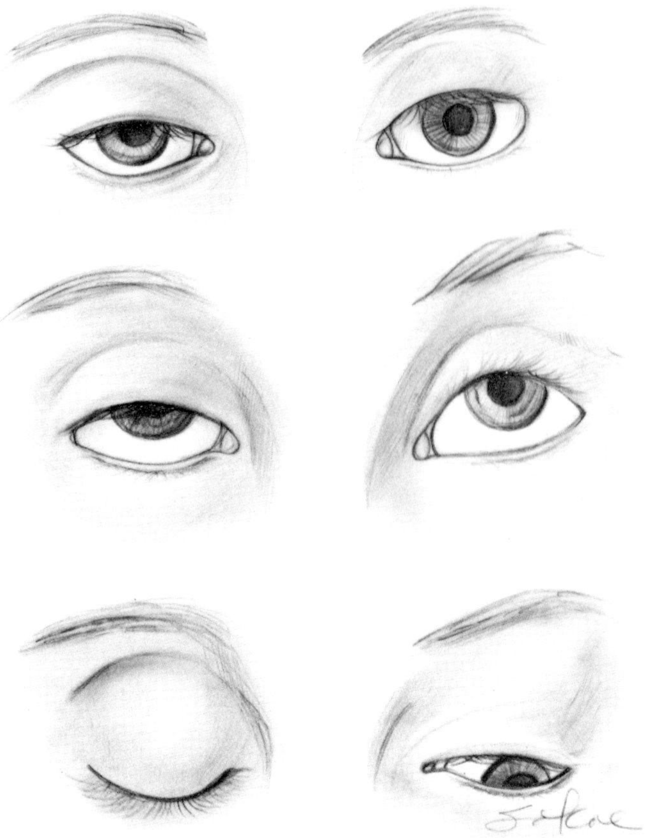

Figure 2.19 *Normal levator function in right eye with senile ptosis. Amount of ptosis is unchanged in primary position, upgaze and downgaze*

Testing for myasthenia gravis

Neostigmine (Prostigmin) or edrophonium (Tensilon) is used to test for myasthenia gravis. In adults, 1 mg of neostigmine injected intramuscularly will dramatically improve the ptosis within 15 minutes if myasthenia gravis is the cause. The edrophonium test uses 10 mg of the drug given intravenously. This is done by first giving 2 mg intravenously over 15–30 seconds. If there are no side-effects within 1 minute, the remaining 8 mg are injected slowly. Improvement in the ptosis occurs after 1–5 minutes if the test is positive. An adverse cholinergic reaction characterized by pallor, perspiration, dizziness and abdominal cramping occasionally occurs. It is treated with atropine sulfate (atropine sulphate) 0.5 mg given intravenously.

Choice of operation

There is considerable difference of opinion among oculoplastic surgeons as to the 'best' ptosis procedure. Although many procedures produce satisfactory results, the surgeon should use the method he feels most comfortable with and which consistently gives the best results. Ptosis surgery is difficult. Many attempts have been made to develop procedures designed to help the occasional ptosis surgeon get satisfactory results. Examples are the Iliff[26] and the Fasanella and Servat[27] procedures.

However, as the field of ocuplastic surgery continues to grow, there is increasing emphasis on understanding the exact cause of ptosis in each case, and on using surgical techniques intended to deal directly with the anatomical defect. We believe that ptosis caused by levator dehiscence should be corrected by repairing the dehiscence. If there is an abnormality of the muscle, the repair should shorten the levator aponeurosis rather than resecting normal tarsus and conjunctiva. A skin approach, with meticulous dissection of the lid structures, is the best way to identify and treat the anatomical defect, and we use this approach for all ptosis surgery except the frontalis sling operation.

Levator resection for congenital ptosis

Mild congenital ptosis (1–2 mm) is usually accompanied by good levator function (8 mm or greater); moderate (3 mm) ptosis has fair levator function (5–7 mm); and severe ptosis (4 mm or more) has poor levator function (less than 4 mm). It is useful to consider levator resection procedures as small (in which 10–13 mm of levator tendon is resected), medium (14–20 mm) and large (21–28 mm) (*Table 2.1*).

Table 2.1 Amount of levator resection in congenital ptosis repair

Amount of ptosis	*Levator function*	*Levator resection*
None	15+ mm	–
Mild, 1–2 mm	Good, 8 mm or more	10–13 mm
Moderate, 3 mm	Fair, 5–7 mm	14–20 mm
Severe, 4 mm	Poor, 5 mm or less	21–26 mm

For mild or moderate ptosis, surgery is based on preoperative measurements and may be modified according to the preoperative findings. If the ptosis is severe and levator function poor, the levator tendon is shortened until the lid level at the time of surgery is in the position where it should be postoperatively (much the way a lid level is set with a frontalis sling procedure). The amount of tendon resection in severe cases is usually 21–26 mm. In severe cases we also modify the position of Mueller's muscle, as described below.

Repair of levator aponeurosis dehiscence

Senile ptosis is caused by dehiscence of the levator tendon[28]. This usually occurs just above the retrotarsal margin. Identification and repair of the area of dehiscence is the preferred method of treatment. A full dehiscence is easily identified because the upper edge of the tendon appears rolled and thickened. In other cases there is diffuse attenuation and stretching of the aponeurosis, and the amount of tendon to be excised or imbricated is harder to determine.

The operation is performed under local anesthesia. Temporary imbrication of the thinned area of tendon is done, and the patient opens his or her eyes so that the sutures can be adjusted to set the optimum lid level.

Levator resection in acquired ptosis

Acquired ptosis, not associated with levator tendon dehiscence, is difficult to treat. Patients with myasthenia gravis, oculopharyngeal syndrome and 'idiopathic' late-onset ptosis are in this category. There is great variability in these conditions.

The operation is done under local anesthesia. The levator tendon is shortened, but no tissue is excised until the patient opens his or her eyes so that the level and contour of the lid can be evaluated and the sutures adjusted if necessary.

Frontalis sling

Congenital ptosis of 4 mm or greater requires a frontalis sling for correction, as does any ptosis in which there is no levator function – such as with 3rd cranial nerve palsy or late cases of progressive external ophthalmoplegia. The frontalis muscle is the secondary elevator of the lid, and slings attached to it provide some movement of the lid.

The jaw-winking phenomenon is best treated by excision of a portion of the levator muscle to eliminate the wink, combined with a frontalis sling to elevate the lid. Beard[29] has suggested excising both levator muscles and doing bilateral frontalis sling procedures for symmetry (*Figure 2.20*). Comparable results can be obtained by not removing part of the levator from the normal eye. We have done several unilateral slings with excellent results. The patient learns to move the one brow to set the lid level close to that of the normal side and to ease the brow on downgaze to minimize asymmetry.

Attempts have been made to use the superior rectus muscle to elevate the lid, but this has caused strabismus[30–32]. Exposure keratitis also occurred as a complication, and we have seen a patient with corneal perforation and blindness due to exposure caused by inability to change the position of the globe relative to the lid.

Recently, Anderson[33] suggested using Whitnall's ligament to elevate the lid. Although the lid can close somewhat because of the elasticity of this ligament, the procedure is not likely to produce even the mild amount of lid movement that is possible with a frontalis sling.

Many materials have been used for frontalis slings, including: suture[34–36], skin[37], silicone[38], sclera[39], collagen[40], autologous fascia[41] and preserved fascia[42]. Autologous fascia lata is now the most popular material for a frontalis sling. However, preserved fascia lata is considered nearly as good and is better than the other materials mentioned. Katowitz[36] reported poor results in 29 per cent of cases when using silicone materials, mainly because of recurrence of ptosis. We have also observed recurrence of ptosis with silicone materials. Skin, although denuded of epithelium, contains dermal elements that occasionally lead to cyst formation. Recurrence of ptosis was a problem when sclera was used[43]; and collagen, as used by Iliff[40], is no longer available.

Crawford[44] reported recurrence of ptosis in 10 per cent of 317 cases operated on over a 20-year period using autologous fascia, and he recommended use of autologous fascia in all cases except in babies and elderly patients[45]. We have achieved a similar success rate with preserved fascia, and feel that the use of autologous fascia (requiring the additional surgery for the harvesting of the material) is not necessary unless there has been previous failure with the preserved material.

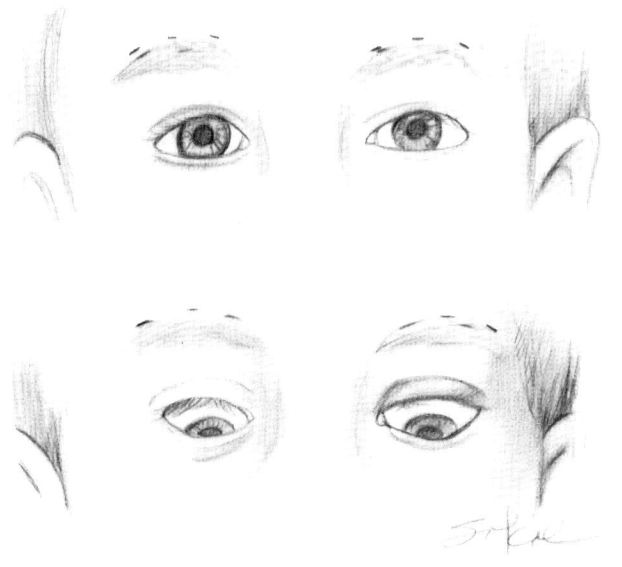

Figure 2.20 *Lid lag in downgaze after sling operation. Lid does not move down in downgaze, resulting in more exposure of superior sclera (lid lag)*

Operative procedures for ptosis

Levator resection

A 2 cm incision through skin is made with a scalpel at the site of the lid crease (or where one will be formed). Skin hooks are used to retract each side of the incision. This elevates the orbicularis, which is opened centrally with sharp iris scissors. One additional cut nasally and temporally completes the incision through the orbicularis and minimizes bleeding. Meticulous control of bleeding with bipolar cautery is essential.

Dissection is continued posterior to orbicularis in a superior direction for about 5 mm. Pressure is applied to the globe to cause forward bulging of the orbital fat behind the orbital septum. This delineates the zone where the septum joins the levator tendon (*Figure 2.21a*). The septum is opened for the length of the skin incision. The septum and orbital fat are then retracted superiorly with a Desmarres retractor.

A small buttonhole is made in the levator tendon at the retrotarsal margin, and with scissors the tendon is divided

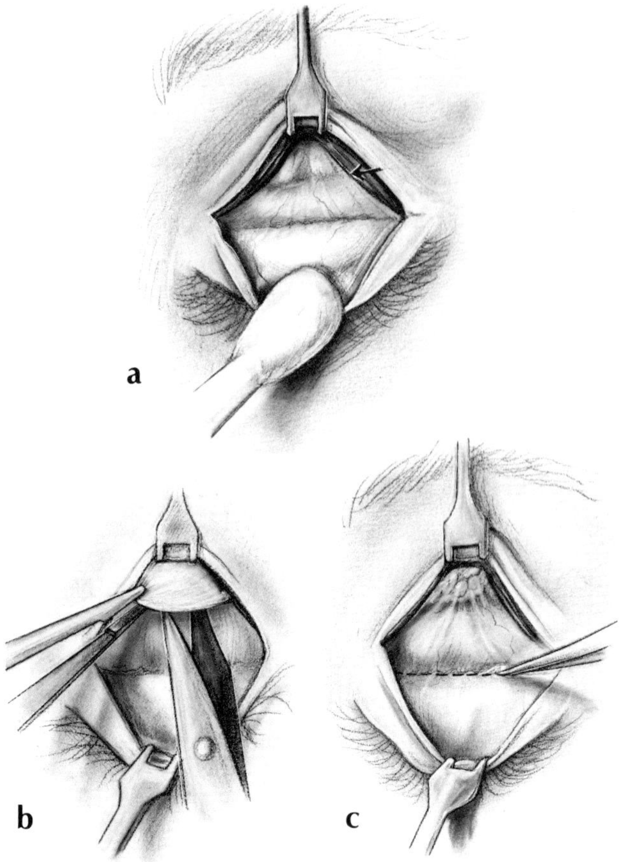

Figure 2.21 *Surgical treatment of congenital ptosis by levator resection through skin approach. Skin is incised at lid crease and orbicularis muscle opened.* **(a)** *Pressure applied to globe causes bulging of orbital fat and demonstrates zone where orbital septum joins levator tendon (arrow).* **(b,c)** *Tendon is divided and dissection extended superiorly to free undersurface of tendon from Mueller's muscle*

across the tarsus for the width of the skin incision (*Figure 2.21b*). The levator aponeurosis is gently elevated with fine 0.12 mm forceps which it is dissected with scissors from the underlying Mueller's muscle. This dissection is continued superiorly until the origin of Mueller's muscle is encountered in the belly of the levator muscle (*Figure 2.21c*). When a small amount of levator resection is planned, no further dissection is necessary. The desired amount of tendon resection is done, and the tendon edge is sutured to the lower tendon remnant with three mattress-type non-absorbable sutures of 5/0 Dacron.

In cases with moderate ptosis and poor levator function and cases with severe ptosis, the origin of Mueller's muscle is separated from the undersurface of the levator muscle using a cautery (*Figure 2.22a,b*). The nasal and lateral horns are cut to allow maximum advancement of levator tendon and muscle (*Figure 2.22c*). Mueller's muscle is then resutured to the undersurface of levator muscle using an absorbable suture (*Figure 2.22d*). The new origin of Mueller's muscle is placed as far proximal as possible (usually 15–20 mm from the retrotarsal margin) (*Figure 2.22e,f*). For moderate ptosis with poor levator function, a levator resection of about 20 mm is performed. For severe ptosis with poor levator function, after resuturing Mueller's muscle, the levator tendon is shortened until the lid level is set at the desired postoperative level (2 mm below the superior limbus with the eye in the primary position). The level of general anesthesia is important because if the patient is in a light anesthetic plane the eye will roll up, making proper setting of the lid level more difficult.

Loss of function of Mueller's muscle results in ptosis, sometimes as much as 2 mm, as can occur with Horner's syndrome. There is no evidence that this muscle is abnormal in congenital ptosis, and use of Mueller's muscle may help to obtain increased mobility in severely affected

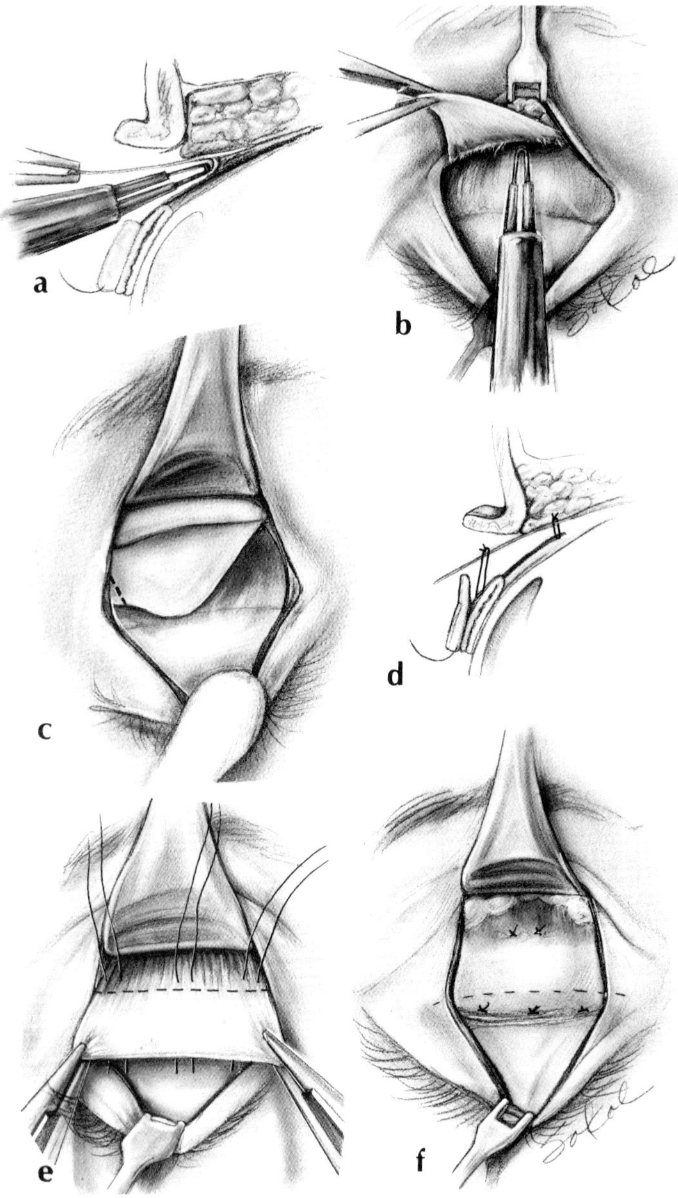

Figure 2.22 *Further steps in levator resection through skin approach for moderate ptosis and poor levator function, and severe ptosis.* **(a,b)** *Dissection to separate levator muscle from origin of Mueller's muscle is done with cautery.* **(c)** *Nasal horn of aponeurosis is cut and then temporal horn (dotted line) is cut to allow maximum advancement of tendon.* **(d)** *Mueller's muscle then resutured to undersurface of levator tendon.* **(e,f)** *Tendon is then advanced the appropriate amount and resutured to site of original insertion on anterior surface of tarsus. Dotted line in* **(f)** *represents superior margin of tarsus*

cases. Beard[46] and Collin[47] believe, as we do, that more attention should be paid to utilizing Mueller's muscle. They modified Jones' levator advancement procedure to allow resuturing of the cut inferior levator edge, and they attached Mueller's muscle under the advanced upper tendon flap. Perivascular sympathetic fibers, especially along the peripheral arcade, supply Mueller's muscle; therefore, separation of the muscle at its origin, or division of the levator muscle just above the origin of Mueller's muscle, does not affect its nerve supply[47].

The skin is closed with 7/0 absorbable interrupted sutures. If a lid crease is needed, several of the sutures include a minute bite of levator tendon with the skin bites. If the patient is old enough so that later suture removal can be done without difficulty, 8/0 black silk is used for closure. A rolled cotton pledget is placed in the superior lid sulcus, and a 6/0 silk suture is passed through the skin just below the lashes of the lower lid and taped to the brow to close the lids. The suture is folded back and forth over three tapes to prevent slippage.

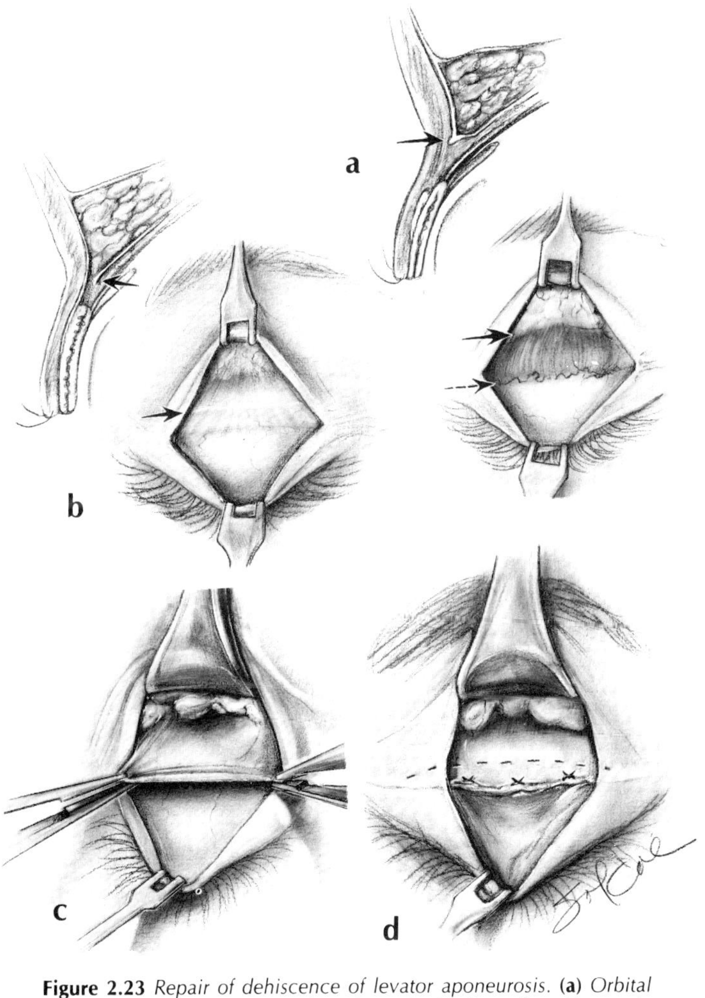

Figure 2.23 *Repair of dehiscence of levator aponeurosis.* **(a)** *Orbital septum may be rolled superiorly and attached to free edge of levator in case with complete dehiscence (arrow). The peripheral arcade of vessels can be seen at the retrotarsal margin on the surface of Mueller's muscle (dotted arrow).* **(b)** *Thin membrane is present at retrotarsal margin in cases with more proximal separation of tendon (arrow).* **(c,d)** *Orbital septum is opened so tendon can be advanced and sutured to anterior tarsal surface. Dotted line in (d) represents superior margin of tarsus*

Repair of levator aponeurosis dehiscence

Local anesthesia is used. We prefer 2 per cent lidocaine (lignocaine), and 0.5–0.75 ml is injected subcutaneously across the lid at the lid crease. The skin incision and dissection through orbicularis muscle are the same as for levator resection. If there is a complete dehiscence, the orbital septum is often rolled superiorly and attached to the free edge of the levator aponeurosis (*Figure 2.23a*). The peripheral arcade is evident on the surface of Mueller's muscle at the retrotarsal margin. Dissection is carried superiorly for 5–8 mm, so that the underlying septum and the dehisced edge of the levator tendon can be identified. Often this edge appears slightly thickened or rolled.

Occasionally a more proximal separation of the tendon has occurred, leaving an attenuated membrane at the retrotarsal margin (*Figure 2.23b*). In such cases the orbital septum is opened to facilitate advancement of the aponeurosis edge (*Figure 2.23c*). Three mattress sutures of 5/0 Dacron are placed at the upper-midportion of the tarsus in the tendon remnant. These sutures can be placed in the anterior tarsus if firm tendon is not present. The sutures are passed through the upper edge of the dehisced tendon and tied temporarily (*Figure 2.23d*). Usually no suture adjustment is necessary, but the patient is asked to open his or her eyes and adjustment made as necessary to obtain optimal lid contour and height.

We find that the best results are obtained with minimal anesthesia and a rapid atraumatic procedure. Postoperatively the lids remain at the level set during surgery or fall slightly. It is important to minimize ocular irritation when the lid levels are set. Tetracaine (amethocaine) drops and turning off surgical lights are helpful. The skin is closed with 8/0 black silk. No lid closure suture is needed. The eye is dressed with a semipressure bandage.

Frontalis sling

Three deep stab incisions are made with a No. 15 Bard-Parker knife just above the cilia of the brow. The lateral and nasal incisions lie above each canthus; the third incision is in the center. These 3 mm incisions extend down to periosteum, and the profuse bleeding that occurs is controlled with pressure. A lid plate is placed under the upper lid to protect the globe, and three 2 mm incisions through the skin and orbicularis are made 2 mm above the lashes. The lateral and medial incisions are about 6 mm from the canthi, and the third incision is placed centrally. A small hemostat is used to make a pocket deep in the temporal and nasal incisions for later placement of the fascial knots.

An empty Wright needle (Storz No. E-954) is inserted through the middle brow incision down to the periosteum. It is angled around the orbital rim to perforate the orbital septum and then passed inferiorly, anterior to the tarsal plate, to emerge through the central lid incision. The fascial strip is threaded through the eye of the needle, and the center of the strip is withdrawn through the incision to emerge from the brow, where it is then divided. Care is taken to prevent cilia from being drawn into the track by depressing the cilia with a cotton swab as the fascia is inserted.

The Wright needle is then inserted from the temporal to the center lid incision, and the fascia is drawn temporally (*Figure 2.24a*). The needle is then passed from the superior temporal incision to the temporal lid incision to draw the fascia superiorly (*Figure 2.24b*). Finally the fascia is drawn from the central to the lateral brow incision so that both ends of the strip emerge from that incision (*Figure 2.24c*) The nasal fascia strip is threaded in a similar fashion so that the ends emerge from the nasal brow incision.

At the nasal and temporal brow incisions the fascial ends are tied with a single overhand knot and are pulled tight enough so that the lid rests just above the superior limbus (*Figure 2.24d*). A full square knot is too bulky, and we use the single overhand throw of 5/0 absorbable suture material to stabilize it, using several firm through-and-through bites. The knots are then placed deep in the temporal and nasal brow wound with a clamp.

Heavy Adson forceps are then used to grasp firmly the tarsus and lid margin and pull downward to seat the fascial strips. The lid should be set at the limbus because there will be some postoperative relaxation, and the lid should have good contour. If the lid position is not suitable, the knots can be externalized, the suture cut, and adjustments made because the fascial ends have not been trimmed. When proper lid position and contour are achieved, the protruding fascial ends are trimmed to about 8 to 9 mm. The Wright needle is passed from the central brow incision to the temporal incision, and the ends of the fascia are threaded a short distance into the eye of the needle. The needle is withdrawn so that the ends bury horizontally in the deep tissue tract and pull free from the end of the needle. The same procedure is used to bury the nasal

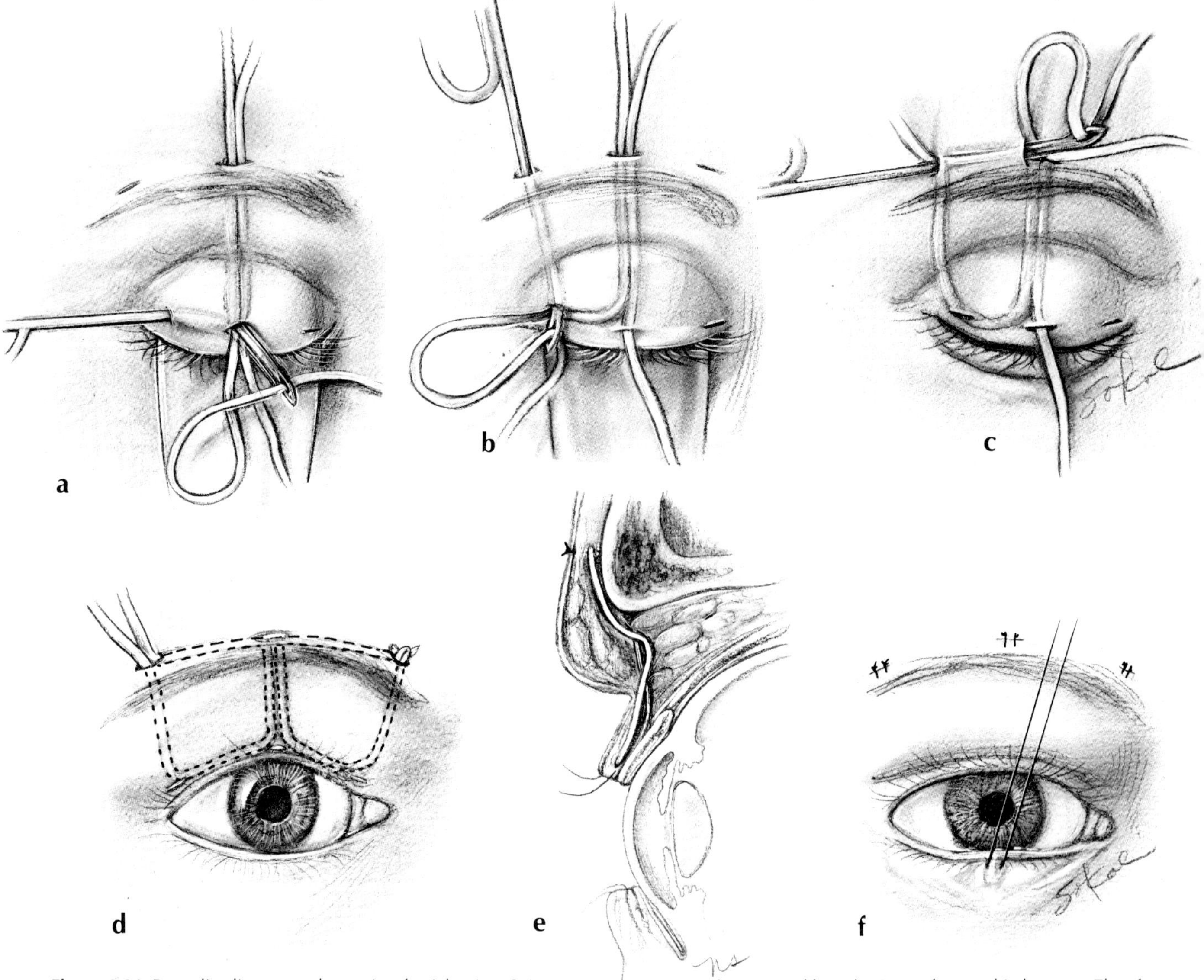

Figure 2.24 *Frontalis sling procedure using fascial strips. Strips are passed vertically from center brow incision to center lid incision.* **(a)** *Wright needle used to pull one strip to temporal lid incision and* **(b)** *then to temporal brow incision.* **(c)** *Same needle then used to bring other end of strip to lateral brow incision where knot is tied.* **(d)** *Each of two fascial loops are tied to elevate lid margin to level of upper limbus.* **(e)** *Vertical portions of fascial strips perforate orbital septum. Therefore traction on tarsus comes from posterior direction and minimizes likelihood of tarsus being pulled away from globe.* **(f)** *Suture used to elevate lower lid and close palpebral fissure during early postoperative period. Suture is placed just below cilia line, lid is elevated and suture taped to forehead above brow*

fascial ends. This is important to minimize the possibility of erosion of the fascial ends through the wound. The tissue tracts are irrigated with gentamicin, and the brow incisions are closed with 7/0 interrupted sutures. The lid skin incisions do not have to be closed.

Use of a double trapezoid procedure allows precise adjustment of lid contour and greater control than a single trapezoid or triangle suspension. Motion of the brow is greatest at the cilia of the brow and attachments higher in the forehead provide less movement of the lid. Passing the sling posterior to the orbital septum helps prevent the tarsus from being pulled away from the globe, which may occur if the strip passes directly from the lid margin to the brow (*Figure 2.24e*). Attachment to periosteum should be avoided for it interferes with mobility. A lid closure suture is used postoperatively for the first 24 hours (*Figure 2.24f*).

Correction of jaw-winking

The only way to eliminate the wink part of the jaw-wink phenomenon is to cut the levator muscle above the levator aponeurosis. Care is taken to remove completely about 1 cm of the levator muscle. The dissection down to the levator is the same as for levator resection. A muscle hook is passed under the levator muscle at the point where it becomes tendinous and begins to fan out into the aponeurosis. A ptosis clamp is placed across the muscle, and the muscle is divided distal to the clamp. The muscle is then advanced with the ptosis clamp and cautery is used to excise 1 cm of the muscle, allowing it to retract into the orbit.

Dissection is performed inferiorly, posterior to orbicularis, to the inferior portion of the tarsus about 2–3 mm above the cilia. Three stab incisions are placed in the brow as described for the frontalis sling operation. Using a lid plate to protect the globe, a Wright needle is passed through the central brow incision, posterior to the septum just below the brow, and then inferiorly into the lid incision. A piece of fascia is passed through the eye of the needle, and the fascia strip is withdrawn through the brow incision and divided. Each of the two fascial strips is sutured with non-absorbable sutures to the levator tendon insertion, so that they lie as though they had been passed with a Wright needle as described for the standard sling procedure. The two fascial ends of each strip are drawn up to the temporal and nasal brow incisions respectively, and the trapezoids are completed. The lid skin is closed with absorbable sutures, and small deep bites through the levator aponeurosis are included in the skin sutures to create a good lid crease. The slings are then adjusted in the usual fashion. The unaffected upper lid is treated with a sling performed as described but without cutting the levator muscle. Bilateral lid closure sutures and semipressure bandages are applied.

Postoperative care

Bandages and the lid closure suture, if used, are removed 24 hours after surgery. Lubricating ointment is used at bedtime, and this may be continued for several months if maximum levator resection was done. Occasionally it is necessary to tape the lids closed to avoid exposure keratitis during the early postoperative period. This is done by using cellophane tape applied to the cheek to elevate the lower lid. The tape is stuck to the brow and forehead.

Sutures in adults are removed in 4–7 days. Many of these tiny sutures fall out; and because only small skin bites are used, suture tracks or epithelial tunnels are never a problem. Antibiotic-steroid ointment is applied to the suture line for the first 2 weeks postoperatively. Patients are asked to keep the incision dry until the sutures are removed.

Complications of ptosis surgery

Undercorrection

Poor surgical technique, failure to identify and resect proper structures, excessive hemorrhage and scarring, and misplaced sutures can lead to undercorrection. These situations can be minimized by choice of the correct procedure and by attention to detail during the operation, although undercorrection can still occur. Unexpected results may occur from an atypical response of the levator muscle.

Inadequate levator resection is the cause of undercorrection in most cases. In other cases undercorrection results from performing a levator resection when a frontalis sling procedure was needed in cases with 3–4 mm of levator function. However, in these cases with minimal levator function a levator resection sometimes gives a good result and can be tried first, because a frontalis sling can be used later if necessary.

If there is adequate levator function postoperatively but the lid is low, further surgery can be done. This is delayed for 2–3 months because often the lids elevate somewhat. Careful re-evaluation of the situation and discussion with the parents or patient will determine whether the amount of undercorrection is considered to be a problem. If further surgery is indicated, and if there is levator function, repeat levator resection is done using the guidelines presented for primary resections. If there is only minimum levator function, it is decided whether further resection or a frontalis sling should be performed. Undercorrection after a frontalis sling procedure is treated by repeat operation, elevating the lid margin to the level of the limbus.

Overcorrection

Overcorrection in treating moderate or severe congenital ptosis is rare. It may occur in cases of acquired ptosis with good levator function. A waiting period is indicated. After the first 3 postoperative days, massage of the lid is started and continued for 2 or more months. Stretching of the lid in the immediate postoperative period can also be helpful. Beginning after an observation period of 3 days, the lid is doubled over a Desmarres retractor and tugged on daily for a few days.

If these methods fail, or if there is a large initial overcorrection, further surgery is essential. During the first postoperative week, the incision can be opened and the sutures moved superiorly on the tarsus or cut altogether. In adults the level of the lid can be reset under local anesthesia.

Levator recession is required if surgery for overcorrection is done several months after the initial operation. A skin incision is made at the original incision site, and dissection is done to the level of the levator muscle above the original operative site. The muscle is isolated on a muscle hook and grasped with a ptosis clamp. The muscle is divided distal to the clamp, and fascia lata is sewn between the cut edges in the fashion described later for correction of lid retraction in thyroid disease. The length of fascia used is equal to the amount of excessive lid elevation plus 3 mm, to allow for suturing.

Poor lid crease

A poor lid crease occurs after ptosis surgery when there was poor levator function preoperatively and the skin sutures did not include a deep bite. Occasionally there is an inadequate lid crease after a frontalis sling procedure. An incision through skin and orbicularis muscle is made across the lid at the level of the desired crease, and the skin edges are resutured using an absorbable suture and taking bites in the deep tissue to cause a mild inversion of the skin edges. If the lid creases are symmetrical, but the lid folds are different because of excess skin hanging over the crease, an ellipse of the excess skin can be removed.

A lid crease can be lowered by incising just above it, making a parallel incision at the desired level for the new crease, excising the intervening skin and closing the incision. It is difficult to elevate the crease, because making a new higher crease exposes the original crease scar. If the scar is faint, however, a new higher crease can be made.

Peaking of the lid

Peaking of the lid is rare after levator resection if the tarsus is left intact, because the width of the tarsus serves to stabilize its contour. Peaking can occur when there is uneven placement of the sutures attaching the resected levator muscle to the pretarsal tissues. Contour problems are more likely if suturing is done directly to the tarsus. Postoperative massage is performed for eyes with peaking of the lid. If massage is not successful, reoperation is necessary, with release or tightening of segments of levator muscle.

Exposure keratitis

Lagophthalmos, in which the eye stays open during sleep and during non-forceful lid closure, may occur after frontalis sling procedures and maximum levator resections. This usually results in exposure keratitis that requires use of lubricating ointments and sometimes taping of the lids at bedtime. Additional lubrication during the day is rarely needed. In children the symptoms usually clear, so that taping can be discontinued within 6–12 months. However, symptomatic corneal drying sometimes persists, and treatment must be continued indefinitely. We always discuss this possibility with the patient or parents preoperatively. Lagophthalmos after surgery for senile ptosis can occur if there has been inadvertent shortening of orbital septum. This should not occur if the operation is done under local anesthesia as described before.

Lid lag

Lid lag, in which the upper lid does not follow the globe on downgaze, occurs in the same situations as lagophthalmos and is mainly a cosmetic problem. Like lagophthalmos, lid lag represents a compromise that must be accepted with certain kinds of ptosis procedures, and this should be discussed preoperatively with the patient or parents. Beard[48] believes that a unilateral frontalis sling produces a more severe cosmetic defect than bilateral sling procedures and should not be done. However, we have had some excellent results with unilateral slings. Children with any kind of sling operation or maximum levator resection are taught to tilt their head down when they look down, not to look down with their eyes alone. If the lid asymmetry is unacceptable, a sling on the normal eye can be done later.

Infection

Infection is rare after levator surgery and is treated with systemic antibiotics and warm compresses. Infection does occasionally occur after frontalis sling procedures, and there can also be a non-infective inflammatory reaction to the preserved fascia. The likelihood of infection seems to be reduced by irrigating the fascial tracts with gentamicin at the end of the procedure. Inflammatory reaction to the fascial knot is reduced by making a smaller (single-throw) knot and burying it deep in the frontalis muscle, which is quite vascular. Frontalis sling operations using foreign substances other than fascia have a higher infection rate of 10–15 per cent[49]. In such cases, removal of the foreign material is necessary, but the fibrous reaction surrounding it may keep the lid elevated, so that the result is not jeopardized.

Entropion and ectropion

Entropion and ectropion do not occur with the levator resection or aponeurosis procedures described above. They can occur after other procedures when the tarsal plate is vertically shortened, causing instability of the lid margin. Posterior lamellar retractor pull and scarring can then cause entropion, and anterior suturing of the levator on an unstable lid margin can cause ectropion. Entropion can be treated by moving the point of attachment of the levator to the anterior portion of the tarsus and, if need be, tightening the skin and muscle above the lashes. Secondary surgery for ectropion requires undermining the skin and orbicularis from the lid crease and moving the levator insertion superiorly, where it is secured to the underlying tarsal remnant to relieve traction on the anterior lid margin.

Loss of lashes

Dissection down to, or incision across, the lash follicles can cause loss of lashes. Postoperative infection can also cause loss of lashes, but this is rare because of the excellent blood supply in that area. Lash grafts can be done, and although not perfect, often give an acceptable result. Artificial lashes are also helpful.

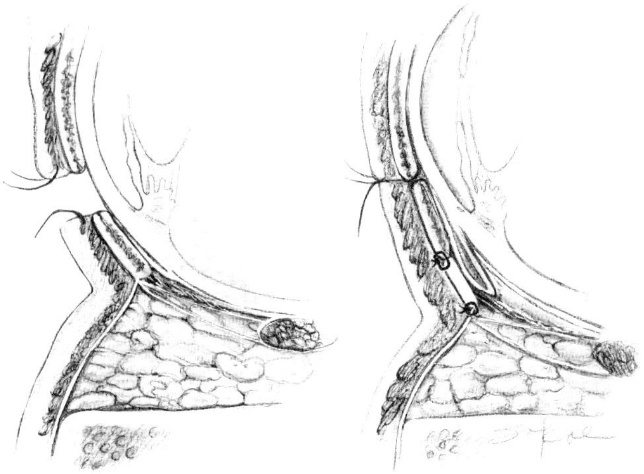

Figure 2.25 *Scleral or cartilage graft for lower lid retraction due to thyroid dysfunction. Retractors of lower lid are incised at inferior margin of tarsus and scleral or cartilage graft sewn between retractors and inferior tarsal margin*

Lid retraction secondary to thyroid dysfunction

Graves' disease can produce severe extraocular problems that are difficult to correct. Extraocular muscles, especially the medial and inferior recti, become thickened and inelastic. Lid retraction and exophthalmos lead to impaired lid function, lagophthalmos, and exposure of the conjunctiva and cornea. Involvement of the eye muscles and orbit can result in a severe cosmetic deformity.

Combinations of strabismus surgery, reduction of lid retraction and orbital decompression are needed to rehabilitate these unfortunate patients. The underlying disease is variable and unpredictable, so that the surgical results also vary from case to case. Still, significant improvement can be achieved in nearly all cases. We are aggressive in operating on these patients, and we believe that early orbital decompression and management of lid retraction is important.

Lower lid retraction

A proptotic eye mechanically depresses the lower lid as the palpebral fissure is forced open by the advancing eye. Fibrotic changes in the orbit play an additional role in lower lid retraction, but not to the extent that they do in the upper lid. Surgery on a tight inferior rectus, even with careful division of the fascial retractors, can aggravate the lid retraction and/or worsen the cosmetic appearance when the eye is returned to a normal position. Tightening the lower lid at the lateral canthus does not elevate it, but actually tends to pull the lid further under the eye. The lid must be pushed up.

An incision across the width of the lid is made just below the lash line. This incision extends through skin and orbicularis down to the anterior tarsal surface. The skin-muscle flap is dissected away from the tarsus and orbital septum for 6–8 mm inferior to the retrotarsal margin. The retractors are incised down to the conjunctiva at the retrotarsal margin. A piece of eye-bank sclera or ear cartilage about 10 mm wide is then sewn between the retrotarsal margin and the retractors of the lid (*Figure 2.25*).

Because cartilage must be obtained from the ear, it is less convenient to use than sclera. However, cartilage is stiffer and tends to retract less, so that the results are better. To obtain cartilage a posteriorly hinged rectangular skin flap 3 cm long and 1.5 cm wide is made on the posterior surface of the ear, extending from the base of the pinna. This location provides flat or gently curving cartilage necessary for the graft. The perichondrium is dissected away from the cartilage as a posteriorly hinged flap. The borders of the cartilage piece are incised with a scalpel without cutting the anterior skin, and the cartilage is separated from the anterior perichondrium by sharp dissection. The incisions in posterior perichondrium are closed with an absorbable suture, and the skin is closed with 6/0 silk or nylon.

Cartilage has a soft, almost soap-like consistency, and must be handled carefully. Suturing at the recipient site is done with 7/0 absorbable suture. The skin is closed with 8/0 silk, and two traction sutures are placed through the lid margin and taped to the brow. These sutures are kept in place at least 1 week, and they are readjusted as needed to keep the lower lid elevated. Passing the sutures over silicone strips helps prevent erosion.

Upper lid retraction

Lagophthalmos, corneal exposure and an unattractive wide-eyed appearance results from upper lid retraction. This usually, although not always, occurs along with exophthalmos. In acute hyperthyroidism, sympathetic stimulation may cause lid retraction. Temporary relief can be obtained with guanethidine drops[50], but this medication is irritating and does not affect the chronic lid retraction that occurs from enlargement and fibrosis of the levator muscle. In these cases, a levator lengthening procedure is required.

Several approaches to levator lengthening have been devised. Recession of the levator tendon on the anterior tarsal surface was suggested by Baylis, Cies and Kayma[51]. Henderson[52] recommended making an incision at the retrotarsal margin through Mueller's muscle and portions of levator aponeurosis, depending on the degree of lid retraction. Cutting the levator aponeurosis and Mueller's muscle and reattaching them to the skin below the brow was sugested by Goldstein[53]. Harvey and Anderson[54] believe Mueller's muscle should be extirpated through an anterior approach after division of the levator aponeurosis. Recently, the recession of the levator aponeurosis by insertion of sclera at the retrotarsal margin has become popular[55]. However, use of sclera is associated with problems in maintaining normal lid contour, and reoperation has occasionally been needed following shrinkage of the implant[56]. For these reasons, we have devised a procedure using preserved fascia lata to lengthen the levator tendon at its narrow portion where it joins the levator muscle. Fascia does not shrink, and lid contour is not affected by the high placement of the graft.

Local anesthesia can be used. A 2 cm horizontal scalpel incision is made in the center of the lid crease. Dissection is done down to the levator tendon and muscle. The levator muscle in the thyroid patient is quite large and easily identified. Blunt dissection is used to dissect under the muscle and allow passage of a muscle hook just distal to Whitnall's ligament. A small ptosis clamp is passed across the tendon at the point there it begins to fan out into the aponeurosis. The tendon is divided distal to the clamp. Two strips of preserved fascia 4 mm wide, or one piece of 8 mm wide fascia if available, are sutured between the cut tendon edges using two 6/0 absorbable mattress sutures at each end (*Figure 2.26*). The length of the implant should be equal to the amount of lid retraction plus 5 mm for suturing and to allow for slight overcorrection.

If there is severe proptosis, the horns and lateral extensions of the levator aponeurosis physically restrict forward motion of the lid as the eye bulges forward. This causes an area of tension at the lateral aspect of the lid, and the aponeurosis should be divided in this area after insertion of the fascial graft. The skin incision is closed and a semipressure bandage is used to keep the eye shut for 2 days. Blepharoplasty, often requested by these patients, should not be done at the time of levator lengthening. It is difficult to predict the amount of skin to remove, and the remaining skin may become abnormally adherent to the area of the graft, giving an irregular sunken appearance to the center of the lid.

The lid may not attain the desired level for several weeks. There is usually ptosis during this time, and the patient should be warned of this possibility. As with all types of surgery for thyroid ophthalmopathy, the result may not be permanent. If progressive disease requires reoperation, there is usually a large amount of fibrous material at the site of the graft, so that addition of another graft is not feasible. Division of the levator tendon inferior to the graft with excision of Mueller's muscle, as described by Harvey and Anderson[54], works well in these cases.

Corneal exposure

Tarsorrhaphy is the procedure of choice to prevent or treat corneal exposure when lid involvement, 7th nerve palsy or proptosis hamper lid closure. Conjunctival drying and inflammation associated with lid retraction and exophthalmos from thyroid dysfunction disease can be improved by lateral tarsorrhaphy which also gives considerable cosmetic improvement. A temporary tarsorrhaphy should be done so there is no sacrifice of lid shape or function when the tarsorrhaphy is later opened.

Marginal tarsorrhaphy

Marginal tarsorrhaphy is a simple, temporary lid closure procedure that can be done laterally, medially or paracentrally. The lid margins are denuded of epithelium for the length of the desired tarsorrhaphy. Mattress sutures of 5/0

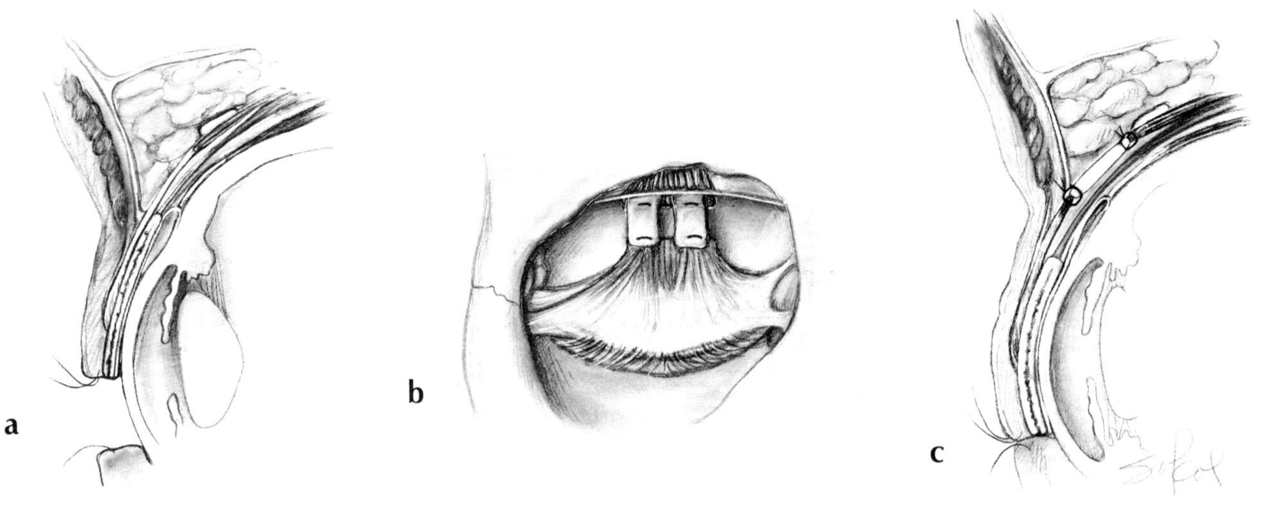

Figure 2.26 *Fascia lata implant to lengthen levator tendon as treatment for upper lid retraction from thyroid dysfunction.* **(a)** *Thickened levator muscle is easily identified. Levator is divided where it fans out into aponeurosis, and* **(b,c)** *two thin pieces of fascia or one wide piece is sewn between cut edges to lengthen tendon and lower the upper lid*

silk are passed through the skin 2 mm above the cilia, down through the grey line of the upper lid, through the grey line of the lower lid and out through the skin 2 mm below the lashes. Passing the sutures over silicone strips or cotton pledgets prevents them from cutting into the skin. The sutures are removed after 10 days. Frequently, the areas of contact between the lids stretch apart after a short time thereby decreasing the effect of the tarsorrhaphy. A modified Elschnig tarsorrhaphy is used for more permanent lid closure.

Modified Elschnig tarsorrhaphy

A variation of the Elschnig tarsorrhaphy method can be used for temporary or permanent closure of the lids. If the tarsorrhaphy is opened later the lids return to their normal appearance, and the lashes are not disturbed. We rotate tarsus from the upper lid to the lower lid in contrast to Elschnig's original procedure in which lower lid tarsus was rotated into the upper lid. This variation avoids possible damage to the lacrimal ducts, and the larger piece of tarsus from the upper lid gives better support to the lower lid if the tarsorrhaphy is later opened.

The skin and conjunctiva of the lateral half of the lid are anesthetized with 1 per cent lidocaine (lignocaine). The upper lid is everted using Adson forceps. The lateral tarsus is divided through the meibomian glands with a Graefe knife for the length of the proposed tarsorrhaphy (*Figure 2.27a*).

A vertical cut to the retrotarsal margin is made through the posterior portion of the tarsus at the medial end of the tarsorrhaphy (*Figure 2.27b*). This mobilizes a lateral triangle consisting of the posterior one-half of the tarsus and the adherent conjunctiva. The conjunctiva along the lid margin edge of the tarsus is trimmed.

The lower lid is everted, and the tarsus is split for a length corresponding to the superior flap. A vertical incision is made through the posterior half of the tarsus corresponding to the medial incision of the upper tarsal flap. The triangle of lower lid tarsus is then excised by cutting along the retrotarsal margin (*Figure 2.27c*). The upper and lower lid incisions are joined at the lateral canthus (*Figure 2.27d*).

A double-armed, 5/0 silk suture is passed through the nasal tip of the superior tarsal triangle. The suture is passed through the lower lid at the inferior nasal corner of the area where tarsus was excised (*Figure 2.27e*). The suture is tied on the skin surface thereby pulling the upper lid tarsal flap into the lower lid defect. The lid edges are sutured together using mattress sutures of 8/0 silk which evert the edges (*Figure 2.27f,g*). The sutures are removed after 1 week.

Opening a tarsorrhaphy

Local anesthesia is injected subcutaneously in the upper and lower lids. Straight scissors are used to make an incision just beneath the lash line of the upper lid. Suturing of the raw edges is usually not necessary. Occasionally the opened tarsorrhaphy will grow partially back together. If this happens, it is reopened and the conjunctival edge is sutured to the skin using 8/0 collagen.

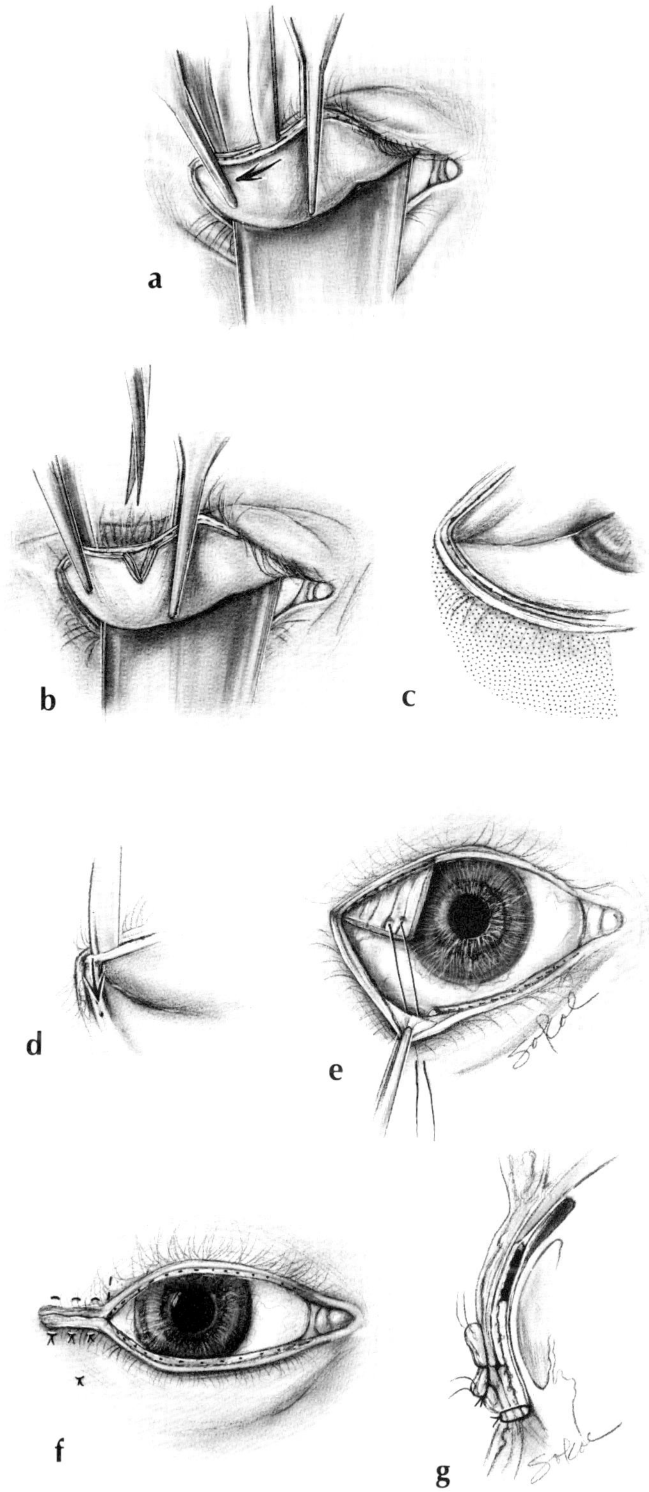

Figure 2.27 *Modified Elschnig tarsorrhaphy.* **(a)** *The upper tarsus is split for the length of the planned tarsorrhaphy.* **(b)** *A vertical incision is made at the nasal aspect of the tarsal-conjunctival flap for the full vertical width of the tarsus.* **(c)** *A corresponding triangle of the posterior half of the lower lid tarsus is excised.* **(d)** *The incisions in the tarsus are connected at the lateral canthus.* **(e)** *The superior tarsal flap is sutured in the inferior lid defect using a 5/0 mattress suture which is tied on the skin surface.* **(f,g)** *The skin edges are everted and sutured with 8/0 silk mattress sutures*

Blepharochalasis

The term 'blepharochalasis' (from the Greek meaning 'eyelid relaxation') was introduced by Fuchs[57] to describe the condition of the lid in a woman aged 20 years who had suffered recurrent bouts of lid edema over several years. There was redness, wrinkling, dilatation of superficial veins, prolapse of orbital fat and ptosis of the skin above the tarsus. Subsequently, however, the use of the term 'blepharochalasis' has been generalized and applied to a diverse group of baggy conditions of the lids. There is still lack of agreement on the medical term for baggy eyelids, but as blepharochalasis is probably the most common descriptive term, we will use it as a general term for the variety of baggy changes that occur in the lids. Modifying phrases such as 'with orbital fat prolapse' will be added to provide more specificity where needed.

Blepharochalasis can occur at any age and can have various causes. Congenital pseudoherniation of orbital fat occurs from attenuation and forward bowing of the orbital septum. (True herniation is not present because there is no defect in the orbital septum.) Atrophy and stretching of lid tissues – including skin, levator tendon and the canthal ligaments – can occur after repeated bouts of allergic lid edema. To a lesser extent, chronic alcohol abuse, periorbital edema associated with the menstrual cycle, and poor sleep habits can aggravate laxity of the skin of the lid. More serious systemic diseases, such as thyroid dysfunction or renal disease, can also produce changes in the periorbital tissues from edema. However, the most common cause of blepharochalasis is aging with loss of elasticity of the tissues.

Although blepharoplasty has become a widely accepted and rather common procedure, it is important to emphasize that it is not a simple 'tuck'. If one considers the great importance of the eyes in the expressiveness of the face, it is apparent that cosmetic surgery on the lids involves interaction with the patient's self-image, a situation that can produce unexpected difficulty even after flawless surgery. The eyes can be, and will be, examined in every detail postoperatively by the patient. With the possible exception of rhinoplasty, in no other cosmetic surgical procedure is the result so apparent to all. Even minor imperfections in the result may cause great patient dissatisfaction.

Although cosmesis motivates most of these patients to seek blepharoplasty, there is a second group of patients who are more likely to come to the attention of the ophthalmologist. The redundant tissues of the upper lids cause a heavy unpleasant draggy feeling, and downward pull on the lower lids leads to further discomfort and epiphora. Superotemporal visual field constriction occurs in severe cases with upper lid skin hanging over the lashes. During sleep the upper lid skin can cross the palpebral fissure and adhere to the lower lid skin. Patients, and occasionally their physicians, do not associate these asthenopic symptoms with what is otherwise considered a purely cosmetic problem of the lids. Blepharoplasty can relieve these symptoms, and the patients are often most grateful. At the same time these patients may be quick to point out any cosmetic imperfection present after surgery.

The patient's expectations have to be addressed when considering blepharoplasty. It is essential that the surgeon explain to the patient the aims and limitations of the procedure. Fine skin wrinkles and crow's-feet creases cannot, for the most part, be removed. Pigmentation cannot be decreased, and it may be worsened. Tightening the tissues is not permanent, and complications can occur.

Preoperative evaluation

Thorough preoperative evaluation includes a complete ophthalmological examination. Measurements of vision, visual fields and extraocular motility, the Schirmer test, and slit-lamp and fundus examination are essential. Vision problems unrecognized preoperatively could later be blamed on the surgery. Visual field tests are important to document peripheral vision loss due to redundant upper lid skin. Decreased tear function is common in women 40 years of age and older. Extraocular muscle or corneal problems and fundus disease must be documented preoperatively.

Evaluation of the lids includes their position, and the amount, texture and color of the skin. Positions of the lid creases are noted. Lower lid laxity, ptosis or drooping of the brow are assessed and may need surgical correction. Lid skin that hangs down in a bag over the upper cheek skin is difficult to remove or flatten. The amount and position of any protruding orbital fat is noted. The position and size of the lacrimal gland is noted, because suspension of the lacrimal gland is occasionally required.

Photographs are required, for documentation for insurance purposes and because preoperative review of the photographs sometimes reveals asymmetries or other problems that were not immediately apparent during the examination. Photographs can protect a surgeon who might be blamed for a defect that was present preoperatively.

Anesthesia

General or local anesthesia can be used. If general anesthesia is used, lidocaine (lignocaine) with 1:200 000 epinephrine (adrenaline) can be injected subcutaneously to aid in separation and delineation of the layers of the lid. However, the tissue distortion caused by this maneuver may counteract the beneficial effects. When local anesthesia is used, we use a 38 mm (1.5 inch) 25 gauge needle to inject subcutaneously. One pass of the needle is made across the lid, expanding the tissues as the needle is advanced. About 1.5 ml are injected in each lid.

Upper lid blepharoplasty

Placement of the suture line in the upper lid is of utmost importance. The final scar should fall in the lid crease across the lid and in a crow's-foot crease temporally. The lower incision should be placed no more than 8 mm from the lid margin at the center of the lid, and should be slightly below the superior crow's-foot at the lateral canthus because the final scar tends to be a little higher than the original incision. The incision can go into, but not across, the hollow just above (or above and nasal to) the medial canthus to avoid a bridging scar. Angling the incision up at this point may be necessary to get a flat closure.

After the lower incision line is marked, fine forceps are used gently to pinch the redundant lid skin to estimate how much can be removed without putting tension on the lid margin (*Figure 2.28a*). The upper incision line is then marked. The planned incision line should be extended temporally to the orbital rim to avoid a residual fold of skin just below the lateral end of the brow. The upper lid is then anesthetized. A scalpel is used to incise the skin along the marks, and the rest of the dissection is done with scissors (*Figure 2.28b*). There may be marked bleeding from orbicularis, and this is controlled immediately with cautery. The skin is closed with 8/0 black silk interrupted sutures, utilizing small bites (*Figure 2.28c*).

An alternative method for skin incision utilizes a blepharoplasty clamp so the lower incision will lie at one arm of the clamp and the upper line at the other. The clamp is left in place for about a minute, and after its removal the skin that stands up in a ridge is excised with scissors. This technique is more difficult to use properly but has the advantage of minimizing bleeding.

If orbital fat is to be removed, pressure on the globe is used to delineate the fat pockets. The overlying orbicularis muscle and the orbital septum are opened, allowing prolapse of the fat. Fine fibrous septae in the fat can be cut with a hot cautery, facilitating the fat prolapse. No traction is placed on the fat, to avoid deep bleeding. The fat is crossclamped with a small hemostat, and the base is cut with cautery (*Figure 2.29*). The clamp is removed and the cut edge is examined for any sign of bleeding. The skin is closed as in *Figure 2.28c*.

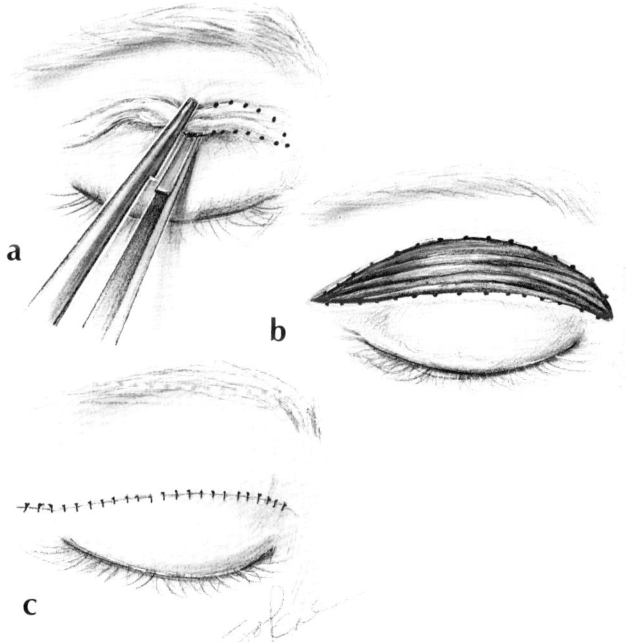

Figure 2.28 *Blepharoplasty technique for blepharochalasis of upper lid.* **(a)** *Forceps are used to determine amount of redundant skin.* **(b)** *This skin is marked and excised.* **(c)** *Skin is closed with interrupted 8/0 black silk sutures after removing orbital fat*

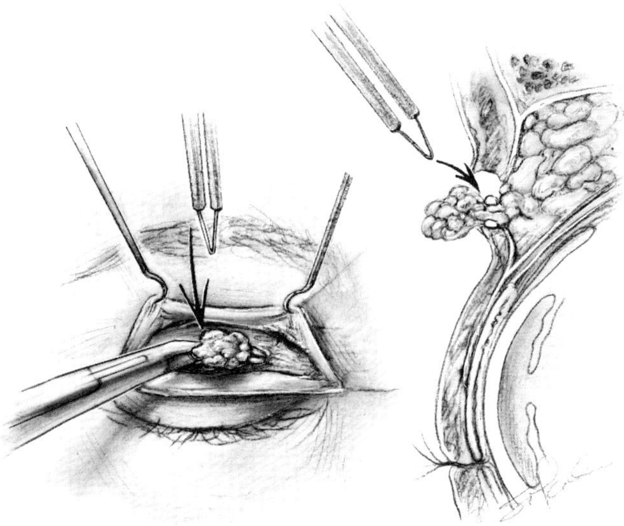

Figure 2.29 *Removal of orbital fat during blepharoplasty. Orbital septum is incised and prolapsing flap is clamped and cut with cautery*

If lid ptosis or brow ptosis is present, it should be repaired at the time of upper lid blepharoplasty. Removal of redundant skin on the upper lid can make ptosis more apparent. If there is ptosis of the brow, it may be aggravated by removal of lid skin and the effect of the lid surgery will be compromised.

Correction of brow ptosis requires removal of an ellipse of skin above the brow. The scar is difficult to hide, even with an incision in the upper cilia line, and the scar is quite obvious for a long time in many patients. This problem has to be discussed with the patient preoperatively.

Lower lid blepharoplasty

Management of the lower lid is more difficult than that of the upper lid as different procedures are used for varying degrees of deformity rather than just enlargements of the same procedure.

For removal of protruding fat in cases with little excess skin, the procedure described by Rees and Dupuis[58] provides excellent results with minimal postoperative reaction. An incision is made 2–3 mm below the cilia line, down through the orbicularis. A skin-muscle flap is then dissected down to the level of the fat pockets, which are evacuated through incisions in the septum as described for the upper lid. A small strip of muscle and skin can be removed if necessary, but this should be done with caution to avoid postoperative contraction of the lower lid. The skin is then closed.

If there is a moderate amount of excess skin, a skin flap is dissected. The incision is made 2 mm below the lashes, and is extended across the lid and about 1 cm farther temporally while angling slightly upward (*Figure 2.30a*). Subcutaneous dissection is then carried out inferior to the incision. The amount of undermining depends on the amount of skin to be removed. Converse[59] recommends little or no undermining when there is only a moderate amount of excess skin. We believe undermining is helpful to get a smooth draping of the skin flap (*Figure 2.30b*). It also allows removal of skin mainly from the temporal area, lessening the chance of vertical tightening and ectropion.

After the undermining, a hook is used to pull the skin flap temporally and to gauge the amount of skin to be removed (*Figure 2.30c*). The skin should drape across the lid without tension. The fold of excess skin is removed with scissors (*Figure 2.30d*). The scissors are angled so that the suture line will fall in an inferior crow's-foot crease.

If fat is to be removed, as is usually the case for the lower lids, pressure on the globe is used to delineate the fat pockets. An incision through orbicularis and septum is made, and the fat is removed as described above. Care is taken not to excise excessive amounts of fat from the temporal pocket, especially in patients with prominent orbital rims or deep-set eyes, to avoid an unattractive depression in the temporal portion of the lid.

The temporal incision is closed so that it lies flat in the inferior crow's-foot crease. A small triangle of skin (2–3 mm at its temporal base and 3 cm long) along the upper edge of the flap is excised to give a flat closure (*Figure 2.30e,f*). If local anesthesia is used, the amount of skin to be removed can be estimated by draping the skin flap up over the lid margin and then having the patient look up and open his mouth. This causes the lid to move up and the skin flap to move down. Only the skin that overlaps the subciliary incision is excised.

A considerable excess of skin that falls in bags over the skin of the upper cheek is difficult to treat. Extensive undermining, past the edge of the bags and often down to the thicker skin just below the infraorbital rim, is necessary. After fat removal, the skin flap is draped over the upper incision and then pulled laterally, trimmed and sutured closed as has been described.

If horizontal lid laxity is present the tarsus should also be shortened. After dissection of the skin flap, a base-up triangle of the remaining lid margin, muscle, tarsus and conjunctiva is removed. The temporal incision is made about 6 mm from the lateral canthus, using scissors. The cut edges are grasped with forceps and are overlapped to estimate the amount of lid tissue to be excised. The nasal arm of the triangle is then cut. The lid margin is reapproximated with 6/0 black silk, and the tarsus is closed with 6/0 absorbable suture such as polyglactin. An additional 6/0 silk suture is added at the cilia line. The skin flap is then draped over the lid, trimmed and sutured.

The lid margin sutures are taped to the brow for 24 hours to maintain upward traction on the lid. After this the sutures are cut to 1 cm and taped to the lower lid. A separate lid closure suture should also be used to elevate the lid for the first postoperative night. A mattress suture passed through the tarsus of the lower lid and taped to the brow (Frost suture) works well. If the lower lid is allowed to retract or if it is pushed down by the bandage during the first night, unwanted adhesions may develop between the skin and the muscle or septal incisions.

Postoperative care

The eye(s) can be bandaged or ice packs applied during the initial postoperative period. Ice packs are preferred by some surgeons because the eye is uncovered and it is easy to check for postoperative problems[60]. However, it is often difficult to keep adequate cold packs on the operative site, and there may be considerable manipulation of the area because of changing the packs. We prefer moderate pressure dressings that provide excellent control of swelling in the immediate postoperative period. The lids are immobile, and this combined with the pressure helps prevent postoperative bleeding. The bandage and lid closure suture, if used, are removed the day after surgery, and the patient is discharged from the hospital.

We believe blepharoplasty should be done as a hospital procedure. The patient can be more readily sedated preoperatively and can remain relatively immobile post-

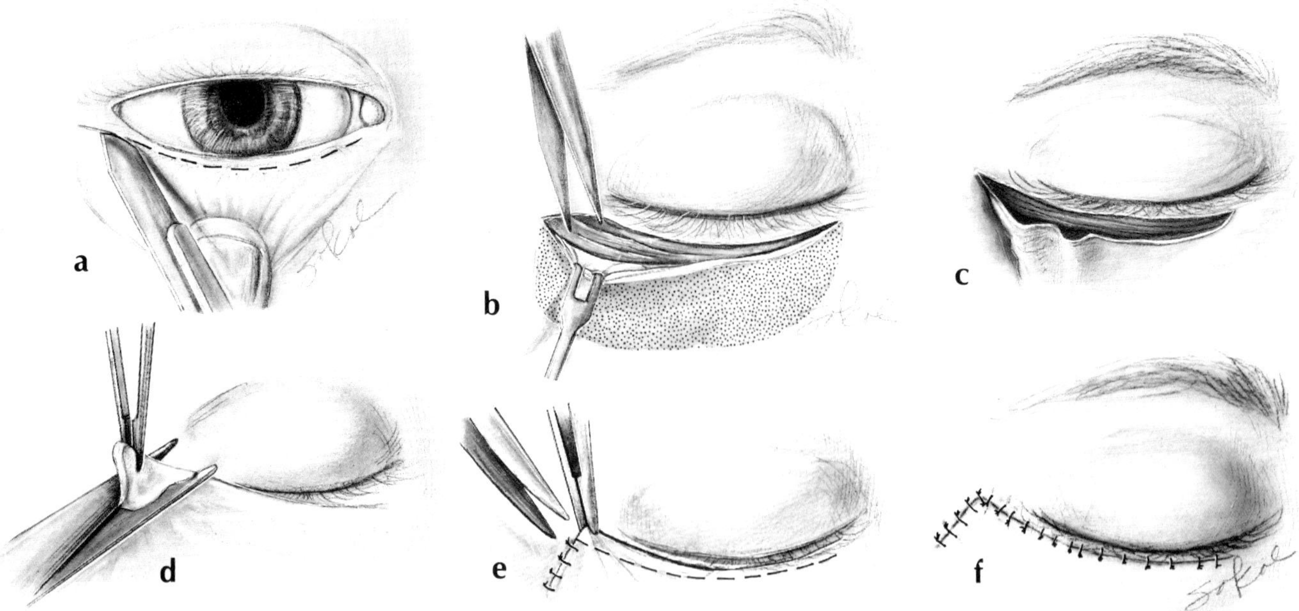

Figure 2.30 *Lower lid blepharoplasty.* **(a)** *Initial incision made 2 mm below cilia and extending across lid to location above and temporal to lateral canthus.* **(b)** *Skin retracted with hook and undermined to produce smooth skin flap. Stippled area indicates extent of undermining.* **(c,d)** *Skin flap is pulled temporally and excess removed.* **(e,f)** *Strip of skin excised along horizontal incision to permit flat closure*

operatively. This may help prevent hemorrhage. If serious hemorrhage occurs, it will be quickly recognized and treated. A patient at home may not recognize a problem and may not contact the doctor promptly.

Ptosis of the brow

Ptosis of the brow produces a redundancy of lid skin, and therefore elevation of the brow minimizes the amount of skin that must be removed from the lid. If the brow is severely ptotic, correction of this problem is necessary during surgery for blepharochalasis. An ellipse of skin must be excised from above the brow. The lower incision lies in the line of the superior cilia. Dissection is not carried into the frontalis muscle, and undermining is not done. The subcutaneous tissue is closed with a deep absorbable suture. A subcuticular suture is used to close the skin incision, and sterile tape is used to reinforce the wound. Bodian[61] has suggested the use of temporary supporting sutures from the brow that are brought out through the skin above the incision and tied over silicone. This he believes is helpful in minimizing the scar by reducing tension on the incision. Despite these precautions, the scar is noticeable for a long time, and cosmetics may be required to conceal it.

Complications

Patient dissatisfaction with the surgical result is a significant problem and can occur despite proper selection and execution of the operation and the absence of complications. This can result from the patient's unrealistic expectations or the surgeon's failure to explain adequately the goals and limitations of the procedure. Some patients, perhaps for psychological reasons, will not be happy with any result, and it is best to identify this type of individual preoperatively and avoid surgery.

A common cause of adverse symptoms after blepharoplasty is insuffucient tear production. Marginal tear production may produce no symptoms preoperatively but may result in pain, burning and reflex tearing postoperatively. This is caused by the slight change in lid dynamics, and occasionally of position, that occurs with blepharoplasty. Frequently a cosmetic blepharoplasty is initially 'tight', causing lagophthalmos. This may cause no symptoms in the presence of normal tear function, but symptoms can be severe in a patient with dry eyes. It is essential that a Schirmer evaluation be done preoperatively. If a tear deficiency is detected, as evidenced by less than 5–7 mm wetting at 5 minutes, the patient is told of possible postoperative problems that would require therapy. Also less skin than usual should be removed. Patients will be more aware postoperatively of any sensation related to the eyes, and minor irritations that may have been present before operation will be attributed to the surgery.

Removal of too little skin can be remedied by further excision, although reoperation should be considered cautiously. Slight overcorrection of the upper lid at the initial surgery usually resolves with time. Massage with a bland ointment aids greatly in the correction of this problem.

Ptosis of the upper lid can be caused by direct injury to the levator or by dehiscence of the aponeurosis due to swelling or lid manipulation. Scarring and adhesion of the levator tendon to the septum can interfere with levator and/or orbicularis function. This occurs only with extensive and excessive manipulation of deep lid structures.

Incisions around the canthi can cause 'webbing' or 'hooding' scars. Likewise, incisions across the hollow at the superior medial canthus area can cause elevated bow-like scars. Asymmetry of lid creases can also be a significant problem. Incisions just below the natural lid crease give the most predictable result. If it is necessary to create or move a lid crease, suturing the orbicularis to the levator tendon at the desired level helps to give the desired result. Sutures in deep structures that also involve the skin, or sutures that invert the skin edges, produce an abnormal-appearing crease which is prominent when the eye is closed.

Overcorrection of the lower lid is difficult to correct. In mild cases there is increased visualization of the sclera and depression of the temporal part of the lid. If lid laxity is a factor, the ectropion can be improved by a tightening procedure as described above. More often, skin grafting is needed. Usually no upper lid skin is available for grafting, and retroauricular or supraclavicular skin is used. The cosmetic result is usually poor. For slight ectropion, massage for several months can cause marked improvement and avoid the need for secondary surgery.

Muscle imbalance is rarely seen postoperatively. This can occur with deep postoperative hemorrhage, in which case it usually improves spontaneously. Muscle imbalance can also be due to involvement of the inferior oblique by scarring caused by excessive manipulation of the inferior orbital tissues during removal of orbital fat.

Blindness after blepharoplasty has been reported in more than 50 cases[62]. This can be due to severe hemorrhage deep in the orbit. For this reason many surgeons prefer not to use pressure bandages because, if hemorrhage occurs, the bandage may limit the ability of the orbital tissues to expand, and also because the problem may not be recognized[62–64]. However, we know of no evidence that there is a higher chance of damage to the globe or optic nerve from retrobulbar hemorrhage in the presence of a pressure bandage than without one. Although the chance of hemorrhage may be less if a semipressure bandage is used, monitoring of vision is more difficult if the eye is covered. A retrobulbar hemorrhage causes a sensation of pressure and pain that is often severe enough to cause nausea. Therefore, it seems unlikely that a significant hemorrhage would go unrecognized if a bandage were used. If a severe hemorrhage occurs, the wound should be reopened and the clot evacuated. If there is elevated intraocular pressure, the retinal vessels are examined. Mannitol is given, and a canthotomy may be needed if there are pulsations of the central retinal artery. If the central retinal artery is closed, an anterior chamber paracentesis may be done, and the surgeon should be prepared to do orbital decompression.

There has been speculation that blindness after blepharoplasty can be related to localized orbital hemorrhage applying pressure on the optic nerve or to the avulsion of the nutrient vesels of the optic nerve[62]. It is thought that this is secondary to vigorous traction on the orbital fat. Fat should not be pulled out; rather, it should be caused to prolapse by pressure on the globe as described above.

Lid reconstruction after tumor removal

Preoperative evaluation

Management of lid lesions requires a careful history and examination, combined with a thorough working knowledge of the appearance and clinical course of the common benign and malignant lid tumors. The ability to do a primary complete reconstruction, regardless of size of the tumor, is essential. The surgeon should not excise a lesion if there is a chance that the excision or reconstruction is beyond his experience or expertise. Prior to definitive surgery, therefore, the probable diagnosis and the chance of inapparent extension of each lesion should be established.

If it is decided that a biopsy should be done, the procedure must be properly executed in order to obtain tissue that will provide the desired information and not mislead the surgeon. When there is doubt as to the clinical diagnosis, a biopsy should always be performed first. This is especially important when the lesion is large and involves the tarsus or canthus.

If a presumably malignant lid tumor has been biopsied elsewhere, the surgeon should obtain the slides from the pathologist and have them reviewed. He should not merely request the previous report, for it may be erroneous. When there is doubt about the diagnosis from examination of the slides, or if the original biopsy material cannot be obtained, rebiopsy should be done before definitive surgery. If possible, the biopsy tissue should be evaluated by a pathologist who is thoroughly familiar with lid lesions.

Small masses that clinically appear benign can be excised without prior biopsy, especially if they are on the skin and away from important lid structures. Only if there is a high clinical likelihood that a mass involving the tarsus or canthus is benign should a localized excision be done without tissue diagnosis.

Biopsy should include adjacent clinically normal tissue. Tissue of adequate size to permit proper analysis should be submitted, because small fragments are difficult to handle and accurate pathological diagnosis is difficult. Great care is needed in handling the specimen, because crush artifacts can obscure important characteristics or make normal tissue appear abnormal. Frozen sections are not as reliable as permanent sections, and so if there is doubt as to a diagnosis that would alter the surgical approach, the surgeon should wait for the results of permanent sections. Frozen sections are often used only to determine whether the lesion is benign or malignant, or whether the surgical margins are normal. In these cases immediate precise characterization of the tumor is not needed because the surgical approach would be unchanged.

The goal of surgery for malignant lesions is to remove the entire tumor with minimum damage to surrounding structures and with restoration of cosmetic and functional anatomy that is as nearly normal as possible. Surgery for benign or presumably benign lesions is done to confirm the diagnosis and to remove masses that interfere with function or cosmesis. Complete removal of benign lesions is often not necessary and is contraindicated if it would interfere with the objectives mentioned above.

Tumors of the lid fall mainly into two groups: those arising from the surface epithelium and those arising from deeper mesenchymal structures.

Benign tumors of epithelial or dermal origin

Papilloma

Papillomas account for about 20 per cent of lid tumors[65]. They can occur anywhere on the lid and can be sessile or pedunculated. Some are compact and raspberry-like; others have long fine fronds. There are varying degrees of pigmentation, and occasionally they present as a cutaneous horn. In adults, papillomas tend to remain stable or to increase in size without spontaneous resolution. In children, papillomas are often caused by a virus. New areas may become infected because of scratching or rubbing of the lesion, and they tend to be multiple. Although papillomas are usually asymptomatic, if the lid margin is involved, a low-grade chronic conjunctivitis can occur[66].

Seborrheic keratosis

This lesion is sharply circumscribed and flat or slightly elevated. It appears as a single or as multiple dirty-yellow or black plaques which often have a pitted oily appearance. The slow growth can be accompanied by inflammation with swelling, oozing and crusting. Although seborrheic keratosis usually occurs as a plaque, pedunculated forms may occur.

Inverted follicular keratosis

Inverted follicular keratosis can be nodular, papillomatous, or verrucous. Rarely it is heavily pigmented. There may be associated symptoms of burning, itching, and bleeding. It is significant that this lesion can be confused with carcinoma both clinically and histologically. There are no specific features that suggest the correct diagnosis prior to excision.

Keratoacanthoma

This lesion may mimic basal cell carcinoma in appearance, because it forms a dome-shaped mass with an umbilicated crusted center. It tends to grow rapidly, often in 2–3 weeks, and this fact helps to distinguish it clinically from carcinoma. Pathologically, keratoacanthoma can be confused with squamous cell carcinoma, especially if only a small section is taken for biopsy. Accurate pathological diagnosis requires a section that is the full width and depth of the lesion at its center. These lesions can be totally excised when they are small, but they can become quite large, making total excision and reconstruction difficult. Curettage can be used, and this is usually followed by regression and healing.

Senile keratosis

These lesions are often multiple and may be associated with a history of prolonged exposure to sunlight. They are slightly pigmented with hyperkeratotic scaly areas that may become inflamed. Senile keratosis is significant because it can develop into squamous cell carcinoma[67]. It can be treated with simple excision.

Tumors of adnexal origin

Sebaceous adenomas and trichoepitheliomas

Sebaceous adenomas are uncommon tumors with no clinically distinguishing characteristics. Trichoepitheliomas are subcutaneous well-defined tiny papules that are firm in consistency and are sometimes associated with telangiectasis. They mainly occur near the lid margin or brow and can become as large as 1–2 cm in diameter, although this is unusual. They are yellowish or bluish in color. Multiple trichoepitheliomas on the forehead, nose and lower eyelids can appear during adolescence as a dominantly inherited condition[68]. They usually remain stable but may grow and ulcerate. Malignant change has been reported[69].

Pilomatrixoma

This mass lesion is a rare benign tumor of hair follicles. It can occur at any time during life but more commonly affects children or young adults. It presents as a slowly growing hard subcutaneous lump in the lid tissue or brow, and it may be mobile or fixed to the overlying skin. Pilomatrixoma may grow to 3 cm in diameter and, although usually single, bilateral lesions have been recorded[70].

Cystic tumors

Epithelial inclusion cysts

Although epithelial inclusion cysts are more common near the canthi, they can occur anywhere on the lids. The cyst is formed by epithelium trapped below the surface, resulting in an island of epithelium which continues to grow and forms a cyst lined with epithelium and filled with keratin debris. There may be episodes of inflammation, especially after trauma. The overlying skin is firmly adherent to the cyst at the site where the epithelium is entrapped, and the skin in that area and the small epithelial tract should be removed with the cyst. The mass may be quiescent for a period of years and then rapidly enlarge. It is important to remove the intact cyst because rupture causes release of the keratin debris that is irritating to the surrounding tissues.

Apocrine hydrocystomas

These are small epithelium-lined cysts of sweat gland origin, and they occur at the lash line of the mucocutaneous junction of the lid. Apocrine hydrocystomas are most common at the canthi. They are usually clear, but rarely pigmentation is present, which may obscure the diagnosis. Simple excision or marsupialization is the treatment of choice.

Milia

Milia are small sharply circumscribed pearly masses that result from obstruction of a pilar shaft, with subsequent build-up of keratin debris. They are usually multiple, about the size of a pinhead and are not associated with inflammation.

Comedones

Comedones, commonly known as blackheads, are caused by obstruction of the pilosebaceous apparatus, and they contain keratin debris and inspissated secretions. The dark color is caused by oxidation products of keratin. Inflammation and swelling may occur around the comedone. A small tube-like extractor is used to apply pressure surrounding the lesion and to extract the central core.

Nevi

Nevi are congenital lesions and have a characteristic pattern of growth. Active development occurs in infancy, followed by a period of slow growth and then quiescence in adult life. Nevi have variable amounts of pigmentation and may be non-pigmented. They can be of any size, but nevi affecting the lids usually measure from a few millimeters to about 2 cm. The dermal nevus is a benign lesion located entirely in the dermis, and it is rarely apparent before puberty. A dermal nevus is usually smooth, elevated and dome-shaped, with a few coarse hairs on the surface.

Junctional nevi are potentially malignant tumors arising in the deep layers of the surface epithelium and the underlying dermis. These lesions are flat and smooth. The compound nevus has both junctional and dermal elements. It may be elevated and may undergo malignant change. Junctional and compound nevi rarely have hair. The presence of hair is therefore strong evidence for the diagnosis of benign dermal nevus[71]. The blue nevus is a slightly elevated blue-gray to black lesion that is usually present at birth or appears soon thereafter and does not change in size. Malignant change, although rare, has been reported[72].

Oculodermal melanocytosis (nevus of Ota) is a unilateral condition presenting as pigmentation of periorbital skin, conjunctiva, sclera and uveal tract. It may be visible at birth or may not become apparent until adulthood.

Oculodermal melanocytosis is associated with an increased incidence of malignant melanoma of the uveal tract[73].

Treatment of nevi is unnecessary if the diagnosis is clear and the patient is not concerned about the cosmetic defect. Increased pigmentation occurring with hormonal changes, such as with puberty or pregnancy, is not a sign of growth. However, in the absence of hormonal changes, alterations in pigmentation or elevation or signs of inflammation suggest malignancy, and excisional biopsy should be done. Nevi can look like basal cell carcinomas, and if the lesion has been present for a long time, excisional biopsy may be necessary to establish the diagnosis. Nevi are usually resistant to radiotherapy.

Xanthelasma

Xanthelasma is a condition in which irregular yellow plaques (xanthomas) occur in and beneath the skin of the lids. The lesions tend to be bilateral and symmetrical and are more common in females. Xanthelasma is most common in the sixth decade, and it may be associated with hypercholesterolemia, hyperlipemia and obesity[74]. The inner canthal area is most often affected. If surgery is done, it is important to remove all of the discolored material to prevent recurrence. Skin grafting may be necessary to fill large defects.

Inflammatory lesions

Hordeola (styes)

These are the most common inflammatory lesions of the lids. They are bacterial infections of the meibomian glands, accessory glands or lash follicles. The typical elevated white tender area may be obscured by diffuse lid swelling. The diagnosis can usually be established from the history of a small tender nodule at the lid margin occurring as the initial problem. Hot compresses and topical antibiotics are the best therapy in most cases, but incision and drainage occasionally are necessary.

Chalazions

These arise as a result of obstruction of the opening of a meibomian gland. Lipid material is trapped within the gland. This causes pressure necrosis and inflammation and subsequent thickening of the tarsus. A pyogenic granuloma of the conjunctiva can form and may be pedunculated.

If it separates from the tarsus, a chalazion may be present as a moveable soft tumor under the skin. Occasionally a chalazion of the lid margin can be umbilicated and have dilated vessels on its surface, thus resembling a basal cell carcinoma. History and response to conservative therapy help to establish the diagnosis, but curettage or biopsy may be needed.

Hemangiomas

Hemangiomas are congenital hamartomatous lesions which occur in several forms. The type, size and location of the lesion determine the management.

Port wine stain

This telangiectatic type of hemangioma consists of dilated capillaries in the dermis. When it occurs in the distribution of the first division of the 5th cranial nerve, there may be associated choroidal and cerebral hemangiomas (Sturge-Weber syndrome). Glaucoma may also occur on the affected side, perhaps due to elevated episcleral venous pressure.

Surgery or irradiation for the skin lesion is not indicated. Cosmetic improvement can be obtained with tattooing methods, and there is some encouraging work being done with the argon laser[75].

Capillary hemangiomas

Small capillary hemangiomas appear as soft, slightly elevated masses. Large capillary hemangiomas produce a considerable cosmetic defect, and they can cause occlusion amblyopia when the lids are severely affected. Permanent astigmatism can be caused by lid pressure on the globe[76].

Capillary hemangiomas appear soon after birth and may grow rapidly for several months. Thereafter, many hemangiomas undergo regression to a cosmetically acceptable appearance. However, amblyopia may occur if there is ptosis obscuring the pupil or if there was significant uncorrected astigmatism prior to regression[77]. Therefore, awaiting regression is not the best treatment for large hemangiomas unless normal vision can be maintained.

Systemic corticosteroids produce dramatic improvement in some cases, and this treatment is used to manage diffuse lesions not amenable to surgery. The initial response is a whitening of the lesion, followed by shrinkage. If a response is not evident after 4 weeks, the steroids should be discontinued. However, steroid therapy can be continued as long as there is continuing improvement and as long as there are no significant side effects from the treatment. Small doses of irradiation can also be quite effective. With a properly shielded eye, the chance of complications from irradiation is minimal. If the lesion continues to cause complete ptosis after medical therapy and irradiation, removal of the angiomatous tissue and ptosis surgery should be done.

Cavernous hemangiomas

Cavernous hemangiomas are subcutaneous lesions made up of large thin-walled vessels. They do not have the red surface component typical of capillary hemangiomas. Although these lesions are congenital, they may not produce symptoms until adulthood. They do not respond to steroid therapy and rarely undergo regression. They often present deep in the lid as a freely moveable mass. Surgical excision is necessary to make a positive diagnosis. They have a distinct capsule, and surgical removal is straightforward.

Lymphangiomas

Lymphangiomas are composed of lymph-filled spaces lined with endothelium. They affect the conjunctiva, orbit and lids. Dilated clear channels in the conjunctiva in the presence of a lid mass help to make the diagnosis. Hemorrhage into the lesion can cause sudden increase in size, simulating rapid growth. The lesion can also increase in size during viral illnesses. Complete removal of these diffuse lesions is impossible. 'Debulking' for cosmetic reasons often requires several operations.

Neurofibromas

Neurofibromas can present in the lid as isolated lesions, or they may be diffuse and massive. Isolated lesions can be completely excised. However, more commonly there is diffuse involvement requiring several small debulking procedures to get the best result.

Malignant tumors

In contrast to the many relatively common benign lesions seen by the ophthalmologist, there are only four malignant tumors that account for the vast majority of malignancies of the lids. These are: (*1*) basal cell carcinoma; (*2*) squamous cell carcinoma; (*3*) sebaceous gland carcinoma; and (*4*) malignant melanoma.

Basal cell carcinoma

Basal cell carcinoma is the most common malignant lesion of the lids. These tumors are slow growing, painless, and may be neglected by the patient until significant lid or ocular damage occurs. Death or loss of vision from this tumor is unlikely with proper management, but both complications can occur if treatment is inadequate[78]. Treatment is total excision with histologically proven normal margins and careful follow-up.

Typically, basal cell carcinomas are small nodular masses with an umbilicated center and elevated pearly margins with dilated blood vessels. The tumor usually enlarges gradually and has repeated bouts of surface ulceration and crusting. When the lid margin is involved, there is usually tarsal distortion and trichiasis or loss of lashes. The lower lid is most frequently involved, followed by the medial canthus and the upper lid. Most basal cell carcinomas are solitary lesions.

Basal cell carcinomas may be cystic, pigmented or papillomatous. There may be an inflammatory component but this is unusual. Children are rarely affected unless they have a tumor diathesis such as xeroderma pigmentosa or the basal cell nevus syndrome. Basal cell carcinomas do not metastasize.

The morphea type of basal cell carcinoma is especially important because the extent of the tumor may not be clinically apparent. This type of basal cell tumor must be treated with wider surgical margins and with pathologic evaluation of the frozen section margins at several levels. In our experience, it is not uncommon for the morphea-type of basal cell carcinoma to involve twice as much lid tissue as is suggested by clinical appearance.

Squamous cell carcinoma

Squamous cell carcinoma more commonly affects the upper lid than the lower lid, and it is relatively rare. It tends to be less elevated and have more keratin debris in the center than basal cell carcinoma. These tumors can metastasize, especially to the preauricular or submandibular lymph nodes. Metastases usually occur late in the clinical course.

Squamous cell carcinoma is treated by wide local excision. Lymph node dissection should be considered if there is a large, longstanding tumor, and should be done if there is a palpable node. Radiotherapy to the area of metastasis is adjunctive treatment.

Sebaceous gland carcinoma

Sebaceous gland carcinomas, including tumors arising in the meibomian glands, may present as a diffuse inflammation of the lid and conjunctiva and may be misdiagnosed as bacterial blepharoconjunctivitis. The lid margin tends to be rounded and there is loss of lashes. Yellowish elevations may be seen at the orifices of affected meibomian glands.

Sebaceous gland carcinomas may initially resemble a chalazion. These tumors have a 30 per cent mortality rate, probably because of their tendency to metastasize, their multicentricity, and because the correct diagnosis is often not made early in their course[79]. Wide excision is needed. Exenteration of the orbit may be required because the bulbar conjunctiva may also be diffusely involved.

Treatment of lid tumors

The size, location and degree of malignancy of a lid tumor determine the surgical approach. There are many different methods of tumor removal and reconstruction. The ones presented here give the best functional and cosmetic results in our experience. Local anesthesia for removal of small lid lesions is obtained by subcutaneous and subconjunctival injection of 2 per cent lidocaine (lignocaine) with epinephrine (adrenaline). About 1–5 ml is required to anesthetize the entire lid. We close all skin incisions with interrupted 8/0 black silk sutures. Running sutures cause distortion and bunching of the thin lid skin. Interrupted sutures provide more control of closure and allow suturing of curvilinear incisions without bowstring distortion. Tiny bites are taken, and most of the skin sutures later fall out spontaneously. Sutures that remain are removed 4–7 days postoperatively.

Excision of chalazions

Chalazions can be drained through the skin or conjunctiva, depending on whether they are more superficial on the anterior or posterior side of the lid. The posterior approach is more common. A chalazion clamp is applied, and a vertical incision with a No. 11 Bard-Parker blade is made through the center of the lesion. Avoiding the lid margin helps minimize contour deformity. The opening can be enlarged by removing a vertical ellipse of tarsus. A small spoon curette is used to remove the content of the chalazion, with care being taken to empty all pockets of the soft material.

In longstanding chalazions there may be a thick fibrous capsule, and this leaves a knot if it is not excised. Extensive dissection in the lid should be avoided, however, because lid deformity can result from scarring. Bleeding tends to be profuse after removal of the clamp, but pressure for a few minutes stops the hemorrhage, and usually no cautery is needed. A drop of phenylephrine can be helpful to constrict the vessels. Inflammation persists for a few days, and warm compresses and antibiotic-steroid drops are used for 5–7 days postoperatively.

Removal of a chalazion through the skin is done through a horizontal incision. Curettage and excision of any capsule are similar to those of the posterior approach. The skin is sutured.

Excision of tumors on the lid skin

Masses thought to be benign can be removed with an elliptical incision whose long axis lies along the natural skin lines. Care is taken to minimize tissue removal in the vertical direction from the lower lid, which could cause ptosis of the lid or ectropion. A free skin graft must be used if the skin cannot be readily approximated after undermining. Lax lower lids will not tolerate any vertical skin shortening, and excision of a mass may have to be combined with horizontal lid shortening. A Z-plasty or Y-V procedure may be helpful, but their use in the lower lid is difficult. A pedicle flap from the upper lid is useful when a large area of skin must be removed from the temporal part of the lower lid.

If malignancy is suspected and a wide excision can easily be done, frozen section examination of the margins may not be essential. However, if there is any doubt as to whether the entire tumor has been excised, or if the lesion is near the canthus, lid margin or punctum, frozen section examination of the margins should be done because secondary surgery would be difficult. Usually only the skin has to be examined by frozen section, but if there is invasion into subcutaneous tissue or orbicularis muscle, a deep margin should also be examined.

Excision of small benign tumors of the lid margin

Removal of benign lid margin tumors is done to minimize damage to the lid contour and the lashes. Nevi of the lid margin may have lashes passing through them. Shaving the mass off flush with the margin is all that is required. This can be done easily by piercing the margin of the mass with a fine sharp blade and cutting to one edge of the lesion. The edge can then be grasped while the cut is made the opposite way. This method gives precise control of the excision. It does not damage the lash follicles, and provides an adequate specimen for the pathologist.

Removal of tumors involving tarsus

When there is question of malignancy with tarsal involvement, a full-thickness lid resection should be performed. Frozen section examination of the margins surrounding the tumor must be done. Full-thickness specimens at least 1 mm wide should be cut from the remaining lid on either side of the area of resection. These margin specimens are put on a small piece of cardboard, such as suture packing material, to keep them flat. From the base of the resection, skin, muscle and conjunctiva are submitted as separate specimens. The extent of involvement at the base of the tumor is usually easier to determine clinically than the extent of tarsal involvement.

Removal of tumors involving up to 25 per cent of the upper or lower lid

Tumors up to 8 mm in length and involving the tarsus can be removed and the defect closed primarily. A pentagonal incision is used (*Figure 2.31a*). The lid margin is then reapproximated with a 6/0 silk suture through the line of the meibomian glands (*Figure 2.31b*). The suture is placed with a deep bite about 2 mm from the cut edge and is tied firmly so that there is some bunching of the margin. A triple surgeon's knot helps to prevent the suture from cutting into the lid margin.

We find it useful to stretch the lid over a lid plate, using the margin suture for traction, while the rest of the closure is being done. The tarsus, conjunctiva and the retractors are closed with interrupted 6/0 absorbable sutures (*Figure 2.31c*). Another 6/0 silk suture is placed with firm tissue bites at the lash line (*Figure 2.31d*), and the skin is closed (*Figure 2.31e*). The end of the lid margin sutures are placed under one of the skin sutures to prevent corneal abrasion.

Excision of lesions involving 25–40 per cent of the upper or lower lid

Release of the lateral canthal ligament extension to the lid allows mobilization of the lateral remnant and primary closure of the incision if the cut lid edges cannot be closed

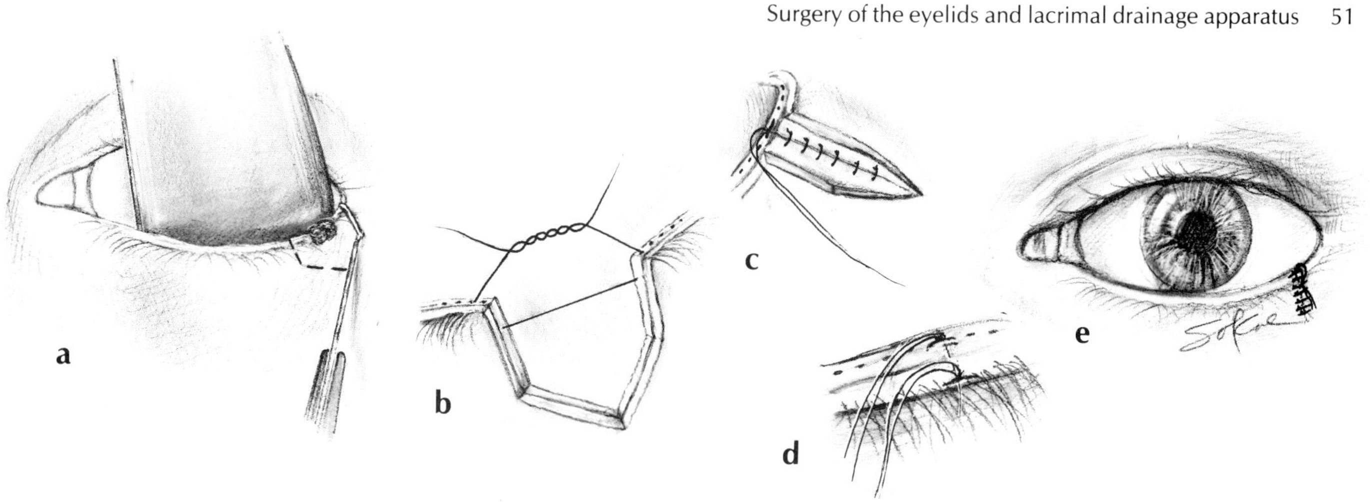

Figure 2.31 *Full-thickness incision to remove tumors involving up to 25 per cent of lid margin.* **(a)** *Pentagonal incision made around tumor.* **(b)** *Lid margin reapproximated with 6/0 silk suture through tarsus.* **(c)** *Tarsus, conjunctiva and lower lid retractors are closed with interrupted absorbable sutures.* **(d)** *Second lid margin suture of 6/0 silk is placed at the lash line.* **(e)** *Lid margin sutures placed under skin suture*

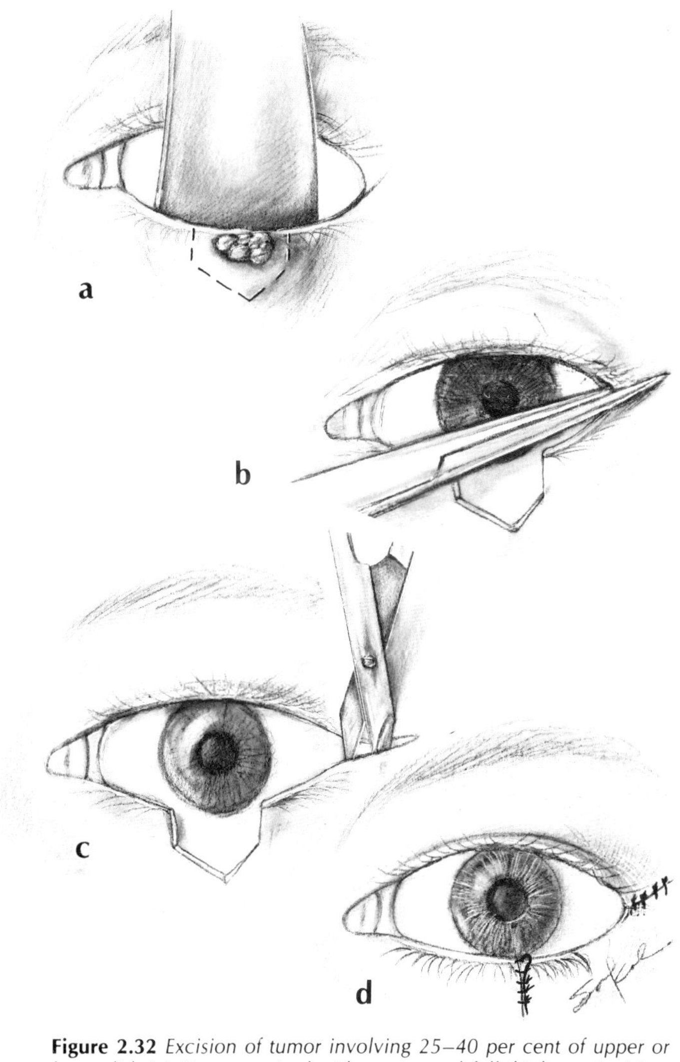

Figure 2.32 *Excision of tumor involving 25–40 per cent of upper or lower lid.* **(a)** *Tumor excised with pentagonal full-thickness incision.* **(b)** *Lateral canthal skin incision is made.* **(c)** *Extension of lateral canthal ligament to lower lid is cut.* **(d)** *This permits movement of temporal portion of lid nasally so that the incision can be closed*

after pentagonal excision of a tumor and if less than 40 per cent of the lid was removed (*Figure 2.32a*).

A lateral canthal skin incision is made at an angle that follows an extension of the line of the involved lid margin (up for the lower lid, down for the upper) (*Figure 2.32b*). This helps prevent postoperative contour defects of the lateral aspect of the lid. Dissection is extended down to the lateral canthal ligament, and the extension of the ligament to the lid is cut with scissors (*Figure 2.32c*). Maximum mobility of the temporal portion of the lid is obtained by dividing the orbital septal attachments to the lid. The incision is then closed as described above (*Figure 2.32d*). Occasionally a small fold of tissue forms at the lateral canthus as the lid is advanced. This fold is excised.

Tenzel and Stewart[80] described a technique whereby a sharply curving incision is made superiorly from the lateral canthus to just below the brow, then down again, creating a semicircular myocutaneous flap. The flap is then advanced following division of the lateral canthal ligament. This method provides support for the lateral portion of the lid, and large defects can be repaired. The incision is initially directed inferiorly, and then superiorly, for repair of upper lid defects.

Lid defects greater than 40 per cent of the lid and those involving more than 10 mm of the temporal part of the lid, when there is no remaining temporal remnant, are best reconstructed using a lid-sharing procedure as described below.

Reconstruction following removal of large tumors of the lower lid

Reconstruction of defects involving more than 40 per cent of the lower lid is best done by a tarsal-conjunctival advancement flap from the upper lid (*Figure 2.33a*). Hughes[81] described a procedure that spared the lid margin by dividing the tarsus 3–4 mm from the margin and advancing the superior part of the tarsus and conjunctiva into the inferior defect. A skin flap or graft was used to cover the tarsal-conjunctival advancement flap.

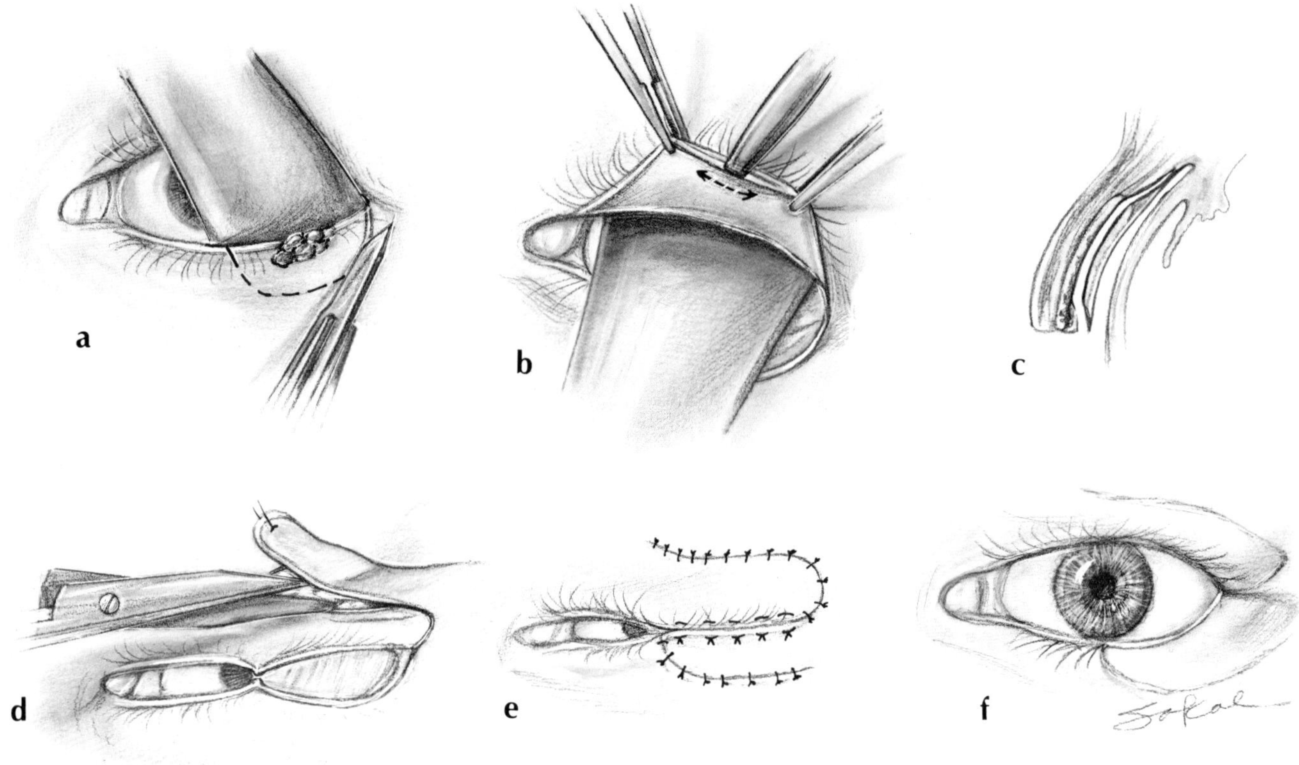

Figure 2.33 *Reconstruction following removal of more than 40 per cent of lower lid.* **(a)** *After excising lower lid tumor,* **(b)** *upper lid is inverted and partial-thickness tarsal incision made along lid margin.* **(c)** *Tarsus split along vertical axis and conjunctiva above tarsus separated from Mueller's muscle.* **(d)** *Tarsal flap advanced and sewn to conjunctiva and retractors in lower lid with* **(e)** *free graft or pedicle skin graft from upper lid used to reconstruct anterior lamella.* **(f)** *Lids are divided 10–12 weeks later*

We have modified the Hughes procedure to reduce the amount of advancement of the flap and to minimize upper lid retraction after separation of the lids by facilitating separation of the advancement flap from the levator tendon. The upper tarsus is split, beginning slightly superior to the posterior edge of the lid margin (*Figure 2.33b*), and sharp dissection is done superiorly through the center of the tarsus (*Figure 2.33c*). Dissection is continued superiorly, separating conjunctiva from Mueller's muscle. Vertical incisions are made to free a tarsal-conjunctival flap (*Figure 2.33d*). This is advanced and sutured to the conjunctiva and retractors in the lower lid defect to form the posterior lamella of the lid. A free skin graft or pedicle flap is used to create the anterior lamella of the lid (*Figure 2.33e*).

We do not alter the upper lid margin. Usually only 50 per cent of the height of the tarsus is advanced so that an adequate amount of full-thickness tarsus is left in the upper lid. The levator tendon, which attaches to the anterior surface of the tarsus, is not altered.

After 10–12 weeks the lids are divided (*Figure 2.33f*). The incision is angled so that the lower lid is left with 1–1.5 mm of tarsus extending beyond the lid margin. This allows for some retraction and seems to encourage coverage of the cut tarsal edge with non-keratinizing epithelium. No suturing of the cut edge is needed.

If the nasal part of the lid has been excised, the remaining temporal part is mobilized and shifted nasally to close the defect. The newly created temporal defect is then repaired by the above procedure (*Figure 2.34*).

Postoperative complications include upper lid retraction, lower lid retraction or ptosis, upper lid trichiasis and upper lid entropion. Upper lid retraction is prevented by careful dissection of the conjunctiva superiorly to a point near the superior fornix to separate the flap from attachments to the levator. Meticulous splitting of the tarsus is also important. An incision too far anterior near the lid margin can damage the follicles of the cilia and cause trichiasis. Upper lid entropion can occur if too much tarsus is removed from the upper lid or if the advancement flap is not completely free from the levator tendon, thus transmitting traction from the tendon to the posterior lamella of the upper lid as the flap is advanced.

Lower lid retraction can occur if a vertical advancement flap of skin and muscle is used from below to cover the lower lid defect. A free graft of inadequate size, or premature opening of the tarsorrhaphy before the reconstructed lid has adequately stretched, can also cause lower lid retraction. Lower lid ptosis results from increased length of the lid.

Correction of the postoperative complications can be difficult. Upper lid retraction requires a levator lengthening procedure. Marginal rotation is used to correct entropion. Additional skin grafting may be needed to correct lower lid retraction. Lower lid ptosis is corrected by a horizontal lid shortening procedure. When secondary surgery is needed, the cosmetic result is rarely as good as it might have been if complications had been avoided through adequate attention to detail during the original operation.

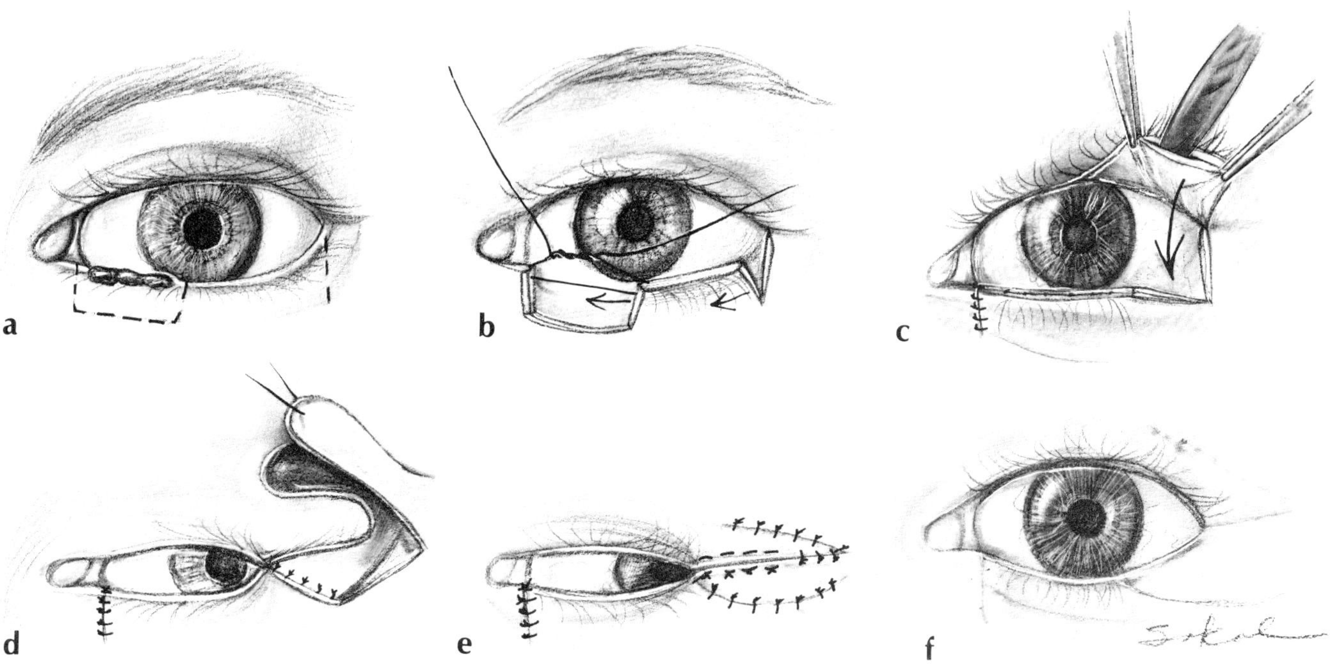

Figure 2.34 *Reconstruction of nasal lower lid defect involving more than 40 per cent of lid margin.* **(a,b)** *Tumor excised and vertical incision made in temporal lid to permit nasal displacement of temporal lid and closure of defect.* **(c–f)** *Temporal lid defect repaired by advancement of tarsal-conjunctival flap for posterior lamella and free skin graft or pedicle flap for anterior defect*

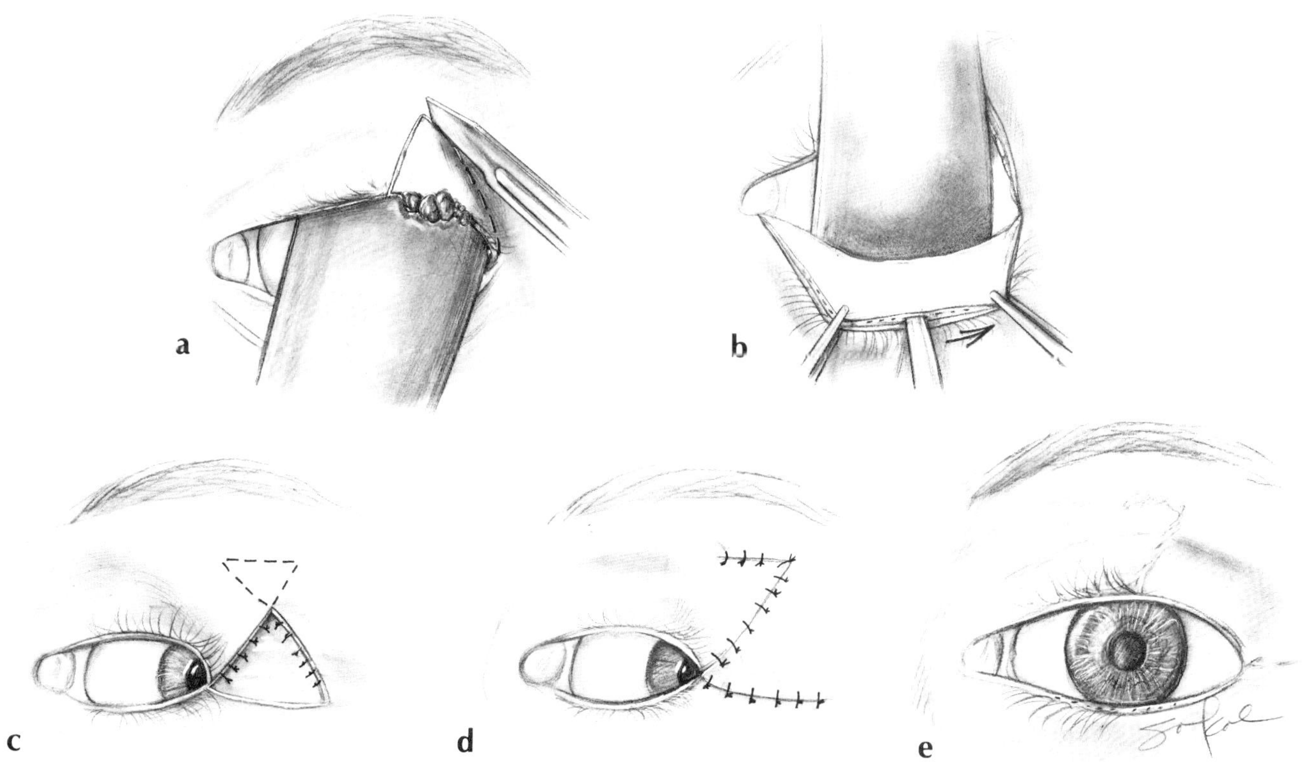

Figure 2.35 *Repair of large upper lid defect.* **(a)** *Lid tumor excised.* **(b)** *Tarsal-conjunctival advancement flap from lower lid prepared by splitting tarsus in vertical dimension through the line of Meibomian glands.* **(c)** *Tarsal-conjunctival flap advanced into upper lid defect and sutured to levator aponeurosis.* **(d)** *Upper lid skin undermined and advanced to fill anterior defect.* **(e)** *Lid margin opened 10–12 weeks later*

Reconstruction following removal of large tumors of the upper lid

Tarsus from the lower lid can be used to repair upper lid defects by using the splitting technique described above. The relative abundance of the upper lid skin aids in reconstruction of the anterior lamella.

For correction of lateral upper lid defects, the lower lid tarsus is split through the center of the meibomian glands, and dissection is done inferiorly to the depth of the cul-de-sac (*Figure 2.35a,b*). A vertical incision through the posterior tarsal flap is made, corresponding to the medial edge of the upper lid defect. The lower lid tarsal-conjunctival flap is then advanced into the upper lid defect and sutured to the cut levator aponeurosis, and nasally to the cut tarsal edge, with 7/0 absorbable suture (*Figure 2.35c*).

The skin and muscle above the defect are undermined and advanced to fill the anterior defect. A triangle of skin is excised to facilitate this maneuver (*Figure 2.35c,d*). As with lower lid reconstruction, the tarsorrhaphy is opened 10–12 weeks postoperatively (*Figure 2.35e*).

Any large upper lid defect can be repaired in this manner. In most cases, myocutaneous advancement flaps can be used to reform the anterior lamella of the lid (*Figure 2.36*). Free skin grafting from the contralateral upper lid or retroauricular area can also be done.

A modification of this procedure uses a conjunctival flap from the retrotarsal margin of the lower lid without disrupting the tarsus (*Figure 2.37a*). The conjunctiva is sutured to the cut conjunctival edge in the upper lid defect (*Figure 2.37b*). Bank sclera or autologous cartilage from the ear is then cut to the shape of the tarsus defect and sutured superiorly to the levator tendon and on either side to the remaining tarsal remnants or canthal ligaments (*Figure 2.37c*). An advancement myocutaneous flap is then mobilized above the graft and is brought down to complete the reconstruction (see *Figure 2.36d,e*). The lower lid margin posterior to the gray line is denuded of epithelium, and the lower edge of the skin flap is sutured to it. The lid margins are separated after 3 months. After division of the lids, the cartilage or sclera graft may have a rough surface at the lid margin that sometimes requires several weeks to re-epithelialize completely. A bandage soft contact lens to protect the cornea is helpful during this time.

The Cutler-Beard procedure[5,19] is also a popular method for repair for large upper lid defects. However, it can cause instability of the lower lid with secondary entropion due to vertical shortening of the tarsus. Lower lid retraction can also occur from excessive shortening of the skin and retractors. Since only a narrow piece of tarsus can be advanced to the upper lid, entropion and contour deformities of the reconstructed lid can occur.

Wesley and McCord[85] have described a modification of the Cutler-Beard procedure in which bank sclera is placed between the lamellae of the split advancement flap from the lower lid. This procedure, which also spares the lower lid tarsus, can be used when there is inadequate upper lid skin. Cartilage from the ear is actually better suited than sclera to replace tarsus, because it shrinks less and heals

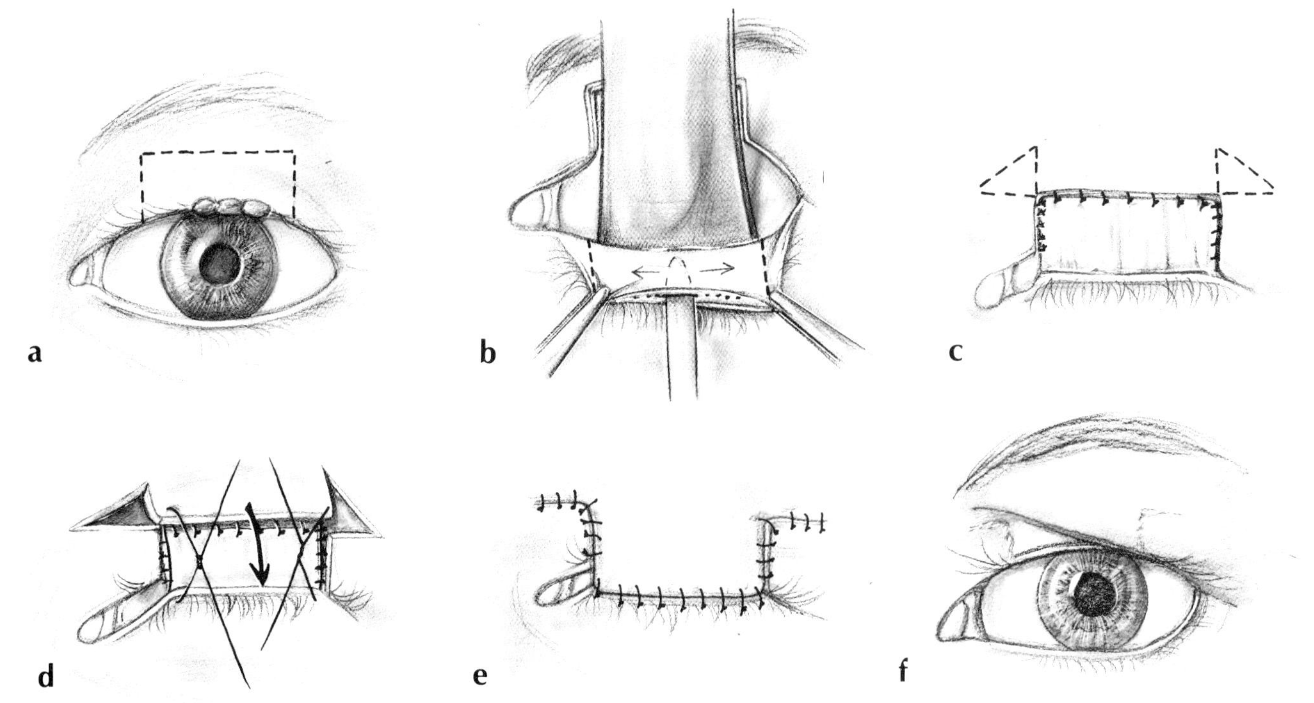

Figure 2.36 *Myocutaneous advancement flap to restore anterior lamella after excision of large upper lid tumor.* **(a)** *Excision of tumor.* **(b,c)** *Tarsal-conjunctival advancement flap from lower lid used to form posterior lamella.* **(d,e)** *Skin and muscle from upper lid undermined and advanced to cover anterior defect.* **(f)** *Lid margin opened 10–12 weeks later*

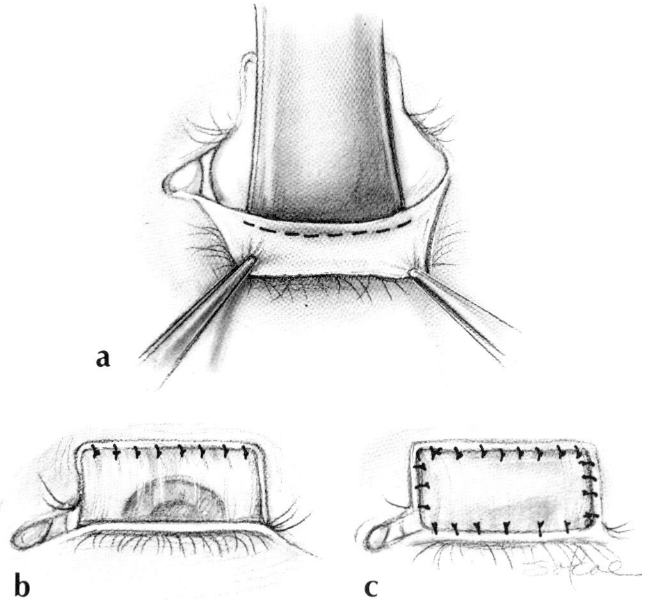

Figure 2.37 *Modified procedure for reconstruction of large upper lid defect.* **(a,b)** *Lower lid conjunctiva from retrotarsal area advanced into upper lid defect.* **(c)** *Free graft of bank sclera or autologous cartilage used to fill tarsal defect*

more rapidly with less inflammation. However, obtaining a cartilage graft is time-consuming and it may be difficult to get a piece of proper contour.

In our experience, secondary problems are minimized by use of a split-thickness full-height tarsal graft. For total and near-total upper lid reconstruction, the smallest chance of complication to the lower lid and the greatest stability of the upper lid are obtained by the cartilage graft technique described above.

Excision of tumors of the inner canthus

Tumors involving only skin can be excised and a free skin graft done if the defect cannot be closed by advancing skin from the upper lid. Deeper involvement by the tumor may mean that the lacrimal apparatus must be sacrificed. Primary lacrimal reconstruction is contraindicated because of the possibility of seeding tumor cells into adjacent bone or the mucous membrane of the nose. Because of already decreased tear production, many older patients have no trouble with tearing postoperatively. A Jones (conjunctival-nasal) tube can be placed as a secondary procedure if needed.

Fox and Beard[83] have recommended allowing granulation and 'healing by second intention' to fill medial canthal defects. Contraction of scar tissue in the area helps to re-establish the medial canthal angle. However, we believe skin grafting speeds recovery and gives superior cosmetic results. If the medial aspect of the lid(s) must be sacrificed, release of the lateral canthal ligament is done to allow medial sliding of the lids and then reattachment of the cut edges to the remnant of the medial canthal ligament or to the periosteum. At a later date a lateral canthotomy is done to enlarge the palpebral fissure.

Lacrimal tract surgery

Blockage of the lacrimal drainage apparatus at any level can cause epiphora or dacryocystitis. However, the cause of the epiphora may be quite unrelated to the lacrimal drainage system, and occasionally this presents a diagnostic problem. A normal eye will tear if exposed to certain common irritants such as smoke or airborne pollutants. Pathological tearing may be intermittent or constant, and often it is profuse enough to blur vision and lead to soreness of the lids from constant mopping. Ascertaining the cause of epiphora takes careful evaluation and use of several simple diagnostic tests. If symptomatic epiphora is due to blockage in the lacrimal drainage system, surgery is indicated.

Dacryocystitis, infection in the lacrimal sac, can occur as the result of blockage of the lacrimal drainage system at any level. Although obstruction of the nasolacrimal tract is the usual causative factor in lacrimal sac infection, blockage of the upper parts of the system – the puncta or canaliculi – can also cause infection. We have treated 3 patients for retrograde dacryocystitis. Two patients had congenitally absent puncta, and the third had prior punctal occlusion for dry eyes. With rare exceptions, dacryocystitis should be treated surgically.

Epiphora

The most common causes of epiphora are ocular irritation and dry eyes. History of redness, itching and burning suggests causes other than lacrimal obstruction. Allergies and the common cold have additional symptoms. Patients with decreased tear formation will (paradoxically) often complain of intermittent tearing, worse in the winter months. This is due to a decrease in baseline tear production followed by ocular irritation and secondary reflex tear production. Such patients tend to be in their midforties or older, and women are affected more often than men. After anesthetizing the eyes with a topical medication, the Schirmer test is done for 5 minutes. Occasionally, there will be several millimeters of immediate wetting of the paper followed by no additional wetting. This may be due to a tear drop in a lax cul-de-sac, and the test should be repeated to get an accurate measurement of baseline tear production. If wetting is less than 5 mm, tear deficiency is the probable cause of the epiphora.

Lid abnormalities – including entropion, ectropion, lid retraction, trichiasis and roughened lid margins – can all cause epiphora. Laxity of the lower lid decreases the effectiveness of the lacrimal pump, and the tears are not properly directed to the puncta. Malpositions of the puncta, especially slight eversion, may not be readily apparent but can be seen with the slit lamp.

If there is no evidence implicating the lids, the ocular tissues or tear production as the cause of epiphora, the problem probably lies with the lacrimal drainage apparatus. Blockage can be partial or total and can involve one or more of the three levels of the system. One or both of the puncta on one side may be congenitally absent; but, in our experience, epiphora is not a problem for patients born with one punctum, and occasionally it is not a problem when both puncta are absent. However, when the puncta are occluded by conjunctival infections, topical medications or trauma, epiphora usually results.

The ampulla of the canaliculi can become blocked by stones and debris and this may be associated with infection by actinomyces organisms. This blockage can be relieved by incision and curettage. Although infections can cause permanent damage and scarring of the canaliculi, the most common causes of canalicular malfunction are trauma and surgery for lid tumors. The relative importance of each canaliculus is uncertain. However, in our experience, epiphora is usually not a problem if either canaliculus is functioning properly.

Blockage at the level of the lacrimal sac can be due to (*1*) infection with mucosal swelling that produces secondary scarring and occlusion; (*2*) lacrimal stones or primary tumors of the sac; (*3*) pressure from adjacent adnexal tumors and trauma.

A deviated nasal septum or nasal trauma can cause blockage of the nasolacrimal duct. In children, a congenital membrane may occlude the nasolacrimal duct where it enters the nose under the inferior turbinate. Atresia of the duct can also occur.

The location and degree of lacrimal obstruction in adults can be evaluated in the office. Slit-lamp examination of the puncta indicates whether or not they are of adequate size. If the puncta are small, and fluid cannot be readily irrigated through the system, surgery is directed at the puncta. Gentle probing of the canaliculi is used to determine whether there is blockage at that level. If irrigation through the upper punctum causes reflux from the lower punctum, blockage is distal to the common canaliculus. If pressure on the sac produces reflux of fluid or mucus, blockage is distal to the sac.

Diagnostic probing of the system distal to the common canaliculus may give a false indication of patency if a soft stone is present, because the probe may pass through it and yet the stone can still act as a ball valve. Therapeutic probing in adults is usually not effective if the obstruction is caused by a stone, because the hole made by the probe in the soft material will quickly close. Edematous or scarred tissue is made worse by probing, and false passages can occur that increase the chance of later infection and generally complicate the situation.

In the presence of partial obstruction, there can be epiphora and yet the tract may irrigate readily. In such cases further testing is helpful. The 'Jones I' test consists of evaluating patency of the system by the passage of fluorescein dye[84]. Two per cent fluorescein is placed in the inferior cul-de-sac. The patient holds his head back for 2 minutes to allow dye passage into the sac and then leans forward to facilitate flow into the nose. After 15 minutes a small cotton swab is used to test for dye under the inferior turbinate. Alternatively, the patient can blow his nose, and the tissue is observed for presence of dye. If dye passes into the nose, it is likely that the epiphora is not caused by blockage of the lacrimal drainage system.

'Jones II' testing is done if dye fails to enter the nose. Following instillation of dye in the cul-de-sac, clear fluid is irrigated through one of the puncta. If fluid entering the nose is clear, it means no dye entered the lacrimal sac, and the partial obstruction lies at the level of the puncta or canalicular system. If fluid entering the nose is tinged with dye, the obstruction is at the level of the nasolacrimal duct, and a dacryocystorhinostomy is indicated.

Dacryocystitis

Acute dacryocystitis causes pain and swelling in the lacrimal area. There may be erythema of the skin overlying the sac. Chronic dacryocystitis may or may not cause pain, and long-term swelling in the lacrimal sac area occurs without erythema. The amount of discomfort often fluctuates.

Mucopurulent discharge from the puncta is occasionally seen, and pressure over the sac often causes reflux of large amounts of material. However, swelling of the sac and common canalicular area can close off the common canaliculus, preventing reflux. In such cases palpation of the sac reveals a smooth, firm, rubbery mass. Occasionally, hard lacrimal stones can be palpated.

Edema can be extensive, obscuring the central problem, but a history of tearing and repeated swelling and soreness in the lacrimal sac area suggests the diagnosis. Perforation through the skin occurs spontaneously in some cases if surgery is not done. Medical therapy for dacryocystitis can be followed by perforation and later recurrence and is therefore not definitive treatment for this disorder.

Infants of less than 2 months and very sick patients can be treated with antibiotics and hot compresses. As mentioned, perforation through the skin often occurs, and there is temporary resolution of the inflammation, only to have infection recur later. In acute cases we treat with antibiotics until surgery is performed, and the surgery is not delayed more than 1 week. Surgery can be done on acute cases, and it is not necessary to wait for resolution of the inflammation in response to antibiotic therapy. Occasionally the situation worsens before surgery and may result in perforation through the skin, causing scarring and making surgery more difficult.

Evaluation and treatment of infants

Although dacryocystitis can be evident soon after birth, tearing is the most common initial symptom of congenital lacrimal tract obstruction. A membrane blocking the nasolacrimal duct where it enters the nose under the inferior turbinate may be present, and this usually opens spontaneously by age 9 months. During the first several months, massage over the lacrimal sac area may be helpful. A finger is placed over the inner canthus to occlude the puncta, and firm intermittent pressure over the sac is exerted in an inward and downward direction to force the fluid contents of the sac against the occluding membrane. If dacryocystitis occurs, antibiotics are started and careful probing of the system is done.

Probing is also done if the membrane obstructing the nasal orifice of the nasolacrimal duct does not open by age 9 months. Probing requires a good working knowledge of the lacrimal system. The slightest motion by the patient can cause failure by producing a false passage. Therefore, all probings should be done under general anesthesia, although insufflation anesthesia without an endotracheal tube can be used and the procedure done on an outpatient basis.

The superior punctum is gently dilated with a sharp punctal dilator. A lacrimal irrigating needle attached to a syringe is gently inserted into the punctum and immediately turned parallel to the lid margin and advanced nasally along the canaliculus. When the medial wall of the lacrimal sac is encountered, the syringe is angled so that the needle is directed inferiorly. The syringe is usually firmly against the brow and approximately parallel to the nose when the needle is in this position. A mildly firm push of irrigating fluid is used in an attempt to break the membrane. If this is successful the obstruction has been cured; otherwise, further probing is needed.

A small-diameter lacrimal probe no larger than a 2/0 Bowman probe is passed through the superior canaliculus and directed nasally until the medial wall of the sac is encountered. Temporal traction on the lid with a finger facilitates passage of the probe. The tip is then directed inferiorly with the probe held against the brow. The tip may need to be directed slightly nasally or anteriorly to pass into the inferior part of the sac, which forms a funnel. As the probe enters the bony canal the tip feels stable, eliminating any wobbling of the probe. The probe can then be advanced into the nose with slight pressure, and the tip observed under the inferior turbinate. The probe is withdrawn and the lacrimal system is filled with antibiotic ointment injected through a lacrimal needle to keep the tract open. If there is bleeding from the punctum the probing has been excessively traumatic, and the procedure may fail.

If blockage is encountered that cannot easily be passed, probing is repeated at a later date. If a second probing is unsuccessful, we recommend that dacryocystorhinostomy be performed during the same operation. This can be done as early as age 6 months but can be delayed until 1 year to reduce the risks associated with anesthesia.

Children with congenitally absent puncta often have a small dimple in the skin at the usual site of the punctum. With the aid of an operating microscope, these areas can be opened with a 25 gauge needle and then enlarged with a punctal dilator.

Surgery for dry eye

Patients with dry eyes benefit by occlusion of the puncta to preserve the tears that are present. It may be uncertain whether all four, or just two, puncta should be occluded; and there are borderline cases with only slightly reduced tear secretion that may have epiphora after punctal occlusion. Thus, temporary occlusion is done first by applying light diathermy to the puncta. This produces closure for only a few weeks. If improvement of symptoms occurs, the punctum and canaliculus are permanently closed by inserting a long diathermy needle into the canaliculus and applying current as the needle is withdrawn. Sufficient current is applied to produce only a blanching of the tissues, and care is taken to avoid a through-and-through burn.

Surgery to enlarge the puncta

Tight puncta can frequently be temporarily improved by dilation, but permanent improvement requires punctoplasty. One-snip, two-snip, and three-snip procedures, done with sharp, pointed iris scissors, are the most popular. Choice of the procedure depends on the degree of obstruction.

One snip with the scissors, directed vertically along the posterior punctal edge into the ampulla of the canaliculus, can open a slightly constricted punctum. A V-shaped incision provides a wider opening in the posterior wall of the punctum. However, we prefer the three-snip procedure because it causes less disruption of the lid margin. A vertical incision is made at the back of the punctum into the ampulla. A second incision, about 2 mm long, is made horizontally in a nasal direction at the base of the ampulla. The upper end of the first incision and the nasal end of the second are connected with a third incision, thereby excising a triangle of tissue.

Dacryocystorhinostomy

Blockage at the level of the lacrimal sac or nasolacrimal duct requires dacryocystorhinostomy (DCR). Before surgery the nose is examined to rule out a severely deviated septum, polyps or other nasal pathology. If possible, any such problems should be corrected prior to the DCR. Likewise, sinusitis should be treated prior to DCR unless there is acute dacryocystitis. If the history of symptoms is not typical of dacryocystitis, or if a firm or irregular mass is palpated that suggests a tumor, orbital X-rays and computerized axial tomography should be done. Radiopaque dye can be injected through a canaliculus to outline pathology in the lacrimal sac.

Use of the Stryker saw with a dacryotrephine and then use of a nasolacrimal catheter have greatly simplified the DCR operation, and a success rate equal to any of the more complex and difficult mucous membrane flap techniques is obtained. The oscillating action of the Stryker saw does not damage soft tissues and can be used in confined areas without danger of wrapping up adjacent tissues as can happen with a mastoid drill. In young children the bone is easily perforated with the tip of a clamp and the opening is enlarged with a sphenoid punch.

The lacrimal sac lies very close to the nasal mucous membrane after the intervening bone has been removed. A medium red-rubber catheter is used as a stent until these two membranes heal together, usually after 10–14 days. Suturing the flaps together is not necessary. In scarred or small sacs, dissection and suturing of mucosal flaps are difficult, and use of the catheter eliminates this problem.

General anesthesia is preferred, but the procedure can be done under local anesthesia. When local anesthesia is used, the nose is packed with gauze soaked in 4 per cent cocaine placed at the level of the middle turbinate. The infraorbital nerve is injected at the infraorbital notch with 2 ml of 2 per cent lidocaine (lignocaine). A second injection is made posteriorly, just inferior to the medial canthal ligament to block the anterior ethmoidal nerve. Subcutaneous injection along the anterior lacrimal crest is also done. The anterior nasal pack is removed after 10 minutes and a posterior nasal pack is placed to prevent aspiration of blood. Use of 1:100 000 epinephrine (adrenaline) in the nasal pack may help reduce bleeding; however, we rarely find this necessary because bleeding stops soon after insertion of the catheter.

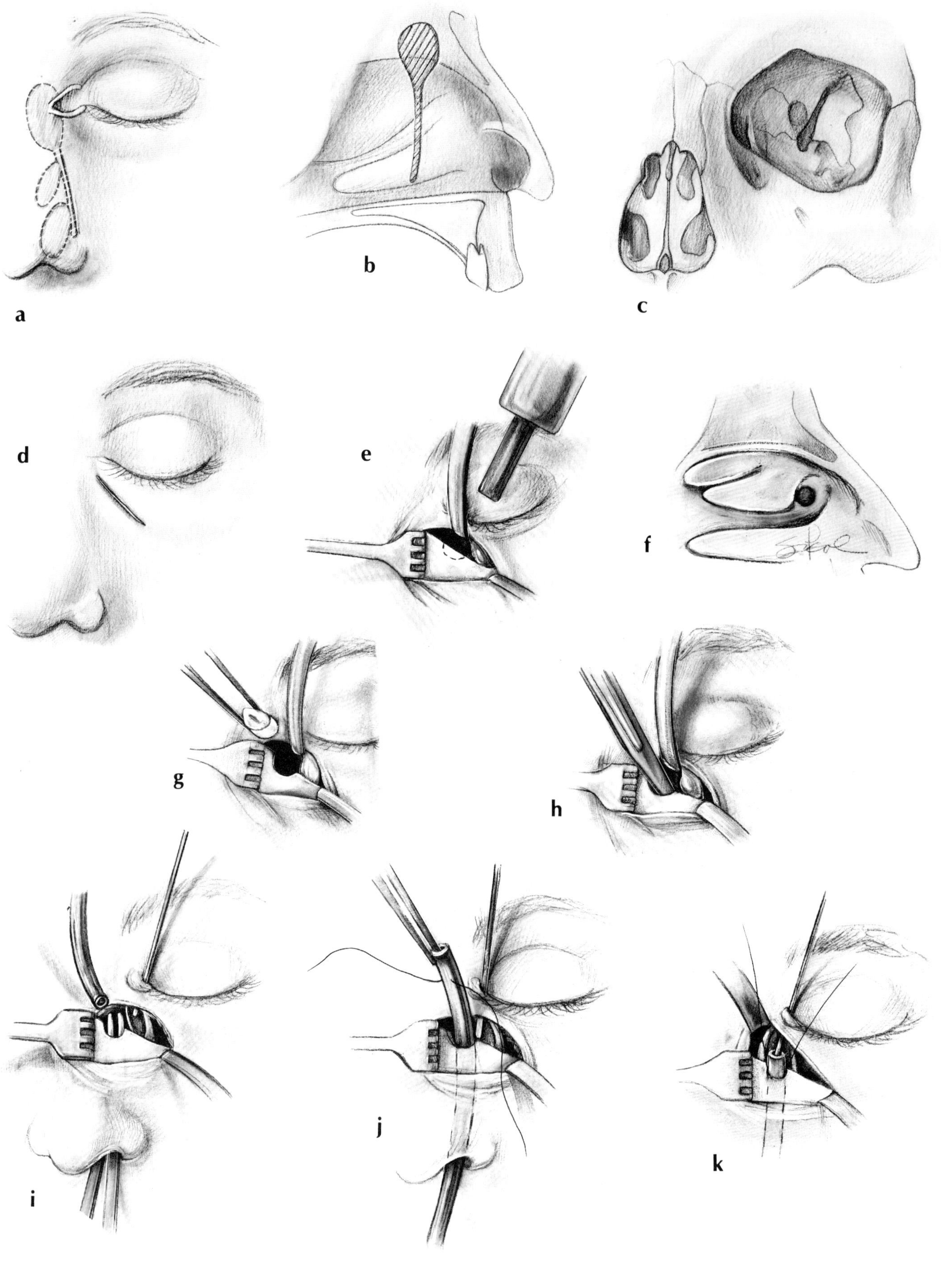
a
b
c
d
e
f
g
h
i
j
k

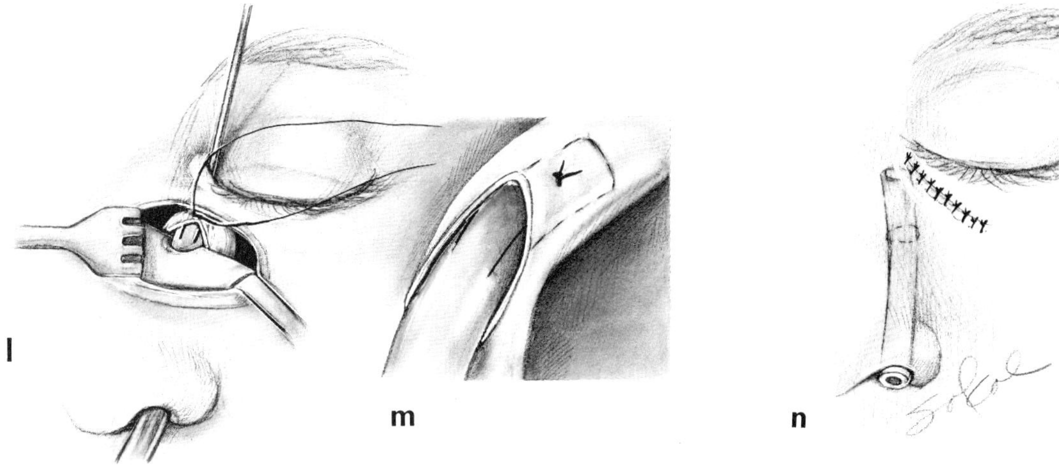

Figure 2.38 *Dacryocystorhinostomy.* **(a–c)** *Lacrimal sac is located posterior to anterior lacrimal crest of orbital rim and nasolacrimal duct extends into nose beneath lower turbinate.* **(d)** *Incision made through skin, orbicularis and periosteum along lacrimal crest.* **(e,f)** *Stryker dacryotrephine, straddling lacrimal crest, makes opening into nose, entering just anterior to middle turbinate.* **(g)** *Plug of bone removed with forceps.* **(h)** *Nasal mucous membrane opened with blade.* **(i)** *Probe placed through superior canaliculus into lacrimal sac, and curved clamp passed up nose into bony defect to grasp rubber catheter.* **(j,k)** *Catheter withdrawn through nose and proximal cut end threaded over lacrimal probe.* **(l,m)** *Catheter sutured to anterior wall of lacrimal sac.* **(n)** *Lower end of catheter is cut flush with nares and sutured to nasal septum*

The patency of the upper and lower canaliculi is confirmed with gentle probing. If the lacrimal sac is markedly distended, it is decompressed with digital pressure to be sure it is not overhanging the anterior lacrimal crest, which would interfere with the incision.

The anterior lacrimal crest and medial canthal ligament are palpated to outline the site of the incision, which should extend for 2 cm below the medial canthal ligament along the crest (*Figure 2.38a–c*). A bold incision down to the orbital rim (anterior lacrimal crest) is made through skin, orbicularis and periosteum (*Figure 2.38d*). The incision should lie in the normal skin crease. The bold incision prevents the sliding of tissues that can occur in a layer-by-layer dissection, and it produces minimal postoperative scarring. Other surgeons have suggested placing the incision on the nose to reduce bleeding[85,86]. In our experience this is not needed, and the chance of unsightly scarring is increased.

Skin rake retractors are used immediately to spread the incision, and pressure from these minimizes bleeding. Suction is used to keep a clear field, and cautery can be used, but usually is not needed. A periosteal elevator is used to elevate the periosteum and anterior wall of the lacrimal sac (which are fused together) from the lacrimal fossa. As these tissues are retracted the lacrimal crest and fossa are exposed.

A Stryker saw with a 7 mm dacryotrephine (Iliff trephine, Storz Instrument Co.) is used to make the bony window. The trephine is placed straddling the anterior crest (*Figure 2.38e,f*), and it is directed nasally, inferiorly and slightly posteriorly. Moderate pressure is applied and the saw is withdrawn when there is loss of resistance, indicating that the tip has penetrated the bone to the nasal mucosa. The bone is cut cleanly and the plug usually comes out in the end of the trephine; if not, it can be removed with forceps (*Figure 2.38g*). The heat from the saw minimizes bone bleeding, but bone wax can be used if needed. Usually the 7 mm trephine hole must be enlarged with a sphenoid punch to provide more direct passage for the catheter from the neck of the sac to the nose.

A cruciate or H-shaped incision is made in the nasal mucous membrane if it is of normal thickness (*Figure 2.38h*). If the mucous membrane is hypertrophic, it is completely excised from the trephine opening. Often there is temporary profuse bleeding from the nasal mucous membrane, and suction through the nose is used to keep the surgical field dry without obscuring visualization.

A probe is passed through the superior canaliculus into the lacrimal sac. This identifies the nasal wall of the sac, which is opened with a vertical incision to expose the end of the probe. A curved clamp is passed up through the nose into the trephine window to grasp the tip of a red rubber catheter (14–16 Fr catheter) which is then drawn into the nose and out the external naris (*Figure 2.38i*). The proximal end of the catheter is cut off, leaving 3 cm projecting from the wound.

A double-armed 3/0 chromic catgut suture with a small half-curved, special needle (Ethicon No. 748G) is placed through the wall of the catheter 1 cm from the cut end (*Figure 2.38j*). The end of the catheter is grasped with toothed forceps and pushed gently into the wound and is then threaded over the probe lying in the lacrimal sac (*Figure 2.38k*). The two arms of the sutures are passed through the anterior sac wall and connective tissue and tied. As they are tied, the catheter tip is advanced into the neck of the sac (*Figure 2.38l,m*). Care is taken to ensure that the edges of the sac are not folded across the end of the catheter. The probe is withdrawn and the skin incision is closed with 8/0 interrupted silk sutures.

The lower end of the tube is cut flush with the external naris (*Figure 2.38n*), and the tube is sutured with 5/0 nylon to the nasal septum. A non-adherent semipressure dressing is applied to the wound. The patient is discharged the next morning. Systemic antibiotics and decongestants are used for 1–2 weeks. The skin sutures are removed in 4 days. The catheter is removed in 10–14 days by cutting the inferior nylon suture in the nasal septum and giving the tube a short, quick tug. This breaks the friable catgut suture between the catheter and the lacrimal sac wall.

Silastic intubation of canaliculi

With canalicular disease and in cases of severely scarred small lacrimal sacs, Silastic cathethers are threaded through the canaliculi and out through the rubber catheter. Occlusion or stenosis of the common canaliculus can be opened with a scalpel, but it must be kept open postoperatively or epiphora may occur despite successful DCR creation of a passageway from the sac to the nose. In these cases, and in reoperations, we use 0.025 inch (0.6 mm) diameter Silastic catheters to provide a long-acting lacrimal stent.

After opening the lacrimal sac during the DRC procedure, a lacrimal probe with an attached Silastic tube is passed through each punctum and canaliculus, out of the sac opening, through the trephine opening and is directed out of the nose with a grooved director. A 6/0 black silk suture is used to tie the two Silastic tubes together at the level of the sac opening. The Silastic tubes loop gently between the puncta. The rubber catheter is then threaded over the tubes and up through the trephine opening. The chromic catgut suture is used to suture the catheter to the anterior sac wall as described above. The Silastic tubes direct the catheter toward the common canaliculus. The catheter and Silastic are cut flush with the external naris.

The rubber catheter is removed in 10–14 days, taking care not to grasp the Silastic tubes at the same time. The 6/0 silk suture prevents the Silastic from being dislodged by accidentally pulling on the loop at the puncta. If the tubes are pulled partially out at the puncta, they can be repositioned by pulling on the ends in the nose or by having the patient blow his nose. The Silastic tubes are left in place for 3–6 months. The loop is then cut between the puncta, and the tubes are pulled out from the nose.

Complications

Drainage of an acute dacryocystitis through the skin, either spontaneously or surgically, can lead to a fistula. A fistula must be excised and closed at the time of DCR, and often there is surrounding scar tissue that must also be excised to give an improved cosmetic result.

The DCR may fail for many reasons. Temporary postoperative failure may ocur if a mucous plug blocks the nasolacrimal opening. This usually can be removed by irrigation. However, irrigation should not be done in the immediate postoperative period, and postoperative manipulation of the lacrimal system is not indicated if the patient is asymptomatic. Later irrigation is done only if there is apparent failure of the procedure. Occasionally mucous membrane overgrows the bony ostium, and probing can readily rupture such a membrane. Rarely, but especially if there was trauma to the nasal bones prior to the DCR, bony overgrowth closes the ostium and requires reoperation.

We have seen 2 children who had unplanned removal of the Silastic tubing used in conjunction with a DCR. A babysitter in one case, an uncle in the second, saw a small 'string' in the child's nose and pulled it out. It is important to show the tubes to the parents and have them inform others who are caring for the child. After removal of the rubber catheter, the tubes should be shortened so that they cannot be easily grasped at the nose. If punctal erosion occurs, the tubes should be removed. We have not seen this, however, and we believe it should not occur if the loop between the puncta is somewhat loose.

Trauma

Lacerations of the canaliculus near the punctum can be repaired using a stainless steel (Veers) rod or Silastic tube as a stent. We prefer Silastic tubes because hard stents produce an unnatural stiff area in the healing lid, and the stent may migrate, extrude or cause inflammation. Lacerations near or involving the common canaliculus are difficult to repair, and often epiphora occurs postoperatively despite apparently successful reanastomosis.

The cut ends of the canaliculus are identified with the aid of an operating microscope. The ends can be seen in nearly every case without special techniques. Occasionally the cut ends, deep in the canthal area, cannot be identified. The canthal area is flooded with irrigating fluid to form a puddle, and air is injected through the puncta to locate the cut ends by observing where bubbles emerge. If a probe can be passed into the nose through the cut canaliculus, a Silastic tube can be threaded on the end of the probe and passed through the canaliculus into the nose. The ends of the Silastic tube can be sutured to the nose and lid and the lacerated tissue repaired. Alternatively another probe can be passed through the intact canaliculus, down into the nose and brought out on a grooved director placed under the inferior turbinate, thereby looping the Silastic tube at the puncta as has been described. The tubes are tied together in the nose.

At times, passage of a probe into the nose is not possible. In these cases we feed the cut end of a piece of silicone tube through the damaged canaliculus and into the sac. A 10/0 nylon suture secures the tube at the cut end of the canaliculus to stabilize it while the lid is repaired. The tube produces an approximation of the canalicular edges, so that no direct suturing is necessary. The end of the Silastic tube is then stabilized at the punctum by suturing it with 8/0 silk in the cul-de-sac or to the lid skin.

Conjunctivodacryorhinostomy

If there is irreparable damage to both canaliculi, a conjunctivodacryorhinostomy is needed. Jones devised various sizes of Pyrex tubes that can be inserted at the medial canthus to drain into the nose[87]. A routine DCR incision is made, and the Stryker saw is used to make the opening into the nose in the manner described earlier. A Graefe knife is used to make a stab incision from the nasal conjunctival cul-de-sac beneath the caruncle, toward the nose and downward at an angle that enters the trephine opening. The Jones tube is slipped into this tract. It should be long enough to enter the nose but not touch the septum. The upper end of the tube is fastened to the conjunctiva with a 6/0 nylon suture. The suture should be placed to prevent conjunctiva from folding over the opening of the tube.

After the tissues heal, the patient is instructed to hold the nose occasionally and breathe in so as to draw air through the tube and keep it patent. Occasionally irrigation is needed to clear a clogged tube. After several months to a year, an epithelialized tract is formed, and the tube can readily be removed, cleaned and replaced. Occasionally the tract is adequate, and so the tube can be left out.

Conjunctivodacryocystostomy

If the lacrimal sac and nasolacrimal duct are normal, and the canaliculi are obstructed, a conjunctivodacryocystostomy can be done to bypass the blocked area. The procedure is usually done under general anesthesia, but local anesthesia can be used. A 16 gauge Angiocath needle with the sleeve removed is used. A No. 160 polyethylene tube is held over an alcohol lamp to produce a 2–3 mm flare of the tip. The tube is cut to a length estimated to be equal to the distance from just under the caruncle to the level of the lower portion of the lacrimal sac (about 2 cm).

The lower one-half of the caruncle and adjacent plica are excised. The polyethylene tube is then placed over the needle which is attached to a 3 ml syringe filled with irrigating solution and fluorescein dye. The needle is inserted through the area just below the caruncle in the direction of the lacrimal sac. When the needle is in the sac, a small amount of dye is injected and the nose is swabbed or suction is applied under the inferior turbinate to confirm passage of the dye. The polyethylene tube is then advanced into the sac. If the needle cannot be passed into the sac or if the polyethylene tube cannot be advanced, a DCR incision, with dissection down to the sac, is necessary.

A 6/0 nylon suture is passed through the lip of the tube and is secured to the conjunctiva and connective tissue under the cut edge of the caruncle. Irrigation through the tube at the end of the procedure confirms its proper placement.

References

1. Iliff, C. E. Exenteration of the orbit. Maryland State Medical Journal 1959; 8:606–611
2. Clemmensen, J. The early circulation in split skin grafts. Restoration of blood supply to split skin autografts. Acta Chirurgica Scandinavica 1964; 127:1–8
3. Smith, J. W., Ringland, J., Wilson, R. Vascularization of skin grafts. Surgical Forum 1964; 15:473–475
4. Converse, J. M., Ballantyne, D. L., Jr. Distribution of diphosphopyridine nucleotide diaphorase in rat skin autografts and homografts. Plastic and Reconstructive Surgery 1962; 30:415
5. Beard, C. H. Ophthalmic surgery, 2nd ed. Philadelphia: Blackston's Son & Co., 1914
6. Feldstein, M. Correction of senile entropion. Ophthalmic Surgery 1970; 1(3):20–23
7. Quickert, M. H., Rathbun, E. Suture repair of entropion. Archives of Ophthalmology 1971; 85:304–305
8. Hecht, S. D. Bowleg's procedure for recurrent and primary senile entropion. Annals of Ophthalmology 1981; 13:119–120
9. Fox, S. A. Streatfield-Snellin 'Tarsoplasty' for cicatricial entropion of upper lid (author's modification). In Fox, S. A., ed. Ophthalmic plastic surgery, 5th ed. New York: Grune and Stratton, Inc. 1976:331–339
10. Beyer, C. K., Carroll, J. M. Moderately severe cicatricial entropion. Archives of Ophthalmology 1973; 89:33–35
11. Iliff, C. E., Iliff, W. J., Iliff, N. T. Oculoplastic surgery. Philadelphia: W. B. Saunders Co., 1979:128
12. Culbertson, W. W., Ostler, H. B. The floppy eyelid syndrome. American Journal of Ophthalmology 1981; 92:568–575
13. Smith, B., Cherubini, T. D. Ocuplastic surgery: a compendium of principles and techniques. St Louis: The C. V. Mosby Co., 1970
14. Smith, B. The 'lazy T' correction of ectropion of the lower punctum. Archives of Ophthalmology 1976; 94:1149–1150
15. Berke, R. N., Wadsworth, J. A. C. Histology of levator muscle in congenital and acquired ptosis. Archives of Ophthalmology 1955; 53:413–428
16. Isaksson, I. Studies on congenital genuine blepharoptosis. Morphological and functional investigations of the upper eyelid. Acta Ophthalmologica 1962; Suppl. 72:1–21
17. Anderson, R. L., Gordy, D. D. Aponeurotic defects in congenital ptosis. Ophthalmology 1979; 86:1493–1500
18. Anderson, R. L., Baumgartner, S. A. Amblyopia in ptosis. Archives of Ophthalmology 1980; 98:1068–1069
19. Beard, C. Ptosis, 3rd ed. St. Louis: The C. V. Mosby Co., 1981:47
20. Iliff, C. E. The optimum time for surgery in the Marcus-Gunn phenomenon. Transactions of the American Academy of Ophthalmology and Otolaryngology 1970; 74:1005–1010
21. Jones, L. T., Quickert, M. H., Wobig, J. L. The cure of ptosis by aponeurotic repair. Archives of Ophthalmology 1975; 93: 629–634
22. Johnson, C. C., Kuwabara, T. Oculopharyngeal muscular dystrophy. American Journal of Ophthalmology 1974; 77:872–879
23. Horner, J. F. Uebir eine Form von Ptosis. Klinische Monatsblätter Augenheilkunde 1869; 7:193–198
24. Cogan, D. G. Current concepts of myasthenia gravis. Archives of Ophthalmology 1965; 74:1–3
25. Beard, C. Ptosis, 3rd ed. St Louis: The C. V. Mosby Co., 1981:87
26. Iliff, C. E. Simplified ptosis operation. American Journal of Ophthalmology 1954; 37:529–533
27. Fasanella, R. M., Servat, T. Levator resection for minimal ptosis; another simplified operation. Archives of Ophthalmology 1961; 65:493–496
28. Jones, L. T., Quickert, M. H., Wobig, J. L. The cure of ptosis by aponeurotic repair. Archives of Ophthalmology 1975; 93:629–634
29. Beard, C. A new treatment for severe unilateral congenital ptosis and for ptosis with jaw-winking. American Journal of Ophthalmology 1965; 59:252–258
30. Young, G. An operation for congenital ptosis. British Journal of Ophthalmology 1924; 8:272–275
31. Jameson, P. C. Surgical management of ptosis with special reference to use of superior rectus muscle. Archives of Ophthalmology 1937; 18:547–557
32. Dickey, C. A. Superior rectus fascia lata sling in correction of ptosis. American Journal of Ophthalmology 1936; 19:660–664
33. Anderson, R. L., Dixon, R. S. The role of Whitnall's ligament in ptosis surgery. Archives of Ophthalmology 1979; 97:705–707
34. Friedenwald, J. S., Guyton, J. S. Simple ptosis operation; utilization of frontalis by means of a single rhomboid-shaped suture. American Journal of Ophthalmology 1948; 31:411–414
35. Henderson, J. W. Tarsal-periosteal frontalis sutures for the correction of palpebral ptosis. Transactions of the American Academy of Ophthalmology and Otolaryngology 1957; 61:701–705
36. Katowitz, J. A. Frontalis suspension in congenital ptosis using a polyfilament cable-type suture. Archives of Ophthalmology 1979; 97:1659–1663
37. Panas, P. D'un nouveau procédé opératoire applicable au ptosis congénital et au ptosis paralitique. Archives d'Ophthalmologie 1886; 6:1–14

38. Tillett, C. W., Tillett, G. M. Silicone sling in the correction of ptosis. American Journal of Ophthalmology 1966; 62:521–523
39. Bodian, M. Repair of ptosis using human sclera. American Journal of Ophthalmology 1968; 65:352–358
40. Iliff, C. E. Surgical management of ptosis. Somerville, New Jersey: Ethicon, Inc., 1963
41. Wright, W. W. The use of living sutures in the treatment of ptosis. Archives of Ophthalmology (1st ser.) 1922; 51:99–102
42. Yasuna, E. Use of prepared fascia lata in correction of ptosis. American Journal of Ophthalmology 1962; 54:1097–1103
43. Helveston, E. M., Wilson, D. L. A suture-reinforced scleral sling. Archives of Ophthalmology 1975; 93:643–645
44. Crawford, J. S. Repair of ptosis using frontalis muscle and fascia lata: a 20 year review. Ophthalmic Surgery 1977; 8:31–40
45. Crawford, J. S. Personal communication, 1981
46. Beard, C. Ptosis, 3rd ed. St Louis: The C. V. Mosby Co., 1981:191–192
47. Collin, J. R., Beard, C., Wood, I. Terminal course of nerve supply to Müeller's muscle in the rhesus monkey and its clinical significance. American Journal of Ophthalmology 1979; 87:234–246
48. Beard, C. Ptosis, 3rd ed. St Louis: The C. V. Mosby Co., 1981:251
49. Beard, C. Ptosis, 3rd ed. St Louis: The C. V. Mosby Co., 1981:2
50. Gay, A. J., Salmon, M. L., Wolkstein, M. A. Topical sympatholytic therapy for pathologic lid retraction. Archives of Ophthalmology 1967; 77:341–344
51. Baylis, H. I., Cies, W. A., Kamin, D. F. Correction of upper eyelid retraction. American Journal of Ophthalmology 1976; 82(5):790–794
52. Henderson, J. W. Relief of eyelid retraction: a surgical procedure. Archives of Ophthalmology 1965; 74:205–216
53. Goldstein, I. Recession of the levator muscle for lagophthalmos in exophthalmic goiter. Archives of Ophthalmology 1934; 11:389–393
54. Harvey, J. T., Anderson, R. L. The aponeurotic approach to eyelid retraction. Ophthalmology 1981; 88:513–524
55. Flanagan, J. C. Eye bank sclera in oculoplastic surgery. Ophthalmic Surgery 1974; 5(3):45–53
56. Dryden, R. M., Soll, D. B. The use of scleral transplantation in cicatricial entropion and eyelid retraction. Transactions of the American Academy of Ophthalmology and Otolaryngology 1977; 83:669–678
57. Fuchs, E. Textbook of ophthalmology. New York: Appleton, 1892:553
58. Rees, T. D., Dupuis, D. Baggy eyelids in young adults. Plastic and Reconstructive Surgery 1969; 43:381
59. Converse, J. M., ed. Reconstructive plastic surgery, Vol. 3. Philadelphia: W. B. Saunders Co., 1964:1333–1336
60. Converse, J. M., ed. Reconstructive plastic surgery, Vol. 3, 2nd ed. Philadelphia: W. B. Saunders Co., 1977:1888
61. Bodian, M. Paper delivered to meeting of American Society of Ophthalmic, Plastic and Reconstructive Surgery, 1975
62. Waller, R. R. Is blindness a realistic complication in blepharoplasty procedures? Ophthalmology 1978; 85:730–735
63. Putterman, A. M. Temporary blindness after cosmetic blepharoplasty. American Journal of Ophthalmology 1975; 80:1081–1083
64. Wiggs, E. O. Blepharoplasty complications. Transactions of the American Academy of Ophthalmology and Otolaryngology 1976; 81:OP603–OP606
65. Welch, R. B., Duke, J. R. Lesions of the lids: a statistical note: American Journal of Ophthalmology 1958; 45:415–426
66. Turtz, C. A. Verruca as cause of unilateral conjunctivitis. American Journal of Ophthalmology 1942; 25:452–453
67. Hogan, M. J., Zimmerman, L. E. Ophthalmic pathology: an atlas and textbook, 2nd ed. Philadelphia: W. B. Saunders Co., 1962:197–198
68. Wolkin, S. H., Spivey, B. E., Blodi, F. C. Hereditary adenoid cystic epithelioma. American Journal of Ophthalmology 1969; 68:26–34
69. Warvi, W. N., Gates, O. Epithelial cysts and cystic tumors of the skin. American Journal of Pathology 1943; 19:765–783
70. Carbone, A., Zingirian, M., Ciurlo, G. Sull' epitelioma calafico denigno di Malherbe. Annali di Ottalmologia 1965; 91:401–409
71. Reese, A. B. Tumors of the eye, 3rd ed. Hagerstown: Harper and Row, 1976:245
72. Braithwaite, F. Melanosis of eyelids. British Journal of Plastic Surgery 1948; 1:206–211
73. Yanoff, M., Fine, B. S. Ocular pathology: a text and atlas. Hagerstown: Harper and Row, 1975:635
74. Pedace, F. J., Winkelmann, R. K. Xanthelasma Palpebrarum. Journal of the American Medical Asssociation 1965; 193:893–894
75. Cosman, B. Experience in the argon laser therapy of port wine stains. Plastic and Reconstructive Surgery 1980; 65:119–129
76. Robb, R. M. Refractive errors associated with hemangiomas of the eyelids and orbit in infancy. American Journal of Ophthalmology 1977; 83:52–58
77. Stigmer, G., Crawford, J. S., Ward, C. M., Thompson, H. G. Ophthalmic sequelae of infantile hemangiomas of the eyelids and orbit. American Journal of Ophthalmology 1978; 85:806–813
78. Payne, J. W., Duke, J. R., Butner, R., Eifrig, D. E. Basal cell carcinoma of the eyelids: A long term follow-up study. Archives of Ophthalmology 1969; 81:553–558
79. Boniuk, M., Zimmerman, L. E. Sebaceous carcinoma of the eyelid, eyebrow, caruncle and orbit. Transactions of the American Academy of Ophthalmology and Otolaryngology 1968; 72:619–642
80. Tenzel, R. R., Stewart, W. B. Eyelid reconstruction by the semicircle flap technique. Ophthalmology 1978; 85:1164–1169
81. Hughes, W. L. Reconstructive surgery of the eyelids, 2nd ed. St Louis: C. V. Mosby Co., 1954:122
82. Wesley, R. E., McCord, C. D. Transplantation of eyebank sclera in the Cutler-Beard method of upper eyelid reconstruction. Ophthalmology 1980; 87:1022–1028
83. Fox, S. A., Beard, C. Spontaneous lid repair. American Journal of Ophthalmology 1964; 58:947–952
84. Jones, L. T., Wobig, J. L. Surgery of the eyelids and lacrimal systems. Birmingham: Aesculapius 1976; 141–145
85. Kasper, K. A. Dacryocystorhinostomy. Survey of Ophthalmology 1961; 6:95–107
86. Dartzbach, R. K. Dacryocystorhinostomy. Ophthalmology 1978; 85:1267–1270
87. Jones, L. T. Conjunctivodacryocystorhinostomy. American Journal of Ophthalmology 1965; 59:773

3

Epibulbar tumors, pterygia, enucleation and evisceration

Lawrence W. Hirst MD

Epibulbar tumors

Introduction

The most common epibulbar mass found in clinical practice is the pterygium. However, other epibulbar tumors that occur less frequently are also important because they must be identified and treated definitively while still small and well circumscribed. Despite the plethora of pathological conditions that may give rise to epibulbar masses, the general treatment consists of complete removal with adequate margins, restoration of the ocular surface and pathological examination of the specimen.

Until recent times, anything larger than the smallest epibulbar tumor was viewed with great concern and might lead to heroic surgery or even loss of the eye. More recently, the limited malignant potential of most ocular surface tumors has been recognized and a more conservative localized excision technique has been used. The role of non-surgical therapy still remains to be established for most types of epibulbar masses, although cryotherapy, radiotherapy and even chemotherapy are sometimes useful for specific epibulbar tumors.

Principles of treatment

Investigative phase

A careful bilateral examination should be completed for a patient with an epibulbar mass. The epibulbar mass should be measured and photographed. Special examinations such as conjunctival scrapings, impression cytology, radionuclear scanning, fluorescein angiography, CT scanning and ultrasonography may be necessary to define further the limits of the tumor, its possible histological nature and the presence of other pathology. After examination and any appropriate tests, it may be decided to observe the tumor over a period of time with repeated measurements. However, early surgical removal may be warranted if there is sufficient evidence of impaired function – e.g. deteriorating vision, muscle involvement or loss of structure – or problems of mass size or possible malignancy.

Operative principles

Once the decision for removal of the mass has been made, the following principles should be kept in mind for the safe and adequate removal of the tumor: (*1*) adequate local anesthesia to control pain and limit eye movement if necessary; (*2*) adequate exposure, hemostasis and microscopic evaluation; (*3*) intraoperative assessment of depth, lateral extension and mobility of the lesion; (*4*) excision of the lesion with surgical margins of adequate peripheral extent and depth; (*5*) reconstruction of the eye wall; (*6*) histopathology of the removed tissue to determine whether the lesion has been completely excised and to establish the pathological diagnosis; and (*7*) careful postoperative follow-up to monitor ocular surface integrity, visual function and tumor recurrence.

Preoperative evaluation

History

Although 'epibulbar tumors' can refer to any tumors lying on the surface of the globe, the term is generally reserved for tumors that are visible on or through bulbar, forniceal or tarsal conjunctiva and do not lie hidden posteriorly in the orbital space. However, this arbitrary definition of epibulbar tumors also includes tumors that, like an iceberg, have a tip visible underneath the conjunctiva but whose mass lies more posteriorly in the orbit.

Because of the visibility of epibulbar tumors, patients are usually aware fairly early of their presence or of changes in existing epibulbar masses. Apart from those patients with bodily neglect or cancerophobia, the patient with an epibulbar tumor is likely to present with a small lesion that is usually treatable.

Although history-taking from the patient is important, it is often equally important to speak with close relatives or friends who may have observed any changes in the tumor. Sometimes the initial appearance of small masses that have escaped the patient's and friends' notice can be seen by the examination of social photographs of the patient in profile or full face.

Except for their visible presence, most epibulbar tumors are asymptomatic. Occasionally, symptoms such as decreased vision occur due to involvement of the optic nerve by intraorbital extension; spread on the corneal surface involving the visual axis; progressive irregular astigmatism from distortion of the corneoscleral tissues; or other ocular involvement.

Pain is an uncommon early symptom of epibulbar tumors and indicates the need for an exhaustive search for other causes or for periocular spread of tumor to involve adjacent sensory nerves or structures innervated by the ophthalmic division of the 5th cranial nerve. Because of the usual location of epibulbar tumors beneath a smooth, distensible epithelial surface, even quite large masses can occur without ocular surface pain. Various tumors, ranging from epithelial dysplasia to squamous cell carcinoma of the limbus, can cause a gritty foreign body sensation because of their irregular and occasionally keratinized surface.

Diplopia is also a rare presenting symptom of epibulbar tumors. It can occur as a result of ocular displacement by the tumor mass, localized extraocular muscle restriction and occasionally of oculomotor nerve involvement.

Rarely, epibulbar tumors may present with bleeding, recurrent swelling and recurrent inflammation in addition to any of the other symptoms, but the most common presenting complaint is an apparent increase in size or color of the mass.

The history-taking should include questions regarding signs and symptoms. A detailed personal medical and surgical history is also essential. In children, questions to the parents regarding ingestion or exposure to parasites, foreign body trauma and congenital anomalies are crucial. For the adult, information on the presence or absence of previous neoplastic disease or surgery for unexplained masses elsewhere must be obtained. Historical evidence of long-term inflammatory disease in the conjunctival sac, or of occupational or recreational exposure to high levels of sunlight, should be obtained.

Particular attention should be paid to family history of neoplastic disease and the outcome. This may help predict the psychological response of the patient to possible observation without treatment, or treatment by radical surgery, as the two ends of the spectrum of epibulbar tumor management.

Ocular and systemic examination

Sophisticated tests cannot substitute for a detailed external and biomicroscopic examination of the tumor. Routine ocular examination of both eyes is also essential to document visual function. Best corrected visual acuity is not only a medicolegal requirement to document pretreatment vision, but it is also necessary to help exclude intraocular or intraorbital involvement by the tumor mass. Any reduction in the corrected visual acuity must be explained and its relation to the tumor mass defined. If anterior global distortion is suspected of causing decreased visual acuity (e.g. pterygium), a diagnostic hard contact lens and over-retraction after keratometry observation of irregular mires may confirm the existence of irregular astigmatism and a normal posterior segment.

Intraocular pressure (IOP) measurement and comparison to that of the fellow eye may disclose possible aqueous-outflow obstruction by the tumor mass. With the involvement of the paralimbal area by an expanding epibulbar tumor, a gonioscopic examination of the anterior chamber angle must be performed to detect possible intraocular penetration (e.g. squamous cell carcinoma). The use of a Zeiss gonioscopic lens will often facilitate this examination if a prominent paralimbal mass prevents examination with larger gonioscopic lenses. Careful slit-lamp examination of the anterior chamber for inflammatory changes or hyphema is necessary to exclude not only intraocular spread of tumor with possible tumor seeding in the anterior chamber but also other intraocular tumors such as juvenile xanthogranulomas. Variations in iris and choroidal pigmentation may be present in ocular or oculodermal melanoses. An indirect and direct ophthalmoscopic examination of the fundus with a fully dilated pupil may reveal localized choroidal folding, exudative retinal detachments or scleral indentation by an extraocular tumor.

Extraocular motility is tested. If limitation of duction of the eye is noted, forced (passive) ductions may be performed.

Examination of the external tumor is best begun using a handlight; the entire conjunctival sac is explored, including eversion of the upper lid to look for signs of other lesions. The tumor is then examined at low and high magnification using slit-lamp biomicroscopy. Special attention is paid to measuring the size of the tumor in both the horizontal and vertical directions using the slit-height calibration system of the Haag–Streit slit-lamp or other technique, and an effort is made to estimate the height of the lesion. Using the slit it is frequently possible to determine the depth of the tumor with respect to the various coats of the eye. The irregular surface of a tumor lying above the conjunctival surface can be readily differentiated from a mass that is distending an overlying smooth conjunctival surface. Flat or elevated lesions may be located in any one of the tissue planes – including conjunctival, episcleral and scleral tissue planes. Encroachment on the limbus or the cornea by a tumor can be readily seen with the slit-lamp, and depth with respect to Bowman's membrane ascertained. The documentation of these features should not be left to photography alone. Careful color drawings should also be made, with measurements noted.

After these examination techniques, it is often useful to anesthetize the anterior ocular surface with a topical anesthetic and gently to apply tangential traction to the tumor mass with a cotton-tipped swab. Impregnation of the swab with cocaine solution can help avoid pain during this maneuver. Gentle traction on the tumor itself or on the layers over the tumor will help define the extent of the tumor within a specific plane and its fixation to or infiltration of overlying or underlying tissue levels. This is especially useful with subconjunctival lesions, in which a movement of the lesion over the sclera may improve confidence in excluding scleral infiltration. Similarly, obvious conjunctival lesions that move freely over the underlying layers generally indicate the absence of any tumor infiltration of the episcleral tissues. Fixation of paralimbal tumors at their limbal edge is not infrequent, and this does not add significantly to information on possible infiltration.

If an epibulbar tumor is found, unless it is obviously benign, the patient should have a detailed physical examination by an internist or an oncologist to exclude tumors elsewhere in the body or generalized infectious disease.

In patients with lesions suspected of being malignant, especially the melanotic and epithelial dysplastic conditions and possible localized lymphoma, an oncological work-up including physical examination, chest X-ray, renal, hepatic and splenic scans, bone surveys and measurement of serum alkaline phosphatase levels, may be indicated. The lymph nodes should be carefully examined for possible tumor spread.

Photographic documentation

External photography should be performed by the ophthalmologist or by a photographer while the ophthalmologist holds the lids and directs the patient's gaze to expose maximum tumor detail. If necessary, Desmarres eyelid retractors may be used to expose the mass. A one-to-one macrophotographic system with a lifelike color film will generally permit good documentation. If stereo photographic equipment is available, macrostereo pictures may aid in documenting height and size of the tumor. Tumors encroaching on the cornea are often also well documented using slit-lamp photography (the Zeiss or Nikon photo-slit-lamp gives the best available background and slit illumination). Similarly, anterior chamber angle involvement can be documented with sequential gonioscopic slit-lamp photographs. Currently the benefit of using anterior segment fluorescein angiography for epibulbar tumors remains speculative[1]. It may occasionally disclose an unexpected vascularity of a seemingly avascular tumor.

Diagnostic tests

The use of P^{32} radioisotope scanning for determining malignancy of lesions that are visible externally and also amenable to fairly simple biopsy is unnecessary.

Ultrasound examination is sometimes useful to exclude orbital extension of epibulbar tumors, e.g. eye-wall distortion by epibulbar tumors may be disclosed by ultrasound to consist of choroidal effusions or thickened sclera.

Conjunctival or corneal cultures are usually not indicated. If an episcleral abscess is suspected, a culture of the abscess fluid is more likely to be positive than that from a conjunctival swab.

Negative cytology results from the ocular surface do not exclude the presence of epithelial tumors. However, especially for the patient in whom there is a suspicion of multifocal epithelial tumors such as epithelial dysplasia or carcinoma *in situ* of the conjunctiva, widespread conjunctival scrapings from both the bulbar and superior and inferior tarsal conjunctiva placed on separate slides may disclose a multifocal tendency[2]. This information is crucial to the management of the condition. A blunt Kimura spatula can be gently scraped across the epithelial surface and the material placed gently on a precleaned glass slide. The slide is methanol-fixed, Giemsa-stained, and examined for abnormal cytology. Material for slides should be taken from each quadrant of the bulbar conjunctiva and from various parts of the superior and inferior tarsal plates, and the slides are marked accordingly.

Impression cytology[3] has been used during the last 10 years to locate areas of possible epithelial dysplasia. This is still a research method with restricted clinical use.

Various other methods may be required in specific cases, such as Hertel examination for possible orbital involvement, maneuvers to attenuate vascular fistulae and communicating cavernous hemangiomas, and neuroradiological studies.

Indications for surgery

Unknown diagnosis

The most frequent reason for surgery of epibulbar tumors is to establish or confirm a diagnosis.

The following facts make the excision of most epibulbar tumors relatively easy and safe: (*1*) the majority of epibulbar tumors are benign or locally spreading only; (*2*) surgical cleavage planes exist above and below the tumor mass; (*3*) except for occasional intrascleral and intraocular involvement, no visually important structures are generally involved; (*4*) the most frequent tissue lost during excision is conjunctiva, and it can usually be readily reapposed; (*5*) careful slit-lamp examination of the surgical area postoperatively makes early diagnosis of recurrence likely; (*6*) most surgery can be performed with either topical or retrobulbar anesthesia; (*7*) the limited size of these tumors usually permits total excision and this is especially important for tumors felt to be malignant. When there is a doubt about the diagnosis, excision by one of the surgical techniques to be described permits a definitive histological diagnosis and further treatment if required, or the patient can be reassured if a benign tumor is found.

Known or presumed diagnosis requiring surgical treatment

Where the clinical appearance or ancillary tests such as smears indicate that the lesion is likely to be malignant, surgery is usually indicated (in preference to other modes of treatment) because of the conditions mentioned above. Where local excision is difficult or impossible because of the extent or the multifocal nature of the tumor, 'debulking' surgery is frequently a prelude to other forms of treatment such as radiotherapy or chemotherapy. In these cases, slightly different surgical techniques are used, as described below. For extensive tumors in which local debulking excision appears impractical, and when retention of the eye is especially important (as in one-eyed patients), small biopsies may be taken from various parts of the tumor and adjacent tissue for histological confirmation of tumor type and extent prior to radiotherapy or chemotherapy.

Occasionally, tumor removal is indicated because of visual or irritative symptoms, despite the evident benign nature of the tumor (e.g. pterygium).

Cosmesis

Only very rarely is cosmesis the sole indication for removal of an epibulbar tumor. Because of the features described above, removal can frequently be accomplished while leaving minimal or no scarring and achieving an acceptable cosmetic appearance. Even in these cases, histological examination should always be performed.

Preparation for surgery

Informed consent

Because most of the patients are asymptomatic preoperatively, it is important to warn them of postoperative pain. Postoperatively discomfort occurs especially from an irregular ocular surface. This may take some weeks to heal completely, such as with bare-scleral closure. The possibility of periorbital hemorrhage should be discussed. Although major hemorrhage and extraocular infection are exceedingly rare, they should be included in any discussion of surgery.

Visual loss is unlikely with localized surface excisions except for rare occurrences such as: intraocular penetration at surgery; disruption of the normal ocular surface defenses and subsequent corneal opacification or perforation; or orbital infection.

It is most important to include in the formed consent a discussion of the possible outcomes of excisional therapy for a tumor of unknown type. With small localized tumors likely to be malignant, the patient must be informed of the possibility of recurrence of the tumor both locally and systemically. It should be made clear that other modes of therapy – including more extensive surgery, chemotherapy or radiotherapy – may be needed.

When the tumor is extensive and probably malignant, and with multifocal tumors when extensive damage to adjacent tissues is likely, a cautious prognosis should be given to the patient. As for all malignant tumor surgery, the patient should be informed that at surgery more extensive procedures may be required because of the operative findings.

Although occasionally enucleation or limited or total exenteration may ultimately be necessary, it is virtually never indicated as an extension of a previously planned local excision. There is usually opportunity for careful reappraisal of the situation after surgery and for routine sectioning and staining of the biopsy tissue (in contrast to frozen sections), and further discussion with the patients to allow time for full consideration of the alternatives before major, additional ocular surgery. However, the need for local excision that is more extensive than anticipated prior to surgery is an ever-present risk. The patient should be prepared to undergo restorative and reconstructive surgery to the eye and adnexa with eye-bank donor tissue or with conjunctiva from the opposite eye. In these cases requiring extensive surgery, the patient should be aware that vision may be altered by corneal visual-axis involvement, anterior segment curvature changes and ocular surface abnormalities (e.g. dellen, corneal vascularization).

Collaboration with ocular pathologist and microbiologist

As described below, frozen section examination of the tumor tissue at the time of surgery may occasionally be indicated. Usually, however, because of localized involvement and the likelihood of successful total excision, it is preferable to wait for stained sections to determine accurately the diagnosis and adequacy of excision. Consultation with the ocular pathologist before surgery will often aid in choosing the optimal method of preservation and orientation of the specimen. This includes the marking of the edges and surfaces of the tumor for proper localization to permit assessment of the surgical margins. The possibility that ultrastructural examination may be helpful affects the choice of fixation media.

If an infective cause of the tumor is suspected, consultation with the microbiological department may allow the choice of the best culture media and handling of the specimen.

Donor tissue

When it is possible that dissection of the tumor may involve the cornea or sclera, donor tissue should be available for reconstruction. It is preferable to obtain fresh material from a local eye bank, and to seek whole-eye material rather than corneoscleral buttons. If fresh material is unavailable, stored corneal and scleral tissue should be available as glycerine-preserved or frozen donor material.

Surgical instruments

Microsurgical instruments and the operating microscope are important for the precise removal of most epibulbar tumors. Although various specialized microsurgical instruments are available for this purpose and are sometimes advantageous, the surgical discussions below will deal only with some of the commonly available instruments.

The operating microscope is essential in the removal of epibulbar tumors. Distinguishing between normal and abnormal tissue is crucial in maintaining adequate surgical margins while conserving the ocular tissues. Microscopes with a zoom magnification system facilitate use of maximum magnification for defining tumor edges, and a lower magnification for the tying of sutures and conjunctival mobilization procedures.

If the epibulbar tumors are located solely on the surface of the globe, lid specula usually suffice for proper exposure. However, when the tarsal conjunctival or forniceal tissue is thought to be involved, lid sutures give better exposure.

Various cutting instruments can be used effectively. If the conjunctival or episcleral tissue is involved, with no scleral involvement, scissors are generally preferable. Sharp Wescott scissors are usually adequate for this portion of the excision, although excisions close to the limbus may require dissection and excision with smaller scissors such as Vannas scissors.

When limbal tissue or scleral tissue is involved, sharp dissection with other instruments is required. The delineation of the peripheral limits of the tumor is best performed using a super-sharp disposable blade, although a razor blade or oscillating knife can be suitable. In these cases of corneal, limbal or scleral involvement, dissection to remove the depth of tumor must be within the tissue involved – e.g. the cornea or sclera. Instruments preferred for this dissection are the Gill dissector or Paufique knife, although an oscillating knife, razor blade or super-sharp blade may be suitable.

Careful intraoperative hemostatis is crucial for adequate localization and removal of tumor with minimal surrounding tissue destruction. Bipolar cautery performed under irrigating fluid is the best method of maintaining hemostasis in these cases. Fine-tipped microsurgical bipolar forceps combined with drop-by-drop fluid irrigation permits controlled closure of individual bleeding vessels.

Anesthesia

Except for removal of localized, superficial lesions such as conjunctival polyps, the use of topical anesthesia or subconjunctival injection is not recommended. General anesthesia is usually not required, except for patients who are unusually anxious, very young, or who require more extensive surgery for larger lesions. Usually, facial nerve block anesthesia together with retrobulbar anesthesia is used for most cases because of the following advantages: (*1*) excellent surface anesthesia is achieved which is important because manipulation of the conjunctiva and corneal surface is very painful — subconjunctival lidocaine (lignocaine) in addition to retrobulbar anesthesia may be a useful adjunct when adequate surface anesthesia has not been obtained, or when separation of the conjunctival tissue plane from the episcleral or scleral plane is needed before tumor excision; (*2*) a steady operating field with minimal eye movements is maintained and this is essential for use of an operating microscope and microsurgical instruments; (*3*) masses not at the limbus or not readily exposed by lid retraction can be best brought into the operating field by rectus muscle fixation by a suture passed through the conjunctiva.

Surgical technique

We will mainly describe the resection or excision of tumors lying on the surface of the globe and not extending onto the lid or into the orbit, and those that are not of multifocal origin. The subject of pterygium removal will be dealt with separately.

Local excision of conjunctival lesions without reconstruction

To excise successfully small conjunctival or episcleral masses with minimal fixation to underlying tissue or to the limbus, it is necessary to have adequate exposure, good hemostasis and correct identification of tissue planes.

The lids are separated with a lid speculum, and further exposure is achieved with a transconjunctival rectus muscle fixation suture of 4/0 silk inserted under whichever rectus muscle is nearest to the epibulbar tumor. The suture ends are held on the surgical drape or around the locks on the speculum in order to position the epibulbar mass in the center and apex of the field of the operating microscope.

Masses that are clearly defined within the conjunctival layer alone are then elevated by injection of 2 per cent lidocaine (lignocaine) with 1:10 000 epinephrine (adrenaline) using a 25 gauge needle on a tuberculin syringe. The bevel of the needle is positioned downward while injecting, and the needle is advanced until the conjunctiva starts to balloon away from the other layers (*Figure 3.1a,b*). This usually results in elevation of both the conjunctiva and the mass, with good separation from the underlying episcleral tissue.

Although the above procedures are performed under low magnification, the magnification is increased to examine carefully the margins of the conjunctival lesion. At this higher magnification, small conjunctival incisions are made with a super-sharp blade to mark beyond the margins of the tumor, with a minimum of 2 mm of normal conjunctiva included on all sides (*Figure 3.1c*). The magnification is now lowered, and an incision is made into the subconjunctival space using sharp scissors. While holding the normal fringe of conjunctiva surrounding the tissue, the sharp scissors are used in a plane parallel to the surface of the globe to separate the conjunctiva from the underlying episcleral tissues (*Figure 3.1d*). The scissors are then used to follow the marked conjunctival edge and to complete the excision of the tumor and a 2 mm margin of normal conjunctival tissue.

The bipolar cautery is used to achieve hemostasis, with the surgeon elevating the conjunctival edges with a fine-toothed forceps and cauterizing bleeding vessels that are seen during constant irrigation by the assistant.

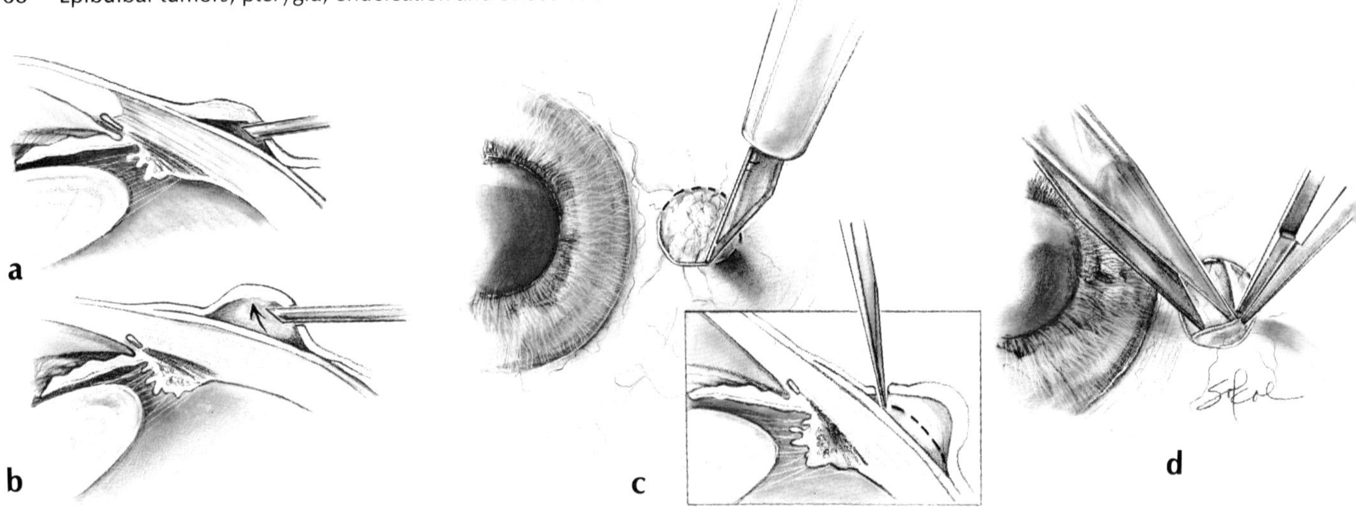

Figure 3.1 *Local excision of conjunctival lesion.* **(a)** *Subconjunctival injection of 2 per cent lidocaine (lignocaine) through a 25 gauge needle with bevel downward.* **(b)** *Elevation of conjunctiva over episclera with bleb of local anesthetic.* **(c)** *Demarcation of conjunctival lesion using super-sharp blade, and side view indicating penetration into subconjunctival bleb.* **(d)** *Dissection with sharp Wescott scissors at subconjunctival level to excise conjunctival lesion*

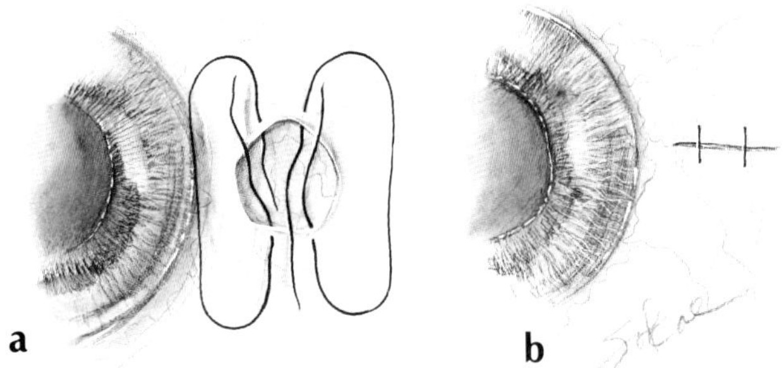

Figure 3.2 *Closures of conjunctival wound with buried sutures.* **(a)** *Technique for burying collagen suture.* **(b)** *Final appearance of sutured incision with knots buried*

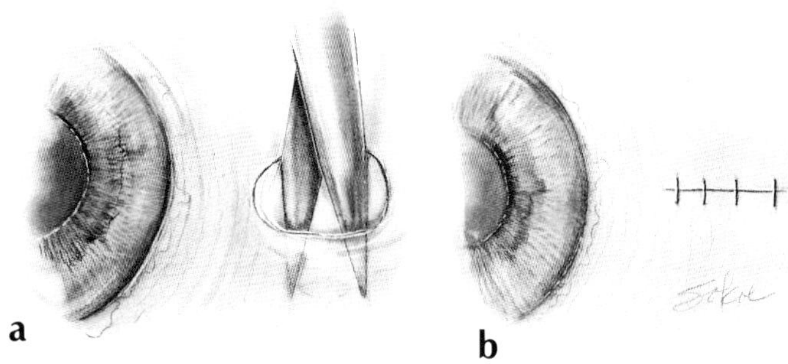

Figure 3.3 *Closure of conjunctival defect by undermining.* **(a)** *Scissors used to undermine the edges of conjunctival incision.* **(b)** *Final suture line*

Conjunctival defects smaller than 5 mm can simply be closed with two or three interrupted 7/0 collagen sutures. Burying the knot of the sutures can help relieve the immediate postoperative discomfort of a roughened ocular surface (*Figure 3.2a,b*). Alternatively, bipolar cautery forceps designed for conjunctival closure may be used in a single application to close this surface defect. Extensive conjunctival excision may require undermining of the free conjunctival edges before closure of the defect (*Figure 3.3a,b*). If a large defect abuts on the corneoscleral limbus, it is often best not to close the conjunctiva, to avoid the formation of elevated tissue at the limbus (which may promote dellen formation and corneal epithelial breakdown), but instead to allow slow epithelialization after closure leaving bare sclera. Alternatively, a conjunctival hood may be fashioned (*Figure 3.4a*), similar to that used for closure of a fornix-based conjunctival incision in cataract surgery. The free conjunctival edges are advanced across the limbus by two interrupted sutures at either end of the conjunctival incision (*Figure 3.4b*). Use of a mild overcorrection, so that the hood lies 1–2 mm over the limbus, will ensure that the early postoperative retraction will align the conjunctiva appropriately at the limbus (*Figure 3.4c*).

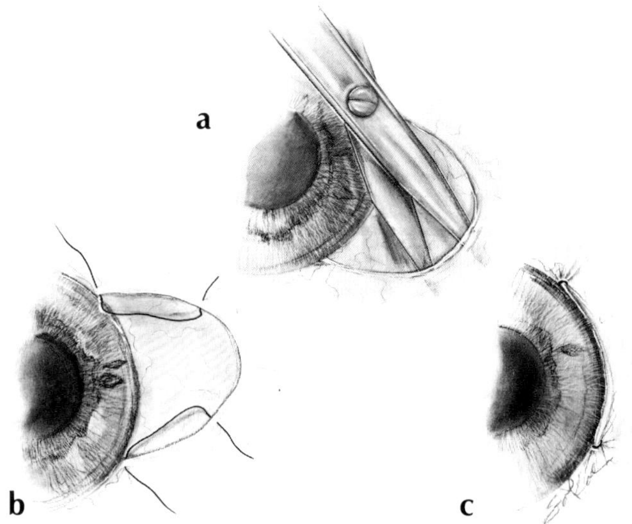

Figure 3.4 *Closure of a conjunctival wound at the limbus.* **(a)** *Undermining the edge of the conjunctival incision.* **(b)** *Use of two interrupted collagen sutures with extended bites to close the conjunctival defect.* **(c)** *Final result of conjunctival closure with the edge of incised conjunctiva at the limbus*

Local excision of episcleral lesions

Excision of episcleral masses that are not fixed to sclera is best performed with the same method as is used for local excision of conjunctival lesions. A 25 gauge needle is inserted beneath the episcleral tissue and local anesthetic is injected to raise the episclera and conjunctiva as one layer. Although it may be possible to spare the conjunctiva when removing small episcleral lesions, the simultaneous removal of conjunctiva overlying the mass is the simplest method.

If conjunctiva moves freely over larger episcleral lesions, it is better to spare the conjunctiva overlying the episcleral mass (*Figure 3.5a*). This is achieved by injection under Tenon's capsule of 1 per cent lidocaine (lignocaine) with epinephrine (adrenaline) (*Figure 3.5b*), as described previously, and use of trapdoor conjunctival incisions (*Figure 3.5c*) that allow adequate exposure of the underlying tumor. Under high magnification the tumor is delineated, with 2 mm of normal tissue on all sides, by incision with a super-sharp blade (*Figure 3.5d,e*). The edge is then elevated gently with fine-toothed forceps, and sharp scissors are used to excise the lesion (*Figure 3.5f*). The conjunctiva is closed with interrupted 7/0 collagen sutures (*Figure 3.5g*).

Local excision, with partial-thickness corneoscleral defects

If superficial tumor infiltration is present at the limbus or 1–2 mm into the peripheral corneal stroma (*Figure 3.6a*), a delineating mark is made that includes a clear 2 mm margin of conjunctiva and episclera but is only just inside the corneal edge of lesion. The mass is then excised, removing the superficial one-third of the involved cornea and sclera, together with overlying conjunctiva. The lesion is approached initially from the corneal side with a Gill dissector (*Figure 3.6b,c*); dissection is extended to the limbus and then the scleral portion is excised. The defect is covered by pulling a conjunctival hood over the sclera (*Figure 3.6d*) as described above (see *Figure 3.4a–c*).

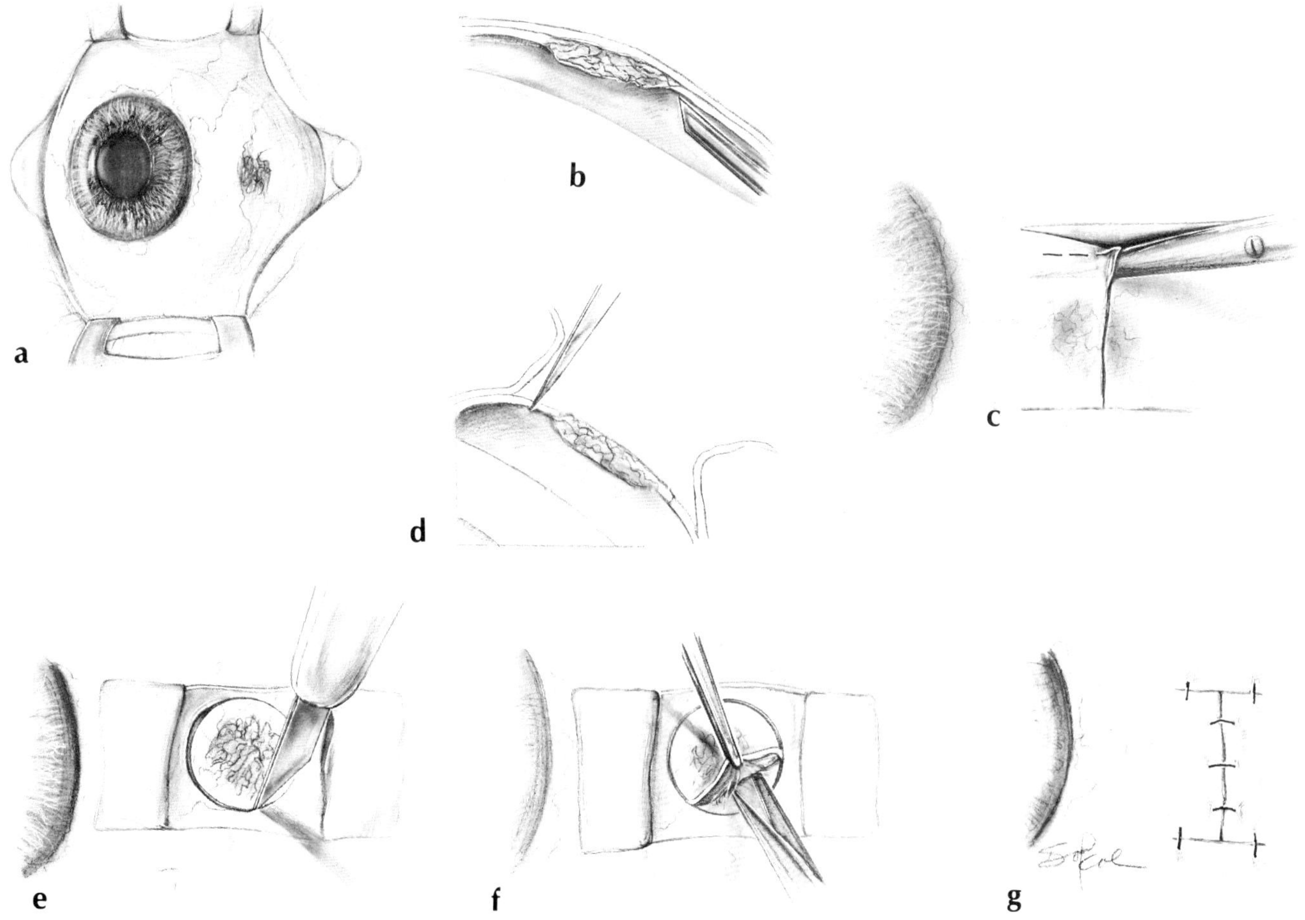

Figure 3.5 *Removal of an episcleral lesion sparing the overlying conjunctiva.* **(a)** *Episcleral lesion.* **(b)** *Elevation of episcleral lesion and conjunctiva by injection beneath Tenon's capsule of 2 per cent lidocaine (lignocaine) through a 25 gauge needle, with bevel downward.* **(c)** *'Trapdoor' incision of conjunctiva overlying episcleral lesion, with sharp scissors.* **(d,e)** *Outlining of episcleral lesion using super-sharp blade.* **(f)** *Dissection of episcleral lesion from sclera, using sharp scissors.* **(g)** *Closure of 'trapdoor' conjunctival incision using collagen sutures and buried knots*

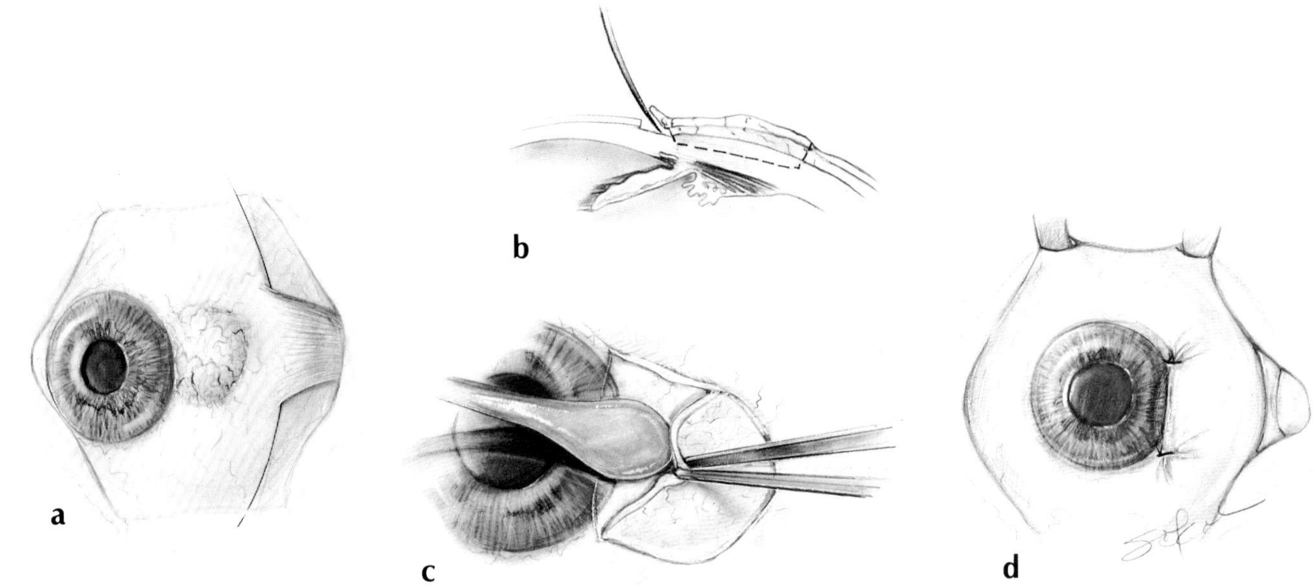

Figure 3.6 *Local excision of episcleral lesion involving the superficial sclera.* **(a)** *Combined episcleral and conjunctival lesion at limbus.* **(b,c)** *After delineating the corneal edge with super-sharp blade, Gill knife dissection is used to remove the episcleral lesion through a plane of superficial sclera.* **(d)** *Hood-like conjunctival closure using two interrupted collagen sutures*

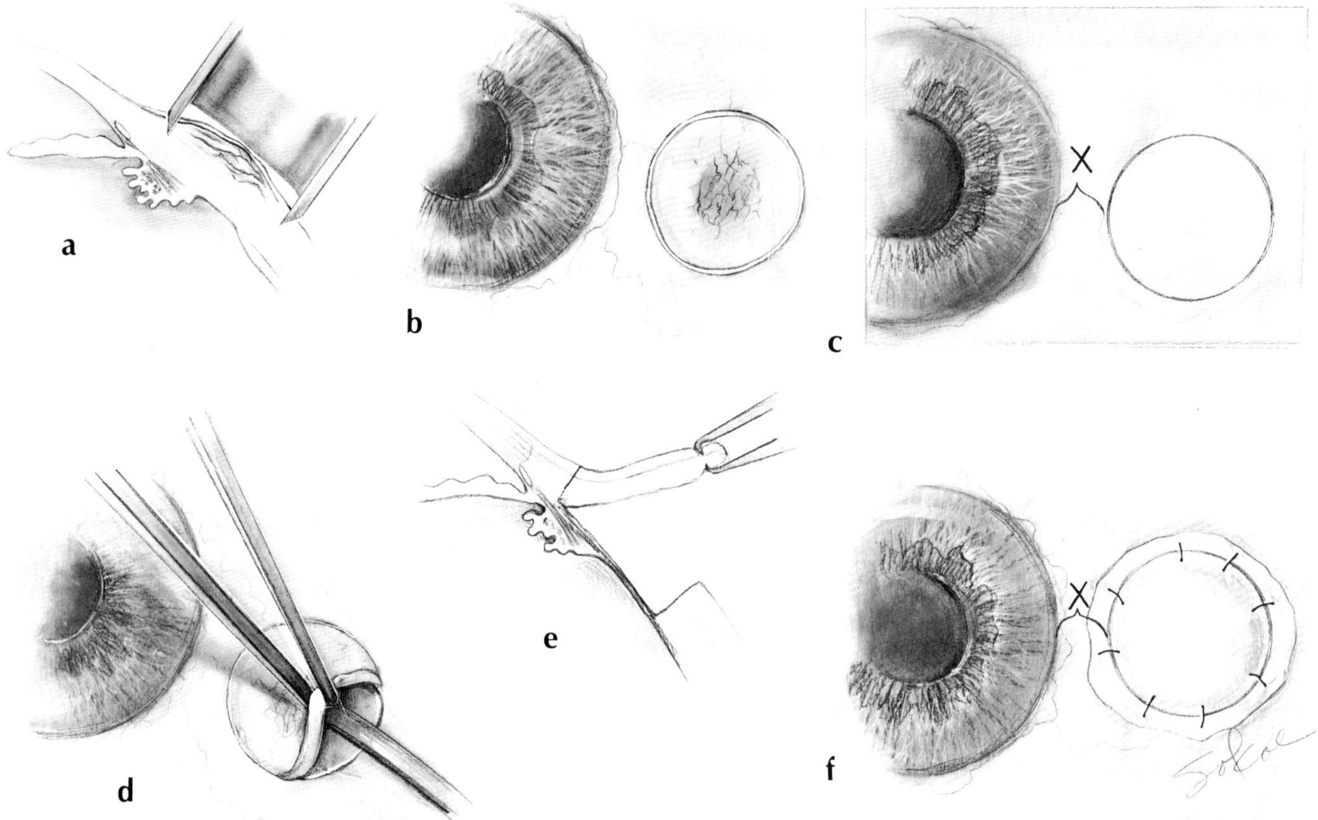

Figure 3.7 *Local excision of lesion involving the full-thickness of the sclera.* **(a)** *Trephine marks the planned margins of excision.* **(b)** *Trephine mark is well clear of scleral lesion.* **(c)** *Full-thickness trephination of sclera on whole donor eye at the same distance (x) from limbus as trephination mark in recipient.* **(d,e)** *Separating scleral lesion from the underlying uveal tissue using cyclodialysis spatula.* **(f)** *Suturing of full-thickness donor scleral patch into recipient bed, using interrupted 10/0 nylon sutures with knots buried*

Local excision with full-thickness scleral reconstruction

Fortunately, full-thickness lesions seldom occur. After removal of such lesions, reconstruction of the defect with donor material is required.

Before surgery, attempts are made to lower the intraocular pressure in order to minimize protrusion of choroid through the trephination site. This is done by use of a Honan intraocular pressure reducer and/or intravenous mannitol begun 30 minutes before anticipated entry into the suprachoroidal space.

In most of these cases the overlying conjunctiva is involved and is removed with the underlying lesion. The lesion is delineated using a corneal trephine that encompasses the tumor mass plus a 1–2 mm margin of normal-appearing tissue (*Figure 3.7a,b*), and the distance of the edge of this mark from the limbus is measured. A whole donor eye is fixated in a donor holder and placed under the microscope. After clearing away the episcleral tissue, a similar distance from the limbus is measured on the donor eye using calipers (*Figure 3.7c*), and a full-thickness trephination is performed through the scleral wall until choroid or vitreous is encountered. The dissection is then completed using corneoscleral scissors, and the inner surface of the donor button is meticulously cleaned of any adherent choroid or vitreous. The donor tissue is kept in normal saline, with the deep surface of the scleral button uppermost for orientation. With the trephine set for a depth of approximately 0.8–1.0 mm, gentle trephination is performed perpendicular to the lesion while maintaining firm fixation on the nearest extraocular muscle. Penetration of the sclera should not be attempted at this stage. After removal of the trephine, the tissue edge is elevated using fine-toothed forceps, and further inward dissection is performed using a super-sharp blade until the choroid is visible. The super-sharp blade is then used to extend the full circumference of the trephination incision to the suprachoroidal space. The choroid can then be teased from the undersurface of the sclera using a cyclodialysis spatula (*Figure 3.7d*). Hemostasis in the suprachoroidal space or sclera is maintained with wet-field cautery. The scleral donor button is now transferred with the uppermost surface (the choroidal surface) placed against the recipient choroid (*Figure 3.7e*). Interrupted 10/0 nylon sutures are used to close the donor-host interface, with the knots cinched into the recipient scleral tissue (*Figure 3.7f*). At the conclusion of the suturing the globe should be firm and no intraocular tissue should protrude through the interface. Conjunctiva is then closed over the scleral graft.

Local excision with full-thickness corneoscleral reconstruction

When a deep or full-thickness mass to be excised involves both scleral and corneal tissue at the limbus (*Figure 3.8a*), a modification of the above method is needed. A large Flieringa ring sutured to the episcleral tissue in an eccentric position is often helpful in preventing the opened globe from collapsing. The mass is excised, beginning the incision with two trephine blades of different diameters to encompass the smaller corneal portions (x) and the larger scleral portion (y) of the mass (*Figure 3.8b–d*). A Ziegler puncture is performed through the limbus opposite the lesion. The trephines are then transferred to the whole donor eye and are used to incise the sclera and cornea partially at the same distance from the limbus, as measured by the demarcation marks on the recipient eye. By angling the trephine, which permits half-thickness incision of the sclera, care is taken not to incise into the limbus or cornea with the scleral penetration. The appropriate trephine for the corneal section of the incision is also angled, permitting a superficial incision of the cornea in a fashion similar to that in the recipient eye as seen in *Figure 3.8b*. The scleral incision is deepened into the suprachoroidal space using a super-sharp blade as for the recipient eye in *Figure 3.8e* and the incision is extended up to the limbus. A cyclodialysis spatula is used to separate the sclera from the underlying choroid and ciliary body, and the spatula is then advanced to enter the anterior chamber and separate the corneoscleral donor tissue from the scleral spur as for the recipient eye in *Figure 3.8f*. Hyaluronic acid injected through a Ziegler puncture helps maintain the anterior chamber. The limbal edges of the scleral incision are made with a super-sharp blade, to the beginning of the corneal mark as for the recipient eye in *Figure 3.8h*. Corneal scissors are then used to excise the corneal portion of the corneoscleral donor button as for the recipient eye in *Figure 3.8i*. An attempt is made to maintain the anterior chamber, so that there is minimal damage to the donor endothelium of the corneoscleral button. The donor tissue is then placed in M–K medium with the deep surface uppermost until use. On the recipient eye the two trephination marks are now deepened, using a super-sharp blade. Entry into the suprachoroidal space is made first at the posterior edge of the scleral incision, and the scleral incision is gently extended to the limbus (*Figure 3.8e*). The sclera is gently elevated and separated from the underlying choroid, ciliary body and scleral spur using a cyclodialysis spatula (*Figure 3.8f*). The spatula is then swept into the anterior chamber beyond the limbal margins of the corneal wound for 1–2 mm superior and inferior to the limbal extent of the incisions. At this stage, the anterior chamber will frequently become shallow. Injection of sodium hyaluronate through the Ziegler puncture keeps the anterior chamber partially formed until incision of the cornea is performed (*Figure 3.8g*). A super-sharp blade is used to join the scleral and corneal incisions along the limbus (*Figure 3.8h*). Corneoscleral scissors are then used to incise the remaining thickness of the corneal button (*Figure 3.8i*). After removal of the corneoscleral mass, cautery is applied to bleeding points on the choroid, ciliary body or iris. A peripheral iridectomy is performed, and sodium hyaluronate is again used to maintain the anterior chamber partially. The corneoscleral donor button is transferred to the recipient, and two 10/0 nylon interrupted sutures are placed at the limbal part of the wound. Interrupted 10/0 nylon sutures are placed through the corneal portion of the wound (*Figure 3.8j*), and the anterior chamber is reformed with air. The scleral portion of the wound is then similarly sutured, the air is replaced with balanced salt solution and the wound tested for its integrity. The knots are buried into the corneal and scleral recipient tissue. A conjunctival hood is brought forward over the limbus (*Figure 3.8k*). Subconjunctival steroids are administered. Postoperatively, intensive therapy with topical steroids and cycloplegic drops is required. The donor cornea usually becomes opacified and vascularized.

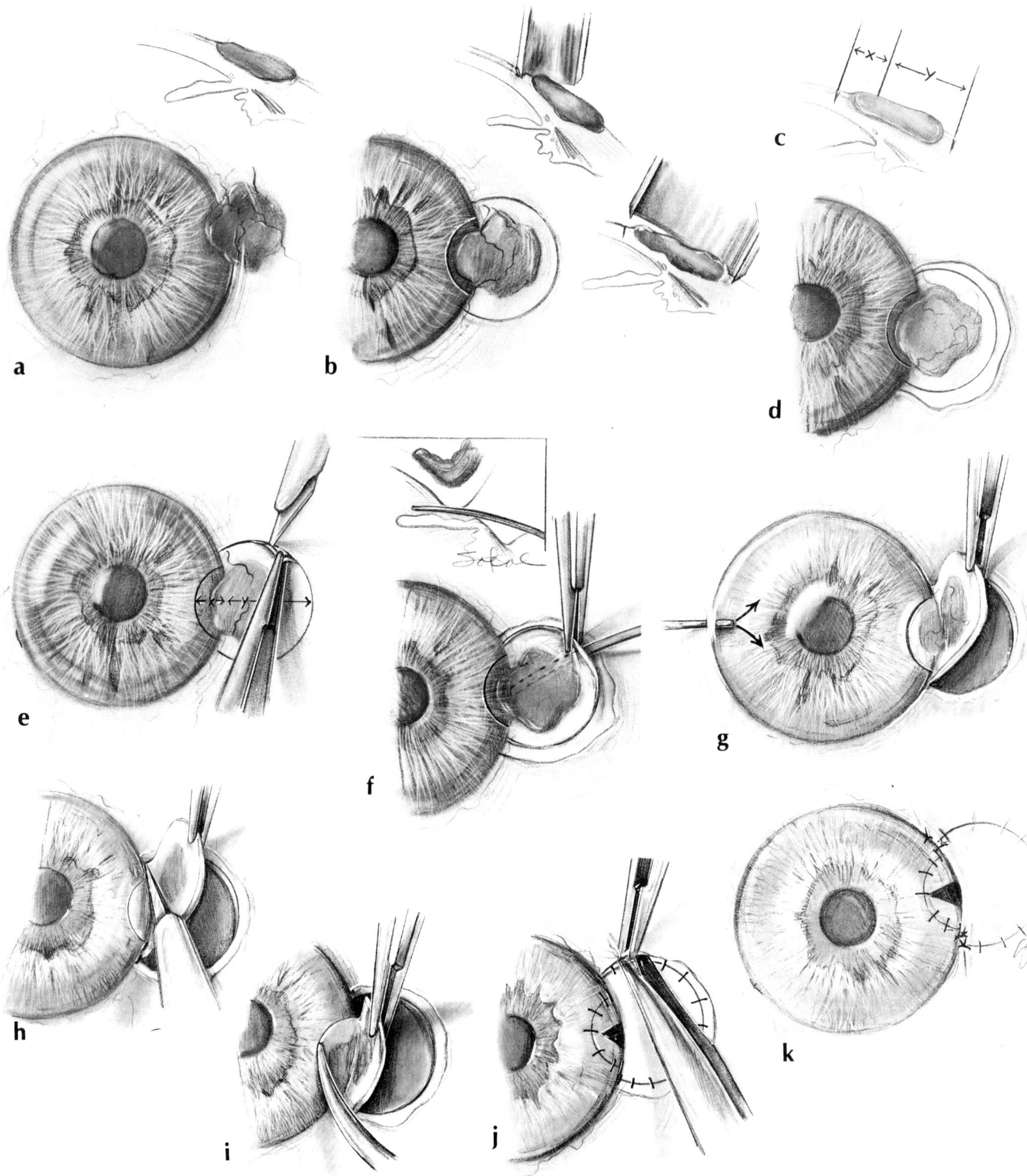

Figure 3.8 *Local full-thickness excision of lesion involving cornea and sclera.* **(a)** *Corneoscleral lesion involving 2 clock-hours of limbus.* **(b)** *The use of two trephines of different sizes to encompass, with adequate margins, the corneal and scleral extent of lesion, angulating the trephines to avoid cutting the lesion.* **(c)** *Corneal extent (x) and scleral extent (y) of lesion to be removed.* **(d)** *Trephination marks delineating the lesion.* **(e)** *Use of a super-sharp blade to deepen trephination marks to suprachoroidal space.* **(f)** *Use of cyclodialysis spatula in the anterior chamber to sweep corneal and scleral tissue from scleral spur.* **(g)** *Injection of hyaluronic acid through Ziegler puncture to maintain partial anterior chamber formation.* **(h)** *Use of super-sharp blade at limbus to join scleral and corneal incisions.* **(i)** *Use of curved corneal scissors to excise corneal extent of lesion.* **(j)** *Similarly shaped corneoscleral patch graft from a whole donor eye has been sutured into place (after peripheral iridectomy) with 10/0 nylon interrupted sutures with knots buried. Conjunctiva is being undermined using scissors.* **(k)** *Conjunctiva is then drawn up in a hood fashion over the scleral portion of the graft with two interrupted collagen sutures*

Surgery for extensive tumor or tumors with eyelid or orbital extension

If radiotherapy and chemotherapy are not to be used in these cases, usually the surgery consists of enucleation, limited exenteration while maintaining lids, or full exenteration including excision of lids. This surgical approach is discussed in Chapter 12.

Pterygium

Pterygia are the most common epibulbar tumors requiring treatment in ophthalmological practice[4,5]. This is especially so in certain geographical areas with a hot, dry environment, where the effect of ultraviolet irradiation and other possible environmental factors are thought to stimulate the growth of pterygia[4,5]. Prevalence rates of pterygia range as high as 1–5 per cent in communities with high-risk environments. Except for use of tinted eyeglasses in these locales, there is no known prophylaxis against this common epibulbar mass.

Indications for removal

The main reasons for removal of a pterygium are: (*1*) impending extension into the visual axis; (*2*) recurrent irritation and vascular injection of the pterygium; (*3*) irregular uncorrectable astigmatism; and (*4*) cosmesis. The two most common reasons for removal are concern that the pterygium will extend to involve the visual axis and recurrent irritation and injection.

Because the growth rate of a pterygium is variable and unpredictable, and because there are few cases[4] that ever involve the visual axis, continuing observation of a pterygium is warranted if it does not cause discomfort and if a safe margin of 3 mm from the visual axis is maintained.

If the decision is made to remove a pterygium, it is currently believed that surgery, with or without postoperative radiation[4,6,7], is the therapy most likely to prevent recurrence. Other methods of treatment have been used in the past, including chemical treatment and radiation treatment alone, but these do not seem as effective. There is still controversy over whether postoperative radiation therapy is beneficial in preventing recurrences. Scattered reports suggest that it is effective, although complications presumably attributable to the radiotherapy have been reported[8,9].

Pterygia are frequently removed under topical anesthesia in the outpatient department without using microsurgery or formal asepsis and the complication rates of this approach seem to be low. However, it does not take much more time to proceed in an operating room using an operating microscope and sterile technique, and this seems suitable to the practice of modern ophthalmology.

Surgical removal of primary pterygium

Surgical removal of a primary pterygium is performed as an outpatient procedure in the ophthalmology operating room with aseptic technique. An operating microscope and microsurgical techniques similar to those described above for epibulbar lesions are used. To obtain maximal exposure and to prevent eye movement, a retrobulbar and facial anesthetic block are given, and a temporal limbal fixation suture with 7/0 silk is placed (*Figure 3.9a,b*). A super-sharp blade is used to superficially incise the cornea just in advance of the pterygium head (*Figure 3.9c*). Because of the necessity for a superficial incision only down to Bowman's membrane, it is advisable to keep the cornea dry with a cellulose sponge so that various light reflections will not interfere with visualization and cause an unduly deep incision. The incision is continued around the entire head of the pterygium to the limbus. If the incision is made just in advance of the pterygium head and only to the limbus bleeding should be minimal. If bleeding occurs, hemostasis is achieved with a Wet-Field cautery before continuing the dissection. After the delineating incision has been performed, the head of the pterygium can be readily dissected from the cornea at a level no deeper than Bowman's membrane by use of the super-sharp blade (*Figure 3.9d*). Between the distal 1–2 mm of the advancing pterygium head and the limbus, there is frequently an area of almost normal cornea in which there is no adhesion between the cornea and overlying pterygium and where minimal or no dissection is needed. After the dissection has been taken back to this midzone, traction alone frequently frees the pterygium from portions of the corneal surface (*Figure 3.9e*). A short 2 mm peritomy is then performed above and below the pterygium using sharp scissors, and from the margins of these two peritomies the pterygium is undermined at the level of the bare sclera using sharp scissors (*Figure 3.9f*). The pterygium is then excised with a circular conjunctival excision close to the origin of the medial rectus muscle (*Figure 3.9g*). Minimal cautery is applied to the bare scleral base of the pterygium. If radiotherapy is to be applied with a strontium applicator at the time of surgery, cautery will frequently not need to be applied at all to the sclera as the pressure of the strontium applicator alone will maintain hemostasis. Avoidance of scleral cautery may minimize the risk of scleral thinning as a late complication[9]. At the end of the procedure the sclera should be bare for an area at least as large as the pterygium, extending almost back to the medial rectus muscle. It is usually unnecessary to suture down the edges of conjunctiva to the sclera, although if unusual mobility of the conjunctiva is present and might cause dellen formation at the limbal edges of the pterygium excision, superficial 7/0 collagen sutures may be used to tack down the conjunctiva to the sclera (*Figure 3.9h*).

If radiotherapy is to be used, it is done at this time in the operating room. The probe and applicator are first cleansed with alcohol. The area of excision is measured

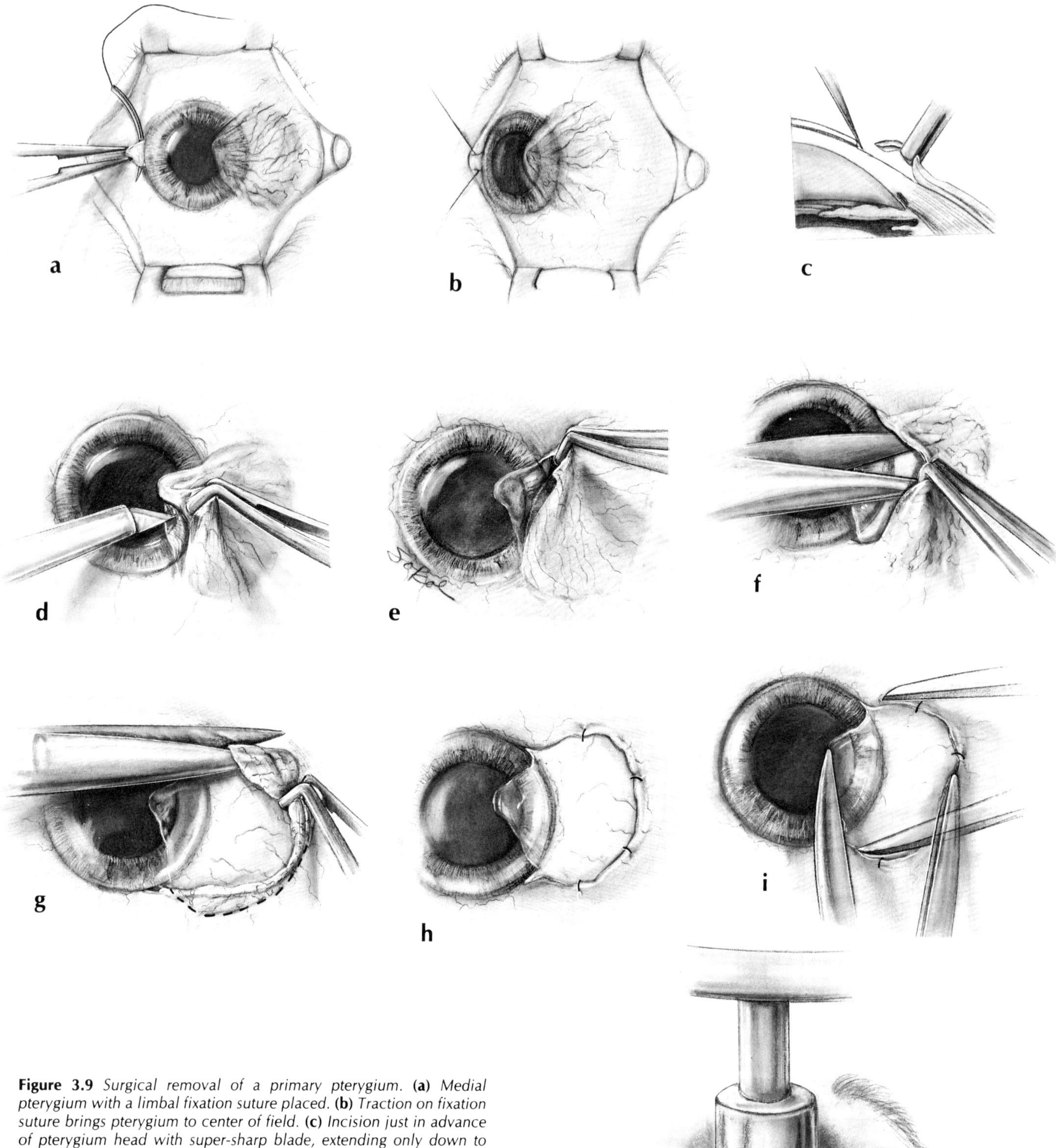

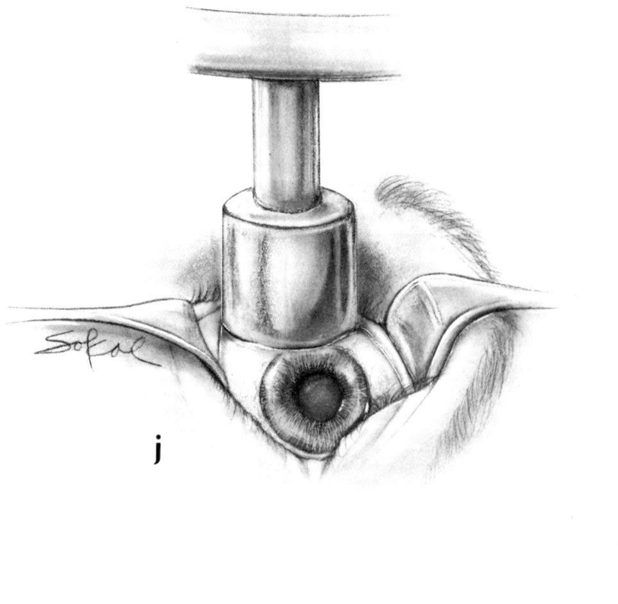

Figure 3.9 *Surgical removal of a primary pterygium.* **(a)** *Medial pterygium with a limbal fixation suture placed.* **(b)** *Traction on fixation suture brings pterygium to center of field.* **(c)** *Incision just in advance of pterygium head with super-sharp blade, extending only down to Bowman's membrane.* **(d)** *Sharp dissection of head of pterygium from the cornea, with traction applied with forceps.* **(e)** *Traction alone may frequently free rest of pterygium from corneal surface.* **(f)** *Undermining of pterygium in the scleral plane.* **(g)** *Excision of pterygium using scissors, with a minimal conjunctival margin.* **(h)** *Suturing conjunctival edge to sclera with interrupted collagen sutures.* **(i)** *Measurement of the area from which the pterygium has been excised to allow selection of the proper size of strontium applicator.* **(j)** *Placement of strontium applicator*

(*Figure 3.9i*) and the base plate of the strontium[90] applicator is selected to cover the extent of the defect. The applicator is applied so that it covers most of the area of pterygium removal from both the cornea and sclera (*Figure 3.9j*). A single dose of between 2000 and 3000 rad can be applied. However, three divided doses, one given immediately postoperatively and two at weekly intervals thereafter (of about 900 rad each) is a preferable method. Antibiotic ointment and a short-acting cycloplegic drop are applied, and the eye is patched for 24 hours. Thereafter, antibiotic eye drops are used and the patient is followed-up at 4 days to confirm that the corneal epithelium has covered the defect.

Surgical removal of recurrent pterygium

The removal of a recurrent pterygium is performed in the same manner as described above, although the actual dissection of the pterygium from the cornea and underlying sclera may be more difficult. The main points again are hemostasis and a careful dissection plane so that no scleral tissue is lost. The use of repeat strontium[90] treatment is dangerous. If the primary pterygium removal, however, was not accompanied by a postoperative strontium[90] application, it can be used after the recurrent pterygium surgery.

Other methods of removal of primary or recurrent pterygium have been used – including avulsion of the pterygium head, transplantation of the head back into the conjunctiva, grafts of skin and conjunctiva, and routine lamellar keratoplasty, but there is no evidence to suggest their superiority over the above method[10,11]. The only other form of surgery that seems to be beneficial in the treatment of recurrent pterygium is a partial lamellar reconstruction of the corneoscleral site of excision. This is performed in the same manner as described above for removal of lesions infiltrating cornea and sclera in which a partial-thickness dissection is performed. The use of free superior bulbar conjunctival grafts has been advocated.

Postoperative management

The postoperative management in cases of epibulbar tumors other than pterygia (*see above*) depends on the type of lesion treated, the extent of surgery required and the presence or absence of operative or postoperative complications.

Patients who have had removal of a simple conjunctival or episcleral mass without reconstruction may be treated as outpatients and released on the same day. Pain is usually not a major problem, and the use of oral analgesics will often suffice to maintain comfort. Conjunctival mobilization and burying of sutures is helpful in maintaining a smooth ocular surface. The only routinely used medication is an antibiotic eye ointment, which usually can be discontinued after 3–4 days.

Those patients in whom a lamellar dissection has been performed with donor tissue transplantation or in whom major conjunctival mobilization has been used should be hospitalized for 2–3 days after the surgery so that adequate analgesia can be given and the eye can be observed more frequently. In these cases, topical steroid and cycloplegic drops are often administered, both to reduce the inflammatory response and to relieve pain. A firm patch also helps to keep these patients comfortable.

For patients who have had penetration of the globe and full-thickness reconstruction, observation must be more frequent and for a longer period, and these patients are often hospitalized for about 5 days, depending on their postoperative course. They are treated in a manner similar to a corneal transplant patient with topical cycloplegics, steroids and antibiotics. They should wear a metal shield or glasses at all times to protect the eye. Their postoperative follow-up is similar to that for corneal transplant patients.

For all patients in whom the histological study reveals a malignant or premalignant tumor, careful follow-up is required to watch for evidence of recurrence. If total tumor excision is evident on histological examination at all edges of the specimen, the early follow-up may depend on the surgical technique used, and the later follow-up to detect tumor recurrence may be at intervals of about 3–6 months for the first 2 years and annually thereafter. When surgical excision was made through planes of tumor itself, the intervals between follow-up should be shorter. For all of these patients, after a satisfactory postoperative surgical result has been achieved with a quiet eye, a standard external photograph and slit-lamp photograph should be taken. This may assist in differentiating a tumor recurrence from a surgical scar.

Operative complications

Inadvertent ocular penetration

Inadvertent penetration of the cornea should be closed like a corneal laceration, using interrupted 10/0 nylon sutures with the knots buried and re-forming the anterior chamber. An inadvertent scleral penetration should be closed with 9/0 nylon or 7/0 polyglactin (Vicryl) sutures. The pupil should be well dilated and careful examination made of the underlying pars plana or retina. Any evidence of retinal damage should be treated with prophylactic cryotherapy, with or without a local scleral exoplant. Ciliary body or choroidal bleeding should be treated with Wet-Field cautery before closure of the wound. Postoperative management is similar to that for intraocular surgery. If a posterior penetration has occurred, the retina should be carefully examined postoperatively.

Surgical incision through known tumor

Operative incision of the tumor sometimes occurs. If this is recognized intraoperatively, and local excision appears feasible, the incision should be enlarged and the remaining tumor excised. The orientation of the two excised specimens submitted for pathological examination should be carefully noted so that the total extent of excision with normal boundaries can be determined at sectioning.

Postoperative complications

Incomplete excision of tumor identified postoperatively

The management of this complication depends mainly on the histological type of the tumor. Usually, further excision of residual tumor is not indicated in the immediate postoperative period. In some cases, depending on the histopathology, radiotherapy is applied; but careful observation is the usual treatment. Malignant tumors, such as melanomas and epitheliomas, may require further surgical removal after the immediate postoperative reaction is over.

Conjunctival flap retraction

This complication is common but it rarely requires treatment because bare sclera is usually soon covered by conjunctival epithelium.

Graft slippage

When this occurs in a lamellar transplant, it can be followed carefully without further surgery (unless dellen formation occurs, as discussed below). Slippage of a penetrating graft of either sclera or cornea is considered an ocular emergency, and the patient should be returned to the operating room for repair of the defect. This is usually done with general anesthesia, because a retrobulbar anesthetic injection cannot safely be given with an open wound.

Dellen formation

This is a common problem after removal of tumors that are close to or across the limbus. Bunching up of conjunctiva during conjunctival reconstruction, or an overlying scleral graft, may not permit adequate wetting of the peripheral cornea and this can result in dellen formation. Because such dellen usually resolve spontaneously, during the gradual reduction of tissue swelling postoperatively, treatment with topical ointments and patching is usually sufficient. If this is unsatisfactory, a soft contact lens can be fitted, but surgical removal of excessive limbal tissue is rarely required.

Poor epithelialization or loose adhesion of corneal epithelium

A firm pressure patch with an ocular lubricant applied for a period of 48 hours generally allows healing of most corneal epithelial defects. If an epithelial defect persists, one should look for causes such as a loose conjunctival suture, an early corneal infection or drug toxicity. The presence of other conditions such as diabetes, familial recurrent corneal erosions and persistent eye rubbing can also delay healing. If healing is progressing but the corneal epithelial defect is still present at 48 hours, patching is recommenced for a further 48 hours. Any defect persisting longer than a week after adequate patching requires an alternative form of therapy, such as a therapeutic soft contact lens for extended wear and the use of topical antibiotics and cycloplegia.

If satisfactory corneal epithelialization is initially obtained but later epithelial breakdown occurs, this is treated in a similar fashion. The use of prophylactic 5 per cent sodium chloride ointment after initial epithelialization seems to prevent recurrent corneal epithelial defects in those patients who are prone to corneal epithelial breakdown.

Corneal and scleral infections

Fortunately, corneal and scleral infections are rare after use of aseptic surgical technique. If they occur, appropriate scrapings and cultures are taken, and antibiotics are begun. Whether these are administered as topical, subconjunctival or systemic antibiotics depends on the severity of the infection.

Staphyloma formation

Scleral staphyloma formation is most commonly seen in epibulbar tumor cases after deep scleral dissection performed without tissue grafting or proper reconstruction, after scleral infection or after local radiation therapy. Perforation of scleral staphylomas is uncommon, but impending perforations should be treated with scleral patch grafts or reinforcement as described earlier in the Surgical techniques section.

Tumor recurrence

The treatment of tumor recurrence depends on the histology of the original tumor, the extent of the tumor recurrence, and the presence or absence of local or systemic spread. Although detailed discussion of therapy for recurrence cannot be undertaken here, it involves careful consultation and coordination of medical treatment between the oncologist and the ophthalmologist. Frequently, further local excision of recurrence together with systemic chemotherapy or irradiation is recommended.

Other modalities of treatment

A brief review of various alternative methods of therapy is available[12]. Two of these are mentioned below.

Radiotherapy

Most sources agree that there is only a limited role for radiotherapy as a primary treatment for most of the epibulbar tumors[13,14]. However, for extensive multifocal epithelial lesions of the conjunctiva, and in treating epibulbar tumor recurrences and the occasional epibulbar metastasis, radiotherapy may be used.

Chemotherapy

Apart from a few isolated reports, chemotherapy has not recently been used in the treatment of any epibulbar tumors. Various reports have appeared on the use of thiotepa and urea[15] in the treatment of such diverse conditions as pterygia and melanosis of the conjunctiva, but there is little evidence that these treatments are justified.

Enucleation

Introduction

Enucleation is one of the oldest procedures known in ophthalmic surgery and was initially reserved for painful eyes. It was performed as a rapid mutilating surgery because of lack of anesthesia, but it is now a controlled cosmetic surgery performed under general anesthesia. With the recognition of intraocular tumors earlier and the increased incidence of badly injured eyes, the indications for enucleation have become wider.

The ophthalmic treatment of the patient requiring enucleation does not end with the immediate postoperative phase but must also include careful fitting of a prosthetic eye, psychological support, and careful follow-up of the remaining eye. Despite the ophthalmologist's inherent dislike of enucleation, this procedure need not indicate any failure of ophthalmic care. In many cases it is a necessary and carefully planned treatment for specific conditions.

Indications

The most common indication for enucleation is an unsightly or painful blind eye. On occasion, the early enucleation of an eye which has been badly traumatized may be indicated to avoid sympathetic ophthalmia in the fellow eye. The next most common reason for enucleation is to treat intraocular tumors, such as retinoblastoma or malignant melanoma of the choroid.

Preoperative evaluation

Because the need to remove a blind badly traumatized eye may erroneously represent for the patient an unexpected failure of previous surgical attempts to save the eye, great care must be taken in explaining not only to patients but also to their relatives the limitations of medical and surgical treatment of severely traumatized eyes. The hazard of sympathetic ophthalmia is explained as the main reason favoring enucleation.

In patients with severe pain and a blind eye, such as with absolute glaucoma, the situation is usually reversed and the patient requests enucleation for relief of pain, and frequently for cosmesis. In these cases, the elective decision by the patient to undergo enucleation usually prevents major psychological problems after surgery. An emotional adjustment is still required, however, and some of these patients may also suffer 'phantom' pain for some time after surgery. Another group of patients is those in whom vision may still be present and may be normal, but in whom an intraocular tumor requires enucleation. Such patients need considerable psychological preparation for the removal of a seeing eye. Eventually, the patient's fear of harboring a growing cancer usually permits acceptance of enucleation.

Nevertheless, enucleation of either a seeing or a nonseeing eye is to most patients a devastating form of surgery that has them worried, frightened, depressed and full of misconceptions. It is critical that care be taken to explain not only the irreversible nature of the surgery, but also the expected postoperative results, together with the mechanics of an implant, the prosthetic eye and its care. The patient must be assured that a full and normal life can be led by someone who has only one good eye. Misconceptions about what a monocular person is capable of doing are widespread, and time and care should be taken in discussing any fears or questions the patient or relatives may have. Especially apprehensive are the parents of children with retinoblastoma, in whom not only one eye may be enucleated but in whom the other eye may suffer severe visual loss or may also require enucleation. Here psychological support is needed from not only the ophthalmologist but also the patient's pediatrician to maintain perspective on the disease process and the resultant quality of life.

For many, the fear of having an empty socket for 2–3 weeks after surgery is in itself a major problem. These patients should be assured that, with either a conformer or a patch, an adequate cosmetic appearance can be obtained until the prosthetic shell is fitted.

Preoperative evaluation should include a general physical examination and routine blood work, and also a chest X-ray and electrocardiogram in older patients, because these patients almost always require general anesthesia for the procedure. Although a local anesthetic block may rarely be used, adequate analgesia by this method alone is usually not achieved. If the circumstances demand local anesthesia, serious consideration should be given to performing evisceration instead of enucleation.

The patient must be questioned with regard to any bleeding diathesis, and any patient with possible sickle cell disease should be tested. If possible, aspirin use should be stopped at least 2 weeks prior to surgery to minimize bleeding.

Very careful examination of the opposite eye should be performed to detect any pathology and also for the feeling of security the patient derives from this, especially if the opposite eye is found to be entirely normal. In the patient who is to have enucleation of an eye that externally appears quite normal (e.g. in choroidal melanoma) an indelible pencil should be used on the day prior to surgery to mark the forehead lightly on that side. This reassures the patient that the wrong eye will not be enucleated.

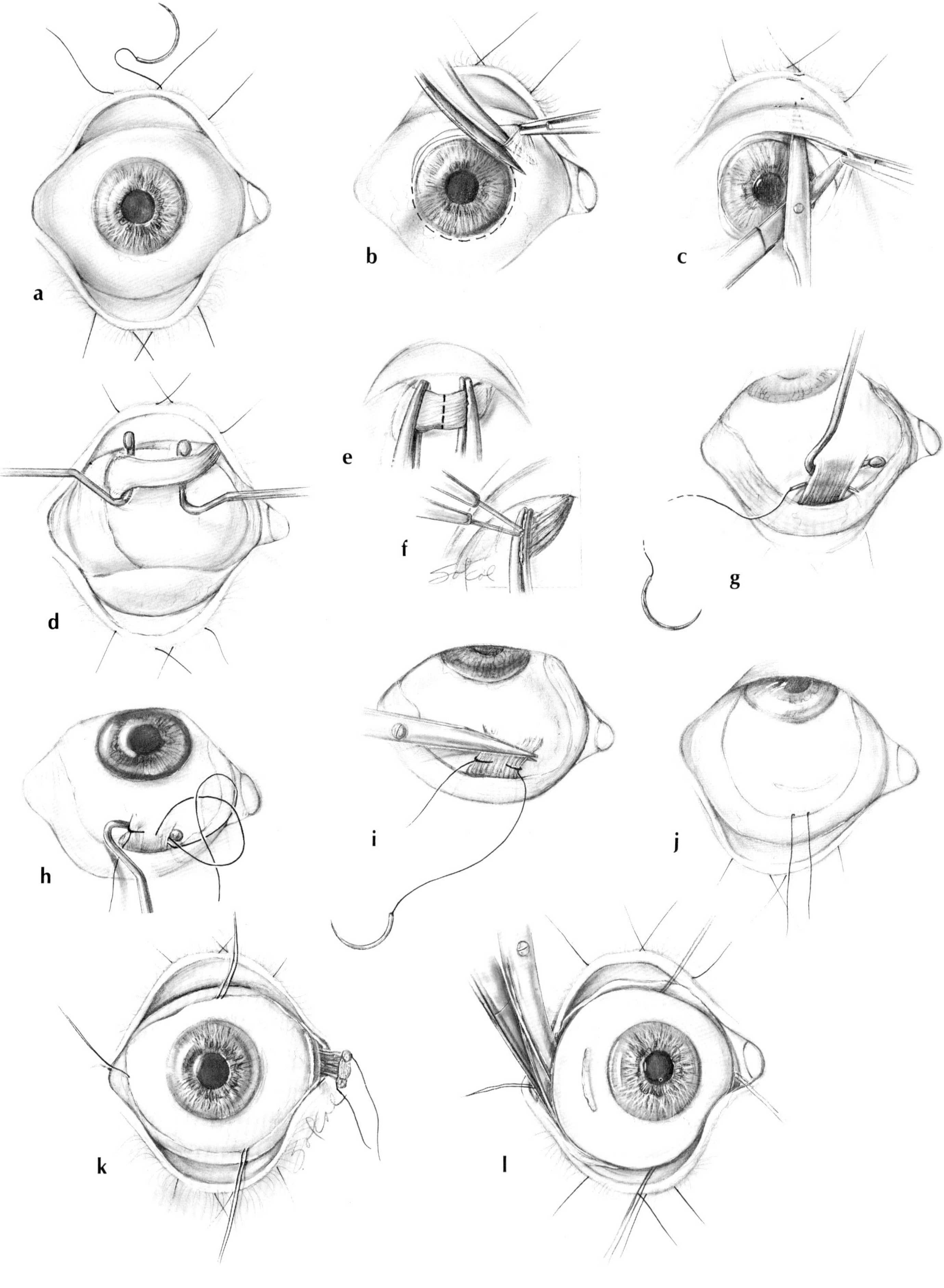
a
b
c
d
e
f
g
h
i
j
k
l

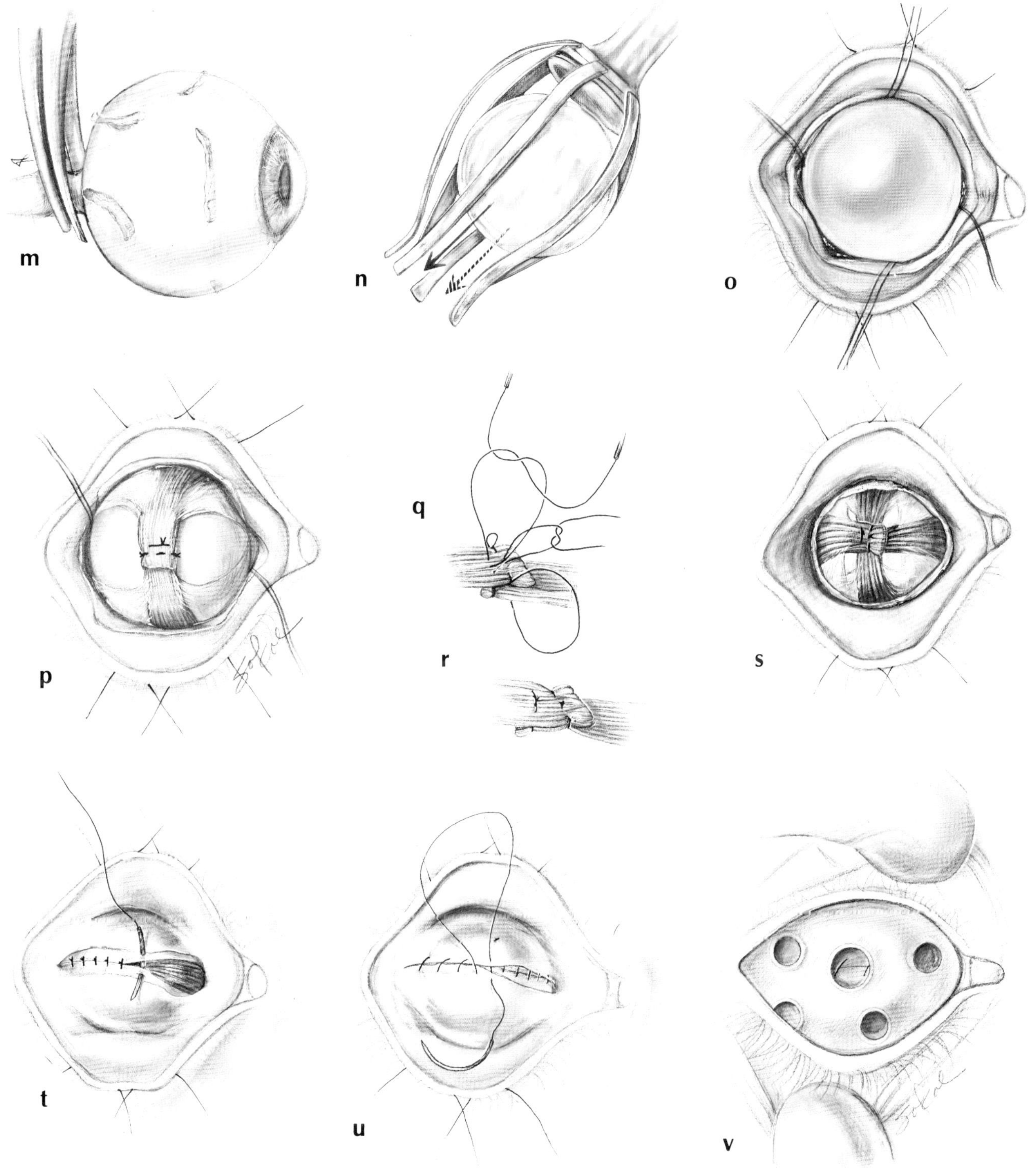

Figure 3.10 *Enucleation of the eye.* **(a)** *Crossover lid sutures for adequate exposure of eye.* **(b)** *Limbal peritomy using sharp scissors.* **(c)** *Undermining of all four quadrants with curved Stevens scissors.* **(d)** *Isolation of inferior oblique muscle with two muscle hooks.* **(e)** *Hemostat clamps across muscle.* **(f)** *Cautery used to prevent bleeding after muscle is cut.* **(g)** *Muscle hook isolation of rectus muscle and passage of transfixation suture.* **(h)** *Locking suture around edge of rectus muscle.* **(i)** *Transection of muscle, leaving small fringe of insertion.* **(j)** *Muscle is allowed to retract.* **(k)** *All four rectus muscles are isolated, sutured, transected and cut from globe.* **(l,m)** *Curved hemostat clamps optic nerve; in front of the hemostat large curved scissors are used to transect optic nerve.* **(n,o)** *Plastic ball implant is introduced into Tenon's capsule cavity.* **(p)** *Superior and inferior rectus muscles are sutured to each other.* **(q,r)** *Overlapping suturing technique.* **(s)** *Horizontal and vertical muscles are sutured across the implant, drawing up intermuscular septa.* **(t)** *Interrupted chromic catgut sutures in Tenon's layer.* **(u)** *Running 7/0 collagen sutures in conjunctiva.* **(v)** *Placement of conformer*

Operative technique

After general anesthesia, the skin of the face is prepared with soap solution followed by an iodine solution. The conjunctival cul-de-sacs are irrigated with sterile saline solution. The area is draped with an adherent plastic drape with the eyelids held open with cotton swabs as the adhesive drape is being fixed to the face. A horizontal incision is made in the middle of the interpalpebral region of the drape, and fixation of the lids is maintained with lid sutures or a lid speculum. The use of two, 4/0 silk crossover sutures on both lids (*Figure 3.10a*) maintains adequate lid separation, and the overlapping plastic drape can be picked up by these sutures to keep the lashes out of the operative field.

A limbal peritomy is performed (*Figure 3.10b*), preserving as much conjunctiva as possible. Gentle handling of the conjunctiva by its edge only is useful to avoid large 'button holes'. Tenon's capsule insertion is then cut and undermined with Steven's scissors (*Figure 3.10c*) in all quadrants, between the muscles. The superior oblique tendon and inferior oblique muscle are each isolated with two muscle hooks (*Figure 3.10d*), clamped with mosquito clamps (*Figure 3.10e*) and then cut. The orbital end is cauterized before release (*Figure 3.10f*). Each rectus muscle is isolated and the insertion well cleared, maintaining as many of the intermuscular septa as possible. A double-arm 4/0 chromic catgut suture is used to transfix the breadth of the muscle near its insertion (*Figure 3.10g*); each arm is double-looped and tied at the side of the muscle (*Figure 3.10h*). Then the muscle is transected near its insertion (*Figure 3.10i*) and bleeding is stopped on the orbital end of the muscle by cautery. After the sutures have been checked for secure muscle fixation they are held with a bulldog clamp and the muscle is then allowed to slip posteriorly (*Figure 3.10j*). All four of the rectus muscles are treated similarly (*Figure 3.10k*), with the lateral rectus insertion stump left longer for fixation.

The globe is gently rotated to look carefully for any further attachments – other than the vortex veins, the posterior ciliary nerves and vessels, and the optic nerve. Any adhesions are cleared, and then a long enucleation clamp is passed from the lateral canthus behind the globe while holding the stump of the lateral rectus forward. Frequently, this can be performed while two cotton swabs are held on either side of the optic nerve so that it can be seen clearly. The optic nerve is clamped at least 10 mm behind the globe. After the clamp has been properly placed, long enucleation scissors are used to slide along the anterior surface of the clamp and then to cut across the optic nerve flush with the clamp (*Figure 3.10l,m*). The eye can now be removed. Cautery is applied to the stump of the optic nerve, and the clamp is carefully released while holding the nerve more posteriorly with a pair of forceps to enable regripping for further cautery, if required. The latter part of the procedure (as seen in *Figure 3.10l,m*) may be replaced by the use of a tonsillar snare, which generally cannot be positioned under direct visualization but can be held back with a hemostat to a more posterior position on the optic nerve before slow tightening is begun. Tightening should be progressive during about 4–5 min. Hemostasis is obtained by the slow compression of the optic nerve vessels, because final transection of the optic nerve by closing the tonsillar snare does not maintain fixation on the optic nerve stump, and therefore cautery cannot be applied readily at a later time.

At this stage, the posterior Tenon's capsule should be carefully examined for any bleeding, which is controlled with cautery. It is vital that enucleation be a virtually bloodless procedure, so that the potential for postoperative extrusion of the implant, swelling and infection is kept to a minimum. The four 4/0 chromic catgut sutures attached to the extraocular muscles are gently pulled into view within Tenon's capsule. A posterior hole in Tenon's capsule can be repaired with a 4/0 chromic catgut purse-string suture. A plastic ball is implanted using a ball introducer, judging the appropriate size of the ball when it is in place (*Figure 3.10n,o*). Starting the fitting with a 16 mm ball is usually appropriate, and if protrusion of the ball seems to be excessive, a smaller ball can be inserted. Similarly, if the ball seems to be too retroplaced, use of a larger ball should be considered (a missed tear in the posterior portion of Tenon's capsule can cause the prosthesis to sink back also). Once the appropriately sized ball has been inserted, the vertical rectus muscles are sutured to each other using all four needles with an overlapping suture technique (*Figure 3.10p–r*). The horizontal rectus muscles are sutured similarly and are imbricated with the already sutured vertical muscles (*Figure 3.10s*). This should bring the intermuscular septi and Tenon's capsule forward around the plastic ball. If any major gaps remain, these oblique defects should be sutured with interrupted catgut sutures. Tenon's capsule is then sutured closed in a horizontal direction with interrupted 4/0 chromic catgut sutures (*Figure 3.10t*). The conjunctiva is closed over Tenon's capsule with a running 7/0 collagen suture (*Figure 3.10u*). An appropriately sized conformer is placed (*Figure 3.10v*), and a semipressure patch is applied over the lids.

Modification of enucleation technique

Various modifications of the enucleation technique have been suggested. The 'no-touch' technique can be used in the case of intraocular tumors, especially choroidal melanomas. A local freezing probe is placed at the site of the melanoma[16] and traction is placed on the globe only after adequate freezing of the intraocular tumor, to help avoid seeding of tumor cells.

Various types of prostheses, either 'semi-integrated' or 'integrated', have been devised. The best known is the Iowa–Allen implant[17]. Use of this implant depends on the skilled prosthetic services that were available in the institute in which this implant was widely used. Usually the cosmetic result and mobility of the prosthesis when using the operative technique described above are satisfactory. Fully integrated prosthetic implant devices have been disappointing in the past because of associated complications such as extrusion of the implant and conjunctival erosion.

Postoperative care and prosthetic management

Adequate pain relief is important in the immediate postoperative phase and may sometimes require systemic narcotics. Severe pain is unusual and should be suspected of being a warning symptom of postoperative bleeding or early infection.

The conformer is left in place until fitting for the prosthesis is started. An antibiotic ointment is used twice a day and is placed through the holes of the conformer to maintain good lubrication. The eyelids are cleaned twice a day, and it is preferable not to apply a patch if the patient can accept the cosmetic appearance of the conformer behind the lids. If not, a light patch is applied. Prosthetic fitting is begun about 3–4 weeks after surgery if the conjunctival wound is adequately healed. The patient should be seen during and after the completion of the fitting to check that it is correct and to make certain that there are no complications such as extrusion of the implant.

It is the responsibility of the ophthalmologist, in the final stages of the patient's preparation during prosthesis fitting, to explain the necessity for wearing protective glasses at all times and especially for using safety glasses and sports glasses during hazardous occupations and sports to protect the only remaining eye. The patient should also be directed to the motor vehicle administration or police department for advice regarding driving and license requirements. In the one-eyed patient, careful examination of the remaining eye should be continued at least at 2-year intervals.

Operative complications

Rupture of globe

Rupture or perforation of the globe, either during initial mobilization of conjunctiva (e.g. over a staphyloma) or during transection of the optic nerve, is a matter of major concern if the eye has an intraocular tumor. If an early penetration of the globe is evident during anterior dissection, closure with sutures or placement of tissue adhesive over the perforation site may prevent the globe from leaking and may maintain its form and pressure. The enucleation may then proceed routinely. The enucleation of a soft globe from which intraocular contents are prolapsed can be extremely difficult. In the case of an inadvertent posterior scleral rupture during transection of the optic nerve, remnants of the scleral envelope and a long piece of attached optic nerve should be removed especially when enucleating for retinoblastoma or choroidal melanoma. In these cases, extreme vigilance must be exercised in the postoperative phase for orbital recurrence of tumor, and postoperative orbital radiotherapy should be considered.

In enucleating infected eyes, rupture of the globe can cause orbital cellulitis, and adequate but gentle irrigation of the operative site should be maintained with an antibiotic solution (e.g. gentamicin and bacitracin) and operative cultures should be performed. Postoperatively, broad-spectrum systemic antibiotics should be used and the regimen modified according to the sensitivities of the organism isolated.

Loss of extraocular muscle

Slippage of a fixation suture from an extraocular muscle, or cutting of a fixation suture during enucleation, frequently results in retraction of the muscle and Tenon's capsule. If Tenon's capsule is intact, the muscle can be found by gentle forceps-over-forceps forward traction on Tenon's capsule in the area of the muscle. This usually exposes the end of the muscle and permits resuturing of the muscle end.

Bleeding

The most common cause of continued bleeding is inadequate hemostasis during dissection around the globe or during sectioning of the optic nerve. Wet-field cautery while the assistant holds Tenon's capsule open may permit cauterization of bleeding points and hemostasis. If hemostasis cannot be maintained by this method, a moist 12–24 inch (30–60 cm) strip of ½ inch (13 mm) gauze pack is inserted into Tenon's capsule, and pressure is applied for a minimum of 5 min over this pad. Gentle removal of the pad at the end of this time should leave a dry operative field. If none of the above procedures maintains hemostasis, microfibrillar collagen may be used sparingly. It is crucial to control bleeding during the enucleation procedure to avoid postoperative complications.

Identification of extraocular spread of tumor at the time of enucleation

Obvious visible extension of retinoblastoma or melanoma beyond the scleral envelope at the time of removal of the eye indicates a poor prognosis. Localized excision of the remaining tumor is considered the most reasonable intraoperative management. Some surgeons feel that an implant should not be placed in this situation, because orbital tumor recurrence might not be observed as soon in the presence of the implant. Others feel that tumor recurrence can be detected earlier in an orbit with an implant by progressive anterior displacement of the implant. After surgery, an oncologist should be consulted regarding possible chemotherapy or radiotherapy.

Postoperative complications

Infection

Postoperative infection should be suspected after enucleation with persistent or increased swelling of lids and conjunctiva, together with increased pain. Any purulent or mucopurulent discharge should be cultured. If infection is suspected, broad-spectrum intravenous antibiotics should be begun, and antibiotic treatment should be modified according to the results of bacterial cultures and sensitivity testing. If an infection does not show clinical improvement over 1–2 days, consideration should be given to reoperation, with opening of conjunctiva and Tenon's capsule to collect a specimen for additional bacterial cultures and for placement of a small drain. For mild infections removal of the implant often will not be required. With an extensive infection the implant may spontaneously extrude.

Extrusion of implant

Extrusion of an implant after enucleation can occur from infection, hemorrhage or breakdown of the conjunctival and Tenon's capsule wound. It is difficult to prevent extrusion once an implant is exposed and protruding through the conjunctiva. Surgery to reapproximate defects over implants or to graft material over defects has been tried with variable success. Usually, if infection and discomfort are not present, small defects should simply be observed. Partially exposed uninfected implants may remain stable for long periods of time without treatment. However, if there is more extensive extrusion, enophthalmos, reduced mobility of the prosthesis or if the implant is already extruded, further surgery may be necessary. Those secondary operations are described elsewhere[18].

Ptosis

Mild upper lid ptosis is not uncommon after enucleation. Moderate or severe ptosis may require surgery to achieve an improved cosmetic appearance and this has been discussed elsewhere[18].

Extrusion of the prosthesis

Extrusion of the prosthesis because of scarring and contracture of the conjunctival cul-de-sac or from lax lids that do not hold the prosthesis in place usually requires surgery. A mucous membrane graft or other surgery may correct a contracted conjunctival cul-de-sac and a small tarsorrhaphy may prevent loss of the prosthesis from lax eyelids. Sometimes, modification of an existing prosthesis may be all that is required to prevent extrusion and to maintain an adequate cosmetic appearance.

Enophthalmos of the prosthesis

Mild enophthalmos of the prosthesis can often be corrected by remaking and enlarging the prosthesis or by wearing a plus lens in glasses over the prosthesis to make the prosthesis appear more prominent. Major enophthalmos requires correction with orbital reconstructive surgery.

Evisceration

Indications

There are few indications for evisceration, and enucleation is preferable in most situations. Evisceration can be performed for treatment of a blind painful eye if a rapid, less traumatic surgery, as compared to enucleation, is preferred. Evisceration is never performed in an eye suspected of having an intraocular tumor. Evisceration is also not performed for the purpose of preventing sympathetic ophthalmia in an eye blinded by trauma. Because an eviscerated eye retains some uveal tissue, sympathetic ophthalmia can develop in the second eye of a patient who has had an evisceration.

Evisceration may be desirable for old or very ill patients in whom general anesthesia is a risk. In the past, evisceration has been said to be preferred to enucleation for cases of advanced, infective endophthalmitis in which sectioning of the optic nerve might allow spread of bacteria through the meningeal spaces to the central nervous system. Enucleation for endophthalmitis, however, avoids contamination of the operative field which can occur while eviscerating infected intraocular contents. Also, the risk of meningitis after enucleation is low if the patient is under treatment with intravenous antibiotics.

It has been held in the past that evisceration permits a better cosmetic result than enucleation and provides a more mobile prosthesis[19]. This is doubtful and enucleation appears to allow as much movement as evisceration.

Lastly, there are some patients who will accept the thought of evisceration but who will not permit enucleation. If not contraindicated for any of the reasons above, evisceration in these patients may be an acceptable method to avoid further psychological trauma.

Preoperative evaluation

The preoperative preparation of the patient for evisceration is the same as enucleation, and this has already been described. Ultrasonography should be performed on eyes with opaque media to make certain no intraocular tumor is present.

Operative technique

Evisceration is preferably performed under general anesthesia, although retrobulbar anesthesia and facial block with 2 per cent lidocaine (lignocaine) and/or bupivacaine can be used. After preparation, exposure of the eye is achieved with a self-retaining lid speculum. A limbal peritomy is performed while maintaining as much conjunctiva as possible (*Figure 3.11a*). The conjunctiva is undermined with scissors so that the sclera around the limbus is free of conjunctiva (*Figure 3.11b*). A keratome entry through the limbus into the anterior chamber is performed (*Figure 3.11c*) and then curved corneal scissors are used to excise the entire cornea (*Figure 3.11d*). An evisceration spoon is used to remove the intraocular contents while the globe is fixed by holding onto the limbal sclera with toothed forceps (*Figure 3.11e*). Large scissors are then used to incise the bare sclera and Tenon's capsule for 5 mm from the limbus at the 3 and 9 o'clock positions (*Figure 3.11f*). The scleral shell is opened by the assistant with two forceps and all uveal tissue is scraped from inside the eye using a gauze square held in a hemostat. Bleeding is controlled with cautery, using suction if necessary to keep the sclera free of blood (*Figure 3.11g*). A plastic ball of suitable size (usually 12 or 16 mm) is inserted inside the sclera (*Figure 3.11h*). The ball should fill the scleral shell but should be small enough so that the

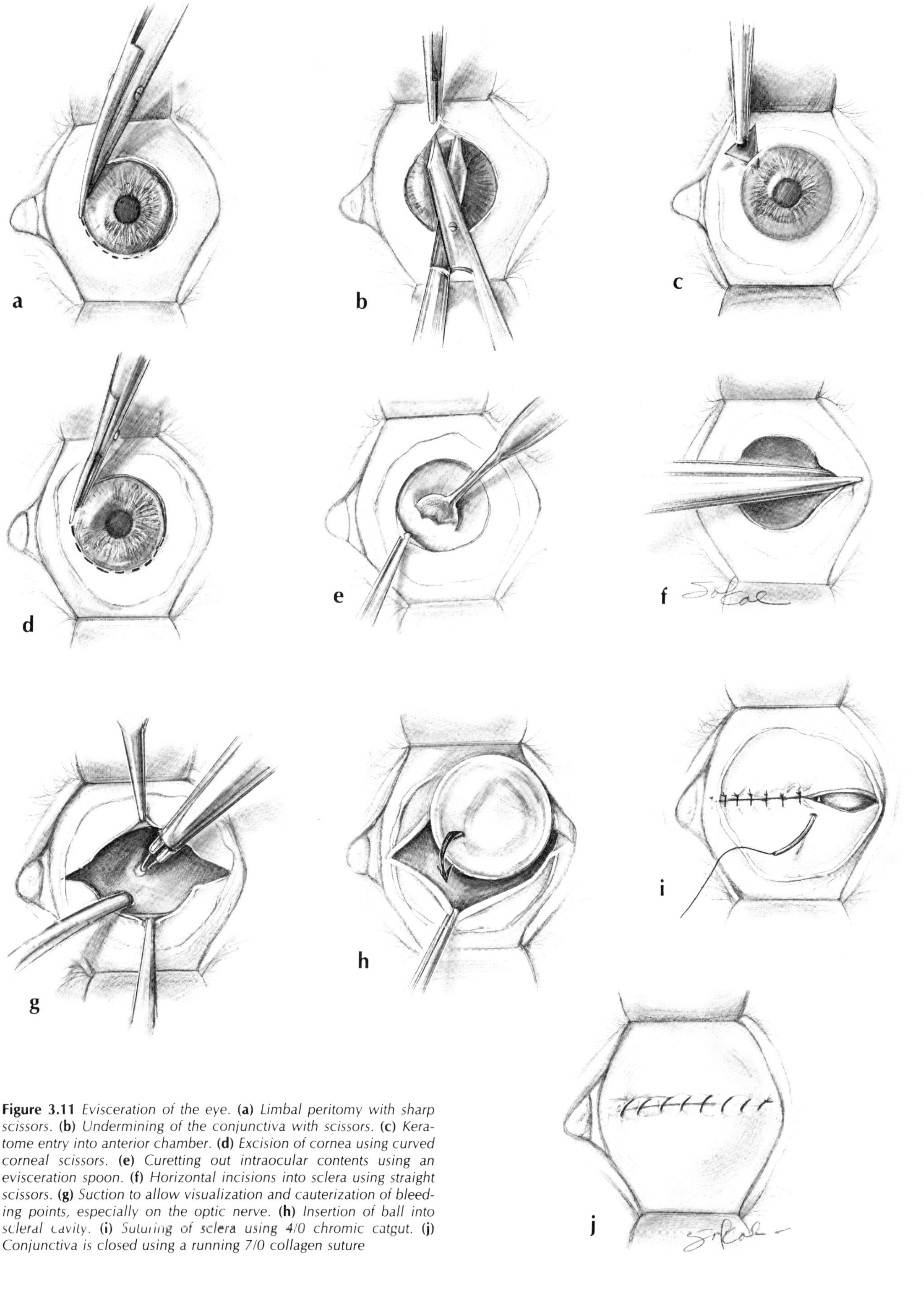

Figure 3.11 *Evisceration of the eye.* **(a)** *Limbal peritomy with sharp scissors.* **(b)** *Undermining of the conjunctiva with scissors.* **(c)** *Keratome entry into anterior chamber.* **(d)** *Excision of cornea using curved corneal scissors.* **(e)** *Curetting out intraocular contents using an evisceration spoon.* **(f)** *Horizontal incisions into sclera using straight scissors.* **(g)** *Suction to allow visualization and cauterization of bleeding points, especially on the optic nerve.* **(h)** *Insertion of ball into scleral cavity.* **(i)** *Suturing of sclera using 4/0 chromic catgut.* **(j)** *Conjunctiva is closed using a running 7/0 collagen suture*

sclera can be sutured closed without tension. Interrupted 4/0 chromic catgut sutures are used to close the sclera horizontally (*Figure 3.11i*). Conjunctiva is closed over the scleral suture line with a running 6/0 collagen suture (*Figure 3.11j*). A conformer is placed over the closed conjunctiva and an eye patch is applied over the lids. Eviscerated contents are sent for pathological examination to exclude sympathetic ophthalmia or tumor.

Postoperative management

The management after evisceration is the same as that for enucleation, except that the prosthesis fitted after evisceration does not usually need to be as large as that used after enucleation.

Special situations

Retention of the cornea at evisceration allows an even larger implant to be placed and perhaps reduces the size of the prosthesis needed. However, if the cornea is not removed and is left exposed, this renders the patient liable to ocular surface problems and pain, which are avoided by excising the entire cornea. If the cornea is retained, however, it is preferable to pull a conjunctival flap over it to avoid some of these problems.

Postoperative complications

Management of infection, extrusion of implant, and ptosis are basically the same as that for similar complications after enucleation.

Summary

The management of epibulbar tumors is dictated by the location, size and fixation of the tumor. The principles of surgical removal rely on defining an adequate tissue plane which will enable removal of the tumor with minimal surrounding ocular tissue destruction. Reconstruction of the globe may be required if significant corneal or scleral tissue has been removed. Inadequately removed tumor, or more malignant tumors, may require additional radiotherapy or chemotherapy.

The surgical removal of a pterygium is indicated if the visual axis is threatened, for irritation and injection, or if the pterygium is unacceptable cosmetically. Surgical removal is best performed after retrobulbar anesthesia in the operating room under microscopic control. The addition of postsurgical strontium radiotherapy would appear to reduce the recurrence rate.

Enucleation for either badly traumatized eyes or for eyes containing intraocular malignancies should be performed only after careful preparation of the patient. These surgical techniques should be bloodless and it is the surgeon's responsibility to follow the patient through the prosthetic fitting phase until an acceptable cosmetic result has been obtained.

Evisceration should be reserved for those blind, painful eyes in which enucleation cannot be performed.

References

1. Kottow, M. H. Anterior segment fluorescein angiography. Baltimore, Maryland: Williams & Wilkins, 1978:78
2. Spinak, M., Friedman, A. H. Squamous cell carcinoma of the conjunctiva. Value of exfoliative cytology in diagnosis. Survey of Ophthalmology 1977; 21:351–355
3. Thatcher, R. W., Darougar, S., Jones, B. R. Conjunctival impression cytology. Archives of Ophthalmology 1977; 95:678–681
4. Cameron, M. E. Pterygium throughout the world. Springfield, Illinois: Thomas, 1965
6. Paton, D. Pterygium management based upon a theory of pathogenesis. Transactions of the American Academy of Ophthalmology and Otolaryngology 1975; 79:603–612
7. Pinkerton, O. D. Surgical and strontium treatment of pterygium: Recurrence and lens changes. Age Statistics. Ophthalmic Surgery 1979; 10(9):45–47
8. Tarr, K. H., Constable, I. J. Late complications of pterygium treatment. British Journal of Ophthalmology 1980; 64:496–505
9. Cameron, M. E. Preventable complications of pterygium excision with beta-irradiation. British Journal of Ophthalmology 1972; 56:52–56
10. Poirier, R. H., Fish, J. R. Lamellar keratoplasty for recurrent pterygium. Ophthalmic Surgery 1976; 7(4):38–41
11. Dake, C. L., Crone, R. A., De Keizer, R. J. W. Treatment of (recurrent) pterygium oculi by lamellar keratoplasty. Documenta Ophthalmologica. 1979; 48:223–230
12. Beard, C., Char, D. H. Prospective views in the treatment of eyelid and adnexal malignancies. Ophthalmic Surgery 1978; 9(4):67–72
13. Lommatzsch, P. Beta-ray treatment of malignant epithelial tumors of the conjunctiva. American Journal of Ophthalmology 1976; 81:198–206
14. Leahey, B. D. Beta radiation in ophthalmology. Indications, technique and complications. American Journal of Ophthalmology 1960; 49:7–29
15. Danopoulos, E. D., Chilaris, G. A., Danopoulos, I. E., Liaricos, S. B. Urea in the treatment of epibulbar malignancies. British Journal of Ophthalmology 1975; 59:282–287
16. Fraunfelder, F. T., Boozman, F. W., Wilson, R. S ., Thomas, A. H. No-touch technique for intraocular malignant melanomas. Archives of Ophthalmology 1977; 95:1616–1620
17. Spivey, B. E. The Iowa enucleation implant. Transactions of the American Academy of Ophthalmology and Otolaryngology 1970; 74:1287–1295
18. Fasanella, R. M., ed. Complications in eye surgery. Philadelphia: W. B. Saunders Co., 1965:390–470
19. Hughes, W. I. (ed.). Ophthalmic plastic surgery, 2nd ed. Rochester, Minnesota: American Academy of Ophthalmology and Otolaryngology, 1964: 193–195, 234–236

4

Strabismus surgery

David L. Guyton MD

Introduction

Of the major types of ophthalmic surgery, strabismus surgery ranks second in frequency only to cataract extraction. Yet many ophthalmologists are uneasy in managing patients with strabismus because of variability in the surgical results, which is seemingly beyond the surgeon's control. Some of this variability can rightly be attributed to unpredictable patient responses to standard surgical procedures. However, a substantial amount of the variability in surgical results is attributable to the surgeon and is caused by measurement error, mistakes in judgment and variations in surgical technique.

Recently there have been important advances in diagnostic methods, in the recognition of different forms of strabismus and in the determination of the best therapeutic options, including the timing of various forms of intervention. Surgical procedures have changed remarkably, especially with respect to the performance of bolder surgery. As the functional interplay between various muscle groups has become better understood, most strabismus surgeons now attempt to correct large deviations, and also combined horizontal and vertical deviations, with one operation rather than planning two or more procedures.

New suture materials and safer needles have lessened the complications from strabismus surgery. Use of adjustable suture techniques now permits bolder, and yet more accurate, surgery in adults. Continued differences in surgical techniques, however, indicate that strabismus surgery is still in a state of evolution. The procedures described in this chapter have been borrowed and modified from many sources, or (in a few cases) newly devised. The techniques described are those currently used by the author and are those which seem to yield the most predictable results.

Indications for surgery

The basic indications for strabismus surgery fall into two groups: cosmetic and functional. Misalignment of the eyes can be a social and emotional handicap of great importance, and strabismus surgery for cosmetic reasons alone is certainly justified. Also, abnormal head postures, even in the absence of obvious strabismus, are often amenable to surgery on the extraocular muscles.

While a successful cosmetic appearance can almost always be obtained with strabismus surgery, functional cures are more difficult and sometimes impossible. Complete functional cure requires that the eyes be freely movable, maintain proper alignment in all directions of gaze, and have single binocular vision and normal stereopsis. Achievement of at least some binocular vision is an important goal, for the better a patient's eyes work together, the more likely they will remain aligned in the future.

It is generally agreed that children with 'congenital' strabismus – that is, strabismus becoming apparent before 6 months of age – should be treated early in life if there is to be any chance of gaining even limited binocular vision. Surgical alignment by 18 months of age is the goal of most strabismus surgeons. When strabismus is 'acquired' – that is, developing after 6 months of age – or when it is intermittent, the chances of regaining at least some binocular vision with appropriate treatment are greatly increased.

The potential for restoration of binocular vision with appropriate treatment decreases, however, with duration of the strabismus. Untreated infants lose this potential quickly, whereas strabismic adults often retain at least some potential for binocular vision for many years.

Although children can adapt to strabismus by the mechanisms of 'suppression' and anomalous retinal correspondence, adults cannot. Therefore functional problems from constant diplopia in the adult with acquired strabismus are often the primary indication for surgical intervention, even in the absence of cosmetic problems.

Preoperative evaluation

History

Past ocular history is often important in determining the potential for binocular vision and thus in determining the goal and expectations for surgical realignment. If there is no potential for binocular vision, a slow drifting outward of the eyes (sensory exotropia) is expected over a 10 to 20 year period. In these patients slight postoperative esotropia is desirable. However, if there is potential for binocular vision, exact alignment immediately after surgery is usually the proper goal.

Factors other than the time of onset of the strabismus are also important in determining binocular potential. These include the fixation preference, the presence of amblyopia, and previous treatment with glasses, patching and miotics. The nature of any previous strabismus surgery should be determined, along with the immediate and long-term results obtained. It is not unusual for an older child with no measurable evidence of binocular vision to obtain at least partial peripheral fusion after strabismus surgery, if the eyes had been straight for at least some time in the past.

Refraction

The refractive state of the patient must always be measured, and any clinically significant refractive error should be corrected. A period of at least several weeks is usually permitted for adaptation to the new optical correction before determining the amount of surgery necessary. Even adults in their 20s and 30s can have a significant component of accommodative strabismus, and cycloplegic refraction is indicated in such patients if there is a suspicion of an accommodative component.

Ocular alignment and motility

Evaluation of ocular alignment and motility includes examination of head posture and of ocular fixation preference. Determination of whether there is limitation of movement in a fixing eye is especially important if the surgical procedure is intended to correct an anomalous head posture. Limitation of movement in the fixing eye *must* be relieved if the head posture is to be corrected.

Examination of ocular motility (ductions and versions) is performed to identify restrictions and limitations, and even minor degrees of paresis. Examination of ductions alone (movement of each eye separately in various directions of gaze) cannot be relied upon to identify muscle pareses, because additional innervation may produce a full range of movement even when muscle paresis is present. However, examination of versions (movements of both eyes together in the various directions of gaze) is a much more sensitive measure of muscle paresis because a paretic muscle is compared directly with its normal yoke muscle in the opposite eye.

Forced (passive) ductions, in which the globe is grasped with forceps and rotated, are helpful in distinguishing a muscle paresis from a mechanical restriction. However, contracture of the direct antagonist of the paretic muscle often complicates interpretation of the findings, and results of forced duction testing may be equivocal. Techniques for forced duction testing of the rectus and oblique muscles are described later under 'Surgical techniques', but gross restrictions of movement can easily be investigated preoperatively using topical anesthesia and forceps.

The muscle force generation test is another method for evaluating possible muscle paresis. Under topical anesthesia the eye is held by forceps in the midline, and the patient is asked to look in the field of action of the muscle suspected of being paretic. With experience in judging muscle strength, the surgeon can determine whether the muscle is weak.

Analysis of saccadic velocities using electro-oculography (EOG) electrodes is occasionally used to help differentiate muscle paresis from restriction. However, not all surgeons agree that saccadic velocity analysis is sufficiently reliable to make the test clinically worthwhile.

Amounts of surgery performed on the extraocular muscles are usually based on measurements of the strabismic deviation in various directions of gaze. These measurements must be estimated in infants by observing the corneal light reflex, using either the Hirschberg test or the Krimsky prism reflex test. More precise methods are used in older children and adults. However, whether or not measurements are made by prism-and-cover testing or by red-green dissociation methods (Hess chart, Lancaster red-green test), it is possible that the measurements do not reflect the true ocular deviations under binocular conditions. Careful testing with the cover-uncover test rather than the alternate-cover test should always be used to confirm the presence or absence of motor fusion ability. When motor fusion ability is present, it is an excellent prognostic sign for a good surgical result.

Analysis of cyclovertical deviations has been complicated in recent years by undue reliance on the Bielschowsky head-tilt test. This test is reliable for uncomplicated superior oblique paresis but may be misleading with other cyclovertical muscle pareses. The Bielschowsky head-tilt test is useless in the presence of primary oblique overaction or with motility restrictions from previous surgery, trauma or thyroid myopathy.

Although while one must always consider the possibility of restrictions, as in Brown's syndrome, and limitations, as in Duane's syndrome, it is usually possible to identify a paretic cyclovertical muscle by having the patient look in the quadrant of greatest hyperdeviation and identifying the underacting muscle. One must remember, however, that secondary overaction of the direct antagonist of a paretic muscle may be responsible for causing the largest hyperdeviation in a quadrant *other than* the field of action of the paretic muscle. This is often seen with inferior oblique overaction developing after the onset of superior oblique paresis. Muscles showing secondary overaction usually must be weakened for an effective surgical result.

Evaluation of cyclodeviations has become especially helpful in recent years in the diagnosis of cyclovertical strabismus. In the inverted indirect ophthalmoscopic view the horizontal position of the fovea should fall within the upper one third of the optic disc. If the fovea is above the upper border of the disc, the eye is extorted; and if the fovea is lower than the junction of the upper and middle thirds of the disc, the eye is anatomically intorted[1]. Because of sensory adaptations to cyclodeviations, which take place mainly in children, the anatomical determination of torsion is more reliable than sensory methods[2]. Sensory methods of torsion measurement, such as the double Maddox rod test, are helpful, especially when dealing with recent onset cyclovertical strabismus in adults.

Sensory tests for fusion and stereopsis are routinely performed in evaluation of patients with strabismus. This is done both to determine the sensory status of the patient and to aid in predicting the surgical outcome. In many strabismic patients, binocular potential, if it is present at all, can only be demonstrated with a haploscope system (amblyoscope, synoptophore). Demonstration of fusional potential by measurement of fusional vergence amplitudes is now the major use for these instruments which were previously used primarily for orthoptic exercises.

General ocular examination

Of prime importance in the evaluation of strabismus, especially in children, is a thorough general ocular examination. This includes measurement of intraocular pressure when possible and examination of the fundus by indirect ophthalmoscopy in all cases. Lesions involving the retina or optic nerve, such as retinoblastoma or retinal detachment, can cause strabismus due to visual loss in one eye. This may not be apparent from the history and will not be overlooked if a thorough examination is done.

Therapeutic methods as adjuncts or alternatives to surgery

The strabismus surgeon should be well versed in methods of strabismus treatment other than surgery. This will avoid unnecessary surgery and also permit treatment of residual or consecutive postoperative deviations.

Optical correction

Prescribing less than the full cycloplegic hyperopic correction will induce some accommodative convergence and may lessen the need for further surgery to treat consecutive exotropia after esotropia surgery. Bifocals are frequently used to treat accommodative esotropia and may also be useful postoperatively in some cases. Prisms, particularly the Press-On™ Fresnel prisms, may be used to advantage for residual or consecutive deviations, especially those which are expected to change during the postoperative period. If the original or residual strabismic deviation can be treated with Fresnel prisms of less than 10^{Δ} to 15^{Δ}, this amount of prismatic correction can usually be ground into permanent glasses, thus avoiding further surgery.

Orthoptic exercises

Orthoptic exercises were widely used in the past but are now seldom used in the treatment of strabismus. However, orthoptic exercises are still useful in certain instances. Problems due to convergence insufficiency respond well to convergence exercises. These often produce more symptomatic relief, even if temporary, than can be obtained with strabismus surgery.

Amblyopia therapy

To increase the likelihood of obtaining binocular function, it has been general practice to treat amblyopia before performing strabismus surgery. There is some question regarding this practice, however, particularly because early surgery may be more effective in promoting development of binocular function. Most strabismus surgeons believe children with amblyopia will never obtain central fusion even if visual acuity in the amblyopic eye can be improved to the level of the other eye. It is unknown whether improved foveal vision obtained by preoperative patching helps achieve a better binocular result after surgery. When early surgery appears desirable, it is now our practice to begin occlusion therapy for amblyopia promptly but not to delay surgery while waiting for visual improvement. Patching is continued after surgery, occluding the sound eye up to 80–90 per cent of the time. Development of whatever binocular function is possible should occur during the 10–20 per cent of the time that both eyes are open.

Design of surgery

As a general rule, surgery is performed as soon as the exact diagnosis is established and the angle of deviation is stable. For functional purposes, surgery should be performed as soon as possible after the onset of the deviation to permit maximum recovery of any binocular function that was present previously.

A frequent question is whether to operate for the angle of strabismus present with distance fixation or the angle with near fixation. Although there is no definite answer to this question, it is generally best to operate for the near measurement when performing medial rectus muscle surgery and to operate for the distance measurement when performing lateral rectus muscle surgery. When performing a recess-resect procedure, a compromise between the two measurements should generally be used.

Recession of a given muscle will usually have more effect in the field of action of that muscle than in the opposite field. Incomitant strabismus, therefore, is best treated by judicious choice of the muscles to be operated on, and often a single large recession is adequate. We find that muscle recessions are usually more predictable than resections, and bilateral recessions of the medial or lateral rectus muscles are preferred to recess-resect procedures. A resection by itself can produce the desired effect initially. However, unless this is combined with recession of the opposing muscle, the effect of the operation is usually lost later with return to the original angle of strabismus.

Previously, it was common practice to correct large deviations, or combinations of horizontal and vertical deviations, with planned, staged procedures. Use of multiple procedures is no longer considered to be necessary, except in unusually complicated cases. Weakening procedures on the superior and inferior oblique muscles usually do not affect the horizontal alignment in primary position[3,4]. Therefore, operations on the oblique muscles are now commonly performed at the same time as surgery for the horizontal deviation. However, if the diagnosis of a vertical imbalance is uncertain, performing surgery for only the horizontal deviation is preferred to avoid unnecessary scarring and to permit later reassessment of any residual deviation.

Many ocular conditions associated with strabismus have previously been thought to influence the response to strabismus surgery. Most of these impressions have not been confirmed by scientific investigation. Several factors, however, do seem to influence the surgical result. With small eyes, for geometrical reasons alone, a larger surgical correction is obtained for a given amount of surgery. Unpredictable results are obtained when the amount of strabismic deviation present preoperatively is variable, as is seen in some children with cerebral palsy. In general, however, neurological problems such as mental retardation, as in Down's syndrome and most types of cerebral palsy, do not influence the surgical result[5]. Lastly, many surgeons believe that the presence of amblyopia predisposes the patient to progressively increasing overcorrections, and initial surgery is planned accordingly.

Strabismus operations are successful 70–80 per cent of the time in achieving the desired result. Reoperation is frequently necessary for the unsuccessful cases, including cases that initially appeared successful but developed progressive esotropia or exotropia during the years after surgery. If it is apparent immediately after surgery that the result is inadequate or that a large overcorrection has been obtained, it is possible to reoperate within several days of the initial surgery. If more than a few days have passed since surgery, reoperation is made more difficult by friable new blood vessels and connective tissue that invade the operative area. Therefore, if repeat surgery cannot be performed within a few days, it is usually best to wait at least 2 months before reoperating in the same location.

The number of times that a muscle can effectively be operated upon depends on the quality of the surgical technique and the particular healing response which occurs. Under ideal conditions, muscles can be operated on three or more times without causing clinically significant restriction or scarring. The fornix approach is particularly valuable to avoid further scarring due to reoperations.

Certain types of reoperation are more effective than others. Further recession of previously recessed muscles is especially effective, with small amounts of additional recession producing large shifts in alignment. Advancement or resection of a previously recessed muscle is less effective in reversing the result of the initial surgery, and recession of the opposing muscle is usually preferred.

Surgical options

Muscles can be weakened, strengthened or transposed to different locations. The basic weakening procedure is recession of the muscle, moving its insertion directly posterior a measured amount. It has been taught that muscles should not be recessed posterior to the point where the muscle belly or tendon is tangent to the globe, to avoid excessive weakening and limitation of movement. However, experience with the faden procedure (posterior fixation procedure in which the rectus muscle is fixed to the globe far behind the point of tangency) indicates that far posterior insertions can be created without producing excessive limitation in the field of action. This suggests that it is acute shortening of the muscle which produces excessive weakening, rather than retroplacement beyond the point of tangency. Therefore, during reoperation, rectus muscles can if necessary be recessed beyond what were previously thought to be 'maximum recession' limits to obtain the needed effect. If sutures cannot easily be placed at the far posterior location, the sutures can be placed anteriorly and the knot tied without pulling the muscle forward to the location of the suture placement ('sling' or 'hang back' suture). This allows the muscle to retract a measured amount to the desired position.

Another method of weakening a muscle is the 'marginal myotomy'. With this technique a Z-type lengthening effect is achieved by making cuts across more than half the muscle width at two or more points along its length. We find that it is difficult to control the effect when using a marginal myotomy, and we prefer instead to recess the muscle further, permitting the muscle to retract on a sling suture if necessary.

The basic strengthening procedure for a rectus muscle is resection and excision of a certain length of muscle and/or tendon measured backward from the insertion. The shortened muscle is then resutured to the original insertion site. Alternatively, the muscle may be advanced anterior to the original insertion site. However, advancement usually produces an unsightly thickening of tissue beneath the bulbar conjunctiva, and advancement anterior to the usual insertion site is best avoided. Still another strenghtening procedure, which is usually reserved for the superior oblique tendon, is 'tucking'. Here the superior oblique tendon is folded and sutured upon itself to shorten its length.

Muscle insertions may be transposed to different locations to alter the functional pull of the muscles. For example, if the insertion of the medial rectus muscle is moved upward, its abducting ability will be lessened in elevation and increased in depression. Transposition of the insertions of the superior and inferior rectus muscles is occasionally used to treat complete sixth nerve palsy. The superior and inferior rectus muscles thereby exert an abducting 'tethering' effect on the eye and oppose the medial rectus muscle, which would otherwise undergo continuing contracture and pull the eye into an adducted position. Another type of transposition operation is the faden procedure (posterior fixation procedure). This is a transposition of the effective insertion of the muscle far posteriorly. In the original faden procedure 'posterior fixation' is performed without disturbing the original insertion of the rectus muscle, and the muscle belly is sutured to the sclera 11–16 mm posterior to the original insertion. This causes only minimal, if any, weakening of the muscle in the primary position but creates a relative paresis of the muscle in its field of action. Therefore the faden procedure is useful when it is desirable to weaken a muscle only in its field of action.

Adjustable sutures allow adjustment of a muscle's position after anesthesia has worn off. Recently, improved techniques have been devised[6] to allow use of adjustable sutures on most adult patients. Adjustable sutures are used most often for recessions, allowing the muscle to hang back in the recessed position. The suture ends are left in an accessible location, and the muscle's position is adjusted the same day or the morning after surgery. Because adjustment of the muscle position can be uncomfortable, this procedure is limited to use in teenage patients or adults, unless rapid-acting anesthesia is easily available for children.

A resected muscle can also be placed on an adjustable suture. However, if the muscle is to be pulled further anteriorly, then excess resection must be done initially so that the cut end of the resected muscle is initially placed posterior to the intended insertion site. The fact that the muscle end is not initially tightened against the globe at the suture site does not seem to cause any problem regarding attachment of the muscle to the sclera. Attachment soon occurs wherever the end of the muscle lies, whether sutured to the sclera at that point or simply suspended against the sclera by the sling suture.

Clinical conditions

Horizontal strabismus

Horizontal strabismus, when persisting after correction of refractive error, is treated by surgery on the medial and lateral rectus muscles. We prefer recessions of the medial rectus muscles for most types of esodeviations, and recessions of the lateral rectus muscles for most types of exodeviations. Incomitance influences the amount of surgery to be done on each side. For example, if an exotropic patient is XT 30$^{\Delta}$ on gaze left and XT 20$^{\Delta}$ on gaze right, the left lateral rectus muscle will be recessed 7 mm and the right lateral rectus muscle will be recessed 5 or 6 mm. If the incomitance is extreme, perhaps only one lateral rectus muscle will be recessed.

Our customary amounts of horizontal rectus muscle surgery are given in *Table 4.1*. These numbers correspond only to the techniques described later. The same amounts of horizontal rectus surgery when used with other techniques may be entirely inappropriate. The amounts of surgery given for exodeviations are designed to produce an initial overcorrection of 5$^{\Delta}$ to 10$^{\Delta}$.

Reoperation for residual horizontal strabismus is often performed by further recession of the previously recessed muscles rather than resection of the opposing muscles.

Table 4.1 Millimeter amounts for initial horizontal rectus muscle surgery

	Esotropia			*Exotropia*		
Deviation (Δ)	*Bilat. MR recession*	*Recess MR*	*Resect LR*	*Bilat. LR recession*	*Recess LR*	*Resect MR*
15	3	3	4	4	4	3
20	3.5	3.5	5	5	5	4
25	4	4	6	6	6	5
30	4.5	4.5	7	7	7	6
35	5	5	8	7.5	7.5	6.5
40	5.5	5.5	9	8	8	7
50	6	6	10	9	9	7
60	6.25	6.25	11	10	10	8

MR = medial rectus; LR = lateral rectus

This is especially true for residual esotropia if the deviation is still greater at near than at distance, and for residual exotropia if the deviation is still greater at distance than at near. We have used resections less frequently in recent years because the results seem less predictable and because of occasional cosmetic problems from the thickened tissue overlying the resection site.

The convergence insufficiency form of exotropia is best treated by orthoptics. If this is not successful, bilateral medial rectus resections are usually performed. We attempt to obtain a moderate overcorrection, with postoperative esotropia at distance. This gradually resolves and can be symptomatically treated by prisms if necessary in the interim. The resected muscles gradually lengthen, however, often allowing the deviation to return to its preoperative state. Therefore, long-term results of surgical treatment of convergence insufficiency are often unsatisfactory.

When an A- or V-pattern is present with horizontal strabismus but without significant oblique overaction, transposition of the horizontal rectus muscles in the appropriate upward or downward direction often gives good results. A useful rule is that medial rectus muscles are transposed toward the apex of the pattern and lateral rectus muscles are transposed toward the base. When performing vertical transposition of horizontal rectus muscles, we transpose the center of the muscle the desired number of millimeters rather than trying to transpose a half muscle-width or whole muscle-width. This is done to avoid variable results from different muscle widths. Between 4 and 6 mm of vertical transposition are usually performed for A- or V-patterns in the absence of oblique overaction.

Cyclovertical strabismus

Many forms of cyclovertical strabismus, such as oblique overaction and dissociated vertical deviation, cannot be attributed to particular cranial nerve dysfunction. These cyclovertical abnormalities are often associated with other forms of strabismus, particularly congenital esotropia, although they may be present alone. Oblique overaction, whether primary, or secondary to paresis of the opposing oblique, nearly always causes significant anatomical torsion of the globe as judged by the position of the optic disc relative to the fovea. However, dissociated vertical deviation, and also pseudo-overaction of the obliques as seen with relative tightness of the lateral rectus muscle, do not cause abnormal torsion of the globe. Therefore, the presence or absence of anatomical cyclodeviation can distinguish true oblique overaction from these other abnormalities or can help determine how much of each problem is present when they are combined.

Overacting inferior obliques are weakened by recession if there is minimal overaction, or by large myectomy for moderate or severe overaction, as illustrated later. Superior oblique overaction is treated by tenotomy of the superior oblique tendon and rarely by tenectomy, as illustrated later. Even large myectomies of the inferior oblique or large tenectomies of the superior oblique do not destroy the function of these respective muscles entirely. The exaggerated traction test of the oblique muscles, as illustrated later, becomes entirely free immediately after transecting the respective oblique, but weeks to months later this test shows essentially normal tightness. This indicates that the residual muscle or tendon stump reestablishes functional connection to the sclera or Tenon's capsule.

Surgical correction of dissociated vertical deviation (DVD) can be difficult. Many methods have been tried, with non-consensus as to the best approach. Large recessions of the superior rectus muscles, large resections of the inferior rectus muscles and recess-resect procedures on the vertical rectus muscles have all been tried with varying degrees of success. Some surgeons use a faden procedure on the superior rectus muscle, combined with a modest recession. However, a faden procedure on the superior rectus muscle should not return the eye all the way to primary position, because the effectiveness of this procedure decreases as the eye approaches primary position. We have not found the faden procedure to be effective in this situation.

We now use large recessions of the superior rectus muscles to treat dissociated vertical deviation. Both superior rectus muscles are recessed if the condition is bilateral, and asymmetrical recessions are done when the DVD is asymmetrical. Typical amounts of recession are 12 mm for the more involved side and 8 mm for the less involved side, with great care being taken to clear away all attachments between the superior rectus muscle and the surrounding tissues before recessing the muscle this large amount on a sling suture. With such careful dissection, no significant lid elevation has been noted.

Pure cyclodeviations are rare because cyclodeviations are usually produced by oblique overaction or muscle palsies which also cause hyperdeviations. The surgery which corrects the oblique overaction or the muscle palsy usually corrects the cyclodeviation also, and special attention need not be paid to the cyclodeviation component. However, there are rare situations when a torsional deviation is symptomatic in the absence of vertical or horizontal problems. This occurs in mild cases of bilateral superior oblique paresis.

When treating symptomatic torsional deviation due to mild bilateral superior oblique paresis, a variation of the so-called 'Harada-Ito' procedure is used on one or both superior oblique tendons. The anterior portion of the superior oblique tendon is moved temporally and anteriorly to create an intorting effect without a depressing effect, as illustrated later. During this procedure the fundus is intermittently examined by indirect ophthalmoscopy to judge the change in torsion produced. Alternatively, the Harada-Ito procedure may be performed using an adjustable suture that can be adjusted postoperatively according to the patient's subjective observations.

Paralytic strabismus

Paralytic strabismus is caused most commonly by fourth nerve paresis or palsy. Many cases are 'congenital', with a compensatory head tilt since childhood. Often such cases decompensate in later life, with the development of frank diplopia. Most acquired forms of superior oblique paresis are caused by trauma, with most of these being bilateral.

With superior oblique paresis from any cause, secondary overaction of the opposing inferior oblique frequently occurs, producing a deviation which is greatest in the field of action of the inferior oblique. Surgical treatment of superior oblique paresis usually includes weakening of the opposing inferior oblique, either alone or in addition to other surgery.

The superior oblique tuck was used in the past to correct the deviation in the field of action of the paretic superior oblique. This is no longer commonly done, however, because if enough of a tuck is done to strengthen the superior oblique, postoperative Brown's syndrome is produced. The preferable procedure is recession of the contralateral inferior rectus muscle, on an adjustable suture if possible.

Sometimes a muscle other than the ipsilateral inferior oblique and contralateral inferior rectus must also be operated on to provide adequate compensation for a superior oblique paresis. This further surgery is determined by the particular pattern of deviation in various directions of gaze. In general, recession of a vertical rectus muscle will affect the deviation most in the field of action of that muscle, but it must be remembered that the rectus muscles have significant vertical action even with the eye out of the abducted position. Resection of the opposing rectus muscle provides increased vertical effect. Weakening an oblique muscle has its major effect in the field of action of the oblique muscle, which is largely restricted to elevation or depression in adduction. The effect of oblique muscle surgery on the vertical deviation in primary position is less than the effect of rectus muscle surgery, but the cyclodeviation effect is greater.

Third nerve paresis or palsy may be difficult to correct surgically because of widespread loss of muscle function. Alignment may be achieved in primary position, but enough limitation of movement is usually present to cause diplopia with change of gaze a few degrees in any direction. Best results are obtained if there is partial recovery of the muscles innervated by the third nerve, particularly the medial rectus muscle. In such cases a large recess-resect procedure on the horizontal rectus muscles of the affected eye is frequently sufficient to return the eye to the midline and to allow recovery of fusion with a restricted horizontal range of gaze.

One congenital form of third nerve palsy involves only the upper division of the third nerve that innervates the superior rectus muscle and the levator of the upper lid.

Vertical rectus surgery may be sufficient to correct this situation, followed by ptosis surgery if necessary. Aberrant regeneration of the third cranial nerve occasionally occurs in a pattern that elevates the lid to a normal position when the eye moves from abduction to the midline. In this situation the preferred procedure is to perform a large recess-resect operation on the horizontal muscles of the opposite eye, turning the normal eye toward the nose. The increased innervation that then occurs to bring the normal eye from the adducted position to the midline brings the paretic eye inward and simultaneously raises the lid. Therefore separate ptosis surgery is avoided[7].

Sixth nerve palsy with weakness of the lateral rectus muscle is frequently seen secondary to hydrocephalus, but it may also occur with a viral illness, after trauma, with intracranial tumors or with diabetes mellitus. Sixth nerve palsy is usually followed by contracture of the ipsilateral medial rectus muscle. A large recession of the medial rectus muscle is essential in any surgical procedure to correct the esotropia that may remain after resolution of the sixth nerve paresis. If lateral rectus muscle function does not return, as indicated by saccadic velocity studies or by the muscle force generation test, a transposition procedure in addition to a large medial rectus recession is necessary. Either temporal transposition of the superior and inferior rectus muscles to the border of the lateral rectus muscle or a Jensen procedure (as described later) is performed. The medial rectus recession used with either of the transposition procedures must be at least 7–8 mm. If partial lateral rectus function returns, a recess-resect procedure alone may be adequate to correct the esotropia resulting from the sixth nerve paresis.

Double elevator paralysis and double depressor paralysis are both quite rare. These conditions are best treated by transposition procedures using the medial and lateral rectus muscles of the involved eye, moving these muscles either up or down depending on the particular problem. Secondary contracture of the opposing depressors or elevators must be evaluated by forced ductions and dealt with accordingly.

Innervational anomalies

Duane's retraction syndrome is the most common innervational anomaly of the extraocular muscles. It is practically impossible to increase the horizontal range of motion of any eye with Duane's syndrome, but the eye can easily be realigned by recession of the appropriate muscle. This corrects the head turn which is frequently present with each of the various forms of Duane's syndrome. Either the medial rectus muscle or the lateral rectus muscle of the eye with Duane's syndrome can be recessed to place the resting position of that eye straight ahead, thereby allowing fusion in primary position. Some of the range of horizontal gaze may be sacrificed by this procedure, but this loss is usually not significant compared to the advantage achieved. We usually avoid resecting a muscle in an eye with Duane's syndrome to avoid increasing the retraction.

Other innervational anomalies include aberrant regeneration after third cranial nerve palsy, as discussed before, and the Marcus Gunn 'jaw-winking' form of ptosis. Correction of the jaw-winking, if necessary, involves dividing the levator tendon on the involved side, combined with bilateral frontalis sling procedures (*see* Chapter 1).

Mechanical limitation strabismus

Several types of strabismus may show mechanical limitations. These include: (*1*) Brown's syndrome, (*2*) the adherence syndrome, (*3*) the tight lateral rectus syndrome, (*4*) thyroid myopathy, (*5*) strabismus fixus, (*6*) limitations from orbital floor fracture and (*7*) congenital fibrosis of the extraocular muscles. Use of forced ductions (the traction test) before, during and after surgery is quite helpful in the diagnosis and management of these cases. In general, limitations must be freed, and tight muscles must be weakened. If this is impossible, adequate alignment can sometimes be achieved by creating a mechanical limitation in the opposite eye to balance the involved eye, but such procedures may be difficult to justify.

Brown's syndrome deserves special discussion. Although there are several varieties of Brown's syndrome, most are caused by a tight or inelastic superior oblique tendon. When significant deviation is present in primary position, surgery is indicated, and the superior oblique tendon is weakened, usually by tenotomy. Because superior oblique paresis frequently occurs after such a procedure, many surgeons perform an inferior oblique weakening procedure at the time of the superior oblique tenotomy. Use of traction sutures after simple 'freeing of the sheath' of the superior oblique tendon has not been effective.

Adjustable sutures are quite helpful in treating many forms of mechanical limitation strabismus, particularly cases of thyroid myopathy. In cases of thyroid myopathy many surgeons wait until the abnormal thyroid condition has stabilized and the myopathy is also stable, although when dealing with lid retraction and proptosis, earlier surgery may be desirable (*see* Chapter 2). The inferior rectus muscle is the muscle most frequently involved in thyroid myopathy, with scarring and contraction. Therefore, a large recession of the inferior rectus muscle is often necessary. However, large bilateral recessions of the inferior rectus muscles may produce enough intorsion to cause troublesome torsional symptoms even though horizontal and vertical alignment is achieved. Temporal transposition of the inferior rectus muscles at the time of recession may help prevent this intorsion effect.

Nystagmus

No practical and effective method has yet been found to decrease significantly the amplitude or frequency of nystagmus. Faden procedures on opposing rectus muscles have been tried but have not been particularly successful. However, when a null position of the nystamus is present, with an accompanying head turn, this null position can be moved to the midline by appropriate horizontal muscle surgery, thus eliminating the head turn. The Kestenbaum-Anderson procedure, performing appropriate surgery on all four horizontal rectus muscles, is used for this purpose, even in the absence of pre-existing strabismus. An estimate is made of the amount of head turn, and each eye is moved in the appropriate direction with a recess-resect procedure on that eye of appropriate amount to equal the amount of head turn. Results have generally been good, but frank strabismus and diplopia can occur as complications.

Patient management

The choice of inpatient versus outpatient surgery depends considerably on cooperation from the anesthetist. Minimizing preoperative medication speeds postoperative recovery, and children under the age of 6 years can usually be discharged within 4–6 h after surgery. Older children and adults do not recover from general anesthesia as quickly, and hospitalization overnight after the operation is often necessary. Adult surgery performed with local anesthesia can easily be performed as an outpatient procedure. However, if an adjustable suture is used, the patient is usually hospitalized until the next morning to permit adjustment of the suture.

It is important that the patient or the parents of the patient be informed preoperatively as to the exact nature of the procedure, the eye or eyes to be operated on and the expected result. The variability of response to strabismus surgery should be discussed before the operation. Therefore, if an unexpected response occurs, the patient or parents are prepared for the possibility and will be more receptive to subsequent recommendations for further surgery to correct the situation.

Preoperative antibiotics are not necessary, but postoperative antibiotics are usually given for 1 week in either ointment or drop form, with or without steroids. Eye patches after strabismus surgery are usually not necessary, especially if a fornix approach is used. We use a patch only when it is necessary to hold down the ends of adjustable sutures. Patients in whom there is a chance of obtaining or losing binocular fusion are examined postoperatively within a few days. In most other cases the first postoperative visit is 6 weeks later. By this time practically all tissue healing has occurred, and the alignment has reached a stable position, permitting further evaluation and decisions for subsequent management.

Operating room procedures

General, local or topical anesthesia may be used for strabismus surgery. With all forms of anesthesia, traction on the eye muscles causes slowing of the heart because of the oculocardiac reflex, although this is less severe with local anesthesia. We prefer local anesthesia for most adult cases because of convenience to the patient and speed of recovery. However, forced duction testing cannot be done as effectively under local anesthesia. Also, repeated local injections are sometimes required.

For local anesthesia we use an equal mixture of 2 per cent lidocaine (lignocaine; Xylocaine) and 0.75 per cent bupivacaine (Marcaine). However, if an adjustable suture is used, we prefer only 2 per cent lidocaine to allow full recovery from anesthesia effects by the time suture adjustment is done. Topical anesthesia is only used in selected cases in which muscle function must be preserved during the operation.

Proper exposure of the operative field and access to all parts of the eye from different directions are important to obtain best results from surgery. The patient's head is placed on a narrow platform extending from the operating table. This allows the surgeon and assistant to be positioned on either side of the patient and to reach easily all portions of the operative field. *Both* eyes are usually 'prepped' to permit comparison of one eye with the other, even though surgery is planned for only one eye. Loupes are used to provide added magnification, and a fiberoptic head-lamp is sometimes helpful with deep surgical dissections.

Sharp, forward-projecting toothed forceps are essential for adequate traction on the globe during strabismus surgery. We prefer 0.5 mm Castroviejo toothed forceps. Blunt Westcott scissors are used for conjunctival incisions, dissection and disinsertion of muscles. We do not use sharp-pointed scissors, to reduce the risk of causing a scleral laceration. Standard locking 'micro' needle holders are used. We prefer two types of muscle hooks – the small Stevens hook and a larger, ball-tipped Jamison muscle hook.

Coated polyglactin (Vicryl) sutures of 6/0 size are used for most muscle surgery including adjustable sutures. If a permanent suture is needed for a superior oblique tuck or a faden procedure, 5/0 Dacron, Mersilene or Supramyd is used. We prefer the Ethicon S-24 spatula needle for most strabismus surgery.

Implantable materials such as Supramyd sheets and sleeves have been advocated by some surgeons to avoid problems from excessive scarring that may occur after reoperations. These materials have not been widely used, however, and may not be as effective as originally hoped. Some experimentation has been performed with tissue adhesives, but these have not yet found a place in strabismus surgery.

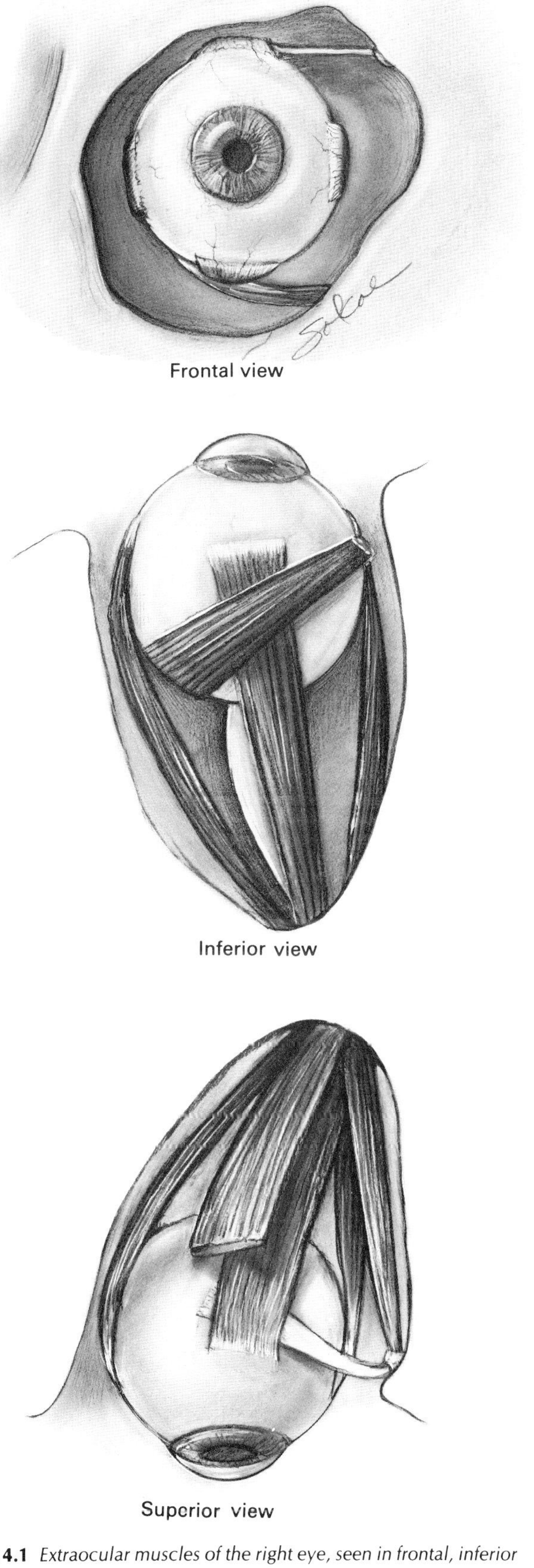

Figure 4.1 *Extraocular muscles of the right eye, seen in frontal, inferior and superior views*

Surgical anatomy

The six extraocular muscles of the right eye, with the other periocular tissues removed, are illustrated in *Figure 4.1*. The nasal orbital wall is nearly parallel to the sagittal plane, and the orbital apex is located somewhat nasally relative to the center of the globe. This relationship between the center of the globe and the somewhat nasal origin of the rectus muscles from the orbital apex is important for two reasons. First, this causes an intorting action by the superior rectus muscle and an extorting action by the inferior rectus muscle. Second, the medial rectus muscle leaves the surface of the globe slightly anterior to the equator, whereas the lateral rectus muscle is tangent to the globe well posterior to the equator. Because of this difference in the point where the muscles become tangent to the globe, the faden procedure (posterior fixation procedure) is much more effective on the medial rectus muscle than on the lateral rectus muscle. In fact, it is difficult to place a posterior fixation suture far enough posterior on the lateral rectus muscle to achieve a good effect.

The superior and inferior obliques pass posterior to the vertical axis of rotation of the eye, which accounts for their abducting effect. Also, the superior and inferior rectus muscles pass slightly nasal to the vertical axis of rotation, explaining their weak adducting effect. The superior and inferior oblique muscles pass inferior to the superior and inferior rectus muscles respectively.

The average locations of the rectus muscle insertions from the limbus are illustrated in *Figure 4.2*. The distance between the limbus and the rectus muscle insertions increases in a spiral-like fashion. The distance is closest nasally and farthest superiorly. This spiral is known as the spiral of Tillaux. The insertions of the superior and inferior rectus muscles are not parallel to the limbus but are closer nasally than temporally. Two anterior ciliary arteries accompany each rectus muscle except the lateral rectus muscle, which usually has only one anterior ciliary artery. These vessels supply most of the blood to the anterior segment of the eye.

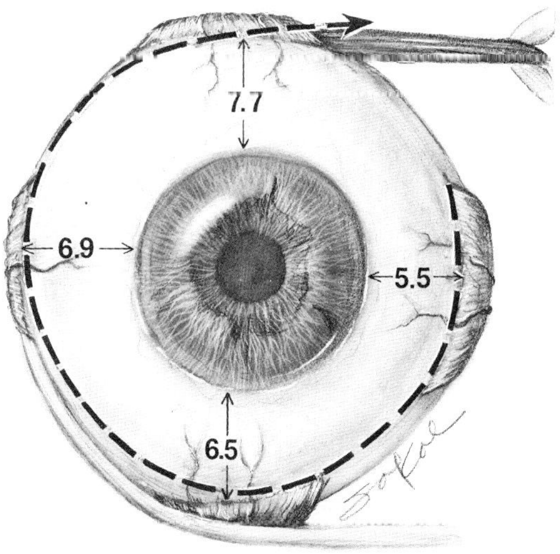

Figure 4.2 *Average locations of the rectus muscle insertions – right eye. Dashed line illustrates the spiral of Tillaux*

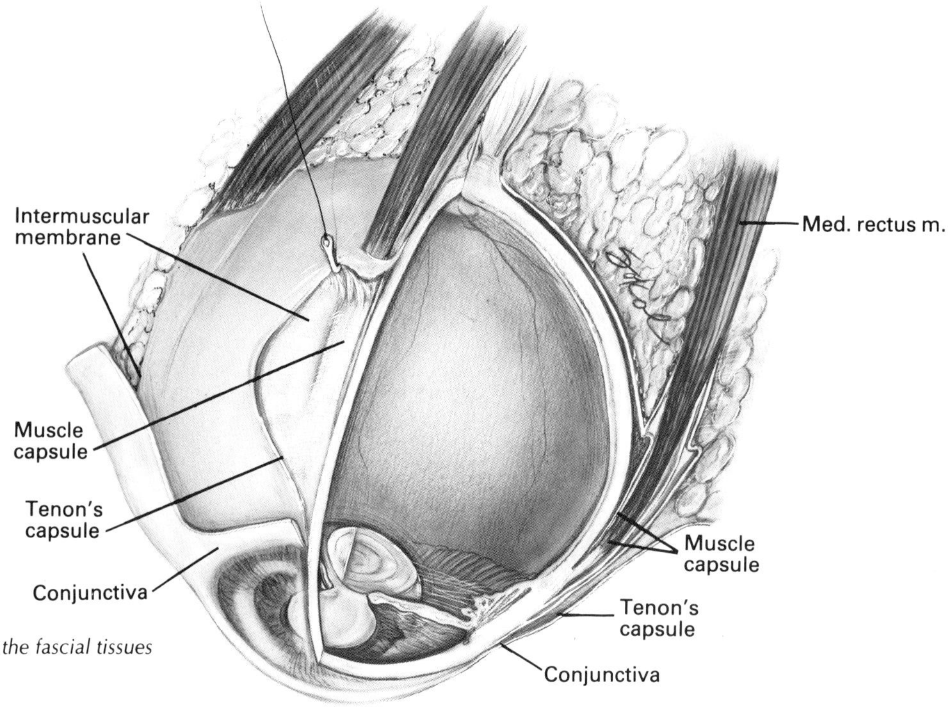

Figure 4.3 *Simplified representation of the fascial tissues surrounding the eye*

The fascial system surrounding the eye is illustrated in simplified fashion in *Figure 4.3*. Closest to the sclera an intermuscular membrane connects the anterior portions of the rectus muscles with one another, and this membrane expands to encapsulate each rectus muscle in a so-called 'muscle capsule'. Fibers from the intermuscular membrane penetrate the sclera in a line connecting the insertions of the rectus muscles. Other fibers extend anteriorly and are inserted loosely into the sclera to within 2 or 3 mm of the limbus. The intermuscular membrane posterior to the eye is not well defined. The surgeon must penetrate the intermuscular membrane to allow easy passage of a muscle hook beneath the rectus muscles, along the surface of the sclera.

Tenon's capsule extends posteriorly beneath the conjunctiva from a location about 1 mm from the limbus and is inserted into the sclera surrounding the optic nerve. The rectus muscles pass through Tenon's capsule slightly posterior to the equator and are attached to Tenon's capsule within a telescoping sleeve-like arrangement. When it is necessary to free a rectus muscle from its surrounding attachments, the attachments between the muscle and the surrounding sleeve of Tenon's capsule are severed by sharp dissection. After this is done, the muscle can be lost posterior to the globe if it slips from the surgeon's grasp or from the suture.

All strabismus surgery should be performed between Tenon's capsule and the sclera because Tenon's capsule separates the space surrounding the globe (sub-Tenon's space) from the extensive cushion of fat surrounding the eye within the orbit. Incisions into the fatty tissue can result in increased scarring and even the severe adherence syndrome that causes postoperative limitation of ocular movement. There is a safe zone extending about 10 mm posterior to the limbus through which Tenon's capsule can be safely incised to gain access to the sub-Tenon's space. Beyond the 10 mm distance, however, no incision should ever be made through Tenon's capsule unless one is prepared to deal with unpredictable scarring and limitation of movement. In addition to the tissues illustrated in *Figure 4.3*, there are numerous fascial planes external to Tenon's capsule, separating lobules of fatty tissue and extending to the periosteum of the orbital wall. These fascial planes are more extensive than was previously believed, as demonstrated by the painstaking work of Koornneef[8].

The thickness of the sclera at various points from the limbus to the posterior pole is shown in *Figure 4.4*. The sclera is thinnest just behind the insertions of the rectus muscles, in the area where sutures are frequently placed during recession procedures. Development of spatula needles was a major advance over the previously used reverse cutting needles in avoiding perforation of the sclera.

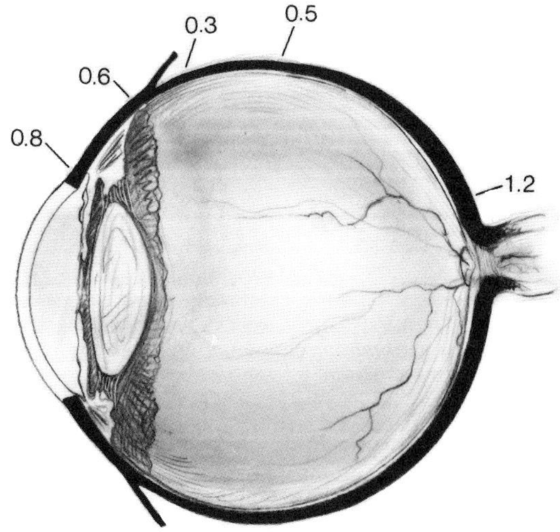

Figure 4.4 *Scleral thickness in millimeters at various locations from the limbus to the optic nerve*

Surgical techniques

Forced ductions

Forced ('passive') ductions should be performed at the beginning of every strabismus procedure. Even if no limitation of movement is suspected, the maneuver is done to aid the surgeon in judging the range of normal forced ductions. Sharp-toothed forceps with forward-pointing teeth are necessary to grasp the globe.

Simple forced ductions of the eye, with the globe in the normal position in the orbit, are not especially useful unless there is gross restriction of movement. An exaggerated form of traction test is necessary to feel minor or moderate restrictions or contractures of muscles. The exaggerated traction test for a rectus muscle is done by grasping the sclera near the limbus adjacent to the rectus muscle and pulling the globe forward as far as possible to put the rectus muscle on maximum stretch. The globe is then moved out of the field of action of the muscle being tested. Tightness of the muscle is indicated if the globe retracts backward before it ordinarily should. Experience is necessary to judge the normal range of movement, but by pulling the globe forward the surgeon can feel lesser degrees of rectus tightness than would otherwise be possible.

Similarly, to feel minor or moderate degrees of oblique muscle tightness, an exaggerated form of traction test must be used[9]. The exaggerated traction test for the left superior oblique muscle is illustrated in *Figure 4.5*. The nasal forceps must have a substantial grasp of sclera, because the key to the procedure is pushing the nasal forceps deep into the superonasal quadrant, then moving the forceps temporally to roll the eye over the superior oblique tendon. To judge inferior oblique tightness, the nasal forceps are pushed into the inferonasal quadrant and the forceps are then moved temporally. The procedure can be performed with only the nasal forceps, but the temporal forceps add better control of the globe. Every normal inferior and superior oblique can be felt with this procedure; if a normal oblique muscle is not felt, the test is not being performed correctly. On a scale of zero to 4+, we judge normal inferior obliques as averaging 1+ tightness and superior obliques as averaging 1.5+ tightness. The superior oblique is more easily felt, because there are no tissues interposed between the superior oblique tendon and the globe, whereas other tissues are present between the inferior oblique muscle and the globe.

A unilateral paretic superior oblique muscle can easily be felt with this exaggerated traction test. Overacting obliques often feel tighter than normal, especially in long-standing cases. The most valuable application of this procedure, however, is in determining whether a complete superior oblique tenotomy has been performed. If only a few posterior fibers remain after attempting to cut the tendon, a tight band will still be felt.

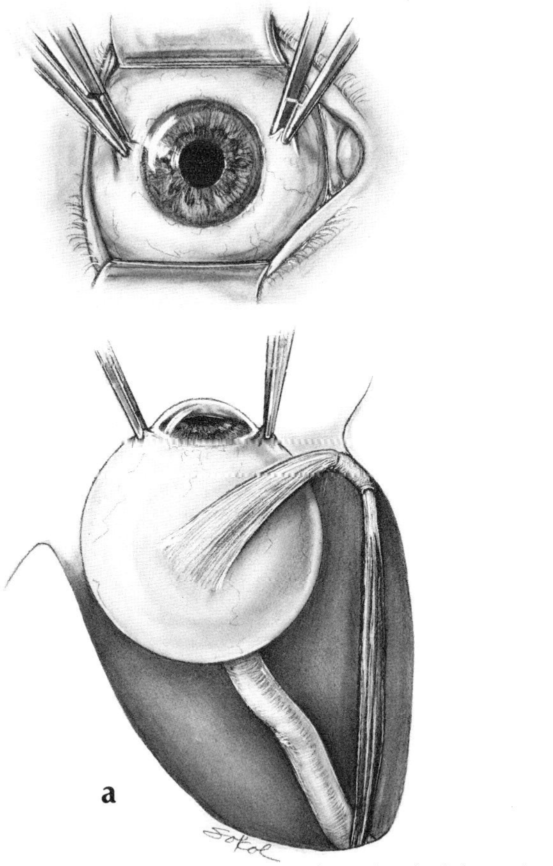

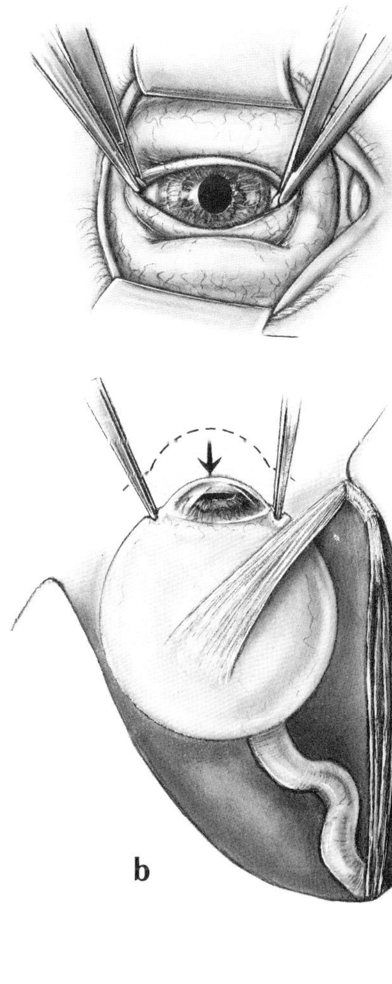

Figure 4.5 *The exaggerated traction test performed on the left superior oblique muscle.* **(a)** *The globe grasped near the limbus at the 3 and 9 o'clock positions using toothed forceps.* **(b)** *Retroplacement of the globe, placing the superior oblique muscle on stretch*

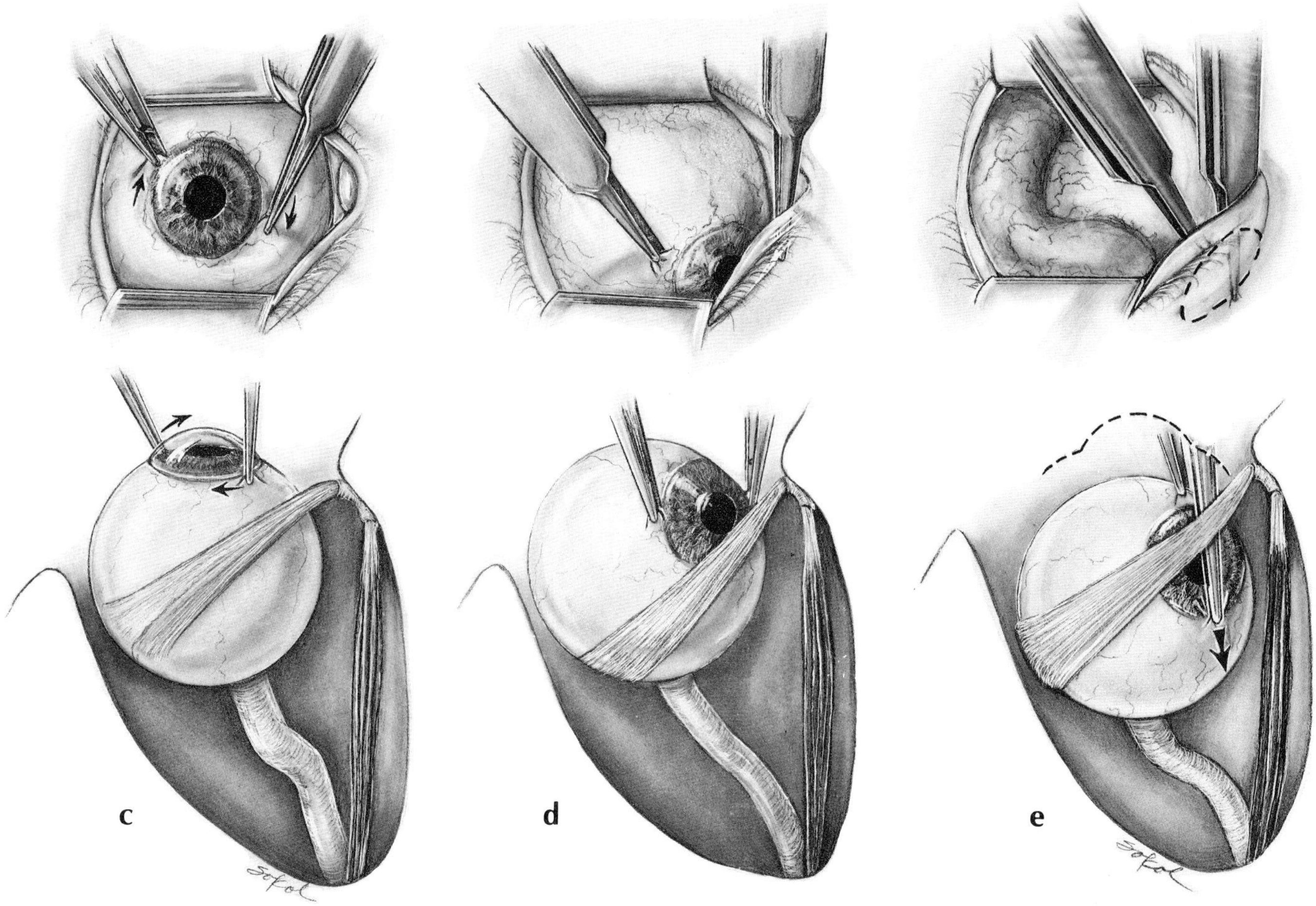

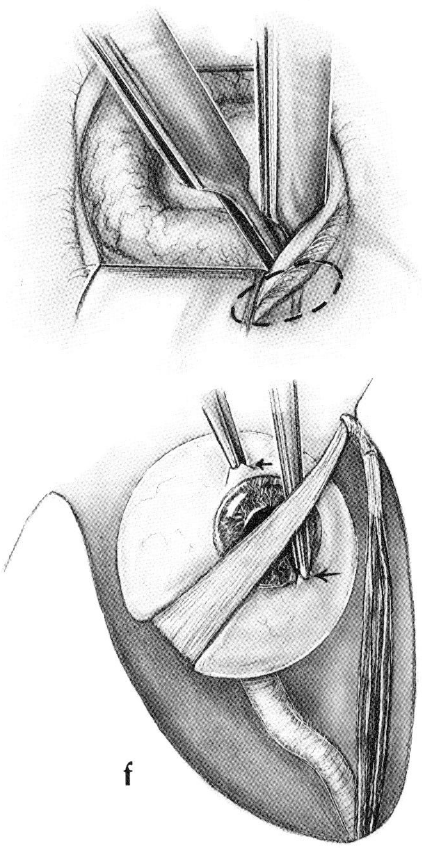

Figure 4.5 (Contd)
(c) *Extorsion of the globe, placing the superior oblique muscle on stretch.* **(d)** *Rotation of the globe superonasally, again placing the superior oblique muscle on stretch.* **(e)** *A maneuver combining the effects of b, c and d, whereby the nasal forceps are plunged superonasally, retroplacing the globe, extorting it and rotating it superonasally. The temporal forceps follow passively.* **(f)** *Both forceps are moved temporally to put the superior oblique muscle on maximum stretch, and tightness of the muscle can be felt easily by the surgeon.* **(g)** *The two pairs of forceps are moved to begin to rock the globe over the taut superior oblique tendon.* **(h)** *The superior oblique tendon slips over the surface of the globe. The amount of this sudden movement is felt by the surgeon and equated with amount of tightness of the superior oblique muscle*

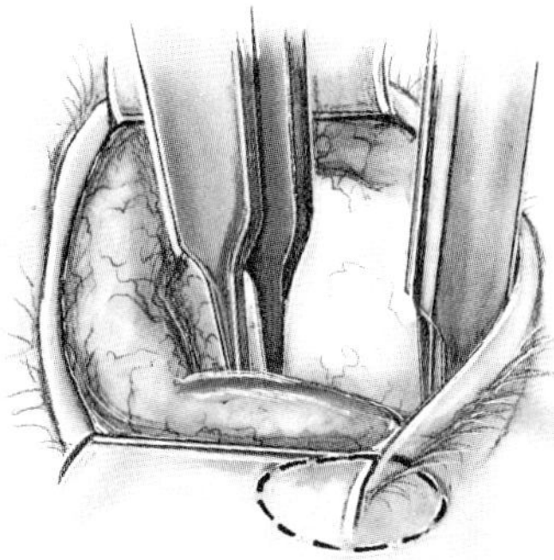

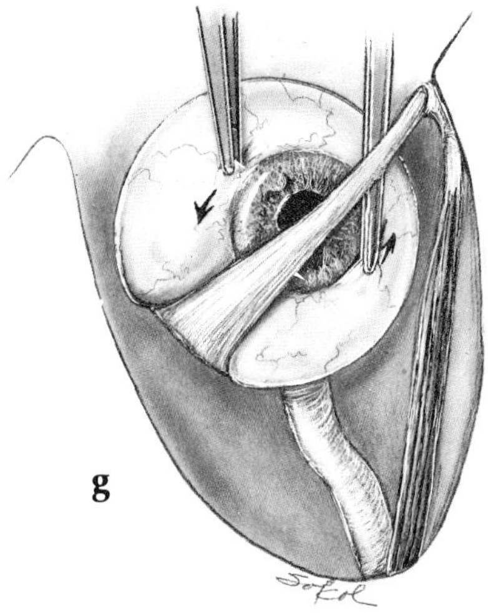

g

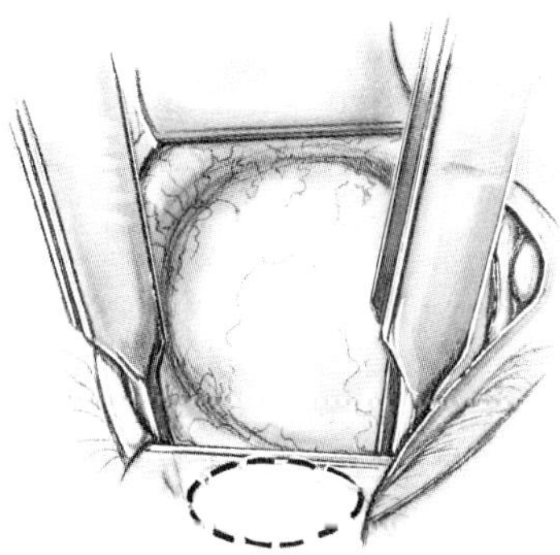

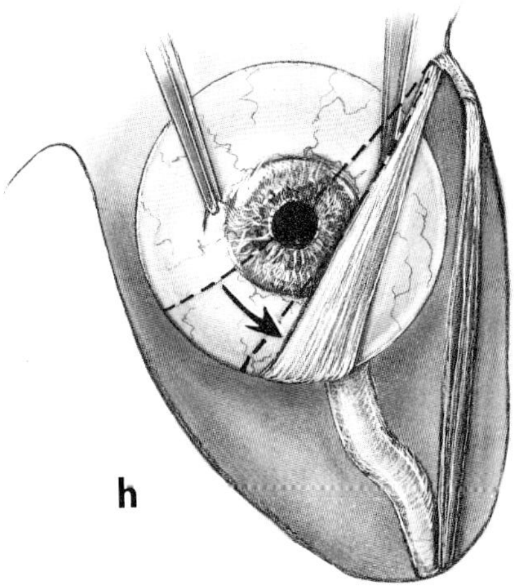

h

Conjunctival incisions

Two forms of conjunctival incisions are used: the limbal incision and the fornix incision. Other conjunctival incisions, those within the palpebral fissure near the insertion of the muscle, often cause excessive conjunctival scarring. Even the limbal incisions (*see Figure 4.6*) can cause noticeable scarring. For this reason, we use the fornix approach almost exclusively (*see Figure 4.8*).

The fornix approach is aesthetically pleasing, more comfortable for the patient postoperatively and may be performed more quickly, for no fixation sutures are needed to hold the globe and usually no closing sutures are necessary. The fornix incision is particularly useful for reoperations, as anterior scarring from previous operations can be avoided completely. Surprisingly little scarring occurs in the area of the fornix incision, and repeat surgery through this area can be done without difficulty.

Recession of a rectus muscle: limbal approach

Recession of a left medial rectus muscle is illustrated in *Figure 4.6*, using the limbal conjunctival approach. Although we rarely use the limbal conjunctival incision, it has the advantages of requiring less skill on the part of the assistant and giving better exposure of the muscle. Therefore it is ideal for initial teaching of muscle surgery.

Fixation sutures placed in midthickness sclera superiorly and inferiorly are used to advantage with the limbal approach to provide optimal exposure. The conjunctiva and underlying Tenon's capsule are incised as close to the limbus as possible to avoid postoperative scarring. The 'wings' of the incision are made rather far superiorly and inferiorly, outside the palpebral fissure, to minimize exposure of scarring which occurs at these sites.

We use a double-armed polyglactin (Vicryl) 6/0 suture to secure the muscle before disinserting it from the globe. The muscle is sutured to the globe in a forward V fashion, bringing the suture ends out of the sclera near one another to improve holding of the suture by the first throw of the knot. Absorbable 8/0 collagen sutures are used to close the wings of the conjunctival incision, and the conjunctiva is pulled slightly over the limbus for optimal wound healing without a visible conjunctival scar near the limbus. If the conjunctiva is tight or if increased effect is desired from the recession, the conjunctiva can be recessed with the edge sutured to the sclera posteriorly, usually at the previous insertion site of the muscle. However, the conjunctiva is rarely tight enough to require recession, and we prefer the fornix approach for most reoperations.

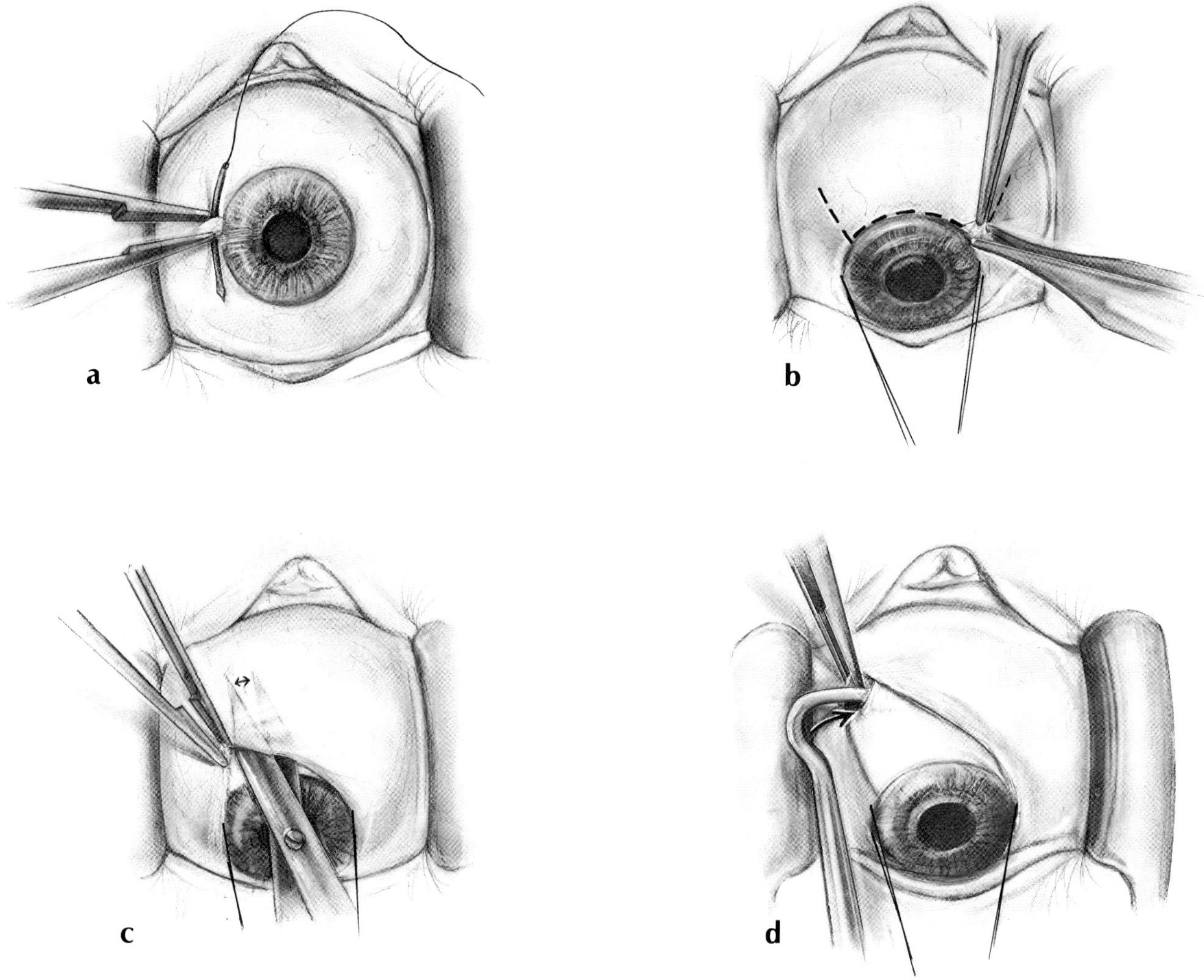

Figure 4.6 *Recession of the left medial rectus muscle by the limbal approach.* **(a)** *Fixation suture of 4/0 silk on a spatula needle is placed in midthickness sclera at 6 o'clock.* **(b)** *Globe held temporally by fixation sutures at 6 and 12 o'clock clamped to the drape. Limbal incision is made with blunt Westcott scissors through conjunctiva and underlying Tenon's capsule. Incision is along the limbus within the palpebral fissue area. Radial relaxing incisions are made at either end under the normal positions of the lid.* **(c)** *Blunt dissection through intermuscular membrane is performed inferior and superior to the medial rectus muscle.* **(d)** *The medial rectus muscle is hooked with a Jamison muscle hook, sliding the hook along bare sclera.* **(e)** *Sharp dissection with the Westcott scissors to cut the 'check ligaments', that is, the attachments between Tenon's capsule and the muscle capsule.* **(f)** *Sharp dissection of the intermuscular membrane from each edge of the muscle. Careful placement of small muscle hooks for retraction by the assistant aids greatly in exposure and proper dissection.* **(g)** *Muscle secured by double-armed 6/0 polyglactin acid (Vicryl) suture (see Figure 4.8j for detail of suture placement).* **(h)** *Muscle disinserted from globe with Westcott scissors, shaving the insertion as flush as possible to the globe.* **(i)** *Minimal cautery applied to insertion site as necessary.* **(j)** *Compression mark from caliper applied to sclera 4 mm posterior to the prior insertion to indicate the intended site for the first needle pass. Measurement is made not from the insertion but from the point where the suture was originally passed through the muscle, about 1 mm posterior to the insertion site.* **(k)** *Needle passes are slanted forward and toward one another to bring the two suture ends out within 1 mm of each other. This provides optimal holding of the first throw of the knot. Ethicon S-24 needles are preferred.* **(l)** *Surgeon's knot is completed with three throws, and suture ends are excised.* **(m)** *Saline is applied to the conjunctiva, and the conjunctiva is 'milked' toward the limbus with a large muscle hook to identify the wings, thereby enabling proper apposition of the wound margins.* **(n)** *Both wings are closed with interrupted 8/0 collagen sutures, placing the sutures so as to stretch the conjunctiva along the limbus, pulling the conjunctiva slightly over the limbal wound margin to ensure proper healing without gape*

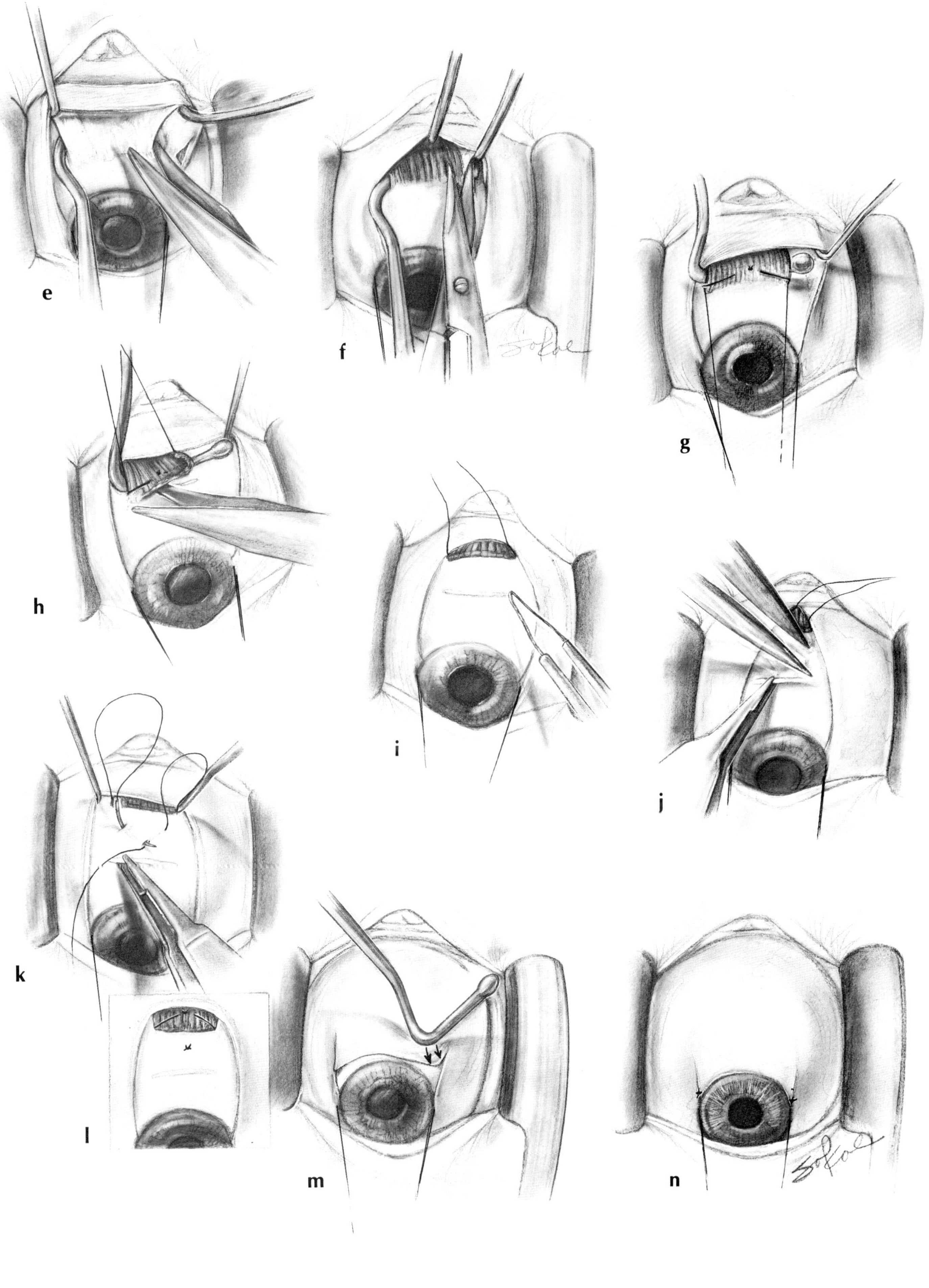
e
f
g
h
i
j
k
l
m
n

Resection of a rectus muscle: limbal approach

Our preferred technique for resection of a rectus muscle is illustrated in *Figure 4.7*. We prefer the fornix approach, but the limbal conjunctival approach is used for convenience in the illustration. A double-armed 6/0 polyglactin (Vicryl) suture is used. When tying the knot after a large amount of resection has been done, the assistant rotates the globe posteriorly by grasping the original insertion with forceps. This allows the surgeon to pull the resected muscle stump anterior for proper apposition of the muscle to the old insertion site.

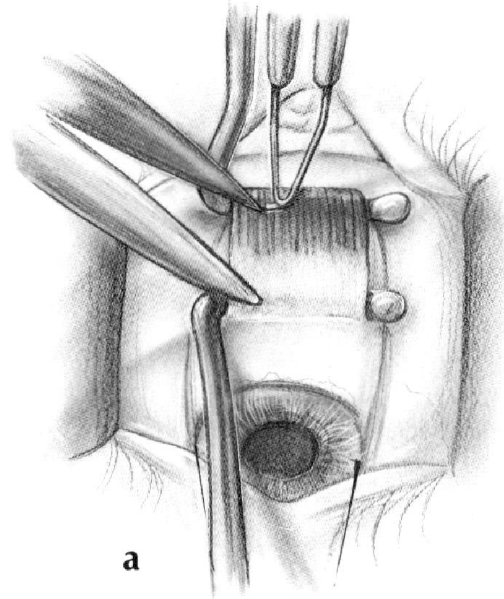
a

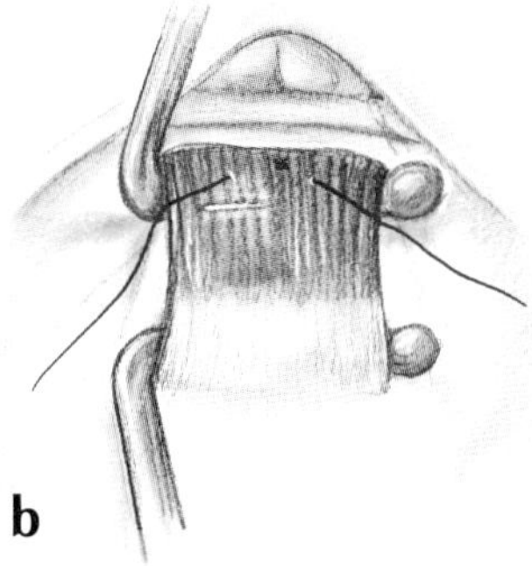
b

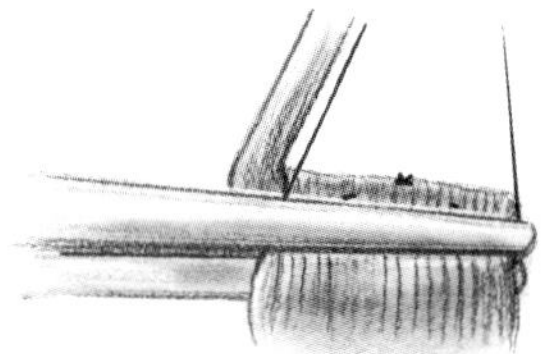
c

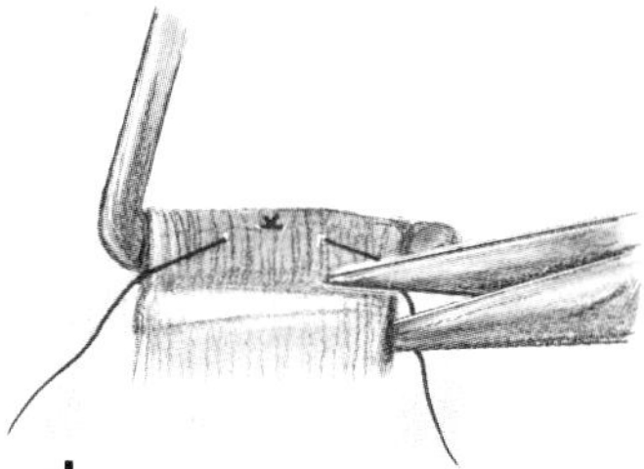
d

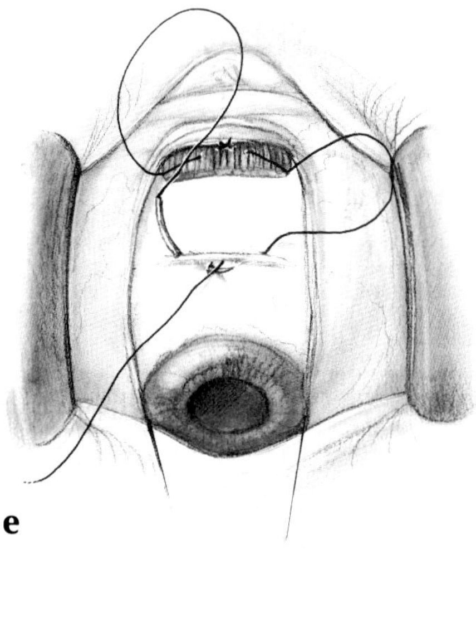
e

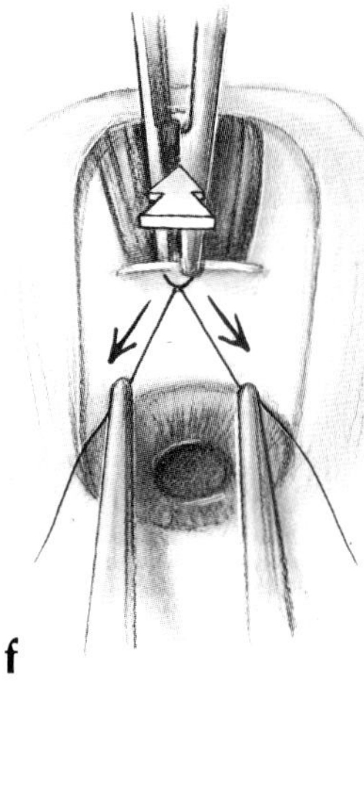
f

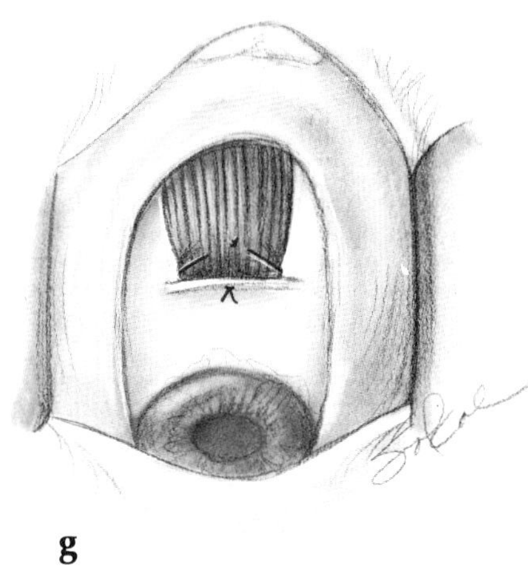
g

Figure 4.7 *Resection of the left medial rectus muscle, using the limbal conjunctival approach illustrated in Figure 4.6.* **(a)** *Attachments between the muscle capsule and overlying Tenon's capsule and to the intermuscular membrane on either side of the muscle are divided far posteriorly to avoid pulling posterior tissue forward with the resection procedure. The assistant holds two Jamison muscle hooks beneath the muscle without causing excessive stretching, and the amount of resection is marked with light cautery. The anterior end of the calipers is placed on top of the anterior muscle hook.* **(b)** *A double-armed polyglactin acid (Vicryl) suture is used to secure the muscle, placing the initial knot in the middle of the muscle 2 mm posterior to the cautery mark. The suture ends are slanted forward on either side so that they exit from the edges of the muscle in line with the cautery mark. This method of suture placement provides support for the middle portion of the muscle and prevents the suture from slipping off the end of the muscle with subsequent 'loss' of the muscle.* **(c)** *The muscle is clamped for a few moments anterior to the suture to aid in controlling bleeding.* **(d)** *The portion of the muscle between the clamp site and the original insertion is excised with Westcott scissors.* **(e)** *The two needles are placed back through the original insertion site while slanting them toward each other. The sutures exit within 1 mm of each other for optimal tying of the knot.* **(f)** *The assistant rotates the eye posteriorly by holding the original insertion with forceps while the sutures are pulled anteriorly to bring the shortened muscle to the insertion without undue stretching.* **(g)** *The muscle stump has been resutured to the insection site. Conjunctival closure is the same as in Figure 4.6m and n*

Recession of a rectus muscle: fornix approach with adjustable suture

The lower fornix is preferable for fornix incisions because the conjunctiva is more redundant there, and the edges fall together easily without the use of sutures. Successful surgery using the fornix approach requires a skillful and experienced assistant to provide proper exposure. Fornix approach surgery has been dubbed by proponents of the limbal approach as 'peek-a-boo' surgery, and indeed such a label is appropriate without proper experience on the part of the surgeon and the assistant. With proper technique, fornix approach surgery is faster, more comfortable for the patient and leaves less scarring. It is now our preferred technique, almost to the exclusion of other approaches.

Recession of a right lateral rectus muscle using the fornix approach and an adjustable suture is illustrated in *Figure 4.8*. Adjustable sutures were first described with a limbal conjunctival incision, and they have not been widely adopted by surgeons using the fornix approach. However, with the technique illustrated in *Figure 4.8*, an adjustable suture can be easily used with the fornix approach, and the final knot is buried completely under the conjunctiva.

The method of suture placement illustrated in *Figure 4.8j* deserves special mention. A central bite is first taken in the muscle tendon several millimeters from the insertion, and a square knot is tied. This initial knot supports the center portion of the muscle which is positioned at the apex of the 'V' formed by later placement of the sutures in the lateral portions of the muscle tendon. It is also a safety knot should other portions of the suture pull out either during or after the operation.

With the adjustable suture technique the muscle is allowed to 'hang back' from essentially a single site of attachment. This has been criticized by those who believe that the muscle should always be splayed out on the sclera in a manner similar to its original insertion. However, to the best of our knowledge, there have been no problems with muscle function associated with this method of using a sling suture.

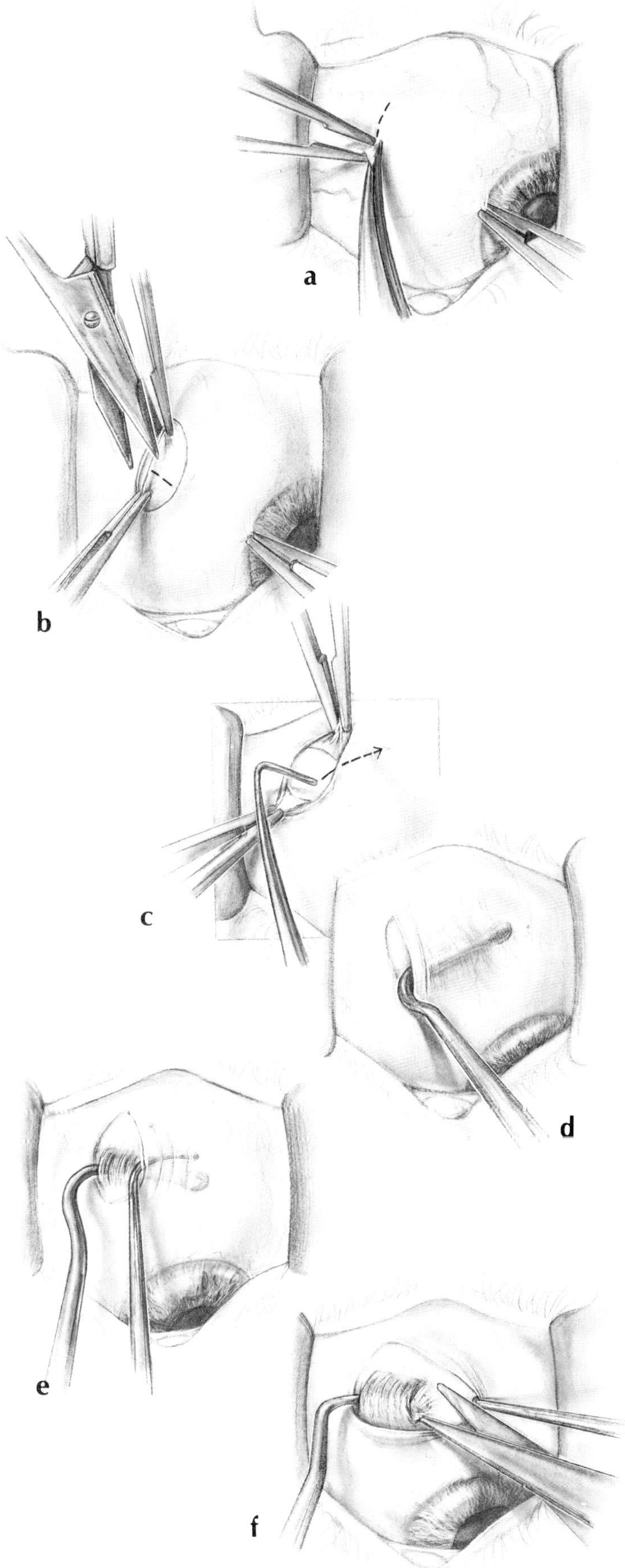

Figure 4.8 *Recession of the right lateral rectus muscle using fornix approach and adjustable suture.* **(a)** *Conjunctival incision is made in the inferotemporal quadrant 8 or 9 mm from the limbus in an arc parallel to the folds of tissue in the fornix. This incision should not be made farther posterior, to avoid the heavy vessels and fat in the fornix.* **(b)** *The assistant holds the eye superonasally with toothed forceps as Tenon's capsule is grasped and incised down to sclera with blunt Westcott scissors. This incision is at a right angle to the original incision to allow better wound closure.* **(c)** *A small muscle hook is placed against the sclera and slid under the lower portion of the muscle insertion.* **(d)** *The small hook is followed by a Jamison muscle hook. A second Jamison muscle hook is passed if there is question as to whether the entire insertion is hooked.* **(e)** *Conjunctiva and Tenon's capsule are reflected with a small muscle hook over the end of the Jamison muscle hook, bringing the muscle out through the incision. Pulling the muscle down toward the incision also helps in this maneuver. The tip of the small hook should be visualized at all times through the conjunctiva and Tenon's capsule to be certain that all portions of these tissues are reflected over the end of the large hook. If a doubling over of these tissues occurs instead, a large buttonhole will be cut in the next step.* **(f)** *As the assistant holds the conjunctiva superiorly with the small hook, a small buttonhole is made with scissors through the intermuscular membrane beneath the ball of the Jamison muscle hook. The closed scissors are introduced into this hole, and remaining tissues are reflected over the ball of the muscle hook.*

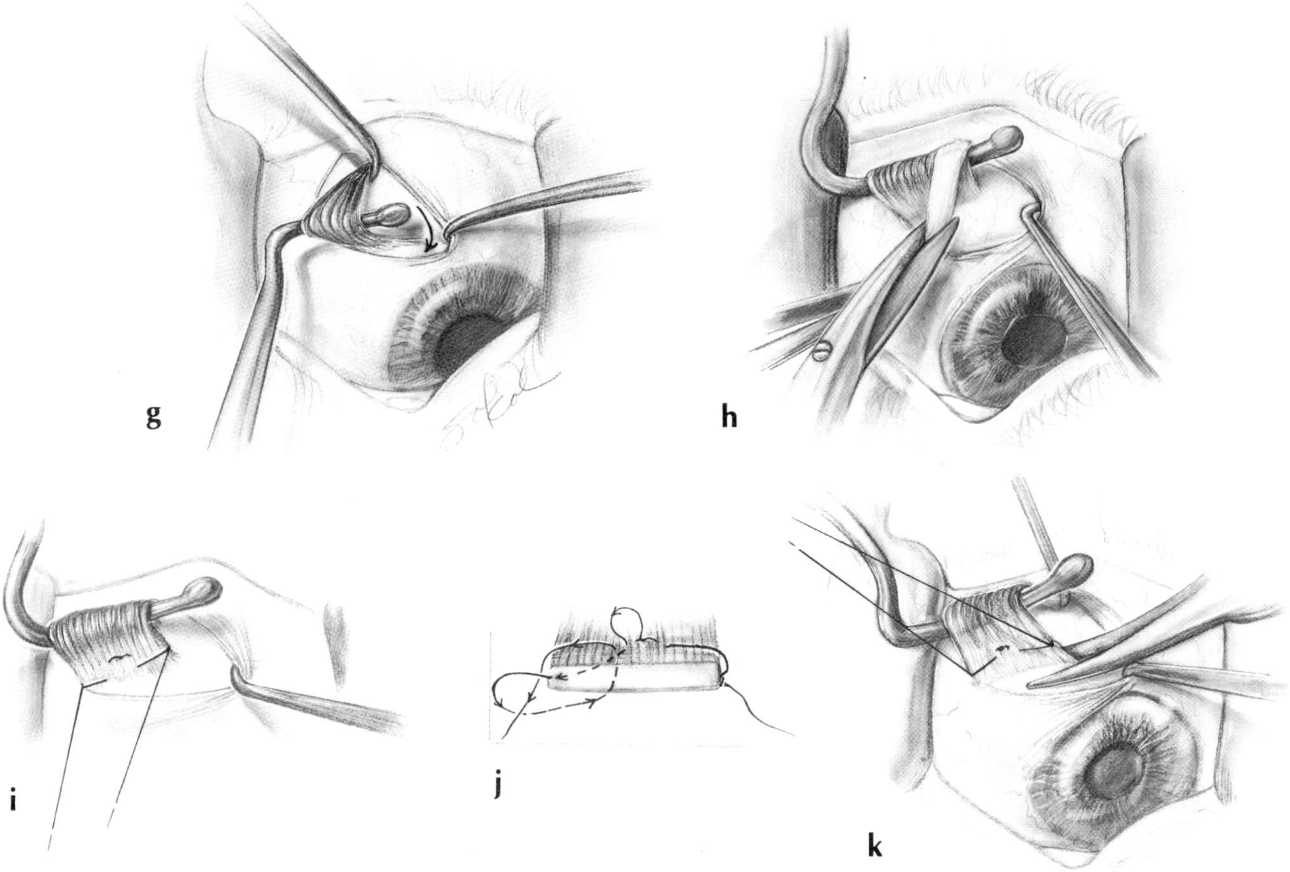

Figure 4.8 (contd)
(g) *The assistant then introduces two small muscle hooks into the perforation through the intermuscular membrane and sweeps the superior hook around the superior border of the insertion, keeping the tip on bare sclera to be certain that all of the insertional fibers have been included on the large muscle hook. This is an important maneuver, for missed muscle fibers can seriously affect the surgical results. Direct visualization is not always adequate to check for missed muscle fibers, and sweeping with the small hook should always be done.* **(h)** *The insertion area is cleared of overlying tissues by sharp dissection while attempting to leave as much of this fascia on the sclera as possible to cover over the insertion site and the thin sclera posterior to the insertion. These areas may show through the conjunctiva and appear grey postoperatively.* **(i, j)** *The muscle tendon is secured with a double-armed 6/0 coated polyglactin (Vicryl) suture. Detail of the suture placement is shown in view (j). A central bite is taken and tied with a square knot 2 or 3 mm from the insertion. Then each end of the suture is passed forward through split-thickness tendon toward the edge of the insertion. The exit site of this split-thickness bite determines the point at which the muscle will be held by the suture when it is reattached. A full-thickness pass is then made from beneath the muscle, bringing the suture through the muscle about one-third the distance across and locking it at the outside corner. Vicryl sutures, even the coated type, tend to catch loose connective tissue and effectively tie upon themselves. The large loops of suture placed around the muscle do not draw up tightly, and therefore the muscle is not bunched up. By placing the suture in this manner, there is never any question as to whether or not the muscle is twisted when it is resutured to the globe.* **(k)** *The muscle is disinserted from the globe using blunt Westcott scissors, cutting the insertion as flush as possible with the globe. Small bites are taken when disinserting the muscle, to avoid including a fold of sclera.* **(l)** *Bleeding points on the insertion site are lightly cauterized if necessary.* **(m)** *With the adjustable suture technique, both ends of the double-armed suture are brought through the center of the old insertion within 1 mm of each other (or in similar manner through another point of the insertion if elevation or depression of the muscle is desired). Alternatively the sutures can be brought through the sclera anterior or posterior to the insertion for better access postoperatively.* **(n)** *While making certain that both suture arms are pulled up equally, the two ends are tied together with a single overhand knot. One suture arm is cut distal to the knot, and this segment of suture is saved to use later for the adjustable noose.* **(o)** *The remaining needle is passed through the conjunctiva just posterior to the scleral exit of the sutures. Bringing this suture through conjunctiva slightly posterior to the scleral exit site allows better coverage of the eventual knot by the overlying conjunctiva.* **(p)** *The cut segment of suture is used to tie a tight noose around the two suture ends exiting from the conjunctiva. A three-throw square knot is used and tied as tightly as possible without breaking the suture. The loose ends of the noose are tied together with a single overhand knot for ease in subsequent handling.* **(q)** *The noose is slid back and forth along the muscle sutures until it slips with moderate ease. Continued back-and-forth movement along the sutures loosens the noose further, so that practically any desired amount of looseness of the noose can be obtained. The noose is positioned at a distance from the conjunctiva equalling the desired amount of recession as measured with calipers.* **(r)** *The muscle is allowed to slip back, the conjunctival incision is retracted and the amount of recession is confirmed with calipers.* **(s)** *A 4/0 silk traction suture on a spatula needle is placed through midthickness sclera near the limbus anterior to the recessed muscle. This suture is tied upon itself with one or two single overhand knots, leaving the ends 8–10 cm long to aid in the later adjustment procedure.* **(t)** *A muscle hook is used to reapproximate the edges of the conjunctival incision. This is best done after the speculum is removed and while the lower lid is retracted from the globe with another muscle hook. Any tags of Tenon's tissue protruding through the incision are excised. Usually no conjunctival sutures are necessary, even though an 'open' wound is seen for days if the lower lid is retracted. The wound eventually heals with only the faintest trace of conjunctival scar. At the end of the operation, the adjustable suture ends and the traction suture ends are brought out temporally and coiled on the surface of the lids beneath an eye patch.*

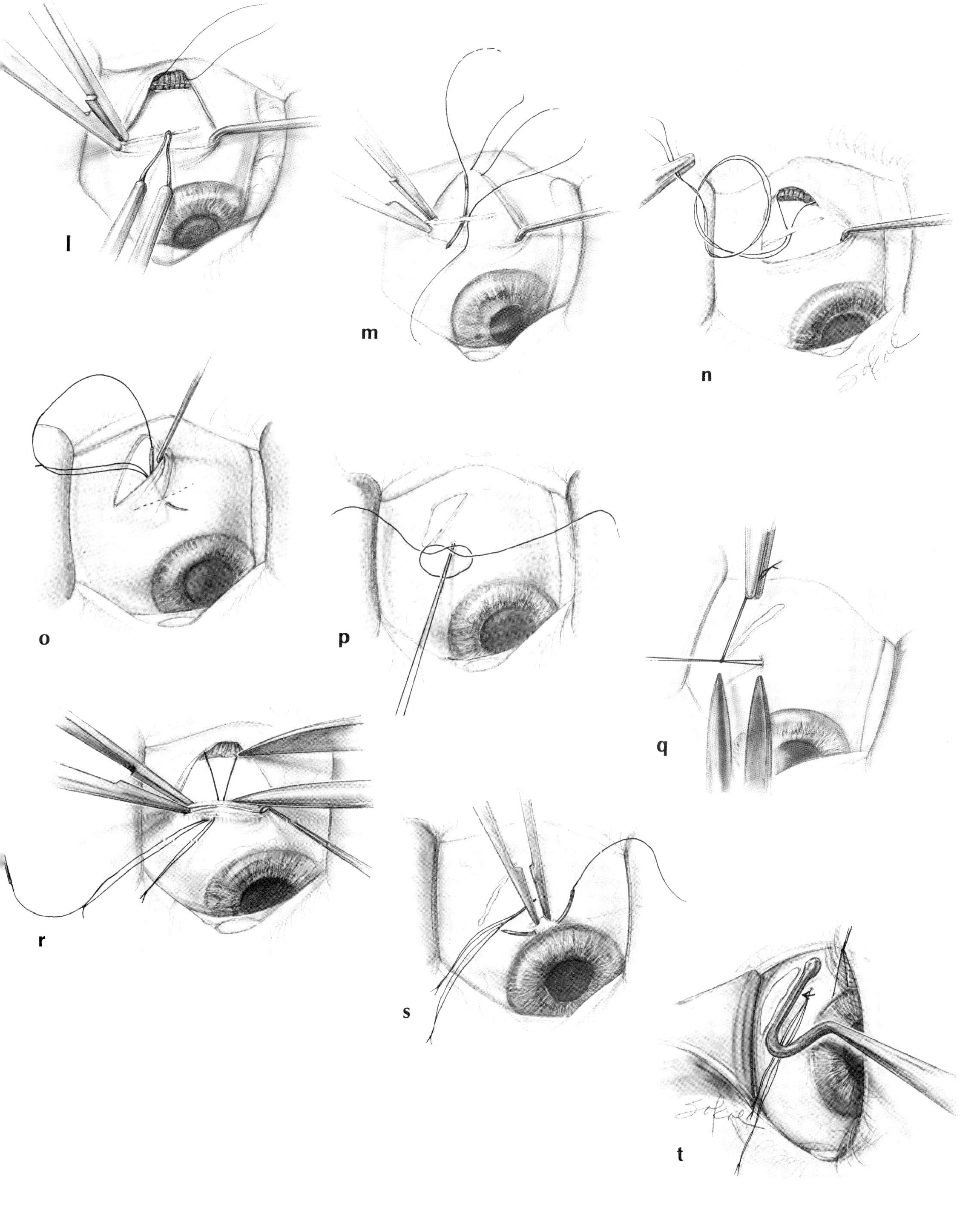
l
m
n
o
p
q
r
s
t

Postoperative adjustment of an adjustable suture

Adjustment of an adjustable suture is usually performed the morning after surgery, although it can be done the evening of the day of surgery if the patient recovers fully from the anesthesia. When local anesthesia is used it is best to wait until the following morning for final adjustment to be certain that all effects from the local anesthesia have worn off.

In our experience adjustment of the suture is necessary in about 50 per cent of cases. It is usually easier to pull the muscle forward than to move it backward. Therefore, the recessed muscle is initially recessed 2 or 3 mm farther than the amount expected to be necessary. Sometimes this added amount of recession gives the desired result, and no further adjustment is necessary. The technique of either tightening or loosening an adjustable suture postoperatively is illustrated in *Figure 4.9*.

Loosening an adjustable suture postoperatively may be difficult because discomfort may limit the patient's ability to cooperate fully in looking in the direction of the field of action of the muscle, to pull the muscle backward. Also, attachments between the muscle and the surrounding tissues may not have been adequately severed, and this may limit backward movement of the muscle. Therefore, if a large recession is needed and use of an adjustable suture is planned, the attachments between the muscle capsule and surrounding Tenon's capsule should be fully divided at the time of surgery. This allows further recession, if necessary, the following morning.

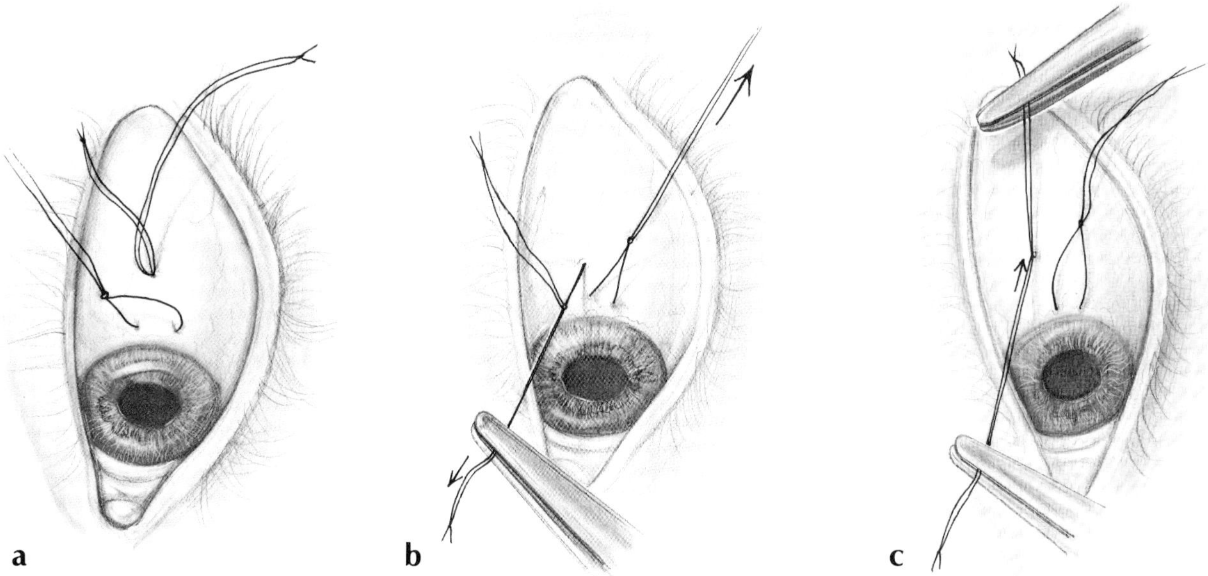

Figure 4.9 *Postoperative adjustment of the adjustable suture on the right lateral rectus muscle after procedures in Figure 4.8. Postoperative alignment is first examined, and the need for tightening or loosening the adjustable suture is determined. Topical anesthesia is used. Proparacaine (proxymetacaine) is usually adequate, but topical cocaine may be needed in some cases.* **(a)** *The muscle sutures, the noose and the traction suture are identified and separated. When the fornix approach is used, a traction suture to hold the globe is preferable to use of forceps because grasping sclera through intact conjunctiva is painful even with use of topical anesthesia. The traction suture avoids this problem entirely.* **(b)** *To tighten the recessed muscle, the muscle sutures and traction suture are pulled in opposite directions.* **(c)** *After the muscle has been pulled forward, a needle holder is used to slip the sliding noose back against the conjunctiva. This holds the muscle in place and alignment is reassessed.* **(b')** *If the muscle must be loosened, the muscle sutures are pulled forward slightly to allow grasping the sutures below the noose with one needle holder, and a second needle holder then slips the noose further forward along the muscle sutures.* **(c')** *To cause the muscle to slip backward, the eye is rotated away from the field of action of the recessed muscle by holding the traction suture, and the patient is asked to look hard in the field of action of the recessed muscle. This may be slightly painful, especially in younger persons, and the patient may not be able to cooperate fully. If necessary, a small muscle hook or forceps may be introduced through the fornix incision to push the muscle farther back. Because this procedure is usually performed at the bedside or in the office, extensive reopening of the wound is to be avoided. The muscle may be advanced, or further recessed, several times by these simple maneuvers to achieve the proper alignment.* **(d)** *After the desired alignment is obtained, the muscle suture ends are tied in a square knot on top of the noose.* **(e)** *All four suture ends are trimmed close to the knot, leaving the noose in place. The traction suture is cut and removed.* **(f)** *The conjunctiva and Tenon's capsule on both sides of the knot are grasped by toothed forceps and pulled away from the globe, allowing the knot to slip through the hole in the conjunctiva and Tenon's capsule, totally burying the suture material. If the knot is not completely buried, it can cause moderate irritation beginning several days after the operation, requiring excision of the knot. Because the healing process is rapid, the adjustable suture knot can be excised 7 days after the operation without slippage of the muscle.*

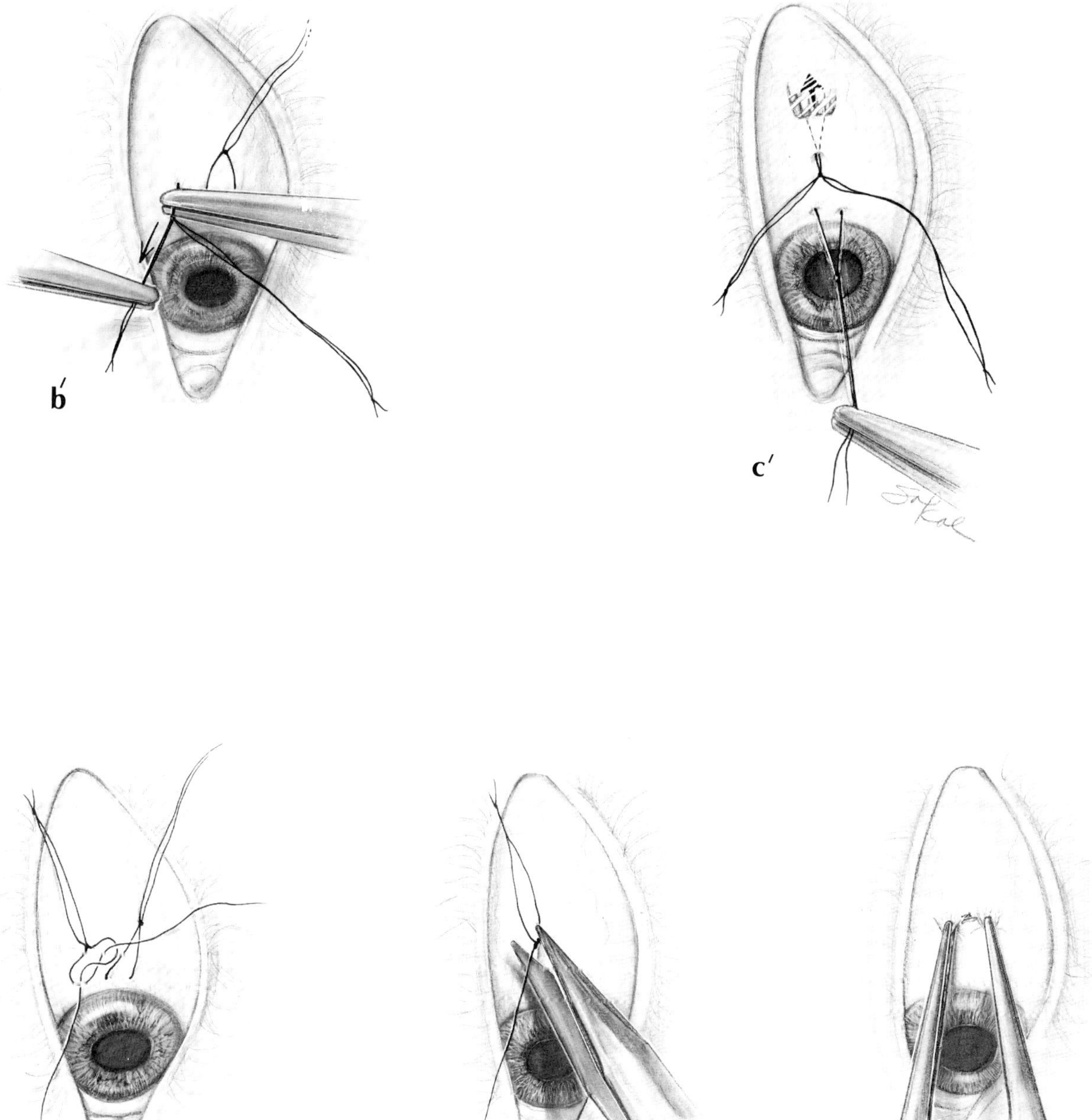
b′
c′
d
e
f

Inferior oblique weakening procedures

The inferior oblique is best approached at its insertion, not only to avoid missing some of the posterior fibers but also to avoid dissecting through Tenon's capsule which could result in prolapse of orbital fat into the wound with excessive postoperative scarring. Thus, whether the inferior oblique muscle is to be recessed or myectomized, the initial approach is the same and is illustrated in *Figure 4.10 a–h*.

Whether the inferior oblique muscle is recessed 8 or 14 mm or whether a large myectomy including denervation and 'extirpation' is performed, residual function of the inferior oblique is to be expected after healing. The exaggerated traction test, described earlier, shows that inferior oblique tightness disappears entirely at the time of the weakening procedure. However, the tightness will have returned to an essentially normal level if the test is performed again several months later, although restriction of movement may be present. This return of function and occasionally minor restriction of movement of the globe as demonstrated by the exaggerated traction test are due to reattachment of the muscle stump to the sclera or to the surrounding fascial tissues. This provides essentially normal inferior oblique function, and persistent underaction of the inferior oblique after weakening procedures is rare.

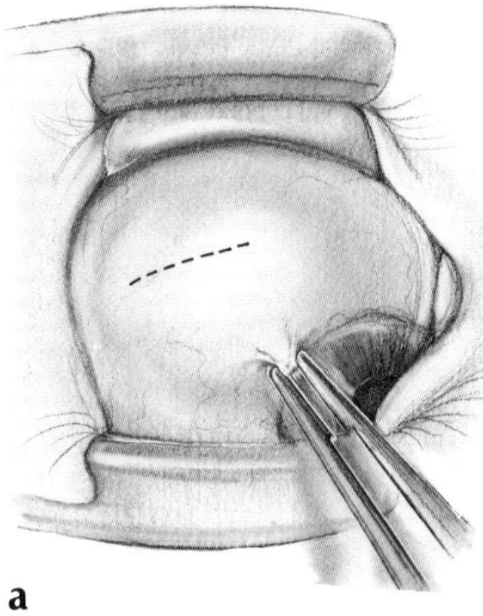

a

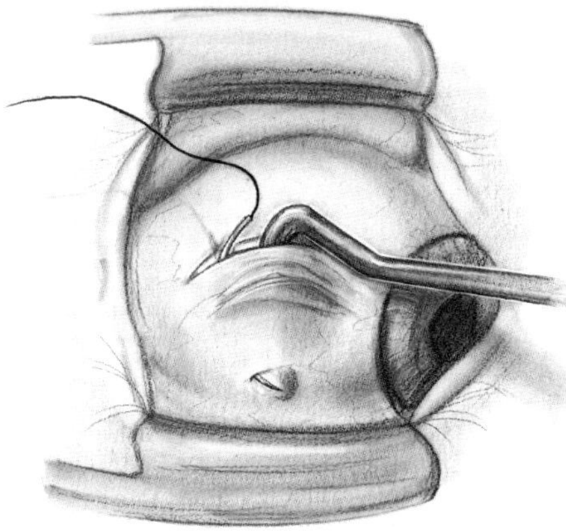

b

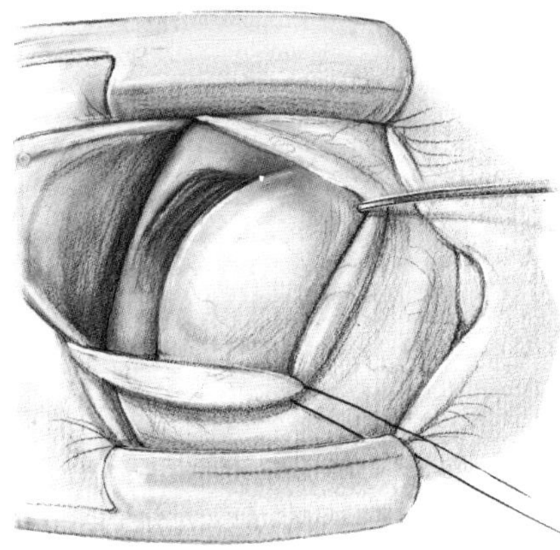

c

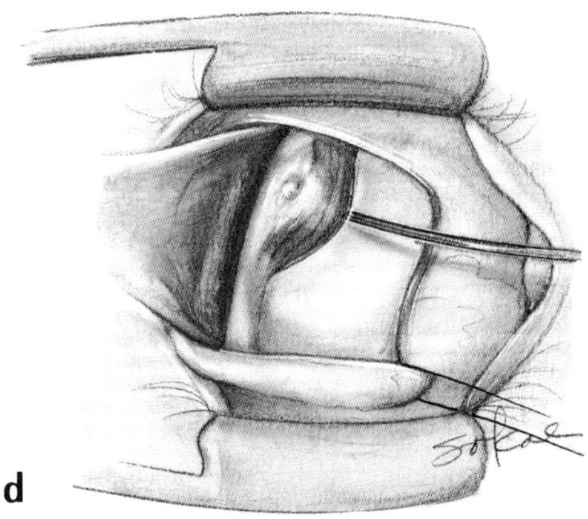

d

Figure 4.10 *Inferior oblique weakening procedures: recession and myectomy.* **(a)** *Viewed from the top of the patient's head, the left inferior oblique is approached through an inferotemporal fornix incision.* **(b)** *A large muscle hook is passed beneath the lateral rectus muscle, and a 4/0 silk suture is placed around the tendon of the lateral rectus to provide traction. The globe is rotated supersonasally, as shown in (c).* **(c)** *Direct visualization of the inferior oblique is obtained with exposure provided by a Desmarres lid retractor held deep in the wound temporarily and a small muscle hook for additional exposure.* **(d)** *The inferior oblique muscle is engaged near its insertion with the small muscle hook. Attachments between the inferior oblique muscle capsule and Tenon's capsule are still present along the temporal border.* **(e and f)** *A small cut is made with scissors along the temporal border of the inferior oblique muscle, allowing the fascial attachments to be reflected over the end of the small muscle hook, as shown in (f). The fold of connective tissue is freed from the hook without allowing the hook to penetrate Tenon's capsule, thus avoiding prolapse of fat into the wound.* **(g)** *The attachments between the inferior oblique muscle and the surrounding tissues are cut by sharp dissection down to the insertion of the muscle.* **(h)** *The muscle is clamped 1–2 mm from the insertion, and the muscle is disinserted from the globe with Westcott scissors. No significant bleeding is encountered at the insertion site, and no cautery is necessary.* **(i)** *If the inferior oblique muscle is to be recessed, the end is cauterized.* **(j)** *To allow placement of a suture in the end of the muscle, the hemostat is placed more posteriorly on the muscle, or a second hemostat is placed posterior to the first and the first is removed. A double-armed 6/0 coated polyglactin (Vicryl) suture is used. A central knot is not necessary for the inferior oblique, and the first suture pass is placed across the entire muscle width at split-thickness depth, with locking bites on either side.*

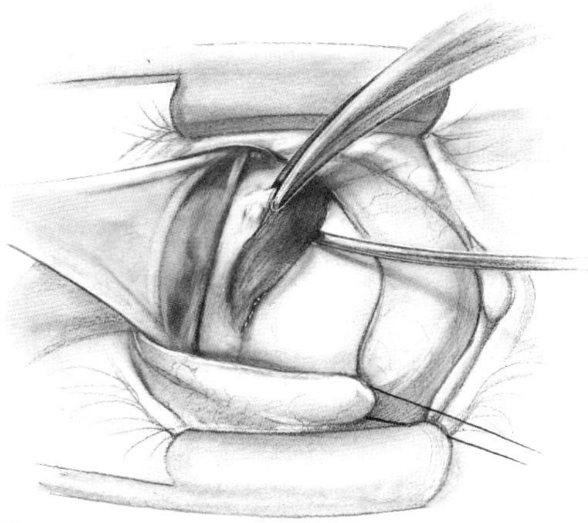

e

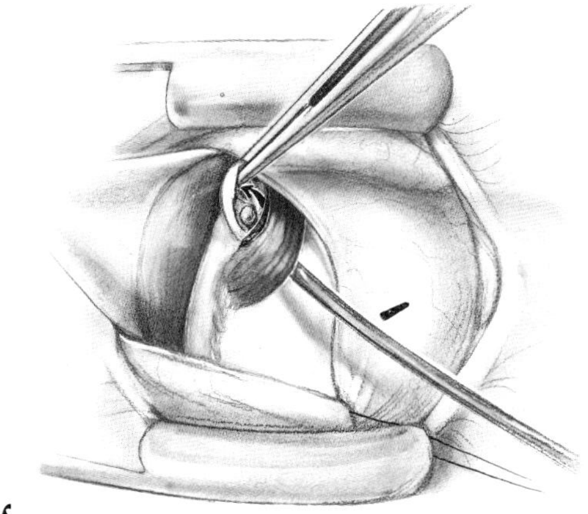

f

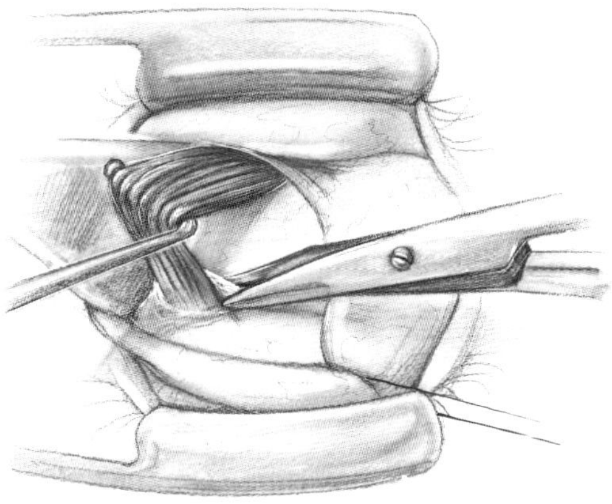

g

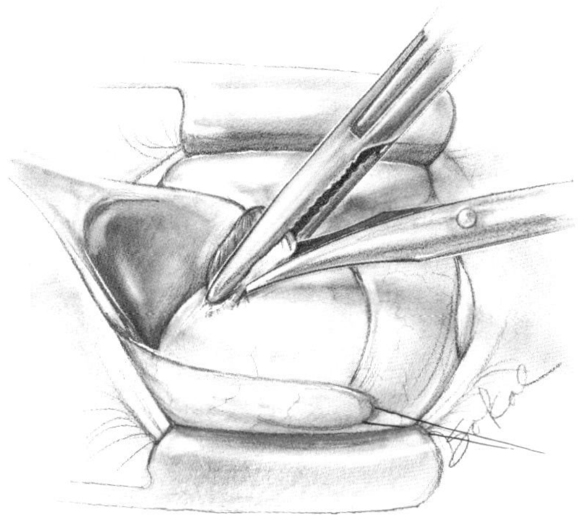

h

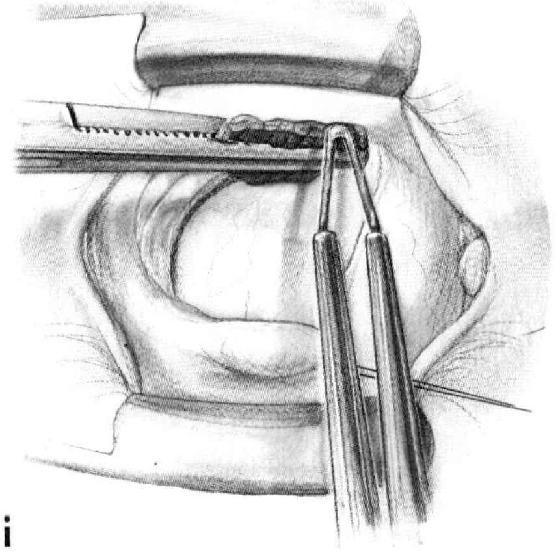

i

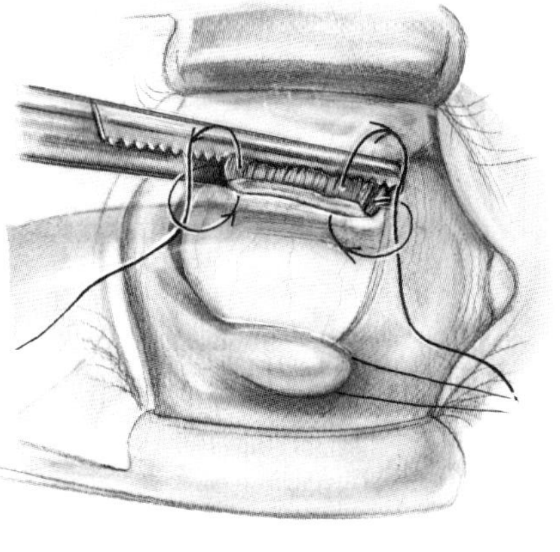

j

Figure 4.10 (contd)

(k) *For an 8–10 mm recession of the inferior oblique muscle, the inferior rectus muscle is engaged with a muscle hook, and the inferior oblique muscle is sutured to the globe with the anterior corner placed 2 mm temporal and 3 mm posterior to the temporal corner of the inferior rectus insertion. For a recession of approximately 14 mm, the inferior oblique muscle is sutured to the globe, straddling the exit of the vortex vein farther posteriorly.* **(i')** *If a large myectomy is to be done, the capsule is first stripped back from the inferior oblique muscle with toothed forceps. The nerve to the inferior oblique can often be visualized coming from posteriorly and entering the internal surface of the muscle.* **(j')** *The nerve to the inferior oblique is tight and prevents the muscle from being pulled far forward. To allow a large myectomy, the nerve is cut, thereby denervating the muscle. The nerve is engaged with a small muscle hook and cut with hot cautery, thereby cauterizing the vessels that accompany the nerve.* **(k')** *The inferior oblique muscle may be pulled farther forward after denervation, and a large portion of muscle is excised by first clamping the muscle and then cutting anterior to the clamp.* **(l')** *Heavy cautery is applied to the muscle stump, otherwise bleeding often occurs from the muscle stump and can cause ecchymosis beneath the skin of the lower lid. The stump is then released and allowed to retract into the sleeve of Tenon's capsule through which it emerges*

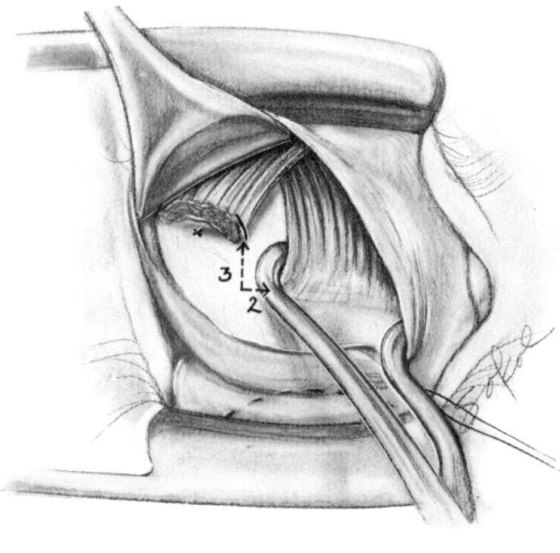

k

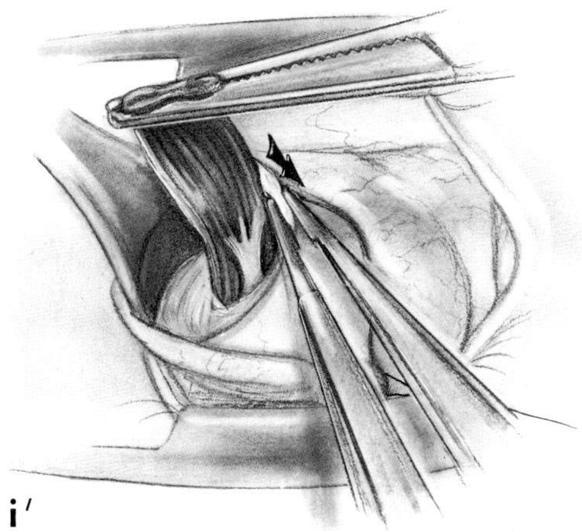

i'

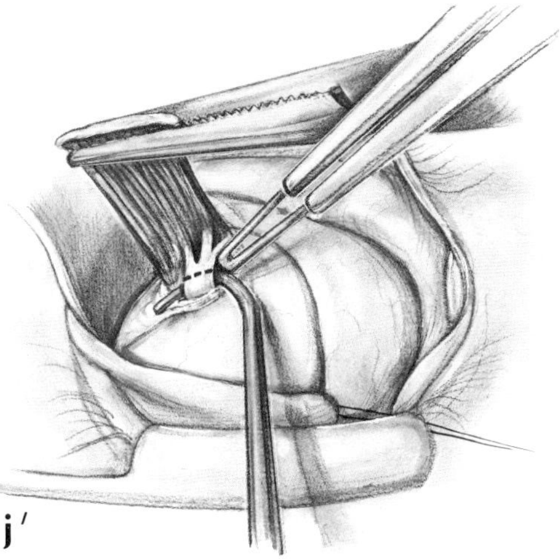

j'

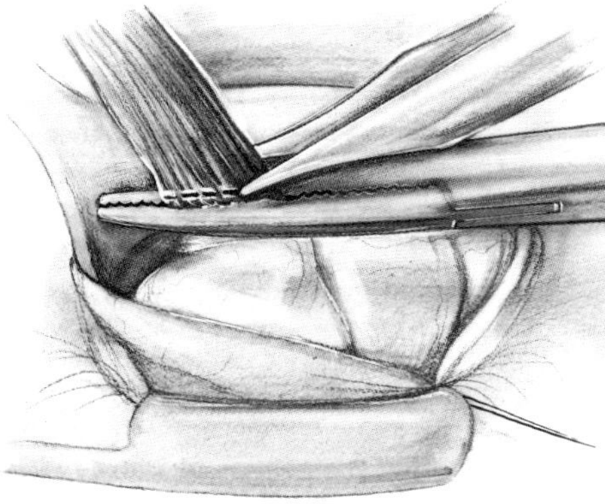

k'

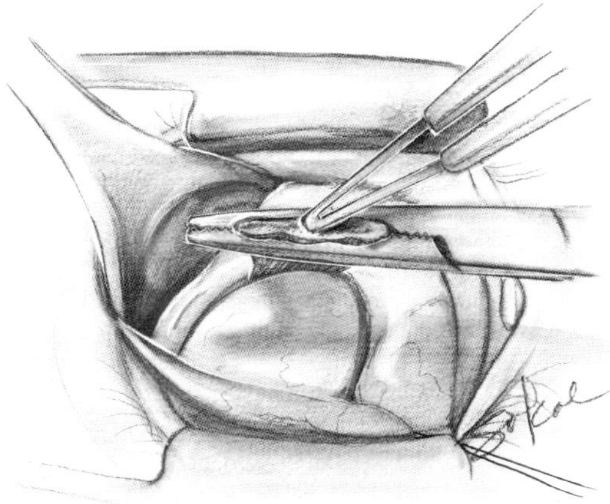

l'

Superior oblique tenotomy

Superior oblique tenotomy may be performed by approaching the superior oblique tendon temporal to or nasal to the superior rectus muscle. We prefer the nasal approach because the most posterior fibers are more likely to be missed with a temporal approach. The superior oblique tendon emerges from the inner surface of Tenon's capsule near the nasal border of the superior rectus muscle. The tendon passes under the superior rectus muscle and fans out to be inserted into the sclera. To avoid unnecessary incisions through Tenon's capsule, the superior oblique tendon is engaged with a small muscle hook near the nasal border of the superior rectus muscle. Our preferred technique for tenotomy of the left superior oblique is illustrated in *Figure 4.11*. The exaggerated traction test is performed both before and after superior oblique tenotomy because a residual tight 'band' can be felt if even a few posterior fibers are missed. This is the most important application of the exaggerated traction test.

Superior oblique strengthening procedures

A tuck of the superior oblique is usually performed temporal to the superior rectus muscle. However, there are few indications for a superior oblique tuck because a Brown's syndrome occurs postoperatively if sufficient surgery is done to strengthen the muscle. A preferable operation is a variant of the Harada-Ito procedure with temporal and anterior transposition of the anterior portion of the superior oblique tendon. Both the superior oblique tuck and this variation of the Harada-Ito procedure are illustrated in *Figure 4.12* for a left superior oblique tendon.

The tightening effect of any procedure on the superior oblique tendon can be judged by performing the exaggerated traction test. In addition, the torsional effect of any superior oblique tightening procedure should be judged intraoperatively by indirect ophthalmoscopy through the dilated pupil. We perform the Harada-Ito procedure as an intraoperative adjustable procedure using the torsional effect on the fundus as a guide to the amount of tightening. A small torsional overcorrection of approximately 5° is desirable at the time of surgery.

Sutures of 5/0 Mersilene or Dacron are often used for these superior oblique tightening procedures. However, absorbable sutures are probably adequate because of the scarring which occurs.

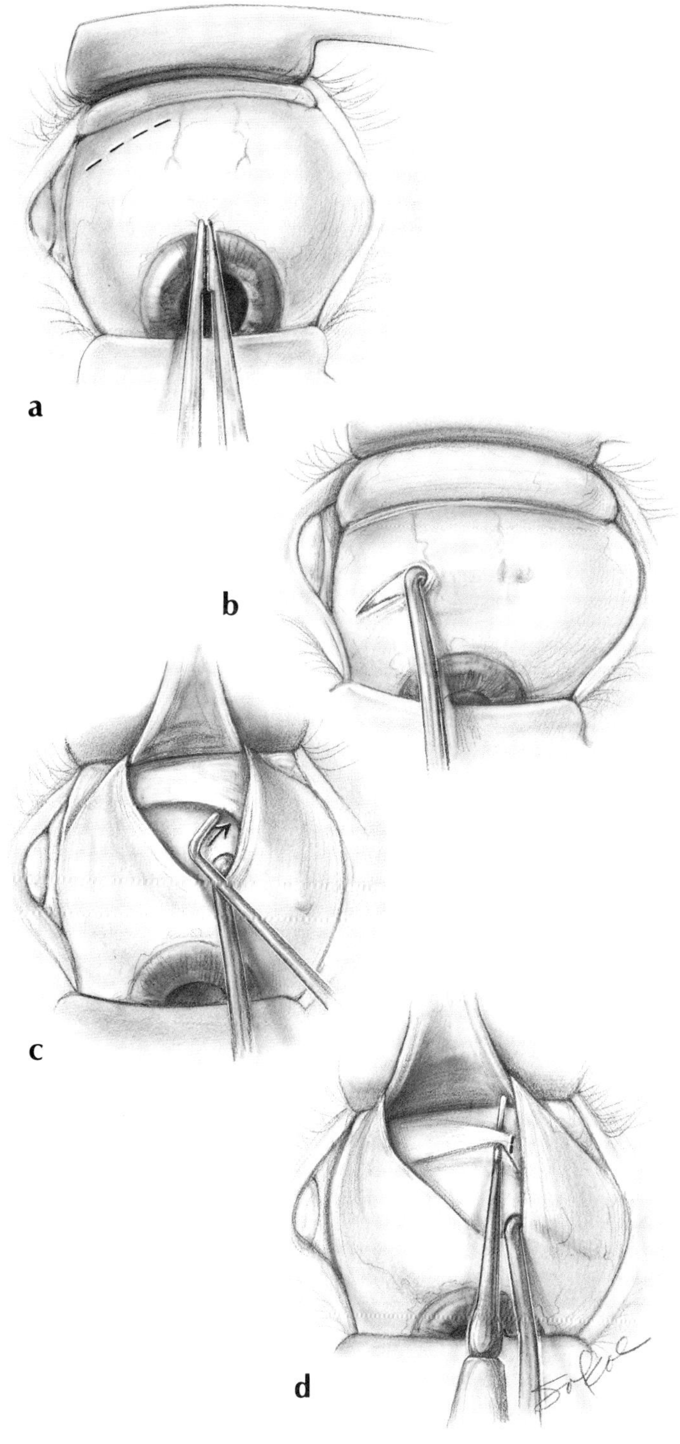

Figure 4.11 *Left superior oblique tenotomy.* **(a)** *The assistant grasps the eye with forceps near the limbus at 12 o'clock and rotates the eye inferiorly. A superonasal fornix incision is made, beginning near the nasal border of the superior rectus muscle (dotted line).* **(b)** *The superior rectus muscle is engaged with a large muscle hook, but the superior rectus is not otherwise exposed.* **(c, d)** *The large muscle hook beneath the superior rectus is used to rotate the globe inferiorly, and a Desmarres lid retractor is placed in the wound superiorly to elevate the undersurface of the intermuscular membrane and Tenon's capsule from the sclera. The superior oblique tendon is visible as a white band passing beneath the superior rectus muscle, partially encapsulated by the intermuscular membrane. The tendon is engaged on a small muscle hook. A small incision is made with scissors through the encapsulating intermuscular membrane, and the tendon is transected. If a greater weakening effect is needed, a tenectomy may be performed. For a tenectomy, the connective tissue surrounding the superior oblique tendon is stripped nasally, and a 3–10 mm portion of the tendon is excised. A tenotomy is usually sufficient, and tenectomy is rarely necessary. No conjunctival closure is needed.*

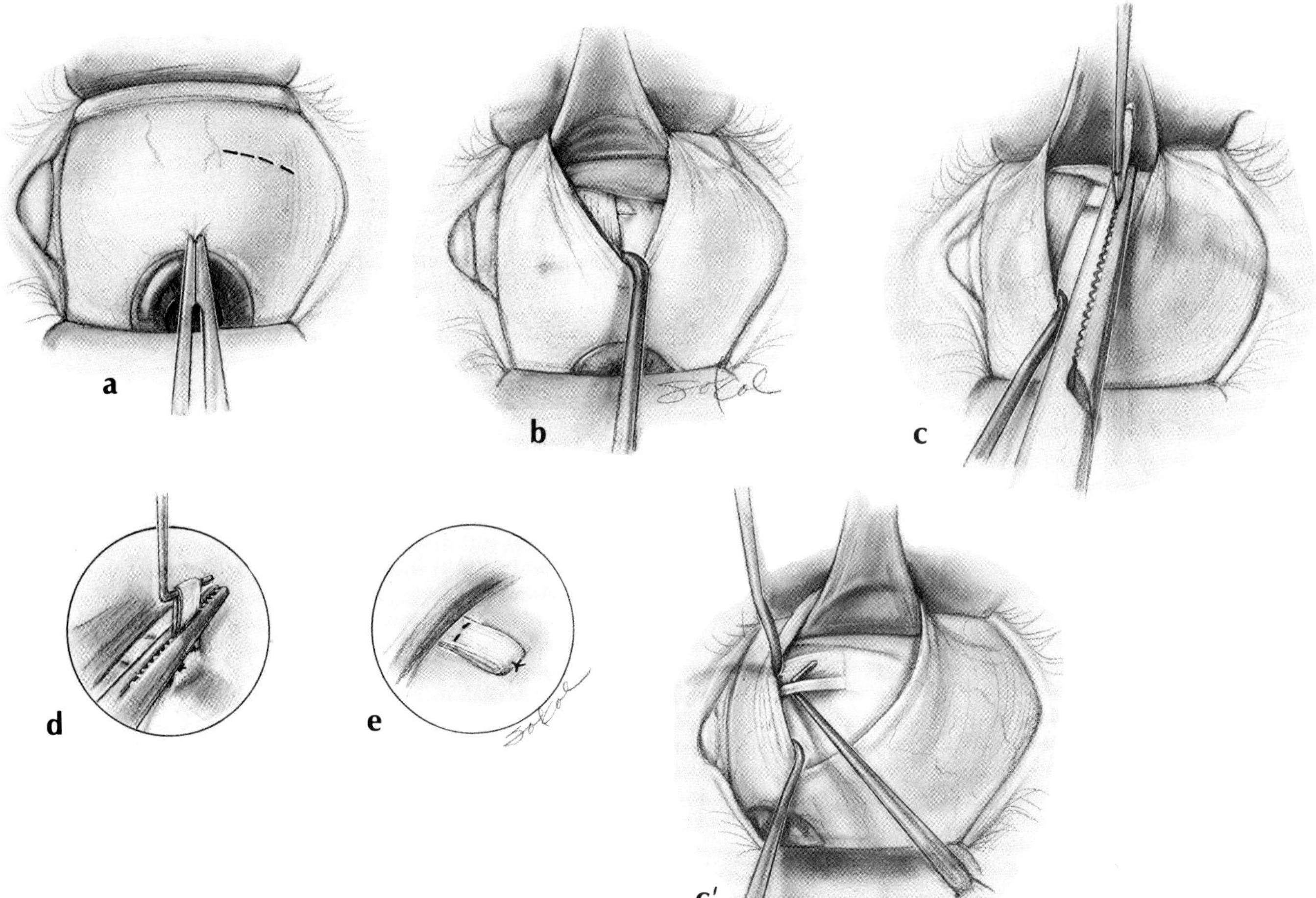

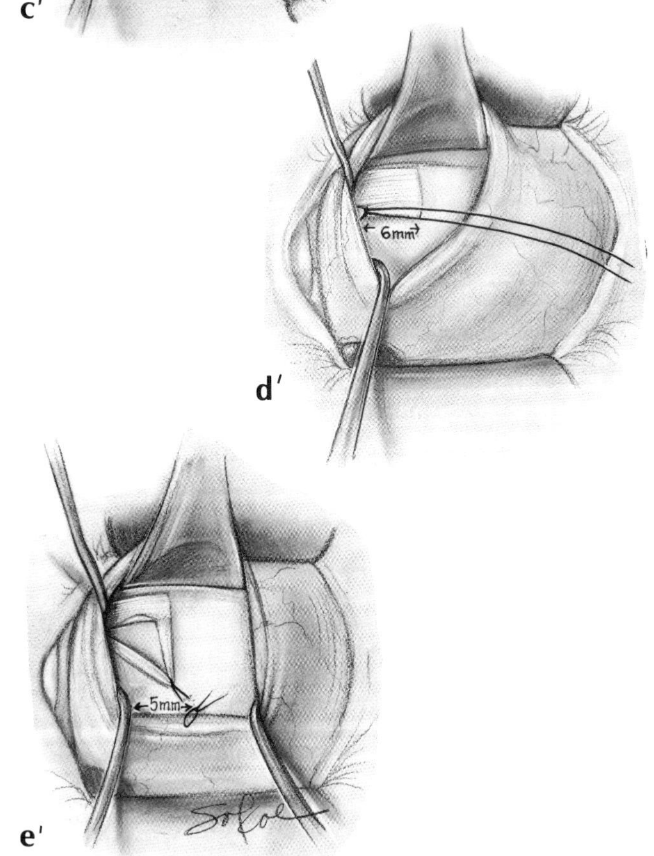

Figure 4.12 *Tightening procedures performed on the left superior oblique tendon.* **(a)** *The superior oblique tendon is approached through a fornix incision temporal to the superior rectus muscle (dotted line). The assistant rotates the eye inferiorly by grasping the limbus at 12 o'clock with toothed forceps.* **(b)** *The superior rectus muscle is engaged on a large muscle hook to rotate the eye inferiorly, and a Desmarres lid retractor is placed in the incision to expose the anterior corner of the superior oblique insertion.* **(c)** *The superior oblique tendon is engaged on a small muscle hook, under direct visualization, and elevated. A hemostat is used to double the tendon upon itself for the desired amount of tuck. No definite numbers can be given for the necessary amount of tuck. Usually the tendon is tucked until moderate resistance is felt to further tightening.* **(d)** *Two interrupted mattress sutures are placed beneath the hemostat to hold the tendon folded upon itself.* **(e)** *Often an additional suture is placed at the apex of the tuck, folding the tendon onto the sclera along its line of action. The amount of tightening achieved and the amount of postoperative Brown's syndrome caused can be judged by the exaggerated traction test.* **(c′)** *If the Harada-Ito procedure is to be performed, the anterior 15–30 per cent of the tendon is split from the rest of the tendon by blunt dissection with a small muscle hook. The greater the amount of tendon included in the transposition, the greater the vertical effect of the procedure. If only the anterior 15 per cent of the tendon is transposed, the vertical effect is minimal.* **(d′)** *A 5/0 non-absorbable suture is tied around the isolated anterior portion of the tendon about 6 mm from the insertion.* **(e′)** *The sutures are passed through partial-thickness sclera about 5 mm directly temporal to the superior rectus insertion. The anterior portion of the superior oblique tendon is pulled toward that point and tied temporarily with a bow knot. After placing the suture but before tightening it, the fundus is inspected by indirect ophthalmoscopy so that the amount of torsional effect induced can be determined after temporarily tying the suture. If the desired amount of torsion has been produced, the temporary knot is converted to a square knot. If the amount of torsion is not correct, suitable adjustment is made. Usually no conjunctival closure is necessary.*

Transposition procedures

Vertical transposition of the horizontal rectus muscles for correction of A- or V-patterns in the absence of oblique overaction has already been mentioned. An additional use for vertical transposition of the horizontal rectus muscles is to correct a small hyperdeviation at the time of horizontal muscle surgery. For example, if the medial rectus muscle is moved upward in addition to recessing or resecting it, a small elevating effect will be obtained, especially in the field of action of that muscle. With a recess-resect procedure on the horizontal muscles of one eye, vertical transposition of both muscles 4 or 5 mm can correct approximately 5^{Δ} of hyperdeviation. We prefer to measure vertical transpositions from the center of the prior insertion to the center to the new insertion, rather than measuring the amount of transposition in terms of muscle width.

Other forms of muscle transposition are illustrated in *Figure 4.13*. For example, transposition of both the medial and lateral rectus muscles superiorly, adjacent to the insertion of the superior rectus muscle, may be performed for double elevator palsy. This operation is usually referred to as the Knapp procedure. The innervation to the transposed muscles does not change because of transposition of their insertions. The transposed muscles simply provide tonic tethering forces to counteract the downward pull of the normal inferior rectus muscle. If the inferior rectus muscle has developed permanent contracture, recession of the inferior rectus muscle is also necessary.

To treat esotropia from sixth nerve palsy the superior and inferior rectus muscles may be transposed temporally (*Figure 4.13b*), and a large recession of the medial rectus muscle is done as well. With other operations such as the Hummelscheim procedure or the Jensen procedure (*Figure 4.13c*) only portions of the superior and inferior rectus muscles are transposed temporally. With any procedure to treat a sixth nerve palsy a large recession of the ipsilateral medial rectus muscle is necessary because contracture has invariably occurred.

In the Jensen procedure the insertions of the superior and inferior rectus muscles are left intact, and only portions of the muscle bellies are transposed temporally and connected to corresponding portions of the lateral rectus muscle. This procedure is intended to maintain a better blood supply to the anterior segment than is possible when the muscle insertions are transposed. Even so, a case of anterior segment ischemia has been reported after a Jensen procedure[10].

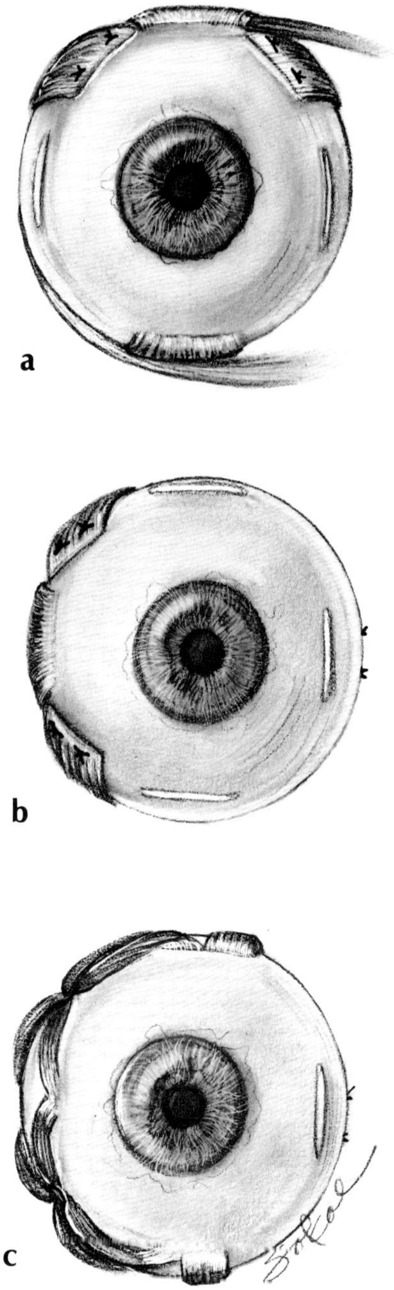

a

b

c

Figure 4.13 *Muscle transposition procedures for correction of muscle palsies.* **(a)** *The Knapp procedure with superior transposition of both the medial and the lateral rectus muscle, performed for double elevator palsy.* **(b)** *Knapp-type procedure performed for right 6th nerve palsy. Both the superior and the inferior rectus muscle are transposed to the border of the lateral rectus muscle, and a large recession of the right medial rectus muscle is done.* **(c)** *Jensen procedure for right 6th nerve palsy. The temporal portions of the superior and inferior rectus bellies are transposed temporarlly, leaving the insertions intact. The transposed muscle halves are tied about 11–12 mm behind the insertions to the respective halves of the lateral rectus muscle. A large recession of the medial rectus muscle is also done, using an adjustable suture if possible.*

Traction sutures

Traction sutures placed under the muscle insertions or through midthickness sclera near the limbus can be used to hold the globe temporarily in a desired position. Traction sutures are used most commonly after extensive surgery, especially reoperations. These sutures are passed through the lids and tied over cotton pledgets. They are left in place for about 1 week to encourage healing of the globe in the desired position. We find little use for traction sutures. They are painful and are rarely, if ever, necessary.

Surgical complications

Anesthesia complications are the most dreaded complications of strabismus surgery because they can result in loss of life. Careful screening for preoperative respiratory illness is important, and cases are postponed if the anesthesiologist detects potential problems. If the patient has been treated with Phospholine Iodide within the previous 6 weeks, the anesthesiologist is alerted to this fact to avoid using succinylcholine, because prolonged apnea may result. Cardiac arrhythmias during surgery caused by the oculocardiac reflex should be detected promptly by the anesthesiologist, and tension on the muscles should be released until normal sinus rhythm resumes.

Postoperative overcorrection and undercorrection are probably the most common 'complications' of muscle surgery. Although full discussion of management of overcorrection and undercorrection is beyond the scope of this chapter, it is not always best to treat an overcorrection by attempting to undo the previous surgery. For example, a consecutive exotropia after medial rectus recessions is best treated by recession of the lateral rectus muscles rather than by resection of the medial rectus muscles. Undercorrections, however, are frequently best treated by surgery on the same muscles as were operated on before. However, significantly more correction will be obtained per millimeter of additional recession than from the original recession.

Persistent diplopia after muscle surgery can be most bothersome. This rarely occurs in young children because of their ability to suppress the second image, but it can occur in older children as in adults. The most symptomatic problems occur with small or moderate overcorrection of either exotropia or esotropia in adults. Prisms can be used to alter the deviation in an attempt to find a retinal area of suppression and thereby relieve the diplopia. However, areas of suppression that existed preoperatively can shrink postoperatively and may be difficult to find. Fortunately, most adults learn to 'ignore' the second image within a matter of months. A useful technique for relief of symptoms is to place a small piece of frosted cellophane tape on the rear surface of one lens of the patient's glasses. The tape may be placed in any specific location to rid the patient of diplopia in that direction of gaze, while allowing binocular vision in other directions of gaze. For example, diplopia in primary position may be abolished while leaving side gaze intact.

Use of partial tape occlusion on the glasses is also helpful in cases of limitation of movement from thyroid myopathy or postoperative scarring if the patient can fuse in some directions of gaze but has diplopia in other directions. The tape is placed in such a way as to allow vision with only one eye in the area of gaze in which diplopia is present.

Operations on the wrong muscles and even on the wrong patient are tragic complications that rarely occur. Each surgeon must develop a method to identify the correct patient and eye, because consecutive cases are often small children of similar size. Some surgeons place an identifying mark on the forehead above the eyes to be operated on during evaluation the day before surgery.

Occasional complications such as scleral perforation or scleral laceration occur from needles or scissors. In these cases examination by indirect ophthalmoscopy should be performed to determine whether retinal damage has occurred. If a retinal tear is present, cryotherapy with ophthalmoscopic guidance is applied around the tear. Occasionally a small sponge episcleral exoplant is placed over the retinal perforation site, but usually this is not necessary. The area of retinal damage is periodically examined postoperatively.

Stay sutures or traction sutures placed near the limbus occasionally penetrate too deeply and cause hemorrhage in the anterior chamber. No treatment is necessary, and the needle tracts are self-sealing. The operation can proceed with the disadvantage that the eye may be softer than usual.

A muscle which is broken or lost posteriorly at the time of surgery may be quite difficult to retrieve. The sleeve in Tenon's capsule through which the muscle emerged from the posterior orbit is located, and the muscle is identified and grasped with forceps through this sleeve using direct visualization. A fiberoptic headlamp aids in seeing deep into the connective tissue recesses.

Occasionally a muscle slips off its attachment to the sclera postoperatively, with apparent muscle paresis after an otherwise uncomplicated operation. The muscle can usually be found on repeat surgery. A limbal incision is used for optimal exposure, and the anterior portion of the muscle is often found attached to Tenon's capsule near the intended scleral insertion site. The muscle only rarely retracts far into the orbit. A CT scan can often help locate a posteriorly slipped muscle.

Anterior segment ischemia can occur if three or more rectus muscles are disinserted. This complication is seen mainly in adults. Iritis is usually present on the first postoperative day, along with corneal edema and hypotony. Topical steroids usually promote partial improvement, but long-term lens and corneal changes may persist.

Allergic reaction to suture material is less common with the synthetic absorbable sutures of polyglactin (Vicryl) and polyglycolic acid (Dexon) than occurred previously with chromic catgut and collagen sutures. Only rare cases of allergic reaction to the new synthetic sutures occur, and such cases are easily treated with topical steroids.

Infection after muscle surgery is quite rare. Lid swelling occurs frequently, but orbital cellulitis is unlikely unless there is moderate or severe tenderness accompanied by erythema. However, if orbital cellulitis is suspected, intravenous antibiotics are used because this can be a life-threatening problem. Consultation with the pediatrician or internist is indicated. Endophthalmitis after muscle surgery has been reported on rare occasions, usually after perforation of the sclera by a needle.

A number of local complications can occur in the area of the surgical wound. These include prolapse of Tenon's tissue through the wound, conjunctival inclusion cysts and dellen formation. Prolapse of Tenon's tissue, appearing as white tissue emerging from the wound, is quite alarming to the parents. This tissue can easily be excised under topical anesthesia. Conjunctival inclusion cysts may gradually enlarge, but often they shrink with time, not requiring excision. Excision of conjunctival inclusion cysts can cause other complications if Tenon's capsule is perforated, with spillage of fat into the wound followed by excessive scarring. Dellen of the cornea or sclera may occur adjacent to the surgical wound. These are easily treated by patching the eye, because increased hydration under the closed lids reverses the changes in the dehydrated areas of tissue.

Conjunctival scarring can occasionally be severe enough to be a cosmetic problem, and the scarred portion of conjunctiva must be excised. The underlying sclera is left initially bare, without conjunctival coverage. It is rapidly covered by proliferation of adjacent conjunctival epithelium. The cosmetic result is excellent.

Changes in the level of either the upper or lower lid often occur after vertical muscle surgery if the muscle capsule is not dissected free from the surrounding tissues. This is a special problem with the lower lid because of extensive attachments between the inferior rectus muscle and the lid structures. Lid complications are best avoided by careful dissection of the tissues, which may be aided by use of a fiberoptic headlamp. Once the lid complications occur, repeat surgery is done to free the tissue attachments causing the problem. If the lid position is severely abnormal, consultation with an ophthalmic plastic surgeon is indicated.

Postoperative limitations of movement may be due to: (*1*) excessive recession of a muscle, thereby weakening it more than anticipated; (*2*) excessive resection of a muscle, thereby creating a tight band; or (*3*) excess scarring associated with fat spillage into the wound. Forced ductions usually establish the correct diagnosis, but further surgery may be necessary, and this is often difficult. Mechanical limitation of movement is best avoided by careful tissue handling, avoiding fat spillage into the wound, and good judgment as to the amount of surgery to be performed on each muscle.

Conclusion

The exact amount of muscle surgery to be performed in various cases is difficult to specify because of differences in surgical technique. Each surgeon must develop his own guidelines for the amount of surgery to be performed for each type and degree of deviation. However, this is only part of successful strabismus surgery. Major factors are accuracy of the preoperative diagnosis and exact measurement of the amount of deviation. Although the results of surgery are somewhat variable even in the most experienced and skillful hands, variability in result can be minimized by attention to detail in preoperative evaluation and surgical technique. The visibility of the results in successful cases can make strabismus surgery most gratifying for both patient and surgeon. Knowing when to operate, how much surgery to perform and the effective application of an intimate knowledge of surgical anatomy should be the goal of every surgeon.

References

1. Bixenman, W., von Noorden, G. K. Apparent foveal displacement in normal subjects and in cyclotropia. Ophthalmology 1982; 89: 58
2. Guyton, D., von Noorden, G. K. Sensory adaptations to cyclodeviation. In: Reinecke, R. D., ed. Strabismus. Proceedings of the third meeting of the International Strabismological Association, 1978. New York: Grune & Stratton, 1978: 399–403
3. Stager, D. R., Parks M. M. Inferior oblique weakening procedures. Effect on primary position horizontal alignment. Archives of Ophthalmology 1973; 90: 15–16
4. Diamond, G. R., Parks M. M. The effect of superior oblique weakening procedures on primary position horizontal alignment. Journal of Pediatric Ophthalmology and Strabismus 1981; 18: 35–38
5. Hiles, D. A. Results of strabismus therapy in cerebral palsied children. American Orthoptic Journal 1975; 25: 46–55
6. Jampolsky, A. Current techniques of adjustable strabismus surgery. American Journal of Ophthalmology 1979; 88: 406–418
7. O'Donnell, F. E., Del Monte, M., Guyton, D. L. Simultaneous correction of blepharoptosis and exotropia in aberrant regeneration of the oculomotor nerve by strabismus surgery: a new, simplified ptosis correction for selected cases. Ophthalmic Surgery 1980; 11: 695–697
8. Koornneef, L. Spatial aspects of orbital musculo-fibrous tissue in man. Amsterdam: Swets & Zeitlinger BV, 1977
9. Guyton, D. Exaggerated traction test for the oblique muscles. Ophthalmology 1981; 88: 1035–1040
10. von Noorden, G. Anterior segment ischemia following the Jensen procedure. Archives of Ophthalmology 1976; 94: 845–847

5

Surgery of the cornea

Walter J. Stark MD
William E. Bruner MD
A. Edward Maumenee MD

Introduction

The first attempts at corneal transplantation in man were made about 150 years ago, but it was not until 1906 that the first successful human penetrating keratoplasty was performed[1]. During the next 75 years, with the advent of the operating microscope, fine suture material and other advances, the procedure evolved to its present state of good technical and visual prognosis. Today keratoplasty is successful in 80–95 per cent of cases in most circumstances

In this chapter on surgery of the cornea, the emphasis will be on penetrating and lamellar keratoplasty. Other surgical procedures involving the cornea, such as the conjunctival flap, repair of corneal perforations and superficial keratectomy, will also be described. Last, the still investigational procedures of refractive corneal surgery will be discussed briefly.

Indications for surgery

Keratoplasty

The indications for penetrating keratoplasty are similar to those for cataract extraction, and they include any opacification or abnormality involving the central cornea that significantly limits visual acuity and cannot be corrected by medical or simpler surgical means. Diseases that can cause such central opacification include: herpes keratitis, corneal dystrophies, keratoconus, trauma, aphakic bullous keratopathy and corneal degenerations. The decision on whether to operate must be made by the patient and the surgeon together, based on the degree of visual disability, the corneal condition and the visual needs of the particular patient.

Lamellar keratoplasty or non-penetrating keratoplasty may rarely be performed to treat a superficial corneal opacity to give more thickness to a thin, diseased cornea. Some corneal diseases that may require a lamellar keratoplasty include Meesmann's dystrophy, Reis-Buckler's dystrophy, corneal dermoid, Saltzman's nodular degeneration, descemetocele and certain cases of keratoconus.

Superficial keratectomy

Superficial keratectomy refers to the removal of superficial cornea without replacement with donor tissue. This procedure may occasionally be useful in certain very superficial corneal problems, such as Saltzman's degeneration and some of the superficial corneal dystrophies.

Corneal perforation repair

Non-traumatic corneal perforation can occur in association with many corneal ulcerative diseases, including infected corneal ulcers, Mooren's ulcer, dry eyes, Stevens-Johnson syndrome and exposure keratitis. Prompt treatment is indicated for corneal perforations in these situations.

The two basic methods of treatment are application of tissue adhesive and use of a lamellar patch graft. Tissue adhesive application remains an investigational (although effective) procedure because the adhesive has not yet been approved by the US Food and Drug Administration (FDA) for this use except under life-threatening or organ-threatening circumstances.

Conjunctival flap

The indications for using a complete Gundersen-type conjunctival flap[2] may include severe non-healing herpetic keratitis, neuroparalytic keratitis and advanced marginal ulcers (such as Mooren's ulcer) that have not responded to patching or the use of a therapeutic soft contact lens. Although therapeutic contact lenses have obviated the need for a conjunctival flap in many corneal problems, the procedure is useful in non-responsive cases.

Refractive corneal surgery

This category includes the procedures of keratophakia for aphakia, keratomileusis for aphakia or myopia, epikeratophakia for aphakia, wedge resection for astigmatism and radial keratotomy for myopia and/or astigmatism. Some of these techniques are still investigational. Because glasses or contact lenses will usually suffice to cure the problems for which some of these operations were developed, there are no absolute indications for these procedures and they should be evaluated and used with care.

Preoperative evaluation

The preoperative evaluation of patients with corneal disease is essentially the same as that described in Chapter 6 on 'Surgery of the lens'. Those factors that are unique to corneal surgery, and especially to keratoplasty, will be described.

Evaluating the recipient

The first steps in evaluating the patient are a careful history and a thorough ocular examination. When the cornea is opaque, additional tests as described in Chapter 6 are useful, such as the entoptic phenomenon, B-scan ultrasonography and the electroretinogram (ERG). The Guyton-Minkowski Potential Acuity Meter™ described in Chapter 6 is useful in predicting visual prognosis.

In evaluating a potential corneal graft recipient, several factors must be taken into consideration. These include the present corneal morphology and condition, the original cause of the disease process and the presence of other ocular problems. The surgeon must consider the patient's reliability and potential for cooperation and compliance. If the patient is phakic and has a cataract, a decision must be made on whether to remove the lens[3]. Also, as in cataract surgery, the visual needs of each patient must be determined.

The corneal morphology and condition of the recipient cornea in the graft zone are important[4]. Normal thickness, normal curvature and absence of vascularization in the recipient-bed area of the cornea are good prognostic signs for grafting, regardless of the status of the central cornea.

One of the most important aspects of the host corneal disease process is whether the disease or inflammatory process is active. If there is active disease present, such as herpetic or bacterial keratitis, the graft prognosis is considerably worse[5,6]. Also the presence of a retrocorneal membrane, iris synechiae and active stromal vascularization worsen the prognosis[7]. Other concurrent ocular diseases such as glaucoma, chronic uveitis, trichiasis, entropion and poor tear production decrease the chances for success. Last, if the patient is unreliable, and is likely to miss follow-up appointments and not use medication, the prognosis is much poorer than for a reliable patient.

Those factors that worsen the prognosis should be treated before surgery. Glaucoma that is unresponsive to medication should be treated with cyclocryotherapy or a filtering procedure before corneal transplantation is attempted. Uveitis must be controlled with steroids. Surgery should be performed for trichiasis and entropion. Moderately dry eyes should be treated with medication or punctal occlusion. For cases with an extremely poor prognosis, such as eyes with severe alkali burn or Stevens-Johnson syndrome, corneal transplantation should be attempted only as a last resort, because the chance of graft failure from complications is high[8].

Evaluating the donor tissue

Careful inspection of the donor tissue is important, and it should be performed by the surgeon before surgery. Abnormalities of the donor tissue, such as moderate to marked corneal edema or striae, endothelial damage or significant epithelial defects, may justify rejection of the tissue for surgery. Although specular microscopy of the donor tissue may be useful[9], careful slit-lamp examination is usually sufficient. This can be performed while the tissue is in the vial of McCarey-Kaufman (M-K) medium (*Figure 5.1*)[10]. It is ultimately the responsibility of the surgeon to determine the suitability of the tissue for grafting. The presence of the following conditions in the donor cornea should generally be considered contraindications to its use: (*1*) excessive time interval from donor death to removal of the eyes (more than 16–18 hours); (*2*) previous intraocular surgery; (*3*) donor sepsis or intraocular tumor; (*4*) unexplained cause of death, or debilitating neurological disease of uncertain etiology.

The following is a more specific list of absolute contraindications for donor corneal use as defined by the Medical Eye Bank of Maryland: (*1*) donor diseases of obscure or unknown etiology; (*2*) Creutzfeldt-Jakob disease; (*3*) rabies; (*4*) congenital rubella; (*5*) subacute sclerosing panencephalitis; (*6*) progressive multifocal leukoencephalopathy; (*7*) subacute encephalitis from cytomegalovirus; (*8*) other disseminated viral infections; (*9*) septicemia; (*10*) hepatitis or jaundice; (*11*) 'blast' forms of leukemia; (*12*) intrinsic eye disease, including retinoblastoma or known malignant tumors of the anterior segment or conjunctivitis; and (*13*) slowly debilitating neurological diseases or mental deterioration.

In addition to the absolute contraindications to donor tissue use, the Medical Eye Bank of Maryland lists the following as possible contraindications: (*1*) leukemia other than 'blast' form, and other blood dyscrasias; (*2*) cancer with metastasis; (*3*) syphilis; (*4*) tuberculosis; (*5*)

Hodgkin's disease and lymphomas; (*6*) chronic debilitating disease; (*7*) history of prolonged terminal life-support or hypothermia, in which unrecognized sepsis may have existed; (*8*) history of immunosuppressive or steroid therapy; (*9*) diabetes mellitus; (*10*) amyotophic lateral sclerosis; (*11*) multiple sclerosis; and (*12*) Reyes syndrome. As mentioned, the surgeon must make the final decision on whether or not to use the donor material available.

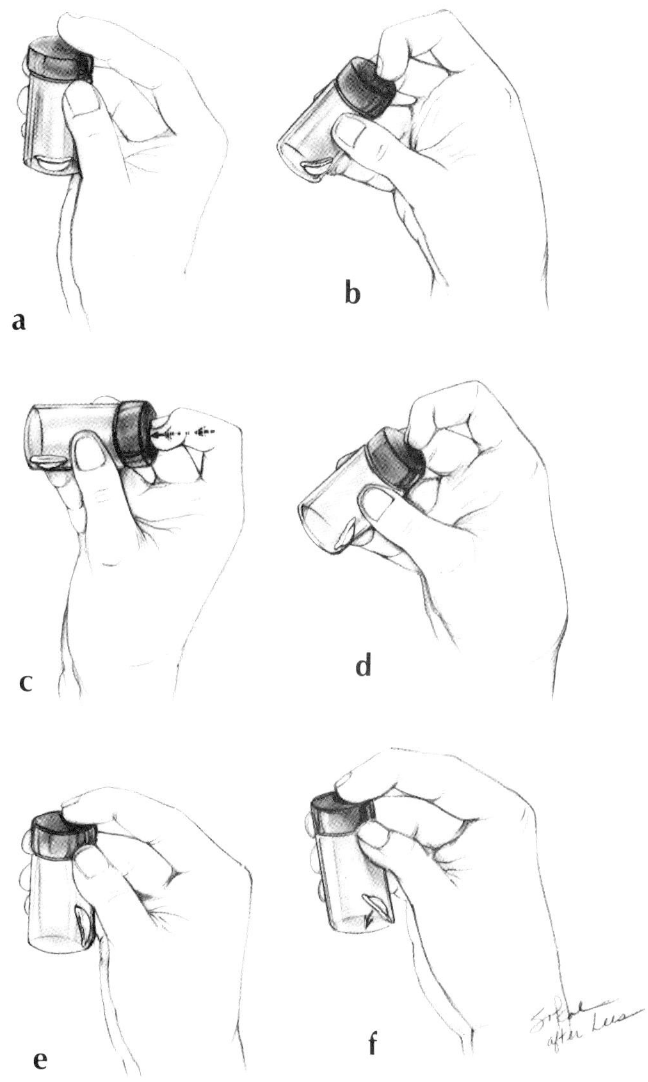

Figure 5.1 *Simple method for turning the donor corneal tissue over in the vial of M-K medium, so that endothelium faces down and can then be examined at the slit lamp*

Age limits for donor use have not been universally established, but surgeons generally prefer tissue that is from a donor younger than 60 years of age, except in emergency situations. An attempt is made to give younger recipients a younger donor cornea. There has not, however, been any documentation to indicate that donor age is a significant factor in graft success. The health of the donor tissue, especially the endothelium, is of prime consideration, and recent specular microscopy studies show a gradual loss of endothelial cells with age.

Surgical anatomy

The cornea forms a protective, transparent cover for the front surface of the eye. It is the main refracting surface of the eye and is normally avascular. The transparency of the cornea depends on several factors, including the smooth and intact epithelial surface, the regular organization of collagen within the ground substance and the absence of blood vessels[11]

When viewed anteriorly, the cornea has a slightly elliptical shape because of the greater extension of limbal tissue onto the cornea superiorly and inferiorly. The vertical diameter is about 10.6 mm and the horizontal diameter is about 11.7 mm. When viewed posteriorly, the cornea is a circle with a diameter of 11.7 mm. The radius of curvature of the cornea is about 7.8 mm, as opposed to that of the eye, which is about 11.5 mm.

Histologically the cornea has five main layers: epithelium, Bowman's layer, stroma, Descemet's layer and endothelium (*Figure 5.2*). Each layer has its particular importance from a surgical standpoint.

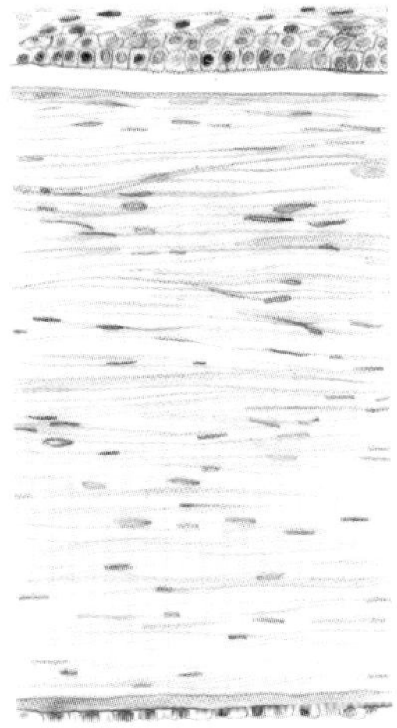

Figure 5.2 *Histological cross-section of normal human cornea*

About 10 per cent of the total corneal thickness is composed of epithelium which heals rapidly after simple abrasion by cell spreading and cell division. The epithelium has a basement membrane, which is thickened and irregular in certain diseases, such as epithelial basement membrane dystrophies and the recurrent erosion syndrome[12].

Bowman's layer consists of collagen and ground substance with no cells. It is significant surgically because, if traumatized, it often leaves scarring. The underlying stroma makes up about 90 per cent of the thickness of the cornea. It comprises collagen, keratocytes and ground substance. The collagen is arranged in lamellae, and this allows the surgeon easily to dissect split-thickness segments of cornea when performing lamellar keratoplasty.

Descemet's membrane is the basement membrane of the endothelial cells, and it grows thicker with age. It is often the last layer to be destroyed by an infectious or other destructive corneal disease. When only Descemet's membrane remains in a cornea, a descemetocele results, which requires surgical treatment in most cases.

The endothelium is composed of a monolayer of hexagonal cells which function to transport osmotically active substances and to maintain corneal clarity. Damage to the endothelium results in cloudiness and edema of the cornea. The endothelium of the donor tissue must not be damaged during corneal transplantation, or the graft may fail and become opaque.

Preoperative preparation and anesthesia

Preparation of patient

It is important that the patient be well informed before keratoplasty. He or she must understand that eyedrops will need to be used for several months or longer and that the best vision may not be obtained until a year or more after surgery, when the sutures are removed. The patient must also be aware of the risks of surgery and the various complications that can occur.

About 1 hour before surgery eyedrops are started if necessary. If the patient undergoing penetrating keratoplasty is phakic and does not have a cataract, pilocarpine drops are begun (4 per cent drops every 10–15 minutes for three doses). If a keratoplasty patient is to undergo simultaneous cataract removal with or without IOL implantation, dilating drops such as tropicamide 1 per cent (Mydriacil) or homatropine 5 per cent with phenylephrine 10 per cent (Neosynephrine) are given every 15 minutes for 3 doses.

About 30 minutes before surgery, phakic patients undergoing any cornea operation that will involve entering the eye may be given intravenous mannitol in a dose of 1.5 g/kg, to lower the intraocular pressure. Mannitol is not used if there are medical contraindications such as a history of heart failure or asthma. Sedation is also given such as meperidine (Demerol) 50–75 mg intramuscularly 1 hour before surgery. Alternatively, diazepam (Valium) may be given orally or intravenously before retrobulbar anesthetic injection.

Anesthesia

We prefer to use local anesthesia for most cases of corneal surgery, except in children and uncooperative adults. Our method of local anesthetic injection is described in Chapter 6. We routinely use the Honan pressure-reducer before keratoplasty (as described in Chapter 6) to ensure a soft eye.

Operative procedures and sequence

Penetrating keratoplasty

Preparation of the donor button

For penetrating keratoplasty, before cutting the recipient cornea, the donor button is cut on a Teflon block, starting the cut from the endothelial side[13]. If the donor tissue has been processed in M-K medium, it can be placed immediately on the trephine block. However, if the cornea must be cut from a whole donor eye, the cornea with some scleral rim must first be excised by an anterior approach. This is done by entering the eye 2–3 mm posterior to the limbus with a sharp blade extending the incision anterior to the uvea for 360° using scissors. The whole cornea with its scleral rim attached is then gently peeled from the eye, leaving iris and lens and other tissues behind.

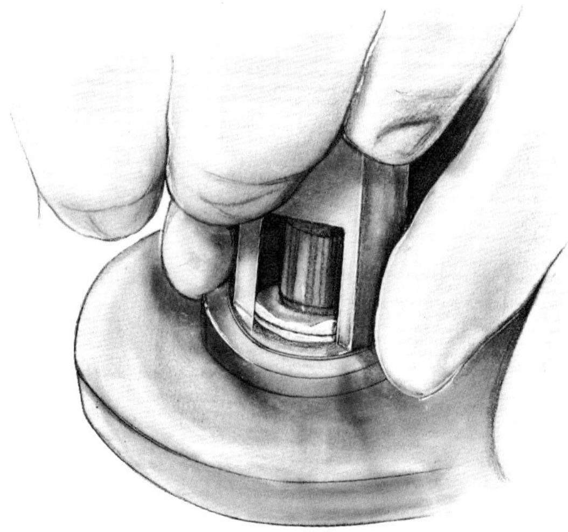

Figure 5.3 *The donor button is cut, using the trephine guide*

The cornea, with its scleral rim, is placed epithelial side down on the trephine block. When cutting donor tissue, we prefer to use a trephine guide, which assures even, perpendicular edges to the donor button (*Figure 5.3*). If a trephine guide is not available, then care must be taken to ensure that the trephine is perpendicular to the cornea when cutting.

We cut the donor button 0.5–0.7 mm larger than the recipient bed for grafts in aphakic eyes; and 0.2–0.25 mm larger than, or the same size as, the recipient bed in phakic eyes. There is evidence that using a donor button that is 0.5–0.7 mm larger than the recipient bed reduces the chance for glaucoma after keratoplasty in aphakic eyes[14]. Also, we prefer the larger donor cornea because sutures do not need to be pulled as tight and there is less postoperative hyperopia. After cutting the donor button, several drops of M-K medium are placed on the tissue to keep it moist. Before placing the cornea on the Teflon trephine block, one must check to make sure the block is cool, because it retains heat after being autoclaved.

Some surgeons prefer to cut the donor button directly from the whole donor eye. This technique is described below and is identical to the technique used to cut the recipient's or patient's cornea.

Cutting the recipient cornea

In aphakic eyes or eyes in which cataract surgery is planned, a single or double Flieringa ring should be sutured into place on the sclera to maintain the shape of the eye and to prevent scleral collapse and vitreous loss after the eye has been entered. The ring may be sutured with interrupted or running 6/0 silk suture. A reverse-cutting or standard cutting needle is preferable to a spatula needle, because it is easier to place a cutting needle through sclera. At least six bites and preferably eight should be taken or a running suture can be used (*Figure 5.4*). The ring should be centered and the suture bites should be evenly placed, so as not to distort the globe and cause astigmatism. While the sutures are being placed to secure the ring, care must be taken not to penetrate the eye with the needle, thereby possibly causing a retinal hole.

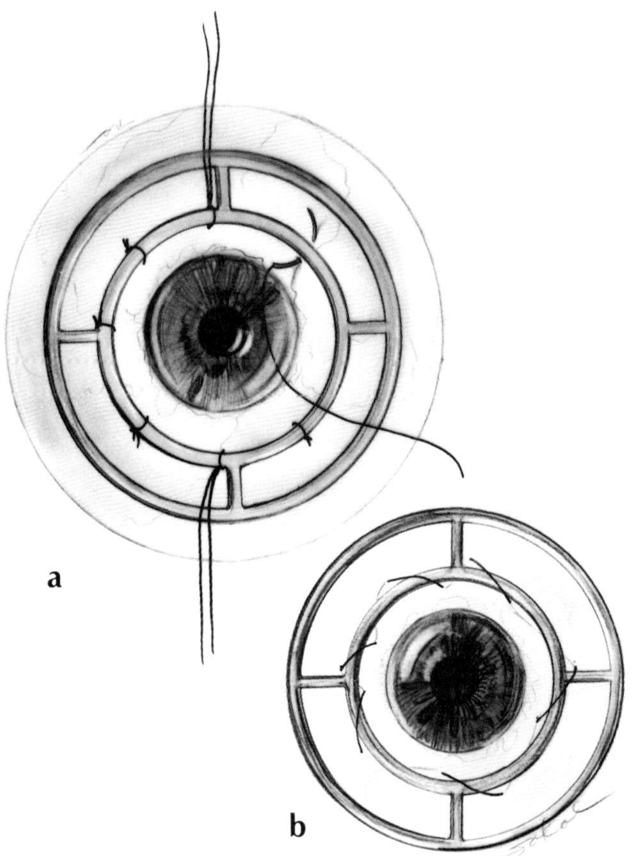

Figure 5.4 *Suturing a double Flieringa ring in position*

Probably the most frequent cause of postoperative astigmatism after keratoplasty is improper technique in cutting the recipient cornea. It is important that the trephine be perpendicular to the cornea and centered for the optical zone, otherwise an eccentric graft with irregular edges will result[15–17]. The recipient cornea should be kept dry at the time of cutting, and the desired trephine placed gently on the cornea to test for size. This procedure will leave a light mark in the epithelium (*Figure 5.5a,b*). The cornea is then cut with the trephine, using gentle downward pressure and a twisting movement in alternating clockwise and counterclockwise directions (*Figure 5.5c*). Several times during the cutting, the trephine should be gently rocked (but not twisted) in the 12–6 and 3–9 o'clock meridians to ensure that it is being held perpendicular to the cornea (*Figure 5.5d,e*). Some surgeons prefer to set the trephine depth to 80 per cent of corneal thickness and then enter the anterior chamber with a knife. With experience, the chamber can be safely entered with the trephine. As soon as the anterior chamber has been entered, a small gush of aqueous fluid will

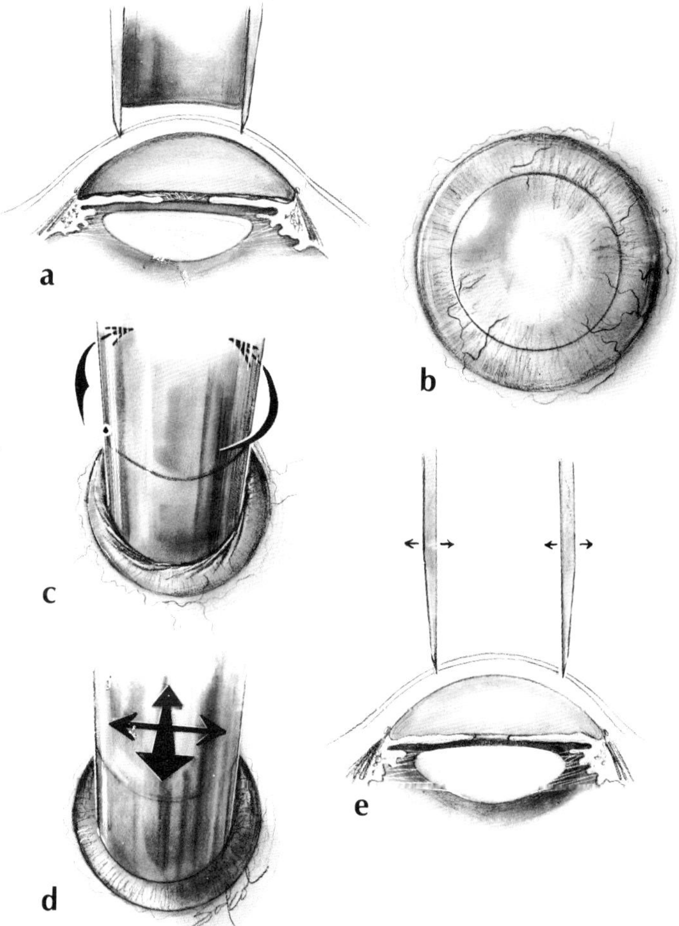

Figure 5.5 **(a,b)** *The recipient corneal bed is marked.* **(c)** *Cutting the recipient cornea with the trephine.* **(d,e)** *Rocking trephine to check that it is perpendicular*

be noted, the chamber will shallow and the trephining must then be stopped. With too much pressure on the trephine at this point, it is possible to cut inadvertently into the iris and even the lens. This can result in hemorrhage and cataract formation. If the lens capsule is inadvertently cut, the lens should be removed.

Once the anterior chamber has been entered, curved corneal scissors are used to complete the incision (*Figure 5.6*). To avoid damage to the peripheral corneal endothelium, the lower blade is introduced into the anterior chamber under the central area that is to be removed, and the blade is then moved into the correct position. The upper blade of the scissors is placed down in the trephine cut, and then cutting is performed by an upward motion of the lower blade. This prevents a double cut to the wound that can occur by cutting down with the upper blade of the scissors. If care is not taken to keep the tip and the lower scissors blade up against the posterior corneal surface, the tip of the scissors may accidentally cut the iris or even the lens capsule (*Figure 5.6c*). Cutting first

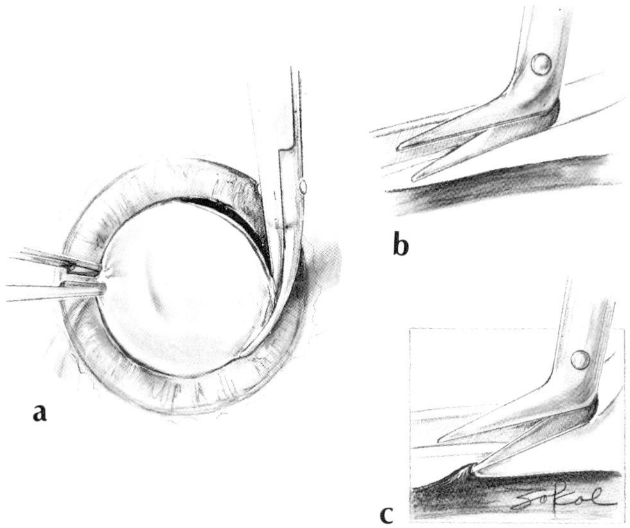

Figure 5.6 (a,b) *Cutting the recipient cornea.* **(c)** *Care must be taken not to cut iris*

in one direction and then the other, the corneal button is excised and removed from the eye. One complication associated with cutting the recipient cornea occurs when part or all of Descemet's membrane detaches from the recipient button and is left in the eye[18]. This is more likely to happen in patients with interstitial keratitis, where there is easy separation of Descemet's membrane. To avoid this problem, one must be certain to cut an adequate opening through Descemet's membrane with the trephine before introducing the corneal scissors into the incision.

When the donor corneal button is cut directly from a whole donor eye in an anterior-to-posterior direction, the trephine cut is made in a similar fashion. The anterior chamber is entered. The lower blade of the scissors is then placed in the eye but is advanced under the peripheral cornea and not under the central cornea. In this way, the lower scissor's blade can cause damage only to the donor endothelium that is not used for the transplant.

Anterior vitrectomy

For keratoplasty on aphakic eyes, an anterior vitrectomy may need to be performed before placing the donor graft, unless the anterior hyaloid face is intact. This can be accomplished using cellulose sponges or a vitrectomy instrument. When using sponges, one touches the vitreous with the tip of the sponge, lifts slightly, then cuts the vitreous flush with the pupil, using scissors (*Figure 5.7*). This process is repeated until the anterior chamber is free of vitreous. Alternatively an 'open sky' vitrectomy

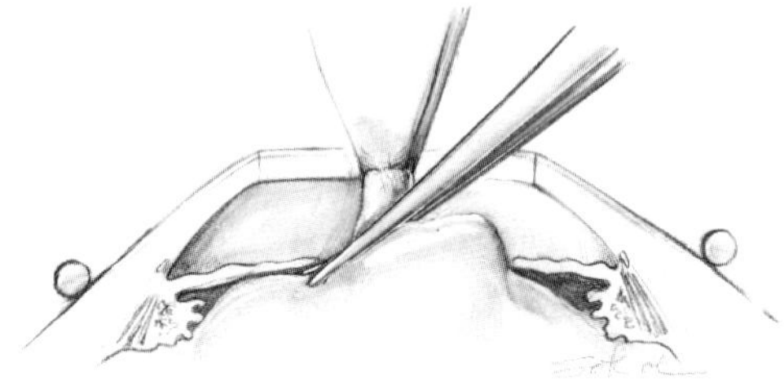

Figure 5.7 *During keratoplasty, anterior vitrectomy performed using cellulose sponges and scissors*

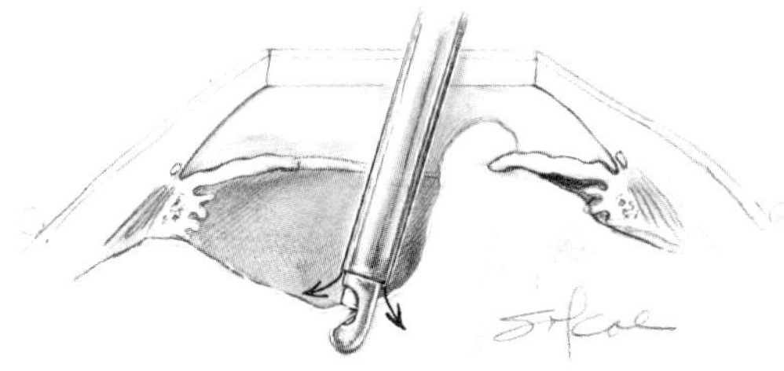

Figure 5.8 *Vitrectomy instrument can be used to remove vitreous during keratoplasty*

may be performed using a vitrectomy instrument. This is accomplished by placing the tip of the instrument through the pupil into the anterior vitreous cavity and gently excising vitreous, using the cutting and suction mode (*Figure 5.8*). If necessary, irrigation can be provided from a bulb syringe with physiological saline.

Suturing the graft

After the recipient corneal button has been removed and the anterior vitrectomy completed if necessary, the anterior chamber is filled with physiological saline or sodium hyaluronate (Healon) and the donor graft is gently placed, endothelial side down, in the recipient bed. The donor cornea is transferred from the Teflon block to the recipient eye by grasping it on the epithelial edge with fine-tooth forceps or by placing a spatula under the epithelial surface. The donor tissue must be handled with extreme care at all times. If too many endothelial cells are injured, this may lead to graft edema and graft failure requiring a regraft.

Once the donor tissue has been placed on the recipient eye, four cardinal sutures should be placed at 90° intervals

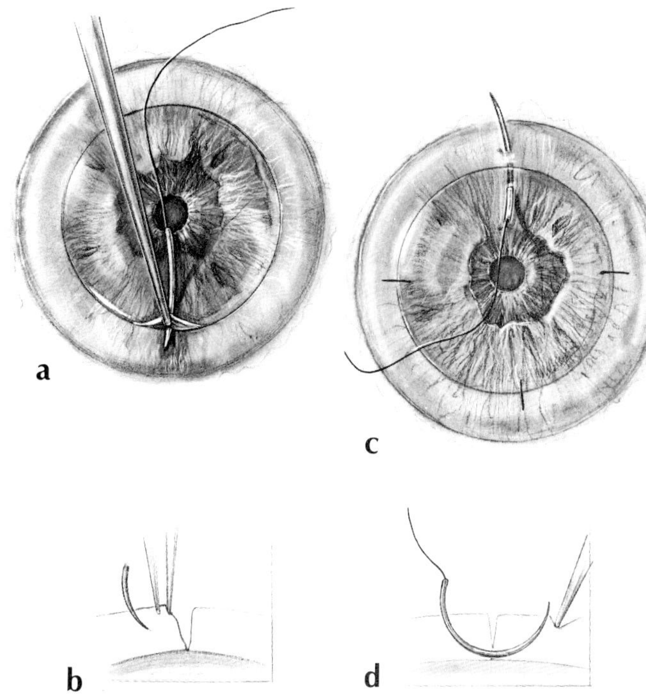

Figure 5.9 *Placement of the four cardinal sutures*

– usually at the 3, 6, 9 and 12 o'clock positions (*Figure 5.9a–d*). When placing the first suture in the graft, usually at 12 o'clock, the assistant can hold the epithelial edge of the graft at 6 o'clock to stabilize the donor cornea. The needle tip should be placed about 1.5 mm from the edge and passed deep, to the level just above Descemet's membrane (*Figure 5.9a,b*). The needle is then passed into the recipient cornea at the same depth and out about 1.5 mm from the bed edge (*Figure 5.9c,d*). Forceps (usually a 0.12 mm forceps) are used to fixate the tissue during suturing. In the graft, the needle is always passed just behind the forceps. In order not to damage corneal endothelial cells, care must be taken not to grab the endothelial surface of the graft, or bend or stretch the donor cornea excessively. In the recipient bed, the forceps can be used to evert slightly the edge so that the proper suture depth can be obtained. After passing the needle, the suture is tied using a triple throw (surgeon's knot) followed by a square knot or by a Dangle slip knot as described in Chapter 6 (*Figure 6.17*).

Once the cardinal sutures have been placed, the suturing can be completed with additional interrupted sutures or with a single running suture. We prefer to use 10/0 monofilament nylon suture for all our graft cases, but some surgeons use 8/0 or 9/0 silk for the cardinal sutures, but then remove them at the end of the surgery.

Interrupted sutures

When the recipient bed is highly vascularized or in corneal melting conditions, interrupted sutures are preferred. If a single interrupted suture breaks or becomes loose, or if it attracts additional vessels onto the graft, it can be removed. This is not the case with a running suture. In placing additional interrupted sutures, the fifth interrupted suture is placed halfway between two of the cardinal sutures and tied. After three more sutures have been placed midway between the other cardinal sutures, eight additional sutures are placed, each halfway between the first eight sutures (*Figure 5.10a,b*). Usually a total of 16 interrupted sutures is sufficient for a 7.0, 7.5 or 8.0 mm recipient bed. It is important to bury the knots of all sutures into the recipient cornea (*Figure 5.10c–e*).

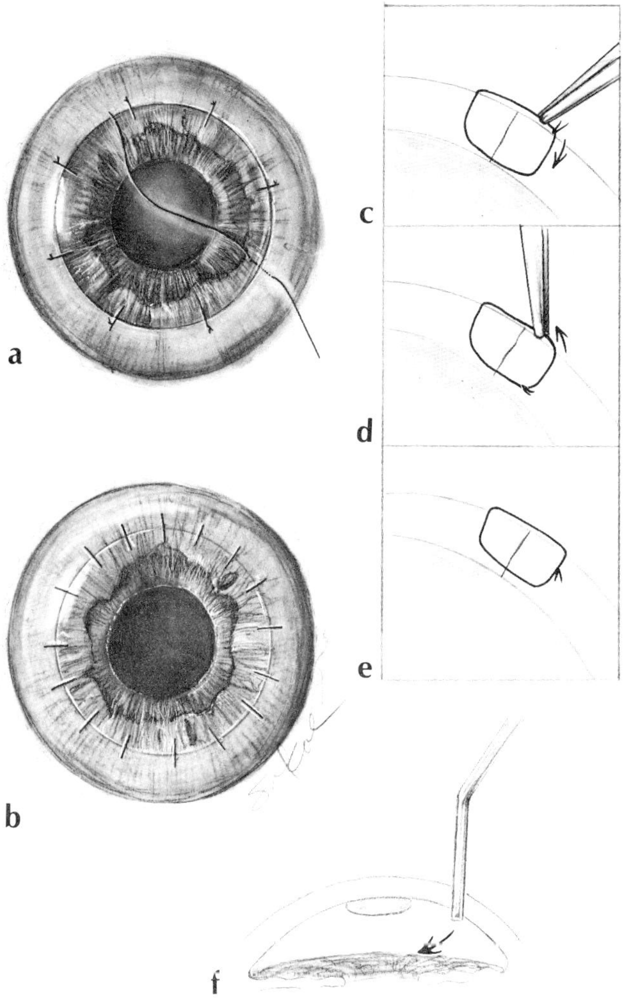

Figure 5.10 *Use of multiple interrupted sutures, with technique for burying the knot in the recipient stroma*

While the sutures are being placed, a formed anterior chamber should be maintained with air. When the suturing is complete, the air can be removed and replaced by physiological saline (*Figure 5.10f*). Some surgeons advocate the use of sodium hyaluronate (Healon) to maintain the chamber[19,20]. If used in phakic eyes, sodium hyaluronate should be removed at the termination of surgery, or else marked elevation of intraocular pressure may develop. One advantage of air over sodium hyaluronate is that it provides a visual aid in determining the correct tension of the sutures. Also, sodium hyaluronate has the appearance and consistency of vitreous and is difficult at times to distinguish from it.

Running suture

In corneal grafts in which the recipient bed is not highly vascularized or unusually thin, a single running suture of 10/0 monofilament nylon is an excellent method of securing the graft. The first passage of the needle on the double-armed, long suture is made between 12 and 2 o'clock. The needle is always placed through the graft first, then through the recipient cornea (*Figure 5.11a,b*). The suturing is continued for 16–24 passes, until it has progressed for 360° around the cornea. While placing the suture, it is much easier to move the microscope (using sterile microscope handles) than it is to bend and contort one's hands to pass a difficult backhand suture. When moving the microscope for better positioning it is best to leave the needle in the wound; it can then be easily relocated when suturing is restarted.

After proceeding for 360° and reaching the first suture bite, a triple-throw surgeon's knot (*Figure 5.11c*) is used to secure the suture while the suture is being tightened with tying forceps (*Figure 5.11d*). Once the running suture has been adequately tightened, the triple throw is taken out and the suture is tied with a single-throw locking knot (*Figure 5.11e–g*) followed by a square knot (*Figure 5.11h,i*). The suture is pulled with tying forceps to bury the knot (*Figure 5.11j,k*). After placing a running suture, the four interrupted cardinal sutures can be removed or left in place with their knots buried.

Fluorescein 2 per cent solution on a cellulose sponge may be used after a running or interrupted closure to check for wound leaks (*Figure 5.11l*). If a leak is found, additional interrupted 10/0 nylon sutures are placed where needed. A small amount of leakage around a suture track can be left alone.

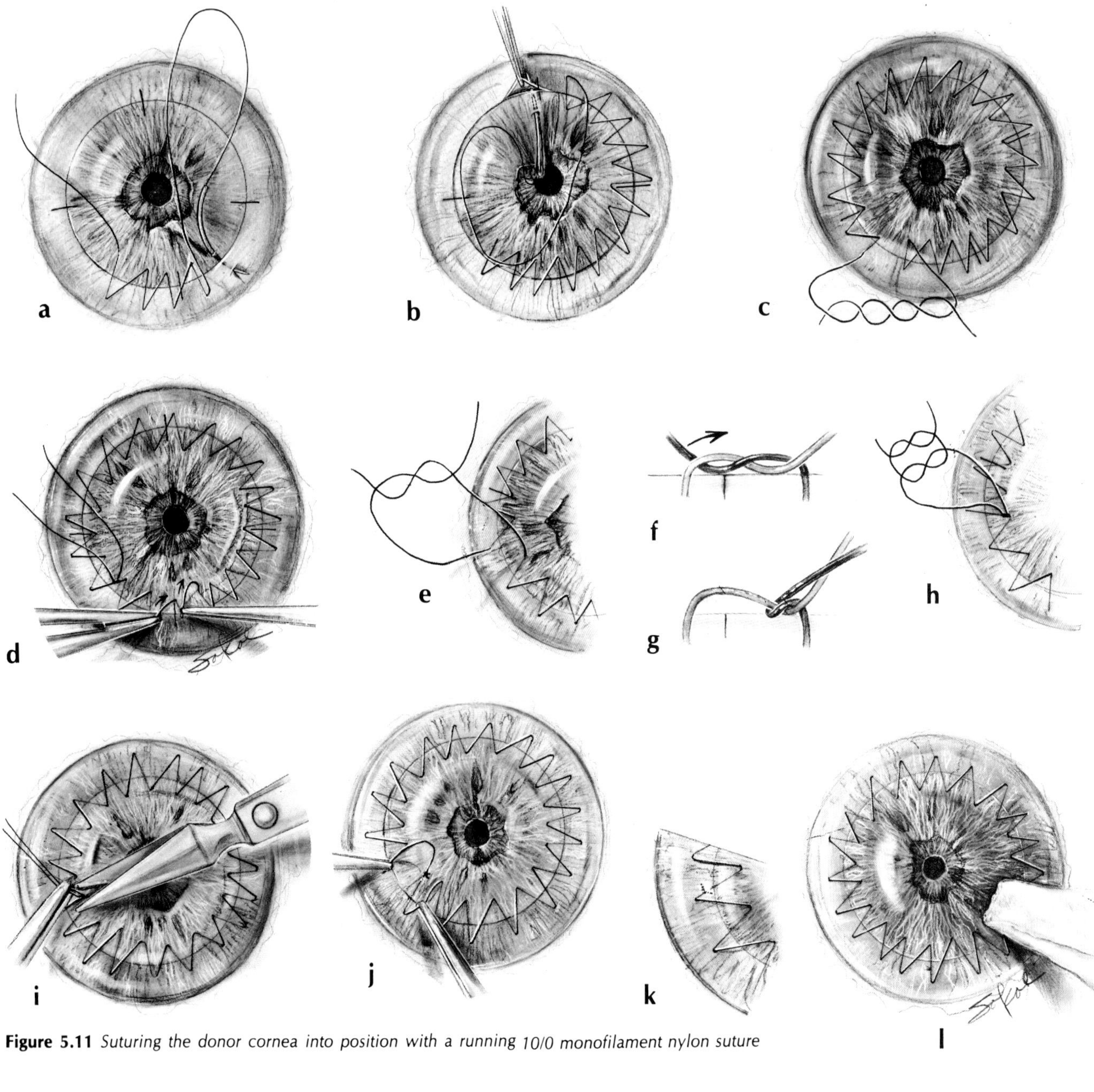

Figure 5.11 *Suturing the donor cornea into position with a running 10/0 monofilament nylon suture*

Keratoplasty combined with cataract extraction

Until the late 1960s the management of a patient with combined corneal clouding and cataract usually required keratoplasty, followed 6–12 months later by cataract extraction. In the early 1970s, the combined procedure of keratoplasty and simultaneous cataract extraction was advocated by some. Data at that time seemed to indicate little difference in results between the combined procedure and keratoplasty followed later by separate cataract extraction[21]. By combining the procedures, the visual recovery period was reduced.

If a patient's eye has a cataract and a corneal opacity, the decision should be made preoperatively on whether to remove the cataract at the time of keratoplasty. There are two options for cataract removal at keratoplasty: intracapsular cataract extraction (ICCE) or extracapsular cataract extraction (ECCE). If ICCE is planned, then the zonular fibers can be released with α-chymotrypsin, or cellulose sponges can be used to strip off the fibers at 6 or 12 o'clock. A cryoprobe is then used to extract the lens (*Figure 5.12*); and an anterior vitrectomy, if needed, is performed as described earlier.

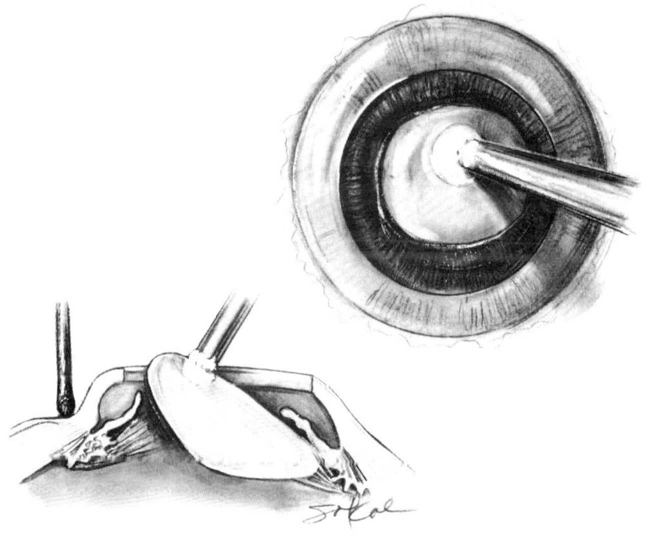

Figure 5.12 *Intracapsular cataract extraction using a cryoprobe, combined with keratoplasty*

Since 1976, some surgeons have advocated ECCE at the time of keratoplasty. Our technique for extracapsular cataract extraction when combined with keratoplasty is as follows[22]: The recipient corneal button is removed, and a razor blade knife or curved Vannas scissors are used to cut the anterior lens capsule for 360° near the pupil margin (*Figure 5.13a*). A cryoprobe is then used to remove the lens nucleus (*Figure 5.13b*). Care is taken not to freeze the peripheral edge of the lens capsule. Cortical material is removed by gentle irrigation, using a bulb and physiological saline solution. The remaining cortical material is gently wiped from the posterior capsule, using dry cellulose sponges (*Figure 5.13c*). A sweeping movement from the peripheral to the central area of the posterior capsule is used, care being taken not to tear the capsule in the process. Alternatively, the irrigating/aspirating tip of the Cavitron or other similar unit can be used in an open-system approach to aspirate lens cortex (*Figure 5.14*). The donor cornea is then sutured into position, using a running or interrupted sutures as described above. During suturing a formed anterior chamber is maintained with air or sodium hyaluronate.

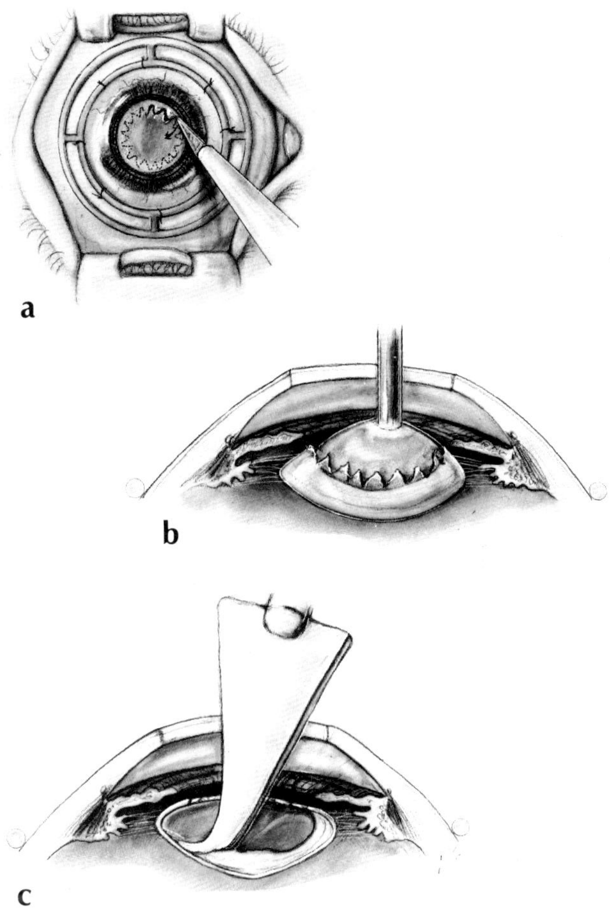

Figure 5.13 *Combined keratoplasty and extracapsular cataract extraction.* **(a)** *Incision in anterior capsule after removal of recipient cornea.* **(b)** *Cross-section of cryoextraction of lens nucleus.* **(c)** *Cellulose sponge used gently to wipe cortex off posterior capsule*

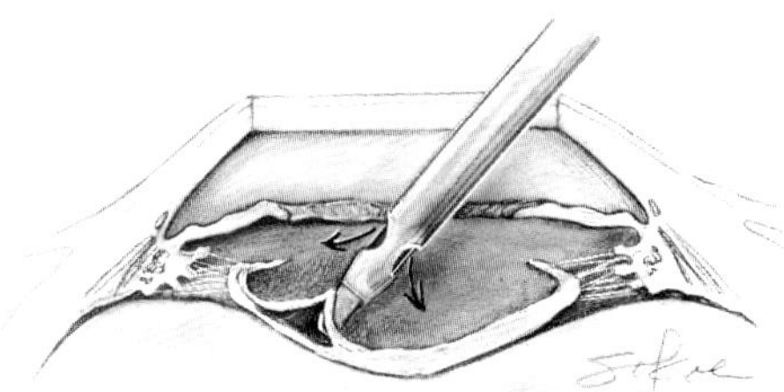

Figure 5.14 *Irrigation/aspiration of lens cortex through keratoplasty incision*

Triple procedure: keratoplasty, cataract extraction and intraocular lens implantation

The combination of keratoplasty, cataract extraction and intraocular lens (IOL) implantation has been called the 'triple procedure'. Since 1976 there have been several reports advocating this method[23–25]. The results of these studies seem to indicate that, in the appropriate circumstances, the triple procedure can give good visual results with a reasonably low risk of graft failure.

Either ICCE or ECCE can be used to remove the cataract, as described above. After an ICCE a flexible anterior chamber IOL or an iris-plane IOL can be inserted (see Chapter 6). If there are no specific contraindications to IOL implantation and it is considered to be in the patient's best interest, we believe there are advantages to a posterior chamber IOL with ECCE at the time of keratoplasty[22]. The theoretical advantages of this method include the following. The posterior capsule is left intact, and there is no need for anterior vitrectomy; this may decrease the incidence of cystoid macular edema[26] and other retinal complications. Second, the IOL is placed at a greater distance from the corneal endothelium, and the iris serves as a protective barrier between the cornea and IOL. Last, the pupil can be maximally dilated after surgery, with minimal risk of complication.

The technique for ECCE is described above. After the posterior capsule has been cleaned of residual lens cortex, a Shearing-type IOL is inspected and irrigated with physiological saline. One loop of the IOL is placed behind the iris and into the lens capsular bag at 6 o'clock (*Figure 5.15a*) or into the ciliary sulcus. The superior loop of the IOL is bent with smooth forceps so that it can be placed behind the iris and into the capsular bag or preferably the ciliary sulcus at 12 o'clock without forcing the inferior loop too far toward 6 o'clock (*Figure 5.15b,c*). After it is positioned behind the iris, the IOL can be gently centered. Acetylcholine or carbachol is instilled to constrict the pupil and protect the donor cornea from the IOL. The donor cornea is then sutured into place with a running or with interrupted 10/0 monofilament nylon sutures (*Figure 5.15d*). Air is used to maintain a formed anterior chamber while the graft is sutured in place.

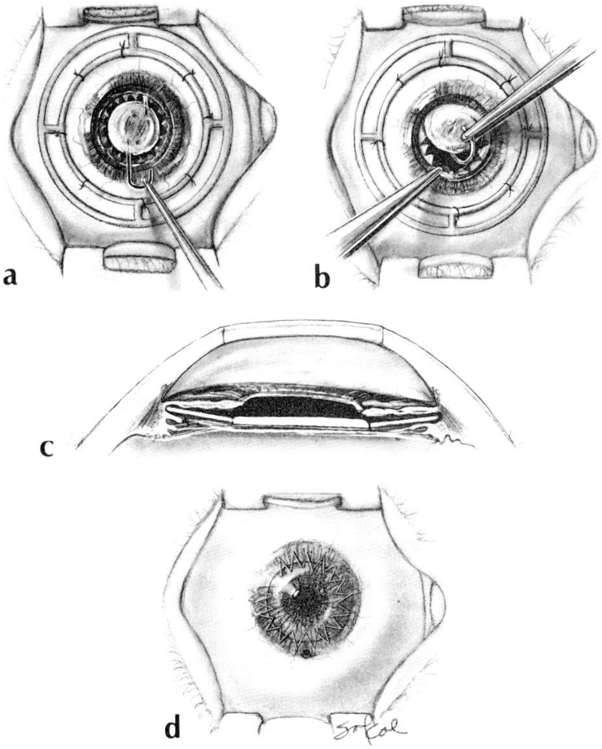

Figure 5.15 *Intraocular lens implantation.* **(a,b)** *Placing a Shearing IOL.* **(c)** *IOL in position.* **(d)** *Donor cornea is then sutured in place*

Lamellar keratoplasty

In lamellar or non-penetrating keratoplasty, the anterior chamber is not entered and only a partial-thickness donor graft is required.

Preparation of recipient cornea

The size of the trephine used will depend partly on the corneal disease process. Usually a 7–8 mm bed is optimal. The trephine guard should be set to the proper depth as determined by preoperative slit-lamp evaluation and corneal thickness measurements. Usually the trephine cutting depth is set no deeper than 90 per cent of the central corneal thickness. As much normal recipient cornea as possible should be left, but the cut should be deep enough to remove diseased tissue.

After a partial-thickness incision has been cut with the trephine (*Figure 5.16a,b*), one edge of the corneal button is lifted with forceps and (using a corneal dissector or an instrument such as the Martinez knife) a lamellar dissection is started (*Figure 5.16c*). A lamellar plane is usually easily obtained, and occasionally the anterior cornea can be peeled from the underlying corneal bed without further dissection. The corneal bed is inspected for further opacifications. If the anterior chamber is inadvertently entered, the wound can be sutured or the procedure can be converted to a penetrating keratoplasty.

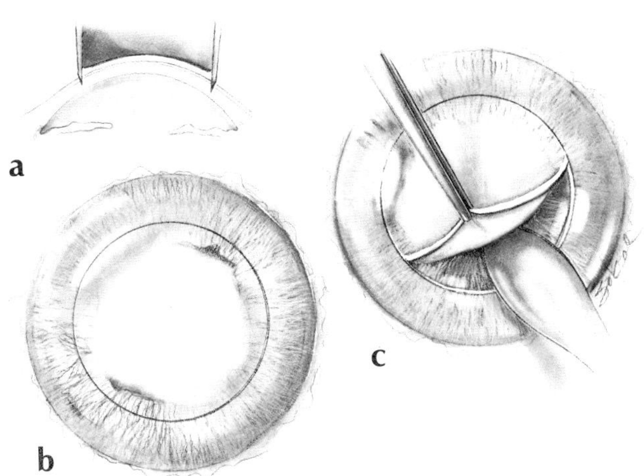

Figure 5.16 *Preparation of recipient bed for lamellar keratoplasty.* **(a,b)** *Partial-thickness cut with trephine.* **(c)** *Dissection of lamellar corneal tissue from recipient*

Preparation of donor cornea

For lamellar keratoplasty the donor tissue is prepared after the recipient cornea has been cut because of the possible need to convert to penetrating keratoplasty. A whole donor eye facilitates cutting of the donor tissue. The donor button for graft is prepared first by starting a lamellar dissection of donor cornea peripherally (*Figure 5.17a,b*). A trephine that is 0.25–0.5 mm larger than that used for the recipient is then used to cut the donor tissue (*Figure 5.17c*).

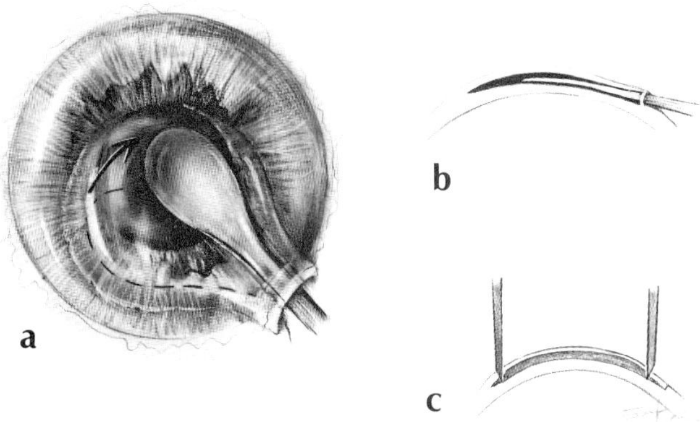

Figure 5.17 *Preparation of donor tissue for lamellar graft*

Some surgeons prefer to use the Barraquer keratome for cutting the donor and the recipient tissue. This microkeratome is designed like a small dermatome and has an oscillating cutting blade that can be set to cut lamellar sections of various thicknesses.

Suturing the graft

The donor graft is secured in position using four interrupted cardinal sutures of 10/0 nylon, as in penetrating keratoplasty. Completion of the suturing can be with additional interrupted sutures or a continuous running suture (*Figure 5.18*). The knots should always be buried into the recipient corneal stroma to reduce irritation and the chance of vascularization of the graft.

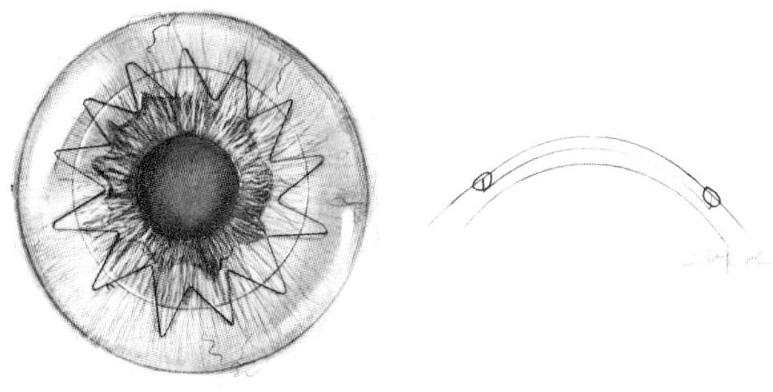

Figure 5.18 *Lamellar graft sutured in position with running 10/0 monofilament nylon*

Superficial keratectomy

Superficial or lamellar keratectomy involves the same preparation and cutting of the patient's cornea as in lamellar keratoplasty. When the corneal disease process is very superficial and involves less than one-quarter of the thickness of the anterior corneal surface, no graft may be required. The area to be excised is cut using the trephine and the superficial cornea is removed with gentle lamellar dissection. Occasionally a small peripheral superficial lesion such as is seen in Bowen's disease can be simply 'shaved off' with a sharp blade without the use of a trephine.

Management of corneal perforation

Tissue adhesive

The use of cyanoacrylate tissue adhesive for sealing small corneal perforations of 3 mm diameter or less and descemetoceles has been shown to be effective[27]. The procedure can often be performed using topical anesthesia and an operating microscope, or, in some cases, the adhesive can be applied at the slit lamp. The edges and base of the area of perforation are first scraped with a blade to remove all epithelium in the area. Cellulose sponges are used to remove any remaining debris and to dry the area to be glued. The anterior chamber is deepened with air or sodium hyaluronate. A drop of cyanoacrylate adhesive is placed on the tip of an iris spatula. The amount of adhesive used will depend on the size of the defect, because the adhesive is applied directly to the base of the defect or perforation. The adhesive usually will spread to fill the defect if enough has been applied. Additional adhesive can be applied if necessary but excessive adhesive is difficult to remove. The adhesive polymerizes on contact with water; therefore if water is applied to the cornea prematurely the adhesive will polymerize in an irregular fashion and not seal the perforation properly. Usually the adhesive dries in 5–10 minutes, and then a therapeutic soft contact lens should be placed over the cornea. The lens prevents lid movement from dislodging the adhesive.

Patch corneal graft

If tissue adhesive is not available or if the perforation is large, a lamellar patch graft may be required. The recipient bed is prepared as described for lamellar keratoplasty. The smallest trephine is used that will enclose the perforation and leave 1–2 mm of normal tissue around it. After the trephine has penetrated to about one-third to one-half corneal thickness, necrotic tissue is removed. Once the bed is cleaned as well as possible, the same size trephine (or 0.5 mm larger) is used to cut and dissect a lamellar graft from the donor eye. The graft is positioned and sutured on the recipient bed with multiple interrupted 10/0 nylon sutures. If the cornea surrounding the recipient bed is severely diseased, tissue adhesive can be applied over the donor graft and surrounding recipient cornea. A therapeutic contact lens is used to protect the cornea if tissue adhesive is used. Sodium hyaluronate can be useful in re-forming the anterior chamber in such cases.

Conjunctival flap

Creation of a Gundersen-style conjunctival flap requires careful surgical technique, because there usually is not enough tissue available for a second attempt. After local anesthesia, a traction suture is placed through the corneal limbus at 12 o'clock. The globe is rotated inferiorly with this suture (*Figure 5.19a*). One to two ml of 2 per cent lidocaine (lignocaine; Xylocaine) mixed with one drop of 1:1000 epinephrine (adrenaline) may be injected beneath the superior conjunctiva to form a bleb. Care is taken not to pass the needle through the portion of the conjunctiva that will be used to cover the cornea (*Figure 5.19a*). The injection helps to separate conjunctiva from Tenon's capsule, but the procedure can be performed without the subconjunctival injection.

Before making the flap, all the corneal epithelium is devitalized by iodine and debrided (*Figure 5.19b,c*). Scissors are used to make a horizontal incision through the bulbar conjunctiva superiorly (*Figure 5.19d*). The conjunctiva is then bluntly dissected from underlying Tenon's capsule, and the dissection is carried down to the limbus (*Figure 5.19e–g*). At the limbus the conjunctiva is cut with a razor blade knife or scissors to free it from the cornea. Care must be taken not to create a button-hole in the conjunctiva (*Figure 5.19h*). A 360° peritomy is made at the limbus by extending the 12 o'clock limbal incision (*Figure 5.19i*). The flap is then spread down over the cornea (*Figure 5.19j*). Two mattress-type sutures of 6/0 silk or gut are placed in the limbus at 5 and 7 o'clock and are passed through the flap (*Figure 5.19k*). The inferior conjunctiva is sutured to the lower border of the conjunctival flap after the mattress sutures have been tied (*Figure 5.19l*). The superior conjunctiva is sutured to the sclera, using interrupted 6/0 or 7/0 silk or gut suture (*Figure 5.19m*).

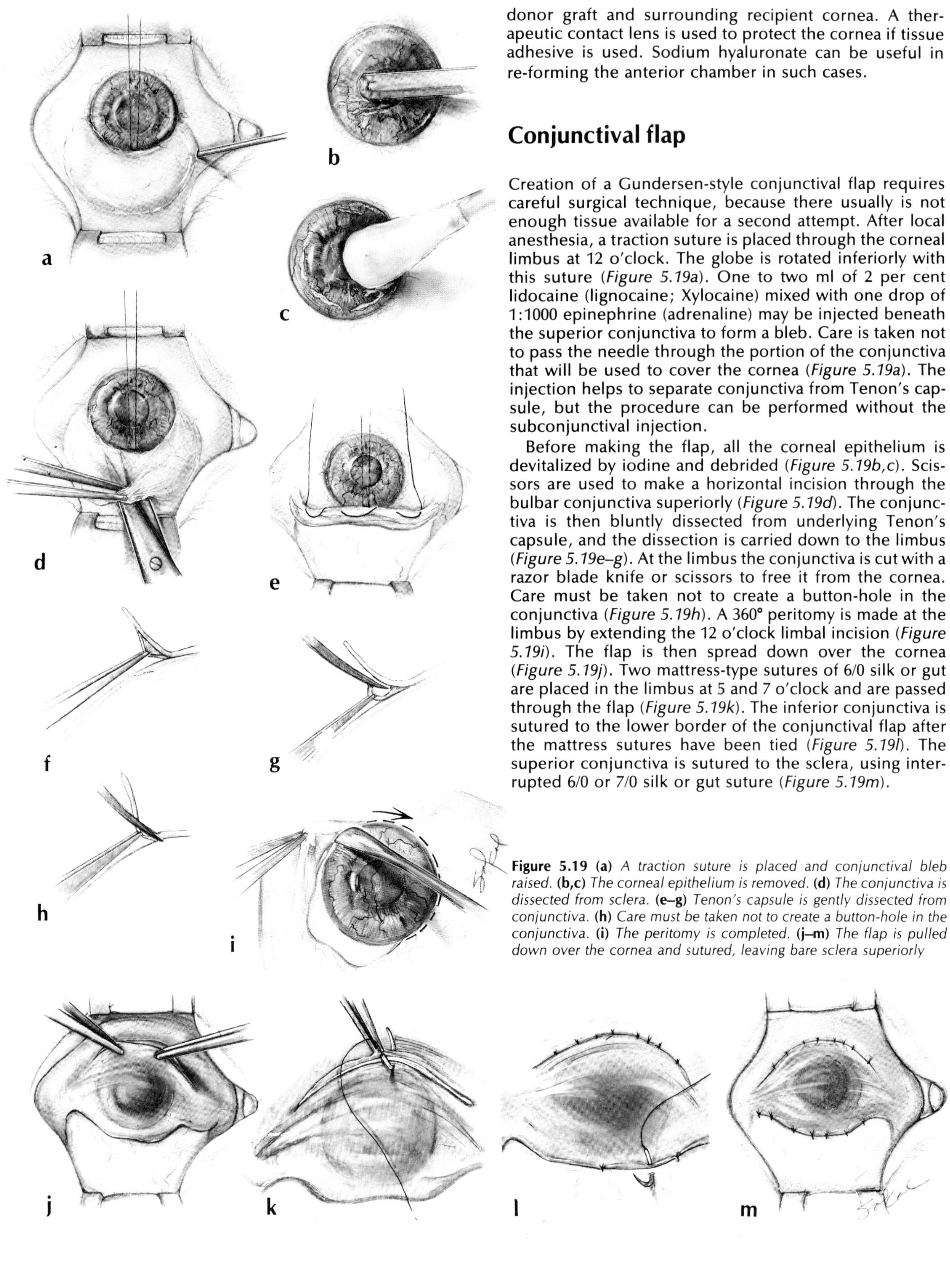

Figure 5.19 **(a)** *A traction suture is placed and conjunctival bleb raised.* **(b,c)** *The corneal epithelium is removed.* **(d)** *The conjunctiva is dissected from sclera.* **(e–g)** *Tenon's capsule is gently dissected from conjunctiva.* **(h)** *Care must be taken not to create a button-hole in the conjunctiva.* **(i)** *The peritomy is completed.* **(j–m)** *The flap is pulled down over the cornea and sutured, leaving bare sclera superiorly*

Refractive corneal surgery

Keratophakia

This technique was developed by Barraquer to correct the refractive error of aphakia. It involves inserting a lathe-cut, corneal lenticule beneath a lamellar dissection of host cornea (*Figure 5.20*). Highly sophisticated equipment is required to cut the lenticule, and a detailed description of the technique will not be given here[28].

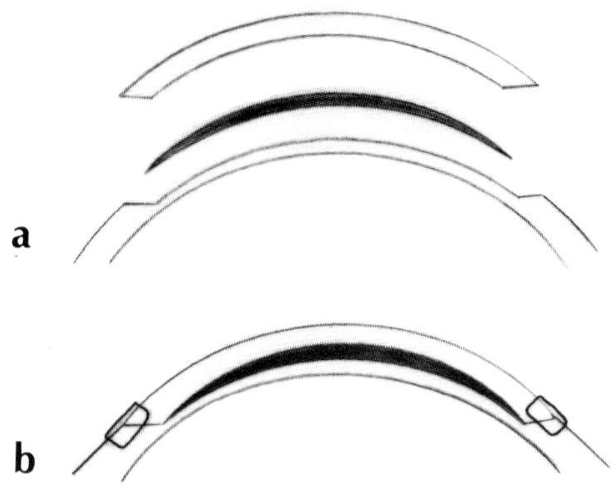

Figure 5.20 *Keratophakia to correct aphakia*

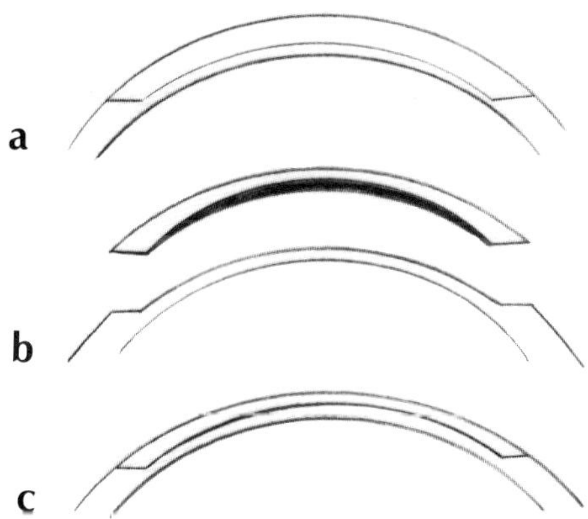

Figure 5.21 *Keratomileusis for the refractive correction of myopia*

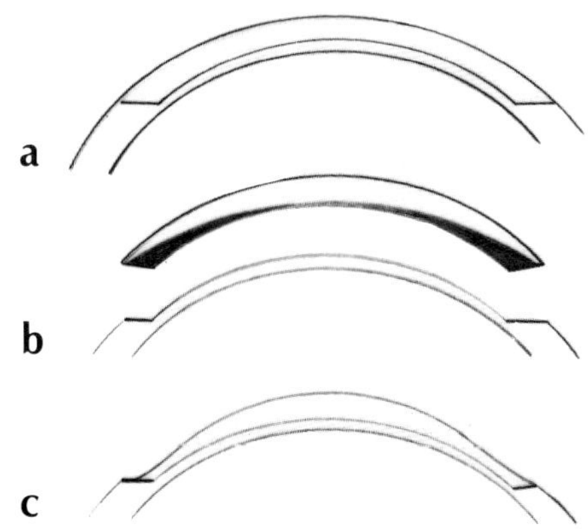

Figure 5.22 *Keratomileusis for the refractive correction of aphakia*

Keratomileusis

This form of refractive surgery, also developed by Barraquer, involves the removal of a portion of a patient's cornea, which is then frozen and lathe-cut to an appropriate plus- or minus-lens shape and reinserted in the patient's cornea (*Figures 5.21, 5.22*). This also requires highly sophisticated techniques and equipment and will not be described further[29].

Epikeratophakia

This form of refractive corneal surgery was first described by Kaufman[30,31]. It involves suturing cryopreserved, lathed donor corneal tissue directly onto the recipient cornea (*Figure 5.23*). Only the epithelium of the recipient is removed, and the risk of damaging the cornea is less than

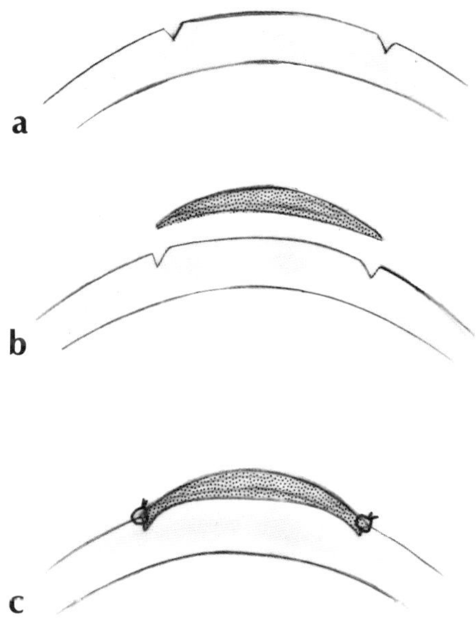

Figure 5.23 *Epikeratophakia for the refractive correction of aphakia*

with some of the other procedures. Another advantage of this procedure is the potential for later changing the donor tissue and hence the power of the lenticule. It may thus be potentially useful after removal of congenital cataracts, where the required correction may change with age. The procedure should still be considered investigational.

Wedge resection

This technique is used in treating high degrees of corneal astigmatism by performing a free-hand, wedge-shaped corneal resection parallel to the limbus in the flatter corneal meridian (*Figure 5.24*). The size and shape of the arc are determined by the amount of astigmatism. After the wedge of cornea has been removed, the resection is

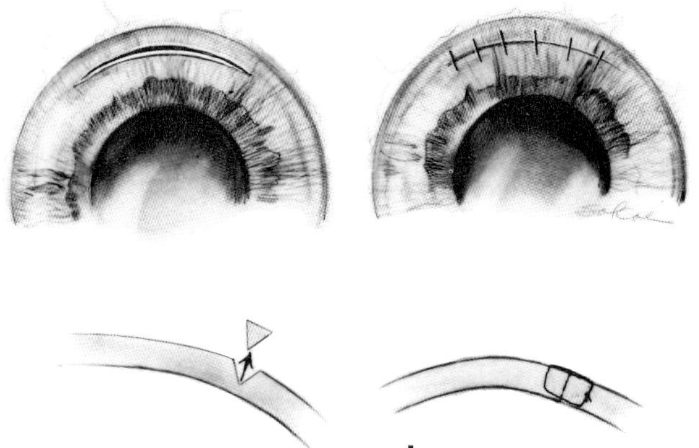

a b

Figure 5.24 *Wedge resection for refractive correction of high astigmatism*

closed with multiple interrupted 10/0 nylon or polypropylene sutures. It is usually necessary to enter the anterior chamber and release aqueous humor to permit tight wound closure. The sutures are removed in a graded fashion 10–16 weeks after surgery or they may be left in place depending on the postoperative refractive error. Final stable vision may not be obtained for several months after suture removal[32]. This corneal steepening technique is especially useful when the corneal curvature is flatter than normal.

Relaxing incision

In cases of high astigmatism, some surgeons prefer a relaxing incision that flattens the steepest meridian, especially if the corneal curvature is steeper than normal. In the case of postkeratoplasty astigmatism, an incision is made in the wound to about two-thirds depth. The incisions are made in the steepest meridians, and the procedure may be performed at the slit lamp under topical anesthetic. The procedure is successful in about 75 per cent of cases, and some surgeons believe it should be attempted first (before a wedge resection) because it is easier and gives more rapid results[32] (*Figure 5.25*). To augment the effect, tightly placed sutures can be used in the flatter corneal meridian. The major disadvantage of this procedure is that it weakens the cornea.

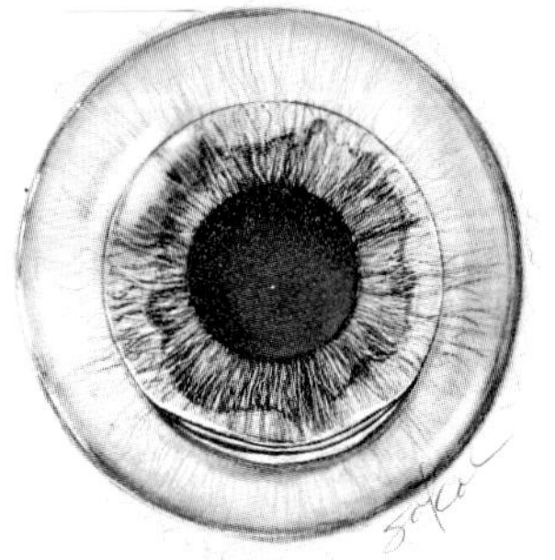

Figure 5.25 *Relaxing incision in graft scar to correct high astigmatism*

Radial keratotomy

This experimental technique for refractive correction of myopia involves making 8 or 16 radial incisions of a 90 per cent depth in the cornea, beginning about 1.5–2.5 mm from the center of the cornea (*Figure 5.26*). The incisions

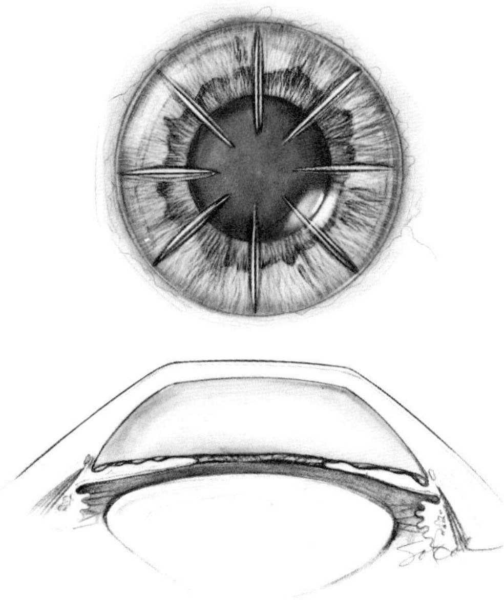

Figure 5.26 *Radial keratotomy, illustrating flattening of cornea*

are extended to, but not through, the limbus. Care is taken not to enter the anterior chamber with the special cutting blade, which has a preset depth setting. The safety and efficacy of this procedure are currently being evaluated by a clinical trial sponsored by the National Eye Institute. The potential complications will be discussed later. Extended-wear contact lenses are a less risky alternative to radial keratotomy.

Postoperative care

Immediately after corneal surgery, most eyes are treated with topical antibiotics and steroid ointment or drops and are covered with a patch and shield. Penetrating keratoplasty patients are usually kept in the hospital 2–4 days after surgery and are examined with a slit lamp daily. Non-penetrating surgical cases and certain cases of penetrating eye surgery can be performed on an outpatient basis if desired. Minimal analgesic medication is usually required after corneal surgery. If more severe pain develops, the possibility of a serious complication such as infection must be ruled out.

After hospital discharge, keratoplasty patients must be followed closely and carefully and should continue to use a topical steroid such as prednisolone acetate 1 per cent and a topical antibiotic such as gentamicin, usually one drop 4 times a day of each. Glasses during the day and a shield at night should be used to protect the eye for 2–3 months after surgery. Unless the recipient cornea is densely vascularized, all drops are discontinued 4–6 months after surgery.

Patients are examined weekly for 2 weeks, then monthly for 4 months, then every 2–3 months for about a year. After that, follow-up examination once a year is probably sufficient. Sutures are usually removed 1 year after surgery, but may be left in place much longer.

Complications

Complications can be divided into operative, early postoperative and late postoperative for each of the procedures described. Complications of keratoplasty have been recently reviewed[33].

Penetrating keratoplasty

Operative complications

In penetrating keratoplasty, it is important to be aware of the following potential intraoperative complications: retrobulbar hemorrhage, vitreous or lens explusion, problems with cutting the donor graft, problems with cutting the recipient bed, anterior chamber hemorrhage, expulsive choroidal hemorrhage, difficulty with suturing the graft and problems with re-forming the anterior chamber.

Retrobulbar hemorrhage

If keratoplasty is to be performed under local anesthesia and a retrobulbar hemorrhage occurs from the local injection, it is important not to proceed with the transplant because further, more serious complications such as expulsive choroidal hemorrhage may occur. After a severe retrobulbar hemorrhage, a lateral canthotomy may be necessary to reduce an elevated intraocular pressure (IOP), and intravenous mannitol may be given if the central retinal artery is pulsating or collapsed from the increased IOP. Surgery can be rescheduled in several weeks, and either local or general anesthesia can be used at that time.

Vitreous or lens expulsion

It is extremely helpful to have a low intraocular and intraorbital pressure before beginning the surgery. Phakic patients who are not having cataract removal at the time of keratoplasty can receive mannitol preoperatively, as mentioned earlier. Pilocarpine drops are routinely used preoperatively in phakic patients to reduce the chance of lens expulsion and to lessen the chance of damage to the lens. We believe that the use of a mechanical pressure-reducer lessens the chance of vitreous loss or lens expulsion when the eye is opened, and it facilitates re-formation of the anterior chamber in phakic eyes. If an anterior vitrectomy is required, vitreous can be removed either using multiple cellulose sponges and scissors (*see Figure 5.7*) or a vitrectomy instrument (*see Figure 5.8*).

Cutting the donor graft

The trephine should be perpendicular to the cutting block in order to avoid cutting the edge obliquely, because such an edge may result in a wound leak or high postoperative astigmatism[16,17]. The use of a corneal punch aids in performing a perpendicular cut. After completing the cut, several drops of sterile M-K medium are placed on the cornea in the Teflon cutting block to keep the donor tissue from drying out while surgery is performed on the recipient eye. The Teflon block must be cool before use or it may damage the donor cornea. These methods have already been discussed more fully under 'Operative procedures and sequence'.

Cutting the recipient cornea

In order to avoid complications it is important to cut the cornea perpendicularly. Some complications have been discussed earlier under 'Operative procedures and sequence'.

Anterior chamber hemorrhage

Often in vascularized corneas, bleeding occurs from the wound edge after the recipient cornea has been cut. Gentle irrigation usually clears the blood. The bleeding almost always subsides when the donor tissue is sutured into place and the IOP is normalized. Bleeding may also occur from the iridectomy site, but this is usually mild and rarely a problem. It is important to avoid performing an iridectomy that is too basal so that it cuts the major iris vessels. Bleeding into the anterior chamber can cause the iris to adhere to the endothelial side of the recipient cornea and make re-formation of the anterior chamber more difficult. Sodium hyaluronate can be used to prevent this adhesion of iris to cornea if bleeding occurs.

Expulsive hemorrhage

The most dangerous period of the operation occurs from the time the recipient corneal button has been removed until the donor corneal button is sutured in place. If the eye is phakic, a sudden increase in IOP can cause extrusion of the lens and vitreous from the eye. In aphakic patients the vitreous may bulge forward, pushing the iris forward beyond the cut edges of the recipient bed. If an expulsive hemorrhage occurs at this time, it may be impossible to save the eye. If this dreaded complication does occur, the surgeon must try to secure the donor button with multiple interrupted 8/0 or 7/0 silk sutures as quickly as possible. These can later be replaced with 10/0 nylon. Once the donor cornea has been secured, scleral incisions may be made to drain suprachoroidal blood. This rare complication usually cannot be successfully managed and results in loss of all useful vision.

Difficulties with suturing the graft

The susceptibility of the donor endothelium to injury with keratoplasty is probably greatest at the time of surgery[34].

Mechanical trauma, toxic effects of medication or even of physiological saline may cause corneal endothelial cell damage[35–37] Glutathione bicarbonate Ringer's solution has been shown to be less toxic to endothelium than other solutions, and it may be preferable for re-forming the anterior chamber[38]. It is also important not to damage endothelium when suturing, by avoiding excessive bending or stretching of the graft.

If a running suture breaks during suturing, it can be removed and a new suture started. Alternatively, a new suture can be attached to the broken end by placing a second needle (with 10/0 nylon) through the wound next to the broken suture and tying a square knot. The new needle and suture can then be used to complete the closure. Another complication that occasionally occurs is suturing the iris to the corneal wound. This can be avoided by careful suture placement under direct microscopic observation, and by maintaining a formed anterior chamber during suturing with air, balanced salt solution or sodium hyaluronate.

Problems with re-forming the anterior chamber

While a graft is being sutured in place the anterior chamber is maintained formed with a small amount of air. If too much air fills the anterior chamber, the air may force its way through the pupil and behind the iris, making it very difficult to re-form the chamber later. Also, when inserting the irrigation cannula into the anterior chamber through the corneal wound, the cannula must be kept perpendicular to the wound edge; otherwise it may cause a detachment of Descemet's membrane. If the anterior chamber cannot be re-formed with air or balanced salt solution, sodium hyaluronate can be used, but it should be removed at the end of surgery to avoid postoperative glaucoma, and this removal is sometimes difficult. Occasionally, to soften the eye, it is necessary to aspirate fluid vitreous with a 20 gauge needle inserted through a pars plana incision 3 mm posterior to the limbus.

Early postoperative complications

Early postoperative complications (during the first week to 10 days after surgery) include wound leak or wound rupture, anterior synechiae, primary graft failure, elevated IOP, hyphema, vitreous hemorrhage, infection and corneal epithelial defects. These complications must be promptly recognized and managed properly to prevent irreversible damage.

Wound leak and wound rupture

Since the advent of modern microsurgical techniques, wound leak after keratoplasty is now less frequent, but it has been reported to occur in up to 10 per cent of cases[39]. Occasionally a mildly positive Seidel test from a suture tract or from the wound may be present 1 day after surgery. Seidel testing should be performed using 2 per cent fluorescein drops rather than a weaker solution. If the anterior chamber is deep and the IOP is normal, no immediate therapy for a leak is needed, or at most a semipressure patch may be applied for 24 hours, or longer if necessary. If the chamber is shallow or flat with a leak and the IOP is low, patching can be used for one day; but if the leak persists, the wound should be reinforced with additional interrupted sutures. Occasionally, a bandage soft contact lens may be used to try to tamponade the leak for a few days without placing additional sutures. A persistent wound leak can lead to other complications such as a persistent fistula, a flat anterior chamber with peripheral anterior synechiae, glaucoma, endophthalmitis or epithelial ingrowth[40].

Shallowing of the anterior chamber within a few days of surgery may be the result of a choroidal detachment rather than a wound leak. This must be considered if there is a negative Seidel test and the IOP is normal or low, with a flat chamber. If the chamber is flat with a high IOP, ciliary- or pupillary-block glaucoma may exist, and a laser iridotomy should be performed if possible (see Chapter 7).

Soon after surgery, while the suture material is still in place, wound rupture or separation is rare. However, this may occur after trauma (*Figure 5.27*) or if the corneal tissue

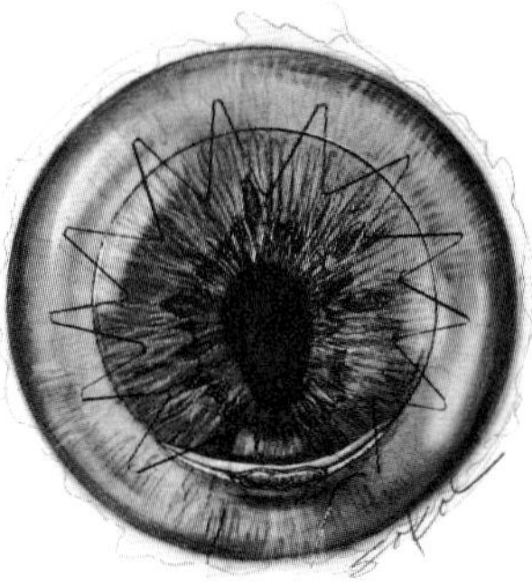

Figure 5.27 *Wound rupture after trauma, with iris in open wound*

is very thin and allows the sutures to pull through[41]. After suture removal wound dehiscence occurs more frequently and Polack and Binder[42] have reported a 9 per cent incidence following suture removal. They also report that these grafts often fail because of a detachment of Descemet's membrane, followed by the development of fibrous membranes. We have not seen this high rate of wound dehiscence or resultant graft failure.

Anterior synechiae

Anterior synechiae usually result from either a wound leak or inflammation, but they may result from incarceration of the iris in the wound during surgery[15] or, in aphakic eyes, from previous iris adhesions. Anterior synechiae are undesirable because they may cause angle-closure glaucoma and may increase the chance of graft edema (*Figure 5.28*)[43]. Anterior synechiae should be treated early to eliminate them before permanent damage to the trabecular meshwork and anterior chamber angle occur. Anterior synechiae can be treated by making a Ziegler knife puncture at the limbus, 180° from the area of involvement. A thin iris spatula or Barraquer sweep can be inserted to free the iris from the wound and peripheral cornea. The chamber can be deepened by injecting a small amount of sodium hyaluronate.

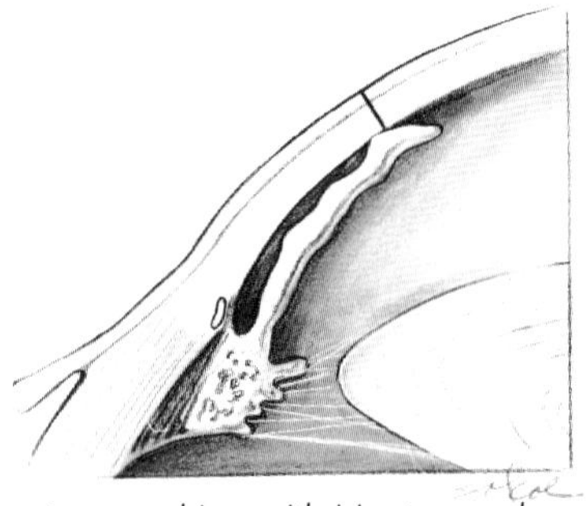

Figure 5.28 *Anterior synechiae, with iris at wound*

The risk of developing anterior synechiae is increased with use of larger grafts and with iritis. Grafts of 7.5–8.0 mm are probably optimal. Operating on a soft eye is also helpful in avoiding this complication. Preoperative and postoperative iritis must be controlled with topical steroids to avoid anterior synechiae. Closure of the anterior chamber angle from anterior synechiae is one of the worst complications that can occur after penetrating keratoplasty.

Primary graft failure

Primary graft failure is manifest by corneal edema that develops within the first day or two after surgery. This is usually a sign of damaged or inadequate endothelial function in the graft. If the edema is severe and persists more than 7 days despite treatment with steroids, glaucoma medications and topical hypertonic saline, then irreversible tissue failure because of poor or damaged endothelium has probably occurred. If there is no improvement, such grafts may be replaced with fresh tissue after 10–15 days. Histological examination of such eyes has shown large areas of bare Descemet's membrane or damaged endothelial cells[44]. Poor donor tissue because of donor tissue deterioration or advanced donor age, the presence of dystrophic changes or improper surgical manipulation of the tissue can lead to corneal edema and graft failure.

Elevated intraocular pressure

The importance of an elevated IOP after keratoplasty has become more evident in recent years[45–48]. With the advent of the pneumatonometer (*Figure 5.29*) and the MacKay-Marg tonometer, measurement of the IOP immediately after surgery has become more practical. Significant elevation of IOP occurs in some patients after keratoplasty. It has been demonstrated that, for aphakic grafts, using a donor button 0.5–0.7 mm larger in diameter than the recipient bed decreases the incidence of elevated IOP after transplant[48]. Unlike many other complications of keratoplasty, permanent damage to the anterior chamber angle structures and glaucomatous optic nerve cupping are irreversible, and every effort should be made to prevent these complications. If a pupillary block is present with high IOP and a flat or shallow chamber, pupillary dilatation should be attempted to break the block. If this is unsuccessful, a laser iridotomy may relieve the block. Elevated IOP not associated with pupillary block is sometimes transient, but the IOP should be measured daily, and if higher than 30 mmHg it should be treated with topical timolol or a carbonic-anhydrase inhibitor.

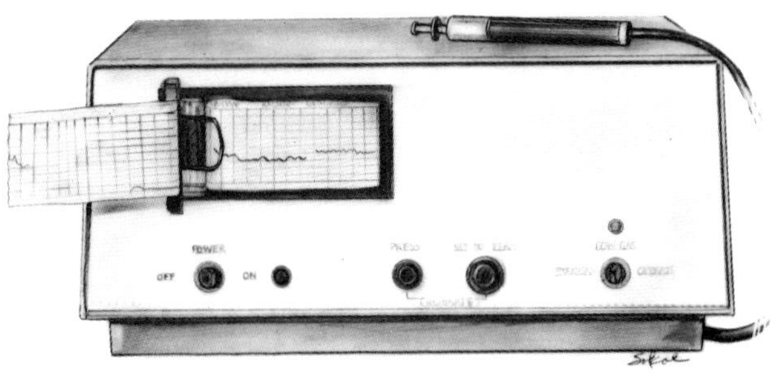

Figure 5.29 *Pneumatonometer, which is useful in measuring intraocular pressure on irregular corneas*

Hemorrhage

A hyphema or vitreous hemorrhage noted after keratoplasty may not be a serious complication and need not be initially treated unless a secondary elevation in IOP occurs. Timolol or a carbonic-anhydrase inhibitor may be used on a short-term basis to control the IOP. Occasionally a large blood clot may form in the anterior chamber and cause endothelial damage and graft edema[49].

Infection and endophthalmitis

External infection soon after keratoplasty is uncommon, and endophthalmitis is very rare after keratoplasty (*Figure 5.30*). Infected ulcers in a graft occur later in the postoperative period and are usually associated with a persistent corneal epithelial defect. When endophthalmitis occurs in the early postoperative period it may be from contamination of the donor tissue[50–52]. Studies of donor corneas have found occasional bacterial contaminants, including Staphylococcus, Pseudomonas and coliform organisms[50]. Therefore, careful donor eye enucleation techniques[53] and the use of antibiotics in the tissue culture storage medium[54] are recommended to reduce the likelihood of bacterial contamination. The Medical Eye Bank of Maryland formerly used 2.5 ml (100 mg) of parenteral-type gentamicin per liter of tissue culture storage medium. However, they now use Garamycin Reagent Solution

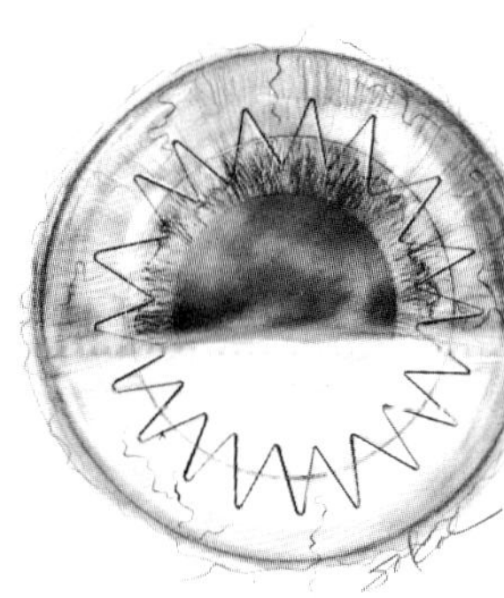

Figure 5.30 *Hypopyon after corneal graft, indicating probable infectious endophthalmitis*

(GRS) made by the Schering Co. This is pure antibiotic without preservatives, and it is added to the M-K tissue culture medium to give a final concentration of gentamicin of 50 μg/ml. Preoperative examination of donor material may show turbid media or a change in color of the phenol red indicator, if used, when bacterial contamination has occurred.

Infection of the graft is usually manifest within 24–48 hours of surgery. Signs of infection include ciliary conjunctival injection, a hazy edematous graft, mucopurulent discharge and sometimes a focus of infiltrate in the graft or around one of the sutures. If there is a 'stitch abscess' and the sutures are of the interrupted type, the affected suture should be removed and topical antibiotics are administered more frequently. If the graft is extensively necrotic and totally involved with infection despite the use of topical, subconjunctival and systemic antibiotics, the graft should be replaced in an attempt to save the eye from endophthalmitis.

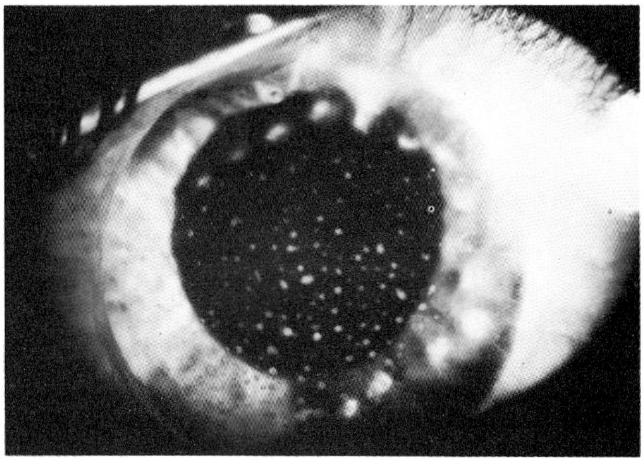

Figure 5.31 *Photograph of keratic precipitates on endothelium of donor cornea*

Corneal epithelial defects

Epithelial defects in the early postoperative course are less frequent now that corneas stored in M-K medium are used more often and the epithelium is not removed from the donor cornea before grafting. If an epithelial defect develops, semipressure patching should be used at first; and if the defect fails to heal after 3–4 days, a therapeutic soft contact lens should be used. Every effort should be made to promote epithelial healing.

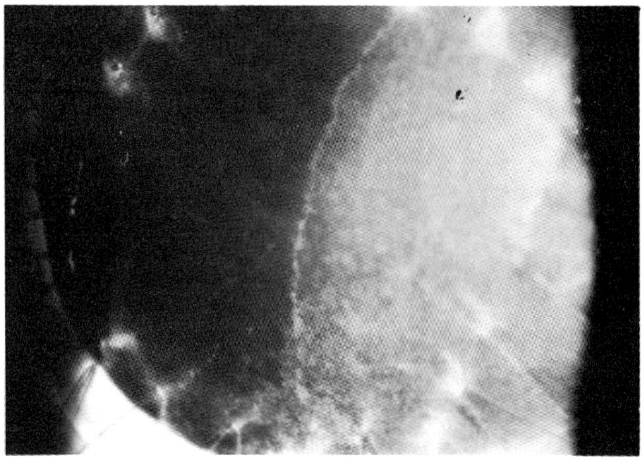

Figure 5.32 *Endothelial rejection line, as seen by direct slit-lamp illumination*

Late postoperative complications

Late postoperative complications of penetrating keratoplasty may occur from 2 weeks after surgery to many years later. These include corneal graft rejection, graft vascularization, retrograft membrane, epithelial ingrowth, complications after suture removal, retinal detachment, astigmatism, recurrence of host disease, problems related to a dry eye and transmission of donor disease.

Graft rejection

The diagnosis of primary immune graft rejection can be made only if the keratoplasty was technically successful and the graft remains clear for at least 7 days after surgery[55,56]. A typical rejection reaction starts with circumcorneal injection, keratic precipitates (*Figure 5.31*) or a rejection line on the endothelium of the graft (*Figure 5.32*). Subepithelial infiltrates have also been described as an early sign of graft rejection[57]. The process of graft rejection may often be reversed by intensive use of topical steroids (prednisolone 1 per cent every 30–60 minutes). Use of sub-Tenon's steroid injections and oral prednisone is recommended if the immune process is severe. If the graft remains clear the process is termed an allograft 'reaction'. If the graft becomes opaque or cloudy despite therapy, the diagnosis is allograft 'rejection'.

Epithelial rejection is characterized by a linear defect in corneal epithelium which progresses across the graft over 3–6 days (*Figure 5.33*). *Stromal* rejection consists of a fairly

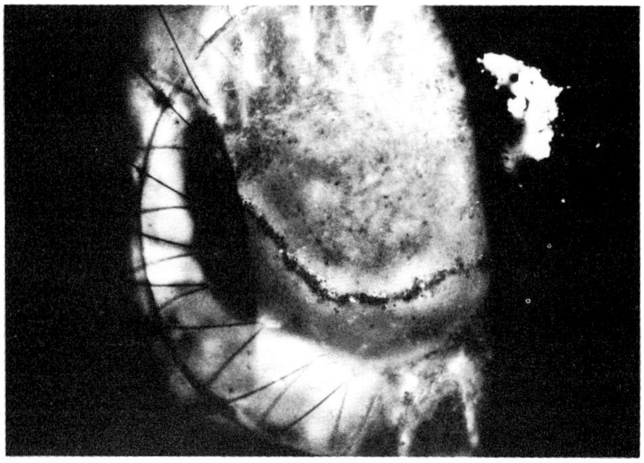

Figure 5.33 *Epithelial rejection line, stained with 1 per cent methylene blue drops*

sudden peripheral, full-thickness haze in a previously clear graft, which often begins as a peripheral arc of haze before progressing centrally (*Figure 5.34*). *Endothelial* rejection typically presents as a thin line of keratic precipitates on the endothelium, often seen best by retroillumination (*Figure 5.35*)[7]. These rejection lines are composed of lymphocytes, which appear histopathologically to be destroying the donor corneal endothelium[58].

The precise role of histocompatibility (HLA) antigens in the immune graft reaction is unknown. However, it has been shown that corneal graft recipients with rejection reactions can develop lymphocytotoxic (anti-HLA) antibodies[59]. It appears that HLA antigens may have a role in corneal graft rejection, and studies are in progress[7,60] to determine whether crossmatch testing for donor selection in recipient cases with high-risk vascularized corneas can provide pairings that will reduce the chance of graft failure from graft rejection. A negative crossmatch test ensures that the recipient does not have a clinically significant level of circulating lymphocytotoxic antibodies that are specific for the prospective donor's HLA antigens. HLA-D (DR) antigen matching studies are also under way to determine if this will reduce graft failure from rejection.

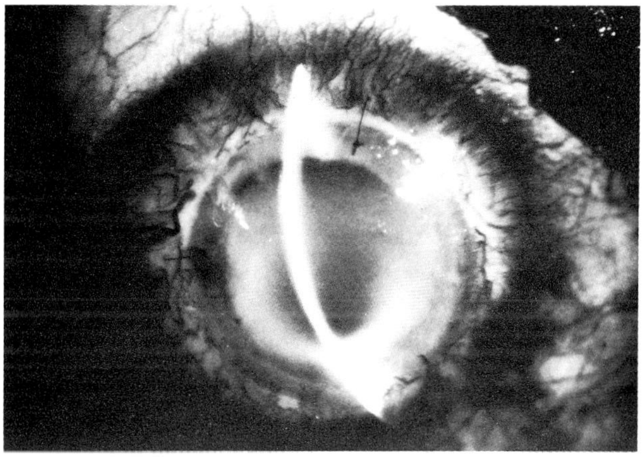

Figure 5.34 *Stromal rejection with peripheral corneal haze*

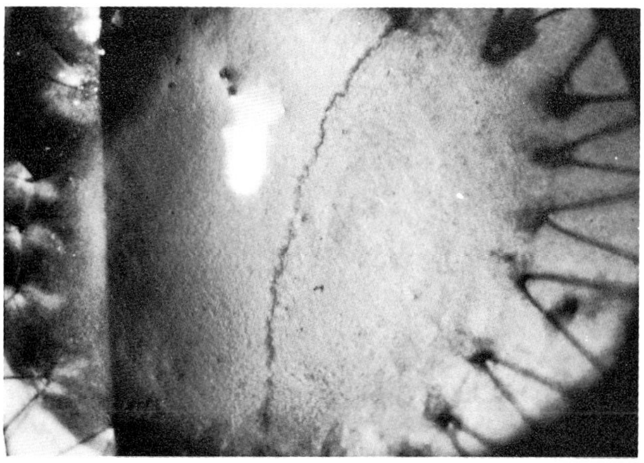

Figure 5.35 *Endothelial rejection line, as seen by retroillumination*

Graft vascularization

Graft vascularization increases the risk of graft reaction and rejection (*Figure 5.36*)[7,61]. When vessels grow into the graft along the suture line, the sutures in the involved area should be removed when possible. Use of 10/0 monofilament nylon suture usually does not stimulate vascular ingrowth, unless the suture is not properly buried and covered by epithelium.

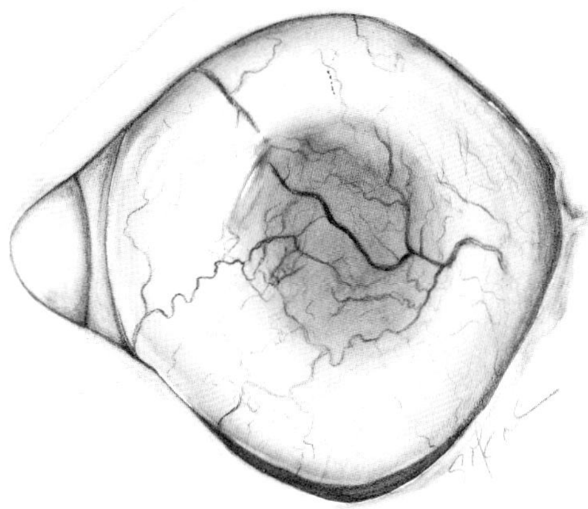

Figure 5.36 *Highly vascularized opaque corneal graft*

Retrocorneal fibrous proliferation

Retrocorneal fibrous proliferation or membrane is seen in a large percentage of opaque grafts[62]. Such retrograft membranes seem to result from damage to the endothelium or from poor wound apposition at surgery. Retrocorneal graft membrane may rarely occur from actual ingrowth of stromal tissue through a dehiscent inner corneal wound. However, the membrane is usually a result of a transformation (fibrous metaplasia) of corneal endothelial cells into fibroblast-like cells, as has been described to occur from herpes keratitis, cryoapplications to the cornea and after vitreous touch[63,64]. Since there is no satisfactory treatment, except regrafting, every effort must be made to prevent fibrous proliferation – by using meticulous surgical technique, minimizing endothelial damage and controlling postoperative inflammation.

Epithelial ingrowth

Epithelial ingrowth is fortunately a rare complication of penetrating keratoplasty[40]. It usually results from poor surgical technique or problems during surgery, with a persistent wound leak, a flat chamber or iris incarceration in the wound. However, epithelial ingrowth has been reported after uneventful keratoplasty[40], and we have seen two such cases. Clinically, it appears as a scalloped line of epithelium growing on the back surface of the cornea. A fine, lacy, white membrane growing over the iris may also be visible. Argon laser photocoagulation can be used to determine whether the iris is involved. When epithelium is growing on the iris, it turns white with laser burns, whereas normal iris turns brown[65]. Treatment of this complication is discussed in Chapter 8.

Complications related to the sutures

With the use of 10/0 monofilament nylon suture, the sutures are left in place for 12 months or longer after keratoplasty. There are several complications that can occur at the time of suture removal. Bacterial endophthalmitis has been reported shortly after suture removal[66]. Graft edema and wound dehiscence have also been noted to follow suture removal[67], and we have seen graft rejection develop in several patients within 2 weeks of suture removal, presumably from stimulation by irritation to the eye. The chance that these problems will develop can be reduced by using aseptic technique and topical antibiotics and steroids for a week after suture removal.

At any time during the postoperative course, protruding broken 10/0 nylon sutures or improperly buried knots can cause inflammation of the eyelid, conjunctiva and cornea[68]. If sutures become loose before healing is complete, irritation and discomfort can be prevented by applying a therapeutic extended-wear soft contact lens. Alternatively, an unburied knot can sometimes be pulled into the stroma at the slit lamp using fine tying forceps.

Retinal detachment

Retinal detachment can occur after any intraocular procedure. Forstot *et al.*[69] found a 5.4 per cent incidence of retinal detachment after keratoplasty that also included vitrectomy. No retinal detachments were reported after phakic keratoplasties, aphakic keratoplasties or combined procedures without vitrectomy. We have had similar experience and therefore prefer to avoid vitrectomy at the time of keratoplasty and cataract removal by performing extracapsular rather than intracapsular cataract extraction if possible.

Postoperative astigmatism

Now that technical advances have greatly improved the prognosis in corneal transplantation, investigative attention is turning toward preventing and treating postoperative refractive error and astigmatism[70]. A high degree of astigmatism in an otherwise successful graft after keratoconus can result in an unhappy patient who continues to need a contact lens for best vision. Jensen and Maumenee[71] reviewed corneal grafts performed at the Wilmer Institute over a period of 3 years and found that 11 per cent of the grafts on phakic eyes required a contact lens postoperatively. For a patient with excessive astigmatism which persists after suture removal and who is unable to wear a contact lens, Troutman[16,17] has advocated a corneal wedge-resection to reduce the astigmatism without affecting graft clarity. He has suggested[72] the use of an operating keratometer at the time of keratoplasty, in an attempt to reduce the astigmatism induced when suturing the graft. Relaxing incisions in the graft wound can also be used as described on p. 128.

Glaucoma

The onset of glaucoma 3 or more weeks after keratoplasty in an otherwise uneventful postoperative course may be a steroid-induced side-effect. Switching to fluoromethalone (FML) for steroid therapy is helpful, because it has less tendency to raise the IOP. If the pressure still remains above 30–35 mmHg, antiglaucoma medications should be used, beginning with topical timolol if there are no contraindications, then progressing to a miotic, then to a carbonic-anhydrase inhibitor. If the IOP cannot be controlled by medical means and by stopping corticosteroid drops, a filtering procedure or cyclocryotherapy should be considered. If the keratoplasty was performed after or in association with extracapsular cataract extraction, then trabeculectomy is frequently successful. If there is vitreous in the anterior chamber, the filtering operation must be combined with a vitrectomy. Cyclocryotherapy is used as a last resort because it causes considerable inflammation and can damage the graft and/or produce hypotony (see Chapter 7).

Recurrence of a host disease

The recurrence of a host disease, such as a corneal dystrophy or herpes keratitis, in the donor graft is a well known complication of keratoplasty. The recurrence of herpetic keratitis in grafts has been reported to be about 25 per cent[73] but this is higher than in our experience. If the graft is performed in an eye with active herpetic keratitis, the recurrence rate may be as high as 75 per cent[6]. Herpes keratitis may recur in typical dendritic fashion (*Figure 5.37*) or it may have a geographical pattern with stromal changes that presents a more difficult diagnostic picture. More frequently, however, herpes keratitis recurs as inflammation with keratic precipitates and can be confused with graft rejection. Patients with a history of previous herpes keratitis may be placed on prophylactic antiviral agents for 2 weeks after keratoplasty. These patients must also be observed closely while on corticosteroids which can induce recurrence; however, our recurrence rate is less than 5 per cent. If herpes keratitis recurs, antiviral medications must be started or increased. Steroids should not be stopped entirely, however, because this increases the risk of inflammation and graft rejection. Trifluridine appears to be the treatment of choice when a patient on topical steroids develops a dendrite.

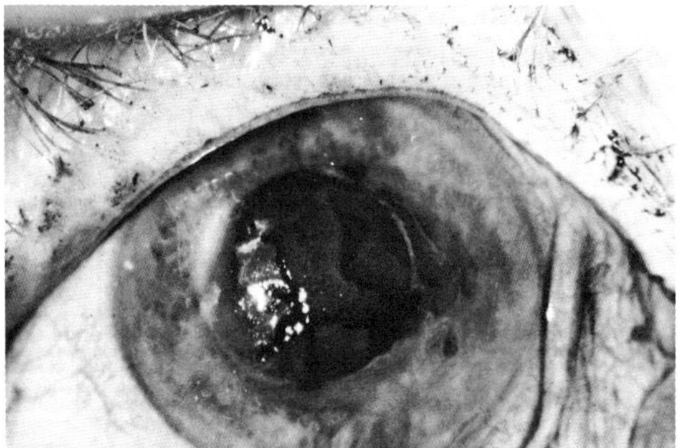

Figure 5.37 *Herpes simplex keratitis in typical dendritic pattern on corneal graft*

Many of the major corneal dystrophies, when present in the recipient, have been reported to recur in the donor graft after keratoplasty. These include lattice, macular, granular[74] and Reis-Bucklers[75] dystrophies. Recently a recurrence of keratoconus has been reported in a graft[76]. Recurrences tend to be gradual over a period of years, and no means of prevention is known. If vision is decreased by such a recurrence, repeat keratoplasty may have to be considered. In some cases, superficial keratectomy may be sufficient to restore vision.

Problems of the severely dry eye

A severely dry eye, such as can occur after an alkali burn or with the Stevens-Johnson syndrome, presents difficult long-term postoperative management problems. Grafts in these eyes often develop persistent epithelial defects that do not heal with patching, and perforations from corneal melting may occur[8]. It is especially important to use a donor cornea with healthy epithelium in a patient with a severely dry eye. Diligent postoperative follow-up is also critical. Many such patients may benefit from a therapeutic soft contact lens to protect the graft epithelium.

Contact lens misuse

The use of contact lenses for refractive reasons after keratoplasty is associated with some risk. Improper fitting or care of the contact lens may lead to severe complications, such as corneal vascularization, infected corneal ulceration and graft failure. If the vision in the fellow eye is good, use of a contact lens for correction of vision in the grafted eye should probably be delayed until sutures are removed at about 1 year. We have recently used high water content extended-wear soft contact lens beginning 2 months after surgery in aphakic eyes, if the other eye has reduced vision. We have had no complications with their use but we advise against the use of lower water-content contact lenses for extended-wear aphakic correction after keratoplasty.

Transmission of donor disease

One reason for strict standards for donor tissue selection, such as outlined earlier, is that some of the diseases listed have been passed on from a corneal donor to a recipient. For example, Creutzfeldt-Jakob disease and rabies have reportedly been transmitted in this manner, in some cases resulting in the death of the recipient[77,78]. For this reason we do not use donor tissue from patients with these and other diseases that were listed under 'Evaluating the donor tissue'.

Lamellar keratoplasty

Many of the complications discussed above regarding penetrating keratoplasty also apply to lamellar keratoplasty. Some of the complications that are unique to lamellar keratoplasty will now be discussed.

Anterior chamber perforation

While cutting with the trephine or during lamellar dissection, the anterior chamber may be inadvertently entered. If this perforation occurs at the periphery and can be repaired with a suture, one can proceed with the lamellar graft. If there is a large or a central perforation, however, the procedure should be converted to a penetrating keratoplasty. For this reason the recipient bed is prepared before cutting the donor eye.

Graft interface problems

After lamellar keratoplasty, most patients will achieve at best 20/30 to 20/40 vision because of light scattering at the interface between graft and recipient cornea. Other problems, such as the presence of foreign material, blood, vascularization or epithelial invasion may occur at the junction between the graft and host, and may diminish vision further. Lamellar keratoplasty is rarely performed because vision after lamellar keratoplasty is usually not as good as that after penetrating keratoplasty.

Wound dehiscence and epithelial defects

These problems may occur in lamellar grafts, and they are managed in the same way as for those occurring after penetrating keratoplasty, as described above. The major difference is that these two complications are usually of less serious consequence after lamellar keratoplasty than when they occur after penetrating keratoplasty.

Conjunctival flap

The major complication that is unique to use of the Gundersen conjunctival flap is the creation of an inadvertent tear or hole in the central portion of the conjunctiva. This often results in failure of the procedure because of retraction of the flap. If a tear does occur, it should be carefully sutured, or tissue adhesive can be applied to the conjunctival hole after the flap is in place.

Refractive corneal surgery

Complications of refractive surgery include unpredictability, inadvertent entering of the anterior chamber, damage to the endothelium (10 per cent endothelial cell loss has been reported in radial keratotomy) and, with the Barraquer procedures, errors in calculating the proper lathing of frozen corneal tissue[79–82]. Recently we have seen one case of cataract formation after radial keratotomy performed elsewhere. Other complications of radial keratotomy include: epithelial ingrowth, corneal vascularization, overcorrection, steroid-induced glaucoma, night glare and fluctuation in vision[83].

Conclusions

Recent advances in microsurgical techniques, use of fine sutures and needles, antibiotic and steroid therapy, and advanced instrumentation have greatly improved the results of all surgical procedures involving the cornea. The success rate for obtaining a clear graft after keratoplasty is now between 80 and 90 per cent, except in highly unfavorable cases[84–86]. In all the procedures discussed herein, proper patient selection, meticulous surgical technique and careful postoperative care are vitally important in obtaining good results.

Acknowledgements

We thank David Andrews, Scarlett Fisher, Donna Optican and Tom Mitchell for assistance during preparation of the manuscript.

References

1. Mannis, M. J., Krachmer, J. H. Keratoplasty: A historical perspective. Survey of Ophthalmology 1981; 25:333-338
2. Gundersen, T. Conjunctival flaps in the treatment of corneal disease with reference to a new technique of application. Archives of Ophthalmology 1958; 60:880-888
3. Arentsen, J. J., Laibson, P. R. Penetrating keratoplasty and cataract extraction: combined vs nonsimultaneous surgery. Archives of Ophthalmology 1978; 96:75-76
4. Paton, D. The prognosis of penetrating keratoplasty, based upon corneal morphology. Ophthalmic Surgery 1976; 7:36-45
5. Langston, R. H. S., Pavan-Langston, D., Dohlman, C. H. Penetrating keratoplasty for herpetic keratitis: prognostic and therapeutic determinants. Transactions of the American Academy of Ophthalmology and Otolaryngology 1975; 79:577-583
6. Polack, F. M., Kaufman, H. E. Penetrating keratoplasty in herpetic keratitis. American Journal of Ophthalmology 1972; 73:908-913
7. Stark, W. J. Transplantation immunology of penetrating keratoplasty. Transactions of the American Ophthalmological Society 1980; 78:1079-1117
8. Brown, S. I., Tragakis, M. P., Pearce, D. B. Corneal transplantation for severe alkali burns. Transactions of the American Academy of Ophthalmology and Otolaryngology 1972; 76:1266-1274
9. Bourne, W. M. One-year observation of transplanted human corneal endothelium. Ophthalmology 1980; 87:673-679
10. Hirst, L. W., Stark, W. J. Donor corneal endothelium: Slit-lamp examination of buttons in storage medium. Ophthalmic Surgery 1978; 9:51-53
11. Hogan, M. J., Alvarado, J. A., Weddell, J. E. Histology of the human eye. Philadelphia: W. B. Saunders Co., 1971: 55-111
12. Fogle, J. A., Kenyon, K. R., Stark, W. J., *et al.* Defective epithelial adhesion in anterior corneal dystrophies. American Journal of Ophthalmology 1975; 79:925-940
13. Brightbill, F. S., Polack, F. M., Slappey, T. A comparison of two methods for cutting donor corneal buttons. American Journal of Ophthalmology 1973; 75:500-506
14. Zimmerman, T., Olson, R., Waltman, S., Kaufman, H. Transplant size and elevated intraocular pressure postkeratoplasty. Archives of Ophthalmology 1978; 96:2231-2233
15. Ainslie, D. Recent advances in keratoplasty. British Journal of Ophthalmology 1974; 58:335-343
16. Troutman, R. C. Microsurgical control of corneal astigmatism in cataract and keratoplasty. Transactions of the American Academy of Ophthalmology and Otolaryngology 1973; 77:563-572
17. Troutman, R. C. Astigmatic considerations in corneal graft. Ophthalmic Surgery 1979; 10:21-26
18. Kurz, G. H., D'Amica, R. A. Retained Descemet's membrane after keratoplasty for old interstitial keratitis. American Journal of Ophthalmology 1973; 76:51-53
19. Pape, L. G., Balazs, E. A. The use of sodium hyaluronate (Healon®) in human anterior segment surgery. Ophthalmology 1980; 87:699-705
20. Polack, F. M., Demong, T., Santaella, H. Sodium hyaluronate (Healon®) in keratoplasty and IOL implantation. Ophthalmology 1981; 88:425-431
21. Kaufman, H. E. Combined keratoplasty and cataract extraction. American Journal of Ophthalmology 1974; 77:824-829
22. Bruner, W. E., Stark, W. J., Maumenee, A. E. Combined keratoplasty, cataract extraction, and intraocular lens implantation: Experience at the Wilmer Institute. Ophthalmic Surgery 1981; 12:657-660
23. Taylor, D. M. Keratoplasty and intraocular lenses. Ophthalmic Surgery 1976; 7:31-42
23. Lee, J. R., Dohlman, C. H. Intraocular lens implantation in combination with keratoplasty. Annals of Ophthalmology 1977; 9:513-518
24. Hunkeler, J. D., Hyde, L. L. The triple procedure: Combined penetrating keratoplasty, cataract extraction, and lens implantation. American Intra-ocular Implant Society Journal 1979; 5:222-224
25. Taylor, D. M., Khaliq, A., Maxwell, R. Keratoplasty and intraocular lenses: Current status. Ophthalmology 1979; 86:242-254
26. The Miami Study Group: Cystoid macular edema in aphakic and pseudophakic eyes. American Journal of Ophthalmology 1979; 88:45-48
27. Hirst, L. W., Stark, W. J., Jensen, A. D. Tissue adhesives: New perspectives in corneal perforations. Ophthalmic Surgery 1979; 10(3):58-64
28. Swinger, C. A., Barraquer, J. I. Keratophakia and keratomileusis: clinical results. Ophthalmology 1981; 88:709-715
29. Barraquer, J. I. Keratomileusis for myopia and aphakia. Ophthalmology 1981; 88:701-708
30. Kaufman, H. E. The correction of aphakia. XXXVI Edward Jackson Memorial Lecture. American Journal of Ophthalmology 1980; 89:1-10
31. Werblin, T. P., Kaufman, H. E., Friedlander, M. H., Schon, K. L., McDonald, M. B., Granet, N. S. A prospective study of the use of hyperopic epikeratophakia grafts for the correction of aphakia in adults. Ophthalmology 1981; 88:1137-1140
32. Krachmer, J. H., Fenzl, R. E. Surgical correction of high postkeratoplasty astigmatism: Relaxing incisions vs. wedge resection. Archives of Ophthalmology 1980; 98:1400-1402
33. Bruner, W. E., Stark, W. J. Complications of corneal transplantation. In: Iliff, N. T., ed. Complications in ophthalmic surgery. Edinburgh: Churchill Livingstone, Inc. (in press)
34. Maumenee, A. E. The Pocklington Lecture 1976. Recent advances in corneal transplantation. Transactions of the Ophthalmological Society of the United Kingdom 1976; 46:462-470
35. Cohen, K. L., Van Horn, D. L., Edelhauser, H. F., Schultz, R. O. Effect of phenylephrine on normal and regenerated endothelial cells in cat cornea. Investigations in Ophthalmology and Visual Science 1979; 18:242-249
36. Edelhauser, H. F., Hine, J. E., Pederson, H., Van Horn, D. L., Schultz, R. O. The effect of phenylephrine on the cornea. Archives of Ophthalmology 1979; 97:937-947
37. McCarey, B. E., Edelhauser, H. F., Van Horn, D. L. Functional and structural changes in the corneal endothelium during in vitro perfusion. Investigative Ophthalmology 1973; 12:410-417
38. Edelhauser, H. F., Gonnering, R., Van Horn, D. L. Intraocular irrigating solutions. A comparative study of BSS Plus and lactated Ringer's solution. Archives of Ophthalmology 1978; 96:516-520
39. Richard, J. M., Paton, D., Gasset, A. R. A comparison of penetrating keratoplasty and lamellar keratoplasty in the surgical

management of keratoconus. American Journal of Ophthalmology 1978; 86:807-811

40. Sugar, A., Meyer, R. F., Hood, I. Epithelial downgrowth following penetrating keratoplasty in the aphake. Archives of Ophthalmology 1977; 95:464-467
41. Raber, I. M., Arentsen, J. J., Laibson, P. R. Traumatic wound dehiscence after penetrating keratoplasty. Archives of Ophthalmology 1980; 98:1407-1409
42. Polack, F. M., Binder, P. S. Detachment of Descemet's membrane from grafts following wound separation: Light and scanning electron microscopic study. Annals of Ophthalmology 1975; 7:47-54
43. Tragakis, M. P., Brown, S. I. The significance of anterior synechiae after corneal transplantation. American Journal of Ophthalmology 1972; 74:532-533
44. Stark, W. J., Maumenee, A. E., Kenyon, K. R. Intermediate-term corneal storage for penetrating keratoplasty. American Journal of Ophthalmology 1975; 79:795-802
45. Binder, P. S., Abel, R., Kaufman, H. E. Cyclocryotherapy for glaucoma after penetrating keratoplasty. American Journal of Ophthalmology 1975; 79:489-492
46. Irvine, A. R., Kaufman, H. E. Intraocular pressure following penetrating keratoplasty. American Journal of Ophthalmology 1969; 68:835-844
47. Thoft, R. A., Gordon, J. M., Dohlman, C. H. Glaucoma following keratoplasty. Transactions of the American Academy of Ophthalmology and Otolaryngology 1974; 78:352-364
48. Zimmerman, T. J., Waltman, S. R., Sachs, U., Kaufman, H. E. Intraocular pressure after aphakic penetrating keratoplasty 'through and through' suturing. Ophthalmic Surgery 1979; 10(7):49-52
49. Leibowitz, H. M., Elliott, J. H. Edema of the graft following penetrating keratoplasty. International Ophthalmology Clinic 1968; 8:697-727
50. Escapini, H., Jr, Olson, R. H., Kaufman, H. E. Donor cornea contamination with McCarey-Kaufman medium preservation. American Journal of Ophthalmology 1979; 88:59-62
51. Keates, R. H., Mishler, K. E., Riedinger, D. Bacterial contamination of donor eyes. American Journal of Ophthalmology 1977; 84:617-619
52. Shaw, E. L., Aquavella, J. V. Pneumococcal endophthalmitis following grafting of corneal tissue from a (cadaver) kidney donor. Annals of Ophthalmology 1977; 9:435-440
53. Goldman, K. N., Centifanto, Y., Kaufman, H. E., Slappey, T. E. Prevention of surface bacterial contamination of donor corneas. Archives of Ophthalmology 1978; 96:2277-2280
54. McCarey, B. E., Kaufman, H. E. Improved corneal storage. Investigative Ophthalmology 1974; 13:165-173
55. Maumenee, A. E. The influence of donor-recipient sensitization on corneal grafts. American Journal of Ophthalmology 1951; 34:142-152
56. Maumenee, A. E. Clinical aspects of the corneal homograft reaction. Investigative Ophthalmology 1962; 1:244-252
57. Krachmer, J. H., Alldredge, O. C. Subepithelial infiltrates – a probable sign of corneal transplant rejection. Archives of Ophthalmology 1978; 96:2234-2237
58. Polack, F. M. Scanning electron microscopy of corneal graft rejection: Epithelial rejection, endothelial rejection, and formation of posterior graft membranes. Investigative Ophthalmology 1972; 11:1-14
59. Stark, W. J., Opelz, G., Newsome, D., *et al.* Sensitization to human lymphocyte antigens by corneal transplantation. Investigative Ophthalmology 1973; 12:639-645
60. Stark, W. J., Taylor, H. R., Bias, W. B., *et al.* Histocompatibility (HLA) antigens and keratoplasty. American Journal of Ophthalmology 1978; 86:595-604
61. Khodadoust, A. A. The allograft rejection reaction: The leading cause of late failure of clinical corneal grafts. In: Corneal graft failure. Ciba Foundation Symposium 15 (new series). Amsterdam: Elsevier, 1973:151-167
62. Kurz, G. H., D'Amico, R. A. Histopathology of corneal graft failures. American Journal of Ophthalmology 1968; 66:184-199
63. Snip, R. C., Kenyon, K. R., Green, W. R. Retrocorneal fibrous membrane in the vitreous touch syndrome. American Journal of Ophthalmology 1975; 79:233-244
64. Michels, R. G., Kenyon, K. R., Maumenee, A. E. Retrocorneal fibrous membrane. Investigative Ophthalmology 1972; 11:822-831
65. Stark, W. J., Michels, R. G., Maumenee, A. E., Cupples, H. Surgical management of epithelial ingrowth. American Journal of Ophthalmology 1978; 85:772-780
66. Forstot, S. L., Abel, R., Binder, P. S. Bacterial endophthalmitis following suture removal after penetrating keratoplasty. American Journal of Ophthalmology 1975; 80:509-512
67. Goldberg, D. B., Schanzlin, D. J., Mondino, B. J., Brown, S. I. Graft edema after suture removal. American Journal of Ophthalmology 1979; 88:165-168
68. Shahinian, L., Jr, Brown, S. I. Postoperative complications with protruding monofilament nylon sutures. American Journal of Ophthalmology 1977; 83:546-548
69. Forstot, S. L., Binder, P. S., Fitzgerald, C., *et al.* The incidence of retinal detachment after penetrating keratoplasty. American Journal of Ophthalmology 1975; 80:102-105
70. Olson, R. J. Aphakic keratoplasty: Determining donor tissue size to avoid elevated intraocular pressure. Archives of Ophthalmology 1978; 96:2274-2276
71. Jensen, A. D., Maumenee, A. E. Refractive errors following keratoplasty. Transactions of the American Ophthalmological Society 1974; 72:123-131
72. Troutman, R. C., Kelly, S., Kaye, D., *et al.* The use and preliminary results of the Troutman surgical keratometer in cataract and corneal surgery. Transactions of the American Academy of Ophthalmology and Otolaryngology 1977; 83:232-238
73. Fine, M., Cignetti, F. E. Penetrating keratoplasty in herpes simplex keratitis. Recurrence in grafts. Archives in Ophthalmology 1977; 95:613-616
74. Lempert, S. L., Jenkins, M. S., Johnson, B. L., Brown, S. I. A simple technique for removal of recurring granular dystrophy in corneal grafts. American Journal of Ophthalmology 1978; 86:89-91
75. Olson, R. J., Kaufman, H. E. Recurrence of Reis-Buckler's corneal dystrophy in a graft. American Journal of Ophthalmology 1978; 85:349-351
76. Abelson, M. B., Collin, H. B., Gillette, T. E., Dohlman, C. H. Recurrent keratoconus after keratoplasty. American Journal of Ophthalmology 1980; 90:672-676
77. Duffy, P., Wolf, J., Collins, G., De Voe, A. G., Streeten, B., Cowen, D. Possible person-to-person transmission of Creutzfeldt-Jakob disease. New England Journal of Medicine 1974; 290:692-693
78. Houff, S. A., Burton, R. C., Wilson, R. W., *et al.* Human-to-human transmission of rabies virus by corneal transplant. New England Journal of Medicine 1979; 300:603-604
79. Aquavella, J. V., Barraquer, F., Rao, G. N., Ruiz, L. A. Morphological variations in corneal endothelium following keratophakia and keratomileusis. Ophthalmology 1981; 88:721-723
80. Hoffer, K. J., Darin, J. J., Pettit, T. H., Hofbauer, J. D., Elander, R., Levenson, J. E. UCLA clinical trial of radial keratotomy: Preliminary report. Ophthalmology 1981; 88:729-736
81. Henkind, P. Cataract and other clouds. Ophthalmology 1981; 88:25A
82. Kaufman, H. E. Unanswered questions about radial keratomy. American Journal of Ophthalmology 1981; 92:292-295
83. Rowsey, J. J., Balyeat, H. D. Preliminary results and complications of radial keratotomy. American Journal of Ophthalmology 1982; 93:437-455
84. Stark, W. J., Paton, D., Maumenee, A. E., Michelson, P. E. The results of 102 penetrating keratoplasties using 10/0 monofilament nylon suture. Ophthalmic Surgery 1972; 3:11-25
85. Barraquer, J. Keratoplasty in Fuchs' dystrophy and bullous keratopathy. American Journal of Ophthalmology 1979; 88:333-341
86. Olson, R. J., Waltman, S. R., Mattingly, T. P., Kaufman, H. E. Visual results after penetrating keratoplasty for aphakic bullous keratopathy and Fuchs' dystrophy. American Journal of Ophthalmology 1979; 88:1000-1004

6

Surgery of the lens

William E. Bruner MD
Walter J. Stark MD
A. Edward Maumenee MD

Introduction

Cataract surgery has been practiced successfully for centuries. The technique of *couching* was replaced by planned extracapsular cataract extraction in the eighteenth century[1] and intracapsular cataract extraction became popular in the early to mid-twentieth century. During the past 20 years, further refinements in cataract surgery have been made possible by the introduction of the operating microscope, finer needles and suture material, and more recently with the development of new modalities such as the phacoemulsifier and vitrectomy instruments.

In this chapter we describe our techniques for performing cataract surgery, including the use of intraocular lenses. We do not present our method as the only acceptable approach to cataract surgery but rather as one that has evolved at the Wilmer Institute during the past 30 years. In addition we discuss the indications for surgery, preoperative evaluation, surgical anatomy, postoperative care and complications.

Indications for surgery

Adult cataracts

The main indication for cataract surgery is decreased vision from a cataract that significantly interferes with a patient's ability to carry out occupational or other regular activities. It is important to assess how disabled a patient is by the visual reduction and to balance this against the expected improvement of vision and function after cataract surgery. In cases of unilateral cataract, surgery may be delayed if the patient is functioning well with good vision in the other eye.

The type of cataract is also an important consideration. Patients with posterior subcapsular cataract can often avoid or delay surgery by using mydriatic drops to dilate the pupil. This allows better vision by permitting light rays to pass through the less cataractous peripheral lens. In addition, elderly patients often function well with the induced myopia resulting from a nuclear sclerotic cataract.

Congenital cataracts

Congenital zonular cataracts probably should not be treated surgically unless it is obvious the child cannot see. Dense bilateral congenital cataracts should be removed during the first few months of life, before the development of amblyopia and onset of nystagmus[2]. Unilateral congenital cataracts present a more complex situation because amblyopia is often a severe problem in these patients. Cataract surgery, if it is to be performed, should be done during the first few weeks of life, and correction with a contact lens and patching therapy for amblyopia should begin immediately. Recent reports suggest that some useful vision may be obtained by this method[3]. Traumatic and juvenile cataracts with onset after the age of 10 years do not carry as high a risk of amblyopia, and the timing of surgery is usually not as critical.

Intraocular lenses

The results of intraocular lens (IOL) correction of aphakia are similar to those of normal aphakic correction in image size and peripheral vision. Aphakic spectacle correction causes a 25–30 per cent magnification and various optical distortions and aberrations. Contact lenses create about an 8 per cent magnification in image size, which is usually small enough to allow binocular fusion in a unilateral aphake. Also, contact lenses provide a full peripheral field as opposed to the narrower field of aphakic spectacle correction. Unlike a contact lens, an IOL has the advantage of not requiring cleaning or change. There are, however, additional surgical risks in IOL implantation, which will be discussed.

Selection of patients for IOL implantation is based on age of the patient and absence of specific contraindications. IOLs may be reserved for older patients but they may be used in younger patients who are not suitable for contact lenses or aphakic glasses. Specific indications and contraindications to lens implantation are described on p. 159.

Special situations

There are several infrequent situations in which a cataract may need to be removed to prevent irreversible damage to the eye, regardless of the visual acuity status of the patient. These conditions include phacomorphic glaucoma, phacolytic glaucoma, phacoanaphylactic endophthalmitis, and the need to apply laser treatment to the retina.

Preoperative evaluation

Needed examinations

The preoperative evaluation should include a thorough ocular examination, including measurement of best corrected visual acuity for both distance and near; external examination of the eyelids, lashes and pupils; slit-lamp evaluation of the cornea, anterior chamber and lens; gonioscopy when indicated; tonometry; and dilated fundus examination with direct and indirect ophthalmoscopy. If the fundus cannot be visualized, B-scan ultrasonography is useful in determining whether there is a retinal detachment or intraocular tumor.

A refraction is performed to obtain the best corrected visual acuity for each eye. Vision should be tested both at distance and near, and in bright and dim illumination. Vision will vary under differing illumination with certain types of cataracts. For example, patients with posterior subcapsular cataract may have poor vision in bright light, but this may improve markedly in dim illumination with a more dilated pupil that allows the patient to 'see around' the central lens opacity, as mentioned earlier.

External examination of the lids and lashes is important to rule out active blepharitis which could increase the risk of postoperative infection. Pupillary evaluation is important in eyes with dense lens opacities. An afferent pupillary defect indicates retinal or optic nerve damage and thus a poor visual prognosis. Slit-lamp evaluation of the cornea and anterior chamber may reveal evidence of keratitis, corneal scarring, iritis or other anterior segment disorders that could influence the visual prognosis. Gonioscopy of the anterior chamber angle may reveal abnormalities such as a narrow anterior chamber angle, abnormal blood vessels or peripheral anterior synechiae that may require a revised approach to surgery. Preoperative gonioscopy is especially important if one is considering implanting an anterior chamber IOL. The intraocular pressure testing may determine the need for further glaucoma evaluation. Slit-lamp evaluation of the lens is useful in deciding on the type of surgery for cataract removal. For example, a dense nuclear sclerotic cataract may be difficult to remove with phacoemulsification.

A dilated fundus examination may disclose retinal, macular, vitreous or optic nerve disease that may alter the visual prognosis. Retinal evaluation of the fellow eye is always an important part of the preoperative evaluation. The Guyton-Minkowski Potential Acuity Meter™ is also useful for predicting visual outcome and will be described in the next section.

Mature cataract evaluation

In eyes in which the cataract is so opaque that fundus examination is impossible, there are ways to estimate the postoperative visual potential. These include determination of the presence of light projection, entoptic phenomena, two-light discrimination and color perception. Other useful tests include ultrasonography, photo-stress testing, laser interferometry, blue-field entoptic phenomenon, the Guyton-Minkowski test and electrophysiologic testing such as the electroretinogram (ERG), the electro-oculogram (EOG) and the visually evoked response (VER).

The absence of correct light projection may indicate a visual-field defect from retinal or optic nerve pathology, but this test can be misleading. The response can occasionally be poor because of a dense cataract alone, without other disease. It may even rarely be correct in the presence of a large retinal detachment.

Entoptic phenomena are demonstrated by moving a penlight or transilluminator against the closed eyelids. If the patient sees dark lines like 'cracked mud' or 'veins of a leaf', corresponding to the image of retinal vessels, this is a sign of good retinal function, as the patient is seeing the shadow of the retinal vessels. However, many patients with no retinal disease cannot experience this phenomenon (*Figure 6.1*). Therefore, the inability to detect the entoptic phenomenon is important only if it can be appreciated in the other normal eye.

The presence of two-light discrimination and color perception suggests that no severe retinal disease is present, but the tests for these are often equivocal. The Maddox-rod test is performed by having the patient look through a Maddox rod at a point light source. If the line seen by the eye is undistorted and continuous, both horizontally and vertically, this is an encouraging sign that there is good macular function. Patients with macular disease may see a break or distortion in the line produced by the Maddox rod. Often, patients with a cataract dense enough to prevent ophthalmic examination of the macula cannot see the red line of the Maddox rod, even with normal macular function, so that the usefulness of this test is limited .

B-scan ultrasonography is useful when the retina cannot be seen ophthalmoscopically. Abnormalities such as a retinal detachment, intraocular tumor or vitreous hemorrhage can occasionally be detected preoperatively using such instrumentation[4]. This test should always be performed when the retina cannot be visualized prior to cataract extraction.

Photo-stress testing is performed by first shining a bright light into the patient's eye and then recording the amount of time it takes for the visual aciuty to recover to the previous level of corrected vision. A delay in recovery of longer than a minute suggests that macular disease is present[5,6].

Laser interferometry is a subjective test that evaluates retinal function in patients with moderately dense cataracts. Interference fringes can be projected onto the retina, using a low-power laser, despite the presence of the cataract. The ability to see various sizes of patterns corresponds to potential visual acuity[7,8]. Drawbacks to this test are that it requires an expensive instrument and is time-consuming. Also, the laser-interferometry test is not useful in eyes with opaque lenses in which the fundus is not visible ophthalmoscopically.

The blue-field entoptic phenomenon, also known as the 'flying-corpuscles phenomenon', refers to the perception of one's own leukocytes flowing in the perifoveal capillaries while looking at a uniformly illuminated blue field. The patient is then asked to count the number of 'flying corpuscles' seen. If many corpuscles are seen (at least 15), this indicates a good prognosis for macular function. This test has been compared with the two-light discrimination test, color perception and the entoptic test, and has been found to be of value[9,10].

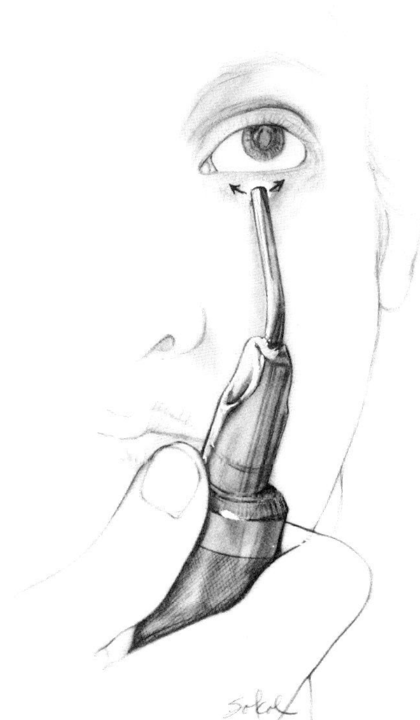

Figure 6.1 *Testing for entoptic phenomenon. The eye being tested may be open or closed as the light is moved back and forth across the lid*

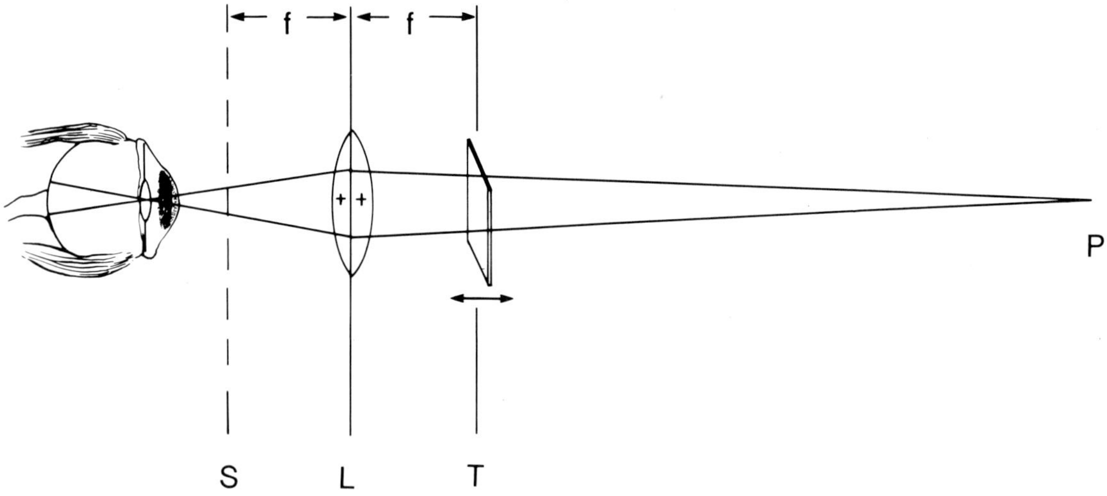

Figure 6.2 *Schematic diagram of the Guyton-Minkowski Potential Acuity Meter*

An instrument recently developed by Minkowski and Guyton[11] projects a standard Snellen chart (T) through a single clear area of the partially cataractous lens. Meanwhile, the spherical refractive error is corrected with an optometer arrangement as shown in *Figure 6.2*. By using a pinpoint light source (P), the image of the pinpoint light source in the patient's pupil may be made quite small, approximately 0.1 mm, thus allowing for a large depth of focus and no loss of illumination. Magnification is controlled by placing the focal point of the lens at the spectacle plane (S) as shown. This instrument is most useful in determining the potential visual acuity in eyes with macular changes (or other posterior pole abnormalities) and a cataract, with vision in the 20/50 to 20/400 range, with clear areas in the cataract through which the image can be projected. However, patients with more severe cataracts can often also be evaluated with this test. If a patient sees the 20/40 line on Potential Acuity Meter testing, then at least 20/40 visual acuity can be anticipated after successful cataract surgery (*Figure 6.3*).

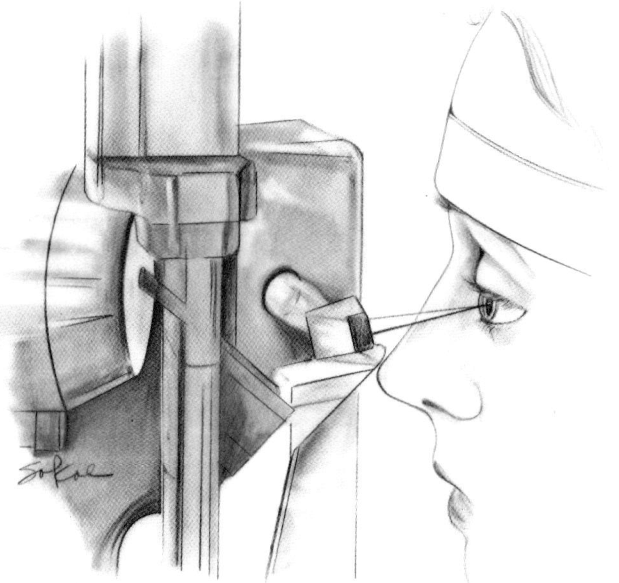

Figure 6.3 *Early prototype of the Guyton-Minkowski Potential Acuity Meter*

The special preoperative evaluation of the patient who is to receive an IOL includes measurement to determine the proper IOL power (*see* p. 159).

Surgical anatomy

Anatomy of the limbus

Knowledge of the anatomy of the limbus – the transition zone between the cornea and sclera – is important in cataract surgery. Physiologically the limbus may contribute to the nutrition of the cornea and the associated trabecular meshwork, and it provides a pathway internally for the drainage of aqueous from the anterior chamber. The anterior anatomical boundary of the limbus is determined by a plane connecting the peripheral termination of Bowman's layer and Descemet's membrane. This corresponds to the furthest anterior point at which a limbus-based conjunctival flap can be reflected. The anterior limbal region extends from this anterior border posteriorly to where the bluish color changes to white. This junction is at the midlimbal line, which lies directly over Schwalbe's line. The posterior limbal zone extends from the midlimbal line posteriorly for about 1 mm to the posterior limbal line, which lies over the scleral spur. The limbus is widest superiorly, where most cataract incisions are made, and narrowest temporally and nasally. This anatomical difference in width of the limbus is important if the cataract incision is to be made other than superiorly – for example, to avoid damaging a filtering bleb from previous glaucoma surgery.

Anatomy of the lens and the zonule

A knowledge of the anatomy of the lens and its zonular attachments is also important in cataract surgery. The human lens is composed of a nucleus, cortex and capsule. The central nucleus is often hard, whereas the cortex tends to be softer. The anterior capsule is thickest along the midperipheral region outside the central area and is thinnest centrally (*Figure 6.4*)[12]. Because the anterior capsule is thinnest centrally, during intracapsular extractions, a cryoprobe tip should be placed off-center to avoid this more fragile area of the lens capsule which is more likely to rupture.

The zonule or suspensory ligament of the lens is a gel-like structure composed of fibers that connect the ciliary body to the lens. The zonular fibers hold the lens in position and allow the ciliary muscle to transmit force to the lens. There are different types of zonular fibers – some connecting the pars plana to the posterior capsule, some leading from the ciliary body to the anterior capsule, others arising from the valley between ciliary processes and attaching to the posterior capsule, and also fibers connecting ciliary valleys to the lens equator (*Figure 6.4*).

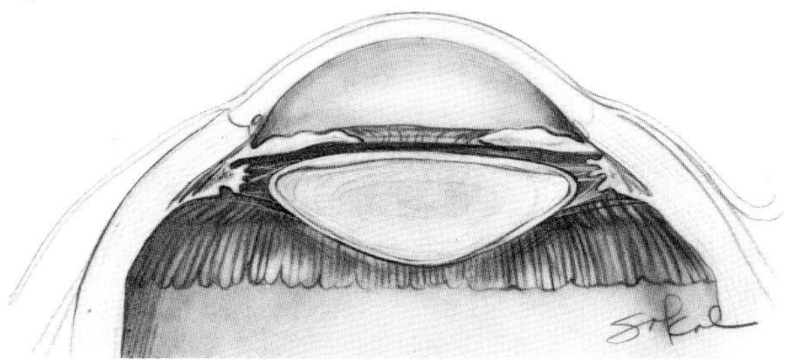

Figure 6.4 *Diagram of cross-section of the anterior segment of the human eye*

The number of zonular fibers declines with age, but the remaining fibers tend to thicken[12]. In intracapsular cataract extraction, the zonular fibers may be dissolved with α-chymotrypsin enzyme to allow easier removal of the cataract. If α-chymotrypsin is not used, the zonular attachments to the lens should be removed from the peripheral portion of the lens where the cryoprobe is likely to freeze. If the ice ball freezes into direct contact with the zonules, the zonular fibers will not break, and pulling on them may put excessive traction on the ciliary body. In extracapsular surgery zonular fibers provide support for the posterior capsule and in cases in which a posterior chamber intraocular lens is used, they help support the IOL[13, 14].

The vitreous is adherent to the posterior surface of the lens during youth, but this attachment weakens with age, making intracapsular cataract extraction without vitreous loss possible after about age 40. Patients under 40 years of age with cataracts should usually not have intracapsular cataract surgery because of this adhesion and the increased chance for vitreous loss and secondary complications[12, 15, 17].

There are many different types of cataract formation. Each type may produce its own visual problem and may have characteristics that will affect or determine the method of management. Congenital cataracts, for example, may appear more severe on slit-lamp examination than the visual acuity would indicate. An anterior polar congenital cataract or lamellar cataract may allow 20/40 or even better vision and usually does not need to be removed. A posterior subcapsular cataract may allow reasonably good vision if the pupil is dilated.

Dislocation of the lens can occur in such diseases as Marfan's syndrome, homocystinuria and Weill-Marchesani syndrome. In Marfan's syndrome the lens is usually displaced superiorly (*Figure 6.5*), whereas in homocystinuria it is usually displaced inferiorly[18]. Other

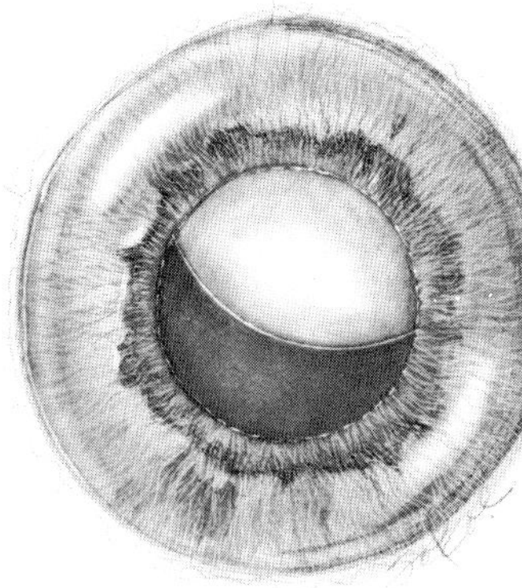

Figure 6.5 *Subluxed crystalline lens as seen in Marfan's syndrome*

causes of partially dislocated (subluxed) or totally dislocated (luxated) lenses include hyperlysinemia, sulfite oxidase deficiency, inherited ectopia lentis and syphilis. Trauma, however, is probably the most common cause of a dislocated lens[19]. In many cases of subluxed clear lenses, surgery is not indicated. Such patients often do well without surgery, wearing aphakic correction spectacles.

When a lens is subluxed, this influences the surgical technique used to remove it, and it makes the chances for vitreous loss much greater. In general an intracapsular extraction is indicated, but excision of the cataract using vitrectomy instrumentation may be required if vitreous is present anterior to the lens or if the lens is dislocated into the vitreous cavity.

Anesthesia and preparation for surgery

Although the risks of general anesthesia have been greatly reduced in recent years[20–23], we prefer local anesthesia unless the patient is a child or an uncooperative adult. The use of local anesthesia gives the patient the added comfort of ocular anesthesia up to 12 hours after surgery. There is less risk of vomiting, and the patient can be ambulant soon after surgery.

About 30 minutes before surgery, we often give intravenous mannitol (20 per cent) in a dose of 1–2 g/kg. Mannitol is not given if there is a history of heart or pulmonary disease or if there are other medical contraindications. The pupil is dilated with phenylephrine 10 per cent and homatropine 5 per cent, using both drops three times every 15 minutes beginning 1 hour before surgery in those eyes undergoing an extracapsular cataract extraction.

Preoperative sedation is useful before either local or general anesthesia to relax the patient. Our choice is either a combination of meperidine hydrochloride (pethidine; Demerol) 50 mg intramuscularly (i.m.) and hydroxyzine hydrochloride (Vistaril) 50 mg i.m. for an adult 60 minutes before surgery or, alternatively, diazepam (Valium) 10 mg orally may be used. Just prior to retrobulbar injection, additional diazepam (usually 2.5 mg) or fentanyl (Sublimaze) 0.05–0.1 mg may be given by slow intravenous (i.v.) injection under the direction of an anesthesiologist. When these methods are used, the patients are sedated, cooperative and do not later remember the local needle injections.

When local anesthesia is used, we prefer a 50:50 mixture of lidocaine (Xylocaine) 2 per cent and bupivacaine (Marcaine) 0.75 per cent with a final concentration of hyaluronidase (Wydase) 3.75 u/ml. A sharp, long (38 mm), disposable 25 gauge needle on a 10 ml syringe is used for a modified Van Lint injection. The sharp needle allows easy tissue penetration and is less painful than a larger, blunt needle. About 1 ml of the anesthetic mixture is injected subcutaneously 2 cm lateral to the lateral canthus. Additional solution is injected at this site into the subcutaneous tissue and muscle toward the tragus of the ear. Then injections are made along the orbital rim, being careful not to balloon the lids with solution. At no time is solution injected directly into the lids (*Figure 6.6a*).

Once the lid block is complete the patient is asked to look up and medially with the eye and the same needle is then inserted through the lower lid into the extraocular muscle cone in a retrobulbar fashion, taking care to avoid the globe (*Figure 6.6b*). The needle is inserted with the bevel toward the globe, so that there is less chance for penetration of the globe by the needle tip, and the syringe is aspirated to be certain the needle tip is not in a vessel. About 3 ml of anesthetic is injected before the needle is removed (*Figure 6.6*). The eye is gently massaged and then checked for akinesia after 2–3 minutes. At this point, eyes undergoing extracapsular extraction have about 0.5 ml of subconjunctival dilating solution injected. Our subconjunctival dilating solution is made of phenylephrine hydrochloride 2.5 g, homatropine hydrobromide 2 g, procaine hydrochloride 5 g, sodium bisulfite 0.5 g, sodium citrate 2 g, benzyl alcohol 5 ml and sodium chloride 1.34 g dissolved in 500 ml of distilled water. This solution is passed through a millipore hydrosol filter, packaged in 10 ml vials, and autoclaved at 121 °C for 20 minutes.

After satisfactory anesthesia and akinesia have been obtained, we prefer to use an intraocular pressure-reducer (such as the Honan Manometer™ intraocular pressure-reducer) on the eye[25]. Gauze is placed over the eye, and care is taken to be sure the eye is closed before the pressure-reducer is applied. The Honan pressure-reducer is set to 30 mmHg and is left on for at least 15–20 minutes (*Figure 6.7*). If such a pressure-reducer is not available, digital massage can be used. This is done by applying constant, even pressure to the globe through the closed eyelids for 10–15 seconds followed by 5–10 seconds of no pressure. This cycle is repeated about 30 times or until the intraocular pressure measures 2 mmHg or less with a Schiotz tonometer.

The sterile operative field is prepared by swabbing the lids and lid margins with a sequence of several cotton-tipped applicators saturated with soap solution, then iodine solution (Ioprep), followed by irrigation of the eye and fornices with sterile saline irrigating solution. It is important, especially before extracapsular surgery, not to get soap or iodine solution on the cornea during the preparation because this may injure the epithelium and prevent a clear view of the anterior chamber during the procedure. A large plastic, adhesive sterile drape is placed over the eye and lids while the lids are kept open with the stick ends of two cotton-tipped applicators. The adhesive portion of the drape is applied to the lids and globe, and then an opening is cut. A lid speculum such as a Maumenee speculum is put in position. This pulls the lashes away from the operative field and covers the lid margins.

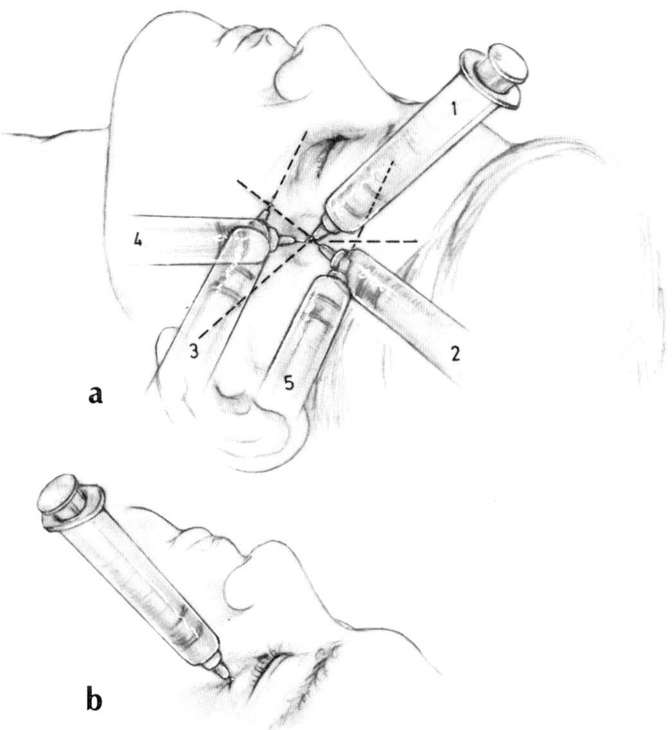

Figure 6.6 *Technique for* **(a)** *modified Van Lint and* **(b)** *retrobulbar injection*

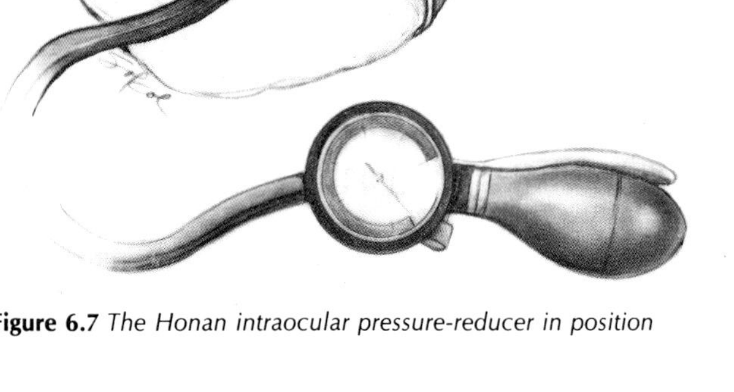

Figure 6.7 *The Honan intraocular pressure-reducer in position*

Operative sequence

Intracapsular cataract extraction

Superior rectus stay suture

For most cataract procedures, a superior rectus stay suture is helpful in stabilizing the eye. A muscle hook can be used to rotate the globe downward by pushing into the inferior cul-de-sac, thus exposing the superior globe. Toothed forceps are used to grasp the superior rectus muscle through the conjunctiva about 2–3 mm from the muscle insertion. A 4/0 silk suture on a cutting needle is passed beneath the forceps and the tendon of the muscle (*Figure 6.8*). The two ends of the suture can be clamped to the drape to stabilize the eye. An alternative method is to pass the needle through sclera anterior to the muscle insertion. To avoid elevation of the intraocular pressure, this clamp should be released just before extraction of the cataract. Care must be taken not to penetrate sclera and enter the globe with the needle.

Conjunctival flap

We prefer a limbus-based flap, although there are no conclusive data showing that this is better than a fornix-based flap.

The limbus-based flap provides the assistant with a convenient tissue to grasp while retracting the cornea rather than having to place a traction suture through the cornea or having to pull on a preplaced suture. A limbus-based conjunctival flap is begun by grasping the superior conjunctiva about 3 mm from the limbus and cutting down with blunt-tipped, spring-type iris scissors (*Figure 6.9a*). It is important to cut through both conjunctiva and Tenon's capsule. The scissors are then passed beneath Tenon's capsule and are spread gently nasally and temporally near the limbus to separate Tenon's capsule from the globe (*Figure 6.9b*). Conjunctiva and Tenon's capsule are cut parallel to the limbus, about 3 mm posterior to the limbus. The flap is reflected downward over the cornea and, using sharp scissors, the remaining Tenon's tissue between conjunctiva and limbus

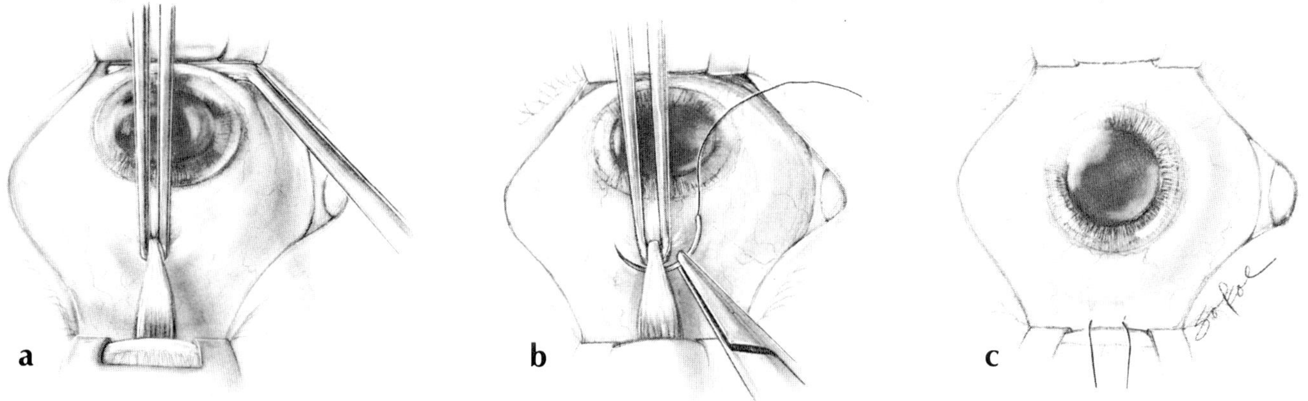

Figure 6.8 *Superior rectus stay suture.* **(a)** *Using a muscle hook to rotate the globe downward aids in grasping the rectus tendon.* **(b)** *Suture needle is passed beneath the muscle tendon.* **(c)** *Stay suture in place*

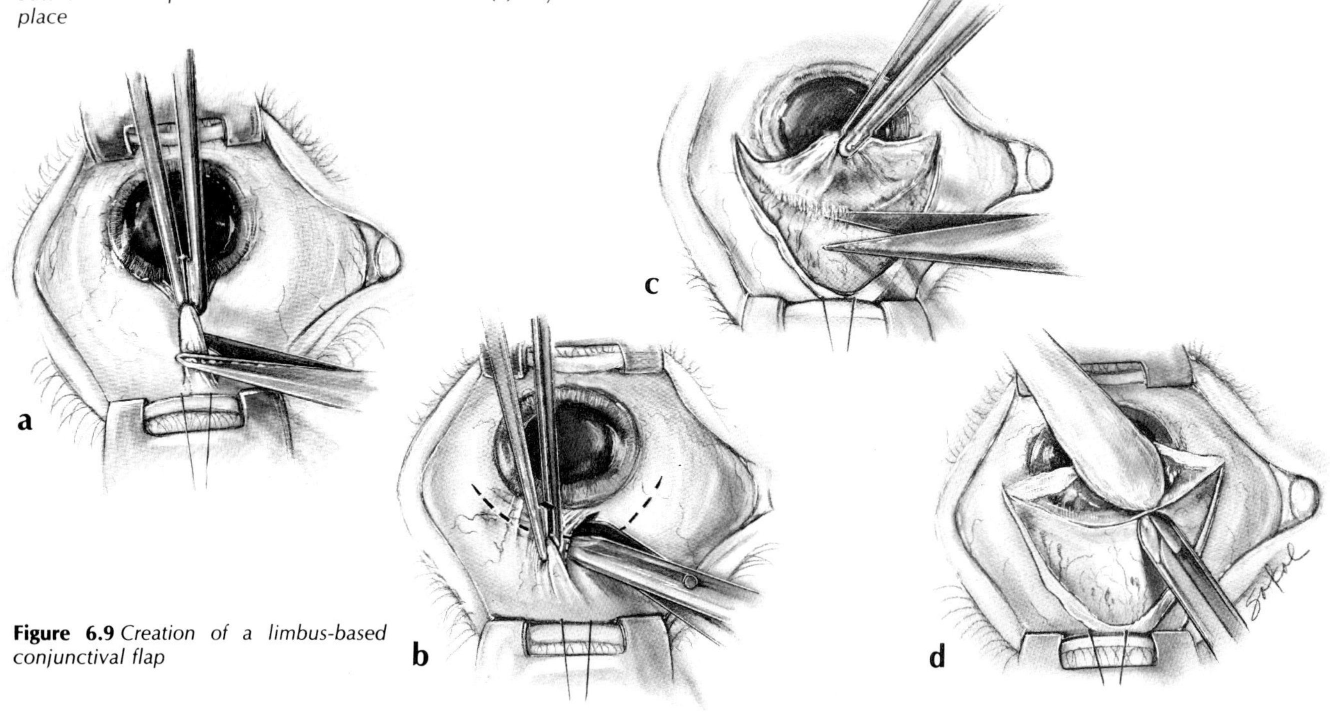

Figure 6.9 *Creation of a limbus-based conjunctival flap*

is cut (*Figure 6.9c*). Next a Tooke knife or Beaver blade is used to clean all remaining Tenon's capsule from the limbal region (*Figure 6.9d*). This is an important step since residual Tenon's tissue at the limbus can interfere with making a groove or placing sutures. When the flap has been completed, light Wet-Field cautery is used to reduce episcleral bleeding.

A fornix-based flap is begun by cutting through conjunctiva and Tenon's capsule at the limbus near the 10 or 2 o'clock position. Blunt dissection is carried out superiorly for several millimeters and the flap is cut flush from the limbus for about 150° superiorly.

Grooved incision

Before making a grooved incision, the superior rectus stay suture should be tightened to increase the intraocular pressure and prevent the eye from moving. A sharp small blade, such as a No. 64 or No. 69 Beaver blade or a razor-blade knife, is used to make an incision that follows the junction between the posterior one-third and the anterior two-thirds of the superior limbus for about 150°. The incision is placed more posteriorly at the 12 o'clock position, and nasally and temporally it is placed more anteriorly. That is, the groove is about 1.5 mm posterior to the conjunctival insertion at 12 o'clock and 1 mm posterior at the 10 and 2 o'clock positions (*Figure 6.10a*). The incision is made at this distance from the conjunctival insertion so that there is enough room to place the sutures in the anterior lip of the wound (*see Figure 6.12*). This first portion of the incision is perpendicular to the surface, and its depth is one-half to two-thirds of the corneal thickness. A razor-blade knife is then used to deepen the incision to three-quarters of the corneal thickness in a beveled fashion (*Figure 6.10b*). This beveled incision allows easy and safe passage of preplaced sutures through the wound, while maintaining a closed eye. Deepening of the groove is facilitated by lifting on the flap with a 0.3 mm toothed forceps. The second beveled portion of the incision creates a shelf which is used as a guide for depth when placing the sutures (*Figure 6.11a*). The 9/0 silk sutures are placed to pass through the junction of the first and second planes of the incision. When the eye is subsequently opened, one has a three-planed, shelved incision (*Figure 6.11b*). The deepened groove also facilitates the looping-out of the preplaced sutures before completing the incision.

An alternative to a three-planed incision is a two-planed incision, which is made by eliminating the second step, in which the groove is deepened with a razor blade. Other surgeons do not make a groove at all but simply open the eye with a knife and extend the incision with scissors. This type of incision makes accurate preplacement of sutures more difficult and does not provide the security of true preplaced sutures.

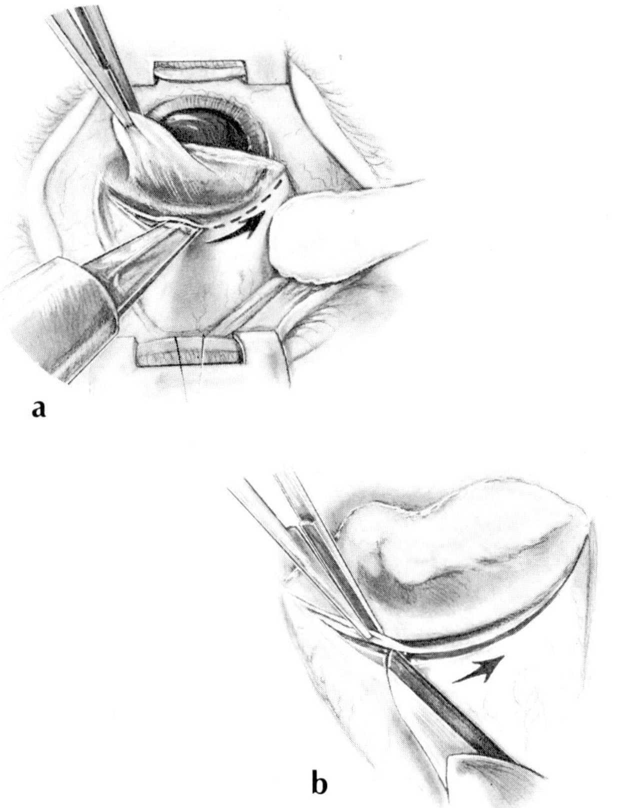

Figure 6.10 *A grooved incision is made in three planes.* **(a)** *The first portion is perpendicular to the surface and* **(b)** *the second is beveled. The third plane is produced on entering the eye*

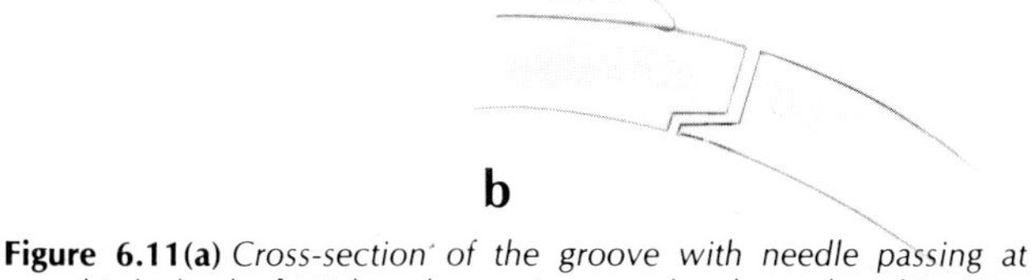

Figure 6.11(a) *Cross-section of the groove with needle passing at two-thirds depth.* **(b)** *When the eye is opened, a three-planed incision results*

Preplaced sutures

The use of true preplaced sutures offers several advantages in cataract surgery. They give added safety during and immediately after the lens is extracted, in that the eye is 'open' the least amount of time. Also, the eye can be closed rapidly if a complication such as increased vitreous pressure or an expulsive hemorrhage develops. If an expulsive hemorrhage occurs with an open eye and no, or only one, preplaced suture, there is little chance of saving the eye. With three preplaced mattress-type sutures, the cataract wound can be closed rapidly and tightly, and there is a chance of saving an eye with an expulsive hemorrhage.

We prefer 9/0 black silk double-armed sutures. Three mattress sutures are placed at the 10, 12 and 2 o'clock positions at about two-thirds depth. The needle bites are placed about 1.5 mm apart, so that very little suture is exposed. The mattress-type suture has an advantage in that the majority of the suture is buried within the sclera; only the anterior loop and the posterior knot are exposed. Also, the three mattress sutures provide the effect of six single sutures across the wound. The sutures are placed at the same depth on both sides of the wound to ensure an even, tight approximation of the wound, with minimal astigmatism (*Figure 6.12*).

Several alternative methods of preplaced suture placement are illustrated in *Figure 6.13*.

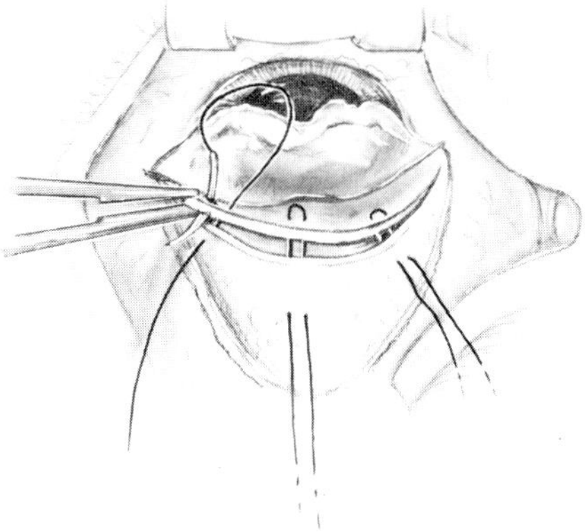

Figure 6.12 *9/0 silk double-armed mattress sutures are placed*

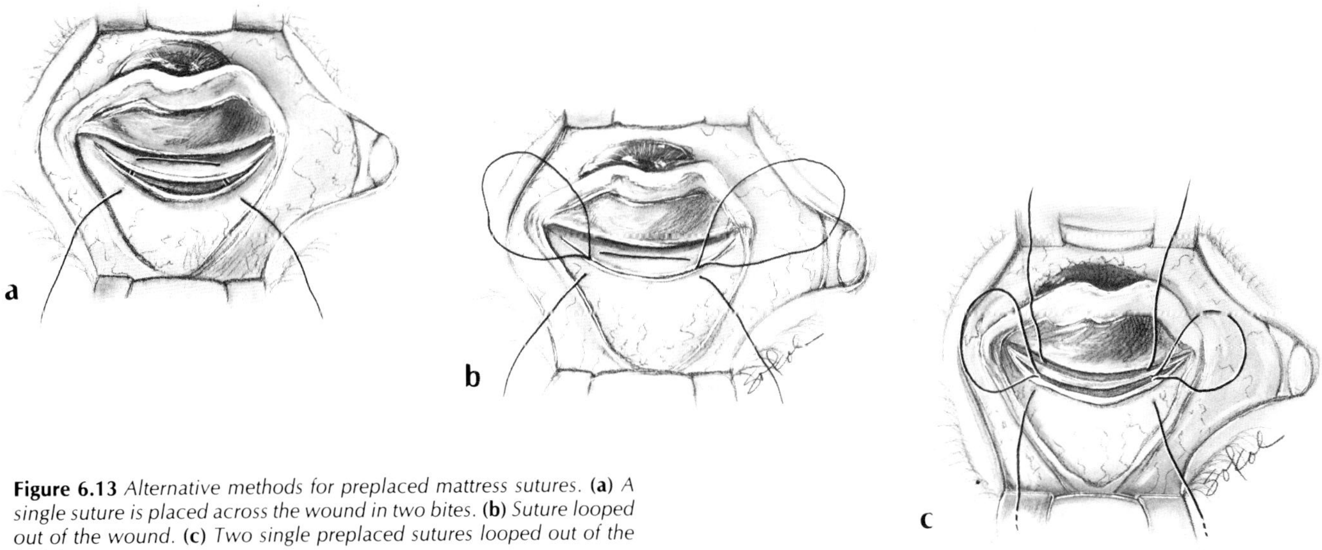

a

b

c

Figure 6.13 *Alternative methods for preplaced mattress sutures.* **(a)** *A single suture is placed across the wound in two bites.* **(b)** *Suture looped out of the wound.* **(c)** *Two single preplaced sutures looped out of the incision*

Entering the eye and the iridectomy

The preplaced sutures are looped out of the wound with smooth jeweler's forceps and fine smooth forceps, care being taken not to fray the silk (*Figure 6.14a,b*). The superior rectus stay suture is loosened. The eye is entered at the 11 to 12 o'clock meridian with a sharp blade such as a Smith-Green knife or a razor-blade knife (*Figure 6.14c*). The incision is extended to the right and left with curved corneal-section scissors. Care should be taken not to detach Descemet's membrane from the back of the cornea, nor cut the iris, nor puncture the lens capsule. The lower blade of the scissors is placed so that it follows the curvature of the limbus and so that the incision does not extend into the cornea or sclera (*Figure 6.14d,e*). If the incision extends into scleral tissue at the 2:30 or 9:30 meridians, there may be excessive bleeding.

After the incision has been completed, the surgical assistant retracts the cornea by grasping the conjunctival flap with fine smooth forceps. The iris is grasped and lifted by the surgeon with fine forceps, and sharp scissors are used to perform a small iridotomy at the 10 and the 2 o'clock positions a few millimeters in from the base of the iris (*Figure 6.14f*). The iridotomies do not need to be large and, if preferred, a single peripheral iridectomy may be performed instead. A sector iridectomy can be performed if the patient has a small fixed pupil.

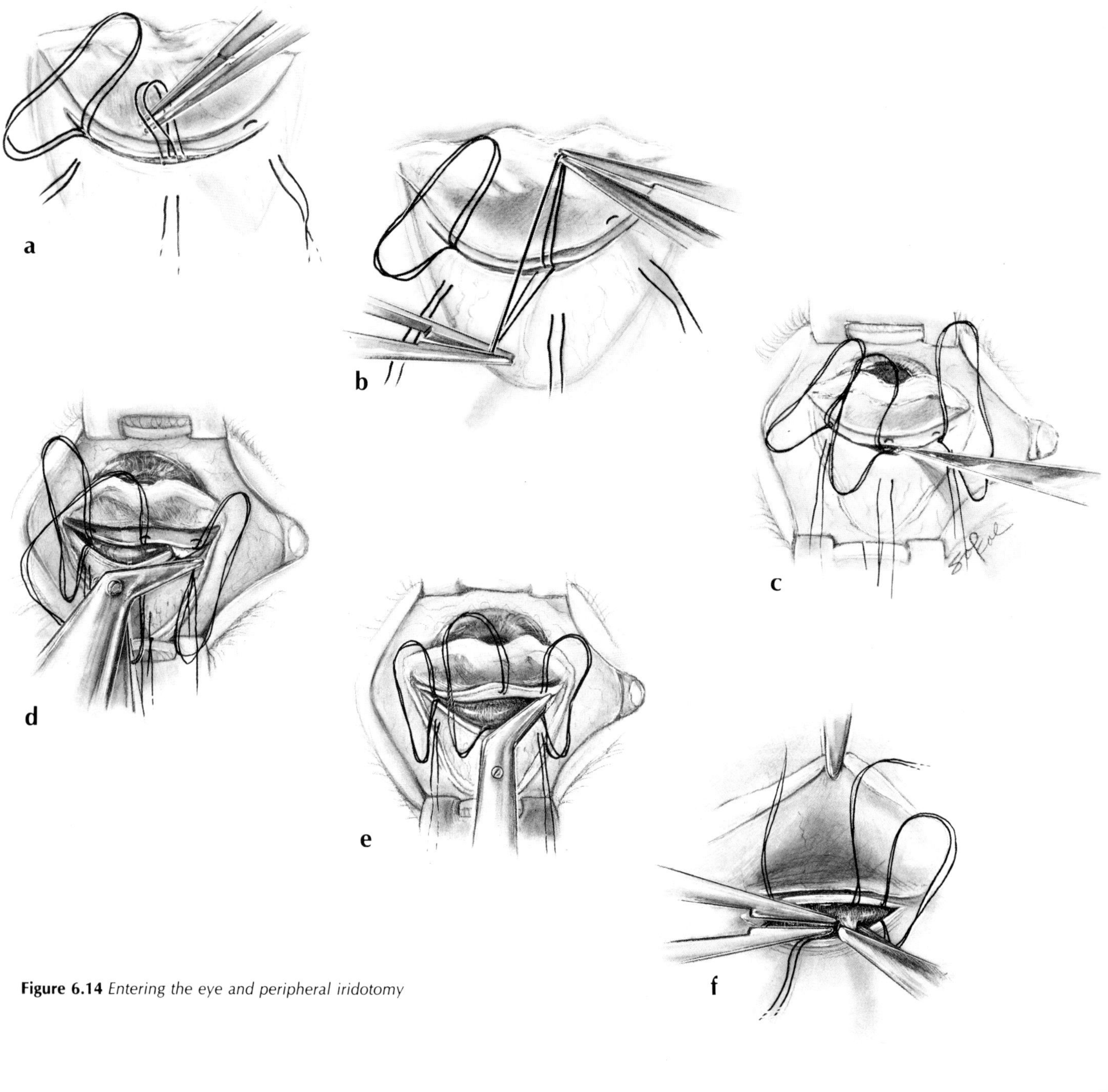

Figure 6.14 *Entering the eye and peripheral iridotomy*

α-chymotrypsin

We do not generally use α-chymotrypsin when doing intracapsular cataract surgery, because it is unnecessary if one properly strips the zonular attachments from the lens before cryoextraction. Use of the enzyme has the following disadvantages: transient elevation of intraocular pressure by temporary blockage of the trabecular meshwork with fragments of broken-down zonular fibers[26–28], more rapid dissolution of absorbable sutures and increased inflammation.

If the surgeon chooses to use α-chymotrypsin, it is prepared as a 1:5000 or 1:10 000 dilution and injected into the posterior chamber through one of the iridotomies prior to the lens extraction. After 2 minutes the anterior chamber is gently irrigated with balanced salt solution and then the lens is extracted.

Cryoextraction of the lens

In cataract extraction zonular attachments to the lens do not break (unless enzyme has been used) – they detach from the lens capsule. Therefore it is essential that zonular fibers be stripped from the lens so that they are not included in the ice ball during cryoextraction.

If α-chymotrypsin is not used, cataract extraction is performed as follows. The assistant retracts the cornea by pulling on the conjunctival flap with fine smooth forceps. Using fine-toothed forceps, such as 0.12 mm, the iris is grasped near the pupillary margin and pulled superiorly toward the 12 o'clock meridian. The zonular fibers are stripped from the lens, using dry cellulose sponges to gently wipe the anterior lens capsule about 3 mm anterior to the equator of the lens (*Figure 6.15a*). This is repeated until the superior fibers are broken from their adhesions to the anterior lens capsule between the 11 and 1 o'clock meridians. The cellulose sponge also absorbs fluid from the anterior chamber, ensuring a small ice ball from the cryoprobe. The cryoprobe is then applied to the superior lens capsule while the surgeon continues the retraction of the iris with forceps (*Figure 6.15b*). The probe tip is placed on the lens before the cryo unit is activated so ice crystals do not form on the probe before it touches the lens. This allows a better adherence between the probe and the lens. Because there is minimal fluid in the anterior chamber because of the use of the cellulose sponges, the ice ball on the anterior surface of the lens does not enlarge rapidly. This allows the cryoprobe to be left on the lens longer and ensures extension of the adhesive freeze well into the cortex and nucleus of the lens before lens extraction is attempted. If the freeze has not penetrated into the depth of the lens, only the lens capsule will be frozen; this will be evident by traction lines in the capsule and is associated with an increased chance of inadvertent capsular rupture. The cataract is removed by initially pulling straight up to free the superior edge of the lens. Then a rotary or rocking motion is used to free the lens from remaining zonular attachments and to pull the lens out of the eye (*Figure 6.15b*). The cornea is released and the preplaced 9/0 silk mattress sutures are pulled down. Millipore filtered air is used to reform the anterior chamber and is injected through the wound using a 27 gauge cannula on a small syringe.

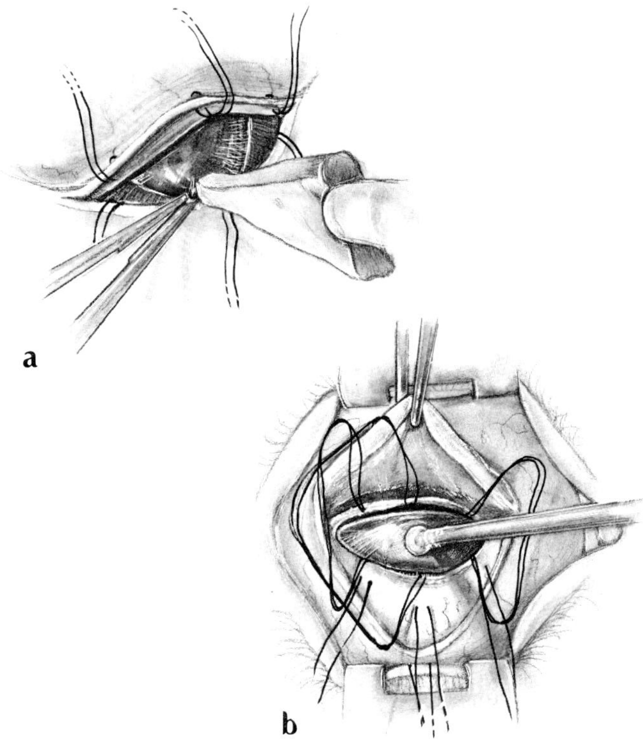

Figure 6.15 **(a)** *Stripping of zonules.* **(b)** *Cryoextraction of lens*

Closure of the wound

The preplaced sutures are tied, using tension lines of the cornea as an indication of proper suture tension (*Figure 6.16a*). Four additional 10/0 monofilament nylon sutures are then placed in interrupted fashion to close the wound securely (*Figure 6.16b*). There are numerous alternative

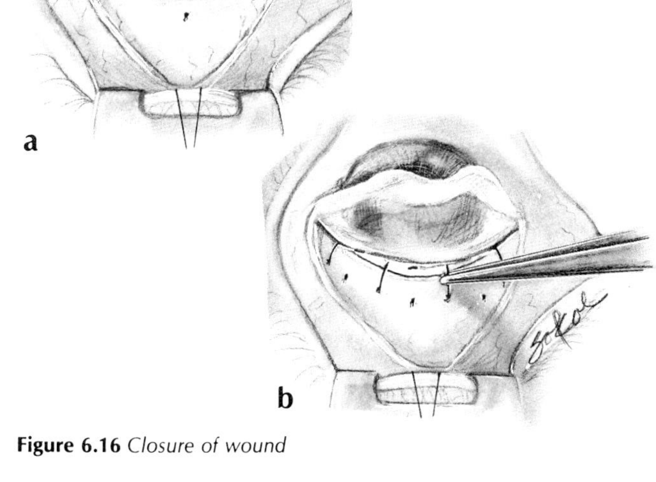

Figure 6.16 *Closure of wound*

methods of cataract wound closure; for example, a running suture for closure of the wound (*Figure 6.17*) or other modifications of mattress or sutures (*Figure 6.18*). The technique shown in *Figure 6.19* is that recently described by Dangle and Keates[29] for use in cataract surgery or keratoplasty. The adjustable slip knot does not show undue slippage and allows more precise wound closure.

Whichever suture technique is used it is important to bury the knot of the nylon or polypropylene (Prolene) suture. This is accomplished by simply pulling the knot into the scleral portion of the wound when using interrupted sutures. The knot for a running or figure-of-eight suture is buried by starting the first bite and ending the last bite within the wound. The surgeon must decide which suturing method works best for him.

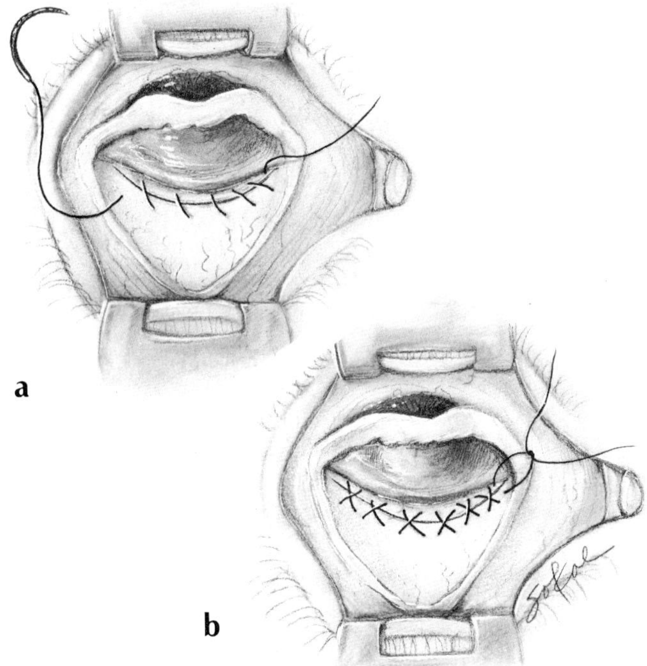

Figure 6.17 *Running shoe-string style suture as alternative method of closure*

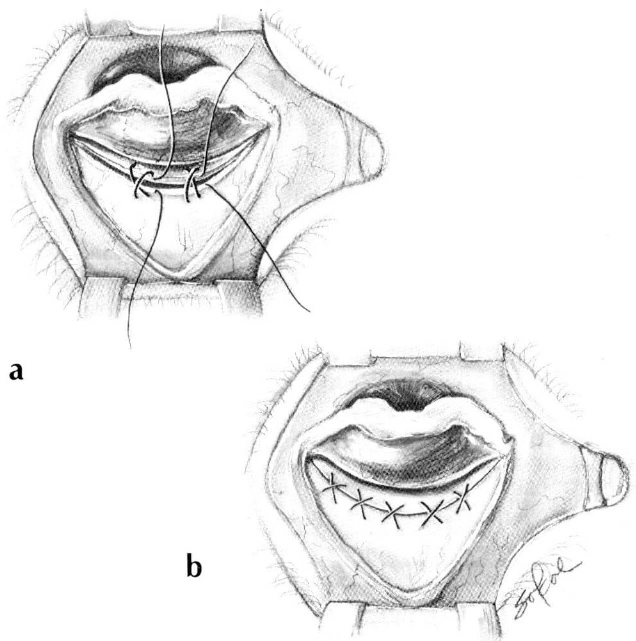

Figure 6.18 *Multiple mattress sutures as alternative closure. Note how suture is placed so that knots are buried in wound*

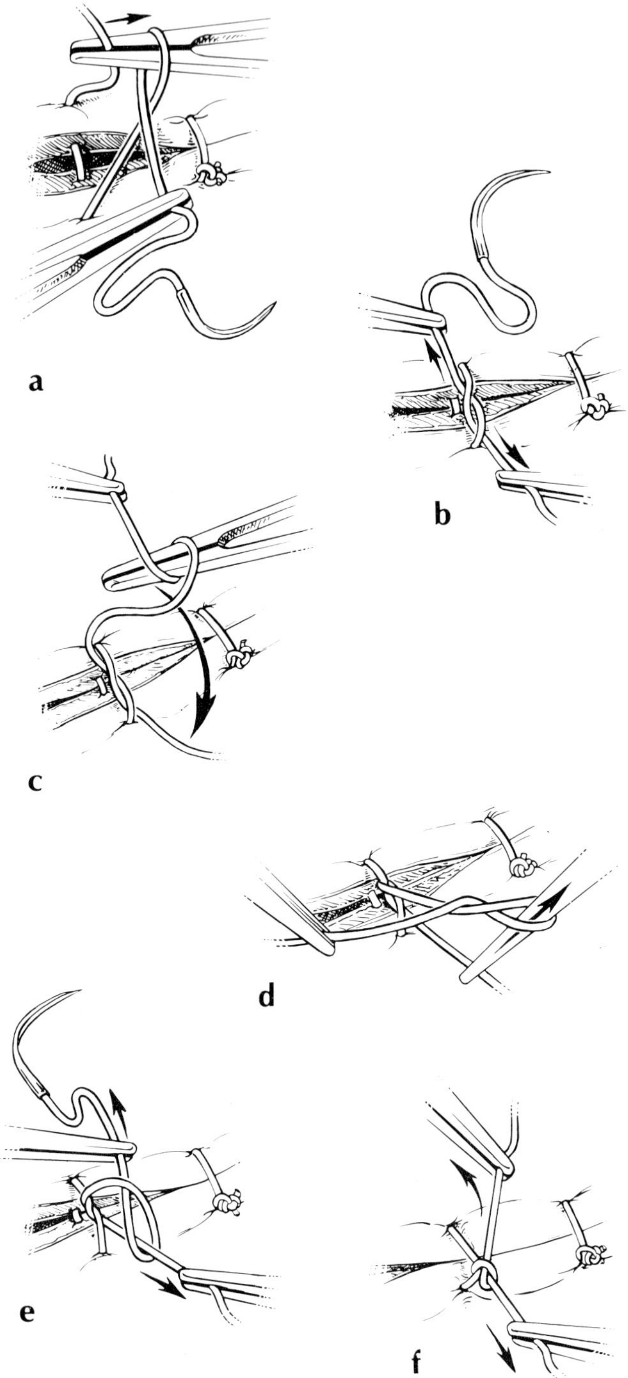

Figure 6.19 *Modified adjustable slip-knot technique for tying nylon suture useful in cataract closure and keratoplasty*

Re-formation of the anterior chamber

After the sutures have been placed, the air in the anterior chamber is removed and replaced with physiologic salt solution (*Figure 6.20*). The wound should then be checked to be sure it is watertight by applying gentle pressure with a cellulose sponge along the posterior lip of the wound. If there is significant leakage of aqueous, another interrupted suture should be placed at the leakage site.

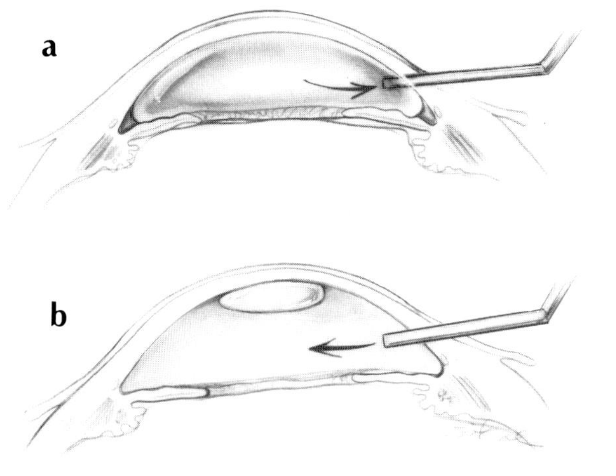

Figure 6.20 *Re-forming the anterior chamber by* **(a)** *removing air and* **(b)** *injecting physiologic saline solution*

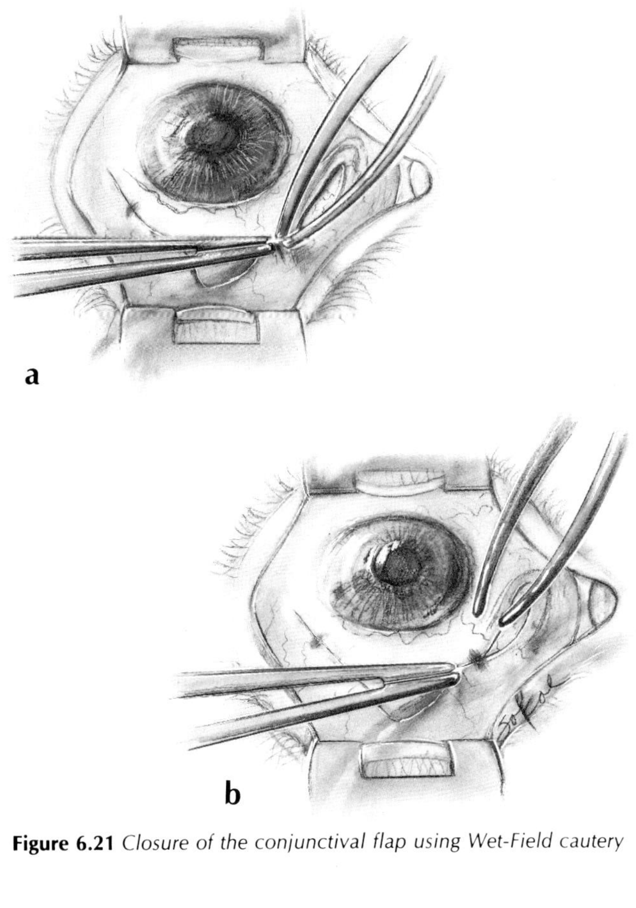

Figure 6.21 *Closure of the conjunctival flap using Wet-Field cautery*

Closure of the conjunctiva

The conjunctival flap is closed with the Wet-Field Coagulator™. The conjunctiva is grasped with a pair of medium-toothed forceps, and the conjunctival cautery forceps are used to grasp and appose the edges of the conjunctiva. The coagulator is activated (*Figure 6.21a*) at a setting of 25 or 30. The coagulator forceps are released first while the two conjunctival edges are held together with the other toothed forceps (*Figure 6.21b*). This maneuver prevents the coagulator forceps, which may stick to the conjunctiva, from pulling the wound open when they are released. It is important not to have Tenon's capsule in between the conjunctival edges which are being cauterized together.

If Wet-Field Coagulator is unavailable, the conjunctiva can be closed using multiple interrupted sutures or a running suture of fine absorbable material such as 8/0 collagen. Closure of a fornix-based flap may be performed with the coagulator or fine absorbable suture. Usually, two interrupted sutures or two cautery burns are sufficient.

At the completion of the procedure, gentamicin 20 mg in 0.5 ml and a short-acting steroid such as dexamethasone (Decadron) 2 mg in 0.5 ml may be injected subconjunctivally. A patch and shield are placed over the eye to protect it.

Planned extracapsular cataract extraction

There have been no prospective controlled studies showing a comparative advantage of either extracapsular or intracapsular cataract extraction in older patients. There is clinical evidence, however, that leaving the posterior capsule intact may decrease the incidence of postoperative cystoid macular edema and also possibly of retinal detachment[30, 31].

We use the following method for extracapsular cataract extraction. A limbal-based conjunctival flap is prepared, a grooved limbal incision is made and 8/0 or 9/0 silk sutures are preplaced as described above for the intracapsular technique. The anterior chamber is entered near 11 o'clock (for right-handed surgeons) with a Smith-Green knife to make a watertight wound for introduction of an irrigating cystotome or a bent 25 gauge needle with the tip bent away from the bevel. The Smith-Green knife is also used to cut the anterior lens capsule at the 11 o'clock position for a right-handed surgeon (*Figure 6.22a*).

The anterior chamber depth is maintained by gravity-type drip irrigation through a cystotome or a bent 25 gauge needle. The capsulotomy is begun at the 6 o'clock position on the lens and is extended clockwise and counterclockwise in a circular fashion. Care is taken to perform a wide capsulotomy and yet to avoid extending the capsular tears through the zonular attachments to the anterior lens capsule (*Figure 6.22b*). The cystotome or bent needle is then removed. Often, the cut anterior capsule will present in the wound and can be removed. The initial cut at the 11 o'clock position will prevent the capsule tearing to the equator when it is removed from the eye. Using scissors, the cataract wound is then enlarged to the left and right for 130° superiorly (*Figure 6.22c*).

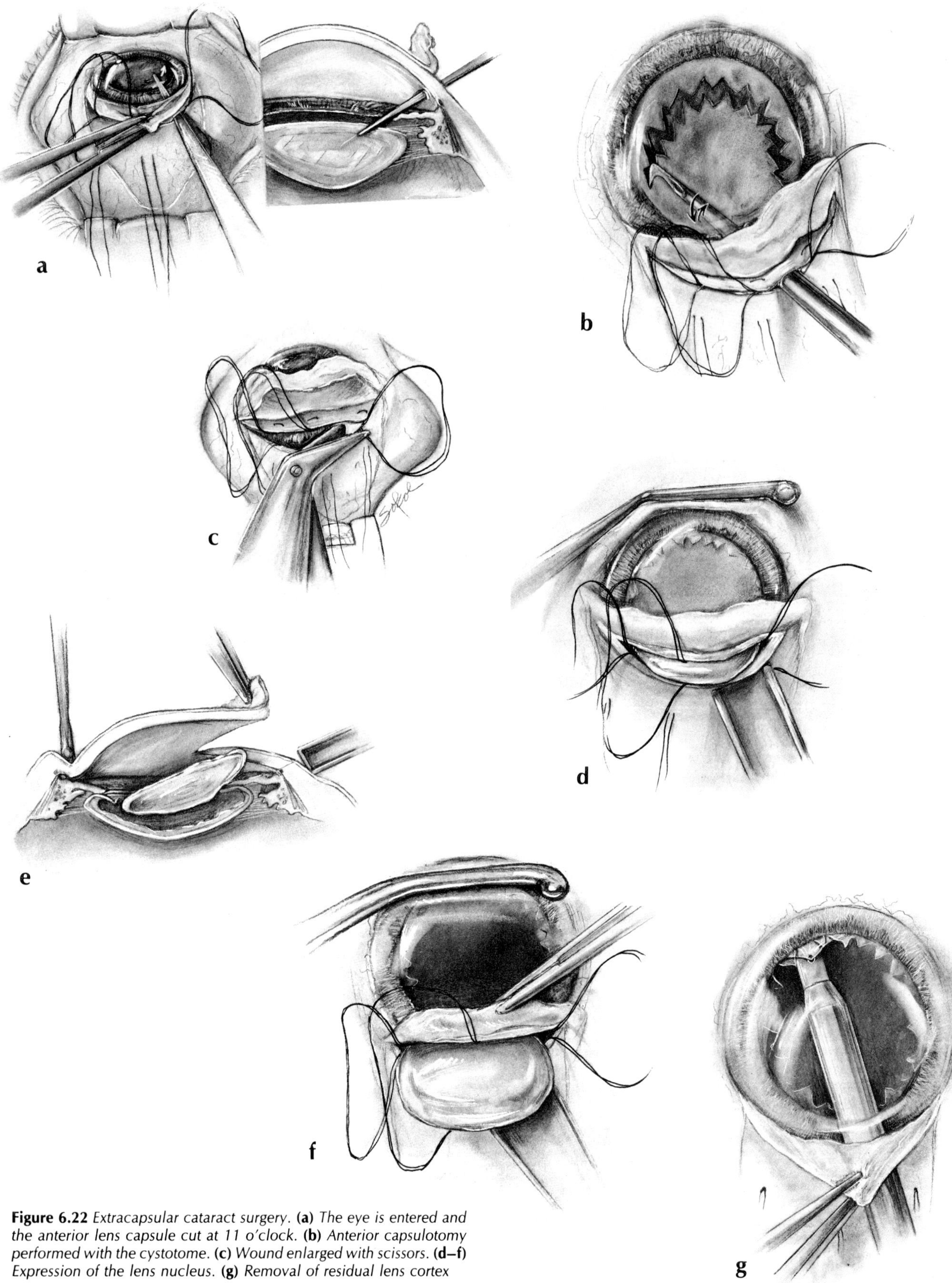

Figure 6.22 *Extracapsular cataract surgery.* **(a)** *The eye is entered and the anterior lens capsule cut at 11 o'clock.* **(b)** *Anterior capsulotomy performed with the cystotome.* **(c)** *Wound enlarged with scissors.* **(d–f)** *Expression of the lens nucleus.* **(g)** *Removal of residual lens cortex*

To remove the lens nucleus, the cornea is retracted and a muscle hook is used to apply pressure at the inferior limbus externally. This tilts the superior pole of the lens anteriorly. While applying gentle downward pressure, a lens spoon is used to depress the posterior lip of the wound at the 12 o'clock position. The lens nucleus is expressed from the eye using the muscle hook and lens spoon to increase the posterior chamber pressure (*Figure 6.22d,e*). Occasionally the nucleus must be rocked completely out of the eye, but it is usually not necessary to put any instrument into the eye.

The three preplaced 9/0 silk mattress sutures are tied securely, using a slip knot so that they can be untied later. The non-ultrasonic 0.3 mm irrigation/aspiration (I/A) unit of the Cavitron Kelman Phaco-Emulsifier^{TM} instrument is used to remove the remaining cortical material. The tip of the I/A unit is inserted into the anterior chamber between two of the mattress sutures, usually at the 11 o'clock position for a right-handed surgeon. Using irrigation only, the tip is inserted into the equator of the capsular bag under the iris. This tends to open the capsular leaves. The irrigation/aspiration mode is then activated, and lens cortex is sucked into the aspirating port as the tip of the instrument is moved into the center of the anterior chamber (*Figure 6.22g*). Thus, one goes 'in' while irrigating and comes 'out' while irrigating and aspirating. The process is begun at the 6 o'clock position and is repeated all the way around the equator of the lens capsule to remove all cortical material. This makes it possible to continue removal of cortex if the capsule is inadvertently ruptured at the 6 o'clock position.

Care must be taken not to tear the lens capsule while aspirating cortex. Aspiration must be stopped immediately if the posterior lens capsule is sucked into the aspiration port. This is evident when radial folds are seen in the posterior capsule (*Figure 6.23*).

All movements must be made while pivoting around the wound so as not to open the wound and allow the anterior chamber to collapse. This principle applies to all extra-capsular surgery no matter which instrument is used.

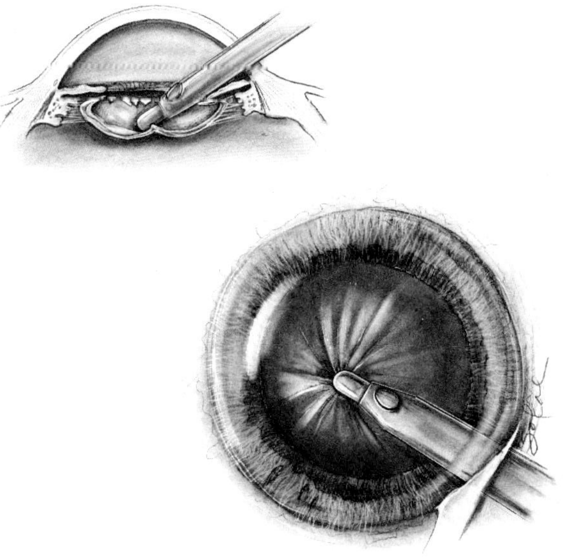

Figure 6.23 *Inadvertent aspiration of posterior capsule causing radial folds and tenting of the capsule*

If a phacoemulsification unit is not available, alternative methods can be used for removing lens cortex. A silicone-rubber bulb with a 19 gauge cannula may be used to aspirate lens cortex. The cannula is inserted through the wound with the bulb partly collapsed. When cortex is against the cannula tip, the bulb is released and cortex is sucked into the cannula. The cortex is gently stripped off the posterior capsule and removed from the eye (*Figure 6.24*).

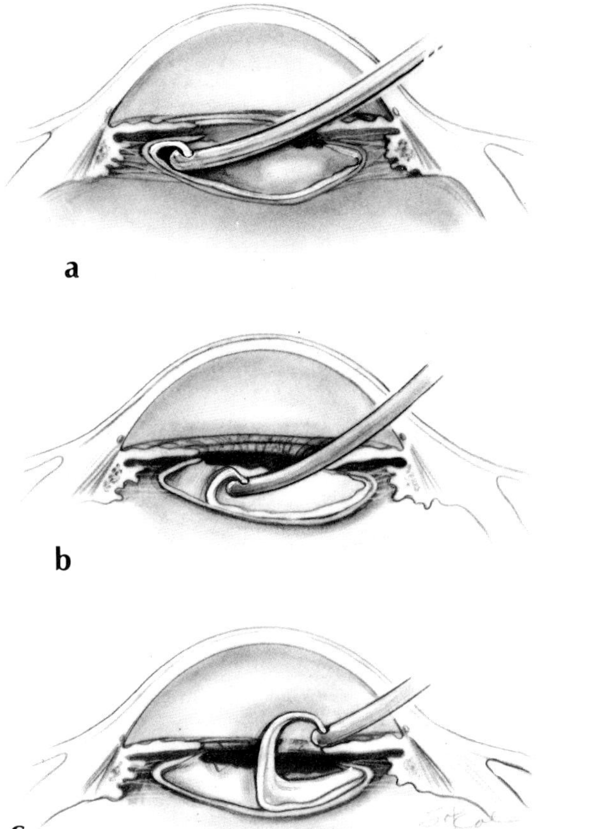

a

b

c

Figure 6.24 *Alternative method of cortex removal using the Simcoe technique*

A third method of removing lens cortex uses the McIntyre needle system. The technique is similar to that described for the I/A unit, except that the suction is produced by a syringe attached directly to the cannula. Irrigation occurs through a sleeve over the aspiration cannula. The McIntyre needle system can be attached to an Ocutome^{TM} console if a more controlled suction is desired.

After the cortex has been removed, and if no intraocular lens (IOL) is to be inserted, an iridectomy or iridotomy is performed. The wound is then closed with the three preplaced 9/0 silk sutures and four interrupted 10/0 monofilament nylon sutures are inserted.

Because the posterior lens capsule becomes cloudy in up to 50 per cent of extracapsular cataract extraction cases[32, 33], we usually cut the posterior capsule at the time of surgery. The exact effect of cutting the posterior capsule on such complications as cystoid macular edema and retinal detachment is unknown. We cut the posterior capsule with a 27 gauge needle with the tip bent away from the bevel. While the irrigation keeps the anterior chamber formed, the needle is inserted through the wound and through one of the iridotomies (*Figure 6.25*). The capsule is hooked with the bent tip several millimeters below the visual axis. The capsule is lifted and torn towards 12 o'clock, creating an adequate (about 3 mm × 3 mm) but not too large an opening in the posterior capsule (*Figure 6.25*). Once the capsule begins to tear, the needle tip is turned horizontally to avoid cutting the anterior vitreous face. To complete the procedure, the conjunctival flap is closed with Wet-Field cautery or sutures, and antibiotics and steroid may be injected subconjunctivally as described for intracapsular cataract surgery.

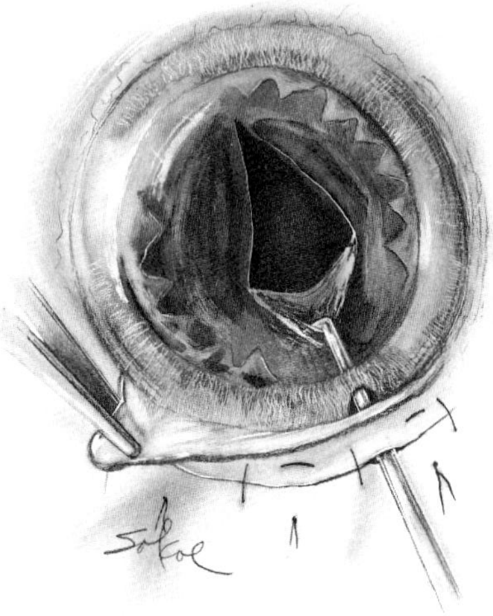

Figure 6.25 *Posterior capsulotomy*

Phacoemulsification

The technique of phacoemulsification as developed by Kelman[34–36] was designed to perform extracapsular cataract extraction through a small incision. The use of a small incision has been advocated to allow patients to resume normal activity quickly after surgery. The small incision is the major advantage this procedure has over standard planned extracapsular surgery, and it is mainly useful in patients without dense nuclear sclerosis.

Preparation for phacoemulsification surgery is the same as that described for standard extracapsular surgery, including preoperative dilation of the pupil and the use of subconjunctival dilating solution (*see* p. 144) 20 minutes before surgery. We also routinely use i.v. mannitol, unless contraindicated, and an intraocular pressure-reducer as described previously. During preparation, care must be taken not to get soap on the cornea, as this may damage the corneal epithelium and prevent a clear view of the lens and anterior chamber. Phacoemulsification surgery requires the use of the operating microscope, and coaxial illumination is preferred so that a red reflex can be seen during surgery.

The Kelman phacoemulsification system consists of a console and three basic handpieces: the irrigation handpiece, the ultrasonic handpiece (*Figure 6.26*) and the non-ultrasonic irrigation/aspiration (I/A) handpiece (*Figure 6.27*). The irrigation handpiece has various tips that can be used, such as the Kratz needle for polishing the posterior lens capsule and a cystotome for performing an anterior capsulotomy. Some surgeons prefer a 26 or 27 gauge needle with a bent tip for the capsulotomy.

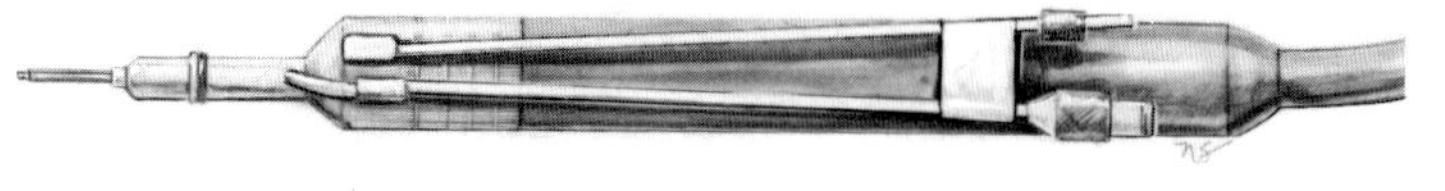

Figure 6.26 *Phacoemulsification handpiece*

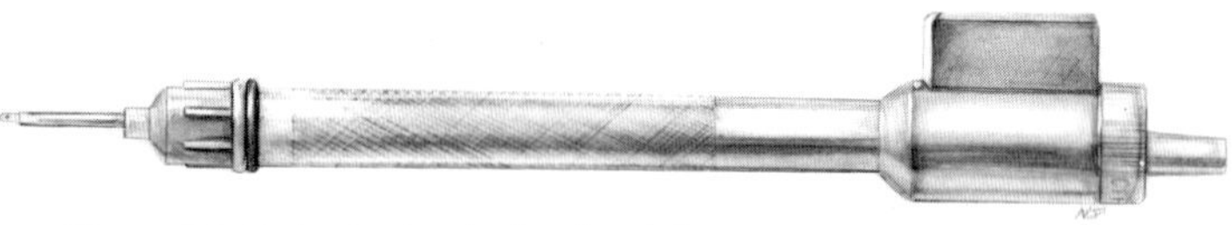

Figure 6.27 *Irrigation/aspiration handpiece*

For phacoemulsification, we prefer a limbus-based conjunctival flap of about 4–5 mm in width. Conjunctiva and Tenon's capsule are entered with scissors, cutting a triangle and dissecting the flap to the limbus. The limbus is cleaned with sharp scissors and a Tooke or Beaver knife. The anterior chamber is entered with a sharp blade, such as a Smith-Green knife, and the superior portion of the anterior capsule is cut as described above (*Figure 6.28a*). The anterior capsulotomy is also performed as described for planned extracapsular surgery (*Figure 6.28b–e*). The incision is enlarged with the keratome to 3.5 mm (*Figure 6.28f,g*). The phacoemulsification tip is then inserted into the anterior chamber, and the ultrasonic mode is used in short bursts to remove the nucleus of the cataract (*Figure 6.28h*). The length of emulsification time required varies considerably with the hardness of the lens nucleus. Much of the lens material in congenital or other soft cataracts can be aspirated with suction and irrigation alone, without using ultrasonic vibration. Senile cataracts with a hard nucleus may require 60–120 seconds of ultrasound-time, or even more, for removal.

Various techniques can be used in performing ultrasonic emulsification of the lens. We usually prefer to emulsify most of the nucleus while it remains in the posterior chamber. This minimizes trauma to the corneal endothelium but is slightly more difficult because there is a greater chance of cutting the posterior capsule. When emulsification is used in the posterior chamber, the phacoemulsifer is used to carve grooves in the anterior lens surface, hollowing or sculpting the lens to about half thickness (*Figure 6.29a–c*). The superior edge of the lens nucleus is then engaged with the instrument tip, and the remaining nucleus is emulsified (*Figure 6.29d,e*). Care must be taken not to engage and tear the posterior capsule.

Alternatively, some surgeons prefer emulsification of the lens nucleus in the anterior chamber. In this technique, before the incision is enlarged to 3.5 mm, the cystotome is used to engage the nucleus, and with a rocking or seesaw movement the nucleus is prolapsed into the anterior chamber (*Figure 6.30*). The corneal incision is enlarged, the ultrasonic tip is inserted into the anterior chamber, the lens nucleus is engaged at its

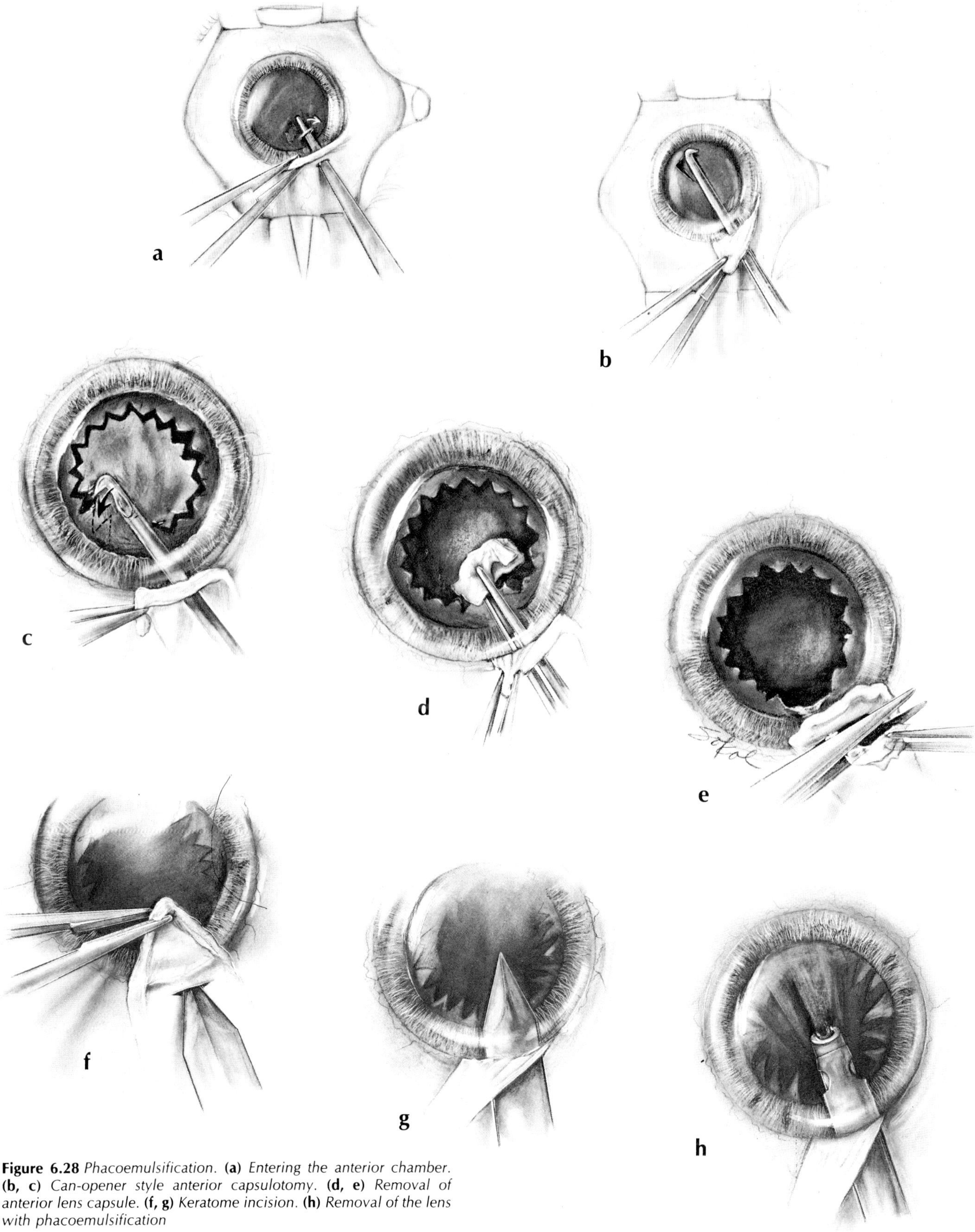

Figure 6.28 *Phacoemulsification.* **(a)** *Entering the anterior chamber.* **(b, c)** *Can-opener style anterior capsulotomy.* **(d, e)** *Removal of anterior lens capsule.* **(f, g)** *Keratome incision.* **(h)** *Removal of the lens with phacoemulsification*

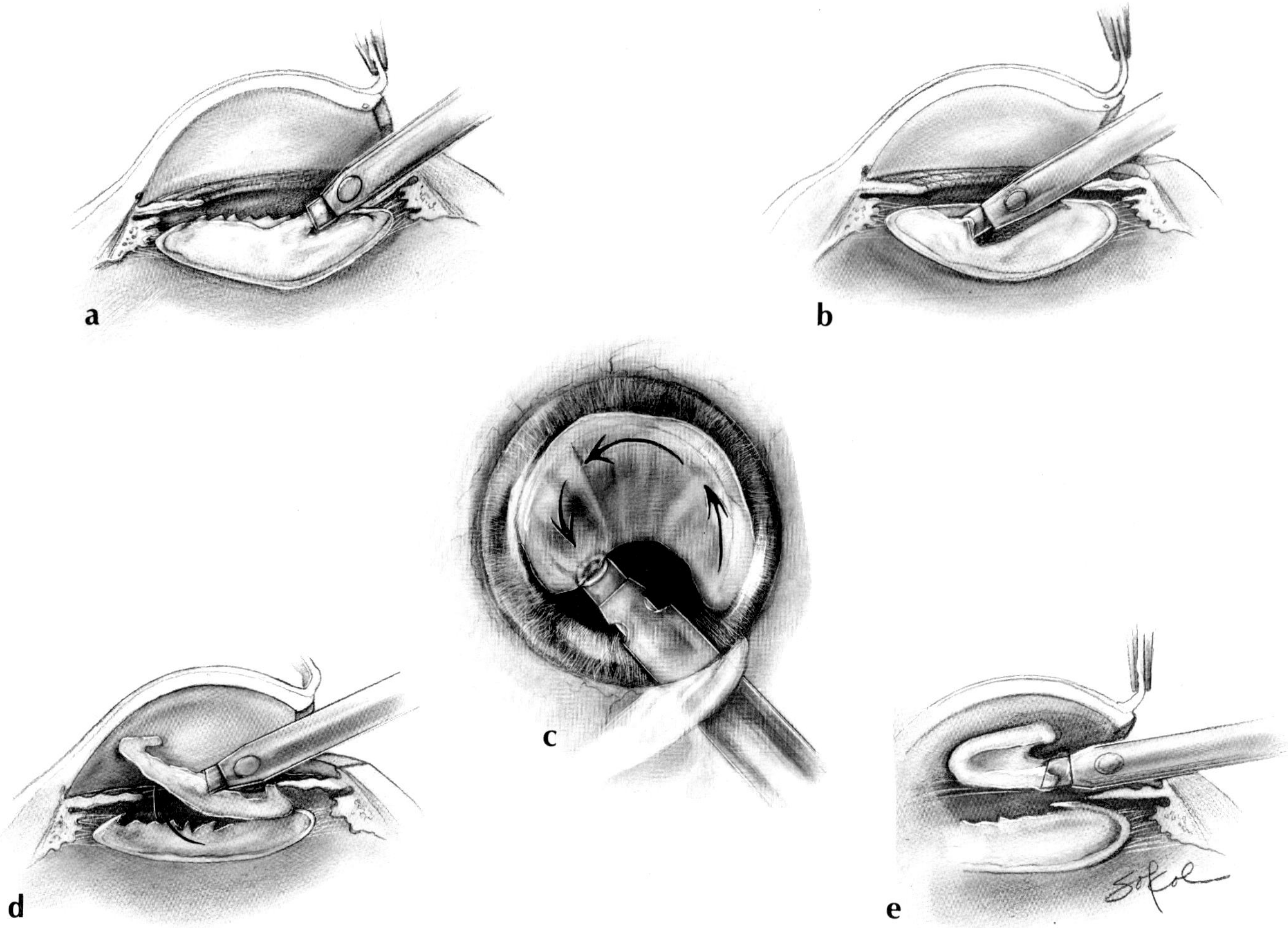

Figure 6.29 *Phacoemulsification. Emulsification of the lens nucleus*

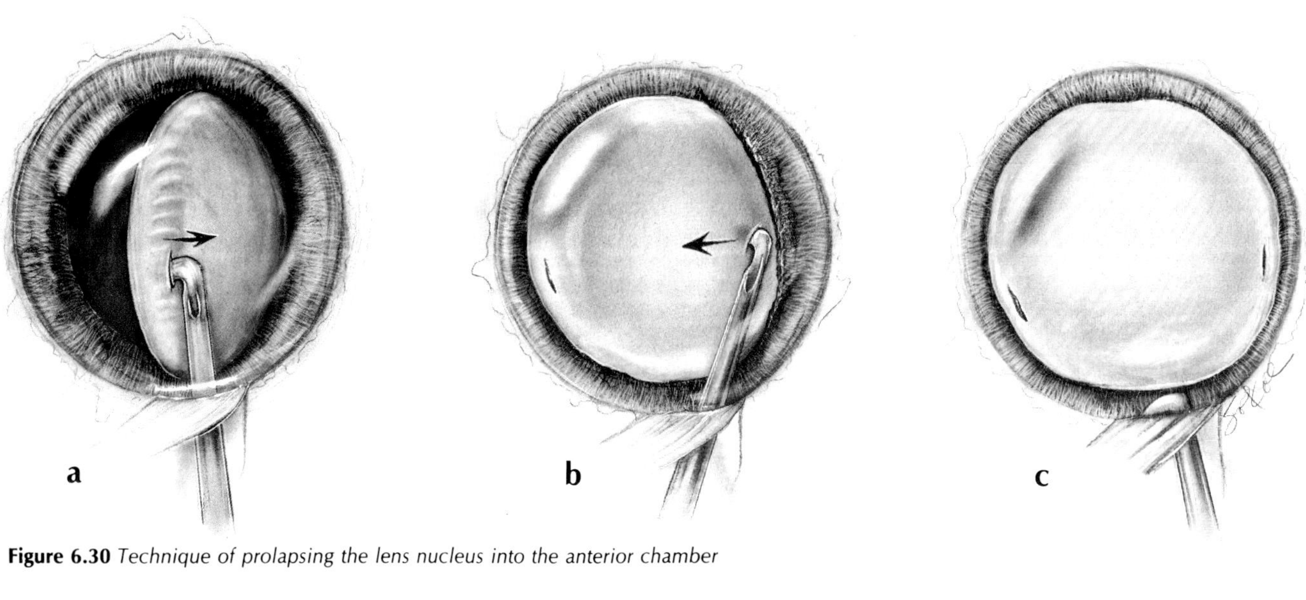

Figure 6.30 *Technique of prolapsing the lens nucleus into the anterior chamber*

equator and, with the tip of the instrument held stationary, the lens is emulsified by 'bursts' (*Figure 6.31*). The phacoemulsifier tip should be kept parallel to the iris plane and in the center of the anterior chamber in the pupillary axis. This is the safest position, where it is farthest from the corneal endothelium and the posterior capsule. Numerous techniques have been described for emulsification of the lens nucleus in the anterior chamber – such as the croissant technique, the sector technique,

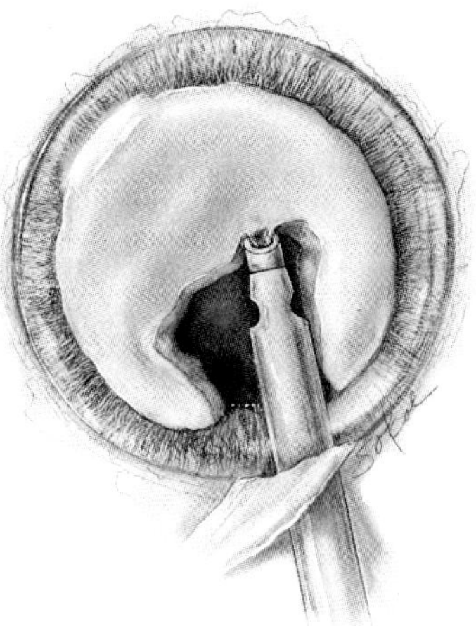

Figure 6.31 *Emulsification of the lens nucleus in the anterior chamber*

the carousel technique[37]. No matter which technique is used, it may be necessary to convert the procedure to a planned extracapsular operation if difficulties arise. These difficulties can include: a constricted pupil that does not dilate in response to 1:5000 intracardiac-type epinephrine (adrenaline) (diluted) instilled into the anterior chamber, inability to maintain a formed anterior chamber, rupture of zonular fibers with subluxation of the lens, mechanical malfunction, and an extremely dense lens nucleus.

Occasionally, while the ultrasonic mode is being used, a piece of hard lens nucleus may become stuck within the phacoemulsifier tip. This can be expelled by having the assistant squeeze abruptly on the aspiration line to force a small amount of fluid and the piece of lens from the tip.

When the dense portion of the nucleus has been removed, the power of the phacoemulsifier is reduced to avoid a rapid penetration through residual soft lens cortex. Reducing the power also helps prevent small pieces of hard nucleus from bouncing off the tip during emulsification.

When all the lens nucleus and hard cortex has been removed, the I/A unit is used to remove remaining cortical material as described under extracapsular surgery (*Figure 6.32a–c*). The posterior capsule is polished (*Figure 6.32d*) and a peripheral iridectomy is performed (*Figure 6.32e*). The small entrance site is closed with a figure-of-eight mattress suture, or two or three interrupted 10/0 nylon sutures (*Figure 6.32f*). The anterior chamber is deepened with balanced salt solution to check whether the wound is watertight. If desired, a posterior capsulotomy may be performed, using a 27 gauge needle with a bent tip introduced through the wound and iridectomy as described previously (*Figure 6.32g,h*).

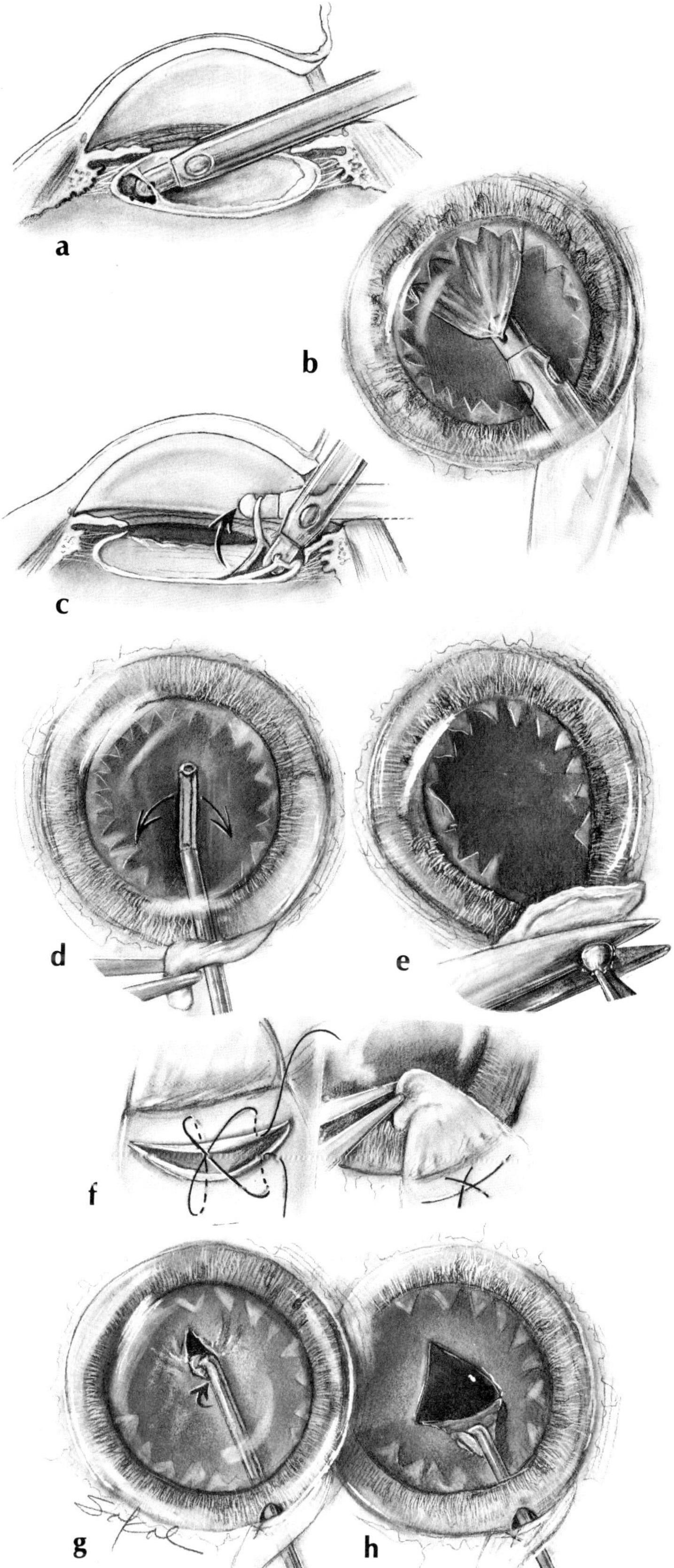

Figure 6.32 *Phacoemulsification.* **(a–c)** *Removal of residual cortex using irrigation/aspiration.* **(d)** *Polishing of posterior capsule.* **(e)** *Peripheral iridectomy.* **(f)** *Closure of the incision.* **(g, h)** *Posterior capsulotomy*

Intraocular lens implantation

There are three basic types of IOLs: (*1*) anterior chamber, (*2*) iris plane (pupillary supported) and (*3*) posterior chamber (*Figure 6.33*). We currently prefer the Shearing style posterior chamber IOL. However, it is important for surgeons who use mostly posterior chamber IOLs to be familiar with insertion of anterior chamber lenses because occasionally the posterior lens capsule will tear prior to lens implantation. In these cases, if no vitreous is lost, another type of IOL may be inserted. We rarely insert anterior chamber IOLs because their use may be associated with an increased risk of complications[38] and poorer visual results[39]. A brief description of anterior chamber IOL insertion will be presented. Our method of inserting a four-loop Binkhorst IOL and a Shearing posterior chamber IOL will be described in more detail, although we now rarely, if ever, insert four-loop iris plane IOLs.

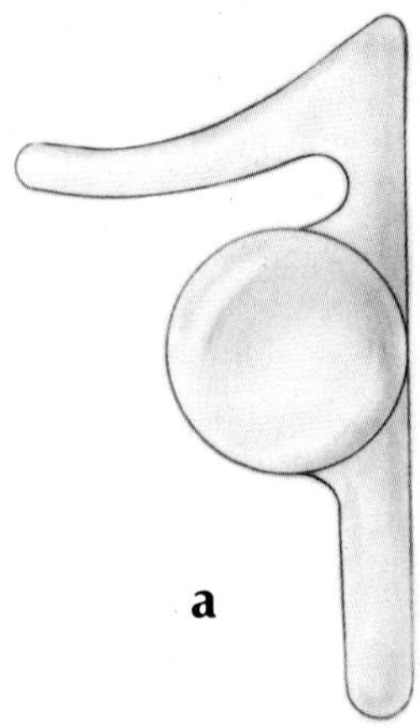

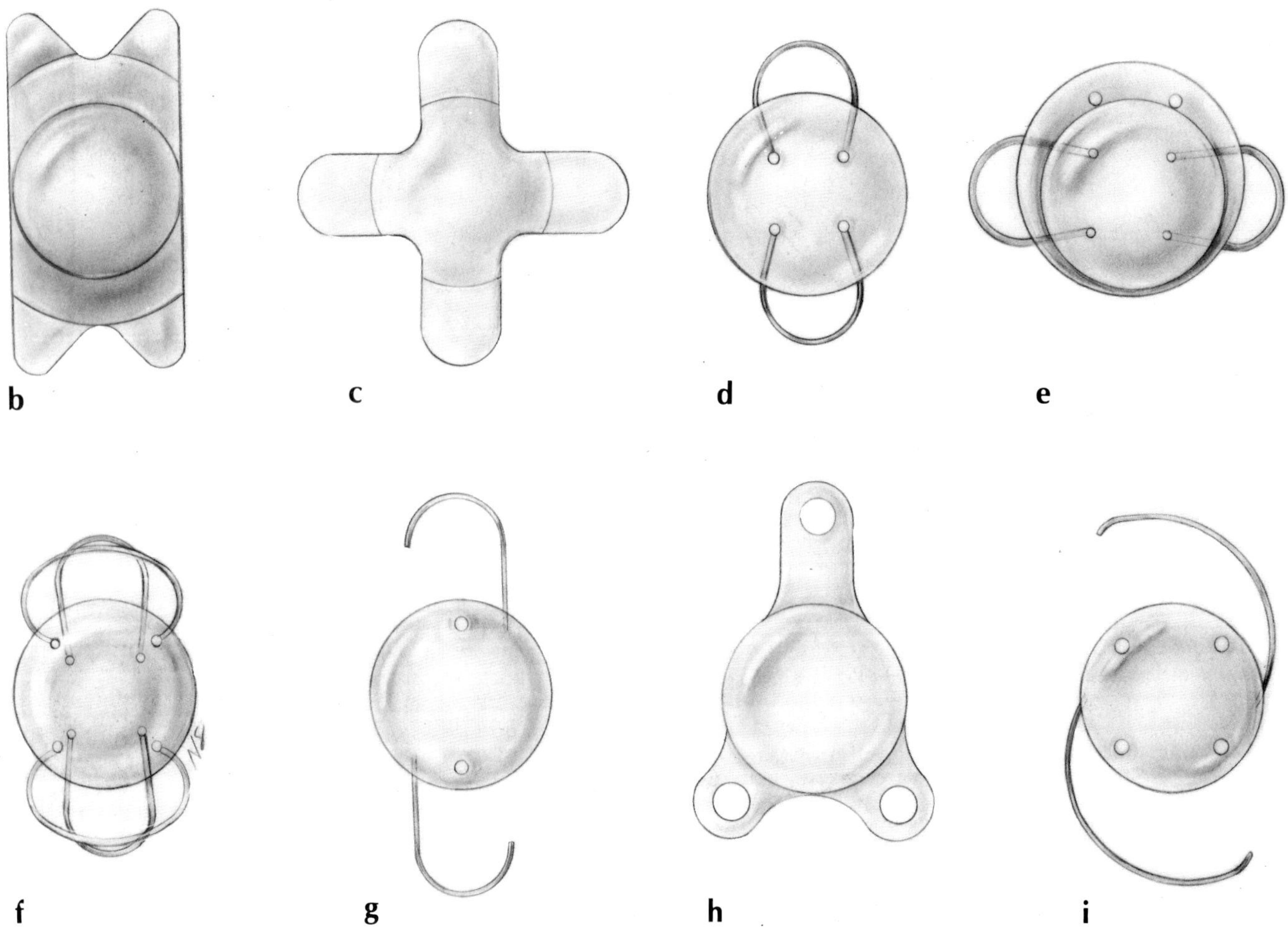

Figure 6.33 *Assorted intraocular lenses including anterior chamber* (**a, b**), *iris plane* (**c–f**) *and posterior chamber* (**g–i**) *style lenses*

Indications

The following can be favorable clinical settings for IOL implantation: (*1*) the patient is not likely to succeed in wearing an aphakic contact lens postoperatively because of poor motivation, dry eyes, corneal epithelial basement-membrane disorders, insufficient manual dexterity, senility or factors of occupation; (*2*) successful aphakic contact lens use in the other eye; (*3*) macular degeneration with dense cataracts; or (*4*) the patient is over 50 years of age.

Contraindications

We reserve IOL implantation for suitable patients when there are no contraindications. We consider the following situations relative contraindications to IOL implantation: (*1*) the patient does not want an IOL; (*2*) high axial myopia – greater than 6–7 diopters (D); (*3*) presence of Fuchs' dystrophy or clinically significant corneal endothelial disease; (*4*) a one-eyed patient (*5*) the patient is less than 50 years of age (except when a contact lens cannot be used); (*6*) the presence of uncontrolled glaucoma, rubeosis iridis, diabetic retinopathy, previous retinal detachment or recurrent uveitis in the operative eye; or (*7*) serious complications at the time of surgery.

Proper patient selection is especially important in IOL implantation cases because of the increased risk of operative and postoperative complications. Also, a surgeon should be capable of inserting various types of IOLs if difficulties arise intraoperatively. For example, if the posterior capsule is broken before placement of a Shearing posterior chamber lens, then a four-loop Binkhorst or an anterior chamber IOL can be placed instead. A posterior chamber lens should be placed only when the posterior capsule is intact. We usually do not implant an IOL if any of the more severe operative complications such as significant vitreous loss occur, although some surgeons disagree with this viewpoint.

IOL power determination

An essential part of the preoperative evaluation of an eye that is to receive an IOL is to determine the proper IOL refractive power. This requires a careful determination of the corneal curvature by keratometer or ophthalmometer measurements, and an ultrasonic determination of the axial length of the eye using A-scan ultrasonography. These measurements, along with an estimation of the expected postoperative anterior chamber depth (which partially depends on the type of IOL inserted), are entered in a computer programmed to calculate the appropriate power of IOL for insertion. The power of IOL selected also depends on the status of the fellow eye. In general we strive for a residual postoperative refractive error of −0.75 D spherical equivalent if the fellow eye is cataractous, aphakic with a contact lens, or is normal with a refractive error between +2.50 D and −3.00 D. This method allows some leeway so that even if our calculations are not perfectly accurate, 90 per cent of patients still have a postoperative refractive error between plano and −1.50 D (−0.75 D ± 0.75 D). If the fellow eye has no cataract and hyperopia greater than +2.50 D, we strive for a plano postoperative refractive error. If the fellow eye has lenticular myopia greater than 3 D and 6/6 to 6/9 vision, we strive for −2.00 D postoperative refractive error.

The four-loop Binkhorst iris fixation IOL

The four-loop Binkhorst iris-clip IOL may be inserted after intracapsular or extracapsular cataract extraction. We have had excellent short-term results using this style of lens, but long-term follow-up data indicate an increase in late-onset corneal edema. Therefore, this lens is used only if the capsule ruptures during extracapsular cataract extraction and then only in eyes of very elderly patients.

Preparation for intracapsular lens surgery with IOL implantation is performed as described on p. 143. Among the more important preoperative goals are akinesia and a 'soft eye'. The surgery is similar to that previously described, except that immediately before cryoextraction, a 10/0 polypropylene (Prolene) suture is placed through the superior iris in a radial fashion, entering about 2 mm above the sphincter and exiting 2 mm from the iris root[40] (*Figure 6.34a*). The IOL, which has been soaking in physiologic saline solution, is examined under the microscope for defects, irrigated with physiologic saline and wiped with cellulose sponges to remove any debris. The cataract is removed with cryoextraction as described on p. 149. The two lateral 9/0 black silk sutures are tied in slip knots to make the wound opening smaller. The pupil is constricted with acetylcholine (Miochol) or carbachol (Miostat), and the anterior chamber is deepened with air. The four-loop IOL is then grasped with a special Binkhorst irrigation-insertion forceps. The inferior end of the 10/0 polypropylene (Prolene) suture (closest to the pupil) is passed through the anterior-superior loop of the IOL (*Figure 6.34b*). The surgeon retracts the cornea, and the IOL is inserted into the anterior chamber while the assistant uses a 20 ml syringe to irrigate balanced salt solution through the irrigating forceps to maintain a deep anterior chamber (*Figure 6.34c*). The IOL is in the proper position when the inferior pupil margin 'squares off' against the posts of the IOL. The IOL is released from the forceps and air is injected into the anterior chamber if necessary. As the assistant gently retracts the cornea, the surgeon grasps the superior loop of the IOL and pushes inferiorly while simultaneously pulling the iris superiorly so that the iris slides in between the two superior IOL loops (*Figure 6.34d–f*).

After the IOL is in place, the anterior chamber is again deepened with air if necessary, and the cornea is retracted by the assistant just enough to expose the superior iris and suture but not enough to lose the anterior chamber air. The 10/0 polypropylene (Prolene) suture, is then tied so that a flat but not taut loop is created (*Figure 6.34g,h*). This loop allows the IOL to move lower when the pupil is dilated postoperatively, which prevents the inferior and superior loops from dislocating. Even if the IOL subluxes, it cannot fall back into the vitreous cavity because of this suture. The eye is then closed as previously described for intracapsular cataract surgery (*see* p. 149).

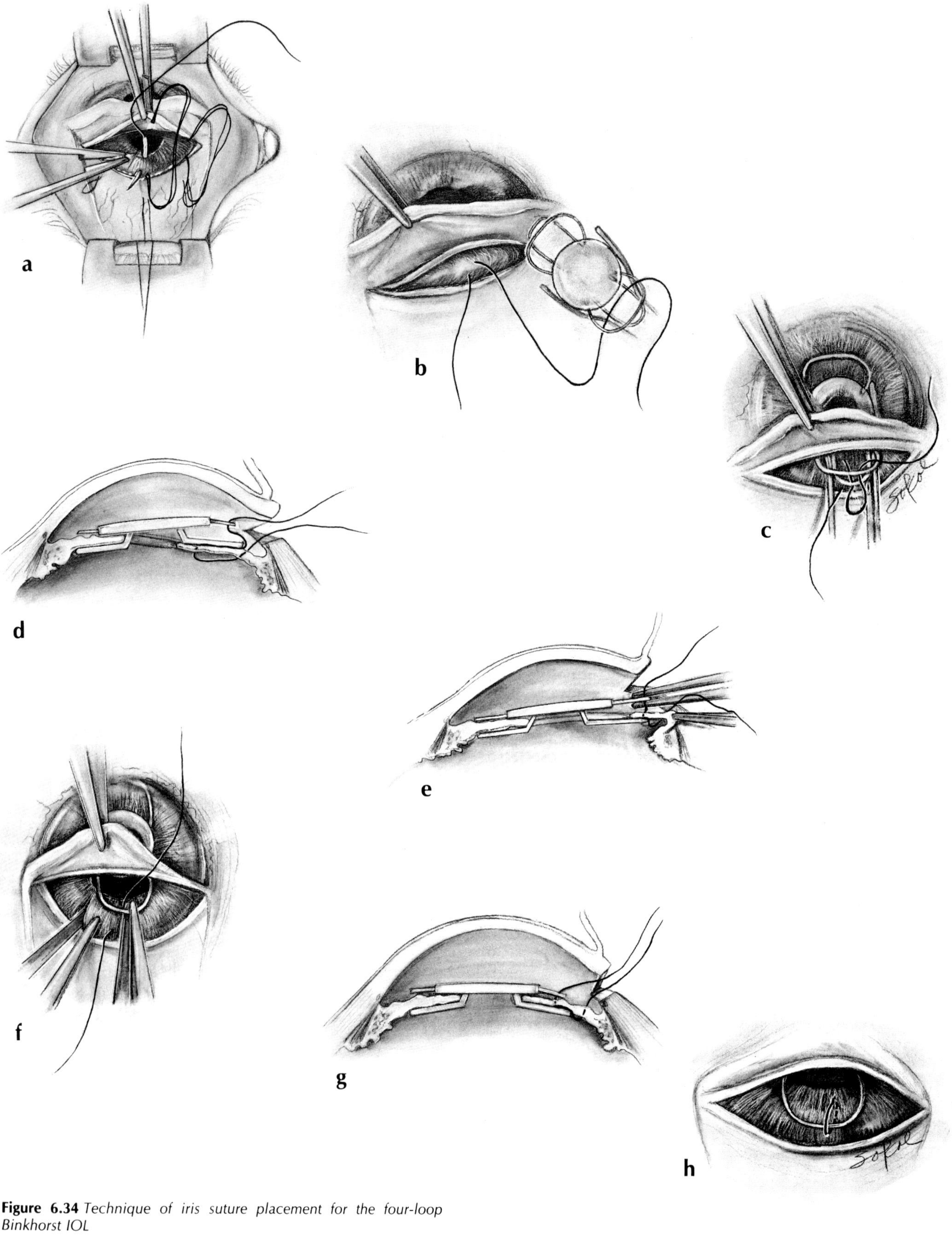

Figure 6.34 *Technique of iris suture placement for the four-loop Binkhorst IOL*

Shearing posterior chamber IOL

We now prefer the Shearing posterior chamber IOL for several reasons. There is evidence that leaving the posterior capsule intact may decrease the incidence of postoperative cystoid macular edema[30, 31]. Also, a recent report found that Shearing-style posterior chamber IOLs gave the highest percentage of patients with 20/25 or better vision, as compared to the Binkhorst two-loop, Binkhorst four-loop and Choyce Mark VIII anterior chamber IOL[41]. Last, posterior chamber IOLs lie farther from the corneal endothelium than anterior chamber or iris plane IOLs and they are prevented from touching the cornea by the iris, even if the anterior chamber becomes shallow or flat.

Preparations for the cataract extraction with placement of a posterior chamber IOL are made as described above

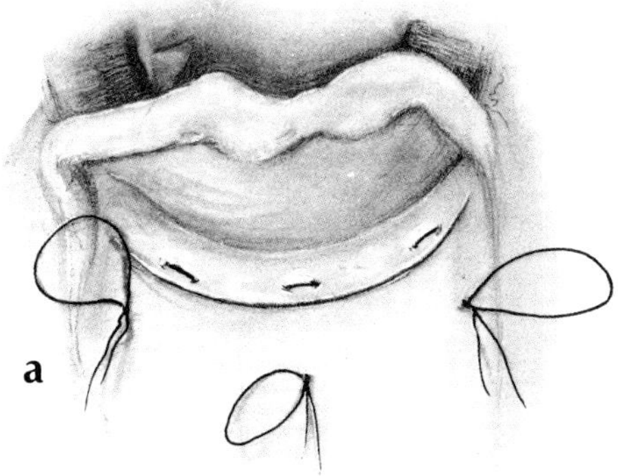

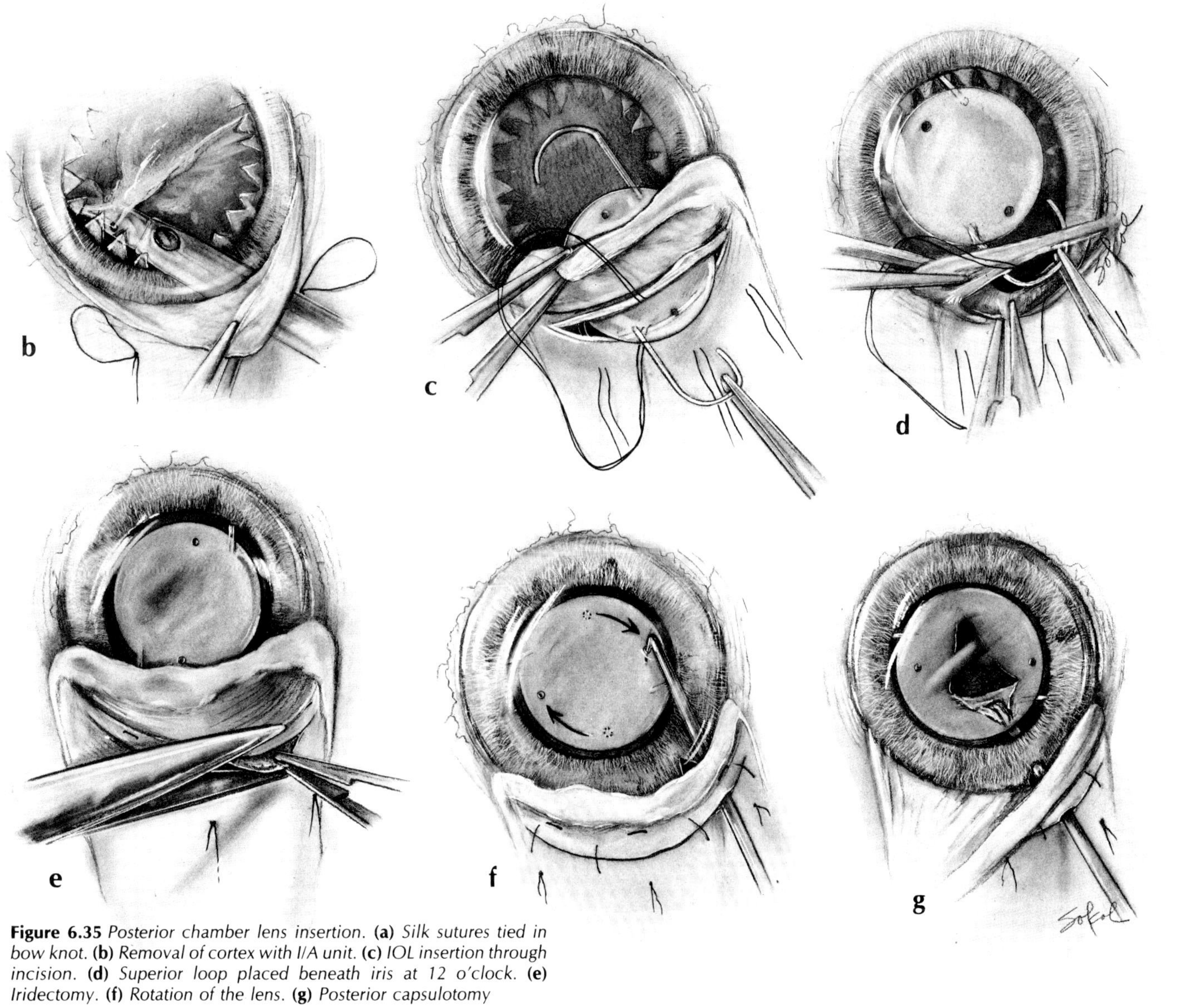

Figure 6.35 *Posterior chamber lens insertion.* **(a)** *Silk sutures tied in bow knot.* **(b)** *Removal of cortex with I/A unit.* **(c)** *IOL insertion through incision.* **(d)** *Superior loop placed beneath iris at 12 o'clock.* **(e)** *Iridectomy.* **(f)** *Rotation of the lens.* **(g)** *Posterior capsulotomy*

under extracapsular surgery (*see* p. 151). After the lens nucleus has been removed, the preplaced 9/0 silk mattress sutures are tied with a single bow knot so that they can be untied easily (*Figure 6.35a*). The cortical remnants are removed with the I/A unit as described on p. 154 (*Figure 6.35b*). The Shearing IOL is then examined under the microscope, irrigated, and wiped with cellulose sponges. The mattress sutures are untied and the 12 o'clock suture is loosened and looped out of the wound in preparation for insertion of the IOL.

The cornea is retracted gently by the surgeon, and the IOL is grasped by the superior loop with tying forceps. The inferior loop is slid into the anterior chamber behind the iris but anterior to the torn anterior lens capsule at 6 o'clock (*Figure 6.35c*). Care is taken not to touch the back of the cornea. The superior loop of the IOL is then placed behind the iris at 12 o'clock while the assistant retracts the cornea. A second pair of forceps is used by the surgeon to retract the iris over the IOL loop if necessary. The IOL should not be forced inferiorly because zonular fibers may be torn from the natural lens capsule in that area. Instead, the superior loop can be bent as illustrated and released behind the iris while the optical portion of the IOL remains near the pupillary axis (*Figure 6.35d*). Previously we used air to form the anterior chamber before IOL insertion, but now we use sodium hyaluronate (Healon). This prevents the posterior displacement of the iris and lens capsule and facilitates insertion of the inferior loop anterior to the capsule rather than within the capsular bag. The sodium hyaluronate is removed from the anterior chamber using the I/A tip after the preplaced sutures are pulled tight and tied. There are various modifications of the Shearing posterior chamber lens. Some have more compressible loops so that tension on the inferior zonular fibers during IOL insertion may be decreased. We prefer the posterior-angulated Shearing lens which lessens the chance of pupillary capture.

The iridectomy (at 11 or 12 o'clock) is performed after IOL insertion, to avoid placing the IOL loop through the iridectomy (*Figure 6.35e*). The 9/0 silk sutures are pulled down and tied, and four additional 10/0 nylon interrupted sutures are placed to close the corneal wound, making it watertight. The anterior chamber is reformed with balanced salt solution, with removal of all air bubbles. Then, a 27 gauge needle with the tip bent away from the bevel is placed on the irrigation unit and inserted into the eye through the wound so that the IOL may be positioned or rotated (*Figure 6.35f*). Usually the lens is rotated 90° so that the loops are horizontal. The needle is then passed through the iridectomy and behind the IOL. A posterior capsulotomy may be performed (*Figure 6.35g*) as described under extracapsular surgery (see p. 154). Care is taken not to cut the anterior vitreous face with the needle. The conjunctival flap is closed after the corneal wound has been checked for leaks.

Anterior chamber IOL

The technique of anterior chamber IOL surgery depends to a degree on the specific type of lens to be inserted. The limbus-to-limbus horizontal diameter is measured from 'white-to-white', with calipers. The lens to be implanted should have a diameter 0.5–1.0 mm greater than the white-to-white measurement.

After the cataract has been removed using either intracapsular or extracapsular techniques, the pupil is constricted with acetylcholine or carbachol. The IOL is then slid through the wound anterior to the iris until the inferior loop or haptic is in the anterior chamber angle. Care must be taken not to touch the posterior cornea. Sodium hyaluronate may be used to maintain the anterior chamber. The superior loop or haptic is then placed behind the scleral lip into the anterior chamber angle at 12 o'clock. If the lens rotates too easily or seems loose, the next larger size lens should be placed. The wound is then closed. Correct placement can be checked by gonioscopy.

Cataract extraction using vitrectomy instrumentation

Vitrectomy instruments capable of excising tissue may be useful for cataract removal in: certain types of congenital cataracts such as rubella cataracts; eyes with persistent hyperplastic primary vitreous (PHPV); eyes with chronic uveitis with extensive posterior synechiae; and eyes with traumatic or membranous cataracts[42]. We prefer the Ocutome™ system. A conjunctival flap is not required. A 1 mm opening is made into the anterior chamber at the 2:30 position through the limbus, using a razor-blade or Ziegler knife. The opening is rounded with a 20 gauge needle. The tip of a long 20 gauge needle on an irrigation line is inserted through the entrance site. Irrigation through the needle maintains the anterior chamber. A second entrance site is then made at the limbus in the 10:30 meridian in the same manner and the vitrectomy instrument tip is inserted. The irrigating needle may be used to open the anterior capsule. Lens material is excised with the vitrectomy instrument, using the cutting and suction mode for harder lens material. Aspiration alone may be sufficient to remove cortical material, and for some soft cataracts little cutting action is required.

In certain cases of complicated cataracts it may be necessary to switch instrument positions and to place the vitrectomy instrument through the 2:30 insertion site.

Persistent bleeding from a cut blood vessel can be stopped using intraocular bipolar diathermy. The leads from the bipolar diathermy are attached to the two metal intraocular instruments, one to the 20 gauge infusion needle and the other to the vitrectomy instrument. The bleeding site is positioned between the two instruments and is cauterized.

A sector iridectomy can be performed with the vitrectomy instrument using cutting and suction. The posterior lens capsule may be excised, along with anterior vitreous if it is opaque, or the posterior lens capsule can be left intact.

After cataract removal the vitrectomy instrument and needle are removed. If an anterior vitrectomy was performed, first air is injected through the irrigation line to keep vitreous out of the entrance wounds (*see Figure 6.43*). The air is injected with a 20 ml syringe connected to the irrigation line through a three-way stopcock. The entrance sites are closed with single interrupted 10/0 nylon sutures and the knots are buried.

Congenital cataract extraction

Irrigation/aspiration

The I/A unit of the Kelman phacoemulsification instrument, or the Ocutome unit using suction and irrigation only, is ideal for removing most types of congenital cataracts[43, 44]. A small limbal conjunctival flap is made followed by a limbal incision. An anterior capsulotomy is performed as described for phacoemulsification (see p. 155). The I/A unit tip is then inserted through the limbal incision, and the cataractous lens material is removed with suction and irrigation. The tip of the I/A instrument is initially held in the center of the pupil, well away from the cornea, with the suction on. Lens material is aspirated into the port without the need to move the instrument tip. The remaining cortical lens material can be removed as described for extracapsular surgery (see p. 155). Care is taken to remove all cortical material from behind the iris. The incision is closed with one or two interrupted sutures. The posterior capsule will usually opacify if left intact, and therefore it is usually cut with a bent 27 gauge needle on an irrigation handle, as described on p. 154.

If an automated I/A unit is not available, an alternative method is simple aspiration of the cataract, after performing an anterior capsulotomy, with an 18 or 20 gauge needle on a syringe. A separate 20 gauge infusion needle may be used to keep the anterior chamber formed (*Figure 6.36*)[45].

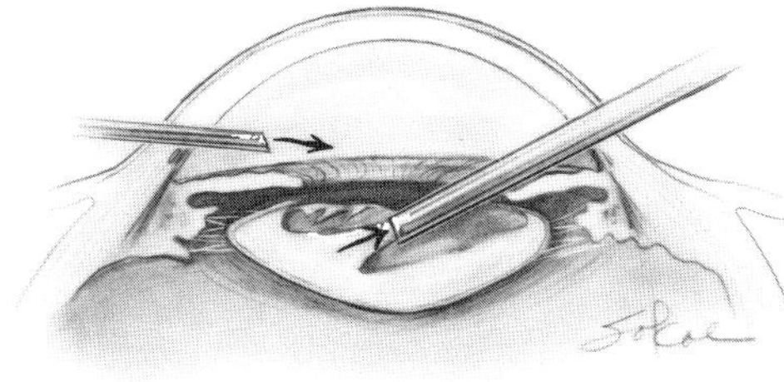

Figure 6.36 *Simple aspiration of congenital cataract with separate infusion*

Vitrectomy instrument excision

A small-diameter vitrectomy instrument may be used to excise certain types of congenital cataracts as described above. The technique for surgery of PHPV differs because the membrane behind the lens is thick[42] and because the peripheral retina is often dragged anteriorly and attached to the membrane. Care must be taken not to tear peripheral retina when making the incision into the PHPV membrane with a Ziegler knife or other sharp instrument. The membrane is then excised in a bite-by-bite fashion (*Figure 6.37a–e*). The cut end of a patent hyaloid artery can be treated with bipolar diathermy (*Figure 6.37f*).

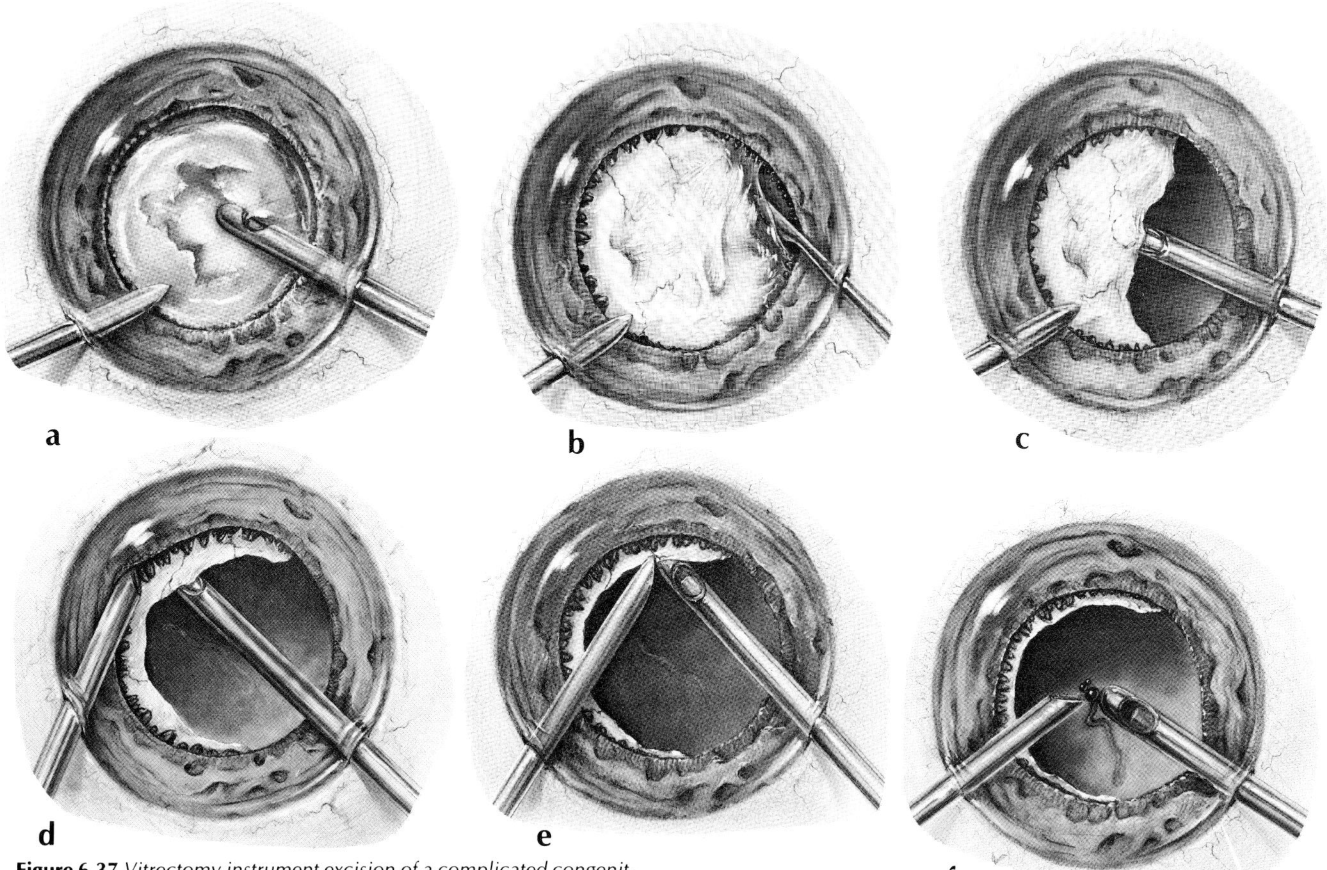

a b c d e f

Figure 6.37 *Vitrectomy instrument excision of a complicated congenital catract (PHPV) using two-instrument technique and a limbal approach*

Postoperative care

Most cataract patients can be discharged on the second day after surgery. We perform a slit-lamp examination 24 and 48 hours after surgery. The intraocular pressure is measured to make certain there is no postoperative glaucoma. The fundus is examined through a dilated pupil. By the time of discharge, an eye patch is usually no longer needed. Patients are told to wear glasses during the day and a shield at night to protect the eye.

Postoperative medication varies, depending on the type of surgery. Patients after an intracapsular extraction are given a topical steroid (prednisolone 1 per cent) and an antibiotic drop (such as chloramphenicol 0.5 per cent or gentamicin) to use four times a day for about 3 weeks. A combination steroid and antibiotic drop can be used instead. Extracapsular extraction patients are given short-acting cycloplegic drops (such as tropicamide 1 per cent and phenylephrine 10 per cent) to use twice a day to dilate and move the pupil to prevent posterior synechiae. After posterior chamber IOL implantation, homatroprine 5 per cent is used for a few days unless there is evidence of pupillary capture of the IOL.

After discharge, patients are seen at 5 days, 3 weeks, 5 weeks and 8 weeks after surgery. If an aphakic contact lens is to be fitted, this is usually done 6–8 weeks postoperatively. After these early postoperative visits, the interval between follow-up visits varies from every 3 months to 12 months, depending on the individual case. Since many of the serious complications of cataract surgery occur during the first 1–2 weeks after surgery, careful follow-up and patient instruction are important to allow early detection of these problems. Patients are told to call immediately if they notice anything unusual – such as increased redness, pain, swelling or a decrease in vision.

Complications of cataract surgery

Complications of cataract surgery can be divided into operative and postoperative complications. Operative complications include retrobulbar hemorrhage, unplanned extracapsular extraction, vitreous loss, expulsive choroidal hemorrhage, and dislocated crystalline lens or lens nucleus. Postoperative complications include wound leak or persistent bleb, endophthalmitis, glaucoma, corneal edema, secondary membranes, flat anterior chamber, hypotony, choroidal detachment, hyphema, vitreous hemorrhage, epithelial ingrowth, retained lens material, and retinal complications such as cystoid macular edema and retinal detachment. Complications of intraocular lens implantation include IOL dislocation, pupillary capture or block, retro-IOL membrane, marked inflammatory response, corneal edema, IOL surface precipitates, synechia as well as complications seen with cataract extraction without IOL implantation.

Operative complications

Retrobulbar hemorrhage

If a retrobulbar hemorrhage occurs as a result of anesthetic injection, cataract surgery should be postponed. In such cases, a lateral canthotomy can be performed if the intraocular pressure (IOP) is very high, especially if the central retinal artery can be seen to be closed. Intravenous mannitol should also be given if the IOP remains elevated. The IOP should be checked periodically during the next 24 hours. Surgery can be rescheduled 10–14 days later, after the hemorrhage has resolved.

Inadvertent extracapsular cataract extraction

The advent of cryoextraction and enzymatic zonulysis has decreased the chance of inadvertently rupturing the lens capsule. However, this complication still occurs, especially in the presence of a swollen hypermature cataract, previous trauma, an inadequate cataract incision, posterior synechiae or a fragile lens capsule. Rupture of the lens capsule usually occurs as the surgeon is delivering the cataract. Often if the capsular tear is anterior and small, the lens can still be removed intracapsularly by placing the cryoprobe on the edges of the capsular tear. If the anterior capsular tear enlarges, then the lens nucleus can be removed as described for extracapsular surgery (see p. 151) or with the cryoprobe. If the posterior capsule is intact, the residual cortex can be removed with gentle irrigation and aspiration with the I/A tip of the phacoemulsification instrument as described on p. 157. If the capsule tears posteriorly it is important not to continue pulling with the cryoprobe because the posterior capsule may be removed without the lens nucleus and the nucleus can slip posteriorly into the vitreous cavity. If a posterior capsular tear occurs it is important to freeze onto the nucleus to remove it, or to express it gently as described on p. 152. It may be necessary to remove the entire capsule if it is opacified, and this can be accomplished by pulling it out with forceps or, if necessary, using a closed-eye system and vitrectomy instrumentation. The nucleus of the cataract must always be removed if possible. However, if the nucleus falls through a tear in the posterior capsule into the vitreous cavity, the eye should be closed and the nucleus removed using pars plana vitrectomy techniques with a closed-eye approach. This can be performed immediately or at a second operation within a few days.

Dislocated lens

Rarely during intracapsular cataract surgery the cataract may partially dislocate after α-chymotrypsin instillation, or it may be slightly dislocated before surgery is begun. If the lens is only slightly subluxed and remains in the pupillary axis, and no vitreous has prolapsed in front of the cataract, a standard intracapsular extraction using cryoextraction may be performed. If, while doing this, the lens falls posteriorly deep into the vitreous cavity, one should not attempt to grab the lens with forceps, extract it with the cryoprobe or perform an open-sky vitrectomy. Instead, as for loss of the nucleus into the vitreous cavity, the cataract wound should be closed and the lens removed using pars plana vitrectomy techniques as described in Chapter 8.

Vitreous loss

Vitreous loss occurs in 2–4 per cent of intracapsular cataract surgery cases[46]. If not treated correctly, it may lead to complications such as an updrawn pupil, the vitreous wick syndrome, vitreocorneal touch with corneal edema, iritis, glaucoma, cystoid macular edema, vitreous hemorrhage, retinal breaks or retinal detachment[47–49]. The risk of vitreous loss can be reduced by lowering the IOP preoperatively with a Honan intraocular pressure-reducer, as described on p. 144, or with digital pressure on the eye[50]. Preoperative intravenous mannitol is also helpful in lowering the IOP, especially in high-risk cases. If vitreous is lost, cellulose sponges and scissors can be used to clean the anterior chamber and wound of formed vitreous, using an open-sky technique. This is performed by touching the vitreous with the tip of the cellulose sponge, lifting slightly, and then cutting the vitreous flush at the level of the pupil (*Figure 6.38*). Each sponge is used only once, then discarded. When the iris and wound have been cleared of vitreous, air can be injected into the anterior chamber to be certain the vitreous has been fully removed from the anterior chamber and surrounding areas. Acetylcholine is then injected into the anterior chamber to constrict the pupil.

Preferably, however, a vitrectomy instrument is used to remove vitreous. This can be done in an open-sky fashion without infusion by inserting the vitrectomy instrument tip into the vitreous just behind the plane of the pupil and excising vitreous in a bite-by-bite fashion using low suction and rapid cutting speed. Probably the safest technique, however, is to close the eye and insert the vitrectomy instrument tip through the sutured wound. A separate infusion with a 20 gauge needle can be used or a Charles infusion sleeve can be placed over an Ocutome vitrectomy instrument as illustrated in *Figure 6.39*. Again, high cutting speed and low suction are used. The anterior segment can be cleared of vitreous in this fashion, and the pupil is then constricted with acetylcholine or carbachol. If a conventional vitrectomy instrument is not available, an open-sky vitrectomy can be done instead using a battery-operated Kaufman Vitrector™ instrument.

Even though these modern techniques for dealing with vitreous loss reduce the risk of complications, vitreous loss remains a serious complication[48]. Any patient who has had vitreous loss at surgery needs to be followed more closely than usual postoperatively, with frequent careful retinal examinations to look for retinal detachment or breaks. The risk of developing cystoid macular edema is also increased in these patients.

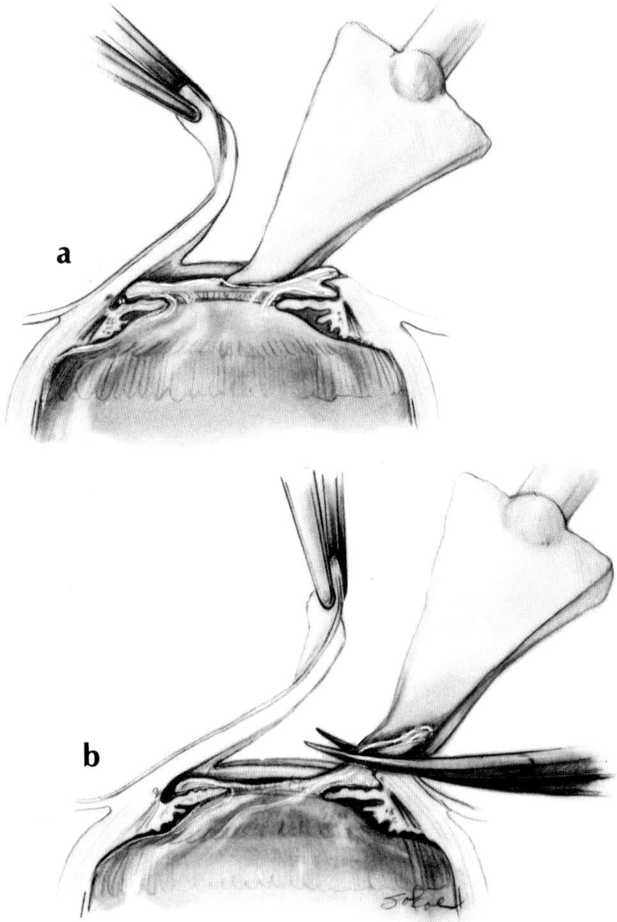

Figure 6.38 *Open-sky anterior vitrectomy following vitreous loss at cataract surgery, using multiple cellulose sponges and scissors*

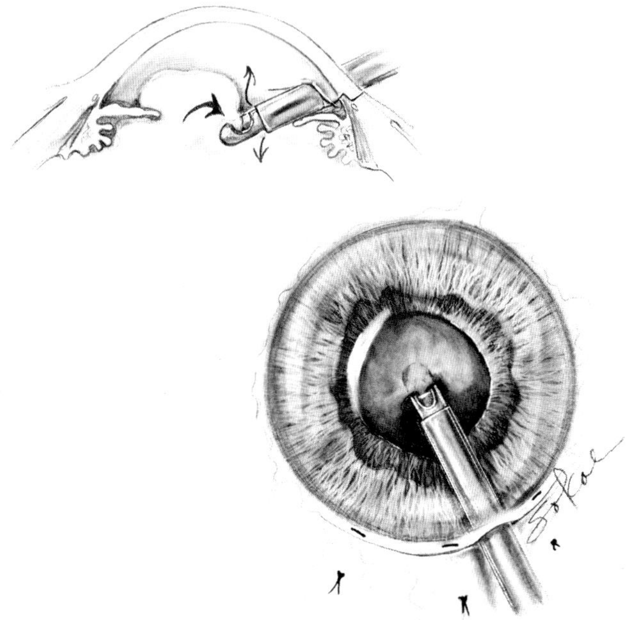

Figure 6.39 *Anterior vitrectomy using Ocutome instrumentation. This can be done on an open eye without infusion, or with a closed eye and the Charles infusion sleeve as shown here*

Expulsive hemorrhage

Expulsive hemorrhage is one of the most serious complications of intraocular surgery, and fortunately it is rare. The incidence during cataract extraction varies from 0.05 to 0.2 per cent[47,51]. It most often occurs during surgery, but rarely it can occur up to one week later. The exact cause of the choroidal bleeding producing expulsive hemorrhage is unknown, but it is more frequent in the presence of diseases such as hypertension, glaucoma and arteriosclerosis[52,53]. If such hemorrhaging occurs during the operation when the corneoscleral wound is open, there is a rapid anterior movement of the iris and vitreous with a gaping of the wound. If the lens has not yet been extracted, it may be forced out through the wound and may be followed by vitreous, retina and blood.

If an expulsive hemorrhage occurs, the preplaced sutures should immediately be pulled down and tied. If there is only a single preplaced suture, or none, it is unlikely that the eye will be saved. Some surgeons have recommended an immediate posterior sclerotomy by cutting down through sclera in any convenient quadrant to release suprachoroidal blood[54]. If this is done, it is important to make a controlled incision in sclera, not a stab incision, because the choroidal hemorrhage may be localized to only one quadrant of the eye. Probably the most important factor in saving the eye, however, is rapid wound closure. This is one reason we prefer several preplaced sutures.

Postoperative complications

Wound leakage and inadvertent bleb

A corneoscleral wound that leaks after cataract surgery may leak externally if it is not covered by conjunctiva, or it may form an inadvertent filtering bleb if covered by conjunctiva (especially if a limbus-based conjunctival flap has been used). The causes of such leaks and blebs include poor wound closure and postoperative complications such as blunt trauma. However, many leaks or blebs occur after uneventful and well-performed surgery without any apparent postoperative complications.

A wound leak that drains externally and persists for several days despite pressure patching should be closed with interrupted sutures. A wound leak should be suspected if the IOP is very low postoperatively. Such eyes should be checked for the presence of a leak using a Seidel test with sterile 2 per cent fluorescein.

When a limbus-based conjunctival flap covers a leaking corneoscleral wound, a bleb may be present and the Seidel test may be negative. Although such blebs can resolve spontaneously and others that do not may cause no problem, complications can arise from those that persist such as endophthalmitis[55], flat anterior chamber, hypotony or macular edema[56]. Various techniques have been described for treating persistent blebs, such as cryotherapy[57], electrocautery[58], chemical cautery[59] and open suturing of the dehiscence[60]. These methods often require several treatments and some carry a risk of serious complication.

We recommend a simple, quick, closed-eye technique for repairing filtering blebs[61] (*Figure 6.40*). First the bleb is collapsed using pressure from a cotton-tipped applicator (*Figure 6.40c*). This allows better visualization of the wound dehiscence through the overlying conjunctiva. Multiple, interrupted 9/0 silk sutures are placed across the wound dehiscence in a radial fashion and are tied externally over the conjunctiva (*Figure 6.40d–e*). The conjunctival flap is never opened. The sutures are removed after 2 weeks. We have had no complications or failures in using this procedure in over 20 cases.

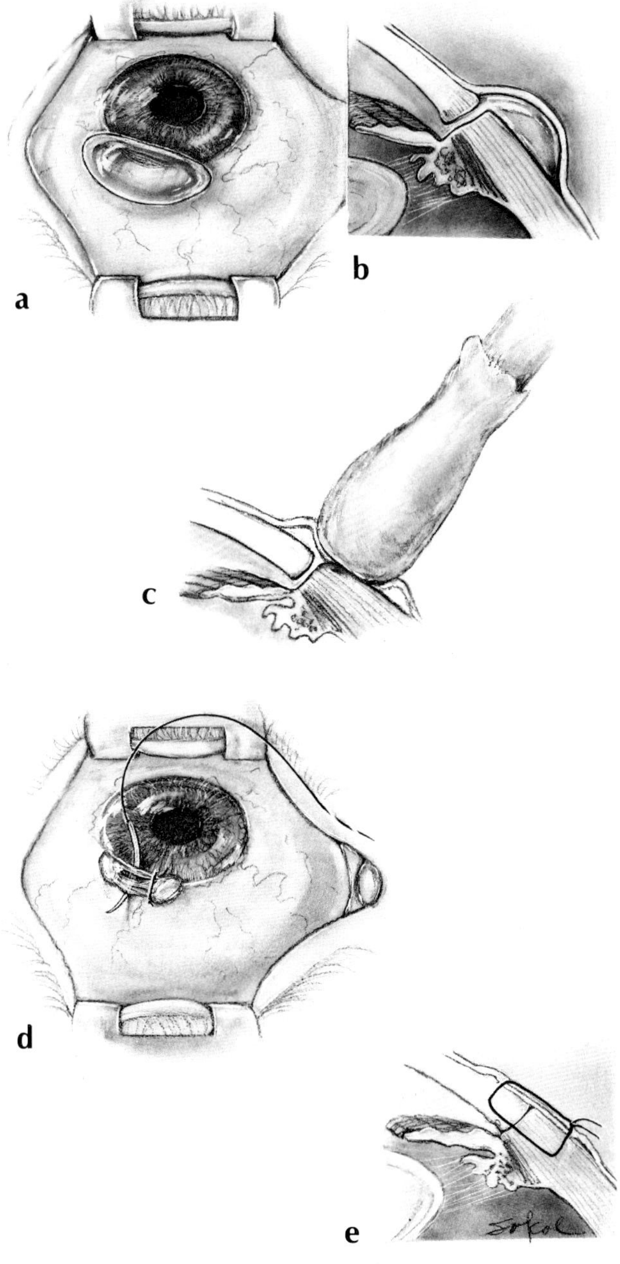

Figure 6.40 *Simple method for closing inadvertent filtering blebs using multiple silk sutures*

Endophthalmitis

Endophthalmitis is probably the most serious postoperative complication of cataract surgery with the possible exceptions of epithelial ingrowth or expulsive hemorrhage (which rarely occurs postoperatively). Endophthalmitis must be recognized and treated promptly if there is to be hope of saving the eye. The reported incidence of endophthalmitis after cataract surgery in the past 20 years varies from 0.02 to about 0.5 per cent[62, 63]. Prevention includes meticulous surgical and sterile technique and use of preoperative and postoperative topical antibiotics.

The management of endophthalmitis will not be discussed in detail here. As soon as endophthalmitis is suspected, cultures should be taken of the aqueous and, more importantly, the vitreous. A paracentesis through the limbus with a 25 gauge needle is performed to obtain fluid from the anterior chamber (*Figure 6.41a*). The same limbal entry site can be used to aspirate vitreous by passing the needle tip into the vitreous cavity. Sometimes a larger bore needle is necessary to obtain a specimen of vitreous. A pars plan approach may be necessary if an IOL is in place (*Figure 6.41b*). Many surgeons prefer the use of vitrectomy instrumentation to obtain an adequate specimen and to remove as much infected vitreous as possible for stains and cultures. Broad spectrum intravitreal, intravenous and subconjunctival antibiotics are administered immediately. When culture and sensitivity reports are available, the antibiotic regimen can be modified. In cases in which paracentesis was used to obtain culture specimens and the vitreous later rapidly opacifies, a diagnostic and therapeutic vitrectomy should be performed to attempt to arrest the fulminant infection. This is described in Chapter 8.

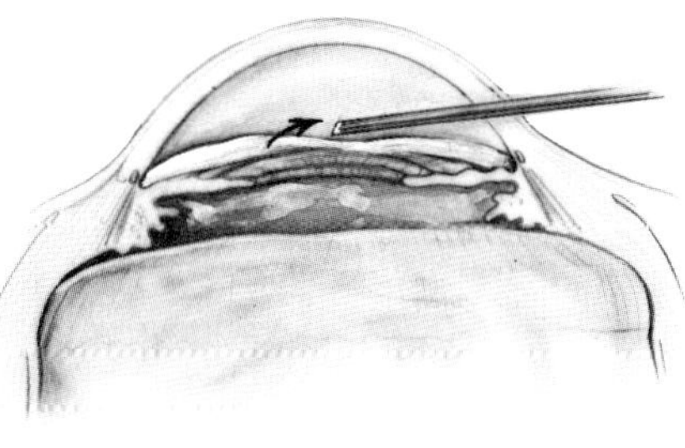

a

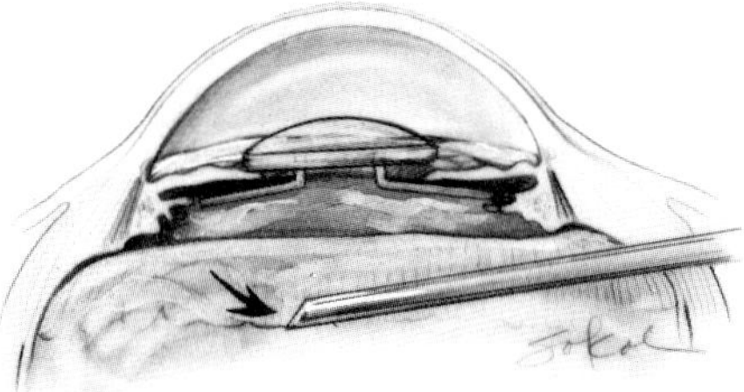

b

Figure 6.41 **(a)** *Anterior chamber paracentesis in endophthalmitis.* **(b)** *Vitreous aspiration done through the pars plana approach in an eye with an IOL*

Glaucoma

There are various causes of elevated intraocular pressure after cataract extraction. These include primary open-angle glaucoma, pupillary-block glaucoma, steroid-induced glaucoma, glaucoma associated with use of intraoperative α-chymotrypsin, inflammatory glaucoma, peripheral iris adhesions, and glaucoma from epithelial ingrowth or fibrous proliferation.

Those patients who have uncontrolled glaucoma prior to cataract surgery should have a combined cataract extraction and filtering procedure as described in Chapter 7. In an eye with glaucoma in which the IOP becomes uncontrolled with medical therapy only after cataract surgery, cyclocryotherapy is probably the best form of surgical treatment, although laser trabeculoplasty and trabeculectomy can be considered instead.

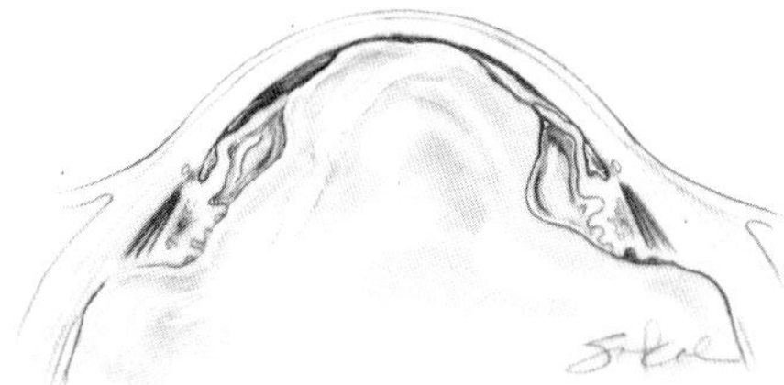

Figure 6.42 *Severe pupillary-block glaucoma with flat anterior chamber. If laser iridectomy fails to cure the problem, anterior vitrectomy may be necessary*

If a pupillary-block mechanism is present as evidenced by a high IOP with a flat or shallow anterior chamber (*Figure 6.42*), dilation of the pupil should be attempted as a treatment. If dilation does not break the pupillary block, a laser iridotomy should be performed[64]. If this is also not successful, pars plana removal of anterior vitreous will relieve the pupillary block.

There are cases of 'ciliary-block' glaucoma in which the aqueous flow is misdirected and becomes trapped behind the vitreous. The vitreous and iris are pushed forward closing the anterior angle. Sometimes pupillary dilation or a laser iridotomy can relieve this type of glaucoma, but often a closed-eye anterior vitrectomy or a total vitrectomy using a limbal or pars plana approach may be necessary (*Figure 6.43*). When the vitreous has been removed and the aqueous has free passage from the posterior to anterior chamber, the anterior chamber will deepen and the glaucoma will be cured.

Steroid-induced glaucoma can be treated with oral acetazolamide (Diamox) or topical antiglaucoma drops, and by stopping the steroid drops or switching to a weaker steroid such as fluorometholone (FML) drops. Glaucoma from enzyme zonulysis is caused by blockage of the trabecular meshwork with fragments of zonular fibers[26–28]. It is transient and can be treated with oral acetazolamide. Some surgeons believe that any patient in whom α-chymotrypsin was used during cataract surgery should be given acetazolamide 250 mg every 6 hours for 2 or 3 days postoperatively as a prophylactic measure against elevated IOP.

Epithelial ingrowth and fibrous proliferation can also cause glaucoma by producing peripheral anterior synechiae, blockage of the anterior chamber angle, or pupillary block[65]. The chance of developing epithelial ingrowth can be minimized by good wound closure at the time of surgery. Management of this complication will be discussed in Chapter 8.

Corneal edema

The causes of corneal edema after cataract surgery include: excessive trauma to the corneal endothelium at surgery, peripheral anterior synechiae, Fuchs' corneal dystrophy, vitreous touch, detachment of Descemet's membrane, epithelial ingrowth or fibrous proliferation, glaucoma and severe iritis. When the cause of postoperative corneal edema is determined, appropriate therapy may result in corneal clearing. For example, if extensive vitreous touch to the endothelium is present after cataract

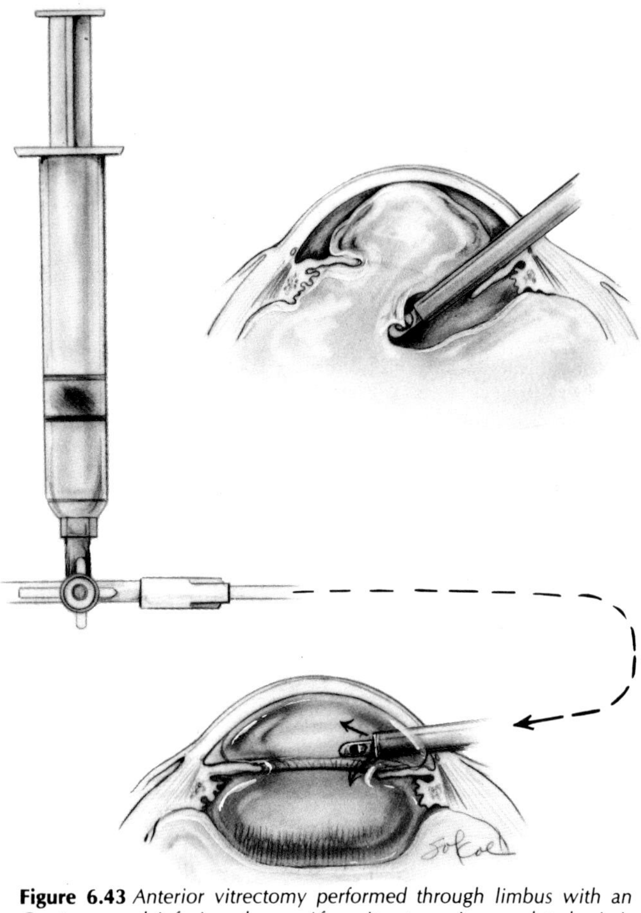

Figure 6.43 *Anterior vitrectomy performed through limbus with an Ocutome and infusion sleeve. After vitrectomy is completed, air is injected through the irrigation line to keep vitreous from the entrance site*

extraction and there is progressive corneal swelling as measured by serial pachometry, we recommend a pars plana, anterior vitrectomy to remove vitreous from the anterior chamber (*Figure 6.43*). Permanent corneal damage from retrocorneal fibrous-membrane formation may result from extensive vitreous touch[66]. If corneal edema persists for more than 6 months and other methods of treatment have failed, a penetrating keratoplasty can be considered for visual rehabilitation (*see* Chapter 5).

Secondary membranes, fibrous proliferation and epithelial ingrowth

The treatment of secondary membranes and opacified posterior capsule are described later in this chapter. Treatment of the vitreous-wick syndrome, fibrous ingrowth, epithelial cyst and epithelial ingrowth are described in Chapter 8.

Flat chamber, hypotony and choroidal detachment

These three complications are often related and may be found simultaneously in an eye. A flat anterior chamber may be from a wound leak, pupillary-block glaucoma, a choroidal detachment or hyposecretion. The IOP must be checked to determine whether hyposecretion (with hypotony) or glaucoma is present, and a Seidel test is performed to look for a wound leak (*see* p. 166). If there is a low pressure with no leak and no sign of choroidal detachment, hyposecretion is probably the cause. If a small wound leak is the cause, the pupil can be dilated and a semipressure patch applied for 1 day. Many eyes with a flat or shallow anterior chamber will re-form without further treatment. If the chamber remains flat for 3–5 days from a wound leak, surgery is done to prevent development of peripheral anterior synechiae and to speed postoperative recovery. The anterior chamber should be re-formed and the leak repaired as follows: fluorescein 2 per cent solution is placed on the eye to locate the site of wound leakage (part or all of the conjunctival flap may need to be opened); the leak is sutured; and the anterior chamber is re-formed with air. This technique is successful in most cases.

If extensive choroidal detachments are present for 7–10 days with a flat anterior chamber, these choroidal detachments should be drained. Chandler and Maumenee[67] have suggested that a serous detachment of the ciliary body associated with choroidal detachment is the cause of hypotension in such eyes. Drainage of the subchoroidal fluid, with simultaneous re-formation of the anterior chamber, is often successful. A posterior sclerotomy is performed to drain subchoroidal fluid, and the anterior chamber is simultaneously re-formed through a limbal puncture[68].

If pupillary block is present as evidenced by high IOP and a flat anterior chamber it must be treated immediately as described on p. 167 and in Chapter 7.

Hyphema and vitreous hemorrhage

Postoperative hyphema and vitreous hemorrhage, if they are mild, usually clear spontaneously without additional surgery. Before performing a pars plana vitrectomy for persistent vitreous hemorrhage, a 6-month period should be allowed for the hemorrhage to clear spontaneously[69–71]. IOP must be monitored closely, and treated when necessary, because of the risk of hemolytic glaucoma[72] If the fundus cannot be seen clearly, B-scan ultrasonography should be periodically performed to make certain a retinal detachment has not occurred. When a vitreous hemorrhage clears, a careful search should be made for retinal tears.

A hyphema after cataract extraction may arise from cut or torn iris vessels, from the ciliary body or from the cataract incision. Most hyphemas absorb spontaneously within several days with the conservative management of bed rest and topical steroids.

Retained lens material

Retained lens material may be present after inadvertent extracapsular surgery as well as after planned extracapsular surgery. A small amount of retained lens cortex in the anterior chamber can be left to resorb spontaneously unless inflammation or glaucoma develops. If the whole nucleus or fragments of it are left in the anterior chamber, they should be removed. This can be done through a small limbal incision using a vitrectomy instrument (*Figure 6.44*), or the cataract incision can be reopened and the lens nuclear material carefully removed with forceps (*Figure 6.45*). If it is necessary to remove residual lens cortex, a closed-eye vitrectomy is the best method[42,73]. A limbal approach can be used, with an irrigating sleeve over the vitrectomy instrument, or a separate limbal infusion site may be used. Frequently soft, swollen cortical material can be removed using irrigation and aspiration alone, but cutting may be necessary (*Figure 6.44*).

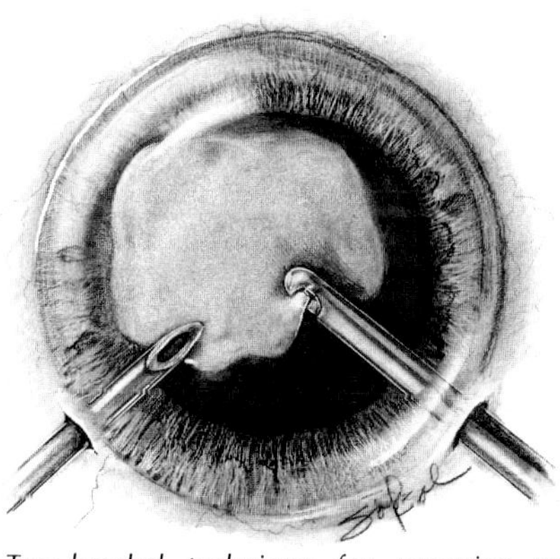

Figure 6.44 *Two-handed technique for removing retained lens material from the anterior chamber with a vitrectomy instrument and an infusion needle*

One of the most difficult and important aspects of extracapsular cataract surgery is the removal of all the lens cortex. If cortex is left behind, posterior synechiae may develop between the iris and lens capsule. If an IOL has been placed, synechiae between the iris and the IOL may occur.

Probably the most serious complication of retained lens material, however, is phacoanaphylactic endophthalmitis. This rare complication can occur if a large amount of lens material is left in the eye. Phacoanaphylactic endophthalmitis is a granulomatous inflammation probably due to autosensitization to lens proteins, with a resultant antigen-antibody reaction[74]. Treatment is the prompt removal of any lens remnants as described above.

Retinal complications

The three major retinal complications after cataract surgery are acute retinal breaks, retinal detachment and cystoid macular edema (CME). After cataract removal the incidence of retinal detachment is 1–3 per cent[75,76]. The incidence of retinal breaks and detachment is increased by intraoperative complications, especially by vitreous loss[77,78]. Aphakic retinal detachment usually occurs within 2 years of surgery, and there appears to be no difference between the incidence of retinal detachment after extracapsular or intracapsular surgery[76]. Because of the risk of retinal detachment, careful indirect ophthalmoscopy after surgery is important and should be performed at each postoperative visit. The diagnosis and management of retinal breaks and detachments is discussed in Chapter 9.

After cataract surgery, the reported incidence of CME ranges from 5 to 50 per cent, depending on the time after surgery and the particular study[31,79,80]. In mild cases of CME, visual acuity is not reduced or improves quickly, but in 5–10 per cent of cases there is a persistent reduction in acuity that persists for several months[31]. There is no evidence proving that any type of medical treatment of

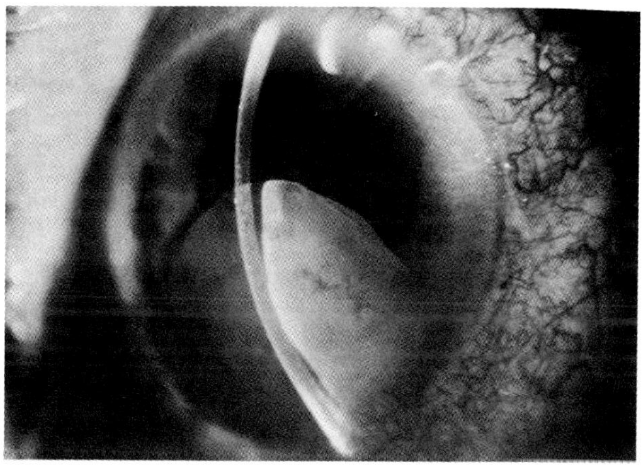

a

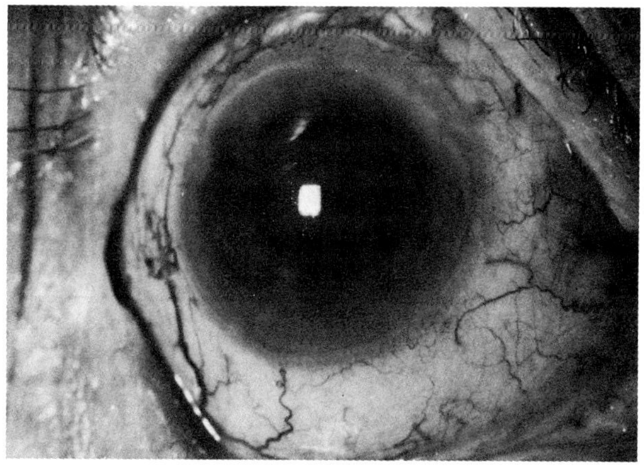

b

Figure 6.45 (a) *Entire lens nucleus in anterior chamber after cataract surgery.* **(b)** *After open-sky removal of lens nucleus*

CME is beneficial, including several studies that have shown systemic indomethacin is ineffective in prevention or treatment[81, 82]. If inflammation is present, we believe topical corticosteroids and atropine are helpful. Pars plana vitrectomy for chronic CME may be beneficial in some cases where there is vitreous incarceration in the cataract wound[83, 84]. Prospective, controlled studies are needed to determine the effectiveness of extracapsular cataract surgery in reducing the incidence of CME.

Postoperative astigmatism

The degree of corneal astigmatism produced by cataract surgery is affected by the surgical technique and the method of suturing. Incisions that are in the anterior limbus or cornea tend to result in more postoperative astigmatism than do those that are more posterior in the limbus. We shall not discuss how the various suturing methods affect astigmatism. Intraoperative monitoring of astigmatism, using special keratometry methods, has been suggested as one way of minimizing postoperative astigmatism[85]. The best means of astigmatism management is prevention. With our use of preplaced sutures and the placement of nylon sutures after cataract removal, postoperative astigmatism is minimal. We occasionally cut one cataract suture 6–8 weeks after surgery to alter the final corneal curvature. Other techniques of treating excessive astigmatism, such as use of corneal wedge-resection, are discussed in Chapter 5.

A simple and useful technique in managing postoperative astigmatism is the proper use of suture removal. If significant astigmatism is present, a suture can be cut in the steepest meridian to lessen the corneal curvature, as mentioned. For example, with plus-cylinder axis at 90°, one or two sutures can be removed (about 6–8 weeks postoperatively) near the 12 o'clock position of the wound. This often eliminates much of the astigmatism. If excessive cylinder cannot be lessened in this way, a hard contact lens or a toric, soft contact lens may be helpful.

Complications of intraocular lenses

IOL dislocation

Dislocation of an IOL occurring after surgery can cause severe corneal or intraocular damage. Because we place an iris suture through one loop of our four-loop iris-fixed IOLs, complete dislocation into the vitreous cavity is not possible. If the lens is not sutured to the iris and it dislocates into the vitreous cavity, the IOL can be retrieved and repositioned properly by using pars plana vitrectomy techniques[86] as described in Chapter 8. Occasionally, because of excessive pupillary dilatation, the lower loops of a four-loop Binkhorst lens may become free of the iris, and both loops can move in front or behind the iris in the 6 o'clock position. When both inferior loops are behind the iris, the IOL can be repositioned properly in the office. This is done by bending the patient's head forward so that the anterior-inferior loop of the IOL passes in front of the iris. The patient is then placed at the slit lamp and pilocarpine drops are administered to constrict the pupil so that the iris lies between the anterior and posterior IOL loops. If repeated dislocations occur, pilocarpine drops can be continued four times a day to keep the pupil miotic.

If pilocarpine fails to keep the IOL in position, the inferior loops of the IOL can be sutured in place using the technique of McCannel[87] or by a technique described by Stark, Michels and Bruner[86] which avoids passing a needle through clear, central cornea (*Figure 6.46*). This technique may also be used to fixate an IOL that has no suture fixation. A CIF needle (Ethicon) with a cutting tip on 10/0 polypropylene (Prolene) is passed through a previously placed limbal incision, then through the iris, and finally between the loops of the IOL to exit through the limbus in the adjacent quadrant (*Figure 6.46a*). An irrigating hooked needle is introduced through the initial limbal incision to retrieve the distal end of the polypropylene (Prolene) suture (*Figure 6.46b*). The suture is tied externally over the IOL loop and is cut flush (*Figure 6.46c, d*).

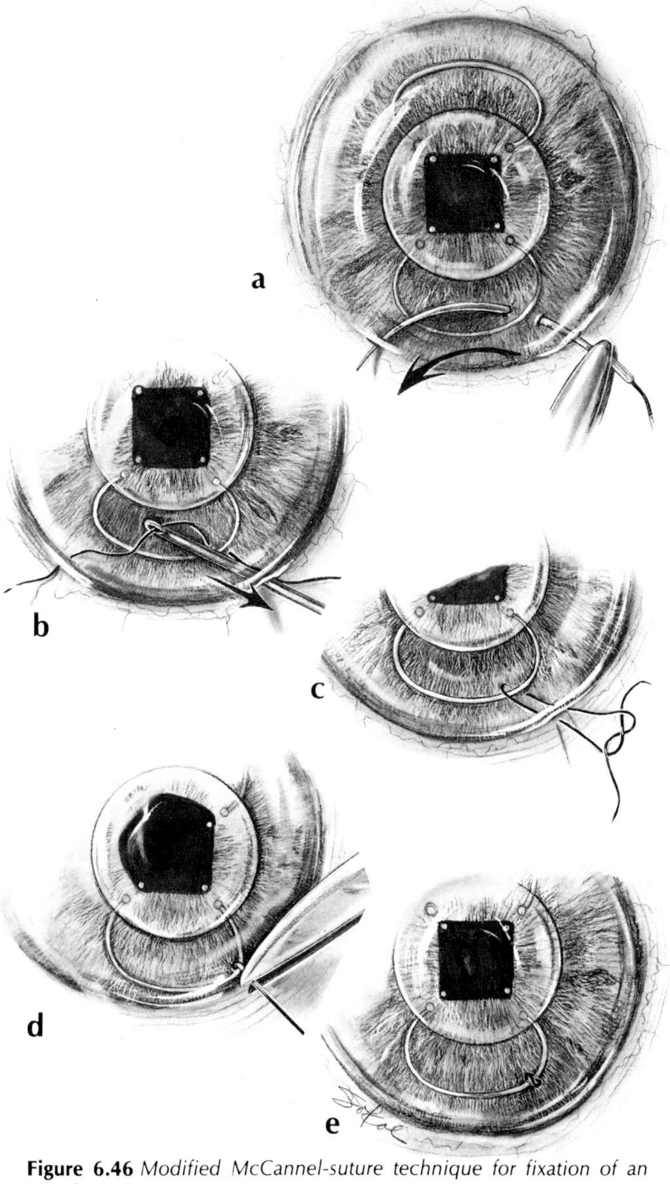

Figure 6.46 *Modified McCannel-suture technique for fixation of an iris-plane IOL*

Dislocation of a posterior chamber IOL into the vitreous cavity is very rare and we have not seen this complication. However, decentration or subluxation of a posterior chamber IOL, when symptomatic or progressive, may require surgery as illustrated (*Figure 6.47*). A modified McCannel-suture technique is used to suture the superior loop of the IOL to the iris after it has been repositioned[88].

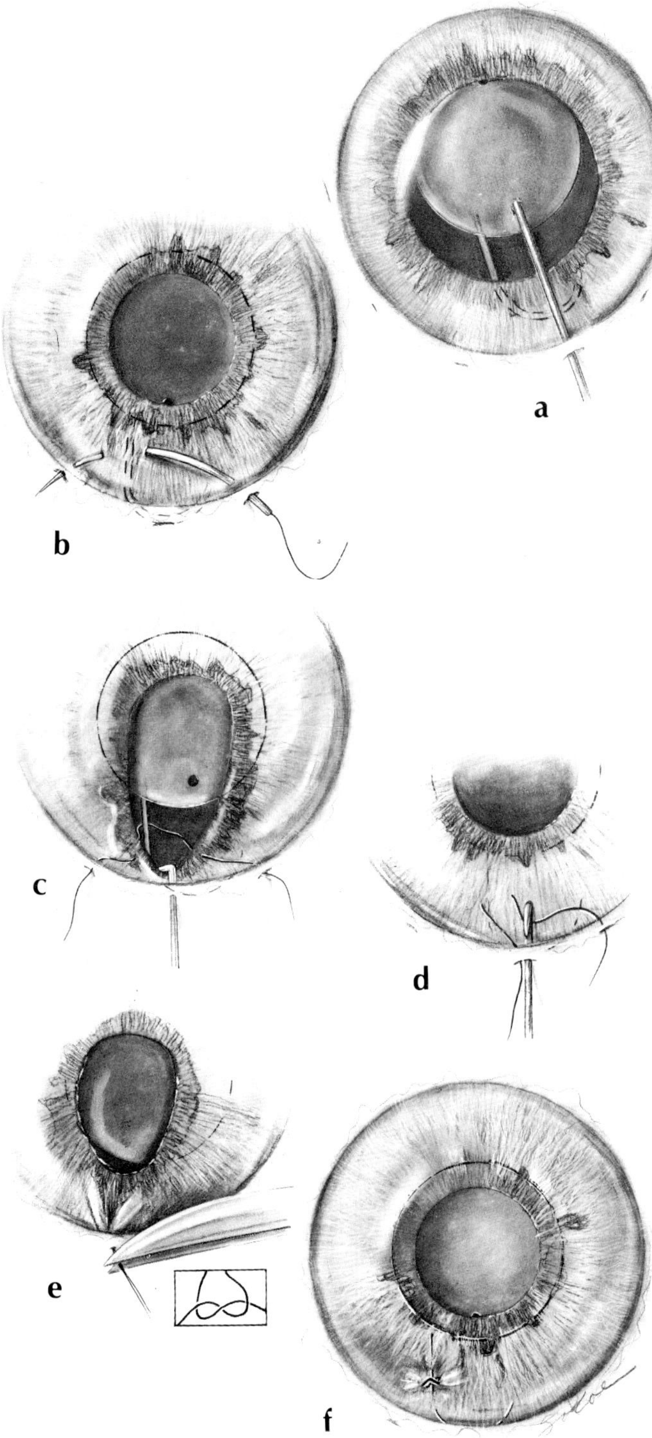

Figure 6.47 *Modified McCannel-suture technique for fixation of posterior chamber IOL*

Pupillary capture of an IOL and pupillary block

Pupillary capture of a posterior chamber IOL is seen occasionally; it occurs when the iris constricts behind the optical portion of the lens but anterior to the lens loops (*Figure 6.48*). This is usually not a serious complication. It is almost always remedied by dilating the pupil with 0.5 per cent tropicamide, having the patient lie supine and then constricting the pupil anterior to the IOL with pilocarpine. On rare occasions it may be necessary to reposition an IOL surgically if it does not move posteriorly using this technique. This is done by dilating the pupil and gently pushing the IOL posteriorly with an irrigation cannula inserted through a small Ziegler knife puncture while injecting acetylcholine (Miochol).

Pupillary block can occur with any type of IOL, and it is manifested by a flat or shallow anterior chamber and an elevated IOP (*Figure 6.49*). If pupillary dilation does not relieve the block, a laser iridotomy[64] or surgical iridectomy should be performed.

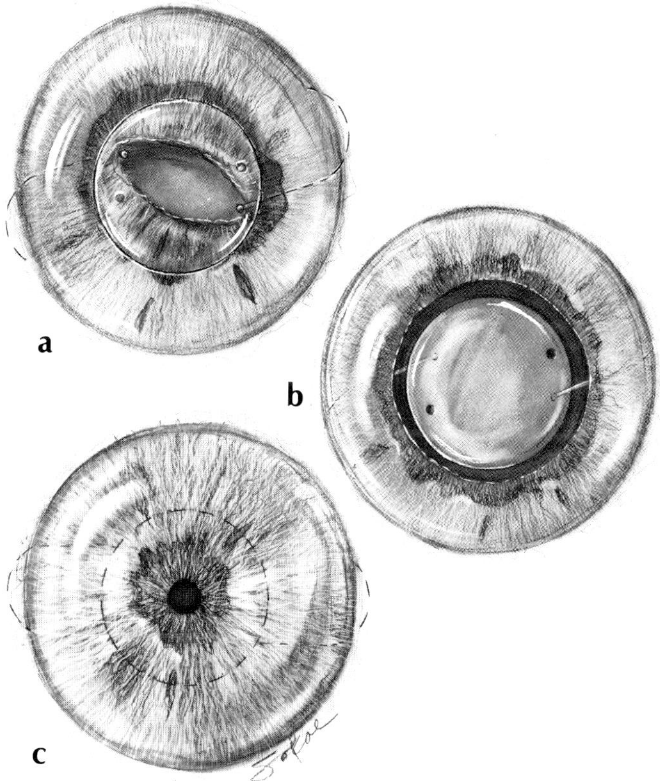

Figure 6.48 (a) *Pupillary capture of Shearing-style posterior chamber IOL.* **(b, c)** *The pupil can often be dilated and reconstricted anterior to the IOL*

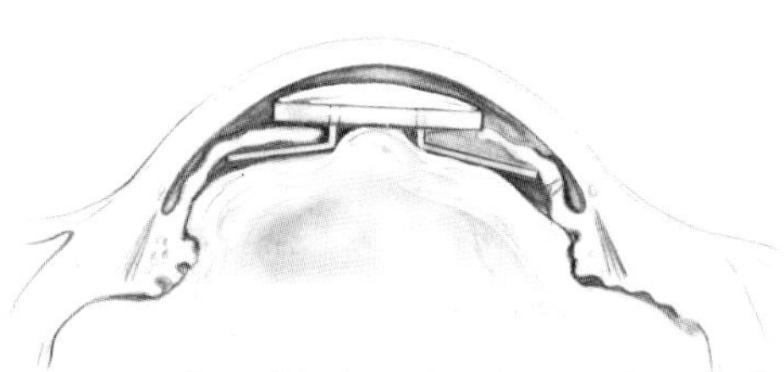

Figure 6.49 *Pupillary block with IOL causing shallow anterior chamber and possible corneal touch*

Retro-IOL membrane and opacified posterior lens capsule

A membrane can develop behind an IOL after intracapsular cataract surgery[89], and the posterior lens capsule may opacify in up to 50 per cent of cases after extracapsular cataract extraction with or without IOL placement[90]. Our surgical technique for management of this problem is as follows[91]. The pupil is dilated with 1 per cent tropicamide, and the tip of a Haab knife with a tapered shaft is inserted through the limbus and then between the IOL and the opacified lens capsule or membrane, if an IOL is present. The capsule or membrane is engaged below the pupillary axis, elevated slightly and then cut through the central pupillary space (*Figures 6.50, 6.51*). Occasionally, it may be necessary to use a pars plana approach with a Haab knife to discise a tough retro-IOL membrane. If these techniques fail to establish an adequate pupillary opening, a pars plana approach with a vitrectomy instrument may be required to excise the membrane, as described in Chapter 8*.

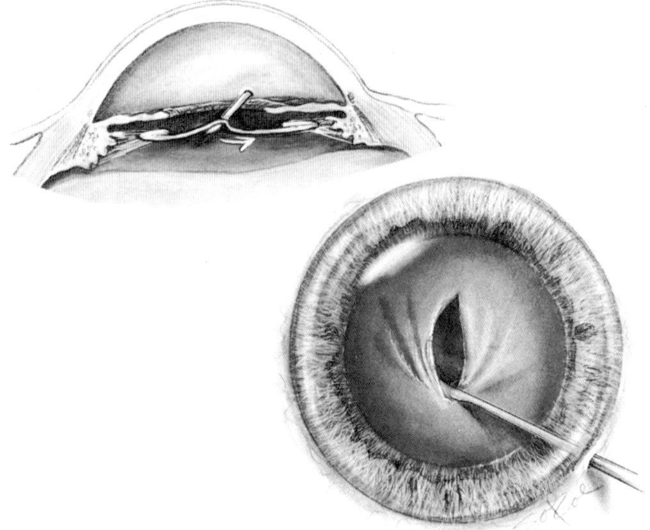

Figure 6.50 *Discission of opacified posterior capsule following extracapsular cataract extraction*

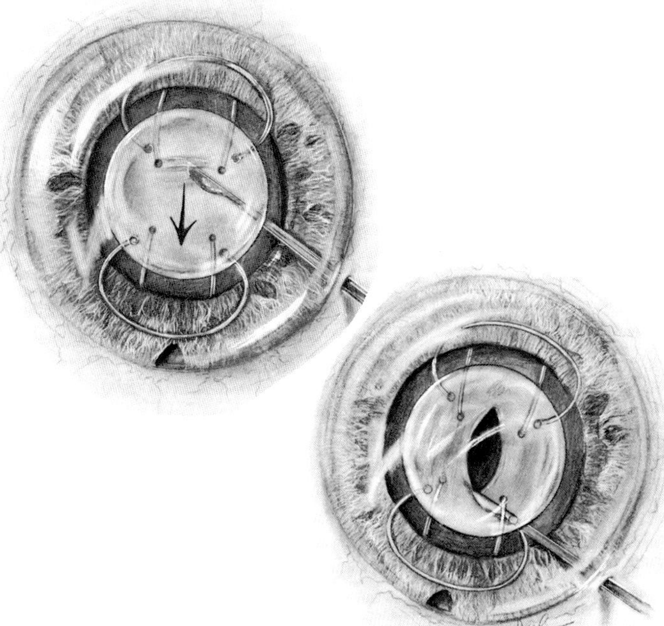

Figure 6.51 *Discission of opacified posterior capsule or retro-IOL membrane after IOL implantation*

Postoperative inflammation

Significant intraocular inflammation after IOL implantation may be from residual IOL polishing compounds that have not been removed before lens implantation[92] or residual ethylene oxide in the IOL[93]. This may be manifest as a sterile hypopyon and severe iritis. A tiny hypopyon 1 day after surgery needs to be followed very closely (*Figure 6.52*). If it has not cleared or improved within 12 hours with topical steroid treatment, a paracentesis should be performed to obtain aqueous and vitreous for cultures so that infective endophthalmitis can be ruled out. If the suspicion of endophthalmitis is high, then a vitrectomy can be done to obtain a vitreous specimen for culture.

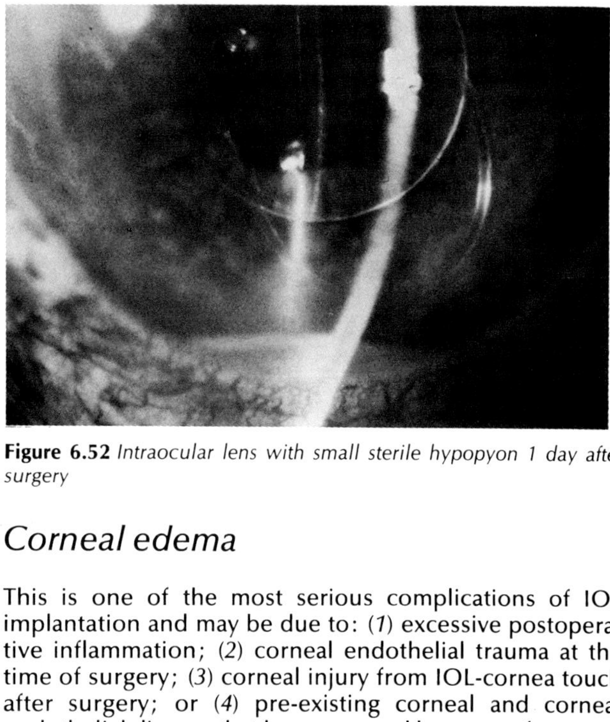

Figure 6.52 *Intraocular lens with small sterile hypopyon 1 day after surgery*

Corneal edema

This is one of the most serious complications of IOL implantation and may be due to: (*1*) excessive postoperative inflammation; (*2*) corneal endothelial trauma at the time of surgery; (*3*) corneal injury from IOL-cornea touch after surgery; or (*4*) pre-existing corneal and corneal endothelial disease that has worsened because of surgery. There is evidence that IOL implantation increases endothelial cell loss[95–97], and there is some evidence that this loss is less with extracapsular than with intracapsular surgery[98, 99].

Problems contributing to localized corneal edema, such as corneal touch by the IOL, should be managed by repositioning or removal of the IOL. If the corneal edema is persistent and has not resolved after 6 months, penetrating keratoplasty can be considered (*see* Chapter 5).

* Subsequent to writing this chapter, the YAG laser has become available, and it can be used in many cases to create an opening in an opacified posterior lens capsule or pupillary membrane

IOL precipitates and synechiae formation

IOL precipitates can consist of inflammatory cells, pigment deposits and/or retained lens material (*Figure 6.53*). Postoperative inflammation should be controlled with topical steroids to avoid inflammatory precipitates.

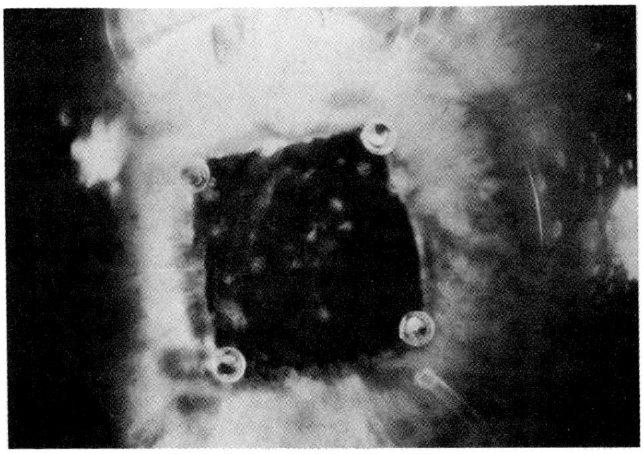

Figure 6.53 *Intraocular lens with pigmented precipitates on the IOL due to low-grade chronic inflammation*

Both peripheral anterior synechiae (PAS)[38] and synechiae between the iris and IOL may develop after IOL implantation. Careful operative techniques and postoperative care may aid in preventing these complications. Topical steroids decrease the inflammation that contributes to PAS, and early postoperative pupillary dilation may prevent or break iris-IOL synechiae.

Retinal complications

The retinal complications after IOL implantation are essentially the same as those described for cataract surgery without IOL implantation (see p. 169). The main difference, when an IOL is present with a retinal detachment, is that the peripheral retina is more difficult to visualize, and therefore the retinal holes are often more difficult to find. This makes surgery more difficult[100]. Although there is some evidence that IOL placement after ECCE may decrease the incidence of postoperative retinal detachment as compared to ICCE with IOL[101], there have been no controlled studies to document this.

The incidence of aphakic CME after ICCE seems to be about the same with or without an IOL implant. However, there is evidence that the prevalence of CME proved by fluorescein angiography at 16–24 weeks after ECCE with implantation of an IOL leaving an intact posterior lens capsule is significantly lower[31]. If a patient develops severe CME after IOL implantation which does not respond to steroid therapy within 6–12 months, surgical removal of the IOL should be considered if there is evidence of chronic inflammation.

Results

There are over 400 000 cataract operations performed each year in the United States. The operation has a high success rate, with more than 97 per cent of patients obtaining visual acuity equal to or better than 20/40[46, 102]. Although complications of cataract surgery can occur, careful patient selection, meticulous surgical technique and proper postoperative care will usually produce results that are successful and gratifying to both patient and surgeon.

Acknowledgements

We thank David Andrews, Scarlett Fisher, Donna Optican and Tom Mitchell for assistance during preparation of this manuscript.

References

1. Duke-Elder, W. S., ed. Cataract: surgical treatment: history. In: System of ophthalmology, Vol. XI, Diseases of the lens and vitreous; glaucoma and hypotony. London: Kimpton, 1969; St Louis: C. V. Mosby, 1969: 248–264
2. Stark, W. J., Taylor, H. R., Michels, R. G., Maumenee, A. E. Management of congenital cataracts. Ophthalmology; 1979; 86: 1571–1578
3. Beller, R., Hoyt, C. S., Marg, E., Odom, J. V. Good visual function after neonatal surgery for congenital monocular cataracts. American Journal of Ophthalmology. 1981; 91: 559–565
4. Purnell, E. W. Ultrasonic interpretation of orbital disease. In: Gitter, K. A., Keeney, A. H., Farin, L. K., Neger, D., eds. Ophthalmic ultrasound. St Louis: C. V. Mosby, 1969: 249–255
5. Chilaris, G. A. Recovery time after macular illumination as a diagnostic and prognostic test. American Journal of Ophthalmology 1962; 53: 311–314
6. Severin, S. L., Tour, R. L., Kershaw, R. H. Macular function and the photostress test. Archives of Ophthalmology 1967; 77: 2–7
7. Green, D. G., Cohen, M. M. Laser interferometry in the evaluation of potential macular function in the presence of opacities in the ocular media. Transactions of the American Academy of Ophthalmology and Otolaryngology 1971; 75: 629–637
8. Green, D. G. Testing the vision of cataract patients by means of laser-generated interference fringes. Science 1970; 168: 1240–1242
9. Sinclair, S. H., Loebl, M., Riva, C. E. Blue field entoptic phenomenon in cataract patients. Archives of Ophthalmology 1979; 97: 1092–1095
10. Loebl, M., Riva, C. E. Macular circulation and the flying corpuscles phenomenon. Ophthalmology 1978; 85: 911–917
11. Minkowski, J. S., Guyton, D. L. Potential acuity meter using a minute aerial pinhole aperture. Ophthalmology 1981; 88 (Suppl.): 95
12. Wolff, E. The eyeball. In: Warwick, R., ed. Wolff's anatomy of the eye and orbit, 7th ed. London: H. K. Lewis, 1976; Philadelphia: W. B. Saunders, 1977: 30–180
13. Olson, R. J., Morgan, K. S., Kolodner, H. The Shearing intraocular lens: Where does it go and what does it do in the eye? Ophthalmology 1980; 87: 668–672
14. Crawford, J. B. A histopathologic study of the position of the Shearing intraocular lens in the posterior chamber. American Journal of Ophthalmology 1981; 91: 458–461

15. Vail, D. Intracapsular extraction: mechanics, technic, variations. Transactions of the American Academy of Ophthalmology and Otolaryngology 1954; 58: 367–370
16. Reese, A. B., Wadsworth, J. A. The adhesion of the lens capsule to the hyaloid membrane and its relation to intracapsular cataract extraction. American Journal of Ophthalmology 1958; 46: 495–498
17. Wolter, J. R. Adhesions of the lens capsule to the anterior hyaloid membrane. American Journal of Ophthalmology 1961; 51: 511–512
18. Jensen, D., Cross, H. E. Surgical treatment of dislocated lenses in the Marfan syndrome and homocystinuria. Transactions of the American Academy of Ophthalmology and Otolaryngology 1972; 76: 1491–1499
19. Jarrett, W. H. II. Dislocation of the lens: A study of 166 hospitalized cases. Archives of Ophthalmology 1967; 78: 289–296
20. Krishna, G., Rao, C. C., Haselby, K. A. Anesthetic considerations for ophthalmic surgery in the pediatric patient. Journal of Pediatric Ophthalmology and Strabismus 1980; 17: 287–291
21. Martin, J. J., Phiffer, J. L., Koch, W. E. The efficacy of general anesthesia for cataract surgery. Ophthalmic Surgery 1976; 7 (3): 89–92
22. Lynch, S. Symposium: anesthesia in ophthalmology: the case for general anesthesia. Transactions of the American Academy of Ophthalmology and Otolaryngology 1973; 79: 559–561
23. Wolf, G. L., Lynch, S., Berlin, I. Intraocular surgery with general anesthesia. Archives of Ophthalmology 1975; 93: 323–326
24. Gills, J. P., Rudisill, J. E. Bupivacaine in cataract surgery. Ophthalmic Surgery 1974; 5: 67–70
25. Martin, N. F., Stark, W. J., Maumenee, A. E., Bruner, W. E., Rosenblum, P. Use of the Honan intraocular pressure reducer at the Wilmer Institute. Ophthalmic Surgery 1982; 13: 101–103
26. Kirsch, R. E. Glaucoma following cataract extraction associated with use of alpha-chymotrypsin. Archives of Ophthalmology 1964; 72: 612–620
27. Kirsch, R. E. Further studies on glaucoma following cataract extraction associated with the use of alpha-chymotrypsin. Transactions of the American Academy of Ophthalmology and Otolaryngology 1965; 69: 1011–1023
28. Kirsch, R. E. Dose relationship of alpha-chymotrypsin in production of glaucoma after cataract extraction. Archives of Ophthalmology 1966; 75: 774–775
29. Dangel, M. E., Keates, R. H. The adjustable slide knot – an alternate technique. Ophthalmic Surgery 1980; 11: 843–846
30. Winslow, R. L., Taylor, B. C., Harris, W. S. A one-year follow-up of cystoid macular edema following intraocular lens implantation. Ophthalmology 1978; 85: 157–163
31. The Miami Study Group. Cystoid macular edema in aphakic and pseudophakic eyes. American Journal of Ophthalmology 1979; 88: 45–48
32. Sinskey, R. M., Cain, W. The posterior capsule and phacoemulsification. Journal – American Intra-Ocular Implant Society 1978; 4:206–207
33. Wilhelmus, K. R., Emery, J. M. Posterior capsule opacification following phacoemulsification. Ophthalmic Surgery 1980; 11: 264–267
34. Kelman, C. D. Phaco-emulsification and aspiration: A new technique of cataract removal. American Journal of Ophthalmology 1967; 64: 23–35
35. Kelman, C. D. Phaco-emulsification and aspiration of senile cataracts: a comparative study with intra-capsular extraction. Canadian Journal of Ophthalmology 1973; 8: 24–32
36. Kelman, C. D. Phaco-emulsification and aspiration. A report of 500 consecutive cases. American Journal of Ophthalmology 1973; 75: 764–768
37. Emery, J. M. Prolapse of the lens nucleus into the anterior chamber. In: Emery, J. M., Little, J. H., eds. Phacoemulsification and aspiration of cataracts. St Louis: C. V. Mosby, 1979: 97–111
38. Rowsey, J. J., Gaylor, J. R. Intraocular lens disasters: Peripheral anterior synechia. Ophthalmology 1980; 87: 645–664
39. Kratz, R. P., Mazzocco, T. R., Davidson, B., Colvard, D. M. A comparative analysis of anterior chamber, iris-supported, capsule-fixated, and posterior chamber intraocular lenses following cataract extraction by phacoemulsification. Ophthalmology 1981; 88: 56–58
40. Taylor, H. R., Stark, W. J. Iris suture fixation for the four-loop Binkhorst intraocular lens. Ophthalmic Surgery 1980; 11: 121–123
41. Kratz, R. P., Mazzocco, T. R., Davidson, B., Colvard, D. M. The Shearing intraocular lens: a report of 1000 cases. Journal – American Intraocular Implant Society 1981; 7: 55–57
42. Taylor, H. R., Michels, R. G., Stark, W. J. Vitrectomy methods in anterior segment surgery. Ophthalmic Surgery 1979; 10(10): 25–58
43. Girard, L. J. Aspiration-irrigation of congenital and traumatic cataracts. Archives of Ophthalmology 1967; 77: 387–391
44. Hiles, D. A., Wallar, P. H. Phacoemulsification versus aspiration in infantile cataract surgery. Ophthalmic Surgery 1974; 5: 13–16
45. Scheie, H. G. Aspiration of congenital or soft cataracts: a new technique. American Journal of Ophthalmology 1960; 50: 1048–1056
46. Meredith, T. A., Maumenee, A. E. A review of 1000 cases of intracapsular cataract extraction: I. Complications. Ophthalmic Surgery 1979; 10: 32–41
47. Vail, D. After-results of vitreous loss. American Journal of Ophthalmology 1965; 59: 573–586
48. Carvounis, E. P., Drance, S. M. The visual results after vitreous loss during cataract extraction. Canadian Journal of Ophthalmology 1978; 13: 237–239
49. Berger, B. B., Zweig, K. O., Peyman, G. A. Long-term results of vitreous loss managed by anterior vitrectomy. In Emery, J. M., Jacobson, A. C., eds. Current concepts in cataract surgery. Selected proceedings of the Sixth Biennial Cataract Surgical Congress, 1978. St Louis: C. V. Mosby, 1980: 274–275
50. Hildreth, H. R. Digital ocular compression preceding cataract surgery. American Journal of Ophthalmology 1961; 51: 1237–1239
51. Owens, W. C., Hughes, W. F., Jr. Intra-ocular hemorrhage in cataract extraction. Archives of Ophthalmology 1947; 37: 561–571
52. Goren, S. B. Expulsive subchoroidal hemorrhage following cataract surgery. American Journal of Ophthalmology 1966; 62: 536–537
53. Shaffer, R. N. Posterior sclerotomy with scleral cautery in the treatment of expulsive hemorrhage. American Journal of Ophthalmology 1966; 61: 1307–1311
54. Vail, D. Posterior sclerotomy as a form of treatment in subchoroidal expulsive hemorrhage. American Journal of Ophthalmology 1938; 21: 256–260
55. Kanski, J. J. Treatment of late endophthalmitis associated with filtering blebs. Archives of Ophthalmology 1974; 91: 339–343
56. Yannuzzi, L. A., Theodore, F. H. Cryotherapy of post-cataract blebs. American Journal of Ophthalmology 1973; 76: 217–222
57. Douvas, N. G. Cystoid bleb cryotherapy. American Journal of Ophthalmology 1972; 74: 69–71
58. Kirk, H. Q. Shallow/flat anterior chamber. Part I. Treatment and prevention of filtering blebs following cataract extraction. In: Emery, J. M., Paton, D., eds. Current concepts in cataract surgery. Selected proceedings of the Third Biennial Cataract Surgical Congress, 1973. St Louis: C. V. Mosby, 1974: 259–261
59. Gehring, J. R., Cicarelli, E. C. Trichloroacetic acid treatment of filtering blebs following cataract extraction. American Journal of Ophthalmology 1972; 74: 622–624
60. Christensen, R. E., Rundle, H. L. Repair of filtering blebs following cataract surgery. Archives of Ophthalmology 1970; 84: 8–11
61. Bruner, W. E., Maumenee, A. E., Stark, W. J. A simple method of repairing inadvertent filtering blebs after cataract surgery. American Journal of Ophthalmology 1981; 794–796
62. Allen, H. F., Mangiaracine, A.B. Bacterial endophthalmitis after cataract extraction. The incidence in 36 000 consecutive operations. Archives of Ophthalmology 1974; 91: 3–7

63. Christy, N. E., Lall, P. Postoperative endophthalmitis following cataract surgery: effects of subconjunctival antibiotics and other factors. Archives of Ophthalmology 1973; 90: 361–366
64. Pollack, I. P. Use of argon laser energy to produce iridotomies. Ophthalmic Surgery 1980; 11: 506–515
65. Stark, W. J., Bruner, W. E. Epithelial ingrowth and fibrous proliferation. In: Rich, R., Shields, M. B., eds. The secondary glaucomas. St Louis: C. V. Mosby, 1982: 381–405
66. Snip, R. C., Kenyon, K. R., Green, W.R. Retrocorneal fibrous membrane in the vitreous touch syndrome. American Journal of Ophthalmology 1975; 79: 233–244
67. Chandler, P. A., Maumenee, A. E. A major cause of hypotony. American Journal of Ophthalmology 1961; 52: 609–619
68. Maumenee, A. E., Stark, W. J. Management of persistent hypotony after planned or inadvertent cyclodialysis. American Journal of Ophthalmology 1971; 71: 320–327
69. Machemer, R. A new concept for vitreous surgery. 2. Surgical technique and complications. American Journal of Ophthalmology 1972; 74: 1022–1033
70. Machemer, R., Norton, E. W. D. A new concept for vitreous surgery. 3. Indications and results. American Journal of Ophthalmology 1972; 74: 1034–1056
71. Michels, R. G. Vitrectomy methods in penetrating ocular trauma. Ophthalmology 1980; 87: 629–645
72. Fenton, R. H., Zimmerman, L. E. Hemolytic glaucoma. An unusual cause of acute open-angle secondary glaucoma. Archives of Ophthalmology 1963; 70: 236–239
73. Michels, R. G., Shacklett, D. E. Vitrectomy technique for removal of retained lens material. Archives of Ophthalmology 1977; 95: 1767–1773
74. Wirostko, E., Spalter, H. F. Lens-induced uveitis. Archives of Ophthalmology 1967; 78: 1–7
75. Scheie, H. G., Morse, P. H., Aminlari, A. Incidence of retinal detachment following cataract extraction. Archives of Ophthalmology 1973; 89: 293–295
76. Wilkinson, C. P. Retinal detachment after phacoemulsification. American Journal of Ophthalmology 1979; 87: 628–631
77. Schepens, C. L. Retinal detachment and aphakia. Archives of Ophthalmology 1951; 45: 1–17
78. Gass, J. D. M. Management of vitreous loss after cataract extraction. Archives of Ophthalmology 1970; 83: 319–323
79. Gass, J. D. M., Norton, E. W. D. Fluorescein studies of patients with macular edema and papilledema following cataract extraction. Transactions of the American Ophthalmological Society 1966; 64: 232–249
80. Gass, J. D. M., Norton, E. W. D. Follow-up study of cystoid macular edema following cataract extraction. Transactions of the American Academy of Ophthalmology and Otolaryngology 1969; 73: 665–682
81. Sholiton, D. B., Reinhart, W. J., Frank, K. E. Indomethacin as a means of preventing cystoid macular edema following intra capsular catract extraction. American Intra-ocular Implant Society Journal 1979; 5: 137–140
82. Yannuzzi, L. A., Klein, R. M., Wallyn, R. H., et al. Ineffectiveness of indomethacin in the treatment of chronic cystoid macular edema. American Journal of Ophthalmology 1977; 84: 517–519
83. Aaberg, T. M. Pars plana vitrectomy for persistent aphakic cystoid macular edema secondary to vitreous incarceraion in the wound. In: McPherson, A., ed. New and controversial aspects of vitreoretinal surgery. St Louis: C. V. Mosby, 1977: 230
84. Fung, W. E. Anterior vitrectomy for chronic aphakic cystoid macular edema. Ophthalmology 1980; 87: 189–193
85. Troutman, R.C., Kelly, S., Kaye, D., et al. The use and preliminary results of the Troutman surgical keratometer in cataract and corneal surgery. Transactions of the American Academy of Ophthalmology and Otolaryngology 1977; 83: 232–238
86. Stark, W. J., Michels, R. G., Bruner, W. R. Management of posteriorly dislocated intraocular lenses. Ophthalmic Surgery 1980; 11: 495–497
87. McCannel, M. A. A retrievable suture idea for anterior uveal problems. Ophthalmic Surgery 1976; 7: 98–103
88. Stark, W. J., Bruner, W. E., Martin, N. F. Management of subluxed posterior-chamber intraocular lenses. Ophthalmic Surgery 1982; 13: 130–133
89. Emery, J. M. Opacified posterior capsule/retroimplant membranes. In: Emery, J. M., ed. Current concepts of cataract surgery. St Louis: C. V. Mosby, 1978: 433–437
90. Sinsky, R. M., Cain, W.. The posterior capsule and phacoemulsification. American Intra-Ocular Implant Society Journal 1978; 4: 206–207
91. Stark, W. J., Bruner, W. E., Michels, R.G. Management of retropseudophakos membranes. American Intra-Ocular Implant Society Journal 1980; 6: 137–140
92. Meltzer, D. W. Sterile hypopyon following intraocular lens surgery. Archives of Ophthalmology 1980; 98: 100–104
93. Stark, W. J., Rosenblum, P., Maumenee, A. E., Cowan, C. L. Postoperative inflammatory reactions in intraocular lenses sterilized with ethylene-oxide. Ophthalmology 1980; 87: 385–389
94. Ellingson, F. T. The uveitis-glaucoma-hyphema syndrome associated with the Mark VIII anterior chamber lens implant. American Intra-Ocular Implant Society Journal 1978; 4: 50–53
95. Bourne, W. M., Kaufman, H. E. Endothelial damage associated with intraocular lenses. American Journal of Ophthalmology 1976; 81: 482–485
96. Forstot, S. L., Blackwell, W. L., Jaffe, N. S., Kaufman, H. E. The effect of intraocular lens implantation on the corneal endothelium. Transactions of the American Academy of Ophthalmology and Otolaryngology 1977; 83: 195–203
97. Rao, G. N., Stevens, R. E., Harris, J. K., Aquavella, J. V. Long-term changes in corneal endothelium following intraocular lens implantation. Ophthalmology 1981; 88: 386–397
98. Irvine, A. R., Kratz, R. P., O'Donnell, J. J. Endothelial damage with phacoemulsification and intraocular lens implantation. Archives of Ophthalmology 1978; 96: 1023–1026
99. Binkhorst, C. D., Nygaard, P., Loones, L. H. Specular microscopy of the corneal endothelium and lens implant surgery. American Journal of Ophthalmology 1978; 85: 597–605
100. Wilkinson, C. P. Retinal detachments following intraocular lens implantation. Ophthalmology 1981; 88: 410–413
101. Binkhorst, C. D., Kats, A., Tjan, T. T., Loones, L. H. Retinal accidents in pseudophakia – intracapsular versus extracapsular surgery. Transactions of the American Academy of Ophthalmology and Otolaryngology 1976; 81: 120–127
102. Meredith, T. A., Maumenee, A. E. A review of 1000 cases of intracapsular cataract extraction. II. Visual results and astigmatic analysis. Ophthalmic Surgery 1979; 10(12): 42–45

7

Surgery of the glaucomas

Harry A. Quigley MD

Introduction

In the last 20 years, glaucoma surgery has undergone significant progress and change due largely to improved technical capabilities. The basic glaucoma entities considered in this chapter are familiar, and their pathogenesis requires little discussion.

Angle-closure glaucoma is considered first, with a brief review of the pathological mechanism of pupillary block. In angle-closure cases, recent development of laser technology has changed the technique of making an iris hole, which can now be done effectively with the laser whereas previously this was produced surgically.

The second section deals with uncontrolled glaucoma, chiefly of the open-angle type. The cause of open-angle glaucoma remains unknown, but the technical advantages of trabeculectomy, as compared to previous filtering operations, are now clear. Interestingly, trabeculectomy was originally developed to function by a different mechanism, but it has become the most popular filtering operation because of a lower incidence of flat anterior chambers postoperatively. In addition, laser trabeculoplasty is now being evaluated as an alternative to filtering surgery.

The third section summarizes the method of cyclocryotherapy. Although cyclocryotherapy has a reputation for possible complications, its efficacy in otherwise uncontrollable glaucoma is established. Not enough attention, however, has been paid to details of technique to maximize its effectiveness and minimize complications.

In the section on the 'combined' cases of cataract and glaucoma, a few practical suggestions are offered. By contrast, there is considerable new information about the causes of congenital glaucoma, and this is presented in the fifth section. Also, the trabeculotomy *ab externo* procedure, as an alternative to goniotomy, is presented.

One of the most perplexing problems for the glaucoma surgeon is the complication of postoperative flat anterior chamber. The factors that aid in deciding when and how to re-form the anterior chamber are reviewed. Last, malignant glaucoma is discussed. This rare condition can rapidly blind an otherwise salvageable eye. Its pathogenesis is reviewed, and advances in vitreous surgery used to treat malignant glaucoma are discussed.

Pupillary-block glaucoma: iridectomy

Indications for surgery

The therapy of pupillary-block glaucoma is simple in concept, and yet it is one of the least understood areas in ophthalmology. Eyes with pupillary-block glaucoma are different from normal eyes in several important ways. Anatomically, they are smaller in axial length, have larger lenses relative to the size of the eye, and have flatter curvature of the posterior cornea[1]. As a result, the anterior chamber depth is shallower than in normal eyes.

As aqueous humor passes from the posterior chamber to the anterior chamber, it must pass between the lens and the posterior iris surface, and then through the pupil (*Figure 7.1a*). In eyes predisposed to pupillary block, the abnormal anatomical features combine to cause difficulty in aqueous passage around the pupillary margin of the iris. The abnormally close apposition between the iris and lens is made tighter when the pupil is mid-dilated or when there is anterior movement and thickening of the lens from physiological or miotic-induced accommodation (*Figure 7.1b*).

When sufficient slowing of anterior movement of aqueous occurs, the pressure behind the iris rises above that in the anterior chamber. Because aqueous can still leave the trabecular outflow pathway through the narrow anterior chamber angle, this higher pressure behind the iris forces more fluid out from the anterior chamber, and the peripheral iris bows forward. If the entire iris were to move forward, the pupillary blockade would end. However, the central iris remains near the anterior lens surface, and the peripheral iris bows further forward until it is in contact with the trabecular meshwork (*Figure 7.1c,d*). Then, no more aqueous can leave the eye, and the intraocular pressure (IOP) rises until aqueous humor formation ceases. Production of a hole in the iris (iridotomy or iridectomy) bypasses pupillary blockade of aqueous movement by providing an alternative pathway for aqueous humor to reach the anterior chamber. (In this chapter, the term 'iridectomy' will sometimes be used to refer to either a surgical iridectomy or a laser iridotomy.)

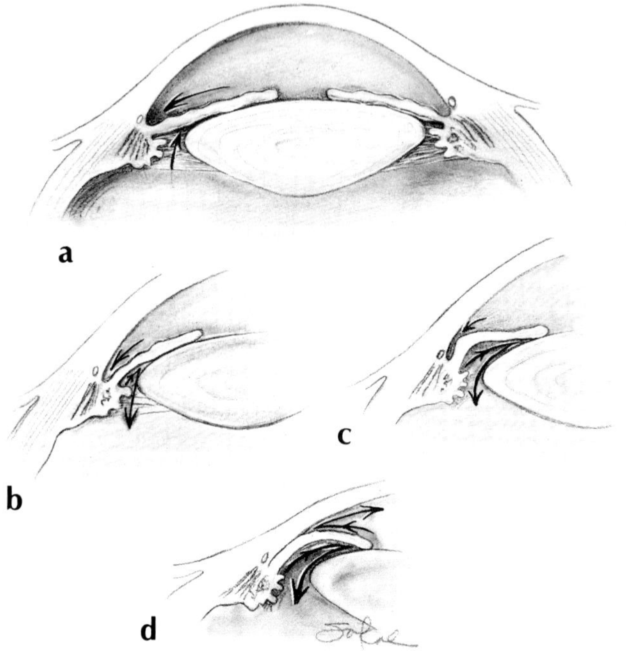

Figure 7.1 **(a)** *In the normal eye, aqueous humor flows from the ciliary body through the pupil (between the iris and lens) and into the anterior chamber where it exits through the trabecular meshwork.* **(b)** *During an angle-closure attack, pupillary block of aqueous movement occurs when the pupil is in mid-dilation where there is maximum iris–lens contact.* **(c)** *The pressure is transiently higher in the posterior chamber, and the iris bows forward.* **(d)** *When the iris comes into contact with the trabecular meshwork, no further aqueous can exit and the IOP rises rapidly*

The misconception commonly encountered is that eyes develop 'angle closure' after pupillary dilation because the iris is bunched up in the anterior chamber angle, directly obstructing outflow through the trabecular meshwork. If this were the case, iridectomy would not cure the problem, since the iris would still be bunched up in the anterior chamber angle. Recurrence of pupillary block after iridectomy only happens in the rare condition of plateau iris which is briefly discussed below. In most eyes, pupillary block initiates an attack of angle closure, and this is cured by creating a hole in the iris.

The size of an iridotomy or iridectomy need only be large enough to accommodate aqueous humor flow of about 2 μl/min or one drop every 20 minutes.

Experience with laser iridotomy holes indicates that even a hole 0.25 mm in diameter is sufficient. The hole in the iris must be located so that the lens cannot obstruct it. While the base of the iris is the best location to avoid lens contact, an iridectomy anywhere in the peripheral one-third of the iris has proved adequate.

Several categories of patients require iridotomy or iridectomy. First are those with acute angle-closure glaucoma. Usually the diagnosis is clear. There is sudden onset of pain, a red eye and a fixed pupil. The anterior chamber angle is closed as seen by gonioscopy, and the IOP is high. This is an ocular emergency that requires prompt attention. Medical measures are used first to lower the IOP, and then iridotomy or iridectomy is indicated.

In the past, one had to consider whether the attack had been prolonged, or whether repeated attacks had occurred that might have caused permanent angle closure. In such cases iridectomy would relieve the pupillary block, but permanent peripheral anterior synechiae (PAS) might cause the IOP to remain high. Hence, anterior chamber deepening procedures were developed to determine whether iridectomy alone would suffice or whether filtering surgery was indicated as a primary procedure[2]. The advent of means to create a hole in the iris with a laser (laser iridotomy) has largely solved this dilemma. We prefer to produce a laser iridotomy in every eye that has an acute angle-closure attack. If the IOP remains uncontrolled, a filtering procedure can be done later; thus, only one intraocular surgical procedure is required.

The fellow eyes of those with acute angle closure also have angle-closure attacks in 75 per cent of cases when no therapy is used. Nearly 50 per cent of fellow eyes have attacks despite miotic therapy[3,4]. Therefore, a prophylactic iridectomy or iridotomy is performed in the fellow eye as soon as possible. Laser iridotomy has reduced the understandable reluctance of patients to undergo a surgical procedure in an asymptomatic fellow eye.

One of the most difficult decisions in glaucoma surgery concerns management of patients with narrow anterior chamber angles as seen by gonioscopy who have not had a documented attack of angle closure. Factors weighing in favor of prophylactic iridotomy are: (*1*) a family history of acute glaucoma; (*2*) symptoms such as pain, blurred vision and redness compatible with intermittent attacks; and (*3*) signs of possible attacks in the past such as iris atrophy and 'glaucomflecken' anterior lens opacities.

Discovery of PAS in an eye with a narrow angle is of special importance. Unless there is clear evidence of past ocular trauma, inflammation or another cause for the PAS, they are thought to indicate past pupillary block with angle closure, and an iridectomy or iridotomy is needed. Provocative testing may also be helpful. Whether this is a darkroom test or a mydriatic-provocative test, a rise in IOP of 8 mmHg, combined with appositional closure of the angle as seen by gonioscopy, confirms the tendency to pupillary block, and an iridotomy or iridectomy is indicated.

Provocative testing fails, however, to detect a significant minority of eyes with angle-closure glaucoma[5]. Likewise, in some eyes the mydriatic test causes IOP elevation (even though the angle is not closed) as a result of other effects of the dilating agent. Despite these false results in some cases, provocative testing is useful. When the advisability of an iridectomy is in doubt, it is best to avoid any therapy. Instead, the patient is re-examined frequently, informed of the symptoms of an acute attack and asked to return immediately if these symptoms occur. Miotic agents are not prescribed because they cause further narrowing of the anterior chamber angle, and this may confuse future gonioscopic evaluation. Miotic agents also have other side-effects, and they occasionally cause an attack of angle closure by inducing pupillary block. Therefore, it is preferable to leave the eye untreated and to observe the natural course before making further decisions.

Eyes with pupillary block but without a history of an acute attack may have various clinical presentations. In some patients, there is a history of intermittent attacks of pain, redness and decreased vision. Others are completely asymptomatic, but there are signs, such as PAS, indicating past pupillary-block episodes. Regardless of whether these cases are called 'intermittent', 'subacute' or 'chronic' angle closure, they all need iridectomy. Previously it was difficult to decide whether iridectomy alone should be done or whether filtering surgery was necessary because of permanent anterior chamber angle damage. These cases are now treated initially by laser iridotomy. If uncontrolled IOP elevation continues and cannot be controlled, filtering surgery is performed.

There are also situations in which iridectomy is indicated but in which pupillary block is not the primary pathological mechanism. Eyes with chronic inflammation, a secluded pupil from posterior synechiae, and iris bombé should undergo prompt iridectomy to prevent permanent PAS. Occasionally an eye with a partially dislocated (subluxed) lens will develop pupillary block when the lens is displaced forward. If removal of the partially dislocated lens is not necessary, but if there is intermittent elevation of the IOP, laser iridotomy is helpful. This is done at a location peripheral to the lens equator. In some aphakic eyes the prior iridectomy is inadequate and vitreous gel occludes the pupillary space. These eyes with aphakic pupillary block are initially treated by iridotomy.

Rarely, what appears to be aphakic pupillary block is actually 'malignant glaucoma' in which increased fluid pressure develops posterior to the vitreous gel, pushing the vitreous forward toward the anterior chamber and pressing it against the ciliary body and iris. This condition can also occur in phakic eyes. The anterior chamber is quite shallow, and the condition may be confused with primary angle closure in the phakic eye. Clues to the diagnosis of malignant glaucoma include: (*1*) high IOP and a shallow anterior chamber but normal depth of the anterior chamber in the fellow eye, and (*2*) failure to respond to usual treatment of acute angle closure. Pilocarpine intensifies the pathological condition in malignant glaucoma. Osmotic agents provide some relief, and the attack can sometimes be broken with systemic use of mannitol or glycerin. When standard 'acute' management using pilocarpine, acetazolamide and osmotic agents does not succeed, the alternative of cycloplegic therapy should be considered to widen the ciliary-body ring.

Often malignant glaucoma is not properly diagnosed preoperatively, and an iridectomy is done in the belief that ordinary pupillary block is present. When malignant glaucoma is present, the IOP does not return to normal after iridectomy, the anterior chamber does not deepen and the anterior chamber angle does not open. The specific surgery for malignant glaucoma is discussed later.

Eyes with *secondary* angle-closure glaucoma are not helped by iridectomy. In conditions such as neovascular glaucoma, traumatic damage to the anterior chamber angle, chronic uveitis and the iridocorneal endothelial syndrome (essential iris atrophy and related disorders), PAS are present but they arise from causes other than pupillary block. Iridectomy should not be performed unless pupillary block is also present. For example, eyes with chronic uveitis often have PAS and secondary glaucoma without pupillary block. However, if posterior synechiae develop the pupil may then become secluded, leading to iris bombé. Only then is iridectomy indicated.

Preoperative management

Regardless of whether iridectomy is to be performed surgically or will be done with a laser, the IOP should be lowered as quickly as possible. Extreme IOP elevation can rapidly damage the anterior chamber angle, lens, cornea, and optic nerve. Therefore, acute angle closure is a true emergency. Pilocarpine drops are given every 5 minutes although, if the IOP is above 50 mmHg, the sphincter muscle of the iris may be unresponsive. Therefore, in eyes with marked pressure elevation timolol drops, acetazolamide and osmotic agents are used. Acetazolamide is best given slowly by intravenous injection during 1 minute, using 500 mg dissolved in sterile saline solution. Nausea associated with acute glaucoma attacks usually prevents use of oral agents. Recently, Anderson[6] has reported that direct pressure on the central cornea with a goniolens can help to relieve some acute attacks.

The choice between laser iridotomy or surgical iridectomy depends on the experience of the surgeon. We now use laser iridotomy instead of surgical iridectomy unless corneal clouding prevents effective use of the laser. Both methods will be discussed.

Surgical iridectomy

Anesthesia

Standard local retrobulbar anesthesia is performed. The IOP is measured before beginning the procedure. If medical therapy has not lowered the IOP, careful decompression of the globe is done during the operation.

Operative technique

A superior rectus suture of 4/0 black silk is used and fastened to the drapes. The initial incision can be made in one of three ways. First, the entire procedure can be done through peripheral clear cornea (*Figure 7.2*). In this approach, a razor blade incision is made to two-thirds of the corneal depth, 1 mm from the superior limbus (*Figure 7.2a*). A preplaced, single-armed 10/0 nylon suture is used (*Figure 7.2b*). Forceps are used to hold this suture and spread the wound for completion of the incision into the anterior chamber along a length of 2 mm (*Figure 7.2c*).

It is important that the internal entry into the anterior chamber be nearly as wide as the external part of the incision, so that the iris will prolapse easily (*Figure 7.2d*).

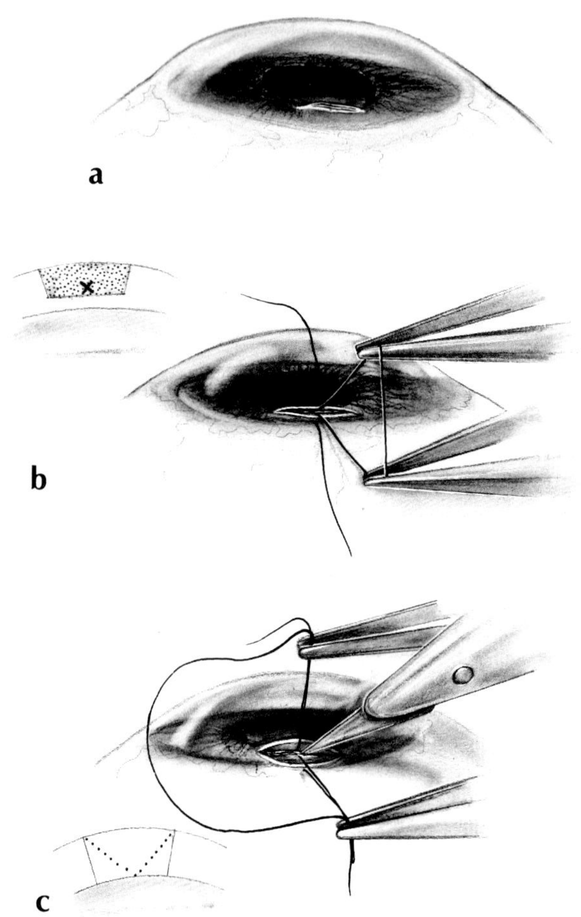

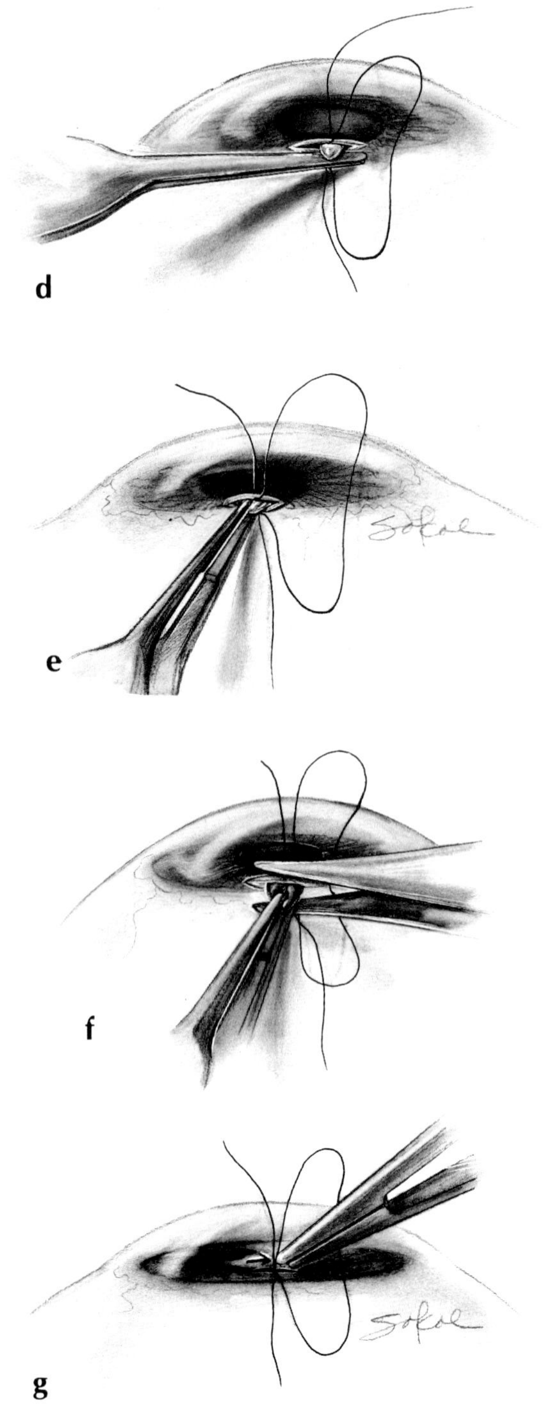

Figure 7.2 *Iridectomy through clear-corneal incision.* **(a)** *Razor blade incision two-thirds the corneal thickness is made in clear cornea for 2–3 mm.* **(b)** *A 10/0 nylon suture is placed across the incision, as deep as possible (see 'x' in corneal cross-section drawing) and is looped out of the wound.* **(c)** *The anterior chamber is entered with the razor blade. The deep portion of the incision should be as long as the external portion (see corneal cross-section), so that the iris will prolapse (an inadequate deep incision, shaped like a triangle, is shown in dotted line).* **(d)** *Pressure on the posterior portion of the wound may cause the iris to prolapse.* **(e)** *Fine forceps can also be used to grasp and externalize the iris.* **(f)** *The iris tissue is cut with scissors.* **(g)** *The anterior margin of the wound is massaged with a smooth instrument to reposit the remaining iris tissue*

However, if the iris does not prolapse spontaneously or with mild pressure on the posterior wound margin, then smooth iris forceps are used to grasp the iris while spreading the wound edges using the preplaced suture (*Figure 7.2e*). Strong traction on the iris is avoided because this can cause bleeding from the iris root and/or cause a cyclodialysis cleft.

The prolapsed iris is cut with scissors (*Figure 7.2f*) and the excised portion is inspected for the presence of pigment epithelium on its posterior surface, to confirm that a full-thickness piece of iris has been removed producing a patent hole. The iris incarcerated in the wound may spontaneously reposit into the anterior chamber, or this can be aided by spreading the wound and gently stroking the anterior margin with a smooth instrument (*Figure 7.2g*). If these measures fail, a smooth repositor may be introduced through the wound. Care is taken to avoid damage to the lens.

The preplaced suture is tightened, tied and cut; and the knot is buried. The anterior chamber should begin to re-form spontaneously. The IOP is measured using a sterile Schiotz tonometer and should be low. If the IOP is high, either the iridectomy is not patent or malignant glaucoma is present. The patency of the iridectomy is evaluated by direct visualization through the operating microscope and/or by transillumination.

Although the clear-cornea approach does not cause scarring of the conjunctiva, and this makes any future filtering surgery more likely to succeed, it may be difficult to produce iris prolapse when an anterior incision is used. Two alternative approaches increase the ease of iris prolapse but cause some conjunctival scarring (*Figure 7.3*).

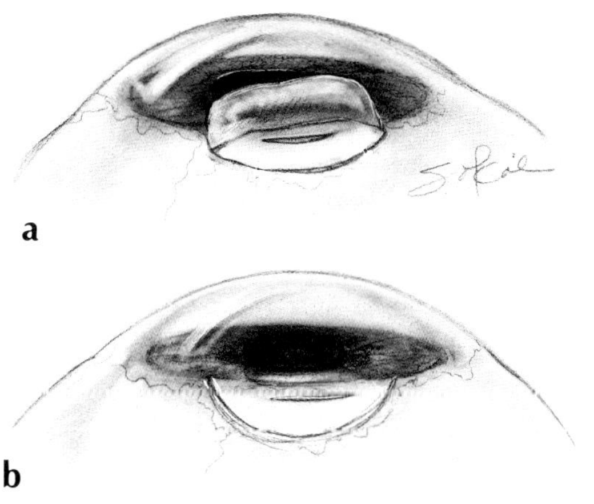

Figure 7.3 *Two limbal approaches for surgical iridectomy.* **(a)** *A limbus-based conjunctival flap can be used.* **(b)** *Alternatively, the conjunctiva can be disinserted at the limbus and displaced posteriorly as a fornix-based flap. With both techniques the incision into the anterior chamber is made in the gray limbal zone*

When these methods are used, the incision should be located either nasal or temporal to the 12 o'clock meridian, so that any later filtering surgery can be performed on the opposite side of the vertical meridian.

One method uses a small limbus-based conjunctival flap (*Figure 7.3a*). The scleral incision is made at the surgical limbus, and a 10/0 suture is preplaced across the wound. The procedure is done as described above. The conjunctiva can be closed with an absorbable suture such as 8/0 collagen or by cautery.

We prefer a small fornix-based conjunctival flap made by disinserting the conjunctiva at the limbus, using a razor blade (*Figure 7.3b*). The scleral incision and 10/0 suture are placed as in the limbus-based flap method, and the iridectomy is done as described before. After tying and burying the 10/0 suture knot, the conjunctiva often returns to a fairly normal position and no conjunctival sutures are needed. Occasionally, one or two interrupted 8/0 collagen sutures at the limbus are needed to pull the conjunctival flap down over the operated area. Rarely, the fornix-based flap interferes with the limbal incision, and a relaxing incision is made perpendicular to the limbus. This requires later suturing and it causes more conjunctival scarring.

Postoperative care and complications

At the end of the operation the eye is treated with dexamethasone ointment and a patch and protective shield are applied. On the first postoperative day, the patency of the iridectomy is reconfirmed. The IOP is checked, and when it becomes normal a short-acting dilating drop is instilled. This prevents formation of posterior synechiae, and also acts as a mydriatic-provocative test. When the pupil is dilated, the IOP should not rise significantly unless the rare 'plateau iris' configuration is present. If plateau iris is present, then long-term pilocarpine therapy is indicated. If the IOP is normal and pupillary dilation produces no IOP rise, the patient is discharged from the hospital on the first postoperative day. Steroid drops are prescribed for use every 6 hours. When surgery on the fellow eye is indicated, this can be done 48–72 hours after the iridectomy for the first eye.

If the IOP is elevated immediately postoperatively, the eye is re-examined to determine the cause. Usually this is from PAS that have formed before the iridectomy and therefore compromise outflow. Gonioscopy shows an approach to the anterior chamber angle that is deeper than before iridectomy but with considerable PAS. Medical therapy is reinstituted to lower the IOP, but miotics are withheld because it is desirable to move the pupil periodically. Long-acting cycloplegics are also avoided because medical therapy might eventually require pilocarpine, and long-acting cycloplegics block the action of pilocarpine.

Another cause of IOP elevation after iridectomy is obstruction of the anterior chamber angle by pigment, inflammatory debris or red blood cells. Postoperative hyphema is uncommon, but when it does occur, gonioscopically the angle is open but the meshwork is hidden by red blood cells. If the IOP remains elevated, the approach to the anterior chamber angle is narrow and the angle is closed, malignant glaucoma may be present. In this case, cycloplegic drops and osmotic agents are tried. As mentioned, persistent angle closure after surgical iridectomy can also result from incomplete removal of a full-thickness piece of iris. This is easily remedied by laser iridotomy through the remaining iris tissue at the same site.

Other disorders can lead to low IOP and a shallow anterior chamber postoperatively. The most common cause is a wound leak. When a clear-cornea surgical approach has been used, a wound leak is detected by placing sterile 2 per cent fluorescein solution on the wound and looking for flow of clear aqueous from the wound through the yellow-green fluorescein dye (Seidel test).

Although minor problems can occur after iridectomy, the most important late complication is development of cataract. Many patients undergoing iridectomy are in the sixth to eighth decades of life, when cataract is common. Also, many have had intermittent or prolonged IOP elevation that predisposes to lens opacity, and many have been treated with medications (such as miotics) that may be cataractogenic. Hence, it is difficult to know whether progressive lens opacities seen in some eyes after iridectomy are because of surgery or from non-surgical factors. At least 25 per cent of eyes lose two or more lines of vision on the Snellen chart within 2 years after iridectomy[7,8]. Most of these cases do not have definite evidence of direct lens trauma from surgery causing cataract. Postoperative endophthalmitis is another complication that can occur after iridectomy but is quite rare.

Laser iridotomy

Anesthesia

Topical proparacaine 0.5 per cent provides sufficient anesthesia. Although the light of the laser is uncomfortably bright during the later stages of treatment, the discomfort is not enough to justify retrobulbar injection.

Instruments and preoperative care

Our experience has been greatest with the continuous-wave argon laser. The krypton red laser is also effective. Pilocarpine drops are instilled 30 minutes before laser treatment. Laser burns cause the iris dilator to contract, pulling the pupil toward the treatment area and making the iris thicker in that location. Pretreatment with miotics decrease this sectoral dilatation. Topical steroids are given before treatment to minimize post-treatment inflammation.

A fundus contact lens is used to prevent lid closure during treatment and to absorb heat energy that would otherwise be delivered to the corneal epithelium (*Figure 7.4*). With an accessory planoconvex button lens (focal length = 15 mm) glued onto the anterior contact lens surface, there is increased focusing of the laser beam and greater penetrating power.

Selection of treatment site

The iris is examined at high power (40×) to find the thinnest spot possible. This is usually at the base of an iris crypt or in an area of atrophy. The upper half of the iris is preferable (*Figure 7.5*). The 12 o'clock position is avoided because bubbles form from treatment and float to this position. The iridotomy site should be as far peripherally in the iris as possible, because this maximizes the chance of eliminating pupillary block and minimizes energy delivered to the patient's lens. However, the far peripheral iris may be difficult to treat because of the presence of corneal arcus senilis. Also, in eyes with a closed or very narrow anterior chamber angle the anterior iris and posterior cornea are so close together at the periphery that

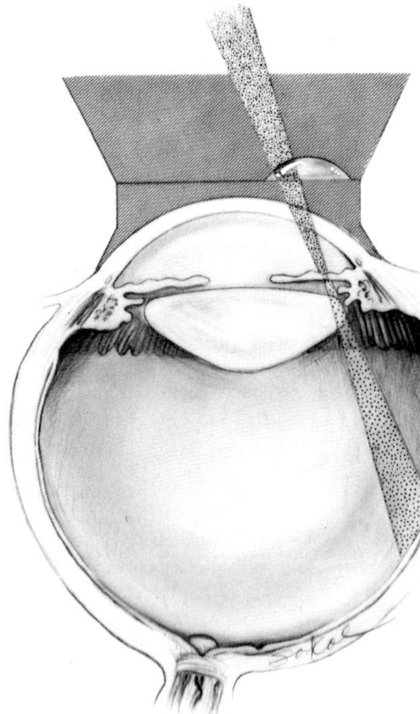

Figure 7.4 *Laser iridotomy using a fundus contact lens with a convex lens glued onto the anterior peripheral contact lens surface. The laser beam is directed away from the fovea. The laser beam is focused to produce the smallest spot possible at the plane of the iris*

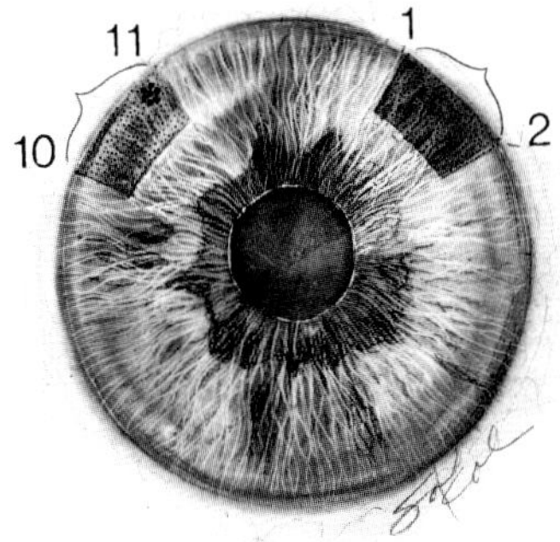

Figure 7.5 *Optimum sites for laser iridotomy are superonasal and superotemporal portions of iris as indicated by dotted zones*

energy applied to the iris will cause a corneal burn and opacity. Because laser burns cause the iris to bow posteriorly in a trough-like zone, preliminary low-energy burns can be applied to the midportion of the iris in such eyes, moving the iris away from the cornea (*Figure 7.6a,b*). Further low-energy burns, along a line leading toward the periphery, may cause enough separation between the iris and cornea to permit safe completion of a peripheral iridotomy (*Figure 7.6c,d*).

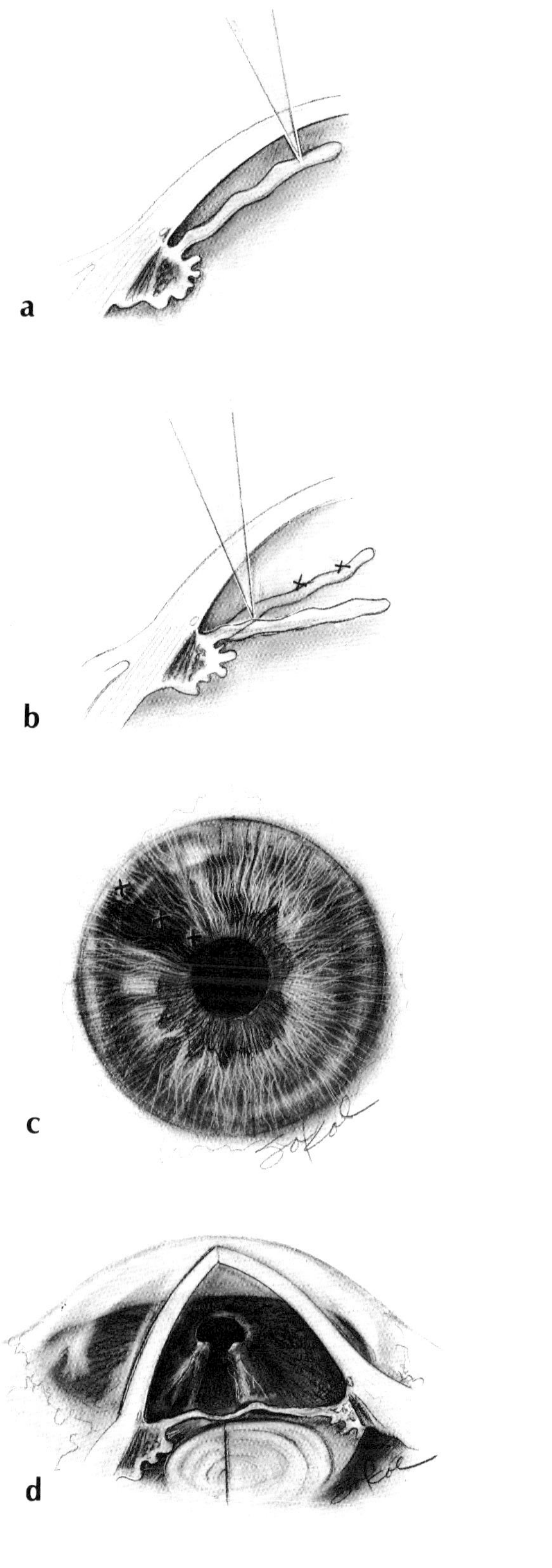

Figure 7.6 *Laser iridotomy in eye with shallow anterior chamber and near apposition between cornea and peripheral iris.* **(a,b)** *Initial low-energy laser treatment is done along a line from the central portion of the iris toward the periphery.* **(c,d)** *This causes the iris to bow away from the cornea, permitting iridotomy in the peripheral iris without corneal damage*

Treatment details

Initial treatment energy should be 500 mW for 0.2 seconds, with a 50 μm spot size. In some irides this is sufficient to produce a hole, and is harmless for most corneas. If there is little effect, the power may be increased to 1000 or 1500 mW. We rarely use power settings higher than this because secondary damage can result. Precise focus of the aiming beam on the iris is important; poorly focused burns are not effective. If the iris stroma is thin, only 8–10 applications will be necessary. More frequently, after application of about a dozen spots, one area within the treatment zone will be thinner than elsewhere; and this area is then treated with increased power (*Figure 7.7*).

The first sign of full-thickness hole formation is often a gush of dark pigment through the hole into the anterior chamber, appearing like a mushroom cloud. One must wait for this pigment cloud to clear before proceeding.

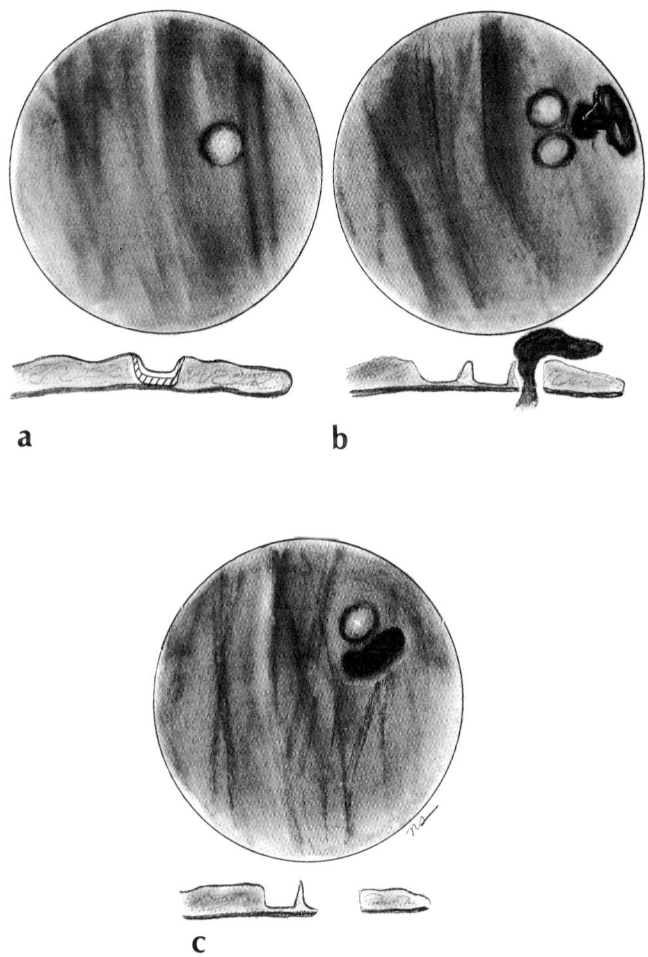

Figure 7.7 (a) *Appearance of iris after initial laser applications during laser iridotomy.* **(b)** *Treatment of nearby areas produces additional zones of thinning until a full-thickness hole is produced, as indicated by a 'mushroom cloud' of pigment.* **(c)** *Further treatment is applied on the remaining bridges of tissue until a larger opening is produced*

From then on, every subsequent laser application should strike iris tissue on the margin of the hole and not pass through the defect. Further applications are used to enlarge the opening and thereby minimize the chance of secondary pigment deposition closing the hole. The greatest danger of inadvertent retinal damage is at this time, and the angle of the laser beam is directed away from the posterior pole while also maintaining precise focus on the remaining margin of iris tissue.

Early descriptions of laser iridotomy advocated placing a circle of laser spots to create a hump in the iris and then burning through the hump center. This method has not proved sufficiently useful to become standard procedure. Often, the limiting factor in completing an iridotomy is transient clouding of the deep cornea. When this occurs, further laser burns do not transmit full energy to the iris, and further laser use can damage the cornea. If the cornea becomes cloudy overlying the area of treatment, the patient is asked to look upward, downward or to the side to allow further treatment through clear cornea adjacent to the opacity (*Figure 7.8*).

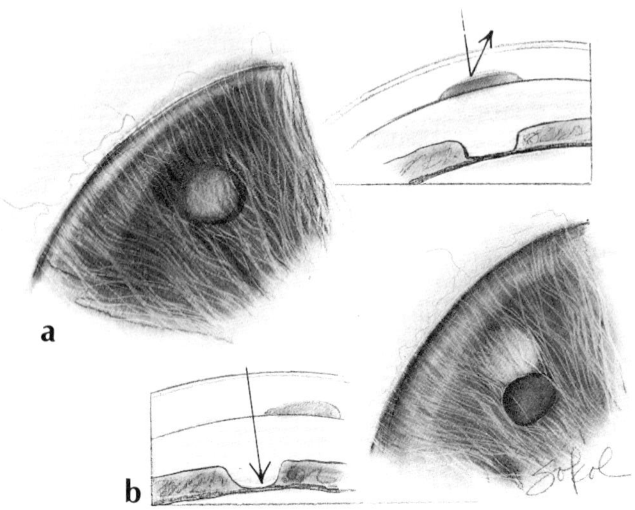

Figure 7.8 **(a)** *Deep corneal opacities may develop during laser treatment, thereby obscuring the view and preventing full delivery of laser energy to the iris.* **(b)** *Ocular fixation is moved slightly so that the opaque corneal zone is moved out of the line of view, permitting further treatment of the same area*

In some eyes, an iridotomy larger than 1 mm in diameter can be readily produced. However, since the amount of aqueous flow necessary to prevent pupillary block is small, holes of 0.25 mm have proved adequate. In eyes that resist enlargement of a small opening, or if no hole is produced immediately, we set a limit of 75 laser deliveries in any treatment session. After about 75 deliveries, the cornea usually has developed enough fine haze that further deliveries do not produce more iris excavation. After a 1- to 2-week interval, pigmented material accumulates in the treated zone, so that a second treatment session is usually needed to produce the desired result. Also, excessive treatment sometimes produces an inflammatory reaction with a fibrin clot over the hole. This can serve as scaffolding for deposition of pigment debris and cellular proliferation that may obstruct the hole.

If the iris in the first area selected for treatment resists hole formation, it may be possible to move to a different area and obtain a better response. If only a tiny hole of 50–100 μm in diameter can be produced, it is advisable to produce a second hole elsewhere to improve the chance of a successful functional result. Another reason for difficulty in producing a hole is pre-existing corneal haze, especially in eyes with recent or persistent IOP elevation. These eyes often have an immediate inflammatory response at the treated site. This appears as fluffy brown material that may be combined fibrin and iris pigment, and it can be difficult or impossible to complete the iridotomy through this material.

Postoperative care

Cellular debris is always present in the anterior chamber at the end of treatment. Topical corticosteroid drops are used four times daily to control inflammation. A few patients have a moderate increase in IOP during the immediate post-treatment period, and therefore any pretreatment glaucoma medications are continued until the eye is quiet and the new IOP level can be determined. The eye rarely requires patching, and vision is slightly blurred for up to 24 hours.

The procedure is routinely performed on an outpatient basis. Both eyes are treated during one session if indicated. The first postoperative examination is performed within 1 week; and if a definite full-thickness iridotomy is seen, the pupil is then dilated. This prevents development of permanent posterior synechiae and provides an improved view of the fundus. Intraocular inflammation is rare at the time of the first post-treatment visit. If the hole is not full thickness or it is too small, retreatment can be done at this time. Usually, less laser energy is required than in the initial treatment session.

Retreatment

Confirming that an iridotomy is full thickness is occasionally difficult. Sometimes the opening is partially obscured by pigmented debris and macrophages that accumulate over the treated zone. The most reliable criterion of a full-thickness hole is direct visualization of structures behind the iris such as the lens capsule, lens zonules or ciliary processes. In dark irides, bright transillumination of the iridotomy, by shining the slit-lamp through the pupil, is a helpful sign. In blue irides, however, there is frequently a large area of transillumination in the treated area from loss of pigment epithelium, even when the iris stroma has not been fully penetrated. We retreat any questionable small iridotomies. Also, another sign of an adequate iris hole is the relief or prevention of pupillary block. The mydriatic or darkroom provocative test should be repeated for confirmation.

Complications

If it is impossible to produce a laser iridotomy after several attempts, surgery is used. Every patient in whom laser iridotomy is recommended should be told of the possible need for surgery if the laser method fails.

Laser iridotomies that are open at 6 weeks post-treatment will usually remain permanently open[9,10]. However, there are rare exceptions. In some eyes a single large opening is not produced, but rather a number of small (50 μm diameter) holes are produced in a cluster with intervening strands of residual stromal tissue. This scaffolding seems to allow regrowth of iris pigment epithelium to cover the hole. We have observed only two such cases in over 1000 treated eyes. These imperfect iridotomies are easily reopened. Also, in eyes with chronic uveitis or rubeosis iridis, later closure of the iridotomy may occur. In these eyes, a larger than normal iris hole should be produced.

The most dangerous potential complication of laser iridotomy is retinal damage. We have not observed loss of visual acuity as a result of this complication. Nevertheless, great care must be exercised in performing the iridotomy.

Nearly every treated eye has some visible change in the deep corneal stroma overlying the treated zone. In most eyes, this clears within 1 week. In a few cases, however, there is a permanent white plaque about 250 μm in diameter in the deep cornea. By comparison a clear-corneal approach for surgical iridectomy produces a much larger peripheral corneal scar. Rarely, more severe temporary changes occur in the cornea after laser iridotomy. If the contact lens moves during treatment or if the laser is incorrectly focused too far anteriorly, superficial white lesions can occur in the cornea. These lesions heal rapidly. Mild striate keratopathy lasting less than 1 week has been observed. Some of these affected eyes had prior acute attacks of angle-closure glaucoma, however, and it is sometimes unclear whether corneal edema resulted from the laser energy or from high IOP.

Other minor changes occur in eyes after laser iridotomy. Every eye has debris floating in the anterior chamber. We presume inflammation occurs in response to treatment, and all patients are treated with topical steroid drops four times daily for 1 week. We have only rarely observed keratic precipitates after laser iridotomy, and the cells in the anterior chamber are almost always gone at the 1 week post-treatment visit. In a small percentage of eyes, posterior synechiae are seen when the pupil is dilated later. Although it is possible that the laser treatment causes posterior synechiae, many such patients have been using chronic miotic therapy, or have had angle-closure glaucoma attacks or chronic uveitis; and it is difficult to know whether the synechiae were present before laser therapy.

Occasionally the IOP has become elevated 10–15 mmHg above the pretreatment level when checked during the 24 hours after the procedure. In our experience, no acute angle-closure glaucoma attack has occurred in an eye with an incomplete laser iridotomy, and no severe elevation of the IOP after treatment has been recognized. With the exception of eyes with iris neovascularization, there has been no hemorrhage during or after treatment.

As with surgical iridectomy, progression of cataract occurs in some eyes after laser iridotomy, but a causal relationship is difficult to prove. A few eyes have small white opacities in the subcapsular lens cortex underlying the iris hole, but none of these localized opacities has progressed to more extensive lens opacity. Instead, we have observed typical progressive senile cataract, decreasing the visual acuity by two Snellen lines or more, in 15 per cent of eyes examined 2 years after laser iridotomy. This occurs in patients with pre-existing lens opacities, and those who have had past acute angle-closure glaucoma attacks and/or who have required antiglaucoma medical therapy, and they are (as a group) statistically older than laser iridotomy patients who do not develop progressive cataract. In patients with pre-existing cataracts, any method of producing an iris hole is associated with cataract progression, and thus far no statistical difference between surgical and laser methods has been shown.

Results

When an iris hole is produced in these patients, pupillary block is relieved. Hence, regardless of whether surgical or laser methods are used, IOP rise from primary angle closure is curable. However, by the time the need for iridotomy or iridectomy is diagnosed, many eyes already have permanent anterior chamber angle damage. Some eyes also have glaucomatous optic nerve damage prior to initial therapy. Thus, the cure rate after surgical iridectomy or laser iridotomy depends greatly on the stage of the disease when the diagnosis is made and the procedure is performed.

Laser iridotomy has a number of potential advantages over the surgical method: (*1*) no retrobulbar anesthesia is required; (*2*) there is no chance of endophthalmitis; (*3*) wound leaks cannot occur; (*4*) intraocular hemorrhage occurs rarely, if ever; (*5*) visual recovery is more rapid; and (*6*) there is no conjunctival scarring that might interfere with future filtering surgery. The disadvantages of laser iridotomy are: (*1*) it cannot be performed in eyes with a hazy cornea; (*2*) several treatment sessions are sometimes necessary; (*3*) late closure of small holes occurs rarely; (*4*) the technique is exacting, and some experience is required before optimal results are obtained; and (*5*) long-term complications of laser iridotomy are less well known than those following the surgical technique.

As we have gained experience, the number of laser applications and treatment sessions required to produce a permanent iridotomy has steadily declined. Now over 85 per cent of eyes are treated in only one session using fewer than 50 laser pulses. Also, iris color greatly affects the ease of producing a hole with the laser. Light brown irides combine the favorable characteristics of good energy absorption (because of their melanin content) and relatively thin stroma, so that iridotomy is easier. Light blue irides absorb laser energy less well, and although they are usually thin, such irides can be resistant to hole formation. Dark brown irides – as in black, Asian and Hispanic patients – absorb the laser energy well, but they are usually quite thick and require more energy and/or more spots to produce a hole.

There is disagreement as to whether the initial step in management of chronic angle closure should be an iridotomy, because some cases have only a mild IOP elevation that is easily controllable with medications. However, we prefer to perform a laser iridotomy because these patients have chronic glaucoma *due to* pupillary block. Without a hole in the iris, an acute attack is possible, progressive PAS often occur and IOP control can become increasingly difficult. Also, without iridotomy, medical therapy must include pilocarpine to guard against acute pupillary blockade. Although pilocarpine is helpful in many eyes, it may produce pupillary block in some, and it is visually debilitating for patients with mild or moderate cataract. Iridotomy improves IOP control and may normalize IOP without medications in some eyes with chronic angle closure[9,11–13].

A second difficult decision in managing chronic angle-closure cases is in those with IOP elevation that is uncontrollable on maximum medical therapy. We prefer to perform a laser iridotomy, and this is followed promptly by filtration surgery if the IOP is not adequately controlled. In a dozen such eyes in recent years, 50 per cent required only iridotomy and use of medications for control of the IOP. The other 50 per cent of cases required filtering surgery despite the iridotomy. It was not possible to predict before or immediately after iridotomy, either from the degree of the anterior chamber angle involved by PAS or from the presence of visual field loss, which eyes would require filtration surgery after iridotomy.

Medically uncontrolled glaucoma without pupillary block

Indications for surgery

Although it is beyond the scope of this chapter to review in detail the pathogenesis of open-angle glaucoma, presumably the system for outflow of aqueous humor in these eyes becomes insufficient during middle or late years of life. The specific anatomical and/or physiological abnormalities that produce this defect and cause excessive IOP elevation are not yet understood. The aim of therapy is to preserve normal visual acuity and the remaining visual field by maintaining the IOP at a low enough level so that it does not damage the optic nerve. This safe level of IOP can vary from patient to patient. In some eyes, statistically high abnormal IOPs can be tolerated for an extended period without optic nerve damage, and in other eyes only a moderate level of IOP elevation can produce damage. Although generally an IOP of 21 mmHg is considered the upper limit of the normal range, in each patient it is essential to make careful observations of the status of the optic disk and visual field, as well as the IOP, to assure preservation of visual function.

The majority of eyes with abnormally elevated IOP that have suffered some visual field loss prior to therapy can be placed in a safe IOP range by medical management, thereby avoiding further field loss. Medical therapy is used until it is determined whether further visual field damage can be prevented. Surgery is needed when progressive optic nerve damage occurs despite maximum tolerated medical treatment.

There are three situations that necessitate filtering surgery.

1. In some patients the IOP cannot be lowered to a safe level despite the simultaneous use of the four types of ocular hypotensive agents: miotics, epinephrine, timolol, and carbonic-anhydrase inhibitors. It is a matter of individual judgment whether echothiophate should also be tried before concluding that medical therapy has failed. Frequently, echothiophate is not accepted by patients and it may hasten cataract development. As newer agents are developed that have an additive effect with the present medications, they will provide additional efficacy and flexibility in medical therapy.
2. Medical treatment fails in some patients because of intolerance or overt allergy to medications that would control IOP if they could be used. Pilocarpine causes a dimming of vision, especially when cataract is present, and can cause induced myopia in younger patients. Either of these side effects can decrease vision too much to justify use of pilocarpine. Epinephrine causes allergic reactions in some treated eyes and may cause cystoid macular edema in aphakic eyes. Carbonic-anhydrase inhibitors can cause a systemic metabolic acidosis that is responsible for a symptom-complex of lethargy, anorexia and paresthesiae. Timolol can potentiate bradycardia, congestive heart failure, asthma or 'dry eye' problems.
3. The largest group of medical-therapy failures are patients who do not comply with therapy but have no demonstrable side effect or allergy. Recent studies with mechanical devices to measure actual eyedrop use indicate that few, if any, patients follow a prescribed four-times-daily regimen. It is difficult for patients to maintain motivation for taking glaucoma medicines whose effect is not to *improve* vision (but rather to prevent further loss) and that also can cause the side effect of decreased vision. Some patients rarely use eyedrops between visits, but restart them just before seeing the ophthalmologist. This may be the most common cause of progressive visual field loss despite apparently normal IOP during therapy. Constant attention to patient compliance is required to achieve the highest level of therapeutic success.

A few patients with consistently high IOP may be considered for surgery despite the absence of progressive visual field damage. When IOP is above 40 mmHg with maximum medical treatment and without a contributing factor that might be expected to improve (e.g. transient uveitis), the level of IOP may be so high that retinal damage is inevitable. In our judgment, eyes with IOP levels above 40 mmHg (and certainly those above 50 mmHg) during treatment are candidates for surgery.

There is controversy over whether filtering surgery without a scleral flap is preferable in patients with lower levels of uncontrolled IOP and in those with so-called 'low-tension glaucoma'. In such cases, some surgeons feel they achieve a lower mean IOP with filtering procedures without a scleral flap, as compared to trabeculectomy in which a scleral flap is used. This will be considered further.

Preoperative evaluation

Progressive optic nerve damage is the most important indication for surgery, and therefore observation of the optic disc through a dilated pupil and also quantitative visual field studies are performed. If filtering surgery or other operations have been performed before, it is best to avoid areas of conjunctival scarring during the next operation, and these areas are detected by slit-lamp examination. The anterior chamber angle is examined by gonioscopy to detect abnormalities that should be avoided during surgery.

Surgery is delayed if active infection of the lids, lashes or lacrimal drainage apparatus is suspected because filtration surgery may be followed by intraocular penetration of bacteria resulting in endophthalmitis. If the IOP is markedly elevated despite medical therapy, it is best to lower it with osmotic agents before surgery to minimize the sudden drop in pressure when opening the globe. Topical steroids are given the day before surgery every 2 hours while the patient is awake to achieve a high steroid level at the time of the operation so as to reduce the inflammatory response.

Anesthesia

Retrobulbar anesthesia with a 1:1 mixture of 2 per cent lidocaine (lignocaine) and 0.75 per cent bupivacaine is preferred. In addition, topical tetracaine (amethocaine) is sometimes useful in providing anesthesia during closure of the conjunctival incision.

Operative techniques

Since the start of this century it has been known that a penetrating hole at the limbus, under a conjunctival flap, can produce a long-term lowering of the IOP by allowing filtration of aqueous into the subconjunctival space. Several procedures of this type will be considered. They differ chiefly in the manner of producing the limbal hole. In the trabeculectomy technique the hole is made under a scleral flap. A scleral flap is not used in the other filtering procedures.

Trabeculectomy

After drawing the conjunctiva anteriorly with smooth forceps, a stay suture of 4/0 black silk is placed under the superior rectus muscle. If the conjunctiva is not held anteriorly, less conjunctival tissue is available for production of a bleb. The eye is then turned so that the operation is centered either superonasally or superotemporally. The former location is preferred for a first operation. This leaves the other superior quadrant unscarred in case a second operation is necessary.

The conjunctiva and Tenon's capsule are grasped with forceps at least 7 mm posterior to the limbus and are incised with scissors until episcleral tissue is reached. Scissors are inserted through the incision, and blunt dissection is done beneath Tenon's capsule throughout the extent of the proposed bleb. The incision in conjunctiva and Tenon's capsule is extended parallel to the limbus for at least 3 clock-hours. The conjunctival flap is handled only with blunt instruments or sponges to avoid causing a hole in the flap (*Figure 7.9a–c*).

The conjunctival flap is dissected anteriorly to expose the area where the gray limbus meets the clear cornea. This dissection is completed with a sharp, rounded blade (*Figure 7.9d*). The conjunctival flap is pulled down over the cornea, so that the flap retracts as each cut is made. Wet-Field cautery is applied to any bleeding episcleral vessels and to the area to be incised for the scleral flap. No cautery is applied to the conjunctival flap.

A razor blade knife is used to make incisions that are two-thirds the scleral thickness, in the desired shape for the scleral flap (*Figure 7.9e*). The flap may be square, triangular or round. The incisions begin just behind the conjunctival flap and extend posteriorly for 3–4 mm. The scleral flap should be at least 3 mm wide at its base. Flaps larger than 4–5 mm have no advantage.

One corner of the scleral flap is grasped with toothed forceps, and a blade is passed under the corner to begin a plane of dissection at a level of one-half of the scleral thickness (*Figure 7.9f*). The dissecting knife is moved side-to-side to establish the plane as the scleral flap is lifted upward. The dissection is extended anteriorly, and the color of the bed turns from white to gray as the limbus is crossed. This indicates the location of the scleral spur which is the posterior limit of the tissue to be excised. At the scleral spur, the angle of dissection is directed farther anteriorly because the corneal curvature is steeper. This avoids premature entry into the anterior chamber. Dissection is stopped when clear corneal tissue is reached, and the sides of the flap can be extended with Vannas scissors (*Figure 7.9g*).

Later, near the end of the operation, it will be helpful to re-form the anterior chamber. This is done most easily through a preplaced peripheral corneal puncture site which is made at this time, while the anterior chamber is still formed and the eye is firm. To stabilize the globe the conjunctiva is grasped at some point other than the location of the future bleb. Sterile fluorescein solution is placed on the tip of the knife blade before entering the anterior chamber, to mark the site of the corneal perforation for later identification. The puncture is made parallel to the iris plane (*Figure 7.9h*). If the IOP is high, decompression of the anterior chamber should be performed slowly.

The scleral flap is then grasped, and the anterior chamber is entered with a razor blade under the most anterior part of the flap. This incision is made from near one side of the bed to the other (*Figure 7.9i*), and care is taken to avoid lens damage because the lens and iris may move anteriorly as aqueous is lost from the anterior chamber. The assistant retracts the scleral flap, and the surgeon grasps the posterior margin of the anterior chamber incision. A razor blade is used to cut posteriorly to the scleral spur, and the deep tissue block is excised (*Figure 7.9j,k*). Extending the incision further posterior than the scleral spur risks damage to the iris root and ciliary body that may cause bleeding.

Usually the peripheral iris prolapses spontaneously through the incision at this time. If it does not, there may

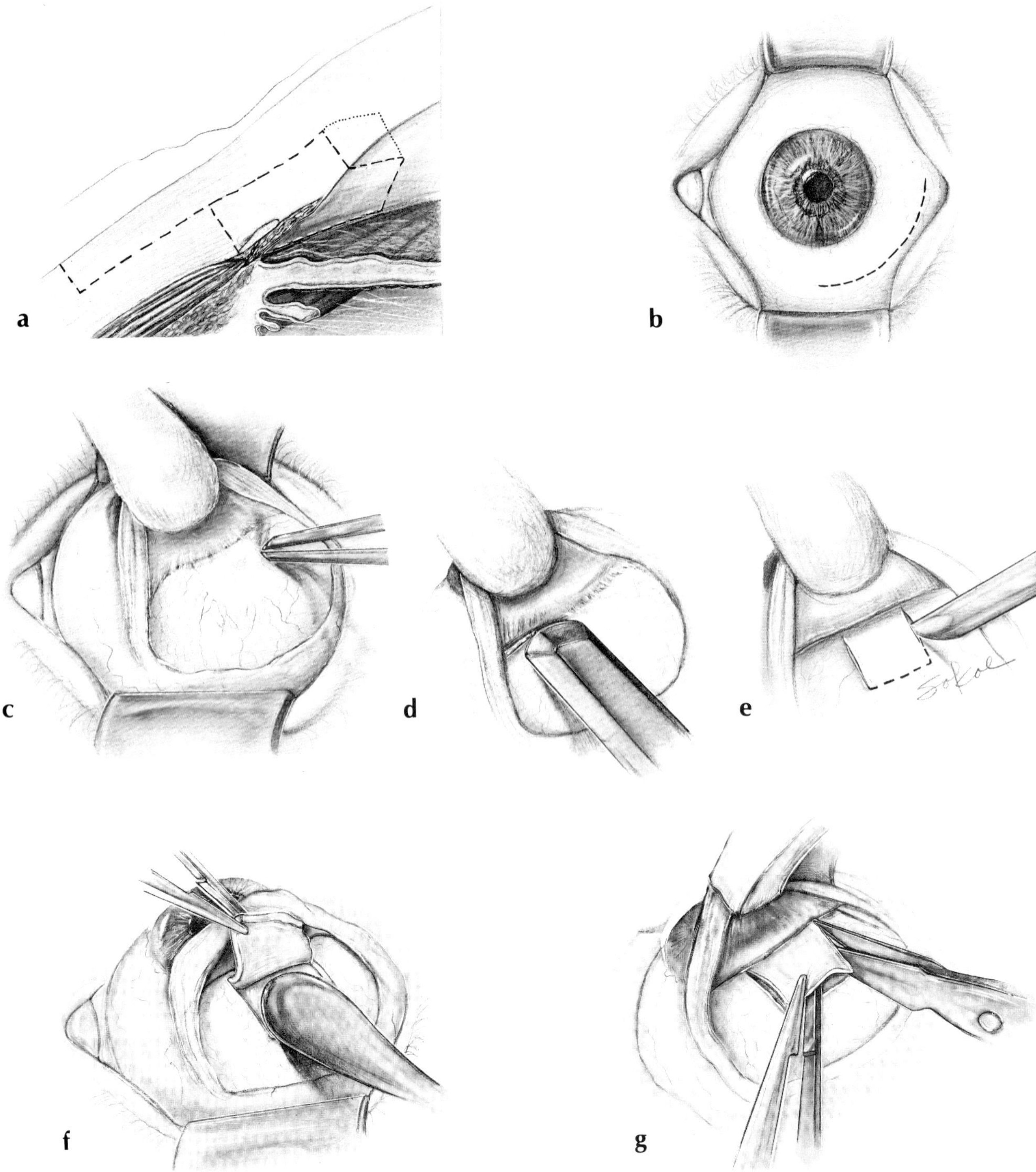

Figure 7.9 *Trabeculectomy technique.* **(a)** *Dotted lines indicate position of scleral flap and zone of trabecular tissue that will be excised.* **(b)** *Conjunctival incision is made 6–7 mm posterior to the limbus in the upper nasal or temporal quadrant.* **(c)** *The cut edge of conjunctiva is retracted with a wet cotton-tipped applicator, and cautery is applied to the episclera to seal bleeding vessels.* **(d)** *Attachments of conjunctiva to the limbus are cut with a Beaver blade.* **(e)** *A limbus-based scleral flap, 3 mm square, is made with a razor blade knife to two-thirds the scleral depth.* **(f)** *Scleral flap dissection is performed with a Gill knife or similar angled blade, and* **(g)** *further anterior extension of the sides of the scleral flap can be done with Vannas scissors.* **(h)** *A shelved puncture incision is made through peripheral clear cornea elsewhere with a Ziegler knife so that the anterior chamber can be re-formed at the end of the operation.* **(i–k)** *The trabeculum is excised with a razor blade knife and scissors and* **(l)** *an iridectomy is performed.* **(m)** *The opening is inspected and ciliary processes and the zonule can often be seen.* **(n)** *Two 10/0 sutures are placed at the corners of the scleral flap, the anterior chamber is re-formed through the corneal-puncture incision, and the amount of leakage is evaluated.* **(o)** *If the anterior chamber does not remain formed for 30 seconds, further sutures are placed in the scleral flap.* **(p)** *The conjunctiva is closed with a running, locked 8/0 collagen suture*

be trabecular tissue remaining, and this may appear as a transparent film. Any such remaining tissue must be excised, for otherwise there will be only a slit-like opening into the anterior chamber. An iridectomy is done to remove iris tissue from the internal limbal opening (*Figure 7.9l,m*) while avoiding excessive traction on the iris that might cause a cyclodialysis or bleeding. After the iridectomy, there is often some bleeding from the iris base, which is stopped with anterior chamber Wet-Field cautery.

Excision of the deep tissue block is difficult in some eyes, such as those with PAS and especially in those with anterior chamber angle neovascularization. In such cases, the conjunctival and scleral flaps are dissected farther anteriorly, to allow greater ease in removing the trabeculum and iris tissue. Also, more bleeding occurs in such eyes, although this rarely requires use of a large amount of cautery. In eyes with high myopia or buphthalmos, the sclera is frequently thinner than normal, and the thickness of the scleral flap should be reduced accordingly, so that the dissection will not damage the ciliary body or enter the anterior chamber prematurely.

The scleral flap is repositioned and sutured at the two posterior corners with single 10/0 nylon sutures, so that the flap is held lightly against the underlying bed (*Figure 7.9n*). The anterior chamber is re-formed through the previously made knife puncture using a 30 gauge cannula. As the anterior chamber deepens, cellulose sponges are placed at the edges of the scleral flap to judge the rate of fluid flow from the eye. If the fluid flows too rapidly and if the anterior chamber flattens within 30 seconds, the anterior chamber will probably be flat on the first postoperative day. To avoid postoperative flattening of the anterior chamber, the two 10/0 nylon sutures can be replaced and tightened or additional sutures can be placed near the limbus (*Figure 7.9o*). The anterior chamber should remain formed at the end of the operation while there should also be slow leakage of fluid through the edges of the scleral incision.

There is disagreement as to whether excision of subepithelial connective tissue (Tenon's tissue) improves the likelihood of obtaining a functioning bleb. Although such excision decreases the amount of tissue that might cause scarring, the wall of the resulting bleb is often quite thin, and the chance of causing an inadvertent hole in the conjunctival flap is increased. We remove the subepithelial connective tissue only in eyes undergoing reoperation, in the eyes of young patients and in eyes with excessive amounts of thick subepithelial tissue. Removal is done just before closing the conjunctiva. The assistant holds the edges of the conjunctiva to elevate the flap, and the tissue to be removed is grasped, pulled toward the operator and cut with scissors held parallel to the flap. Excision is not needed within 2–3 mm of the limbus where Tenon's capsule is thin.

We use a running, locked 8/0 collagen suture to close the conjunctiva (*Figure 7.9p*). Use of a topical anesthetic, such as tetracaine (amethocaine), may be necessary to prevent pain while closing the incision. The anterior chamber is again re-formed, to be certain that the bleb inflates and the anterior chamber remains at least partially formed. The eye is treated with topical steroid ointment and 1 per cent atropine drops, and a patch and shield are applied.

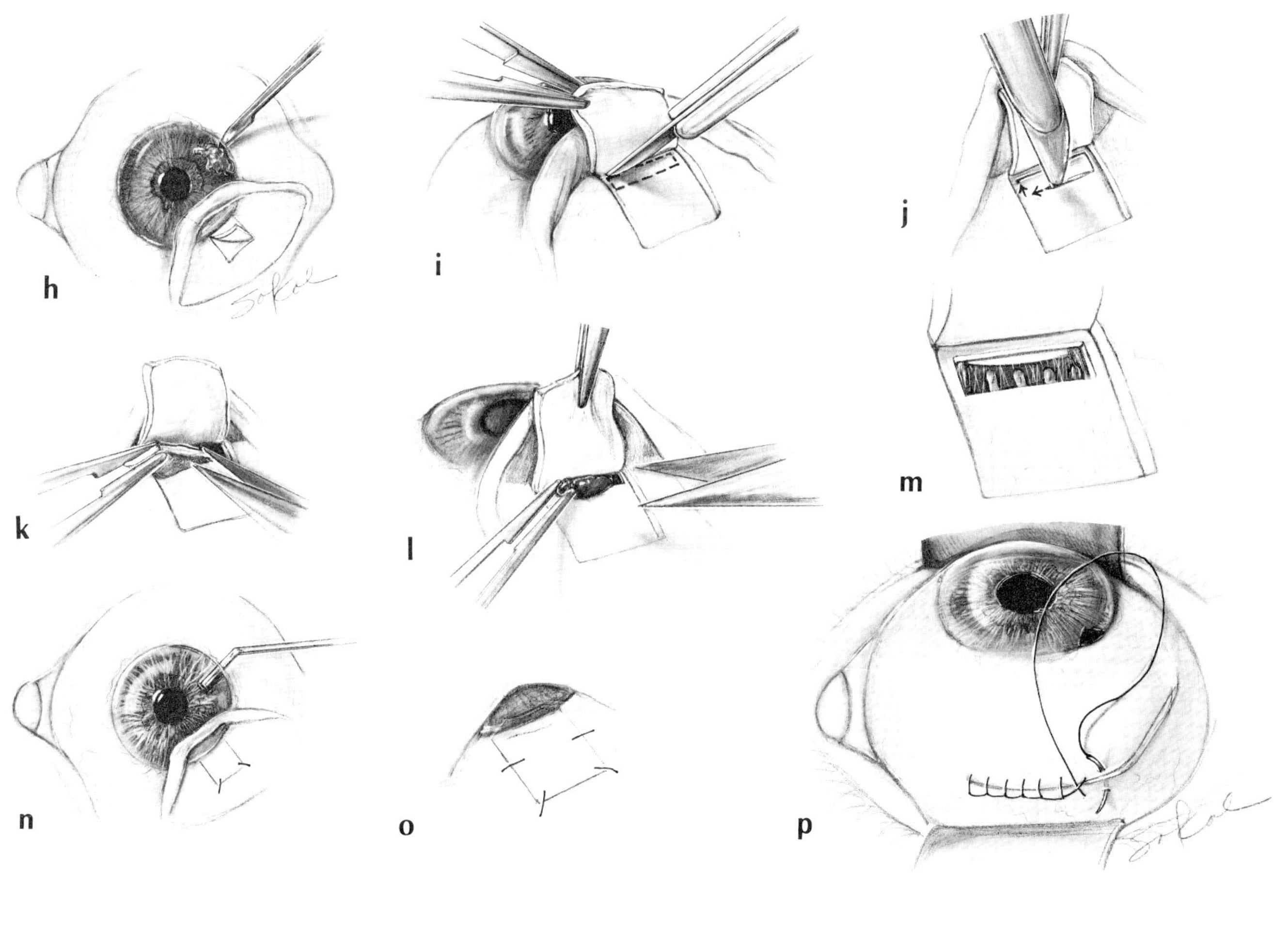

Filter without scleral flap

The conjunctival flap is prepared in the same manner as described for a trabeculectomy. A variation of conjunctival-flap preparation for any filtration procedure is a fornix-based flap. Although it may be easier to perform the operation using this approach, external wound leakage sometimes occurs and requires postoperative resuturing.

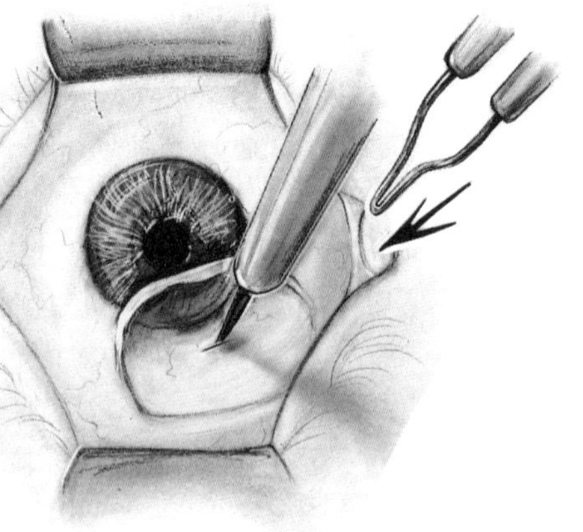

a

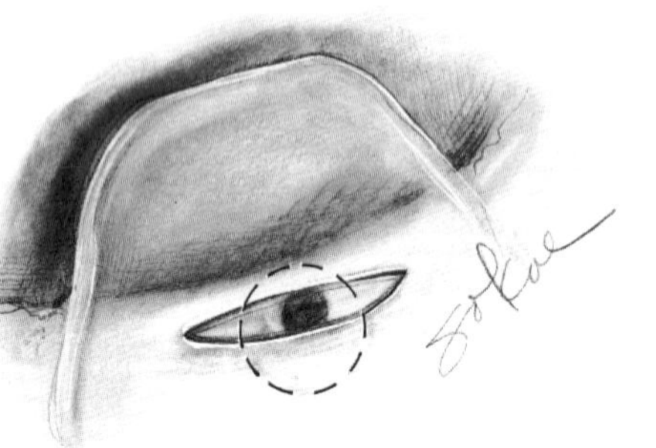

b

Figure 7.10 *Filtering operation without a scleral flap, using a limbus-based conjunctival flap.* **(a)** *For Scheie-type procedure a razor incision is made at the posterior limit of the limbus. Alternating use of cautery and the blade is used to deepen the incision and to enter the anterior chamber.* **(b)** *Position of either a Scheie-type opening or trephine placement (dotted line) is shown*

For the *Scheie-type procedure*, a partially penetrating razor blade incision is made at the posterior limit of the limbus for a depth at least two-thirds of the scleral thickness (*Figure 7.10a*). Cautery is then applied to either or both wound edges until there is outflow of aqueous humor. Alternating use of the razor blade and cautery may facilitate entry into the anterior chamber. Usually there is a spontaneous prolapse of the iris, and an iridectomy is performed.

For a *trephine procedure*, the limbus is cleaned well onto clear cornea. A 1.5 mm trephine is applied anterior to the scleral spur, which is marked by the junction of the white and gray parts of the limbal zone (*Figure 7.10b*). The trephine is used with a rotating motion, to cut at an equal depth all around the incision. A slight 'give' is felt when the anterior chamber is entered and again when the trephine is withdrawn. If one edge of the tissue button remains attached, it is cut free with scissors. The iris usually prolapses, or it can be easily grasped with smooth forceps, and an iridectomy is performed. The conjunctival incision is then closed as in a trabeculectomy, but it is not helpful to reform the chamber in a filtration procedure without a scleral flap.

Postoperative care

Topical 1 per cent steroid drops are begun on the day before surgery. Postoperatively, steroid drops are given every 2 hours from 8 a.m. to 8 p.m., and steroid ointment is applied at bedtime. Atropine 1 per cent drops are used twice daily. The patient is allowed full activity the day after surgery, and discharged on the second day if the anterior chamber is formed. If the anterior chamber is not formed, further inpatient observation is needed. Slit-lamp examination and IOP measurement by applanation tonometry are done each day. Usually the IOP is between 5 and 15 mmHg for the first 2 weeks.

If the IOP is higher than 25 mmHg for 2 consecutive days, gonioscopy is performed to examine the internal opening in the sclera. Blood or iris plugging the hole is sometimes detected. If so, light pressure is applied to the cornea through the lower lid. Often this pressure causes the IOP to drop rapidly and the bleb enlarges. Daily, or more frequent, ocular massage is only occasionally helpful, however, in preserving the function of a filtering procedure, although this can be tried whenever the IOP rises above normal.

Excessive pressure during ocular massage is avoided because this can cause a flat anterior chamber, rupture of the bleb and/or hyphema. If the patient is to massage the eye at home, it is wise to give instructions on how to apply pressure through the lower lid. The lid is pressed for 10 seconds at a time and then released. This is repeated two or three times but stopped if there is severe discomfort. Ocular massage is done first in the office, to determine whether the bleb enlarges and the IOP decreases.

After filtering surgery, it is desirable to have enough aqueous passing through the scleral opening to produce an effective conjunctival bleb. Therefore, drugs that suppress aqueous secretion are discontinued, including acetazolamide and related compounds. If the unoperated fellow eye has glaucoma, this may cause the IOP to rise to a dangerous level. For such a patient, the eye with the higher preoperative IOP is operated on first; and surgery for the second eye, if indicated, is done soon thereafter, usually within 3 days.

Steroid drops are gradually discontinued (tapered) while monitoring the degree of anterior chamber reaction and the redness of the conjunctiva in the area of the bleb. Ordinarily, the drops are decreased to 4 times daily by 1 week after surgery, and discontinued entirely (by stepwise reductions) after 2 months. A shield is taped over the eye each night for 2 weeks to prevent accidental trauma.

Full activity of the patient is possible within 2 weeks, depending on the rapidity of recovery of visual acuity. In some eyes, hypotony leads to decreased vision due to retinal edema. The conjunctival suture causes a mild foreign body sensation for the first few days, but this suture is no longer visible by 3 weeks.

Complications

The two most troublesome problems after filtering surgery are excessive elevation or excessive lowering of the IOP. The problem of failure of filtration with high IOP is discussed below in the 'Results' section. A combination of hypotony, flat anterior chamber and choroidal detachment is the most common serious problem after filtering surgery. Various methods are used to manage this problem. Although many flat anterior chambers re-form spontaneously, some do not and serious damage may occur. Fortunately, use of a scleral flap (trabeculectomy) has markedly decreased the occurrence of flat anterior chambers and the need for re-formation. Fewer than 5 per cent of cases require further surgery to re-form the anterior chamber after trabeculectomy.

The first step in managing an eye with a very shallow or flat anterior chamber postoperatively is to measure the IOP. If it is above 25 mmHg, malignant glaucoma is likely. If the IOP is less than 10 mmHg, causes for hypotony are investigated. Also, IOP measurement may be unreliable in eyes with a flat anterior chamber. Sometimes the IOP measured by applanation tonometry is between 10 and 20 mmHg, but the globe is obviously soft by tactile assessment. Presumably, in such eyes, the lens is so close to the cornea that the cornea and lens make contact during the applanation measurement, accounting for the incorrect higher value.

Hypotony may be caused by direct leakage through a hole in the conjunctiva, a cyclodialysis cleft or a choroidal detachment. A direct leak is detected by placing sterile 2 per cent fluorescein solution on the bleb and observing flow of clear aqueous fluid (Seidel test). Direct leaks are treated by tight patching or by placement of a soft corneal contact lens large enough to cover the hole. Unless other complications are developing because of the low IOP, we wait for spontaneous improvement rather than resuture the wound. If low IOP persists and the anterior chamber is formed, gonioscopy is used to search for a cyclodialysis cleft. These clefts appear as dark areas just posterior to the scleral spur, and they are usually near the iridectomy. Topical cycloplegic treatment may close the cleft by relaxing the ciliary muscle so that the ciliary body lies against the sclera. If this is not effective, the cleft can be closed by laser coagulation applied through a gonioprism or by surgery as described later.

The most common cause of hypotony and a shallow anterior chamber after filtering surgery is a choroidal detachment. It is not known whether hypotony precedes choroidal detachment or vice versa. The sequence probably begins, however, with intraoperative lowering of IOP, followed by partial choroidal detachment. This causes the ciliary body, lens and iris to rotate anteriorly, thereby flattening the anterior chamber. In the opinion of some surgeons, the choroidal detachment causes reduced formation of aqueous humor, perpetuating the low IOP. A low IOP with choroidal detachment may not actually be due to reduced production of aqueous humor. Rather, choroidal detachment may increase the less common routes of aqueous outflow (uveoscleral outflow) via the suprachoroidal space and out through the vortex veins. If aqueous enters the suprachoroidal space this would tend to perpetuate the choroidal detachment, causing the cycle to continue until the situation is altered by natural forces or surgery.

Eyes with a flat anterior chamber, low IOP and no direct leak through the conjunctiva are initially followed without surgery. The pupil is maximally dilated. If the anterior chamber remains flat and there is enlargement of the choroidal detachment, then surgical re-formation of the anterior chamber and drainage of choroidal detachments is done (*see* p. 202). If the choroidal detachment becomes smaller each day, it is unlikely that further surgery will be needed. If the cornea is clear, the eye is quiet and there is enough aqueous humor present so that the lens is not touching the cornea, then we wait as long as 10 days before performing surgery to deepen the anterior chamber. However, if there is striate keratopathy, cornea–lens touch, or an inflamed eye, prompt intervention is indicated.

Other complications of filtering surgery can include cataract development, hyphema, infection and reduced vision. As discussed regarding iridectomy, eyes undergoing filtering surgery are sometimes predisposed to cataract for reasons other than the glaucoma surgery. However, manipulations associated with the operation, postoperative hypotony and use of topical steroids can also contribute to progression of lens opacities. The incidence of decreased vision after filtration surgery varies, but 10–25 per cent of eyes lose two or more Snellen lines of visual acuity within 2 years after surgery.

Although trabeculectomy has reduced the incidence of postoperative flat anterior chambers, and although this might lessen the development of cataract, there is no definite evidence that use of a scleral flap during filtering surgery has improved the visual results.

Mild hyphemas occur often after trabeculectomy, but less frequently than after filtering procedures without a scleral flap. A hyphema is seldom a major problem, and the blood clears spontaneously in most cases. If a filtering operation is done inferiorly because of past surgery on the superior limbus, hyphema can occlude the internal opening of the scleral defect, and the patient must be positioned to avoid such obstruction.

Endophthalmitis soon after filtering surgery probably occurs less often than after cataract surgery, but the exact incidence has not been established. A special problem after filtering surgery, however, is late endophthalmitis. This may result from relatively easy access of bacteria to the anterior chamber through the thin wall of the conjunctival bleb and the scleral opening. Both trabeculectomy and filtering procedures without a scleral flap have about a 1 per cent incidence of late endophthalmitis. Patients with a filtering bleb are reminded that redness, pain and/or decreased vision require immediate examination because of possible infection.

Results

Glaucoma therapy is considered to be successful when no further optic nerve damage occurs. Yet the majority of reports of surgery give only the IOP lowering effect[14–19]. Although in most eyes return of the IOP to the normal range assures stable vision, it is preferable to judge the success of filtering surgery on stability of the visual acuity and visual field as well as on normalization of the IOP. In some eyes with a seemingly successful trabeculectomy and good postoperative IOP, there is progressive visual field loss postoperatively[20]. This may be due to fluctuations in the IOP that are characteristic of glaucoma and are not entirely eliminated by filtering surgery. Therefore, patients with normal postoperative IOP still require periodic evaluation of the optic disc and visual field testing.

The reported success rates of filtering surgery, as judged by postoperative IOP levels of 21 mmHg or less, vary from better than 95 per cent to less than 50 per cent. The highest success rates have been reported from Europe, where surgery is often done after a less vigorous attempt to control the IOP medically. Thus, European results may include more eyes with less severe glaucoma. Studies from university centers in the United States indicate that, in eyes without IOP control using maximum tolerated medical therapy, the success rate is 75–80 per cent as determined 1–2 years after surgery. Of the successful surgical cases, at least one-third require continued use of medications for control of the IOP.

The success rates of trabeculectomy using a scleral flap and of other types of filtering procedures are quite similar. Comparisons of the two types of operations in consecutive or alternate case studies have found that the rate of successful IOP control is similar[21–23]. In some series, the mean postoperative IOP level is comparatively lower after filtering procedures without a scleral flap, although other series find the same mean IOP results. There is a lower incidence of postoperative shallow or flat anterior chambers and a reduced need for surgical re-formation of the anterior chamber after trabeculectomy. The long-term comparative results as to whether there are fewer progressive cataracts and better visual results have not been established, however.

The conjunctival bleb after trabeculectomy tends to be flatter and broader than with other types of filtration procedures. A reliable sign of filtration in eyes with a low, diffuse bleb is a fine microcystic appearance of the conjunctiva which is seen best by retroillumination using a thin slit-lamp beam. The microcystic spaces have the appearance of oil droplets. They are about the diameter of large episcleral vessels and correspond histologically to channels within the connective tissue through which aqueous humor flows from the eye.

Several factors influence the success of filtering surgery regardless of the procedure chosen. Since the operation depends on imperfect tissue healing to allow long-term drainage of aqueous, any factor that increases local scarring lowers the success rate. Thus, young persons have a lower success rate than elderly patients. Among patients in the seventh or eighth decade, 80–90 per cent of filtering procedures are successful; but in the teenage or younger group, long-term filtering success is rare. Also, in eyes with previous surgery on the conjunctiva, successful filtering procedures are less likely, and this is also true of eyes with prior inflammatory disease or active anterior segment neovascularization.

The success rate of filtering surgery may be increased by efforts to minimize formation of new connective tissue in the subepithelial conjunctiva. Corticosteroids hinder formation of new connective tissue by fibroblasts, and this is the rationale for use of steroids during and after filtering surgery. There have not been controlled studies evaluating the effect of steroid use, however. Although topical steroids are commonly used during the postoperative period, systemic or periocular 'depot' steroid injections are reserved for eyes with a high risk of failure.

In some eyes there is an IOP rise into the 20–35 mmHg range at 4–6 weeks after trabeculectomy. This may be a response to use of topical steroids, or the IOP rise may occur because aqueous humor formation returns to normal before the conjunctival bleb is capable of handling the increased flow. In many eyes the IOP decreases again below 20 mmHg without requiring long-term use of hypotensive agents.

A small percentage of successful filtering blebs cease to function after 1 or more years. Although late failures are infrequent, all patients must be followed up indefinitely by optic disc and visual field examinations as well as measurement of the IOP.

Reoperation

If the IOP becomes elevated again and medical therapy fails to achieve control, a second filtration procedure is indicated. Since the previously operated site is likely to have considerable conjunctival scarring, the nonoperated superior quadrant is preferred for repeat surgery. Rarely, if bleb failure is recent, separation of the conjunctiva from the episclera by knife dissection may salvage the prior procedure. Also, passing a needle across the anterior chamber and through the internal scleral opening, or treating the internal part of the scleral defect with laser energy delivered through a gonioprism, may salvage the bleb in rare cases.

When a second filtration procedure is attempted, some surgeons switch from trabeculectomy to other types of operations. Others add resection of Tenon's tissue, systemic steroid therapy, or leave the scleral flap loose at the end of the second operation. Although such changes seem appropriate, none is of proven value, and the success rate for a second filtering procedure is considerably less than for first operations. It is possible to achieve control of the IOP with a second filtering procedure, however, and this attempt is preferable to permitting the IOP to remain uncontrolled or to alternative procedures now available. After two failed filtration procedures, cyclocryotherapy may be tried.

Filters with setons or artificial materials

Various methods have been tried that utilize artificial materials in filtering surgery to hold the drainage channel open and/or to control the rate of fluid outflow. Previously, these attempts did not increase the success rate of standard glaucoma surgery. Artificial materials placed at or near the limbus erode through the conjunctiva and may increase scarring because of the foreign-body reaction. Furthermore, most failures after filtering procedures are due to scarring in the subconjunctival tissues and not to closure of the scleral drainage channel. Clinical trials are needed to compare surgery using artificial materials versus conventional methods.

Laser trabeculoplasty as an alternative to filtering surgery

Introduction

In the last 10 years, a number of investigators have applied laser energy to the trabecular meshwork to treat glaucoma[24–26]. Favorable results have been obtained in some otherwise uncontrolled patients. The mechanism by which laser trabeculoplasty lowers the IOP is unclear. Histological studies indicate that permanent holes are not made in the trabecular meshwork; instead, laser treatment causes localized zones of scarring. The procedure will undoubtedly evolve further in the future, and optimal parameters of laser energy will be determined. No long-term results of treating large numbers of patients are yet available. This section presents our current approach and experience.

Preoperative evaluation

A complete eye examination is done, with particular attention to gonioscopy. The anterior chamber angle 'approach' must be wide enough to permit a good view of the filtering meshwork structures. The degree of pigmentation is important in choosing laser energy levels. If a few PAS are present, these areas are avoided during laser treatment. If most of the angle is covered by PAS, laser trabeculoplasty is probably futile.

Treatment technique

Treatment is done after topical anesthesia, and a drop of topical steroid is applied to minimize later inflammation. Either the argon blue-green or the krypton red laser can be used. We prefer the one-mirror Goldmann-type goniolens. The lens has a coated anterior surface to reduce the possibility of laser beam reflection that might damage the eye of an observer.

The most important aspect of treatment is precise aiming of the laser beam. The aiming beam is focused using the smallest spot size and checking to see that it appears round, not ovoid. Treatment is begun only when both the view of the angle structures and focus of the laser are perfect, because the desired effect of treatment requires a high density of energy. Eyes with cloudy media are impossible to treat. Patients with nystagmus or those who cannot hold still require retrobulbar anesthesia.

The laser is aimed at the junction between the pigmented and non-pigmented trabecular meshwork. In eyes with heavy pigmentation, there may be a pigmented trabecular band between Schwalbe's line (anteriorly) and the scleral spur (posteriorly). In such eyes we treat the anterior edge of the pigmented trabecular band. A 50 μm spot size is used and is aimed to 'bridge' this junction of non-pigmented and pigmented tissue. In eyes with little or no pigment in this area, we intend to treat that same location, but the landmarks are less certain. Even in lightly pigmented eyes, however, the more-posterior zone often looks grey as compared to the white anterior meshwork. There has been no clear evidence, as yet, that this is the ideal zone to treat, but more-posterior treatment seems to cause higher IOP pressure elevations afterward.

Viewing is best at a magnification between 16× and 40× with the slit-lamp delivery system. We use 50 μm spot size and 0.1 second burn duration. The power setting, however, is different for different eyes, and must be changed during therapy in the same eye. The laser energy is probably absorbed mainly by melanin, and the amount of melanin varies from eye to eye. Also, the inferior anterior chamber angle is usually more pigmented than the superior angle and so the power setting must be changed when treating different parts of the angle. In a lightly pigmented eye initial treatment is begun with about 750 mW, and in heavily pigmented eyes a setting of 300–500 mW is used. The objective is to produce a visible effect without causing large bubbles due to focal tissue explosion. If no effect is seen after the first two shots, the power is increased in steps of 100–200 mW until a visible effect is noted. Rarely, power settings as high as 1.5 W are needed. In lightly pigmented eyes a whitening of the tissue is seen, whereas in heavily pigmented angles there is pigment dispersion after each application. If bubbles larger than the 50 μm aiming beam occur, the power setting is reduced.

About 100 burns are applied evenly spaced around the 360° of the anterior chamber angle. To judge the proper spacing between burns, after a 50 μm spot is applied one should skip four or five widths of the aiming beam before the next application. After finishing the first quadrant, the number of burns is counted and should be about 25. In eyes with markedly elevated IOP, and those with visual field loss threatening fixation, only 180° of the angle is treated during each session. This seems to minimize the chance of developing high IOP after treatment.

In eyes with a narrow anterior chamber angle, laser trabeculoplasty may be difficult. If the view is not adequate for treatment, then the base of the iris can be treated first using low-energy, 100 μm size, 0.1 second burns. Often this bows the iris backward, thereby improving the view and permitting treatment of the trabecular meshwork.

Postoperative care

Unless there is a corneal abrasion, no patch is necessary. Topical steroid drops are used every 6 hours for 1 week. All prior glaucoma medications are continued during the immediate post-treatment period. The IOP is measured 3 hours after treatment and again after 24 hours, 1 week, and 2–4 weeks.

Results and complications

After laser trabeculoplasty, the majority of patients have a beneficial response with lowering of the IOP. Some patients achieve a sufficient response so that some or all of the glaucoma medications can be stopped. These medications are not discontinued for 1–2 months after treatment, during which time the response of the IOP to the laser treatment is determined.

About 20 per cent of patients have no significant lowering of the IOP after laser trabeculoplasty. Also, in a few eyes the IOP is temporarily or permanently higher after treatment. High IOP pressure 10 mmHg or more greater than the pretreatment IOP can occur, and therefore the IOP must be periodically measured after treatment. Since laser trabeculoplasty is reserved for eyes that cannot be controlled medically, filtering surgery is necessary if trabeculoplasty does not produce a favorable response or if the IOP is higher after treatment. We do not know the likelihood of late elevation of the IOP in patients with an initially successful trabeculoplasty.

In patients with primary open-angle glaucoma, laser trabeculoplasty lowers the IOP an average of 7–9 mmHg in about 75 per cent of eyes. The effect of lowering the IOP is sustained in most eyes for at least 1 year. Therefore the need for filtration surgery can be avoided or delayed in 75 per cent of eyes, although nearly all patients continue to require medical therapy. The medication required may decrease, and sometimes it is possible to stop carbonic-anhydrase inhibitors or miotics. In some eyes, treatment of only 180° of the anterior chamber angle lowers the pressure enough so it is not necessary to treat the remainder of the angle.

Patients with secondary glaucoma or those who have had filtering surgery previously respond less well. Eyes that have had one laser trabeculoplasty treatment and are re-treated have a reduced chance of further lowering of the IOP. As yet, there are no long-term studies of the visual fields after laser trabeculoplasty.

Medically uncontrolled glaucoma without pupillary block: cyclocryotherapy

Indications and pathophysiology

Cyclocrytherapy has a destructive effect on ocular tissues and is therefore reserved for eyes that are unmanageable by other means. This includes eyes with repeated failures after filtration surgery or those in which the chance of successful filtration surgery is so low that it should not be tried. The latter category includes many eyes with secondary glaucoma, such as some cases with neovascular glaucoma or elevated pressure due to inflammation or epithelial ingrowth. Cases of infantile glaucoma in which goniotomy or trabeculotomy fail to control the pressure may also be treated by cyclocryotherapy. Cryotherapy is also useful in eyes with elevated IOP that require penetrating keratoplasty[27].

The aim of cyclocryotherapy is to decrease aqueous humor production (inflow) by destroying part of the pars plicata of the ciliary body. Experimental work in lower animals and early clinical trials demonstrated the general feasibility of damaging the pars plicata by cryo-applications[28–34]. More recently, there have been experiments in primates[35–36] and histopathological study of human eyes after cyclocryotherapy[35,37].

Experimental data using an internal electronic temperature-measuring probe indicate that with an external freezing-probe temperature of −60 °C to −80 °C, the lowest temperature obtained at the ciliary-body pars plicata is only −10 °C[35]. With external temperatures lower than −100 °C, it is possible to reach lower internal temperatures but this causes severe damage to the ocular tissues[33]. In enucleated eyes the internal ciliary body temperature is lower during external cryotreatment than in clinical application[35]. This indicates that the uveal blood flow is the main factor preventing marked freezing of the ciliary body.

The time needed for the pars plicata to reach the minimum-effective internal temperature is about 20 seconds[35]. Therefore, it may be more effective to maintain each application for 60 seconds rather than applying two applications of 30 seconds each. The extent of treatment needed can also be judged from experimental data. When 180° of the ciliary body is treated in monkey eyes, the untreated portion remains relatively normal and normal IOP is maintained. However, when a 360° portion is treated there is severe persistent hypotony[36,38] and the likelihood of anterior segment ischemia and phthisis bulbi is increased.

A retinal cryoprobe of 2–3 mm diameter is used for cyclocryotherapy, and it is placed 2–3 mm posterior to the visible limbus. Placing the probe farther posterior fails to treat the pars plicata effectively[37]. In monkey eyes the histological effect of a freeze of 60 seconds duration using a 2 mm diameter probe extends posterior to the ora serrata. Larger probes probably achieve no greater effect on the pars plicata and only unnecessarily damage more retinal and choroidal tissue.

Operative technique

Retrobulbar anesthesia is ideal for cyclocryotherapy. This can be combined with systemic sedation if the patient is apprehensive. The procedure can be done on an outpatient basis, but we often hospitalize the patient overnight after treatment because there may be moderate pain requiring narcotic analgesics. Also, hospitalization is needed if heavy sedation is used. Severe postoperative discomfort can be minimized by use of a mixture of short-acting and long-acting retrobulbar anesthetic agents, such as a 1:1 mixture of 2 per cent lidocaine (lignocaine) and 0.75 per cent bupivacaine.

Because of the factors discussed above, there is inherent variability in the effect of cyclocryotherapy; and no single method is applicable for every eye. The greatest danger is an excessive response – with hypotony, anterior segment ischemia and phthisis bulbi. Therefore, cyclocryotherapy is done as a staged procedure, and more than one treatment is often necessary before the desired IOP level is reached.

We treat only 180° of the circumference of the globe at one time, usually with 8 applications. The conjunctiva is dried, and the probe is centered 2–3 mm posterior to the limbus (*Figure 7.11a*). Transillumination can be used if the location of the ciliary body is in doubt (*Figure 7.11b*). The 2 mm diameter probe is cooled to between −60 °C and −80 °C, and each application is maintained for 60 seconds after a temperature of −60 °C is reached. The probe is allowed to thaw free from the conjunctiva before being moved.

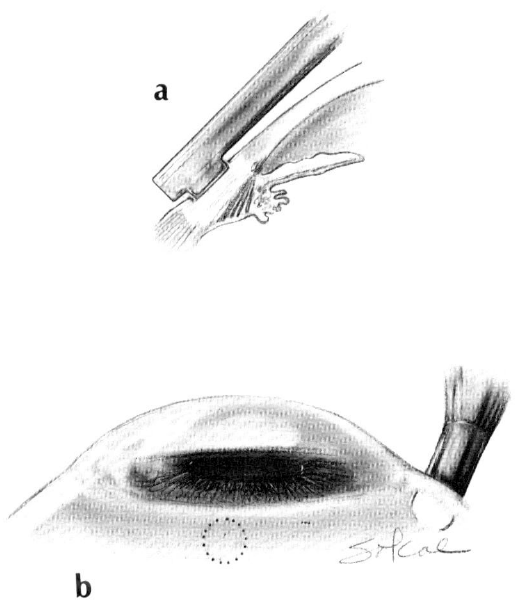

Figure 7.11 *Cyclocryotherapy.* **(a)** *Cryoprobe is centered over the pars plicata of the ciliary body. Firm pressure on a dry surface indents the sclera.* **(b)** *To ensure proper localization of the probe, transillumination can be done to identify the zone of the ciliary body before applying the cryoprobe*

Postoperative care

During the first week after treatment, the IOP can remain high or become elevated further. This is probably a result of inflammation and obstruction of the trabecular meshwork by debris and red blood cells. Frequent topical steroid drops and cycloplegics are used to treat the inflammation.

In eyes with profound visual loss in which the purpose of cyclocryotherapy is to decrease the IOP in order to relieve discomfort, a 2 ml retrobulbar injection of 50 per cent ethanol can be made at the time of the procedure[39]. This is usually effective in relieving ocular pain, although it may be followed by persistent ptosis.

If the IOP is not decreased after 1–2 months of follow-up, the treatment is repeated. When retreatment is done there is an increased chance of causing phthisis bulbi. The second treatment is done in a fashion identical to the first. A 180° portion of the circumference of the eye is treated, overlapping 90° of the previously treated part of the ciliary body and treating 90° that was not treated before.

Complications

Hyphema is common during the immediate postoperative period. Bleeding probably occurs from ruptured capillaries of the ciliary pars plicata. This complication is unavoidable, although the anterior chamber blood usually clears in 1–2 weeks. About 5 per cent of eyes may have persistent blood in the vitreous cavity[40,41].

The most serious complication after cyclocryotherapy is severe persistent hypotony leading to phthisis bulbi. The incidence of persistent IOP of less than 10 mmHg varies from 0 to 30 per cent[40,42–44]. Treatment of the entire circumference of the ciliary body at one time is very likely to cause hypotony and phthisis[38]. Choroidal detachment associated with hypotony occurs in some eyes after cyclocryotherapy[27,44]. In these cases vigorous treatment with topical, subconjunctival, and/or systemic steroids may help achieve IOP normalization.

Cryotherapy can damage all of the anterior structures of the eye. Iris atrophy, accelerated cataract development and persistent corneal opacity sometimes occur. There is usually a long-lasting aqueous flare due to damage to the blood–aqueous barrier. This alteration of the blood–aqueous barrier cannot be eliminated by topical steroid treatment. Steroid use is discontinued after cellular inflammation in the aqueous humor has subsided.

Follow-up studies indicate that light perception is eventually lost in many eyes after cyclocryotherapy[42,43]. This is partly due to the severity of the ocular conditions being treated. If the pressure can be controlled, however, cyclocryotherapy affords the best chance for maintaining useful vision in these desperate cases.

Results

The results of cyclocryotherapy are difficult to judge because a variety of techniques has been used to treat a diverse group of conditions. The IOP can probably be reduced to less than 20 mmHg in 50–75 per cent of eyes with otherwise uncontrolled glaucoma[27,41–45]. Up to 50 per cent of patients require more than one treatment before adequate control is achieved. Lack of permanent pressure control is probably due to inadequate destruction of pars plicata tissue rather than regeneration of normal ciliary body structure[35].

Improved use of cyclotherapy might be possible if one could judge accurately the capacity of aqueous inflow in the eye to be treated. This would allow more precise planning of the amount of treatment necessary for pressure control.

Combined cataract and glaucoma

Indications

Simultaneous glaucoma and cataract surgery should be performed in eyes with functionally inadequate visual acuity because of lens opacity in association with optic nerve damage from uncontrolled IOP on the maximum tolerated glaucoma medications. Often, however, the clinical indications are less certain. Some eyes with progressive glaucomatous damage and uncontrolled IOP have early or moderate cataract changes decreasing the visual acuity to 20/40 or 20/50. In such eyes, the lens opacity may progress rapidly after uncomplicated filtration surgery, and later cataract surgery might cause the prior filtering operation to fail. In such cases it may be best to wait, if the glaucomatous damage is not progressing rapidly. Then the natural course of the cataract can be better assessed. If vision is being rapidly lost because of progressive lens opacity, then a combined cataract extraction and filtration procedure is preferred.

In other eyes, there is an advanced cataract requiring surgery and also glaucoma that *is* controlled medically. In such eyes, combining filtering surgery with cataract extraction may also be desirable. This reduces the need for medical therapy and reduces the side-effects of medical therapy such as topical epinephrine (adrenaline) drops that can cause cystoid macular edema in aphakic eyes. There are no confirmed clinical data to support the belief that cataract surgery alone has a significant and long-lasting beneficial effect on glaucoma management[46,47]. While the IOP may be lower for several months after cataract extraction, this seems to be due to transient reduction in aqueous formation.

Operative technique

Trabeculectomy combined with intracapsular cataract surgery has been our procedure of choice in the past. Recently, however, combined extracapsular lens extraction (using phacoemulsification or non-ultrasonic

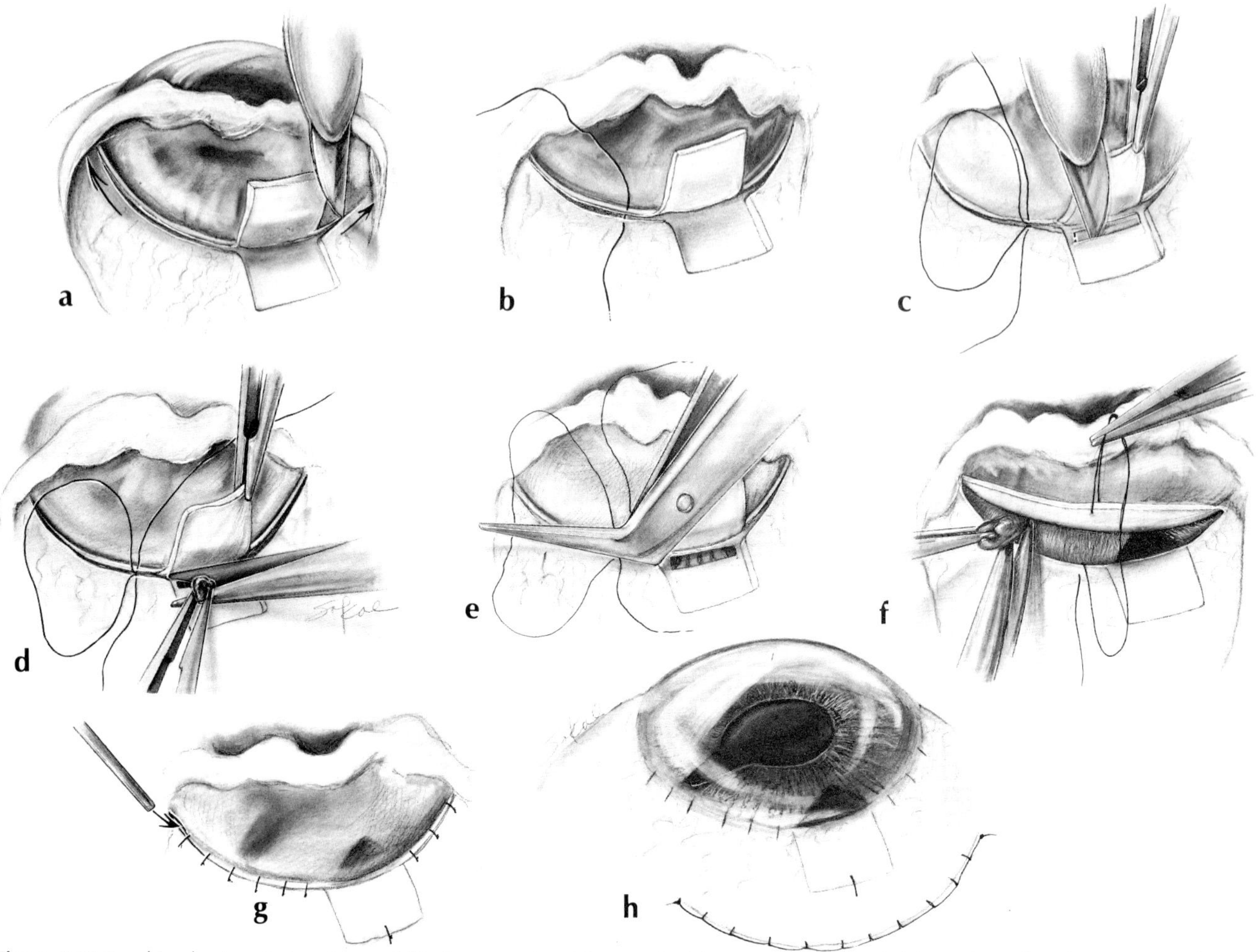

Figure 7.12 *Combined cataract extraction and filtering operation.* **(a)** *Conjunctival and scleral flaps are prepared as in trabeculectomy, and scleral flap is placed either temporal or nasal to the 12 o'clock meridian. A partially penetrating corneoscleral groove is then made, extending from either side of the scleral flap.* **(b–d)** *One preplaced 9/0 silk suture is placed at the 12 o'clock meridian, the trabeculectomy excision is completed and an iridectomy is done.* **(e)** *The limbal incisions are then extended from the trabeculectomy site.* **(f)** *If the pupil will not dilate, a sector iridectomy is performed on the side opposite the scleral flap.* **(g)** *The lens is extracted with a cryoprobe, and the preplaced suture is tied. Interrupted 10/0 nylon sutures are placed to achieve watertight wound closure, and one or two sutures are placed in the scleral flap.* **(h)** *The conjunctiva is closed with a running 8/0 collagen suture*

methods) and trabeculectomy has been used, and this offers certain advantages. Maintaining an intact posterior lens capsule prevents vitreous from entering the internal opening of the filtration tract. Remaining cortical lens material has not obstructed the filtration opening in our experience or caused additional inflammation that has been a problem. We illustrate the combination of intracapsular surgery and trabeculectomy, but the 'combined' technique can also be used with extracapsular surgery.

When performing combined trabeculectomy and cataract surgery, a limbus-based conjunctival flap is used. The conjunctival flap is started 6–8 mm posterior to the limbus. After dissecting the conjunctiva to the limbus, a square limbus-based scleral flap measuring 3 mm by 3 mm is prepared with a razor blade and Gill knife. This scleral flap is placed on either the nasal or temporal side of the 12 o'clock meridian. A one-half to two-thirds depth corneoscleral groove is then made with a razor blade for about 120° total extent, beginning at the anterior edges of the scleral flap (*Figure 7.12a*). A single-armed suture of 9/0 silk is preplaced in the vertical meridian, and the suture is looped out of the wound (*Figure 7.12b*). The anterior chamber is entered at the anteriormost portion of the bed of the scleral flap, and the tissue under the flap excised back to scleral spur (*Figure 7.12c*). A peripheral iridectomy is performed (*Figure 7.12d*). Alternatively, the tissue excision and iridectomy can be done after the lens extraction.

The corneoscleral incision is extended from the scleral flap nasally and temporally with straight corneoscleral scissors (*Figure 7.12e*). If the pupil is not sufficiently dilated, a sector iridectomy is performed in the superior quadrant opposite the trabeculectomy site (*Figure 7.12f*). In patients on long-term miotic therapy, posterior synechiae may be present and these are broken with an iris sweep prior to removing the lens.

The cataract is extracted with a cryoprobe aided by application of counterpressure inferiorly, and the preplaced 9/0 suture is tied with a single throw. Approximately eight interrupted sutures of 10/0 nylon are used to close the incision (*Figure 7.12g*). After the first two sutures are placed, the anterior chamber can be filled with air to restore the normal shape of the globe and to assist in accurate placement of the remaining sutures.

The scleral flap is sutured with one 10/0 nylon suture on each posterior 'corner', and these sutures are tied loosely. Air in the anterior chamber is replaced with balanced salt solution, and leakage at the filtering site is confirmed. The conjunctiva is closed with a running, locked 8/0 collagen suture tied at each end (*Figure 7.12h*). If a filter without a scleral flap is to be performed, a piece of the corneoscleral wound margin can be removed with a punch, or cautery can be applied to the wound margins to produce a leak.

Cataract extraction in eyes with a filtering bleb

When removing a cataract in an eye with a filtering bleb, an incision is made in clear cornea in front of the bleb[48]. The corneal incision is placed 1 mm anterior to the bleb and is extended for 150–180° (*Figure 7.13a*). A clear corneal incision must extend farther to each side than is necessary for a more-posterior limbal incision, in order to provide a sufficient opening for safe lens extraction. The incision is made perpendicular to the corneal surface using a razor blade knife and is cut to two-thirds the corneal thickness. A suture of 10/0 nylon is preplaced in the vertical meridian and looped out of the wound (*Figure 7.13b*). The posterior exit of the needle of this suture should not penetrate the bleb, and all subsequent sutures should also avoid the bleb. The anterior chamber is entered with a knife, and the incision is enlarged to its full extent with corneoscleral scissors (*Figure 7.13c*). Shelving of the incision toward the visual axis is avoided.

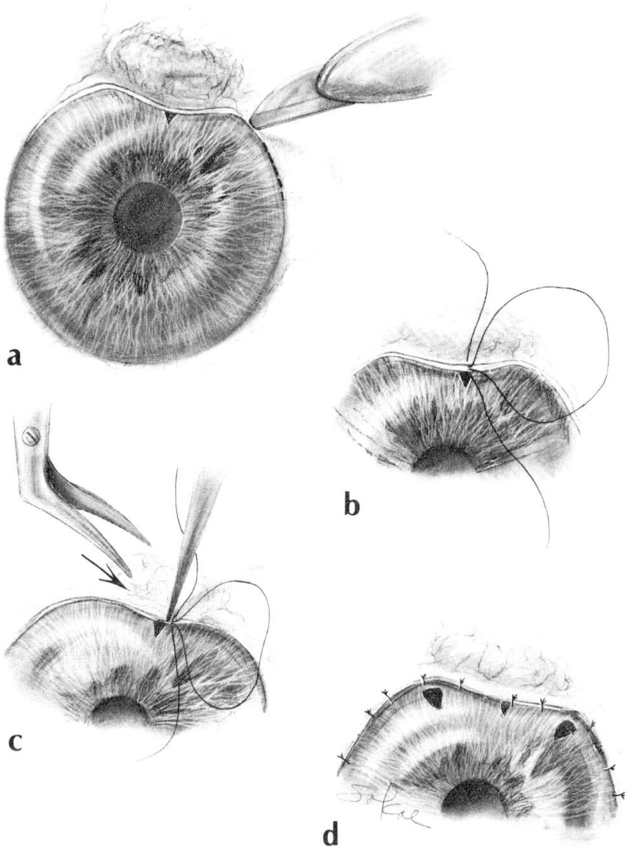

Figure 7.13 *Cataract extraction in an eye with a filtering bleb.* **(a)** *A corneal incision is made with a razor blade 1 mm in front of the bleb, conforming to the shape of the bleb.* **(b)** *A suture is placed at 12 o'clock and* **(c)** *the corneal incision is extended with corneoscleral scissors.* **(d)** *A sector iridectomy or further peripheral iridectomies are performed, the lens extracted and the preplaced suture is tied. Further sutures are placed to achieve watertight closure*

If the pupil is widely dilated, the lens is removed with a cryoprobe without an additional iridectomy. If the pupil is small and/or if posterior synechiae are present, a sector iridectomy is done in a meridian other than that of the filtering opening, and the synechiae are lysed before removing the lens. The preplaced suture is tied after removing the lens, and several additional interrupted 10/0 nylon sutures are placed to achieve watertight closure (*Figure 7.13d*). The knots of these sutures are buried. The anterior chamber may be filled with air during placement of the sutures, and the air is replaced with balanced salt solution at the end of the operation.

Postoperative care and complications

As with other types of filtering surgery, frequent topical steroids and cycloplegic drops are used postoperatively. The complications encountered are identical with those discussed previously under trabeculectomy. Although in these aphakic eyes a flat anterior chamber presents no risk of causing lens opacity, there is the possibility of vitreocorneal contact and corneal damage if a shallow anterior chamber persists. Vitreous obstructing the internal filtering opening is uncommon, especially if a round pupil is maintained and vitreous prolapse does not occur.

Results

Our experience with combined filtering surgery and intracapsular cataract extraction has been favorable[49]. More than half the cases have not required further glaucoma medications to control the IOP. Other surgeons have reported a similar success rate[50]. The results of separate cataract extraction and filtering operations are slightly less favorable. The success rate for trabeculectomy is about 80 per cent with the postoperative IOP controlled at 21 mmHg or less. When cataract extraction through a clear corneal approach is done later, about 50 per cent of the blebs fail, resulting in loss of control of the IOP or the need for increased medications. Hence, the final result is somewhat less than 50 per cent for control of the IOP with the two separate operations.

Infantile glaucoma: goniotomy and trabeculotomy

Pathogenesis

Glaucoma in infants and children differs from adult glaucoma in its pathogenesis, clinical manifestations and accepted therapy. Infantile glaucoma, in this discussion, includes both congenitally affected eyes and glaucoma developing in childhood. It is unclear whether glaucoma appearing in the second or third decade should be classified as 'delayed infantile' or 'early adult' glaucoma.

As in adult glaucoma, infantile glaucoma has a variable hereditary tendency that is not consistent with a strict Mendelian classification. Ten per cent of patients with infantile glaucoma have a similarly affected family member[51], and the incidence of an affected sibling is 2–10 per cent[51,52]. Thus, the large majority of cases are sporadic; and although there are several ocular and systemic syndromes associated with childhood glaucoma, most cases are isolated abnormalities of aqueous humor dynamics without other associations.

The primary management of infantile glaucoma is surgical, because surgical procedures are often successful whereas medical therapy usually fails. Medications seem to be relatively ineffective in treating infantile glaucoma. Also, careful evaluation of IOP, the optic disc and visual field are often impossible, making it difficult to determine the effectiveness of medical therapy.

Conventional glaucoma filtering surgery is considerably less effective in children than in adults, and a number of different surgical methods have been tried. Barkan[53] popularized the technique of goniotomy, an incision of the trabecular meshwork, and demonstrated excellent results. Allen and Burian[54] advocated an external approach to incising the trabecular area, and Harms and Dannheim[55] developed instrumentation and an effective procedure for satisfactory trabeculotomy *ab externo*.

The rationale for these surgical approaches is based on the gonioscopic and histological findings in infantile glaucoma and knowledge of the normal development of the anterior chamber angle. At about 5–6 months' gestation, the iris begins to assume its final appearance, but the attachment to the anterior chamber angle is anterior to the adult location[56]. Usually the insertion of the iris becomes progressively more posterior. By 9 months' gestation, the iris root is posterior to Schlemm's canal and is located at the posterior part of the trabecular meshwork. Then, during the first years of life, there is a further posterior movement of the iris root, so that a concavity develops at the junction of the iris and the anterior chamber angle called the angle recess. The progressive posterior movement of the iris attachment occurs by rarefaction and rearrangement of the angle tissues rather than by splitting of the tissues[56]. Thus, the anterior chamber angle in normal infants is different from adult eyes because there is an iris insertion with more extensive connections between the iris stroma and the uveal trabecular meshwork.

A second important feature is development of the trabecular endothelial cells. At 5 months' gestation, the trabecular meshwork is covered by corneal endothelial cells[56,57]. These endothelial cells develop into cells which line the trabecular sheets in the adult eye. Between 8 and 9 months' gestation, spaces normally appear between these cells, and this occurs first in the posterior meshwork[56]. This increased porosity probably facilitates outflow of aqueous humor to Schlemm's canal.

While performing goniotomies in eyes with infantile glaucoma, Barkan[53] noted that the angle tissue split *as if* a membrane was being cut. This observation suggested that the cause of infantile glaucoma was an imperforate membrane over the angle. However, specimens of the trabecular area and whole-eye specimens with infantile glaucoma examined by light microscopy and by scanning and transmission electron microscopy have failed to show an imperforate membrane over the angle[59–61]. Instead, the anterior chamber angle structures resemble the 7–8 month stage of fetal development. Therefore, the beneficial effect of goniotomy may be due to a release of the abnormal pull of the ciliary muscle on the trabecular meshwork, rather than to incision of a membrane over the anterior chamber angle.

In normal adult eyes, ciliary muscle contraction causes an increase in outflow facility, perhaps by physically pulling the meshwork open[62]. Similarly, the improved outflow facility caused by pilocarpine seems to depend on ciliary muscle traction on the trabecular meshwork[63].

Preoperative evaluation: examination under anesthesia

The usual symptoms of glaucoma in children are photophobia and tearing although signs of increased IOP, including an enlarged cornea and hazy cornea, are often recognized first[64,65]. Examination under anesthesia (EUA) is often necessary to examine the eye properly and to measure the IOP accurately.

Intramuscular ketamine is used as an anesthetic agent because it does not significantly change the IOP. If an examination is begun with ketamine and surgery is necessary, anesthesia with halothane can be used immediately.

The corneal diameter is measured. The normal diameter at birth is 9–10 mm, and this increases by 1 mm at age 1 year. Shaffer[66] considers corneal diameter greater than 11 mm at birth or 12 mm at 1 year of age indicative of abnormal corneal enlargement. Large, clear corneas not due to glaucoma also occur in megalocornea and occasionally in high myopia. These conditions are distinguished from infantile glaucoma by a normal intraocular pressure and the absence of optic disc cupping. Striae in Descemet's membrane occur in infantile glaucoma from rupture of the membrane by corneal enlargement. Corneal haziness from infantile glaucoma has a diffuse, ground-glass appearance from stromal edema. This is easily distinguished from other causes of corneal clouding that have a normal IOP and corneal diameter.

Accurate measurement of the IOP in infants is difficult. The Schiotz and applanation instruments are relatively large compared to the width of the palpebral fissure, so that considerable force may be needed to open the lids widely unless anesthesia is used, and this force may cause a falsely high IOP reading. Inhalation anesthesia with halothane is sometimes used, but this alters several physiological variables and usually causes a change in the IOP. Hetherington and Shaffer[67] measured the IOP in normal children's eyes and demonstrated variability, depending on the depth of the anesthesia. The IOP was lower at deeper planes of anesthesia. Sampaolesi[68] also found relatively low IOP in normal children under anesthesia. We also find that halothane anesthesia usually lowers the IOP level, and that the amount of lowering is unpredictable.

Measurement of the IOP with a Schiotz tonometer is unreliable because scleral rigidity in children's eyes, especially buphthalmic eyes, is not the same as in normal adult eyes. We prefer a handheld applanation tonometer. Sometimes in infants under 1 year of age the IOP can be measured without systemic anesthetic agents[69]. After eating, the child may fall asleep and the IOP can be measured with a pneumatonograph after gently elevating the upper eyelid. However, eye 'squeezing' by the patient can raise the measurement by 10–20 mmHg, and so anesthesia must be used if the child is not completely quiet.

Gonioscopy can be done with a 16 mm Koeppe lens, a handheld illuminator, and the standard binocular gonioscope. However, we prefer a one-mirror or four-mirror goniolens, used with the operating microscope. Often in eyes with infantile glaucoma but without associated anterior chamber anomalies, the appearance of the angle is quite similar to that of normal infants[66]. We find that gonioscopy is most helpful in identifying eyes with anterior chamber cleavage anomalies such as Axenfeld's syndrome or Rieger's syndrome. Although the therapy of these disorders is the same as for idiopathic infantile glaucoma, the natural course and response to therapy may be different, and genetic counseling is different.

Because of enlargement of the globe in buphthalmos, eyes with infantile glaucoma frequently become myopic and astigmatic. The refractive error in the two eyes of such patients is frequently quite different, and severe amblyopia is common, especially in cases of unilateral glaucoma[70]. Therefore, it is important to measure accurately the refractive error by retinoscopy.

Examination of the optic disc frequently influences the final decision regarding therapy. In an infant with slight corneal enlargement and equivocal IOP elevation when tested under general anesthesia, a significantly cupped optic disc indicates the need for prompt surgery, whereas surgery may be delayed if the optic disc is normal. In normal infants, the optic disc cup is rarely larger than one-fifth the diameter of the disc. In infants an increased cup size can return to a normal size if the glaucoma is detected early and the IOP is normalized by treatment[71,72]. This early reversibility of abnormal nervehead cupping probably results from incomplete development at birth of the structural connective tissue of the optic nervehead[73]. Thus, abnormal cupping is an important sign in the initial diagnosis, and a return to normal cup size may be an important sign of successful therapy.

It is rare to be able to measure visual fields accurately in patients with infantile glaucoma because of their young age. However, an attempt is made by confrontation testing after age 3 years, and 5- to 6-year-old patients can sometimes be tested with a perimeter.

Indications for surgery

Medical therapy is used in infantile glaucoma only as a temporary measure preceding surgery or for eyes in which repeated surgery has been unsuccessful. Surgery is recommended in eyes with an enlarged cornea, IOP greater than 30 mmHg and abnormal optic disc cupping. If the optic disc has abnormal cupping and the cornea is enlarged, surgery is indicated even though the IOP is between 20 and 30 mmHg when measured under general anesthesia, because the anesthetic agent may artificially lower the IOP. If only one of the three criteria is abnormal, it is best to observe the disease course by repeat examinations every 1–2 months and not to operate immediately. If the IOP is markedly elevated to 40 mmHg or greater, however, it is probably best to proceed with surgery even if no corneal or optic nerve damage is evident yet.

Choice of surgical procedure

The choice of surgical procedure for infantile glaucoma depends on the experience of the surgeon and the clinical findings. Goniotomy is usually the procedure of choice when the cornea is clear and there is a good gonioscopic view of the anterior chamber angle. Trabeculotomy is preferable when the cornea is cloudy and goniotomy cannot be performed properly.

Goniotomy

General anesthesia is nearly always required. When ketamine sedation is initially used for examination under anesthesia before deciding whether a goniotomy is needed, an inhalation anesthetic agent is later used for the operation.

The head is turned about 45° away from the surgeon, and the eye is fixated by an assistant with locking forceps grasping the superior and inferior rectus muscles through the conjunctiva. This also usually eliminates the need for a lid speculum. Alternatively, traction sutures can be used under the superior and inferior rectus muscles, but the forceps method allows better control of the eye position.

A Barkan goniolens is used and is held by the surgeon. We prefer the operating microscope for visualization because it provides a wide range of magnification and excellent illumination through its lighting system. Some surgeons who are experienced in goniotomy use operating loupes to provide magnification, combined with a headmounted illuminator. This system provides more flexibility but the magnification is less. If the view is poor because of corneal epithelial edema, use of topical glycerin drops or removal of the epithelium may improve visualization. The pupil is constricted with dilute pilocarpine eyedrops.

We prefer a Barkan or Swan goniotomy knife because the shaft is slightly tapered near the tip but elsewhere of constant diameter. This makes it easier to pass the knife across the anterior chamber. The knife tip is introduced through the peripheral cornea 1–2 mm anterior to the limbus in the inferotemporal quadrant, and the goniotomy incision is made through approximately 4 clock-hours of trabecular meshwork on the opposite side of the eye in the superonasal quadrant (*Figure 7.14a,b*). If a second goniotomy is needed later, the corneal entry is made superotemporally, and the trabeculum is incised in the inferonasal quadrant. A third goniotomy, when necessary, is done through a nasal incision to incise the trabeculum temporally.

The knife is passed across the anterior chamber, avoiding contact with the iris, and the trabecular meshwork is engaged just below Schwalbe's line. If the exact location of anterior chamber angle structures is uncertain, compression of the jugular veins in the neck is done to reflux blood into Schlemm's canal, which is located in the midtrabecular area. The knife is passed about 60° around the angle in one direction, and usually the iris drops back away from the angle (*Figure 7.14c*). A gritty feeling of resistance to the knife blade indicates an excessively deep incision. After passing the knife in one direction, the blade is turned, and the incision is extended for about 60° in the opposite direction.

After the incision, a thin white line of tissue separation should be visible. The knife is then removed from the eye, and some bleeding from the anterior chamber angle may occur at this time. The anterior chamber occasionally requires re-formation with balanced salt solution through the corneal incision. The anterior chamber should not be re-formed with air, because this can lead to pupillary block and flattening of the anterior chamber. If a suture is necessary to close the corneal incision, 10/0 monofilament nylon is used. The suture is removed when examination under anesthesia is done later.

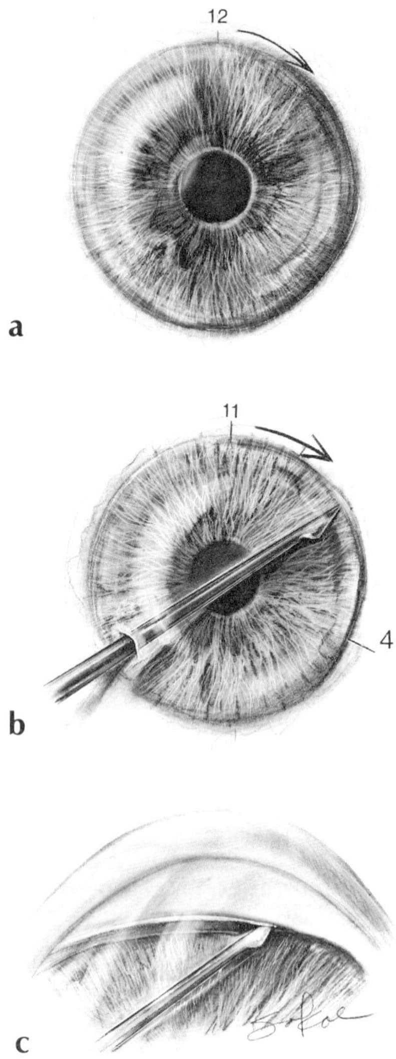

Figure 7.14 **(a)** *Goniotomy in a right eye performed in superonasal quadrant.* **(b)** *The eye is rotated clockwise using traction sutures, gonioknife is introduced at 7 o'clock and the trabeculum is cut from 11 to 3 o'clock.* **(c)** *If a second operation is needed, it can also be performed from the temporal side by rotating the globe counterclockwise and introducing the knife at 11 o'clock. The knife tip engages the trabecular meshwork, and the peripheral iris seems to fall away from the angle when the cut is made*

The patient is positioned postoperatively so that the area of the anterior chamber angle incision is uppermost. Any blood then tends to accumulate on the opposite side of the anterior chamber, away from the area of the goniotomy. Antibiotic drops are used postoperatively, but neither miotic nor cycloplegic medications are used. If surgery is indicated for both eyes, bilateral goniotomies are done during the same operation to reduce the risks associated with general anesthesia[86]. Each eye is cleaned and draped separately to reduce the chance of bilateral endophthalmitis.

Trabeculotomy

An operating microscope is necessary for trabeculotomy. A traction suture is placed under the superior rectus muscle and fastened to the drapes. The operation is centered on the nasal side of the 12 o'clock meridian. A limbus-based conjunctival flap is made, and a limbus-based scleral flap about 3 mm by 3 mm in size is made with a razor blade knife, similar to the flap used in a trabeculectomy. A thick scleral flap aids in identification of Schlemm's canal; a flap three-quarters the thickness of the sclera is ideal. The flap is dissected toward the limbus until the underlying tissue changes color from white to gray. At the limbus, the plane of dissection anteriorly is angled slightly upward to follow the steeper curvature of the cornea.

The sulcus containing Schlemm's canal lies in the zone between the white sclera and the gray limbus. A radial incision 1–2 mm long is made bridging this transition zone (*Figure 7.15a*). The incision is made deep enough to transect Schlemm's canal without entering the anterior chamber, and aqueous humor may be seen leaking from the incision.

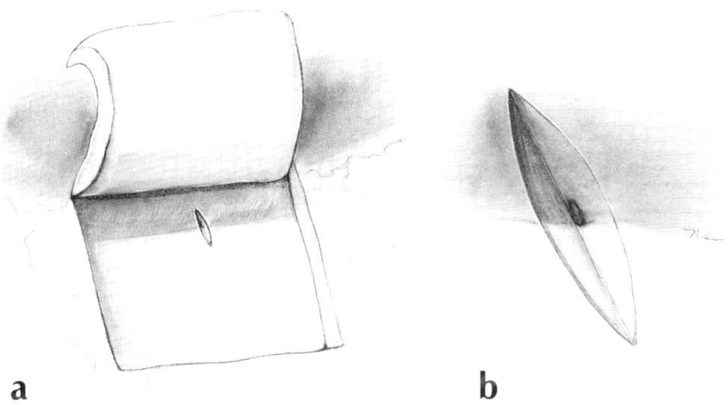

Figure 7.15 *Trabeculotomy technique. Limbus-based conjunctival flap is prepared, and three-quarter thickness scleral flap is made showing the location of the scleral spur at the junction between white sclera and the darker, gray limbal zone.* **(a)** *A radial incision is made across this border and* **(b)** *on high-power inspection the lumen of Schlemm's canal can sometimes be observed in the deep part of the incision*

If a distinct lumen of Schlemm's canal is visible within the cut edge of the radial incision (*Figure 7.15b*), a Harms trabeculotomy-probe tip is inserted into the lumen. If the location of Schlemm's canal is uncertain, a stiff 4/0 or 5/0 nylon suture held by forceps is used to probe gently the cut edge and search for the lumen (*Figure 7.16a*). After the lumen has been identified, the trabeculotomy probe is inserted and advanced (*Figure 7.16b*). When the probe has been advanced for about one-quarter of its length, gentle pressure is applied to rotate the advancing end posteriorly, using the radial incision as the fulcrum. If the probe is in the proper location within the scleral sulcus, it cannot be rotated posteriorly. However, if the probe is in a more posterior location, it can be rotated easily, indicating that it is in the supraciliary space. In this case the probe is withdrawn and reinserted more anteriorly.

The probe is inserted for nearly its entire length, and the handle is then rotated to move the distal end toward the

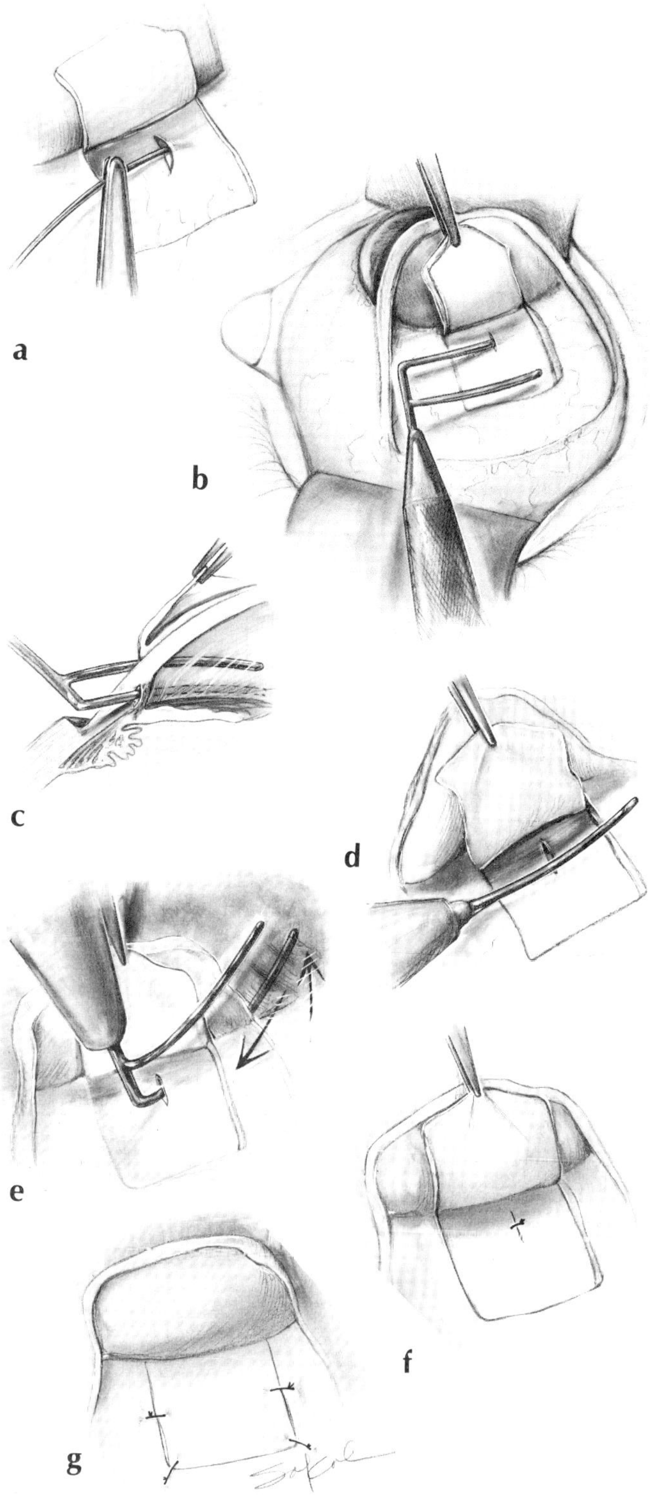

Figure 7.16 **(a)** *If the lumen of Schlemm's canal cannot be seen, a stiff nylon suture is inserted into the radial scleral incision to probe for the canal.* **(b–d)** *The trabeculotomy probe is then inserted, and* **(e)** *the probe is rotated so that the inner arm of the probe enters the anterior chamber. A probe curved in the opposite direction is then used.* **(f)** *If there is marked aqueous leakage and a flat chamber persists, the radial incision is closed with a single 10/0 suture.* **(g)** *The scleral flap is closed with four interrupted 10/0 sutures, and conjunctiva closed with 8/0 collagen*

anterior chamber (*Figure 7.16e*). A slight amount of resistance is common, but if excessive force is required this suggests that the probe is too far anterior and will strip Descemet's membrane rather than disinserting the trabecular fibers from their attachments to the scleral spur. The probe is rotated until about nine-tenths of the arm enters the anterior chamber. If the probe is rotated a full 90°, the trabeculum underlying the radial incision will be torn, and the anterior chamber may collapse before the second probe can be inserted in the opposite direction. A second probe is inserted, and a trabeculotomy is made in the opposite direction. The total extent of the trabecular opening is about 4 clock-hours.

Often there is some bleeding after the trabeculotomy, but the blood usually absorbs during the early postoperative period. The scleral flap is repositioned and sutured with four 10/0 nylon sutures placed at the corners of the flap and on either side near the limbus (*Figure 7.16g*). The conjunctiva is closed with a running, unlocked suture of 8/0 collagen that is tied at each end.

Pilocarpine drops (1 per cent) are used 3 times daily for 3 weeks postoperatively. Contraction of the ciliary muscle caused by the pilocarpine may displace the ciliary muscle away from the trabeculum during the healing phase. If significant inflammation occurs the miotic is discontinued to prevent development of posterior synechiae. Pilocarpine is stopped within 1 month to allow measurement of the IOP level off antiglaucoma therapy. If the IOP remains elevated for 2 months postoperatively, the trabeculotomy is repeated.

Complications

Goniotomy is nearly free of complications if done by an experienced surgeon [86]. Rarely, anterior chamber hemorrhage persists and leads to fibrous organization or blood-staining of the cornea. Trabeculotomy can also be associated with postoperative anterior chamber hemorrhage, and this may be severe enough to require removal of the blood[55]. During trabeculotomy, inadvertent damage to other anterior chamber structures can occur, such as separating Descemet's membrane from the corneal stroma. After trabeculotomy a temporary filtering bleb may be present for up to 3 months.

Results

Success in glaucoma surgery should properly be judged by prevention of progressive optic nerve damage, as mentioned before. Since visual fields usually cannot be measured in small children, the success of goniotomy or trabeculotomy is judged by a lack of progression, or an improvement, in optic disc cupping. In eyes in which the optic disc cannot be seen, lowering of the IOP is the most important criterion of success.

A survey of goniotomy results suggests that the IOP is lowered to normal in about 50 per cent of cases after one operation[53,64,70,74–77]. IOP control is achieved in 75–85 per cent of eyes after one to three goniotomies. Although most published series do not indicate how many patients had idiopathic infantile glaucoma and how many had glaucoma associated with ocular or systemic syndromes, there is evidence that eyes with other ocular abnormalities are more difficult to control. Grant and Walton[78] reported no successes after one to three goniotomies in 12 eyes with aniridia.

Once the IOP is controlled, most eyes retain satisfactory IOP control for a long period of time. However, a small number of eyes, perhaps 5 per cent, have recurrent IOP elevation after several years of control following surgery[75]. Therefore, these cases must be followed up indefinitely.

Assessment of reported trabeculotomy results is also difficult because various criteria are used for success. However, lowering of the IOP to below 24 mmHg is achieved in about 85 per cent of eyes with infantile glaucoma[55,79–85]. About one-third of such cases require two operations before pressure control is achieved. After two unsuccessful trabeculotomies, few eyes have a good response if the same operation is performed a third time. Eyes with a cloudy cornea or other associated abnormalities also have a less favorable prognosis.

Re-formation of the anterior chamber and revision of filtering procedures

Indications

Surgical re-formation of a flat anterior chamber after filtering surgery is indicated if iridocorneal contact has been present for 7–10 days, if corneal or lens opacities have developed, or if visible choroidal detachments have appeared and are not decreasing in size. The anterior chamber does not always re-form spontaneously, and additional surgery is required in some cases[87]. There are no exact guidelines as to when chamber re-formation should be done. Reoperation causes further trauma and inflammation and may decrease the chance of successful filtration. However, failure to re-form a persistently flat anterior chamber may be complicated by permanent secondary angle closure and corneal and/or lens damage.

Preoperative evaluation

Before performing surgery to re-form the anterior chamber, careful examination is done to determine the cause of the flat chamber. First the IOP is measured. Elevation of the IOP suggests malignant glaucoma, and vitreous surgery may be required. If the IOP is low, then the filtering bleb is examined to identify any defect in the conjunctiva. Sterile 2 per cent fluorescein solution is placed on the bleb, which is then examined with blue light to detect leakage of clear fluid. If the anterior chamber is sufficiently deep to permit gonioscopy, the chamber angle is examined for a possible cyclodialysis cleft.

Operative technique

A 4/0 black stay silk suture is placed under the inferior rectus muscle and is grasped with a clamp to position the eye. A traction suture beneath the superior rectus muscle can also be used (*Figure 7.17a*). The eye is then grasped with forceps near the limbus, avoiding the area of the conjunctival bleb. A knife, such as a Ziegler knife, is passed obliquely through the peripheral cornea to form a passage for re-formation of the anterior chamber (*Figure 7.17b,c*). A cannula is inserted through this knife tract, and balanced salt solution is injected to deepen the chamber (*Figure 7.17d*). Air can also be injected into the anterior chamber, but we prefer to use balanced salt solution.

The conjunctival bleb is then examined, and any needed revision is made. If a small defect in the conjunctiva is leaking and contributing to the flat anterior chamber, the defect is closed with sutures. Size 10/0 nylon is used for closure if there is sufficient subepithelial connective tissue to be included between the suture bites. Excessive tightening of the suture, however, may cause further tearing of the conjunctiva. The 10/0 nylon suture requires later removal; and if several sutures are needed, we sometimes use a fine absorbable suture such as 8/0 collagen.

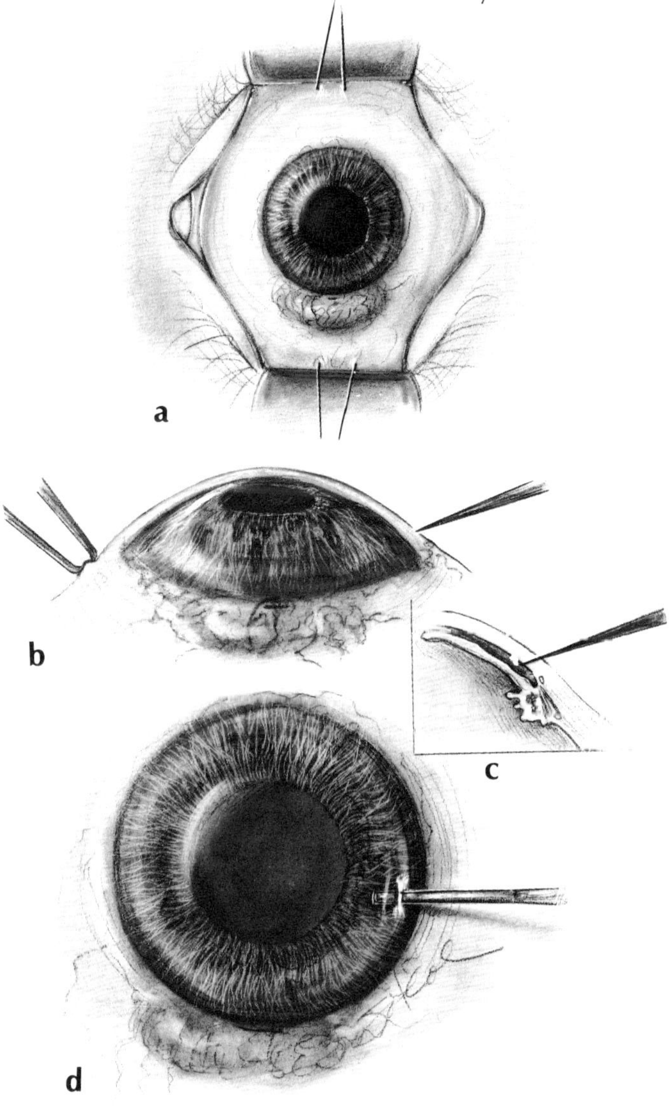

Figure 7.17 *Re-formation of the anterior chamber.* **(a)** *Traction sutures are placed under the superior and inferior rectus muscles.* **(b,c)** *The eye is also stabilized with forceps, and a small corneal incision is made with a Ziegler knife without injuring the iris or lens.* **(d)** *The anterior chamber is then filled with balanced salt solution*

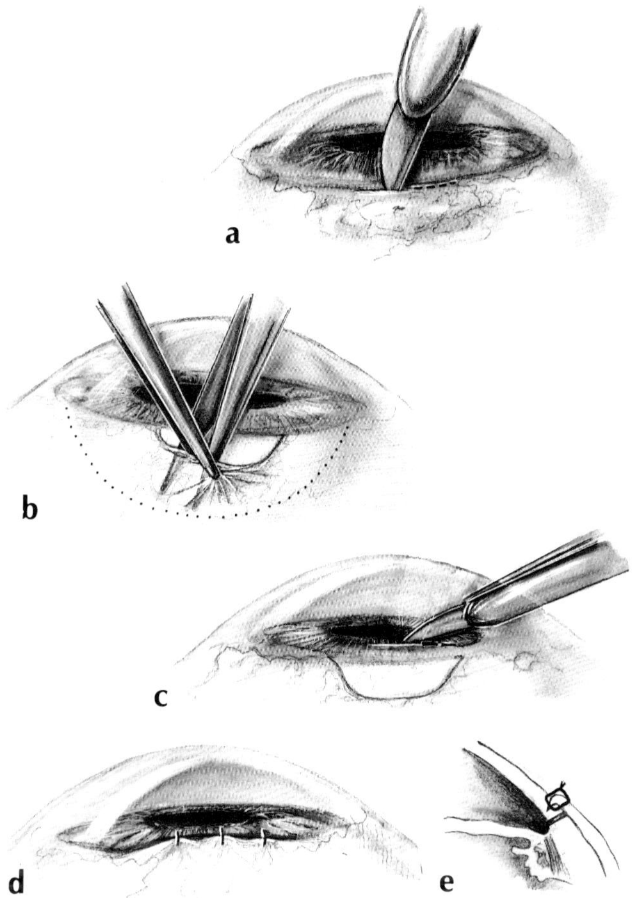

Figure 7.18 *Repair of conjunctival bleb with diffuse leakage.* **(a)** *Excision of the leaking area of conjunctiva is started with a razor blade knife.* **(b)** *Blunt dissection with scissors is done posteriorly so that the conjunctiva can be advanced.* **(c–e)** *A partial-thickness corneal incision is made, and the conjunctiva is sutured into the corneal incision*

A large leak in the bleb, surrounded by friable conjunctiva, is not amenable to direct suturing; and the leaking area must be excised. This is sometimes necessary in cases with old blebs that become thin and cystic near the limbus and then develop a leak. The thin area of conjunctiva is removed with scissors and a razor blade knife (*Figure 7.18a*). The conjunctiva posterior to this area is freed from the underlying sclera by blunt dissection and relaxing incisions are made under the epithelial surface (*Figure 7.18b*). Then, a slightly shelved, half-thickness corneal incision is made with a razor blade parallel to the area of excised conjunctiva (*Figure 7.18c*). The cut edge of the conjunctiva is placed in the corneal incision and sutured in place with 10/0 nylon (*Figure 7.18d,e*). The suture knots are pulled into the corneal incision. This provides watertight closure of the conjunctiva at the limbus, and later retraction of the flap is avoided.

When a cyclodialysis cleft is suspected, intraoperative gonioscopy is performed after deepening the anterior chamber. Gonioscopy is done with a four-mirror goniolens and an operating microscope. Such clefts are most often found at the site of an iridectomy, and they are probably caused at surgery by undue traction on the iris root.

If a cyclodialysis cleft is suspected but cannot be visualized, sterile fluorescein solution is injected into the anterior chamber, and a scleral incision is made into the suprachoroidal space. If fluorescein dye is found in the suprachoroidal fluid, this indicates a direct communication between the anterior chamber and the suprachoroidal space through a cyclodialysis cleft (*Figure 7.19a*). Fluorescein is injected into the anterior chamber through a corneal puncture on the opposite side of the eye from the scleral incision. Otherwise, fluorescein may leak from the corneal puncture site and flow over the scleral incision, thereby confusing the interpretation. A cobalt blue filter is used to confirm the presence of fluorescent dye in the fluid coming from the scleral incision because suprachoroidal fluid usually also appears yellow.

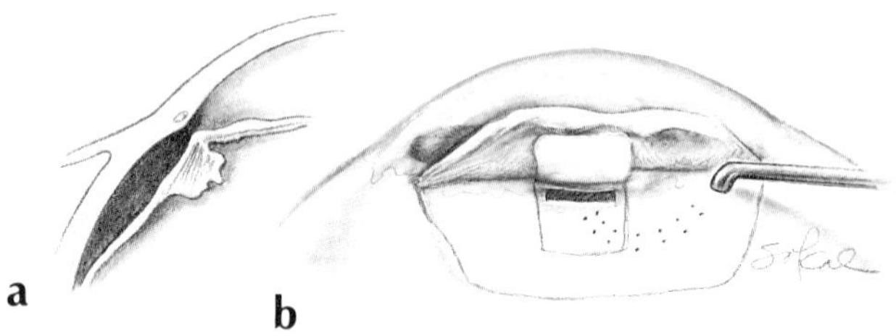

Figure 7.19 *Treatment of cyclodialysis cleft.* **(a)** *Direct communication between anterior chamber and fluid in the suprachoroidal space.* **(b)** *Conjunctival and scleral flaps are reopened, and a double row of penetrating diathermy is placed around the area of the cleft*

If a cyclodialysis cleft is identified, it is best treated by argon laser photocoagulation using a gonioprism. This technique is effective in most cases, and the cieft closes after a week or two. However, if recurrent flattening of the anterior chamber precludes laser treatment, surgical methods can be used to seal the cleft. The original conjunctival incision for the filtering bleb is reopened, and a double row of penetrating diathermy is applied from limbus to limbus in a horseshoe pattern surrounding the area of the cleft (*Figure 7.19b*). This is done using a diathermy pin with a 1.5 mm long tip, and an energy setting intense enough to cause mild scleral shrinkage. If a trabeculectomy flap is present, this is elevated and the diathermy is applied to the deep scleral bed. The scleral and conjunctival flaps are resutured.

Suprachoroidal fluid is drained in almost all cases undergoing surgical deepening of the anterior chamber. Conjunctival incisions are made about 4 mm posterior to the limbus in the inferior quadrants (*Figure 7.20a*). A scleral incision 2 mm long is made parallel to the limbus, into the suprachoroidal space. When the suprachoroidal space is entered, clear or yellow fluid flows out. Holding the lips of the incision open with forceps improves drainage of the fluid (*Figure 7.20b*). This can be further facilitated by applying pressure to the opposite side of the globe using cotton applicators (*Figure 7.20c*). Balanced salt solution is injected into the anterior chamber to restore the intraocular volume.

A second conjunctival and scleral incision is made in the other inferior quadrant to search for further suprachoroidal fluid. Adequate time should be allowed for drainage of all the fluid, because it leaks out intermittently. Finally, indirect ophthalmoscopy is done to see whether the choroidal detachments have completely flattened. The scleral incisions are left unsutured, and the conjunctival incisions are closed with interrupted sutures of absorbable 8/0 collagen (*Figure 7.20d*).

The superior conjunctival bleb is not disturbed during drainage of suprachoroidal fluid unless there is reason to suspect that a problem with the bleb or the scleral-filtration defect has caused the persistent flat chamber. For example, in eyes after trabeculectomy, if fluid injected into the anterior chamber immediately enters the bleb and the chamber will not remain formed, then leakage through the trabeculectomy defect is excessive. In such eyes the conjunctival incision is reopened and the scleral flap is tightened. This is done only if absolutely necessary, however, because increased inflammation and scarring from further surgical manipulations decrease the chance of successful filtration.

The eye is treated with topical steroid ointment and cycloplegic drops, and a semipressure patch and shield are applied. Topical steroids are also used frequently during the postoperative period.

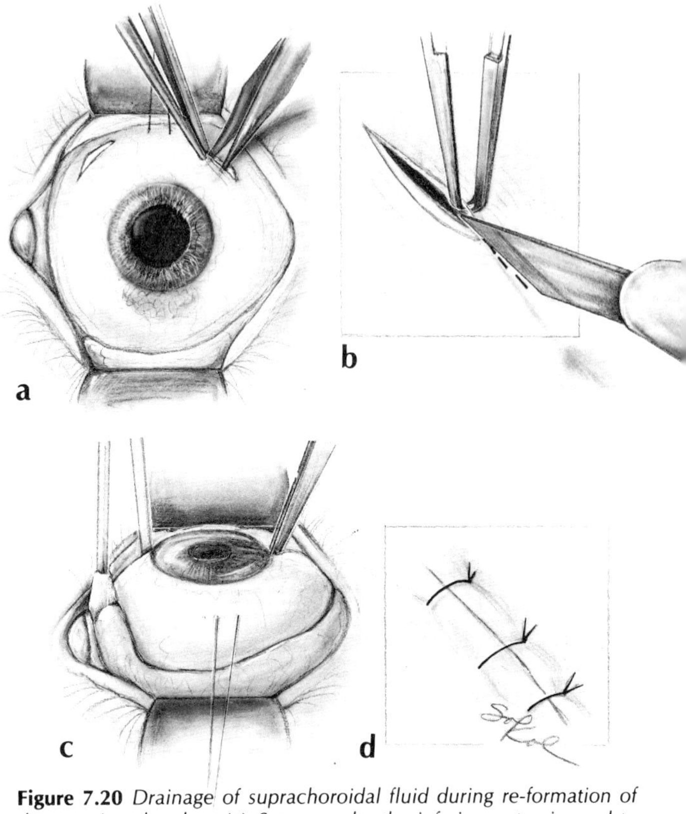

Figure 7.20 *Drainage of suprachoroidal fluid during re-formation of the anterior chamber.* **(a)** *Suture under the inferior rectus is used to expose the inferior bulbar conjunctiva, and incisions are made through conjunctiva 4–6 mm posterior to the limbus.* **(b)** *Razor blade incision parallel to the limbus is made through sclera into the suprachoroidal space.* **(c)** *To facilitate outflow of fluid, the eye is rotated inferiorly and cotton-tipped applicators are used to place external pressure on the globe while the incision is held open with a forceps.* **(d)** *The conjunctiva is closed with interrupted 8/0 collagen sutures, although the scleral incisions are not sutured*

Complications and results

Failure of the anterior chamber to remain re-formed, together with recurrence of choroidal detachment, is the most common postoperative problem, but it is infrequent. If it does occur, the operative steps to re-form the chamber are repeated, and the possible cause of the flat anterior chamber are reassessed. As mentioned before, corneal damage, progressive cataract, secondary angle closure and failure of filtration all occur after a prolonged flat anterior chamber. These further complications are also more likely to occur in eyes in which the flattening is recurrent or includes corneolentricular touch.

Malignant glaucoma

Pathogenesis

The puzzling condition known as malignant glaucoma is usually recognized after surgery for glaucoma. Occasionally malignant glaucoma occurs in eyes that have not undergone prior surgery, and it can occur in either phakic or aphakic eyes[88,89]. The clinical picture is that of a markedly shallow or flat anterior chamber with a high IOP. In phakic eyes the clinical features resemble acute pupillary-block glaucoma. In patients with malignant glaucoma, however, the fellow eye usually has a deep anterior chamber, whereas the anterior chamber is shallow in both eyes of patients with pupillary block causing angle closure. Also, eyes with malignant glaucoma respond poorly to medical therapy that is used to treat acute angle closure resulting from pupillary block, especially pilocarpine which makes the malignant glaucoma worse[90].

In malignant glaucoma the initial event seems to be a transient elevation of the pressure in the fluid behind the detached posterior surface of the vitreous gel, as compared to the pressure in the anterior and posterior chambers[91–93]. In eyes that develop malignant glaucoma after iridectomy or filtering surgery, transient elevation of the retrovitreal IOP probably occurs when the anterior chamber is opened. In eyes that have not had prior surgery, the initiating event is unknown.

Two changes then seem to occur because of the increased pressure posteriorly. First, the vitreous gel, lens and iris move forward, and the anterior chamber shallows. Then, the vitreous gel seems to become compressed, and this decreases fluid passage through the vitreous gel from the posterior 'fluid vitreous' space behind the gel to the posterior chamber. A vicious cycle is thus begun. The higher pressure posteriorly compresses the vitreous gel further, causing more shallowing of the anterior chamber and angle-closure glaucoma. Unlike angle-closure glaucoma due to pupillary block, in malignant glaucoma the vitreous gel, rather than the pupillary block, is the barrier to fluid movement within the eye. Shaffer has called this condition ciliovitreolenticular block[91]. In aphakic eyes, malignant glaucoma is due to ciliovitreal block.

The IOP rises until it eventually reaches a level that suppresses further aqueous humor secretion. It is unknown why such a cycle of events occurs in just a few eyes and not in others: many eyes have transiently elevated pressure behind the vitreous gel as compared to the pressure in the anterior chamber and yet do not develop this problem. Perhaps some eyes are especially susceptible to malignant glaucoma because of abnormally low vitreous-gel permeability. Further study is necessary to improve understanding of this condition.

The principles of surgery for malignant glaucoma are straightforward. Since the pathological cycle involves compression and forward displacement of the vitreous gel, disruption or removal of the vitreous should interrupt this cycle and prevent recurrence. Previous operations to treat malignant glaucoma included removal of the lens allowing anterior prolapse of the vitreous gel in phakic eyes, or cutting the anterior vitreous surface with a knife in aphakic eyes. Since the development of vitrectomy instruments used to cut and remove vitreous gel, malignant glaucoma is now treated by excision of the vitreous using these instruments.

Preoperative evaluation and medical therapy

Phakic eyes with a shallow anterior chamber and high IOP are usually diagnosed as having pupillary-block glaucoma. If medical therapy with miotics and a carbonic-anhydrase inhibitor and/or surgical therapy by iridotomy or iridectomy fail to cure the problem, then malignant glaucoma should be suspected. Osmotic agents may lower the IOP in eyes with either angle-closure or malignant glaucoma[94]. Therefore, malignant glaucoma may not be recognized until after an iridotomy or iridectomy has been performed that is unsuccessful in controlling the IOP.

If malignant glaucoma is suspected, medical therapy is attempted with cycloplegics[95]. Although a mid-dilated pupil results in maximum iris–lens contact that may cause pupillary block, if the pupil is dilated further the attack of malignant glaucoma may be relieved by relaxing the ciliary muscle. Relaxation of the ciliary muscle expands the diameter of the ciliary ring and provides a larger surface area for anterior movement of intraocular fluid. Also, expanding the ciliary ring may tighten the lens zonules and thereby partially reverse the forward displacement of the lens and iris.

In most cases of malignant glaucoma the diagnosis is not evident until after an iridectomy has been performed for suspected angle-closure glaucoma. Therefore, after an iridectomy the IOP is measured immediately to determine whether it is lower. In eyes undergoing surgical iridectomy the IOP is measured on the operating table. If the iridectomy is patent but the IOP remains elevated and the anterior chamber cannot be easily deepened, then malignant glaucoma is likely instead of pupillary-block glaucoma. Similarly, after laser iridotomy malignant glaucoma is diagnosed if the anterior chamber remains shallow and the IOP remains high, unless the elevation of IOP is due to PAS seen by gonioscopy.

Surgical technique

Either local or general anesthesia can be used. In phakic eyes surgery is done through a pars plana approach, and in aphakic eyes either a limbal or pars plana approach can be used. The technique of vitreous surgery is described in Chapter 8. In phakic eyes, as much of the vitreous gel is excised as possible without damaging the posterior surface of the lens. A posterior vitreous detachment is present in these cases, and so the posterior vitreous gel and cortex are easily removed. This usually results in deepening of the anterior chamber; but if the chamber does not deepen spontaneously, balanced salt solution is injected through a limbal incision. If the anterior chamber remains flat, then the lens is removed through a pars plana approach (*see* Chapter 8). Lens removal is rarely necessary to treat phakic malignant glaucoma, although a combined pars plana lens removal and vitrectomy may be planned in eyes with malignant glaucoma and a visually significant preoperative cataract. In aphakic eyes the anterior vitreous surface is excised as well as the vitreous gel and the posterior vitreous cortex. We prefer a pars plana approach in aphakic eyes although a limbal approach can also be used.

Postoperative care

Topical steroid and cycloplegic drops are used postoperatively. The IOP is measured frequently and gonioscopy is done. In many eyes, the vicious cycle of anterior displacement of the lens and flattening of the anterior chamber is ended by vitrectomy, and the anterior chamber is restored to a normal depth. PAS may have formed, however, and secondary angle-closure glaucoma may be present. This may require medical therapy to control the IOP, later filtering surgery, or cyclocryotherapy in severe cases. In aphakic eyes cycloplegics are discontinued soon after surgery. In phakic eyes or those in which the attack was broken with cycloplegic and osmotic agents without vitrectomy, atropine or homatropine drops are continued. Later the cycloplegics are discontinued during a period of careful observation to detect possible recurrence of malignant glaucoma.

Results

Malignant glaucoma is a rare condition, and no large studies are available detailing the results of surgery. Our experience has been greatest in treating malignant glaucoma in aphakic eyes, and in 10 such cases the pathological mechanism was interrupted. Approximately 50 per cent of these eyes required prolonged medical or later surgical therapy for glaucoma because of permanent PAS after an undue delay between the onset of the attack and vitreous surgery. In phakic eyes we have successfully treated malignant glaucoma by vitrectomy alone, and by combined pars plana lensectomy and vitrectomy in eyes with malignant glaucoma and pre-existing cataract.

References

1. Lowe, R. F. Primary angle-closure glaucoma: a review of ocular biometry. Australian Journal of Ophthalmology 1977; 5:9-17
2. Chandler, P. A., Simmons, R. J. Anterior chamber deepening for gonioscopy at time of surgery. Archives of Ophthalmology 1965; 74:177-190
3. Bain, W. E. The fellow eye in acute closed-angle glaucoma. British Journal of Ophthalmology 1957; 41:193-199
4. Lowe, R. F. Acute angle-closure glaucoma. The second eye: an analysis of 200 cases. British Journal of Ophthalmology 1962; 46:641-650
5. Wand, M. Provocative tests in angle-closure glaucoma: a brief review with commentary. Ophthalmic Surgery 1974; 5:32-37
6. Anderson, D. R. Corneal indentation to relieve acute angle-closure glaucoma. American Journal of Ophthalmology 1979; 88:1091-1093
7. Krupin, T., Mitchell, K. B., Johnson, M. F., Becker, B. The long-term effects of iridectomy for primary acute angle-closure glaucoma. American Journal of Ophthalmology 1978; 86:506-509
8. Floman, N., Berson, D., Landau, L. Peripheral iridectomy in closed angle glaucoma – late complications. British Journal of Ophthalmology 1977; 61:101-104
9. Quigley, H. A. Long-term follow-up of laser iridotomy. Ophthalmology 1981; 88:218-224
10. Pollack, I. P. Use of argon laser energy to produce iridotomies. Transactions of the American Ophthalmological Society 1979; 77:674-706
11. Pollack, I. P. Chronic angle-closure glaucoma. Diagnosis and treatment in patients with angles that appear open. Archives of Ophthalmology 1971; 85:676-689
12. Gelber, E. C., Anderson, D. R. Surgical decisions in chronic angle-closure glaucoma. Archives of Ophthalmology 1976; 94:1481-1484
13. Playfair, T. J., Watson, P. G. Management of chronic or intermittent primary angle-closure glaucoma: a long-term follow-up of the results of peripheral iridectomy used as an initial procedure. British Journal of Ophthalmology 1979; 63:23-28
14. Scheie, H. G. Filtering operations for glaucoma: a comparative study. American Journal of Ophthalmology 1962; 53:571-593
15. Sugar, H. S. Limboscleral trepanation. Eleven years' experience. Archives of Ophthalmology 1971; 85:703-708
16. Cairns, J. E. Trabeculectomy. Preliminary report of a new method. American Journal of Ophthalmology 1968; 66:673-679
17. Schwartz, A. L., Anderson, D. R. Trabecular surgery. Archives of Ophthalmology 1974; 92:134-138
18. Jerndal, T., Lundström, M. 330 trabeculectomies – a follow-up study through 1/2–3 years. Acta Ophthalmologica 1977; 55:52-62
19. Wilson, P. Trabeculectomy: long-term follow. British Journal of Ophthalmology 1977; 61:535-538
20. Werner, E. B., Drance, S. M., Schulzer, M. Trabeculectomy and the progression of glaucomatous visual field loss. Archives of Ophthalmology 1977; 95:1374-1377
21. Drance, S. M., Vargas, E. Trabeculectomy and thermosclerectomy: A comparison of two procedures. Canadian Journal of Ophthalmology 1973; 8:413-415
22. Spaeth, G. L. A prospective, controlled study to compare the Scheie procedure with Watson's trabeculectomy. Ophthalmic Surgery 1980; 11:688-694
23. Blondeau, P., Phelps, C. D. Trabeculectomy vs thermosclerostomy. A randomized prospective clinical trial. Archives of Ophthalmology 1981; 99:810-816
24. Worthen, D. M., Wickham, M. G. Argon laser trabeculotomy. Transactions of the American Academy of Ophthalmology and Otolaryngology 1974; 78:371-375
25. Wise, J. B., Witter, S. L. Argon laser therapy for open-angle glaucoma. Archives of Ophthalmology 1979; 97:319-322

26. Schwartz, A. L., Whitten, M. E., Bleiman, B., Martin, D. Argon laser trabecular surgery in uncontrolled phakic open angle glaucoma. Ophthalmology 1981; 88:203-212
27. West, C. E., Wood, T. O., Kaufman, H. E. Cyclocryotherapy for glaucoma pre- or post-penetrating keratoplasty. American Journal of Ophthalmology 1973; 76:485-489
28. de Roetth, A., Jr. Cryosurgery for the treatment of advanced chronic simple glaucoma. American Journal of Ophthalmology 1968; 66:1034-1041
29. Vannas, S., Palkama, A., Keikola, J., Mali, A. Effect of cryosurgery on the ciliary processes. Annals of Ophthalmology 1970; 2:460-465
30. Polack, F. M., de Roetth, A., Jr. Effect of freezing on the ciliary body (cyclocryotherapy). Investigative Ophthalmology 1964; 3:164-170
31. Sudarsky, R. D., Hulquist, R., Chi, H. H. Cryogenically induced iris atrophy, iridectomy and cataract in rabbits. American Journal of Ophthalmology 1965; 60:217-231
32. Howard, G. M., de Roetth, A., Jr. Histopathologic changes following cryosurgery of the rabbit ciliary body. American Journal of Ophthalmology 1967; 64:700-707
33. Lincoff, H., Cavero, R., Nadel, A., McLean, J. M. Cryosurgery of the ciliary body. Part 2. Archives of Ophthalmology 1968; 79:196-204
34. Scullica, L. Giraldi, J. P. Modificazione della circolazione del corpo ciliare dopo trattamenti criogenici. Bollettino de Oculistica 1969; 48:302-311
35. Quigley, H. A. Histological and physiological studies of cyclo-cryotherapy in primate and human eyes. American Journal of Ophthalmology 1976; 82:722-732
36. Minckler, D. S., Tso, M. O. Experimental papilledema produced by cyclocryotherapy. American Journal of Ophthalmology 1976; 82:577-589
37. Ferry, A. P. Histopathologic observations on human eyes following cyclocryotherapy for glaucoma. Transactions of the American Academy of Ophthalmology and Otolaryngology 1977; 83:90-113
38. Krupin, T., Johnson, M. F., Becker, B. Anterior segment ischemia after cyclocryotherapy. American Journal of Ophthalmology 1977; 84:426-428
39. Michels, R. G., Maumenee, A. E. Retrobulbar alcohol injection in seeing eyes. Transactions of the American Academy of Ophthalmology and Otolaryngology 1973; 77:164-167
40. de Roetth, A., Jr. Cryosurgery for the treatment of advanced chronic simple glaucoma. American Journal of Ophthalmology 1968; 66:1034-1041
41. Binder, P. S., Abel, R., Kaufman, H. E. Cyclocryotherapy for glaucoma after penetrating keratoplasty. American Journal of Ophthalmology 1975; 79:489-492
42. Boniuk, M. Cryotherapy in neovascular glaucoma. Transactions of the American Academy of Ophthalmology and Otolaryngology 1974; 78:337-343
43. Feibel, R. M., Bigger, J. F. Rubeosis iridis and neovascular glaucoma. Evaluation of cyclocryotherapy. American Journal of Ophthalmology 1972; 74:862-867
44. Bellows, A. R., Grant, W. M. Cyclocryotherapy in advanced inadequately controlled glaucoma. American Journal of Ophthalmology 1973; 75:679-684
45. de Roetth, A., Jr. Cryosurgery for the treatment of glaucoma. Transactions of the American Ophthalmological Society 1965; 63:189-202
46. Randolph, M. E., Maumenee, A. E., Iliff, C. E. Cataract extraction in glaucomatous eyes. American Journal of Ophthalmology 1971; 71:328-330
47. Bigger, J. F., Becker, B. Cataracts and primary open-angle glaucoma: the effect of uncomplicated cataract extraction on glaucoma control. Transactions of the American Academy of Ophthalmology and Otolaryngology 1971; 75:260-272
48. Scheie, H. G., Muirhead, J. F. Cataract extraction after filtering operations. Archives of Ophthalmology 1962; 68:37-41
49. Maumenee, A. E., Wilkinson, C. P. A combined operation for glaucoma and cataract. Transactions of the American Ophthalmological Society 1969; 67:116-130
50. Johns, G. E., Layden, W. E. Combined trabeculectomy and cataract extraction. American Journal of Ophthalmology 1979; 88:973-981
51. Sorsby, A. Ophthalmic genetics, 2nd ed. London: Butterworths, 1970
52. Merin, S., Morin, D. Heredity of congenital glaucoma. British Journal of Ophthalmology 1972; 56:414-417
53. Barkan, O. Surgery of congenital glaucoma. Review of 196 eyes operated by goniotomy. American Journal of Ophthalmology 1953; 36:1523-1534
54. Allen, L., Burian, H. M. Trabeculotomy ab externo. A new glaucoma operation: techniques and results of experimental surgery. American Journal of Ophthalmology 1962; 53:19-26
55. Harms, H., Dannheim, R. Epicritical consideration of 300 cases of trabeculotomy ab externo. Transactions of the Ophthalmological Society of the United Kingdom 1969; 89:491-499
56. Smelser, G. K., Ozanics, V. The development of the trabecular meshwork in primate eyes. American Journal of Ophthalmology 1971; 71:366-385
57. Hansson, H. A., Jerndal, T. Scanning electron microscopic studies on the development of the iridocorneal angle in human eyes. Investigative Ophthalmology 1971; 10:252-265
58. Worst, J. G. F. The cause and treatment of congenital glaucoma. Transactions of the American Academy of Ophthalmology and Otolaryngology 1964; 68:766-788
59. Maumenee, A. E. The pathogenesis of congenital glaucoma: a new theory. Transactions of the American Ophthalmological Society 1958; 56:507-570
60. Maumenee, A. E. Further observations on the pathogenesis of congenital glaucoma. American Journal of Ophthalmology 1963; 55:1163-1176
61. Anderson, D. R. The development of the trabecular meshwork and its abnormality in primary infantile glaucoma. Transactions of the American Ophthalmological Society 1981; 79:458-485
62. van Buskirk, E. M., Grant, W. M. Lens depression and aqueous outflow in enucleated primate eyes. American Journal of Ophthalmology 1973; 76:632-640
63. Kaufman, P. L., Barany, E. H. Loss of acute pilocarpine effect on outflow facility following surgical disinsertion and retrodisplacement of the ciliary muscle from the scleral spur in the cynomolgus monkey. Investigative Ophthalmology 1976; 15:793-807
64. Scheie, H. G. The management of infantile glaucoma. Archives of Ophthalmology 1959; 62:35-54
65. Robin, A. L., Quigley, H. A., Pollack, I. P., Maumenee, A. E., Maumenee, I. H. An analysis of visual acuity, visual fields and disk cupping in childhood glaucoma. American Journal of Ophthalmology 1979; 88:847-858
66. Shaffer, R. N., Weiss, D. I. Congenital and pediatric glaucomas. St. Louis: C. V. Mosby, 1970
67. Hetherington, J., Jr, Shafer, R. N. Tonometry and tonography in congenital glaucoma. Investigative Ophthalmology 1968; 7:134-137
68. Sampaolesi, R. La pression oculaire et le sinus camérulaire chez l'enfant normal et dans le glaucome congénital au dessous de l'age de cinq ans. Documenta Ophthalmologica 1969; 26:497-515
69. Radtke, N. D., Cohan, B. E. Intraocular pressure measurement in the newborn. American Journal of Ophthalmology 1974; 78:501-504
70. Richardson, K. T., Jr, Ferguson, W. J., Jr, Shaffer, R. N. Long-term functional results in infantile glaucoma. Transactions of the American Academy of Ophthalmology and Otolaryngology 1967; 71:833-837

71. Hetherington, J., Shaffer, R. N., Hoskins, H. D. The disc in congenital glaucoma. In: Etienne, R., Paterson, G. D., eds. XXII Congrès International D'Ophthalmologie, International Glaucoma Symposium, Albi, France, 1974. Diffusion Générale de Librairie, 1975: 127–151
72. Quigley, H. A. Childhood glaucoma. Results with trabeculotomy and study of reversible cupping. Ophthalmology 1982; 89:219-226
73. Quigley, H. A. The pathogenesis of reversible cupping in congenital glaucoma. American Journal of Ophthalmology 1977; 84:358-370
74. Haas, J. S. Symposium: congenital glaucoma. End results of treatment. Transactions of the American Academy of Ophthalmology and Otolaryngology 1955; 59:333-341
75. Douglas, D. H. Reflections on buphthalmos and goniotomy. Transactions of the Ophthalmological Society of the United Kingdom 1970; 90:931-937
76. Bietti, G. B. Contribution à la connaissance des résultats de la goniotomie dans le glaucome congenital. Anales d'Oculistique 1966; 199:481-496
77. Leydhecker, W., Dardenne, U., Willome, J. Goniotomie bei 200 Hydrophthalmieaugen. Angulozision, eine neue Operationstechnik. Klinische Monatsblätter für Augenheilkunde 1969; 154:12-19
78. Grant, W. M., Walton, D. S. Progressive changes in the angle in congenital aniridia, with development of glaucoma. American Journal of Ophthalmology 1974; 78:842-847
79. McPherson, S. D. Jr. Results of external trabeculotomy. American Journal of Ophthalmology 1973; 76:918-920
80. Bechetoille, A., Brachet, A., Saraux, H. Microchirurgie des glaucomes. Bulletin de la Société Ophtalmologie de France 1976; Numéro special: 1-179
81. Asseman, R., Corbel, M., Leser, C. Résultats comparés de la trabeculotomie et de la goniotomie chez le buphtalme. Bulletin de la Société Ophtalmologie de France 1972; 72:241-244
82. Dubois-Poulsen, A., Brachet, A. Les indications de la trabeculotomie ab externo. Année Thérapeutique et Clinique en Ophtalmologie 1971; 22:371-385
83. Urrets-Zavalia, A., Jr. Indications et resultats de la trabeculotomie. Annales d'Oculistique 1972; 205:647-666
84. Meixner, N., Ricci, A., Babel, J. Indications et resultats de la trabeculotomie ab externo. Ophthalmologica 1975; 170:124-129
85. Luntz, M. H. and Livingston, D. G. Trabeculotomy ab externo and trabeculectomy in congenital and adult-onset glaucoma. American Journal of Ophthalmology 1977; 83:174-179
86. Litinsky, S. M., Shaffer, R. N., Hetherington, J., Hoskins, H. D. Operative complications of goniotomy. Transactions of the American Academy of Ophthalmology and Otolaryngology 1977; 83:78-79
87. Cohen, J. S., Shaffer, R. N., Hetherington, J., Jr, Hoskins, H. D. Revision of filtration surgery. Archives of Ophthalmology 1977; 95:1612-1615
88. Shaffer, R. N. A suggested anatomic classification to define the pupillary block glaucomas. Investigative Ophthalmology 1973; 12:540-542
89. Schwartz, A. L., Anderson, D. R. 'Malignant glaucoma' in an eye with no antecedent operation or miotics. Archives of Ophthalmology 1975; 93:379-381
90. Rieser, J. C., Schwartz, B. Miotic-induced malignant glaucoma. Archives of Ophthalmology 1972; 87:706-712
91. Shaffer, R. N. Role of vitreous detachment in aphakic and malignant glaucoma. Transactions of the American Academy of Ophthalmology and Otolaryngology 1954; 58:217-231
92. Epstein, D. L., Hashimoto, J. M., Anderson, P. J., Grant, W. M. Experimental perfusions through the anterior and vitreous chambers with possible relationships to malignant glaucoma. American Journal of Ophthalmology 1979; 88:1078-1086
93. Quigley, H. A. Malignant glaucoma and fluid flow rate. American Journal of Ophthalmology 1980; 89:879-880
94. Weiss, D. I., Shaffer, R. N., Harrington, D. O. Treatment of malignant glaucoma with intravenous mannitol infusion. Archives of Ophthalmology 1963; 69:154-158
95. Chandler, P. A., Grant, W. M. Mydriatic-cycloplegic treatment in malignant glaucoma. Archives of Ophthalmology 1962; 68:353-359

8

Vitreous surgery

Ronald G. Michels MD

Introduction

Modern vitreous surgery has developed rapidly to provide generally accepted and widely practiced methods that now have an important place in ophthalmic surgery. Vitreous surgery permits effective treatment of certain blinding disorders for which no therapy was previously available, and it provides alternative methods to manage other conditions. Surgical procedures to treat abnormal vitreous conditions date from as early as the mid-nineteenth century, but modern vitreous surgery techniques have been developed since about 1965. This development followed (and also promoted) a change in attitude toward excision of the vitreous gel, and the later development of specialized instrumentation and techniques to perform vitreous surgery through small incisions in the pars plana.

Kasner[1], during the 1960s, advocated excision of damaged or diseased vitreous gel using scissors and forceps or cellulose sponges while working through a large limbal incision or a corneal wound (open-sky approach). This was done to minimize later complications in situations such as severe penetrating injuries and vitreous prolapse during cataract extraction. Kasner[2] demonstrated that the eye can tolerate excision of portions of the vitreous gel, and the technique of open-sky vitrectomy was also used in a few cases to remove opaque vitreous gel after extraction of the crystalline lens.

Machemer[3] pioneered development of vitreous surgery through a pars plana approach using specialized instruments introduced through watertight incisions. This method of closed-eye vitreous surgery allows treatment of selected posterior segment disorders while minimizing damage to the anterior segment, maintaining normal or slightly elevated intraocular pressure during the operation and permitting precise control during intraocular manipulations and excision of abnormal tissue. Machemer and co-workers[3–6] designed the first clinically effective instrumentation for pars plana vitrectomy, and Machemer also developed the fundamental surgical principles.

Many other surgeons and investigators have contributed to the refinement of vitreous surgery instrumentation and operative techniques, and these methods have been applied to a number of different clinical conditions. Thus, the field of vitreous surgery has changed rapidly. Enough clinical experience has now accumulated to indicate the effectiveness and limitations of these methods, even though further refinements in both instrumentation and surgical technique are continuing.

Instrumentation

Specialized instrumentation is required for vitreous surgery, including: (*1*) an appropriate operating microscope and a head-support for the patient; (*2*) illumination and surgical probes for visualization within the eye and for cutting and removal of intraocular tissues; and (*3*) various accessory instruments for special functions such as removal of firm lens material, application of diathermy, sectioning of fibrovascular tissue, separation of epiretinal membranes, treatment of retinal breaks and introduction of intraocular gas. Several instruments of different design are available for each of these purposes, and each instrument can be used effectively. Therefore, only the principles of instrumentation are presented as they relate to surgical techniques.

Operating microscope and patient head support

Vitreous surgery is usually performed using a multifunctional operating microscope. The binocular indirect ophthalmoscope has been tried as the main viewing system during the operation, and it is still used during certain stages of the procedure to evaluate peripheral vitreoretinal pathology. However, an operating microscope is preferred as the primary method to provide visualization because it: (*1*) provides a wide range of magnification; (*2*) presents an upright image; and (*3*) permits the surgeon to use both hands to control surgical instruments. The microscope should have motorized functions for focusing, zoom magnification and two-dimensional movement of the microscope head in a horizontal plane[7]. These functions are controlled by a foot pedal and/or chin switch in order to free both of the surgeon's hands (*Figure 8.1*).

The patient's head is supported on a platform extending beyond the end of the operating table. This provides additional room beneath the table for the surgeon's legs and for convenient placement of the foot controls needed for the microscope and mechanized surgical instruments. A padded, horseshoe-shaped ring of adjustable height is attached to the head support. This ring can be used as a wrist support for the surgeon. However, its primary function, when covered with sterile drapes, is to form a trough that can be used for temporary placement of surgical instruments and to prevent water used in the operative field from draining onto the floor and damaging the electric foot pedals.

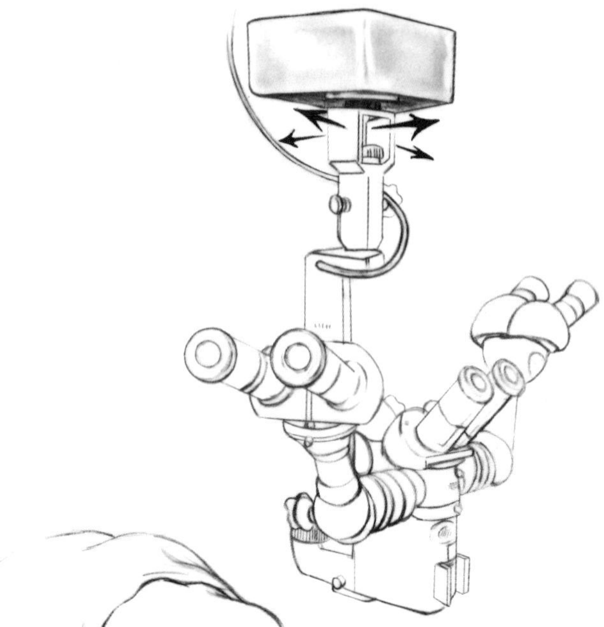

Figure 8.1 *Operating microscope and special patient head support used during vitreous surgery. Microscope has motorized functions for focus, zoom magnification and two-dimensional movement of microscope head in horizontal plane (arrows). Head support includes padded, horseshoe-shaped ring that can be adjusted in height*

Basic vitrectomy instrumentation

Vitreous surgery requires specialized instruments with small-diameter tips that are capable of excising intraocular tissue a bite at a time, removing the abnormal tissue from the eye and simultaneously replacing the excised tissue with a clear physiological solution. These functions of cutting, aspiration and infusion are usually combined with fiberoptic intraocular illumination which provides optimum reflex-free illumination of the operative field while work ensues within the vitreous cavity[9]. Instruments have been designed that combine these four functions in a single tip (full-function probes)[3]. In other instruments these functions are divided among two or more probes and cannulae (divided-system instrumentation)[10].

Full-function vitrectomy probes

Full-function vitrectomy probes usually combine cutting, aspiration and infusion features in the housing of the instrument tip, and fiberoptic illumination is added as a sleeve around the tip (*Figures 8.2* and *8.3*). Such probes usually have a tip diameter of 2.2–2.5 mm, requiring a pars plana incision of about 3.5 mm for safe introduction. Instruments of this type, such as the Machemer VISC (Vitreous-Infusion-Suction-Cutter), were the most commonly used instruments during the first 5 years of modern vitreous surgery. The several commercially available instruments differ in design features, including the type of cutting mechanism and the location and diameter of the aspiration and infusion systems. Cutting mechanisms with oscillating or guillotine-like movement of the blade were found to be safer than those with a continuously rotating blade because the latter could cause excessive traction due to vitreous strands being wrapped around the rotating part.

Divided system instrumentation

Divided system instrumentation has become increasingly popular, and it is now used more commonly than are full-function probes. The four instrument functions are divided among different probes and cannulae, each of the same diameter, as exemplified by the O'Malley Ocutome system[10]. Usually the cutting and aspiration functions are contained in one probe, illumination is provided by a separate fiberoptic probe, and infusion is provided by a

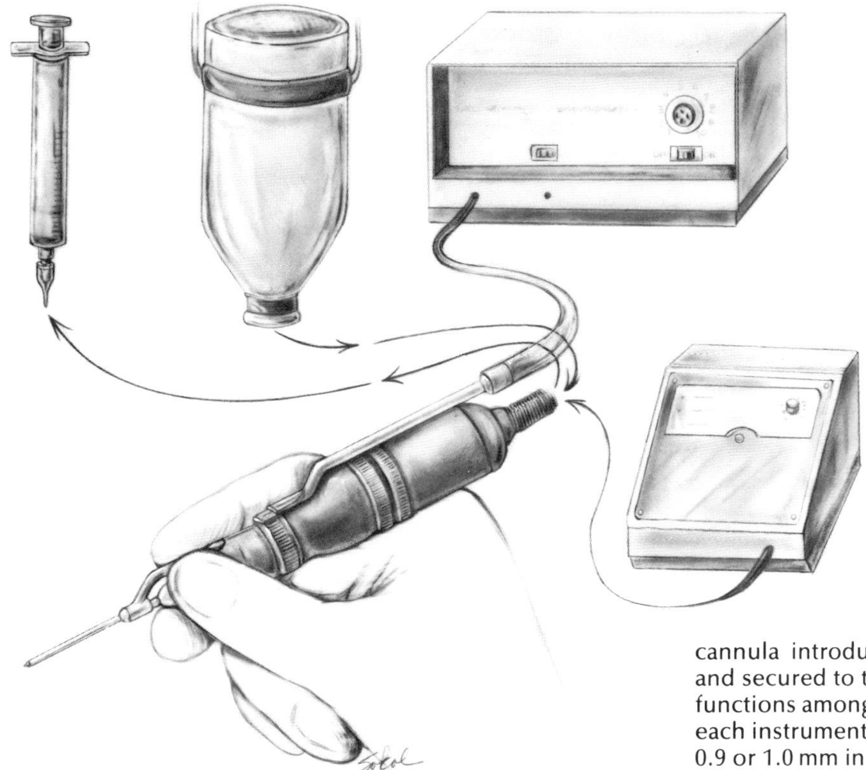

Figure 8.2 *Vitrectomy probe combining multiple functions in a single handpiece. Infusion is indicated by bottle of irrigating solution. Suction is indicated by syringe. Cutting capability is indicated by power device attached to micromotor in the instrument handle. Illumination is provided by fiberoptic sleeve around instrument tip and attachment by fiberoptic cable to light source*

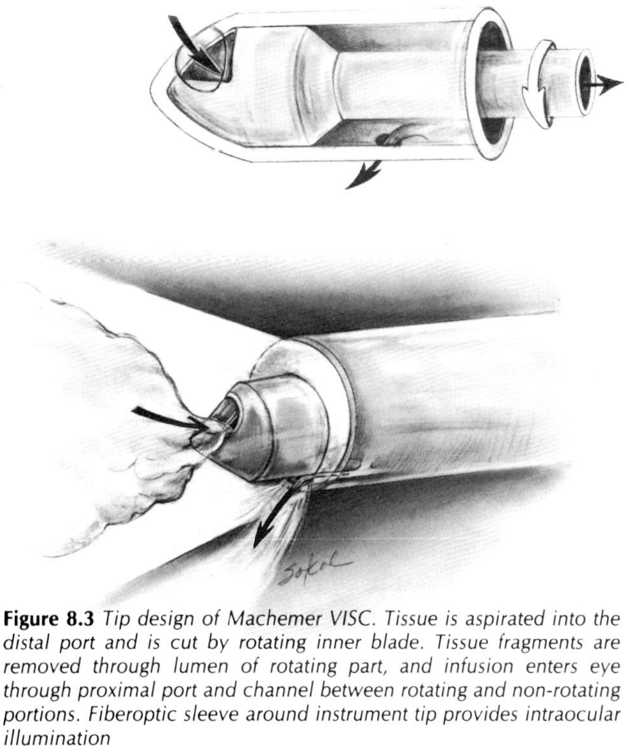

Figure 8.3 *Tip design of Machemer VISC. Tissue is aspirated into the distal port and is cut by rotating inner blade. Tissue fragments are removed through lumen of rotating part, and infusion enters eye through proximal port and channel between rotating and non-rotating portions. Fiberoptic sleeve around instrument tip provides intraocular illumination*

cannula introduced through a third pars plana incision and secured to the sclera (*Figure 8.4*). By dividing the four functions among different instruments, the tip diameter of each instrument is reduced. These instruments are usually 0.9 or 1.0 mm in diameter and require pars plana incisions of 1.4 and 1.5 mm in length, respectively.

Divided system instrumentation has several advantages compared to full-function probes, and this accounts for its current popularity. The smaller instruments are easier to handle. Obligatory bimanual techniques facilitate rotation of the globe during the operation when this is needed to improve visualization in different quadrants. The small-diameter instruments can be safely introduced through either the temporal or nasal quadrants. The surgeon can therefore use his most dextrous hand for difficult manipulations, and the positions of the instruments can be exchanged to permit access to intraocular tissues from the opposite direction. The separate illumination probe provides improved visualization because it permits variations in the direction and intensity of light and because it does not have a fixed relation to the vitrectomy cutting probe.

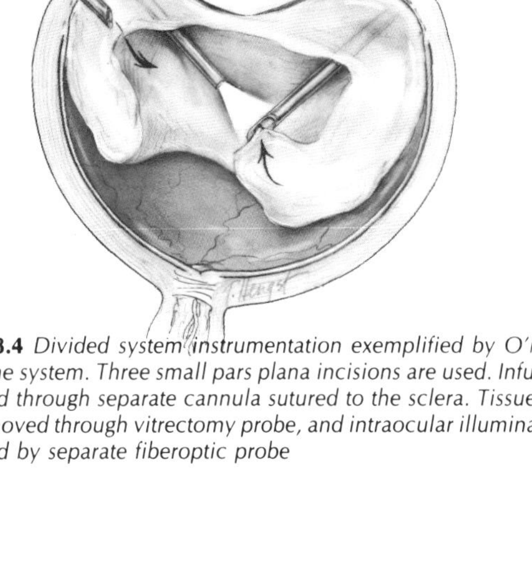

Figure 8.4 *Divided system instrumentation exemplified by O'Malley Ocutome system. Three small pars plana incisions are used. Infusion is provided through separate cannula sutured to the sclera. Tissue is cut and removed through vitrectomy probe, and intraocular illumination is provided by separate fiberoptic probe*

The separate infusion cannula has a large enough diameter, so that an adequate rate of infusion can be maintained even if a low intraocular pressure is selected. The separate cannula can be left in place while the other instruments are temporarily withdrawn and/or while procedures such as scleral buckling are performed. The separate infusion cannula also facilitates techniques for removal of non-clotted blood and for introduction of an intraocular gas bubble. Finally, the small-diameter probes can be easily exchanged for other specialized instruments during surgery. Divided system instrumentation provides considerable flexibility, and it is well suited for specialized techniques needed to treat complex cases.

Infusion and aspiration systems

The infusion system is under hydrostatic control, mostly determined by the height of a hanging bottle of clear physiological solution. Other more sophisticated mechanisms have been tried for controlling infusion, but these have been abandoned in favor of the simple and reliable hydrostatic method. The rate of infusion is dependent on a combination of factors, including: (*1*) the height of the fluid column in the infusion system; (*2*) the length and diameter of the connecting tubing and the lumen size of the infusion cannula; and (*3*) the rate of outflow from the eye through the aspiration system. In practical terms, the rate of flow through the infusion system is usually rapid enough to keep pace with outflow through the instruments so that, in most situations, the height of the column of infusion fluid above the eye is the main factor controlling the intraocular pressure.

The amount of suction force within the aspiration system is of considerable importance because this controls the entry of fluid and tissue into the aspiration-cutting port of the vitrectomy probe. Originally, suction force was controlled by a surgical assistant using a hand-held syringe while viewing the operative field through the operating microscope equipped with a beam splitter.

Automated devices are now preferred to provide the precise levels of suction force desired and to permit the surgeon to control the application of suction force using a footswitch or a device on the handpiece of the vitrectomy probe. Some instruments also permit the surgeon to alter the amount of suction force, although with many other instruments changes in the amount of suction force are made by other operating-room personnel adjusting the console panel. Even so, vitreous surgery is performed with considerable safety using automated devices to produce suction force, because only low amounts of suction force are usually needed and because the surgeon can instantly start and stop the suction force.

The amount of force acting to suck tissue into the cutting port is a complex matter determined by: (*1*) the amount of suction force in the aspiration system (difference between the higher intraocular pressure and the lower pressure in the cutting probe); (*2*) the distance the tissue is from the cutting port; and (*3*) the flow through the suction-cutting probe. However, once the height of the infusion bottle is selected, and if the infusion system is capable of rapid flow, changes in the amount of suction force in the aspiration system correlate directly with differing effects on intraocular tissue(s).

Accessory instruments

Accessory instruments used during vitreous surgery include: (*1*) a contact lens to permit visualization of the vitreous cavity; (*2*) an ultrasonic device to emulsify firm lens material; (*3*) needles, picks, probes and scissors for removing non-clotted blood, dissecting tissue planes and sectioning certain tissues; (*4*) forceps for removal of intraocular foreign bodies and for grasping tissue; and (*5*) separate probes and devices for transvitreal application of diathermy, cryotherapy and xenon photocoagulation. The tip diameter of each accessory instrument is the same as that of the basic vitrectomy illumination and cutting probes so that these instruments can be exchanged during the operation.

Corneal contact lenses

A planoconcave contact lens is needed to permit visualization deep in the vitreous cavity while using the operating microscope. Lenses of various designs are available, including self-retaining lenses, those with a surrounding ring that is secured to the sclera and those attached to a handle held by the surgical assistant. Some lenses contain an infusion system to irrigate fluid between the posterior lens surface and the cornea. We prefer a small (10 mm) lens to minimize contact with the shaft(s) of the intraocular instruments. Lenses with an infusion system and a handle seem to provide optimum visualization, and the position of the lens is easily adjusted as the eye is tilted and rotated during the operation (*Figure 8.5*).

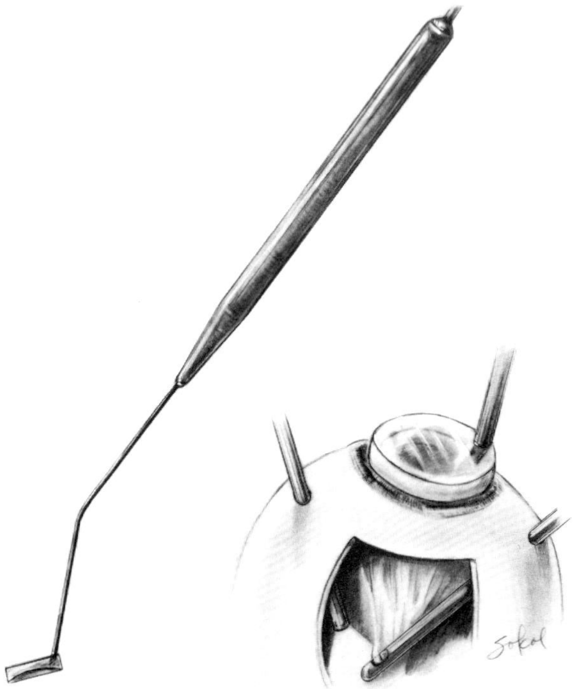

Figure 8.5 *Hand-held planoconcave contact lens used to permit visualization deep within vitreous cavity. Handle contains infusion channel for constant irrigation of fluid between lens and cornea*

Ultrasonic phacofragmenter

Removal of a cataractous lens during vitreous surgery is done effectively through a pars plana incision using an ultrasonic needle to emulsify and remove lens material of firm consistency[11]. Several devices are available for this purpose (*Figure 8.6*). When using divided system instrumentation with a separate infusion cannula, a second infusion system attached to the ultrasonic needle is not necessary. Therefore, an ultrasonic needle that is the same diameter as the vitrectomy probe is used, and the emulsified lens material is removed through the lumen of the needle as described later.

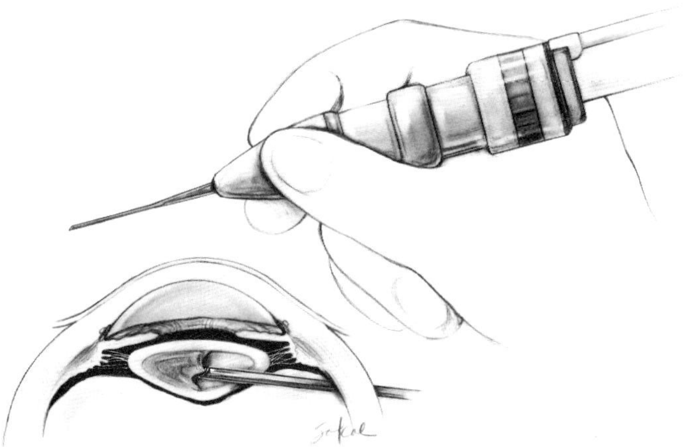

Figure 8.6 *Ultrasonic device, illustrated as Fragmatome component of Ocutome system, to remove firm lens material during combined cataract extraction and vitrectomy. Needle tip is introduced into lens through pars plana, and infusion is provided by separate needle or cannula (not shown)*

Aspiration, dissection, cutting and grasping instruments

Needles, picks, probes, scissors and forceps are used for specialized purposes during vitreous surgery. A blunt needle with a handle containing a channel and side port that is vented externally (Charles flute needle; *Figure 8.7a*) is used to evacuate non-clotted blood by permitting intraocular fluid to flow out of the eye through the needle and handle. This flow is the result of the pressure difference between the intraocular pressure and the lower atmospheric pressure outside the eye when the side port of the flute needle is not covered, as described later[12]. Vitreoretinal picks, hooked-tip needles and illumination probes with angulated metal tips are used to dissect tissue planes and separate epiretinal membranes from the inner retinal surface (*Figure 8.7b*). A series of such instruments with different tip designs of varying degrees of angulation, contour and sharpness is advantageous to permit dissection from different directions and to engage tissues of different consistencies. Vitreoretinal scissors are especially useful to section tissue near the inner retinal surface while causing only minimal traction on adjacent vitreoretinal attachments. Both motor-driven and finger-activated scissors are available. The most effective tip design places the blades at about a 90° angle to shaft, so that tissues along the plane of the inner retinal surface can be engaged between the blades (*Figure 8.7c*). Specialized forceps are used to grasp intraocular tissue during certain manipulations and to extract selected intraocular foreign bodies (*Figure 8.7d*). Forceps with different tip sizes, contours and design of blade surfaces are available for grasping foreign bodies of varying size, shape and consistency.

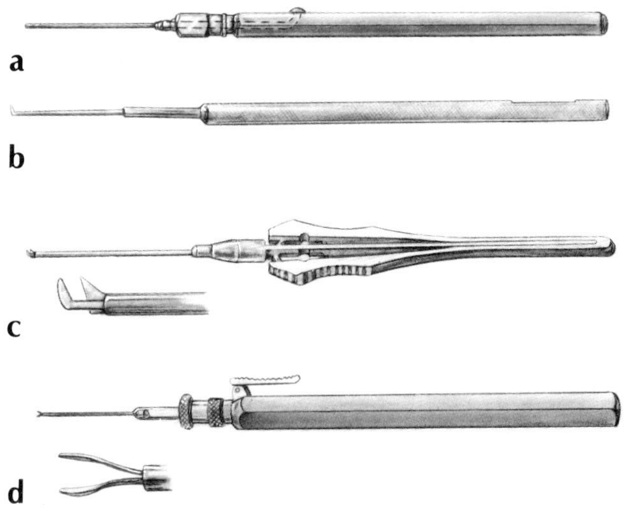

Figure 8.7 *Accessory instruments commonly used during vitreous surgery.* **(a)** *Blunt needle with 'flute handle' to permit rapid evacuation of intraocular fluid* (see also Figure 8.31). **(b)** *Vitreoretinal pick used to dissect tissue planes and separate epiretinal membranes from inner retinal surface.* **(c)** *Vitreoretinal scissors with blades oriented about 90° to instrument shaft and used mainly to cut tissue membranes parallel to inner retinal surface.* **(d)** *Intraocular forceps used to grasp selected foreign bodies or abnormal intraocular tissue*

Intraocular diathermy

Intraocular diathermy is used frequently during vitreous surgery to control bleeding and, less frequently, to cause shrinkage of fibrovascular tissue. Diathermy can be applied using a unipolar or bipolar system, but the bipolar method is preferable to minimize stray current that might be conducted by the optic nerve. Bipolar diathermy can be applied using a single coaxial probe containing two electrodes separated by suitable insulation. However, a more frequently used method is to attach diathermy leads to each of two surgical instruments within the eye, so that the instrument tips serve as electrodes (bimanual bipolar diathermy)[13,14]. Vascular tissue is positioned between the instrument tips, and current is conducted through the tissue to produce the coagulation effect (*Figure 8.8*). Bleeding sites on the inner retinal surface are more safely and easily treated with a single bipolar coaxial diathermy probe. This creates a small elliptical field of current around the end of the tip so that tissue can be treated without touching the probe to it.

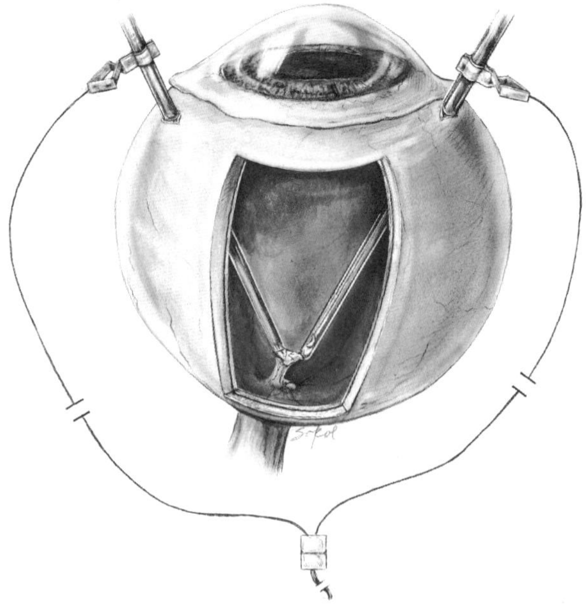

Figure 8.8 *Bimanual bipolar diathermy used to treat elevated fibrovascular tissue. The vitrectomy and illumination probes are connected to diathermy leads, and instrument tips serve as electrodes. Diathermy is conducted through fibrovascular tissue positioned between instrument tips*

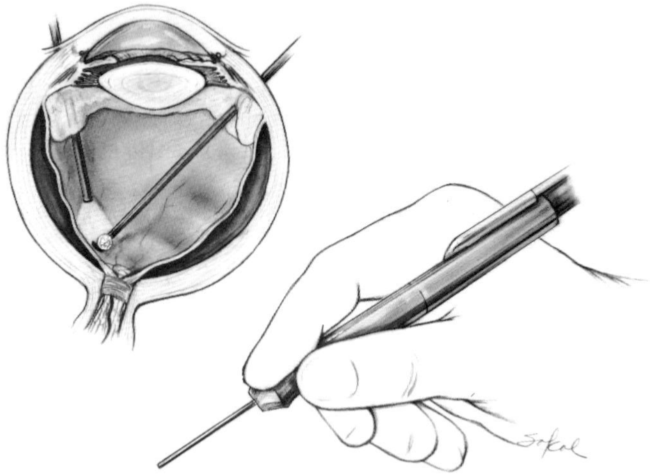

Figure 8.9 *Straight cryotherapy probe used for transvitreal treatment of posterior retinal breaks. Iceball formed on the instrument tip damages the retina and underlying pigment epithelium*

Intraocular cryotherapy and photocoagulation

Cryotherapy and xenon photocoagulation can both be applied in intravitreal fashion using special probes. Intraocular cryotherapy is sometimes used to treat posterior retinal holes. A straight cryoprobe with a diameter the same as the vitrectomy instrument is used. Tissue to be treated is touched with the end of the probe, and an iceball develops surrounding the tip (*Figure 8.9*). Transvitreal photocoagulation can be applied using a special fiberoptic probe attached to a xenon light source (*Figure 8.10*)[15]. This is used to coagulate bleeding sites, to treat selected retinal breaks and to apply panretinal (scatter) retinal photocoagulation. The light emitted from the fiberoptic probe is divergent, so the probe must be positioned near the area of retina to be coagulated. Both intraocular cryotherapy and photocoagulation permit precise, effective treatment of posterior retinal breaks located near the macula or optic nerve and limit the amount of adjacent tissue damage.

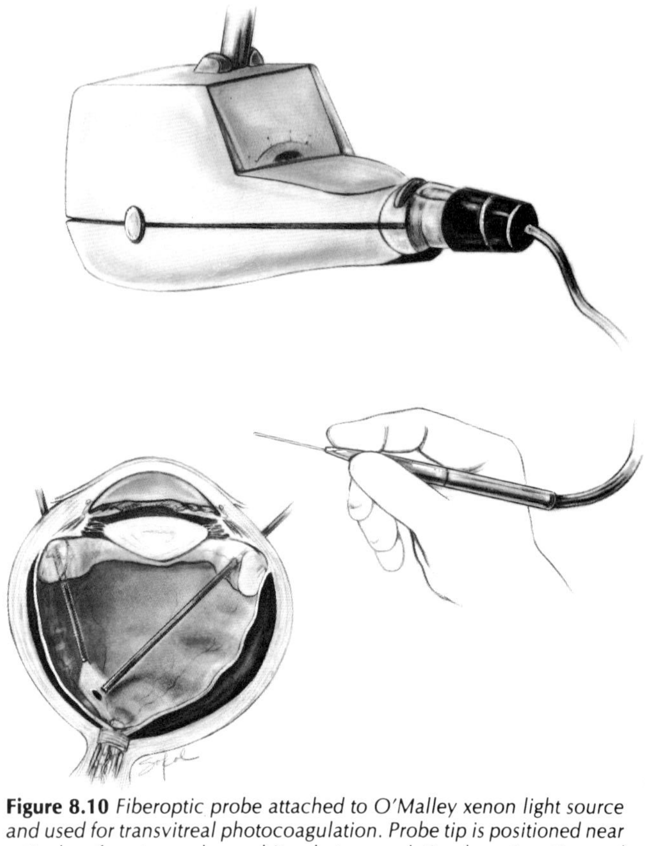

Figure 8.10 *Fiberoptic probe attached to O'Malley xenon light source and used for transvitreal photocoagulation. Probe tip is positioned near retinal surface to produce white photocoagulation burn in retina and pigment epithelium when treating posterior retinal break*

Preoperative evaluation

Preoperative evaluation of patients considered for vitreous surgery requires detailed history-taking and ocular examination and use of special tests in many cases. Thorough knowledge of the pathophysiological changes encountered in different disease conditions is also necessary to enable the physical findings to be interpreted correctly. Vitreous surgery is more complex and potentially more hazardous than most other ophthalmic surgical procedures, so that detailed preoperative evaluation is especially important to assist in proper case selection, to plan details of the operation, and to permit realistic discussion with the patient of potential benefits and risks.

Ophthalmic history

A complete ophthalmic history is taken, including any previous conditions that might limit postoperative vision and also those conditions currently affecting each eye. Specific aspects of history-taking depend on the underlying disease process. For example, details of the previous visual acuity, vitreoretinal anatomy and any photocoagulation therapy are especially important in diabetic patients with vitreous hemorrhage. This information helps in predicting the potential postoperative visual acuity, interpreting ultrasonographic findings and gauging the complexity of the anticipated surgical procedure.

Symptoms and physical findings in the fellow eye are also important in patients with proliferative diabetic retinopathy because of its often rather symmetrical clinical course. By aiding prediction of the further course of the disease in the other eye, this information may influence the decision on whether to recommend vitreous surgery. For example, if rapidly progressing fibrovascular proliferation is present in the fellow eye, vitreous surgery may be considered earlier in the eye with vitreous hemorrhage to prevent inoperable structural damage. However, if mild non-progressive background retinopathy or stable fibrotic-appearing proliferative tissue is present in the fellow eye, vitreous surgery may be delayed to await spontaneous clearing of the opacities.

In eyes with vitreous hemorrhage the length of time vision has been impaired is important. Vitrectomy is considered to remove the blood if there is no evidence of clearing after 6 months and if the fellow eye is also blind. If nearly normal vision is present in the fellow eye, we usually wait a minimum of 1 year, hoping for spontaneous clearing, unless early restoration of binocular stereoscopic vision is needed or unless there are signs of progressive damage that would cause irreversible visual loss. Surgery is usually deferred if there has been significant recent visual improvement although opacities may have been present for many months.

When the cause of vitreous hemorrhage is unknown, an attempt is made to identify medical conditions that may have affected the eye or to detect symptoms that are characteristic of a specific disorder. Diabetes mellitus with proliferative retinopathy is the most common cause of dense vitreous hemorrhage. Hemoglobin sickle-cell disease and other hemoglobinopathies should be considered in non-diabetic black patients. Prolonged systemic hypertension may be associated with retinal branch vein obstruction, followed later by neovascular proliferation and subsequent vitreous hemorrhage. However, in these eyes there is usually a history of pre-existing partial visual loss because of macular involvement by the vein obstruction. Patients with chronic leukemia occasionally develop vitreous hemorrhage, and in patients with Terson's syndrome (vitreous hemorrhage following subarachnoid hemorrhage) the history is diagnostic. When vitreous hemorrhage is due to a primary ocular condition, the history of antecedent symptoms may be diagnostic. For example, when an acute vitreous hemorrhage is preceded by severe photopsia, it is likely that vitreous traction on the retina causing a retinal tear is the pathogenetic mechanism.

Ocular examination

Both eyes are examined, including best corrected visual acuity, external evaluation, tonometry and slit-lamp examination. Detailed examination of the vitreous cavity and vitreoretinal relations by binocular indirect ophthalmoscopy is performed, and fundus biomicroscopy with a three-mirror contact lens is done when possible.

The best corrected visual acuity is measured quantitatively, including low levels of vision of less than 20/200. When visual acuity is less than 1/200, the presence of light perception and projection and the ability to perceive hand motion are determined and measured at the farthest distance the patient can recognize them. Light projection is evaluated in each quadrant, and the accuracy and rapidity of subjective responses are recorded. In our experience, brisk and accurate light projection is the most important preoperative finding corresponding favorably with visual improvement after vitrectomy in eyes with dense vitreous hemorrhage.

Brisk pupillary constriction to light is also a good prognostic sign in eyes with vitreous opacities. However, the pupillary response is often sluggish in patients with proliferative diabetic retinopathy, especially if extensive retinal photocoagulation has been performed. Dense vitreous hemorrhage alone can also cause a detectable afferent pupillary defect.

Examination of the iris and pupil is also important for other reasons. The size of the pupil after maximum dilation is measured to determine whether intraoperative visualization will be adequate, taking into account the location of the vitreoretinal pathology that must be approached by the vitrectomy instruments. The presence of preoperative iris neovascularization is a poor prognostic sign. It may influence the decision on whether or not to recommend vitreous surgery and/or the technique to be used, such as combining intraoperative panretinal photocoagulation with vitrectomy in eyes with active proliferative diabetic retinopathy and rubeosis iridis.

The intraocular pressure is measured and correlated with other physical findings. Intractable pressure elevation may be an indication for surgery in selected eyes with hyphema or blood-induced glaucoma complicating vitreous hemorrhage. In other cases, glaucoma influences intraoperative decisions such as whether to use an intraocular gas bubble that would expand postoperatively. Low intraocular pressure may be a sign of retinal detachment and/or suprachoroidal effusion. The latter is especially important because it makes introduction of vitrectomy instruments hazardous. These cases are investigated by ultrasonography if dense lens or anterior vitreous opacities are present, and drainage of suprachoroidal fluid is performed before making pars plana incisions through the uveal tissue into the vitreous cavity.

Slit-lamp examination of the lens is performed to evaluate the optical significance of opacities and to decide whether lens removal should be combined with vitreous surgery. The degree of firmness of the lens nucleus is estimated, and this finding influences the method chosen for lens removal. Lenses with a slight or moderate amount of nuclear sclerosis are removed through the small pars plana incision using ultrasonic emulsification. If brunescent nuclear opacities are seen that suggest a hard lens consistency, intracapsular or extracapsular extraction may be performed through the limbus and combined with vitreous surgery during the same operation.

Examination of the vitreous gel and vitreoretinal relations is the most important part of preoperative evaluation, and this is done both by indirect ophthalmoscopy and by biomicroscopy using a three-mirror contact lens. Three-dimensional relations of the vitreous gel and retina are recorded, including cross-sectional views and a conventional fundus drawing (*Figure 8.11*). Of special importance are the relations between the posterior vitreous surface and the retina, including (*1*) areas where the posterior vitreous surface is separated from the retina; (*2*) the size, location and characteristics of vitreoretinal adhesions; (*3*) optical and structural density of membranes involving the posterior vitreous surface; (*4*) areas of vitreoretinal traction; (*5*) areas of retinal detachment, including both traction and rhegmatogenous types; and (*6*) the exact location of any retinal breaks. Proper interpretation of the physical findings requires a thorough knowledge of the pathophysiological features of each separate disease entity.

Fortunately as regards surgery, certain patterns of vitreoretinal relations occur repeatedly in different clinical disorders, and recognizing these patterns facilitates preoperative evaluation. For example, in eyes with proliferative retinopathies, fibrovascular tissue grows along the posterior vitreous surface. Therefore, elevation of the margin of fibrovascular tissue indicates that the posterior vitreous surface is partially separated from the retina (*Figure 8.12*). This characteristic helps to identify a transparent posterior vitreous surface. Similarly, in eyes with massive periretinal proliferation, there is typically a transvitreal sheet in the midvitreous cavity, and abnormal tissue on the inner retinal surface is evidenced by fixed retinal folds and other features of distortion of the inner retinal surface.

Preoperative identification of all retinal breaks is especially important when rhegmatogenous detachment is present, so that details of the operation can be planned accordingly. The location of any breaks and the complexities of the related vitreoretinal anatomy determine such decisions as whether scleral buckling will be needed as an

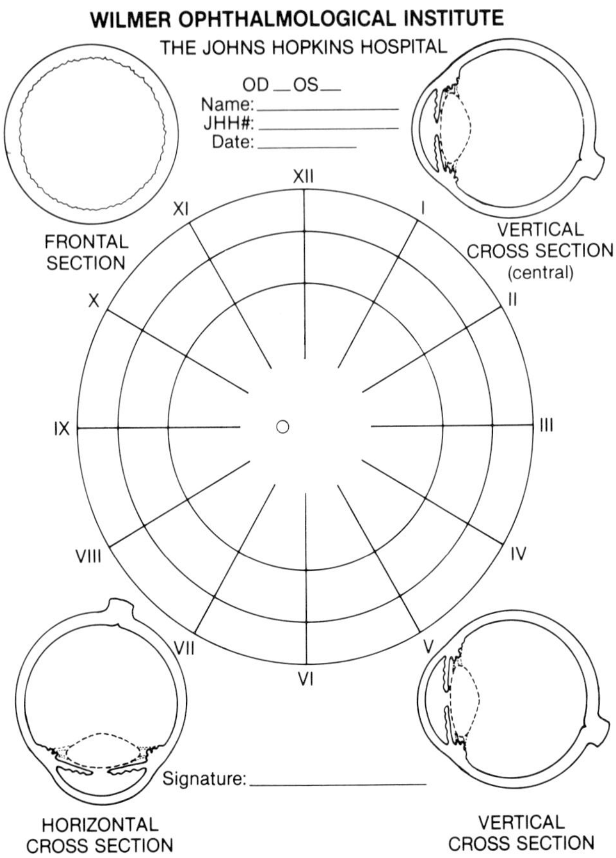

Figure 8.11 *Vitreoretinal drawing chart with space for usual large retinal drawing and cross-section representations of vitreoretinal anatomy*

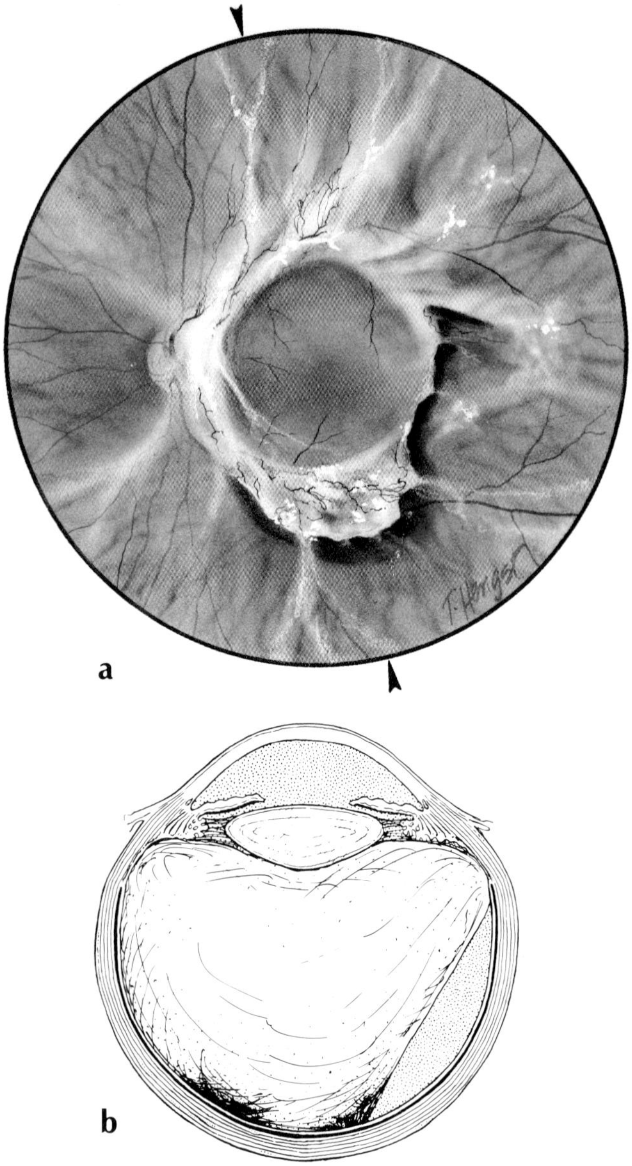

Figure 8.12 **(a)** *Proliferative diabetic retinopathy with epiretinal fibrovascular tissue having elevated peripheral margin inferiorly.* **(b)** *Elevated edge of fibrovascular tissue indicates detachment of adjacent posterior vitreous surface on which the abnormal tissue is growing*

adjunct to vitreous surgery, whether transscleral or transvitreal treatment of the retinal breaks will be performed, and whether an intraocular bubble will be needed. When the exact location of each retinal break is known preoperatively, this also influences the sequence of events during the operation. For example, retinal breaks may first be localized regarding their position in relation to the sclera, so that sutures can be placed for later scleral buckling before performing intraocular portions of the operation.

When vitreous opacities are present, visualization of the retina may be limited or impossible. However, the vitreous gel is examined despite the presence of opacities, and this can give important information about the underlying vitreoretinal anatomy. The degree of mobility of the vitreous gel is determined. The presence of visible transvitreal membranes and/or restricted mobility suggests that there is peripheral vitreoretinal traction. Often the vitreous gel is cone-shaped because the posterior hyaloid surface is partially separated from the retina and extends in an anteroposterior direction from the vitreous base to areas of posterior vitreoretinal attachment. Frequently, opacities in the vitreous cavity involve mainly the posterior vitreous surface, or blood may be present primarily in the preretinal space behind the partially separated

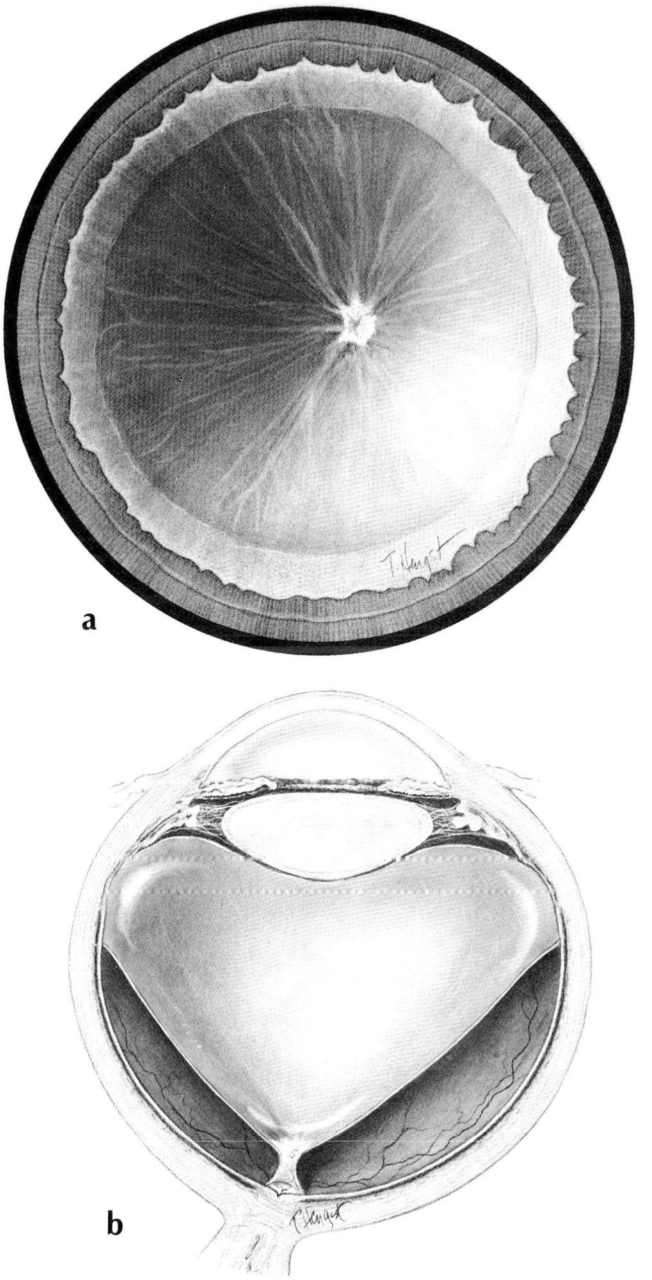

Figure 8.13 **(a)** *Cone-like shape of an opaque posterior vitreous surface inserting into a small, moderately elevated fibrovascular stalk coming from the region of the optic nerve.* **(b)** *Narrow base of the fibrovascular stalk causes minimal damage to the posterior retina*

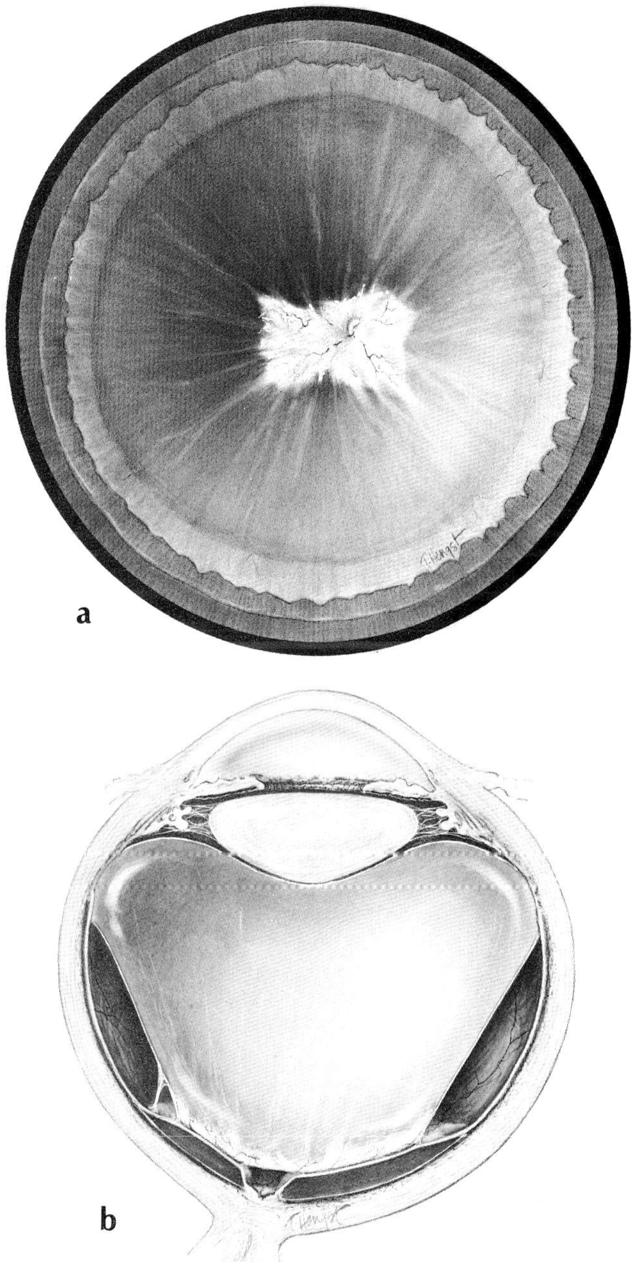

Figure 8.14 **(a)** *Cone-like shape of an opaque vitreous surface inserting into the peripheral margin of a large sheet of epiretinal fibrovascular tissue covering much of the posterior retina.* **(b)** *Often the underlying retina is detached by traction*

posterior vitreous surface. The structural anatomy of the vitreous may therefore be visible despite the presence of opacities that obscure details of the retina.

The size, location and other features of posterior vitreoretinal adhesions provide important clues to the probable underlying vitreoretinal anatomy. For example, when the cone-shaped posterior vitreous surface inserts into a pedicle of fibrovascular tissue with a narrow base, the effect of this vitreoretinal complex on the underlying retina may be mild (*Figure 8.13*). However, when the posterior vitreous surface inserts into the peripheral margins of an extensive sheet of epiretinal fibrovascular tissue, the underlying and surrounding retina is likely to be severely involved (*Figure 8.14*). Identification of these features also aids in interpreting ultrasonographic findings.

Special ophthalmic tests

Additional tests, including combined A- and B-scan ultrasonography and electroretinography, are valuable in the preoperative evaluation of certain patients. Radiographic examination of the orbit is performed if a retained intraocular foreign body is suspected, and CT scan localization is of particular value in such cases. Fundus and/or iris fluorescein angiography are sometimes performed.

Diagnostic ultrasound

Diagnostic ultrasound performed with ultrahigh frequency sound waves is used to localize, outline and characterize intraocular tissues and foreign material – including their configuration, interrelations, tissue density features, and response to external stimuli. A beam of ultrahigh frequency sound is passed through the eye, and the acoustic-impedance interfaces along the pathway of the beam cause differential reflection of the sound waves back to the transducer. This reflected information is then displayed on cathode-ray tube.

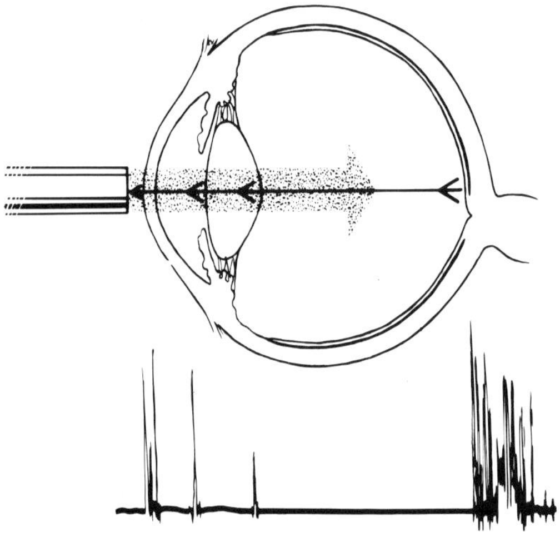

Figure 8.15 *Principle of A-scan ultrasonography. Sound waves emitted by a transducer are reflected by the ocular tissue surfaces, and the reflected waves are displayed on cathode-ray tube. The amplitude of each reflected wave is proportional to the acoustic-impedance interface, and this characterizes the ocular tissue*

Anatomical features of ocular tissues provide reflective interfaces that can be spatially localized and characterized. Because sound waves travel through soft tissue at a nearly constant velocity, the elapsed time between the emission of the wave and reception of the various reflected waves by the transducer is directly proportional to the distance travelled. The amount of sound reflected at each acoustic-impedance interface characterizes the density of the ocular tissue (A-scan ultrasonography) (*Figure 8.15*).

By moving the transducer back and forth in a single plane and displaying the echo pattern as a composite representation, features of the globe can be demonstrated in horizontal, vertical or oblique cross-section (B-scan

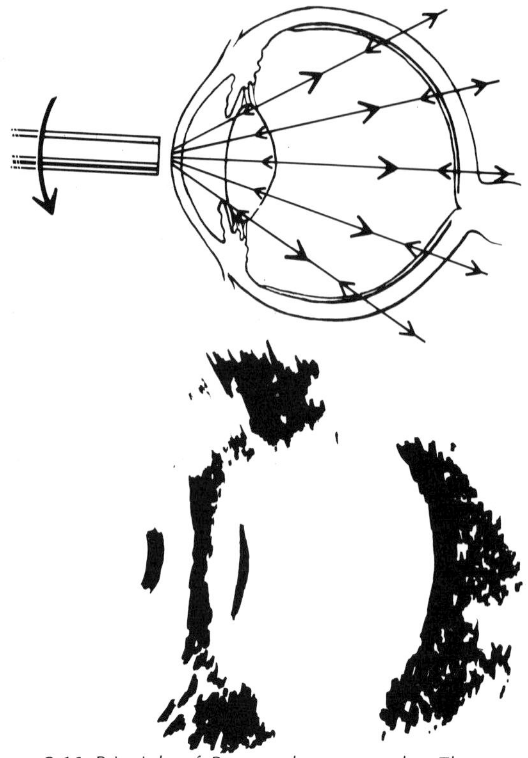

Figure 8.16 *Principle of B-scan ultrasonography. The transducer is moved in a plane and the reflected sound waves from each tissue interface are displayed as single dots, giving a composite representation of the globe*

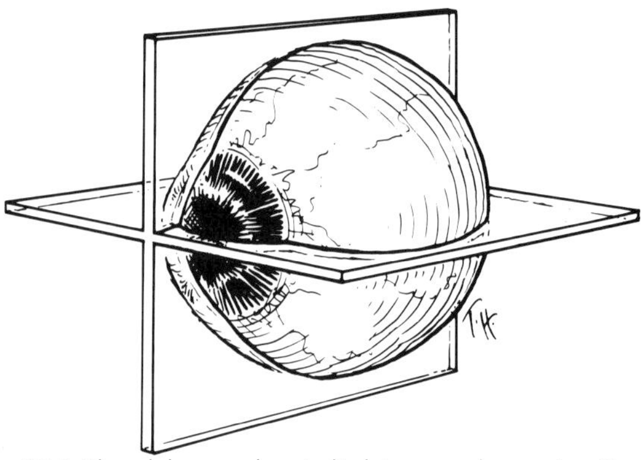

Figure 8.17 *The globe can be studied in any plane using B-scan ultrasonography although vertical and horizontal anteroposterior sections are used most commonly because these are easily interpreted*

ultrasonography) (*Figures 8.16* and *8.17*). The B-scan method provides a graphic representation of various ocular tissues which are identifiable by their morphological characteristics. Ultrasound examination is a kinetic procedure in which the examiner moves the transducer and simultaneously observes the image displayed on the screen. Varying the position of the eye and the transducer probe permits examination of different portions of the globe.

Diagnostic ultrasound is important in preoperative evaluation of patients with opaque ocular media. Ultrasound examination occasionally discloses unsuspected pathology such as a choroidal tumor. Its primary value, however, is in studying the extent and complexity of posterior vitreoretinal adhesions that cannot be visualized directly and in determining the location and extent of retinal detachment. For example, traction retinal detachment that is thought to involve the macula constitutes an indication for immediate vitrectomy even though vitreous hemorrhage has been of short duration and may be expected to clear spontaneously.

Electroretinography

The electroretinogram (ERG) is an external recording of the summated electrical responses of the retinal cells to a standardized light-flash stimulus. The clinically significant portion of the recording has a characteristic waveform composed of an initial downward deflection generated by the outer segments of the receptor elements (a-wave) and a subsequent upper deflection generated by the bipolar cells and/or the Mueller cells (b-wave) (*Figure 8.18*). The ERG thus provides information about two different

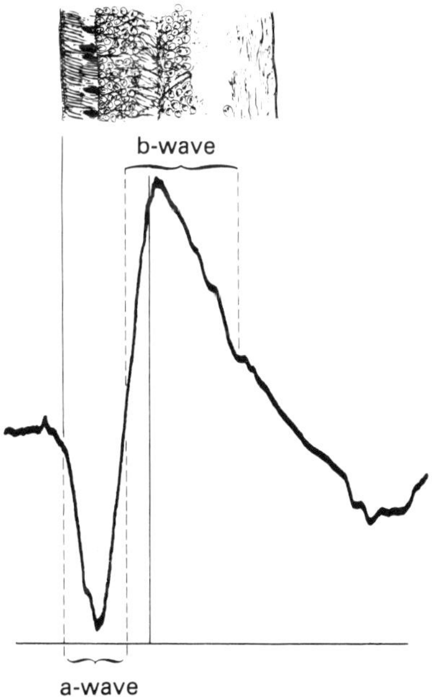

Figure 8.18 *Normal ERG wave form composed of an initial downward deflection (a-wave) generated by the outer segments of the receptor elements and a later upward deflection (b-wave) generated by the Mueller cells and/or the bipolar cells. The latter portion of the initial downward deflection is obscured by the larger upward deflection*

populations of cells within the retina with separate vascular supplies, and it can be analyzed with regard to alterations in the wave form and/or variations in the amplitude of deflection.

The ERG is dependent on the light-flash stimulus reaching the retina, and opacities of the media can filter or block the light. When dense intraocular opacities are present, a brighter light-flash stimulus can be used to penetrate the opaque media and elicit an electrical response (bright-flash ERG) (*Figure 8.19*).

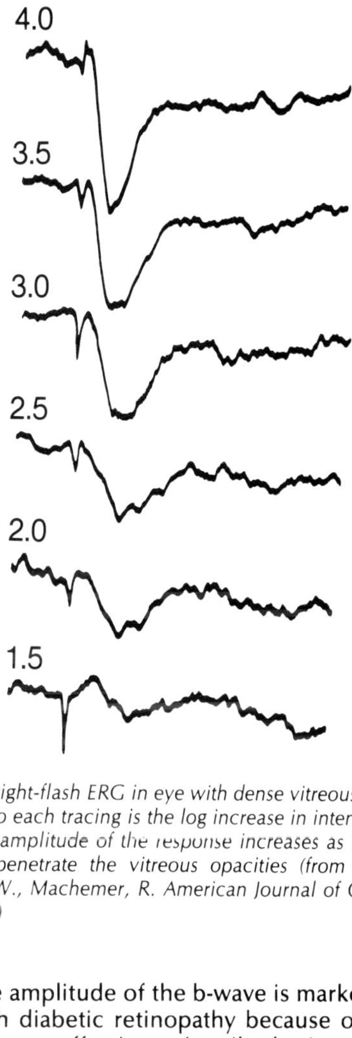

Figure 8.19 *Bright-flash ERG in eye with dense vitreous opacities. The number next to each tracing is the log increase in intensity of the light stimulus. The amplitude of the response increases as brighter stimuli are used to penetrate the vitreous opacities (from Fuller, D. G., Knighton, R. W., Machemer, R. American Journal of Ophthalmology 1975; 80:214)*

Often the amplitude of the b-wave is markedly reduced in eyes with diabetic retinopathy because of intraretinal vascular disease affecting primarily the inner half of the retina. Therefore even though a markedly reduced b-wave, with a good amplitude a-wave, may be recorded in eyes with diabetic retinopathy and vitreous hemorrhage, vision may still improve considerably after removing the vitreous opacities (*Figure 8.20*).

The most useful application of electroretinography is in helping to differentiate between a total retinal detachment and a thickened opaque posterior vitreous detachment. Usually an ERG response cannot be recorded in eyes with total retinal detachment. This ERG correlation is especially helpful when ultrasonography shows a funnel-shaped echo pattern extending from the optic nerve to the region of the ora serrata, because this pattern may be caused either by retinal detachment or by a partially separated

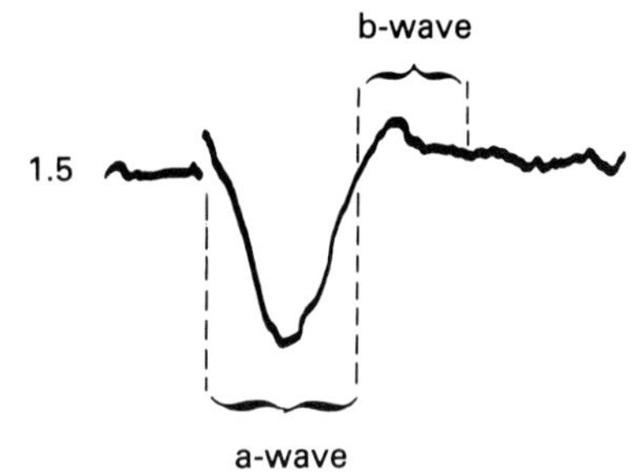

Figure 8.20 *ERG in eye with clear media and advanced proliferative diabetic retinopathy with a reduced b-wave amplitude suggesting severe intraretinal vascular disease affecting the inner half of the retina. The a-wave is prominent when a light flash 1.5 log units brighter than the usual stimulus is used, whereas the b-wave is of low amplitude (from Fuller, D. G., Knighton, R. W., Machemer, R. American Journal of Ophthalmology 1975; 80:214)*

and thickened posterior vitreous surface. When this ultrasonographic echo pattern is associated with a recordable ERG response, it is likely that the retina is not detached and that the echo pattern is caused by vitreous membranes instead.

Surgical principles and techniques

Vitreous surgery methods are now used to treat a wide variety of conditions, ranging from thin, opaque pupillary membranes to complicated types of rhegmatogenous retinal detachment with severe vitreous traction and extensive epiretinal membranes[16]. Therefore, the objectives of surgery vary widely, and different techniques are used in various combinations and sequences. Many types of instrumentation are used, each with different capabilities and limitations. Finally, differing surgical approaches can be used, including limbal or pars plana incisions or a combination of both approaches.

Despite the variations introduced by different indications and instrumentation, and also the individual features of each case, the basic principles of vitreous surgery are well established. The operation is performed through watertight incisions, so that the intraocular pressure is maintained in a suitable range throughout the procedure and yet needed movement of the instruments is not restricted. The pupil is dilated widely to permit optimal visualization, and care is taken to avoid damage to the corneal epithelium from direct trauma or from drying changes. Minimum levels of suction force are used throughout the operation to avoid creating retinal breaks. Various instruments are used, one after the other, or in various combinations, to perform special tasks. The procedure is completed as rapidly as safely possible, and damage to adjacent normal tissues is avoided.

The anatomical and mechanical objectives of the operation are achieved in a sequential fashion. This minimizes the risks associated with certain complex maneuvers, and it facilitates prompt treatment of any complication that may occur. When treating anterior segment conditions such as a pupillary membrane or vitreous complications in the anterior chamber, the primary objectives are often to create a clear pupillary space and to leave the anterior chamber free of vitreous gel. When dealing with posterior segment conditions, the objectives are usually to remove any intravitreal opacities, to excise the posterior vitreous surface, to stop any active bleeding, and to remove or segment epiretinal membranes or preretinal proliferative tissue that is distorting and/or damaging the retina or that is likely to cause postoperative complications. These surgical objectives in posterior segment conditions are usually achieved in the following sequence: (*1*) removal of axial opacities; (*2*) release of anteroposterior vitreoretinal traction by excising the posterior vitreous surface, which is often partially separated from the retina and extends between the vitreous base anteriorly and the optic nerve and/or areas of posterior vitreoretinal attachment; (*3*) release of transverse or tangential vitreoretinal traction by excision of remaining portions of the posterior cortical vitreous and/or elevated tissue membranes that bridge one area of retina and another; and (*4*) separation or segmentation of epiretinal membranes that are adversely affecting the peripapillary retina or macular area.

Surgical anatomy

Safe performance of vitreous surgery requires knowledge of the anatomical features of the pars plana and its adjacent structures. The pars plana ciliaris is the flat part of the ciliary body; it extends between the posterior margin of the pars plicata ciliaris, which is about 2 mm posterior to the limbus, and the ora serrata which varies in position as regards the nasal and temporal sides of the globe (*Figure 8.21*). The pars plana zone is approximately 4.5 mm wide in the temporal quadrants and 3 mm wide in the nasal quadrants. Transillumination through the pupil can

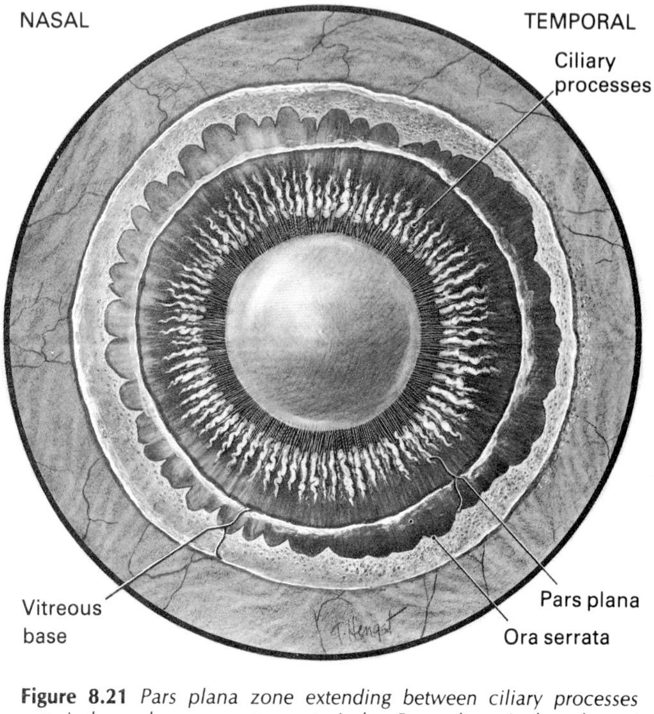

Figure 8.21 *Pars plana zone extending between ciliary processes anteriorly and ora serrata posteriorly. Pars plana is broader on temporal side and vitreous base extends onto pars plana for variable distance*

be used in eyes with normal pigmentation to aid in identifying the pars plana, which is bounded anteriorly by the more heavily pigmented pars plicata ciliaris and posteriorly by a ring of increased pigmentation at the ora serrata (*Figure 8.22*). The position of the ora serrata can

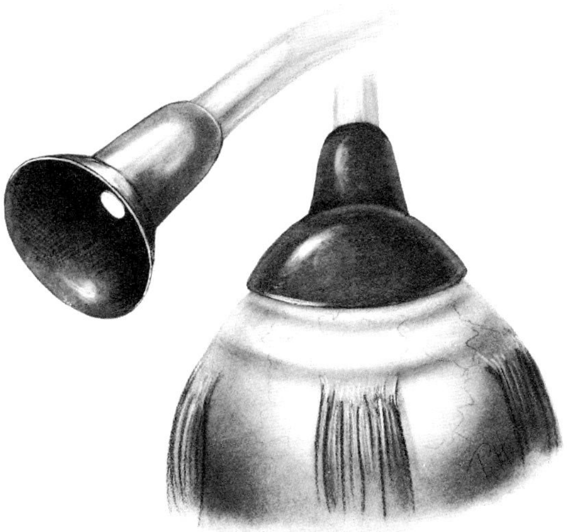

Figure 8.22 *Fiberoptic transillumination used to demonstrate ora serrata when choosing location for pars plana incision. Corona ciliaris and ora serrata appear as concentric dark circles on either side of pars plana zone*

usually be ascertained externally by identifying the rectus muscle insertions, which correspond closely to the location of the ora serrata in adult non-myopic eyes. In myopic eyes the ora serrata is often located posterior to the rectus muscle insertions and it is best to use transillumination.

The pars plana sclerotomies are prepared in the mid or anterior part of the pars plana to avoid the vitreous base – a zone 3–4 mm wide straddling the ora serrata, where the vitreous is firmly adherent to the underlying retina and to the ciliary epithelium anterior to the ora serrata (*Figure 8.23*). The posterior extent of the vitreous base is variable.

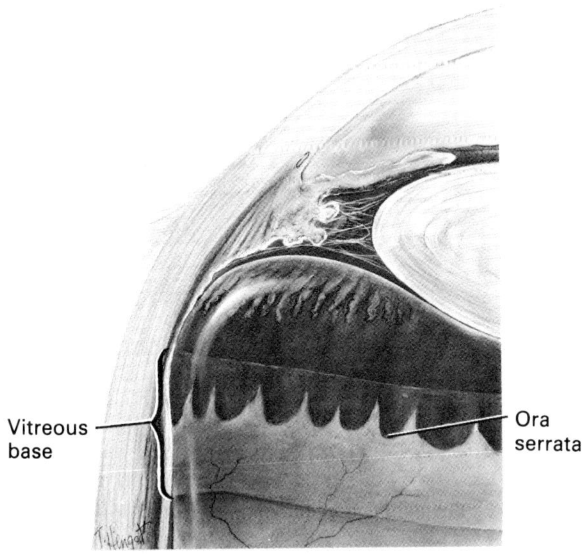

Figure 8.23 *Region of vitreous base straddling ora serrata. Vitreous is firmly adherent to peripheral retina and ciliary epithelium in this 3–4 mm zone*

It usually extends farther back on the nasal side than on the temporal side. The concentration of collagen fibrils is especially high in the region of the vitreous base, and these fibrils have a radial orientation rather than the circumferential orientation of collagen fibrils in the posterior vitreous cortex. The radially oriented collagen is interwoven with a complex of multilaminar basement membrane and cell processes from the adjacent retinal and ciliary body epithelial cells. This accounts for the zone of firm attachment of the vitreous base. Traction on the region of the vitreous base may cause retinal breaks along its posterior margin.

Other important features of intraocular surgical anatomy depend on posterior vitreoretinal relations and secondary changes in the vitreous gel. These features, in turn, are affected by the specific disease process. Normally the cortical vitreous is in contact with the internal limiting membrane of the retina, and there are relatively firm adhesions between these surfaces at the optic disc and along the peripheral margins of any zones of lattice degeneration. Less firm vitreous adhesions may be present in the macular area and along some retinal vessels.

Separation of the cortical vitreous from the retina (posterior vitreous detachment) may occur as a result of aging changes that affect the hyaluronic acid macromolecular structure of the gel or as a result of secondary changes in various diseases. For example, in proliferative retinopathies bleeding may occur into the vitreous gel causing liquefaction, and/or extraretinal fibrovascular tissue may grow along the posterior vitreous surface and contract. These features result in vitreous detachment, although the vitreous usually remains adherent posteriorly in the areas of fibrovascular tissue growth (*Figure 8.24*). Secondary changes in the vitreous gel may lead to further alterations such as posterior traction retinal detachment or retinal break formation resulting in rhegmatogenous detachment and dispersion of pigment epithelial cells into the vitreous

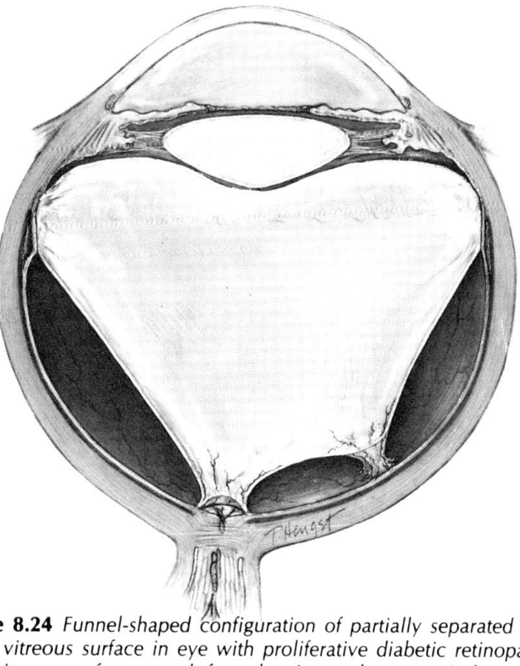

Figure 8.24 *Funnel-shaped configuration of partially separated posterior vitreous surface in eye with proliferative diabetic retinopathy. Taut vitreous surface extends from the vitreous base anteriorly to areas of fibrovascular proliferation posteriorly and bridges between separate areas of proliferation*

cavity. This cellular dispersion may be followed later by cell proliferation on vitreous surfaces and along the inner retina, causing membranes that contract and distort and/or elevate the retina further. It can be seen that the anatomical features of the vitreoretinal relations can vary widely, and these features are mentioned later when surgical management of specific clinical conditions is discussed.

Anesthesia and preparation for surgery

Ordinarily, either local or general anesthesia can be used for vitreous surgery, and the choice is often left to the patient. General anesthesia is necessary for children, and this is also preferred for reoperations and procedures that will require more than 2 hours. Some patients become restless when local anesthesia is used, and general anesthesia minimizes the risk of sudden movement.

Occasionally it is desirable to use local anesthesia so that the patient can change his position during the operation to assist in performing certain maneuvers. For example, when epiretinal fibrovascular proliferation extends far toward the fundus periphery, it is helpful if the patient can slowly rotate his head from side to side, or elevate or lower his chin when requested by the surgeon to improve visualization of the midperipheral fundus in various quadrants. In treatment of eyes with giant retinal tears that require intraoperative fluid-gas exchange in a face-down position, use of local anesthesia permits the patient to assist the surgeon by assuming a prone position at the appropriate time during the operation. Lastly, use of local anesthesia may minimize the likelihood of postoperative nausea and vomiting and severe metabolic disequilibrium in diabetic patients. This, in turn, may lessen the likelihood of postoperative intraocular bleeding.

When local anesthesia is selected, we prefer 4 per cent lidocaine (lignocaine) mixed in equal parts with 0.75 per cent bupivacaine to which hyaluronidase is added. We first inject this mixture just posterior to the earlobe to block the facial nerve; then we infiltrate the region of the lateral canthus if a canthotomy is needed; finally a retrobulbar injection is given into the extraocular muscle cone (*Figure 8.25*). This combination of anesthetic medications

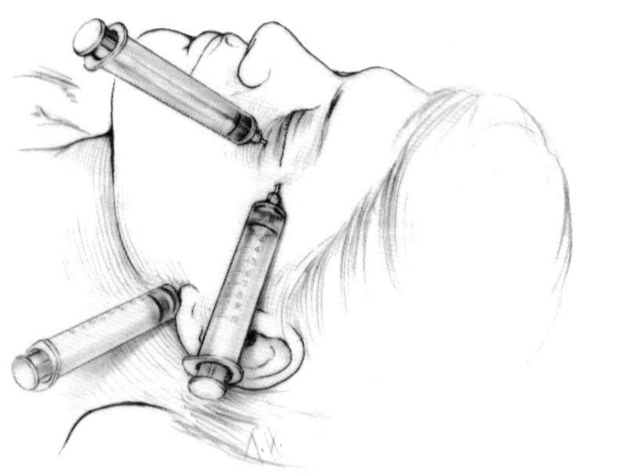

Figure 8.25 *Injections of medications for local anesthesia, including facial nerve block posterior to earlobe, infiltration of lateral canthal area and retrobulbar injection into extraocular muscle cone*

usually provides adequate analgesia and akinesia for about 3 hours. The retrobulbar injection can be repeated if some of the extraocular muscles remain active after 20 minutes or if the patient experiences pain later during the operation. Systemic medications to provide a sedative effect are administered intravenously.

The head is rotated so that the eye is in a suitable position before cleaning the operative field and applying the drapes. Usually we rotate the head slightly away from the eye to be operated on, to minimize mechanical restrictions caused by the nose. The eye is oriented in a straight-ahead position to permit equal rotation in all directions later. The viewing axis of the operating microscope is oriented vertically to permit equal viewing in all quadrants of the vitreous cavity (*Figure 8.26*).

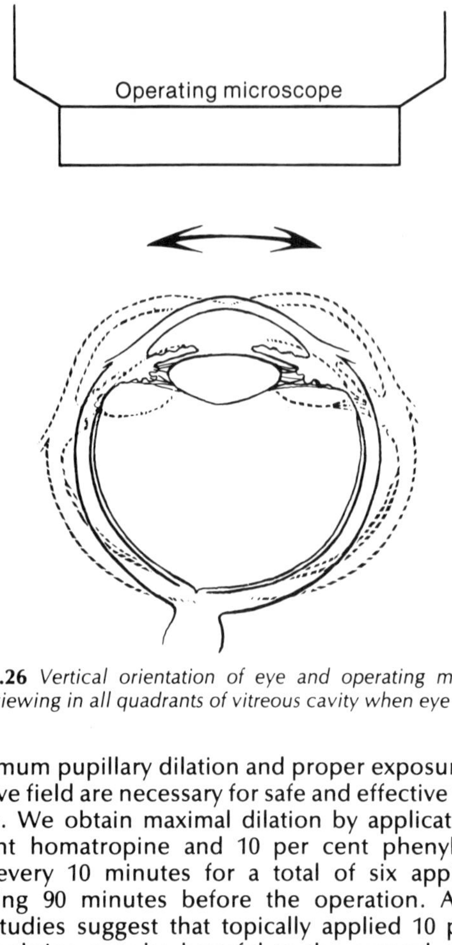

Figure 8.26 *Vertical orientation of eye and operating microscope permits viewing in all quadrants of vitreous cavity when eye is rotated*

Maximum pupillary dilation and proper exposure of the operative field are necessary for safe and effective vitreous surgery. We obtain maximal dilation by application of 5 per cent homatropine and 10 per cent phenylephrine drops every 10 minutes for a total of six applications beginning 90 minutes before the operation. Although some studies suggest that topically applied 10 per cent phenylephrine may be harmful to the corneal endothelium, we have not noted this effect if the corneal epithelium is normal when the medication is applied. The patient is instructed to keep both eyes closed between application of these mydriatic drops because phenylephrine may cause mild opacities, irregularities and other drying changes of the corneal epithelium if the lids remain open after the medication is applied.

A 0.2 ml subconjunctival injection of a mydriatic compound containing 0.4 per cent homatropine, 0.5 per cent phenylephrine, and procaine in an isotonic solution may be given before beginning the operation. This may dilate the pupil further, and it also seems to maintain maximal pupillary dilation throughout the operation despite brief periods of hypotony and possible contact with the iris by the surgical instruments. If the pupil constricts during the operation despite these precautions, various methods may be used to enlarge it, such as excision of portions of iris tissue in aphakic eyes, topical application of mydriatic drops and intraocular injection of dilute mydriatic solutions such as 1:10 000 epinephrine (adrenaline).

A lateral canthotomy is often performed to permit especially wide separation of the lid margins. This permits use of a conventional lid speculum, and it minimizes difficulties caused by contact between the vitrectomy instruments or corneal contact lens and the lid speculum when the eye is rotated superiorly or inferiorly. Eyes with marked enophthalmos may also be a problem because of contact between the instruments and the bony orbital rim. A supplemental retrobulbar injection can be given to cause some proptosis of the eye, although this is rarely necessary.

Pars plana and limbal incisions

Pars plana incisions are made parallel to the limbus in the mid or anterior portion of the pars plana zone. Incisions for small diameter vitrectomy instruments are made 3–4 mm posterior to the anterior margin of the limbus. Therefore, each incision is well anterior to the region of the vitreous base. Usually three incisions are made: one just inferior to the meridian of the lateral rectus muscle for introduction of the infusion cannula, and the others just superior to the meridians of each horizontal rectus muscle for introduction of the vitrectomy probe and the separate fiberoptic illuminating probe (*Figure 8.27*). When a full-function vitrectomy probe with a fiberoptic sleeve is used, the incision is made 5 mm posterior to the limbus in the superotemporal quadrant where the pars plana is widest. This provides adequate clearance between the crystalline lens anteriorly and the ora serrata posteriorly. Each incision is made with a knife that has a blade of suitable width to permit easy introduction of the surgical instruments through the scleral incision while maintaining a watertight seal around the instrument shaft. When a larger incision is

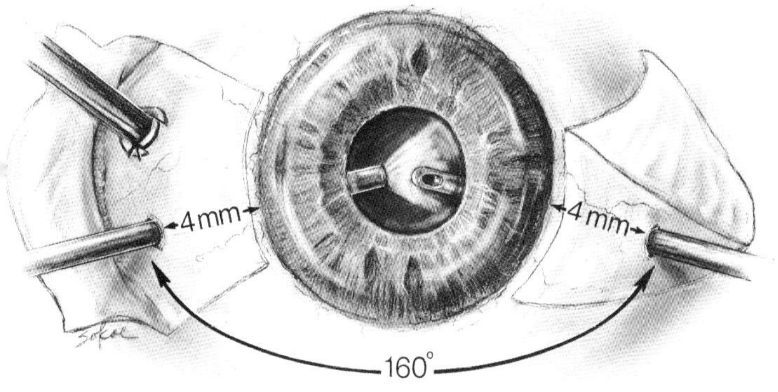

Figure 8.27 *Surgeon's view of left eye with three pars plana incisions made for divided system vitrectomy instrumentation. Infusion cannula is sutured to sclera inferior to lateral rectus muscle. Vitrectomy and illumination probes are introduced about 160° apart through incisions just superior to horizontal rectus muscles. Each incision is about 4 mm posterior to the anterior margin of limbal zone*

made for use of a full-function vitrectomy probe, the interior opening in pars plana uveal tissue is inspected before introducing the surgical instrument to make certain the opening in this elastic tissue is as large as the scleral incision. If it is not, the uveal incision is enlarged with scissors.

When a limbal approach is chosen, the incisions are made parallel to the plane of the iris to facilitate introduction of the instruments for manipulations in the pupillary space and the anterior portion of the vitreous cavity. Incisions may be made through peripheral clear cornea anterior to the limbal zone or through the limbus after creating a small, limbus-based conjunctival flap. These incisions are made with a knife that has the correct blade-width to produce a watertight incision for the surgical instruments. Excessively long limbal incisions are troublesome because if leakage occurs around the instrument shaft, the anterior chamber, which has a small volume, will collapse and damage to the corneal endothelium may occur.

Lens removal

The crystalline lens is removed if cataractous changes are severe enough to limit the visualization needed for safe completion of the operation or to reduce significantly the postoperative visual acuity. Rarely, it is necessary to remove a clear lens to facilitate special techniques when treating complicated forms of retinal detachment. We remove a cataractous lens through the small pars plana incision that is made for the vitrectomy instrument unless the lens nucleus is exceptionally hard, in which case intracapsular cataract extraction through a limbal approach is done before beginning vitreous surgery during the same operation.

A lens of soft consistency is fragmented and aspirated using the vitrectomy cutting probe. A lens of firm consistency is removed by ultrasonic emulsification. The ultrasonic needle is introduced into the lens through an incision in the equatorial portion of the lens capsule, and care is taken to avoid rupture of the anterior or posterior lens capsules while the nucleus is being emulsified. The portion of the nucleus nearest the needle entry site is emulsified first. Side-to-side and anterior-to-posterior motion of the needle tip is used until the lens nucleus is completely removed (*Figure 8.28*)[11].

The emulsified lens material is evacuated through the lumen of the needle, which is attached to an aspiration line. When a separate pars plana infusion cannula is used, this provides enough inflow so that the lens capsule usually does not collapse as emulsification proceeds. An infusion needle can be introduced into the vitreous cavity through another pars plana location or introduced into the lens through the opposite side if a separate infusion cannula is not used. Minimal suction force is used to evacuate the emulsified lens material through the ultrasonic needle. Often, the tubing attached to the needle is merely vented to the atmosphere so that the suction force is determined by the difference between the intraocular and atmospheric pressures.

After removing the lens nucleus, the surrounding soft cortical material is then emulsified, or it can be aspirated and excised with a vitrectomy cutting probe. The posterior

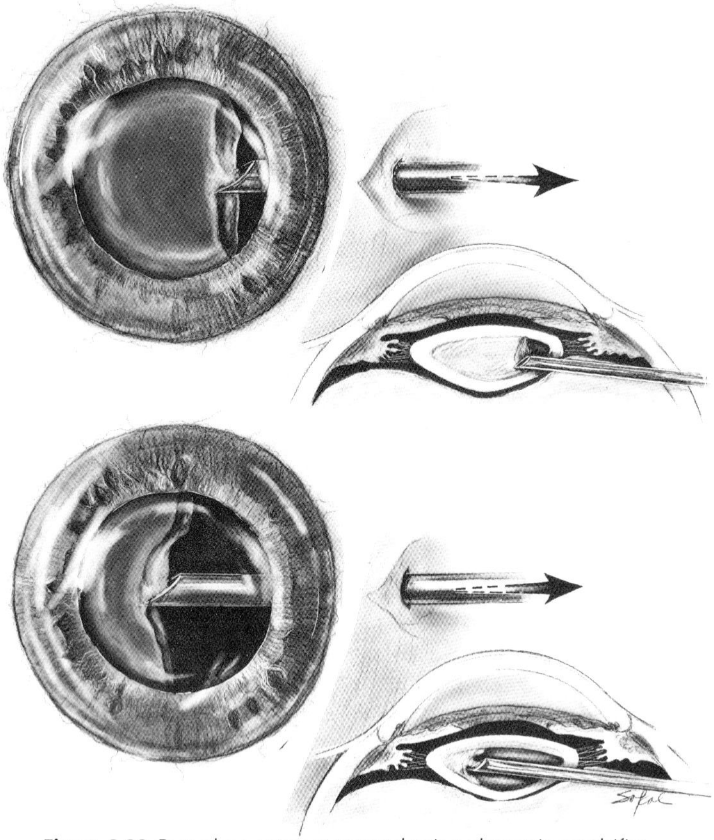

Figure 8.28 *Pars plana cataract removal using ultrasonic emulsification. Proximal portion of lens nucleus is emulsified first, using side-to-side and anterior-to-posterior motion of needle tip. The entire lens nucleus is emulsified before removing cortical material. Infusion is provided by separate pars plana cannula (not shown)*

lens capsule is excised, but the anterior lens capsule is left intact until after completing the vitrectomy procedure. Leaving the anterior lens capsule intact minimizes damage to the corneal endothelium and anterior chamber tissues. The anterior lens capsule is excised with the vitrectomy probe at the end of the intravitreal portion of the operation.

Excision of vitreous gel

The central portion of the vitreous gel is excised first, using a low suction force. A fluid space is created, and during this time the cutting efficacy of the vitrectomy probe is assessed. In aphakic eyes the anterior vitreous gel is then excised, but in phakic eyes with clear anterior vitreous some vitreous gel is left undisturbed behind the posterior lens capsule. The remaining vitreous gel is then excised in an anterior-to-posterior direction to remove intravitreal opacities and to allow identification of the posterior surface of the vitreous body. If a complete posterior vitreous separation is present, the cortical vitreous is easily excised and the operation is terminated after removing the axial opacities (*Figure 8.29*).

Often the cortical vitreous has partially separated from the retina and has a funnel-shaped configuration extending from the vitreous base anteriorly to posterior areas of vitreoretinal attachment. The posterior vitreous surface is incised in a safe location away from vitreoretinal attachments and/or areas of underlying retinal detachment. Any non-clotted blood present in the preretinal space is evacuated using a blunt needle with a flute handle, as described later[12]. With this technique the loose blood usually does not swirl into the fluid-filled vitreous cavity and interfere with visualization of the instrument tips.

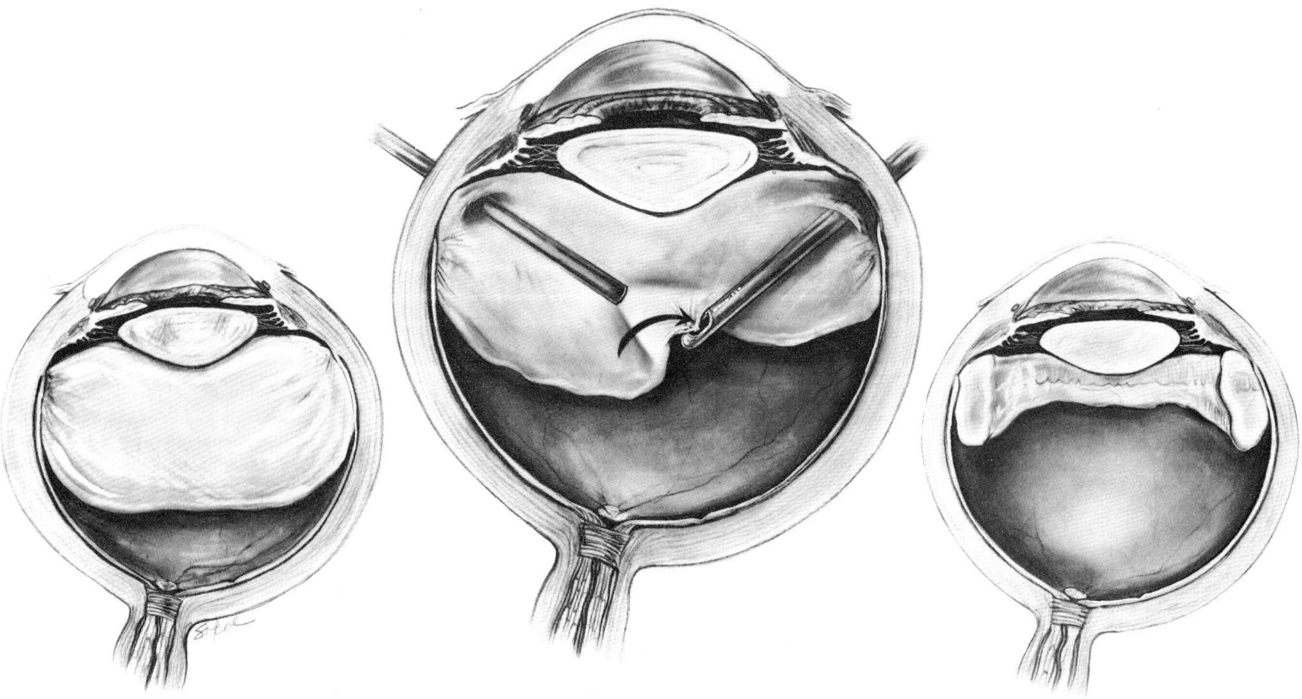

Figure 8.29 *Excision of opaque vitreous gel in phakic eye with complete posterior vitreous separation. Opaque gel is excised to clear the optical pathway, leaving anteroperipheral vitreous adjacent to vitreous base*

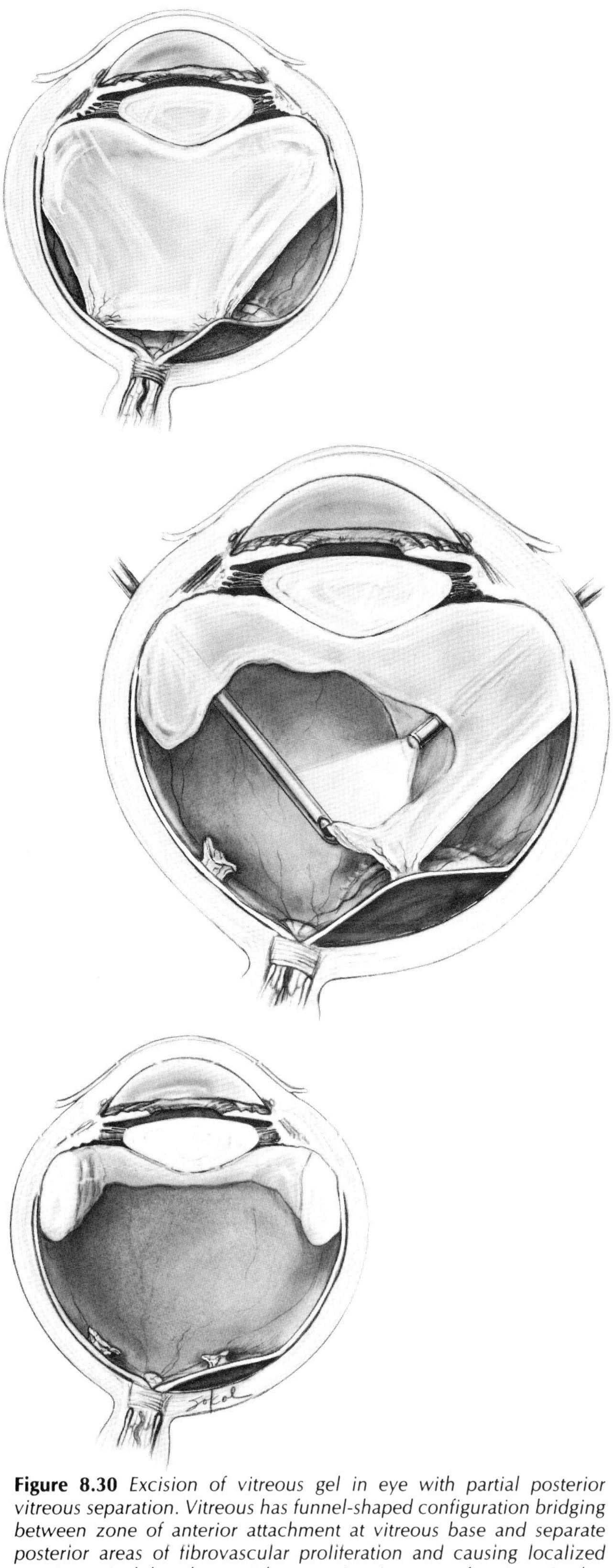

Figure 8.30 *Excision of vitreous gel in eye with partial posterior vitreous separation. Vitreous has funnel-shaped configuration bridging between zone of anterior attachment at vitreous base and separate posterior areas of fibrovascular proliferation and causing localized traction retinal detachment. The posterior vitreous surface is excised to relieve anteroposterior traction between the vitreous base and the posterior retina, and to relieve transverse traction between the separate areas of fibrovascular proliferation*

After removal of non-clotted blood from the preretinal space, the posterior vitreous surface is excised around the circumference of its cone-like structure to relieve traction between the vitreous base and the posterior retina. As much of the cortical vitreous is excised as possible, except for anterior portions adjacent to the vitreous base and posterior remnants near areas of vitreoretinal attachment. Other portions of the posterior vitreous surface are then excised where they form a sheet or membrane extending between one area of the posterior retina and another. This situation is often seen in eyes with proliferative diabetic retinopathy, because fibrovascular tissue grows along the posterior vitreous surface after originating from the retina in different locations (*Figure 8.30*).

After completing excision of the posterior vitreous surface, selected epiretinal membranes are separated from the retina or segmented into smaller islands as described later. Portions of the anteroperipheral vitreous are then excised if this part of the vitreous gel is opaque. Enough vitreous is removed to permit visualization of the peripheral retina by indirect ophthalmoscopy so that the retina midway between the equator and the ora serrata can be seen.

Special techniques

Special techniques are used during vitreous surgery to: (*1*) remove non-clotted blood; (*2*) separate or segment epiretinal membranes; (*3*) apply intraocular diathermy; (*4*) perform transvitreal removal of subretinal fluid; (*5*) treat retinal breaks; and (*6*) perform fluid-gas exchange. Vitreous surgery methods may also be combined with scleral buckling techniques. These special techniques are performed with accessory instrumentation described earlier, and they often permit successful treatment of complex situations and effective management of intraoperative complications.

Removal of non-clotted blood

Non clotted blood is evacuated using a blunt needle and flute handle containing an internal channel and side port (see *Figure 8.7a*). Fluid and dispersed blood will flow out of the eye when the side port is uncovered because of the pressure gradient between the vitreous cavity at the needle tip and the lower atmospheric pressure at the side port of the flute handle[12,17]. This method minimizes the amount of fluid needed to flush opacities from the vitreous cavity because the tip of the blunt needle can be placed close to any preretinal blood that has to be removed. The high flow rate possible with this needle also allows rapid clearing of blood dispersed through the vitreous cavity, and blood can be evacuated from the preretinal space after incision of the posterior vitreous surface as mentioned earlier (*Figure 8.31*).

After excision of the posterior cortical vitreous any non-clotted blood that remains on the inner retinal surface is removed. This is evacuated from the surface of attached retina using the blunt needle and flute handle (*Figure 8.32*). Removal of blood from the surface of detached retina is more hazardous because of the possibility of incarcerating this more mobile retina in the needle tip, and blood on detached retina is usually washed up with a gentle infusion stream. A modified probe combining both fiberoptic illumination and an infusion channel is convenient for this purpose, so that the fluid can be simultaneously evacuated through a blunt needle positioned in the midvitreous cavity.

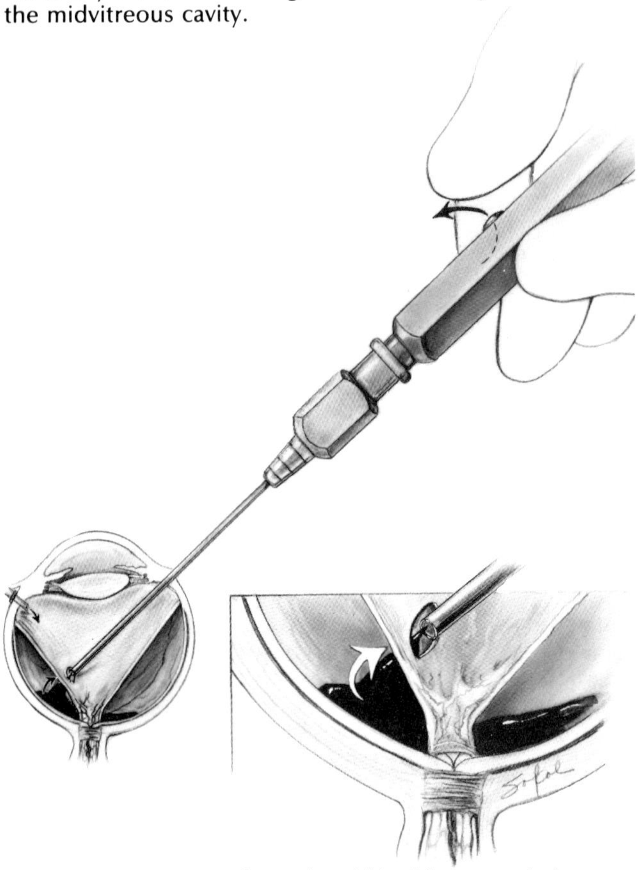

Figure 8.31 *Evacuation of non-clotted blood from preretinal space, using blunt needle with flute handle. Posterior vitreous surface is incised and preretinal blood removed while maintaining clear view of needle tip*

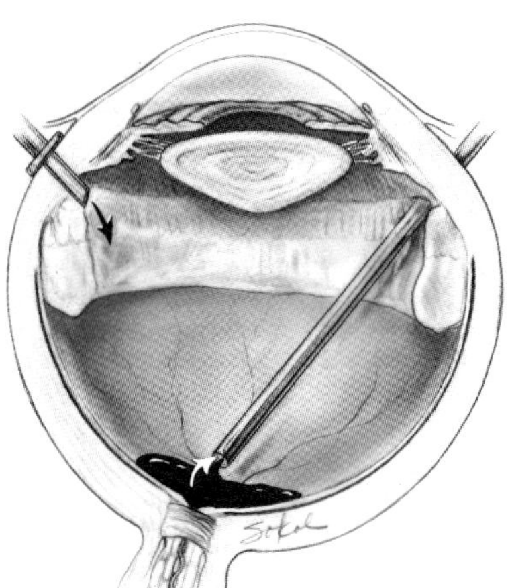

Figure 8.32 *Removal of non-clotted blood from inner retinal surface, using blunt needle with flute handle as illustrated in* Figure 8.31. *Residual blood is easily removed after excision of posterior vitreous surface*

Separation and/or segmentation of epiretinal membranes

Epiretinal membranes and fibrovascular tissue growing along the inner retinal surface may be removed or divided into smaller separate islands to relieve traction on the posterior retina and to minimize postoperative complications. Often, avascular membranes can be engaged with a vitreoretinal pick and gently separated from the retina. Vascularized membranes are usually firmly adherent to the retina in locations where the proliferative tissue originated and along the peripheral margin of large fibrovascular tissue sheets. In such eyes, a hooked needle or vitreoretinal pick is used to identify a cleavage plane between the retina and the epiretinal tissue in different locations (*Figure 8.33a*). Vitreoretinal scissors are then

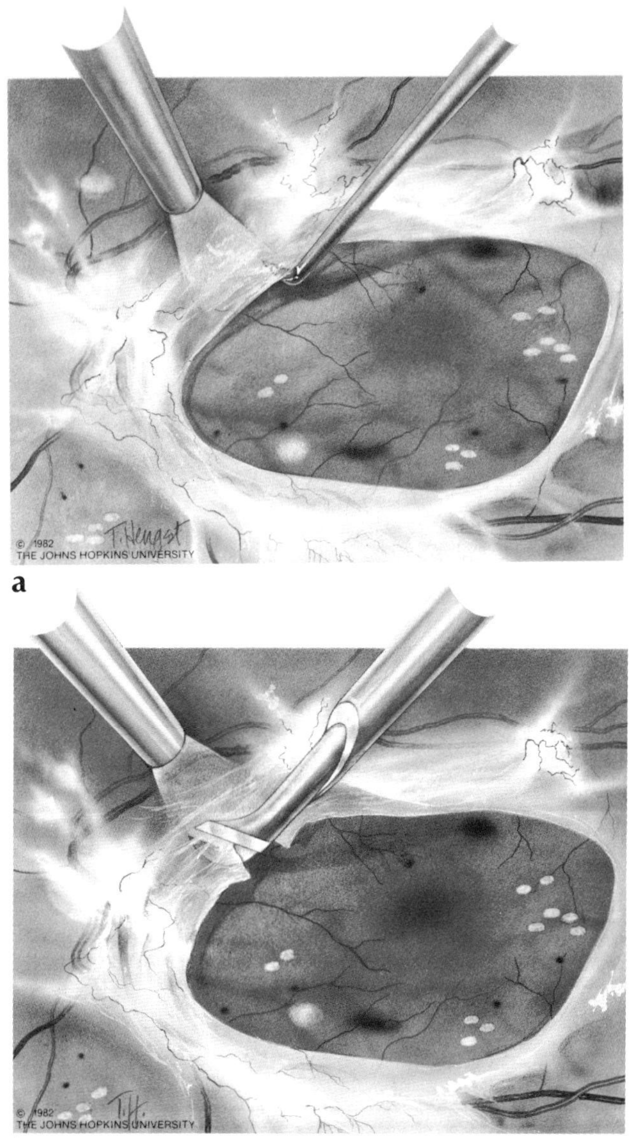

Figure 8.33 *Dissection and segmentation of epiretinal fibrovascular tissue in diabetic eye.* **(a)** *Vitreoretinal pick is used to identify cleavage plane between fibrovascular tissue and underlying retina.* **(b)** *Abnormal tissue membrane is then cut with vitreoretinal scissors*

used to divide the membrane into separate islands while avoiding traction on adjacent retinal attachments (*Figure 8.33b*)[18,19]. Often the edges of epiretinal membranes separate widely after being cut, thus demonstrating that the membrane was causing considerable traction.

Intraocular diathermy

The cut edges of vascularized tissue are usually treated with diathermy, either prophylactically or to stop active bleeding. A bimanual bipolar technique is preferred, as described earlier, using the fiberoptic light probe and the vitreoretinal scissors or vitrectomy probe as electrodes (*Figure 8.34*). Diathermy can also be applied to vascularized tissue before it is cut, and this is done if the tissue bridge is partially elevated. However, diathermy causes some shrinkage of tissue, thereby increasing traction on adjacent vitreoretinal attachments and sometimes making introduction of the vitrectomy probe or scissors blade between the membrane and the underlying retina more difficult.

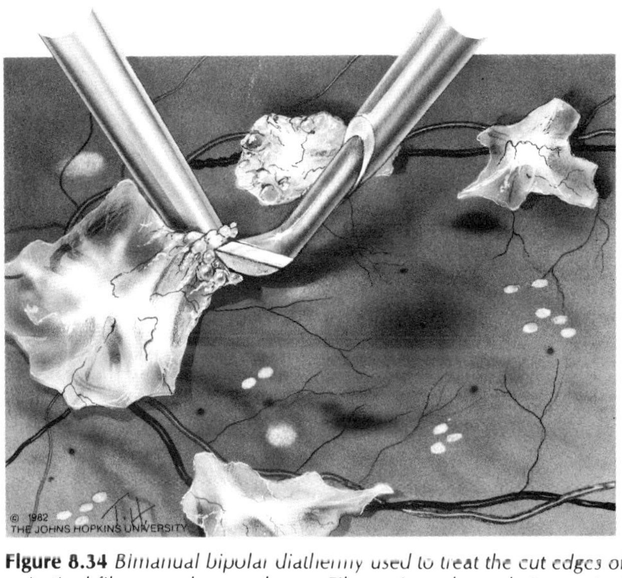

Figure 8.34 *Bimanual bipolar diathermy used to treat the cut edges of epiretinal fibrovascular membrane. Fiberoptic probe and vitreoretinal scissors serve as electrodes to apply diathermy after cutting tissue*

Evacuation of subretinal fluid

Subretinal fluid is removed through suitable posterior retinal breaks using a transvitreal approach with the blunt needle and flute handle. After relieving all vitreous traction, the blunt needle is passed through a posterior retinal break, and the side port on the handle is uncovered to vent the needle to the atmosphere[13,17]. The pressure in the infusion system causes subretinal fluid to drain out of the eye, and the retina settles against the pigment epithelium (*Figure 8.35*). This technique also demonstrates whether all vitreoretinal traction has been relieved, which is necessary for the retina to settle. If the retinal hole is large or if multiple holes are present, subretinal fluid may

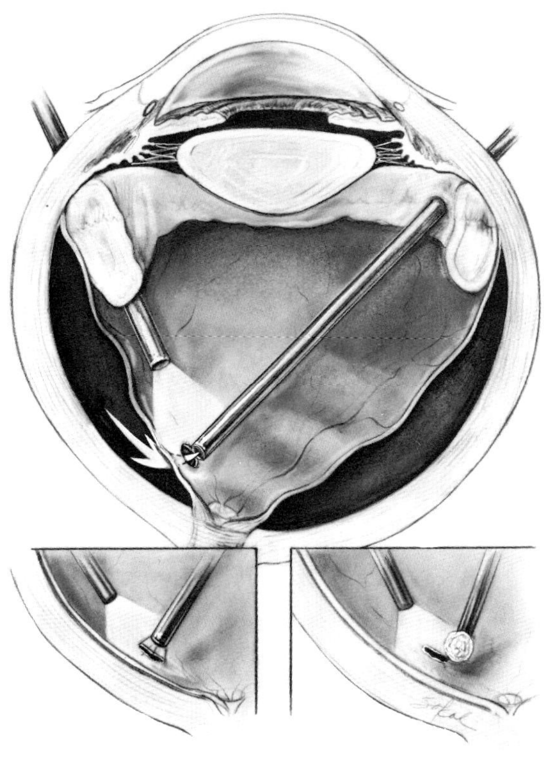

Figure 8.35 *Transvitreal methods to manage retinal detachment associated with posterior retinal break. Subretinal fluid is first evacuated using blunt needle with flute handle as illustrated in* Figure 8.31. *Photocoagulation or cryotherapy (lower insets) are then used to treat edges of retinal break and underlying pigment epithelium*

rapidly reaccumulate. In these cases, transvitreal drainage of subretinal fluid may be combined with simultaneous fluid-gas exchange as described later.

Treatment of retinal breaks

If the edges of a posterior retinal break are near the pigment epithelium the break can be treated with transvitreal cryotherapy or photocoagulation to create a postoperative chorioretinal adhesion. Cryotherapy is applied with a straight cryoprobe. The retina is gently pushed against the pigment epithelium, and then the freeze is initiated so that the pigment epithelium is damaged by the iceball on the probe tip (*see Figures 8.9* and *8.35*)[20]. Several applications may be required to surround the retinal hole. After each application the tip must defrost completely before the probe is moved, to avoid causing a choroidal hemorrhage.

Photocoagulation is applied using a fiberoptic probe attached to a xenon light source as described earlier. The tip is positioned near the retina to produce a coagulation effect from the diverging light beam (*see Figures 8.10* and *8.35*). This technique produces a typical whitening of the retina, and it is most effective if the edges of the retinal break are flat against the pigment epithelium.

Fluid-gas exchange

A gas bubble may be introduced into the vitreous cavity to assist in transvitreal drainage of subretinal fluid, to stop intraocular bleeding that cannot be controlled by other means or to provide tamponade of retinal holes during the early postoperative period. Sterile air is used most often, although sulfur hexafluoride (SF_6), in various dilutions mixed with air, may be used if a postoperative bubble is needed for more than 5 days or if expansion of the bubble is desirable during the early postoperative period[21,22]. The bubble is usually introduced through the infusion system, and the expanding bubble displaces portions of intravitreal fluid from the eye through the aspiration system of the vitrectomy probe or through a separate needle which is vented to the atmosphere (simultaneous fluid-gas exchange) (*Figure 8.36a*).

The gas bubble immediately fills the anterior chamber in aphakic eyes and partially neutralizes the refractive power of the cornea. The instrument tips in the vitreous cavity can therefore be visualized during the fluid-gas exchange using the operating microscope alone with illumination provided by the intraocular fiberoptic probe. The needle tip is moved farther posterior until a bubble of desired size is obtained (*Figure 8.36b*). With this technique, all of the preretinal fluid can be removed and the entire eye can be filled with a gas bubble.

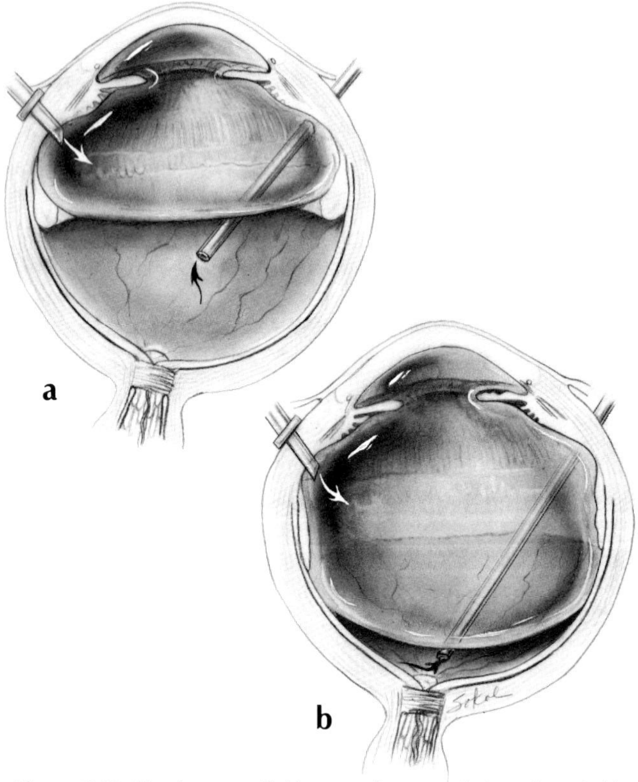

Figure 8.36 *Simultaneous fluid-gas exchange technique in aphakic eye, using divided system instrumentation.* (**a**) *Gas is injected through infusion cannula, and expanding bubble displaces intraocular fluid out of eye through blunt needle.* (**b**) *Needle tip is moved farther posterior until bubble of desired size is obtained. Visualization is through operating microscope, with intraocular illumination provided by fiberoptic probe (not shown). Intraocular bubble neutralizes refractive power of cornea, and contact lens is not necessary*

In phakic eyes, when a gas bubble is present posterior to the crystalline lens the instrument tips cannot be visualized using the operating microscope without the use of a special biconcave contact lens. In these cases, visualization during fluid-gas exchange is usually achieved by indirect ophthalmoscopy. With this method, manipulation of the needle is more difficult because of the minified, inverted and reversed image seen by the surgeon. The needle tip is therefore usually positioned in the midvitreous cavity before gas injection is started and is held immobile until the posterior surface of the bubble extends back to the needle tip (*Figure 8.37*). With this technique, 50–75 per cent of the vitreous cavity can be safely filled with a bubble without requiring movement of the needle tip within the vitreous cavity.

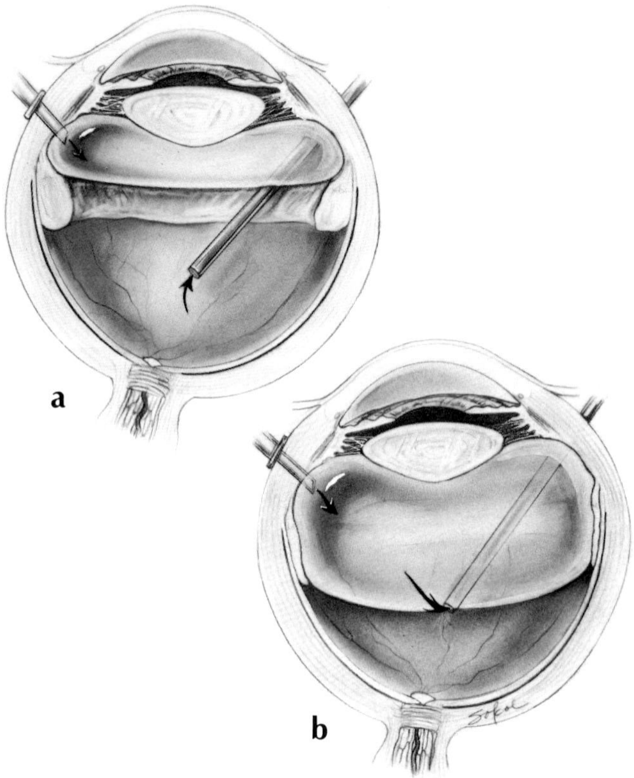

Figure 8.37 *Simultaneous fluid-gas exchange in a phakic eye, using divided system instrumentation. Combination of crystalline lens and intravitreal bubble limits visualization of needle tip through operating microscope, and visualization is provided by indirect ophthalmoscopy.* (**a**) *Needle tip is positioned in proper anteroposterior location and* (**b**) *held immobile until posterior bubble surface reaches needle tip*

Simultaneous fluid-gas exchange is often combined with transvitreal evacuation of subretinal fluid in aphakic eyes with suitable posterior retinal breaks. The gas bubble assists in flattening the retina if large or multiple retinal holes are present. Transvitreal evacuation of the subretinal fluid is performed first to flatten the retina as much as possible, and then the gas bubble is injected through the infusion cannula as preretinal fluid is removed (*Figure 8.38a, b*). The expanding bubble displaces remaining subretinal fluid posteriorly, and this fluid is then removed through the most posterior retinal break as additional gas is injected (*Figure 8.38c, d*). With this technique, the retina can often be completely reattached and held against the

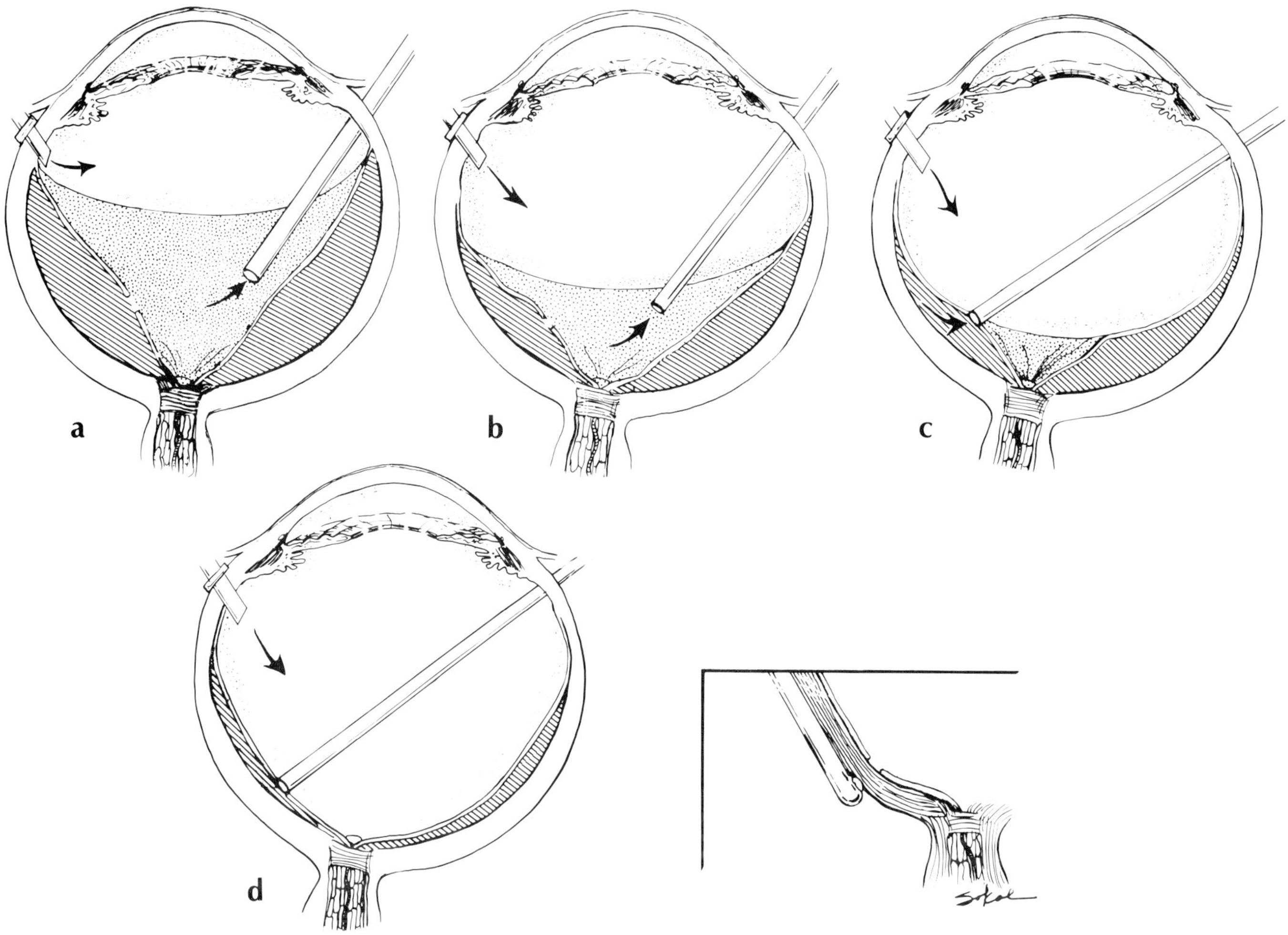

Figure 8.38 *Simultaneous fluid-gas exchange combined with transvitreal evacuation of subretinal fluid in an aphakic eye with retinal detachment and a posterior retinal break.* (**a, b**) *Preretinal fluid is displaced out of eye through blunt needle as gas bubble is injected.* (**c, d**) *Residual subretinal fluid is then removed through posterior retinal break until retina is flattened against pigment epithelium by intraocular bubble. After withdrawing instruments, transscleral cryotherapy (inset) is used to create chorioretinal adhesion around posterior retinal break*

pigment epithelium by the intraocular gas bubble. After closing the sclerotomies, transscleral cryotherapy (as monitored by indirect ophthalmoscopy) can be used to treat the retinal breaks if transvitreal methods were not used previously (*Figure 8.38 inset*).

Closure of sclerotomies

Each pars plana incision is closed so that it is watertight, using several suture bites. We prefer a running shoestring suture technique using 7/0 polyglactin to close the 20 gauge size incisions. Four scleral bites are taken to produce a double figure-of-eight configuration (*Figure 8.39*). The separate infusion cannula is left in place until after any scleral buckling procedure is performed. Then the cannula is removed, and this last incision is closed using the same technique.

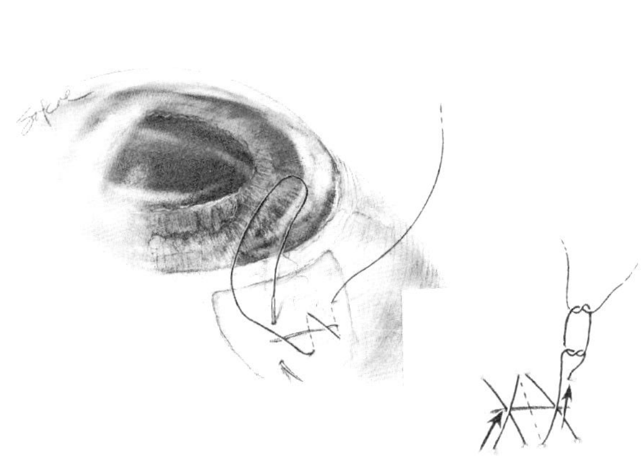

Figure 8.39 *Suture technique for closure of small pars plana incisions. Running shoestring technique with 7/0 polyglactin suture creates double figure-of-eight configuration and gives watertight closure without distortion of wound edges*

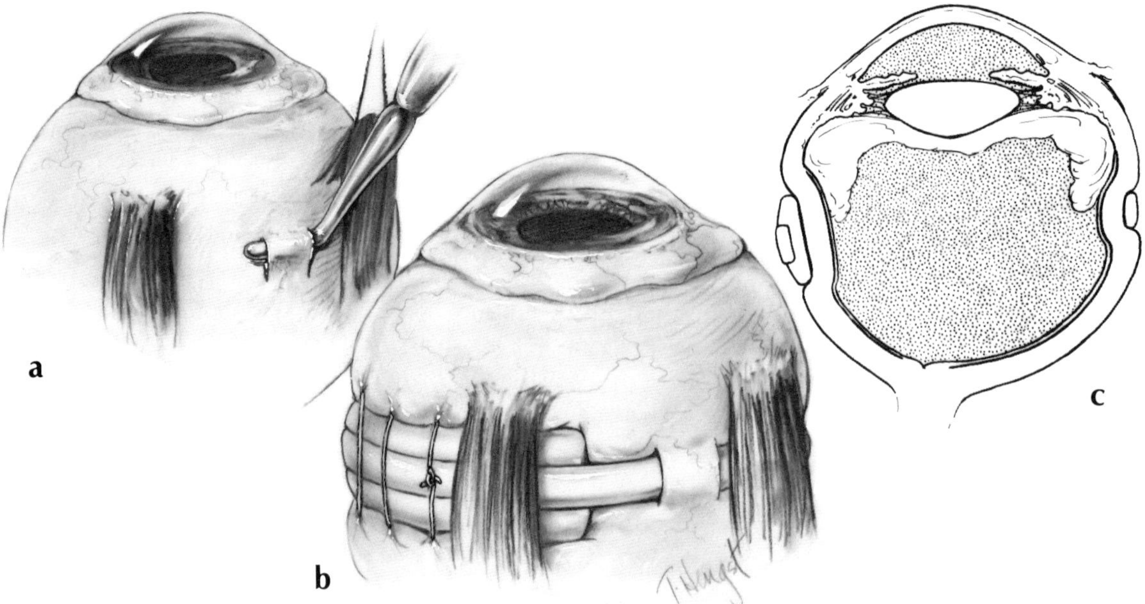

Figure 8.40 *Scleral buckling technique combined with vitrectomy to treat anterior retinal breaks. (**a**) Scleral tunnels are made to accept an encircling band. (**b, c**) Retinal breaks and adjacent retina are supported on a broader buckle created by grooved silicone-rubber exoplant and mattress-type episcleral sutures. Encircling band, secured in other locations by scleral tunnels, creates narrower zone of indentation and maintains permanent buckling effect*

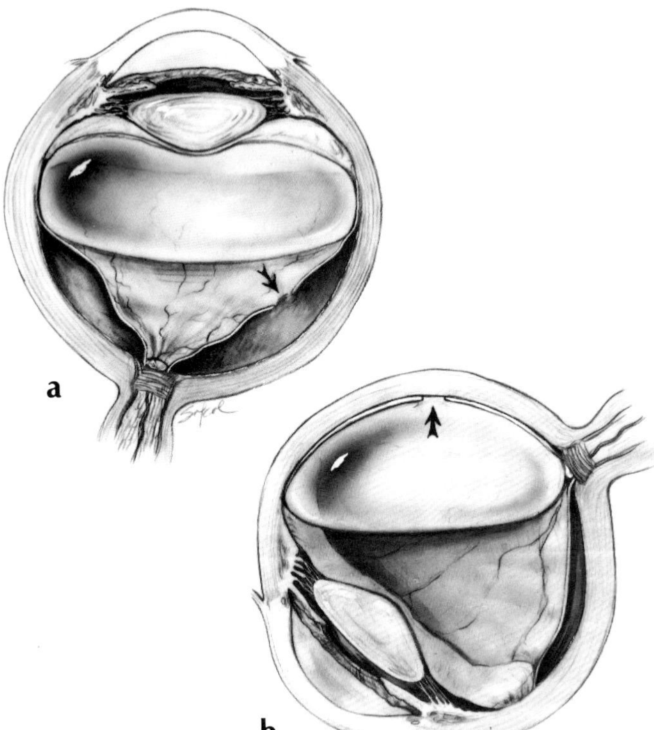

Figure 8.41 *Treatment of posterior retinal break (arrow) in phakic eye, using intravitreal bubble and postoperative face-down positioning. (**a**) Air bubble in eye with retinal detachment before face-down positioning. (**b**) With proper face-down positioning, surface of bubble occludes retinal break, permitting absorption of subretinal fluid. This brings edges of torn retina into apposition with pigment epithelium, and chorioretinal adhesion occurs in response to previous cryotherapy, diathermy or photocoagulation (not shown). This technique is used when all vitreoretinal traction has been relieved*

Scleral buckling

Scleral buckling is combined with vitreous surgery in some eyes to treat selected retinal breaks and areas of persistent vitreoretinal traction. Retinal breaks located anterior to the equator are supported on a scleral buckle. Usually an encircling band is used in combination with a broader piece of grooved silicone rubber to support the retinal break(s) and adjacent retina. The piece of grooved silicone rubber is sutured to the sclera with mattress-type sutures, and the partial-thickness scleral bites are spaced wide enough apart to produce moderate indentation of the silicone rubber when the sutures are tightened. In quadrants where the broader exoplant is not needed, a smaller encircling silicone-rubber band passes under partial-thickness scleral tunnels which maintain the band in the proper anteroposterior location (*Figure 8.40*).

Retinal breaks located posterior to the equator, without residual traction from vitreous sheets or epiretinal membranes, are usually treated without a scleral buckle. Cryotherapy or photocoagulation is used to treat the retinal break, and this is combined with temporary intraocular gas tamponade. Appropriate positioning is used postoperatively to place the bubble against the retinal break and to avoid prolonged contact between the bubble and the lens if the eye is phakic (*Figure 8.41*).

When there is persistent traction on the retina in the area of the retinal break because of remaining vitreous sheets or an epiretinal membrane, a localized scleral buckle is used to support the posterior retinal break. A short, radially oriented piece of silicone-rubber sponge is usually sutured to the sclera with a single mattress-type suture (*Figure 8.42*) or is placed in an intrascleral pocket after careful localization of the retinal break relative to the adjacent sclera.

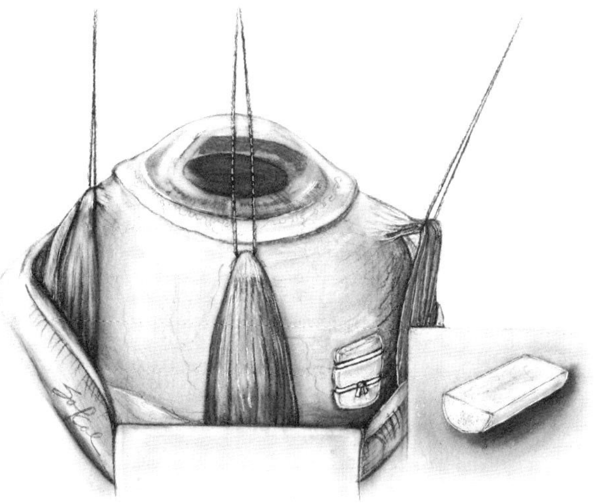

Figure 8.42 *Radially oriented exoplant used to create localized scleral buckle beneath posterior retinal break associated with persistent vitreoretinal or epiretinal membrane traction. Half-thickness silicone-rubber sponge indents sclera and is secured with mattress-type suture*

Indications, results and special techniques

Vitreous surgery is used to treat the following conditions:

1. Non-clearing vitreous opacities
2. Proliferative retinopathies
   (*a*) Non-clearing vitreous hemorrhage
   (*b*) Traction retinal detachment with recent macular involvement
   (*c*) Complicated combined traction and rhegmatogenous detachment
   (*d*) Progressive fibrovascular proliferation causing visual loss
   (*e*) Progressive rubeosis iridis with vitreous hemorrhage
3. Selected retinal detachments
   (*a*) Traction retinal detachment
   (*b*) Rhegmatogenous detachment with dense vitreous hemorrhage or severe vitreous traction
   (*c*) Giant retinal tears
   (*d*) Retinal detachment with posterior retinal breaks
   (*e*) Massive periretinal proliferation (MPP)
   (*f*) Inadequate pupillary space
4. Ocular trauma
   (*a*) Corneoscleral laceration with disrupted lens and/or vitreous in anterior chamber
   (*b*) Severe posterior segment penetrating injury with dense vitreous hemorrhage
   (*c*) Selected reactive intraocular foreign bodies requiring specialized extraction techniques
5. Diagnostic vitrectomy
   (*a*) Reticulum cell sarcoma
   (*b*) Endogenous fungal endophthalmitis
   (*c*) Phacoanaphylactic endophthalmitis
6. Anterior segment disorders
   (*a*) Inadequate pupillary space
   (*b*) Vitreous complications in the anterior segment
   (*c*) Retropseudophakos membranes
   (*d*) Epithelial ingrowth
   (*e*) Complicated and congenital cataracts
   (*f*) Hyphema
7. Secondary open-angle glaucoma
   (*a*) Blood-induced glaucoma
   (*b*) Phacolytic or phacoanaphylactic glaucoma
8. Retained lens material causing secondary complications
9. Infective endophthalmitis
   (*a*) Bacterial endophthalmitis
   (*b*) Fungal endophthalmitis
   (*c*) Parasitic endophthalmitis
10. Vitreopapillary and vitreomacular traction
11. Epiretinal membranes involving the posterior pole

Some of these abnormalities, such as non-clearing opacities and epiretinal membranes, cannot be directly treated by other surgical means. Vitreous surgery is an alternative means of treatment in conditions such as pupillary membranes and selected retinal detachments. In still other conditions, such as infective endophthalmitis, vitreous surgery provides capabilities that are combined with conventional medical or surgical management. The objectives of vitreous surgery vary according to the specific indication for the operation and the particular features of each case. The results achieved and the complications encountered therefore also vary considerably. Even so, enough experience has accumulated to permit evaluation of the role of vitreous surgery in various conditions.

Non-clearing vitreous opacities

Non-clearing vitreous opacities are an important indication for vitreous surgery, and the large majority of such eyes are blinded by vitreous hemorrhage. This may be associated with various underlying conditions, ranging from idiopathic cases, to those following ocular trauma or associated with proliferative retinopathies. The complexity of the vitreoretinal anatomy therefore varies considerably. Treatment of vitreous opacities associated with other structural abnormalities in the posterior segment will be discussed later.

Surgery is considered when vitreous hemorrhage does not clear after 6 months. During this time, the eye is examined regularly, and diagnostic ultrasound is used to determine whether additional abnormalities such as retinal detachment are present. Immediate surgery may be necessary if complications such as posterior retinal detachment or severe blood-induced glaucoma occur. Otherwise, surgery is delayed for at least 6 months. The final decision about vitrectomy is dependent on the patient's visual needs, the status of the fellow eye, the likelihood of a successful result and the underlying condition – which may influence the amount of vision to be expected after removal of the opacities.

The surgical technique depends on the location of opacities within the vitreous cavity and the structural anatomy of the posterior vitreous surface. Often the anterocentral portion of the vitreous gel is clear, and this is left undisturbed behind a clear crystalline lens. Opaque vitreous gel is easily excised if a complete posterior vitreous separation is present (*see Figure 8.29*). When a partial vitreous detachment is present, the posterior vitreous surface is resected except at areas of firm attachment to the retina (see *Figure 8.30*). Blood in the retrovitreal space is usually not clotted, and this blood is removed by lavage or by suction with a blunt needle and flute handle as described earlier. Successful results are achieved in 80–90 per cent of eyes that have no other serious pre-existing posterior segment complications[16,23–25]. The postoperative vision is rarely normal, however, because of underlying conditions affecting the retina or secondary changes from damage by the hemorrhage and/or surgery – such as effects from hemosiderosis, cystoid macular edema, or an epiretinal membrane involving the macula.

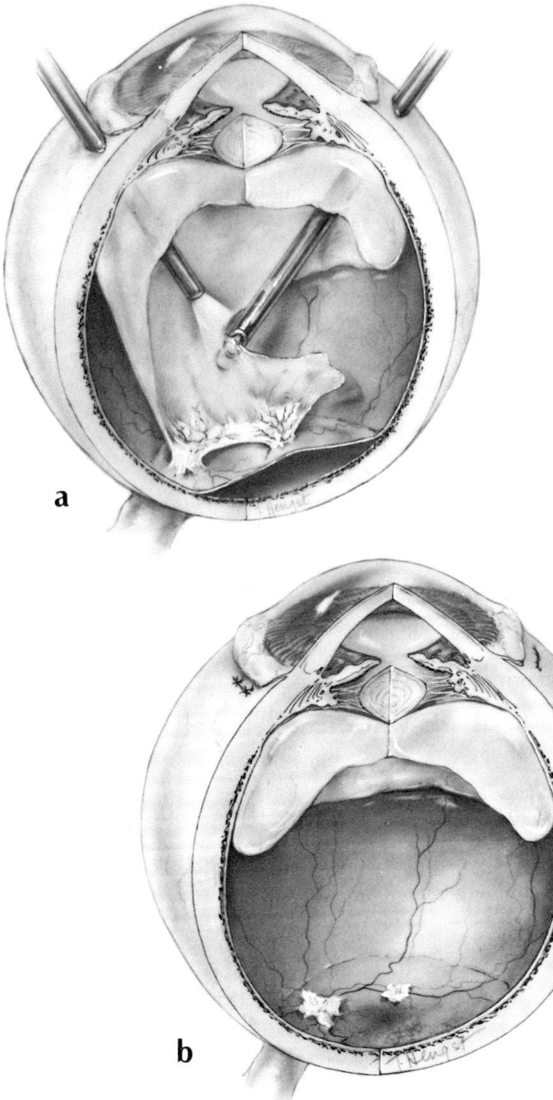

Figure 8.43 *Treatment of traction retinal detachment complicating proliferative diabetic retinopathy.* **(a)** *Anteroposterior traction is relieved by cutting cone-like posterior vitreous surface, and portions of posterior fibrovascular proliferation are excised (not shown).* **(b)** *Postoperatively, clear vitreous remains anteriorly, and separate islands of fibrovascular tissue remain posteriorly. Subretinal fluid gradually resorbs*

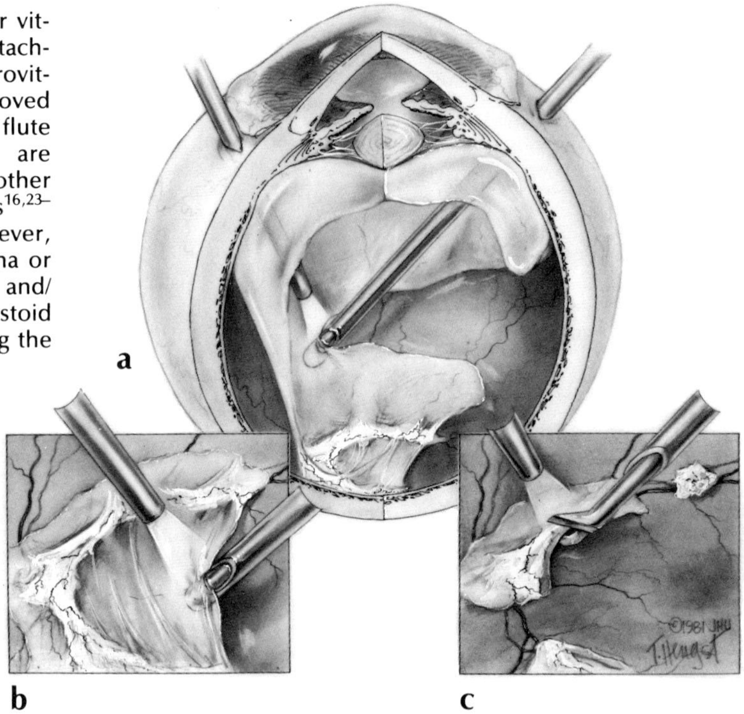

Figure 8.44 *Treatment of diabetic retinopathy with advanced fibrovascular proliferation.* **(a)** *Portions of the vitreous gel are excised and posterior vitreous surface is cut to relieve anteroposterior traction.* **(b)** *Remaining portion of the posterior vitreous surface bridging across the macula is excised.* **(c)** *Fibrovascular tissue bridging between one area of retina and another is cut with scissors*

Proliferative retinopathies

Proliferative retinopathies cause complications that may require vitreous surgery. These conditions have in common certain basic pathological mechanisms, and therefore the principles of surgery are similar. Proliferative diabetic retinopathy is the most common cause of complications requiring vitreous surgery, and such cases compose 40–50 per cent of all vitrectomy cases.

Extraretinal fibrovascular proliferation grows along the posterior vitreous surface. When portions of the posterior vitreous separate from the retina, the fibrovascular tissue may continue to proliferate, covering parts of the retina or causing secondary complications such as vitreous hemorrhage and traction or rhegmatogenous retinal detachment. Certain structural changes causing visual loss can be modified or reversed by vitreous surgery.

The indications for vitreous surgery in eyes with diabetic retinopathy are: (*1*) non-clearing vitreous hemorrhage; (*2*) traction retinal detachment with recent macular involvement (*Figure 8.43*); (*3*) combined traction and rhegmatogenous detachment that cannot be treated by conventional scleral buckling techniques; (*4*) progressive fibrovascular proliferation with distortion of the macula or traction on the optic nerve and/or peripapillary retina (*Figure 8.44*); and (*5*) early neovascularization of the iris and anterior chamber angle in eyes with vitreous hemorrhage. In the latter condition, vitreous surgery is done to clear opacities to permit use of scatter retinal photocoagulation which causes regression of iris neovascularization in some eyes[26]. For each of these indications, the surgical objectives are the same (*see* p. 220) although in each case different aspects are emphasized, depending on specific pathological features of the vitreoretinal relations.

Management of the lens must also be considered because many diabetic patients develop early cataracts, and lens opacities can also occur as a secondary complication of hemosiderosis from longstanding vitreous hemorrhage. A clear lens is preserved whenever possible because this reduces the incidence of postoperative rubeosis iridis in diabetic patients[27]. Lens removal, when necessary, is usually performed with the aid of ultrasonic emulsification.

Although the results of vitrectomy in diabetic eyes vary according to the specific indication for surgery, 50–75 per cent of cases achieve a successful result with vision of 5/200 or better and stable long-term anatomical relations[18,28–31]. The results are more favorable in eyes with only vitreous hemorrhage, with a successful result being obtained in up to 80 per cent of such cases. When vitreous hemorrhage is combined with either traction or rhegmatogenous retinal detachment, successful results are obtained in 35–50 per cent of cases. Eyes with clear media and traction or rhegmatogenous retinal detachment are successfully treated in 50–75 per cent of cases[32].

Resection of the posterior vitreous surface and isolation of separate islands of epiretinal and preretinal fibrovascular proliferation is followed by atrophy of the remaining fibrovascular tissue and absence of further preretinal (elevated) fibrovascular proliferation[18,29,33]. Also, the postoperative occurrence of additional epiretinal (flat) fibrovascular tissue growth is rare if the early postoperative course is uncomplicated and an initially successful result is obtained. Therefore, successful achievement of the surgical objectives, regardless of the specific indication for surgery, has a beneficial effect on the visual acuity and the pre-existing vitreoretinal abnormalities, and it dramatically changes the otherwise progressive course of the posterior segment disorder. More than 90 per cent of eyes with an initially successful result maintain about the same level of vision during ensuing years[34].

Selected retinal detachments

Vitreous surgery, often combined with other retinal reattachment methods, provides an important means of treating selected retinal detachments that have a poor prognosis when treated by only conventional methods. Vitreous surgery permits removal of intraocular tissue and it allows the surgeon to: (*1*) improve visualization by clearing intraocular opacities such as vitreous hemorrhage; (*2*) cut vitreous bands and sheets causing traction on the retina and remove epiretinal membranes covering, distorting or immobilizing the retina; (*3*) provide a fluid space in the vitreous cavity from which fluid can be removed to assist in creation of a scleral buckle and/or placement of an intravitreal gas bubble; and (*4*) perform other intraocular manipulations such as unfolding the flap of giant retinal tears, applying transvitreal cryotherapy or photocoagulation, and performing transvitreal drainage of subretinal fluid with or without simultaneous fluid-gas exchange.

These capabilities permit successful treatment of several types of complicated retinal detachment, including: (*1*) traction retinal detachment recently involving the macula; (*2*) rhegmatogenous detachment complicated by dense vitreous hemorrhage or severe vitreous traction; (*3*) selected giant retinal tears; (*4*) retinal detachment with posterior retinal breaks; (*5*) retinal detachment complicated by massive periretinal proliferation (MPP); and (*6*) aphakic eyes with retinal detachment and an inadequate pupillary space.

Traction retinal detachments

As mentioned earlier, traction retinal detachments occur most commonly in eyes with proliferative retinopathies, although they can also occur after penetrating injuries, intraocular inflammation, and cataract extraction with loss of vitreous. Surgery is recommended when the macula becomes involved and vision is reduced to less than 20/100. Vitrectomy is usually not performed if the posterior retina has been detached for longer than 6 months, although visual improvement has been documented as late as 18 months after involvement of the macula when this area of detachment was not highly elevated. Vitrectomy methods have virtually replaced scleral buckling techniques in the treatment of traction retinal detachment, because vitreous surgery permits direct treatment of the pathogenetic mechanism causing the detachment.

Dense vitreous hemorrhage or severe vitreous traction

Vitreous hemorrhage is often seen in eyes with proliferative retinopathies and also either traction or rhegmatogenous detachment, but severe vitreous hemorrhage is unusual as a complication of primary retinal detachment in eyes without other underlying abnormalities. Still, in eyes with dense vitreous hemorrhage, vitrectomy can be performed to clear the media and to relieve vitreoretinal traction, thereby permitting identification of specific retinal breaks and so appropriate scleral buckling can be used (*Figure 8.45*). When dense hemorrhage and possible retinal detachment coexist, special care must be exercised during vitrectomy to avoid cutting the mobile detached retina. When severe vitreous traction prevents successful treatment of a rhegmatogenous detachment by scleral buckling alone, vitreous surgery is used in conjunction with scleral buckling techniques. In such cases, vitreous surgery is used to relieve the traction, and this is usually combined with an intravitreal gas bubble for internal tamponade of the retinal break(s) and placement of a scleral buckle.

Giant retinal tears

Vitrectomy methods are especially useful to treat certain giant retinal tears in which the retinal flap is inverted and cannot be positioned against the pigment epithelium by other means because of vitreous traction, obstruction from vitreous gel, or secondary retinal changes causing an immobile flap. In such cases, vitreous surgery is used to relieve the traction, to excise as much of the vitreous gel as possible, and to remove epiretinal membranes causing contracture of the retinal flap or the inner retinal surface in other locations (*see* Chapter 9).

After the flap has been mobilized, an air bubble is placed in the vitreous cavity using simultaneous fluid-gas exchange techniques. If the retinal tear is less than 180°, an air bubble filling about 50 per cent of the vitreous cavity is often used. This is combined with postoperative rotation of the patient's head, using the air bubble to unfold the retinal flap and position it against the pigment epithelium which has been treated with cryotherapy or diathermy (*Figure 8.46*)[35].

When the giant retinal tear is greater than 180°, a technique for fluid-gas exchange with the patient in a

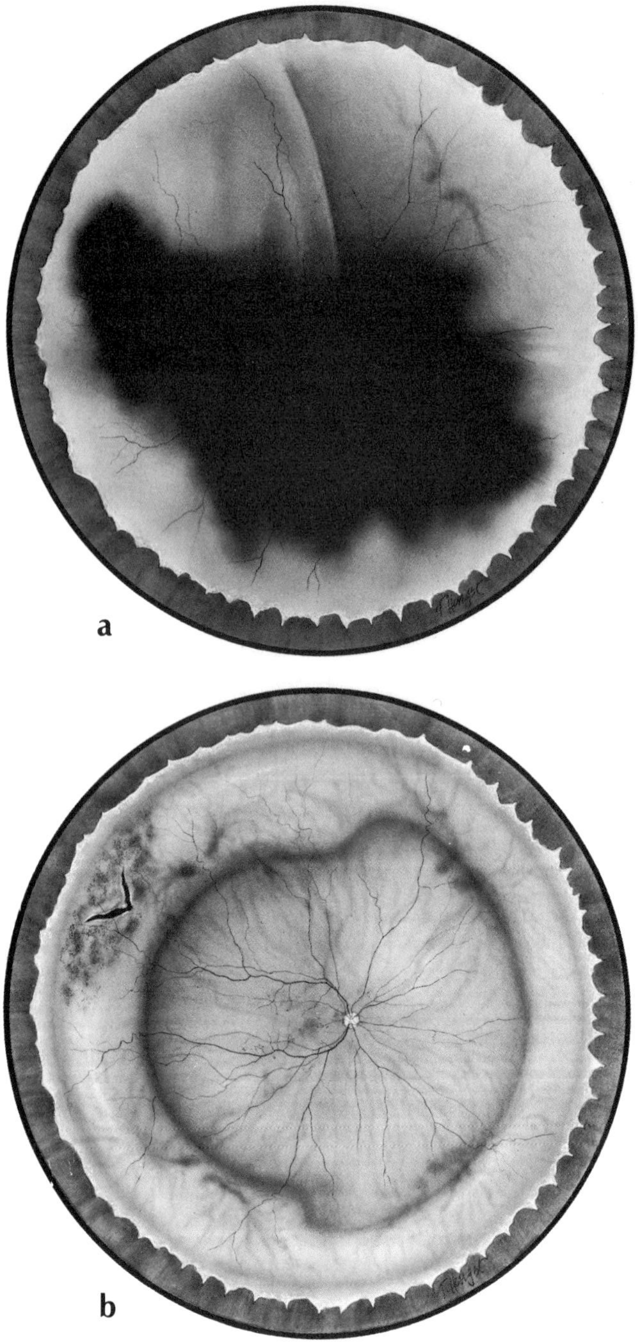

Figure 8.45 **(a)** *Dense vitreous hemorrhage obscuring rhegmatogenous retinal detachment in right eye following blunt injury from rock thrown by a lawn mower. Only peripheral portions of the detachment are visible, especially in the superotemporal quadrant.* **(b)** *Postoperative appearance after removal of vitreous hemorrhage and treatment of retinal detachment by cryotherapy, scleral buckling and intravitreal air injection. Temporal retina had been detached from 5 to 12 o'clock because of large retinal tear in superotemporal quadrant*

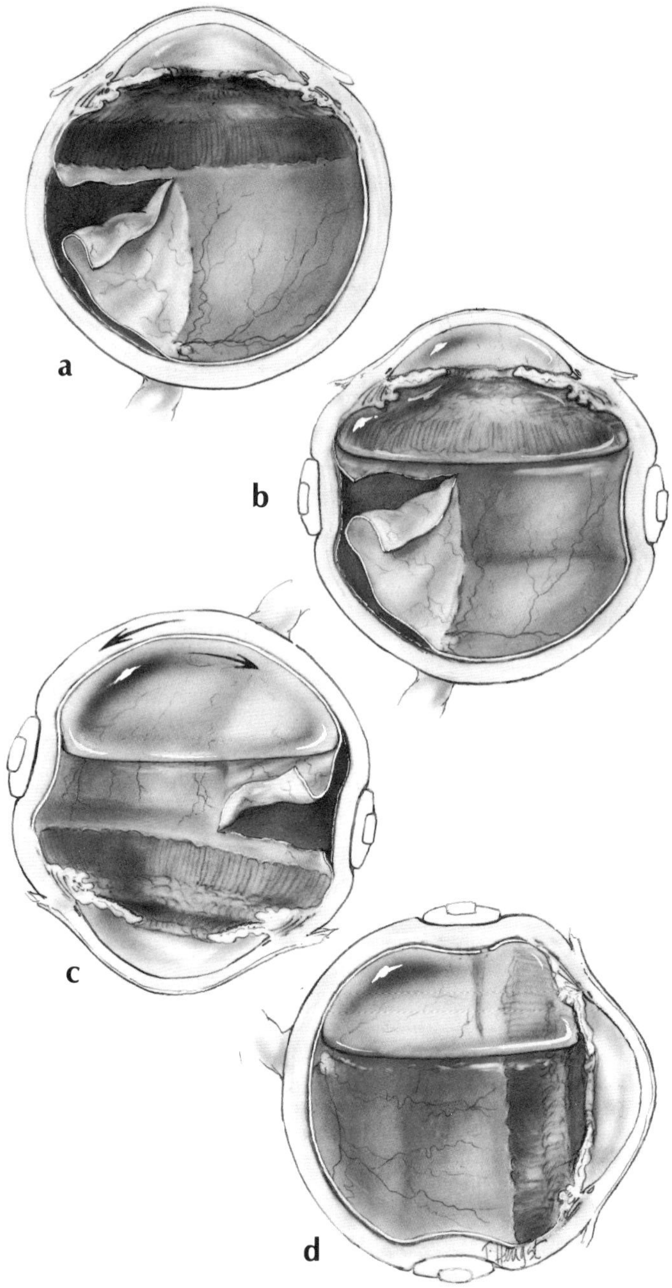

Figure 8.46 **(a)** *Giant retinal tear less than 180°.* **(b)** *Initial treatment includes vitrectomy, peripheral cryotherapy, broad encircling buckle and partial fluid-air exchange.* **(c)** *Postoperatively the patient rotates so the bubble unfolds the retinal flap and* (**d**) *positions it against the treated pigment epithelium and scleral buckle*

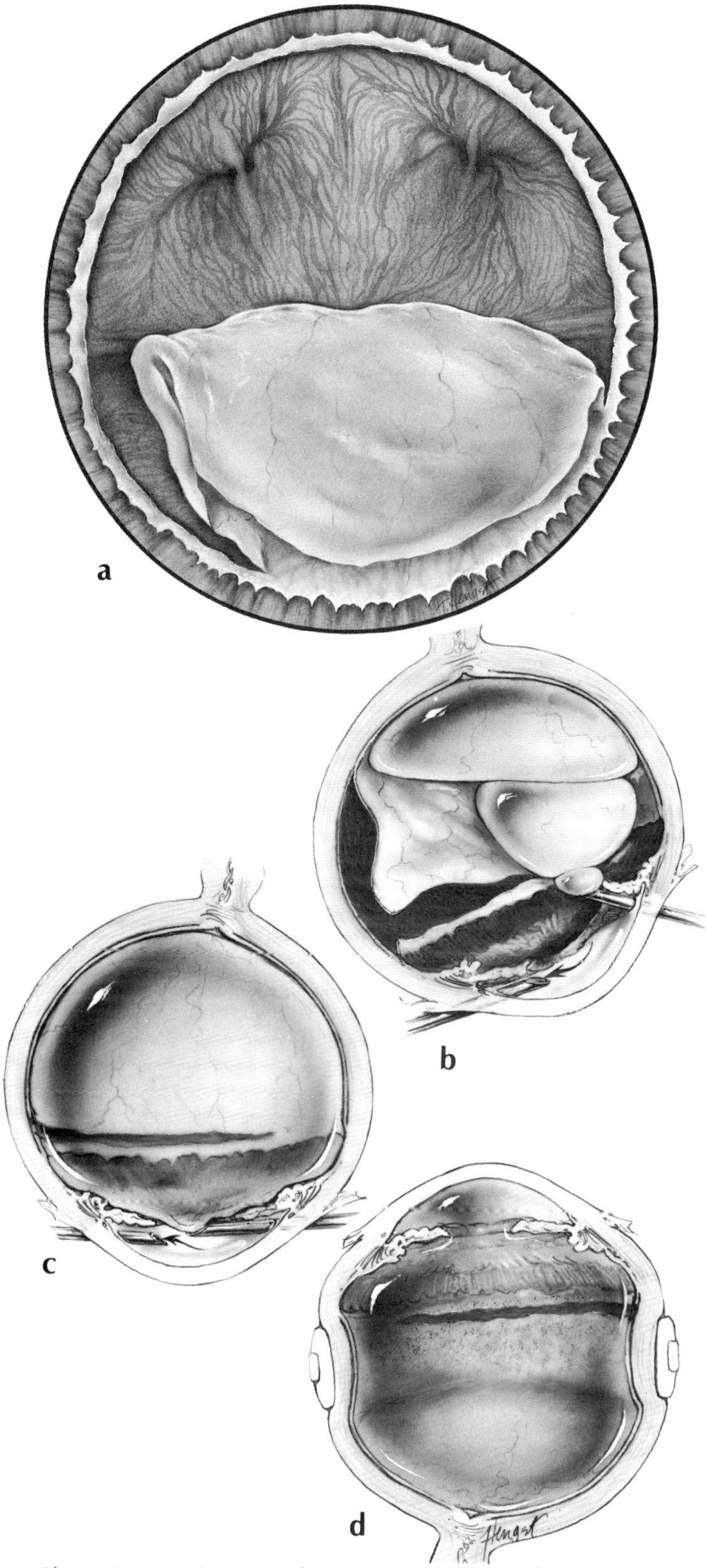

Figure 8.47 **(a)** *Giant retinal tear greater than 180°.* **(b)** *After lens removal and vitrectomy, gas is injected with patient in face-down position.* **(c)** *Expanding bubble unfolds retinal flap and flattens it against pigment epithelium as intraocular fluid is displaced through separate needle.* **(d)** *Pigment epithelium is treated with cryotherapy or diathermy and a broad encircling scleral buckle is used*

prone position is preferred[36]. In such cases, the crystalline lens is removed, and the bubble is injected so that it floats toward the optic nerve and/or toward the portion of the retina that is not torn. Therefore, as further gas is injected, the bubble positions the detached retina and retinal flap against the pigment epithelium while simultaneously displacing the preretinal and subretinal fluid from the eye through a separate needle positioned in the anterior chamber. With this technique, the eye is completely filled with gas, and the retina is unfolded and flattened against the pigment epithelium (*Figure 8.47*).

In all eyes with giant retinal tears, we prefer to use a broad and high scleral buckle for 360°, together with cryotherapy or diathermy treatment to the pigment epithelium throughout the limits of the buckle. Usually the cryotherapy or diathermy treatment is applied before the vitrectomy and fluid-gas exchange are performed. The scleral sutures and silicone-rubber elements for the scleral buckle are also positioned before the vitrectomy, so that the buckle can be elevated by tying the scleral sutures immediately after completing the fluid-gas exchange and returning the patient to a supine position.

Laser photocoagulation may be necessary postoperatively if portions of the retinal flap begin to separate from the surface of the buckle. With these techniques, nearly all retinas with recent giant retinal tears can be anatomically reattached, although about 50 per cent of these cases develop recurrent detachment later, usually from development of massive periretinal proliferation (MPP)[36].

Retinal detachment with posterior retinal breaks

Retinal detachments caused by posterior retinal breaks are difficult to manage by conventional techniques because of difficulty in accurately localizing the break by transscleral methods, difficulty in obtaining optimum treatment with cryotherapy or diathermy, failure of the retinal break to settle on a scleral buckle, damage to short posterior ciliary vessels, and an increased risk of optic nerve or macular damage during treatment with diathermy or cryotherapy or from later migration of external material used for the scleral buckle.

Vitreous surgery methods provide an alternative approach using techniques for transvitreal evacuation of subretinal fluid, transvitreal application of cryotherapy or photocoagulation and methods for fluid-gas exchange, as described earlier. These techniques are combined with a scleral buckle if traction on the posterior retinal break cannot be completely relieved. This is often the case in eyes with proliferative retinopathies when tangential traction persists because of remaining areas of epiretinal fibrovascular proliferation in nearby locations. Occasionally, an eye with a macular hole or retinal break near the macula can be treated with vitrectomy, evacuation of subretinal fluid, and fluid-gas exchange without using cryotherapy or other treatment to create a chorioretinal adhesion. In such cases, laser photocoagulation can be applied postoperatively if the retina does not remain reattached. This is done before the bubble completely absorbs, to permit temporary tamponade of the retinal break by the remaining bubble after application of the photocoagulation energy[16].

Massive periretinal proliferation

Massive periretinal proliferation (MPP) is the most common cause of failure after surgery for rhegmatogenous retinal detachment. This condition is caused by proliferation of cellular membranes within the vitreous gel, on the inner retinal surface, and (to a lesser degree) on the outer retinal surface in the subretinal space[37–39]. These cellular membranes contract, causing rigid immobile retinal folds. New collagen is secreted by myofibroblasts. This further strengthens the membranes and results in a fixed funnel-shaped configuration of the detached retina.

Vitrectomy techniques are used to relieve vitreous traction and to mobilize the retina by separating epiretinal membranes from the inner retinal surface[40] (*see* Chapter 9). A vitreoretinal pick is used to engage the epiretinal membrane and separate it from the inner retina and/or the membrane may be divided with scissors where it bridges between folds of retina. This results in increased mobility of the retina so that it can flatten against the pigment epithelium after closure of the retinal breaks. Usually, some portions of the epiretinal tissue cannot be completely removed; this is especially common for membranes near and anterior to the equator. Therefore, vitreous surgery is usually combined with a broad and high scleral buckle extending from the ora serrata to a location posterior to the equator. Cryotherapy or diathermy is used to treat each retinal break, and an intraocular gas bubble is used to ensure flattening of the retina during the early postoperative time.

Depending on the complexity of the initial vitreoretinal abnormalities, about 75 per cent of these cases can be anatomically reattached during the early postoperative period. However, a long-tern successful result is obtained in less than 50 per cent of eyes with advanced MPP, because there is a high incidence of recurrent epiretinal membranes causing further traction or rhegmatogenous detachment[40].

Inadequate pupillary space

Aphakic eyes with retinal detachment and a small pupillary opening can be treated using vitrectomy instruments to excise portions of iris tissue and/or pupillary membrane to create a larger pupillary space and improve visualization of the posterior segment[17] (*see* Chapter 9). This is usually performed through a limbal approach, although a pars plana approach is used and combined with excision of posterior vitreous gel when vitreous traction, vitreous opacities, epiretinal membranes or other anatomical abnormalities require vitreous surgery as an adjunct to conventional retinal reattachment techniques.

Ocular trauma

Vitreous surgery techniques now allow treatment of selected eyes after severe penetrating injuries (*see* Chapter 13). Each injury is characterized by a variable amount of initial tissue damage, and secondary complications can occur, including: (*1*) hemorrhage; (*2*) infective endophthalmitis; (*3*) toxicity from retained foreign body material; (*4*) intraocular fibrosis and cyclitic membrane formation; and (*5*) vitreoretinal traction causing traction or rhegmatogenous retinal detachment. Secondary complications causing severe visual loss occur most commonly in eyes after penetrating injuries of the posterior segment.

The pathogenesis of blinding secondary complications due to intraocular fibrosis and vitreoretinal traction has been studied by review of clinical material and also by laboratory animal experiments. This pathological process seems to be mediated by an inflammatory reaction, and the damaged vitreous gel serves as a scaffold on which myofibroblasts proliferate. These proliferating cells then contract, causing vitreoretinal traction and/or traction on the ciliary body. Collagen is secreted, forming intravitreal sheets and accentuating the traction on the retina and ciliary body[41–43]. These pathological changes occur most commonly after penetrating injuries directly involving the vitreous gel, combined with severe intravitreal hemorrhage (*Figure 8.48*).

Vitreous surgery may interrupt this pathological process by removing portions of the scaffold on which myofibroblasts proliferate, and perhaps also by reducing the stimulus to cellular growth by excising portions of the damaged vitreous gel together with intravitreal blood and inflammatory debris[42,44]. If infective endophthalmitis is present, excision of the vitreous gel provides material for culture and microscopic study, permits bulk removal of microorganisms and probably reduces enzymatic damage to ocular tissues by removing inflammatory cells and necrotic debris. Certain complicated reactive foreign bodies can also be removed using vitreous surgery methods to minimize secondary inflammatory and/or ionic damage.

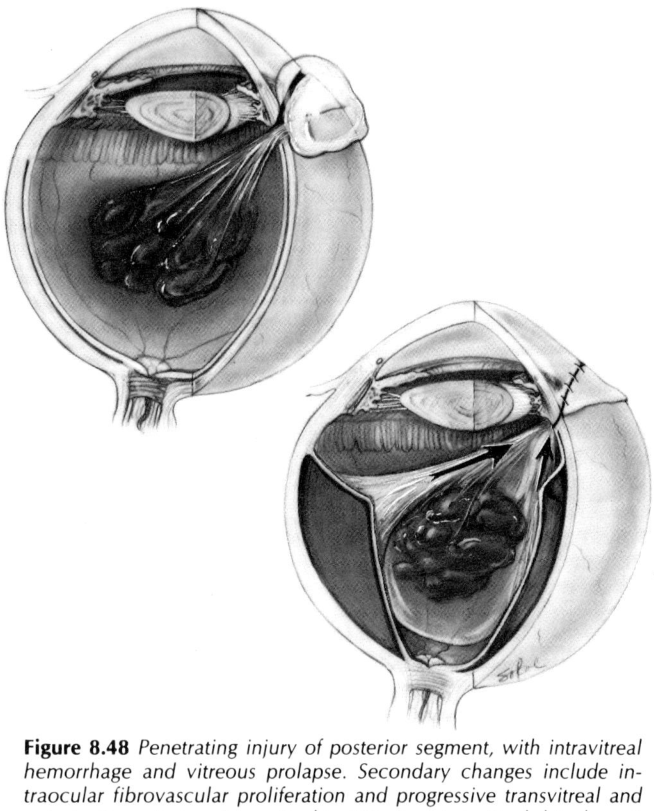

Figure 8.48 *Penetrating injury of posterior segment, with intravitreal hemorrhage and vitreous prolapse. Secondary changes include intraocular fibrovascular proliferation and progressive transvitreal and anterior-to-posterior vitreoretinal traction causing retinal detachment*

Vitreous surgery is reserved for eyes with injuries that have a poor prognosis when managed by conventional methods. These cases include eyes with: (*1*) vitreous gel, iris tissue and/or lens material incarcerated in a corneal wound; (*2*) a disrupted lens and admixed lens material and vitreous gel; (*3*) reactive non-magnetic foreign bodies or certain magnetic foreign bodies that cannot be safely removed with a magnet; (*4*) penetrating injuries of the posterior segment with vitreous prolapse and dense intravitreal hemorrhage; and (*5*) traction and/or rhegmatogenous retinal detachment with vitreous hemorrhage or severe vitreous traction.

When the injury involves mainly the anterior segment, the surgical objectives are to: (*1*) remove vitreous gel and/or lens material incarcerated in the corneal wound; (*2*) leave the anterior chamber free of vitreous; and (*3*) remove damaged tissue from the pupillary space that could result in a secondary membrane. These objectives can often be achieved through a limbal approach (*see Figure 13.12*).

When severe posterior segment damage has occurred, an extensive vitrectomy is performed (*see* Chapter 13). This includes, when possible, separation of the posterior cortical vitreous from the inner retinal surface posterior to the equator to prevent later traction. Certain foreign bodies are grasped and extracted with special forceps introduced through the pars plana (*see* Chapter 13). The foreign body may be withdrawn through the pars plana incision or through a separate limbus incision if it is large and the lens was damaged and removed. A broad encircling scleral buckle, extending from ora serrata to the equator, is used in most eyes with severe posterior segment injuries and vitreous hemorrhage. This is especially useful if the anteroperipheral retina and/or adjacent ciliary body were damaged. Secondary fibrosis and vitreous traction often occur in this area, and the scleral buckle reduces the chance of posterior retinal detachment occurring from traction and/or retinal breaks involving the area near the ora serrata (*Figure 8.49*).

The timing of vitreous surgery and proper case selection are both important in eyes that have suffered severe trauma. The objective is to minimize secondary complications, and therefore surgery is desirable before these complications cause permanent structural damage. Immediate vitrectomy, performed at the time of repair of the penetrating wound, is considered when vitreous surgery techniques are needed to remove a reactive intraocular foreign body, when advanced infective endophthalmitis is present, and when it is necessary to excise vitreous gel and extracapsular lens material from the anterior chamber and pupillary space after repair of a corneal laceration.

In other cases, prompt repair of the penetrating wound is performed, and any small magnetic foreign bodies are extracted by conventional means. Broad-spectrum antibiotics are given intravenously after the operation. Vitreous surgery is performed as a secondary procedure 5–7 days after the injury if vitreous gel remains incarcerated in a central corneal wound or if lens material and vitreous gel in the pupillary space are likely to cause a secondary membrane. Posterior vitrectomy is performed 5–14 days after the injury in eyes with severe penetrating injuries of the vitreous and vitreous hemorrhage, double-perforating injuries with vitreous hemorrhage, and cases with dense vitreous opacities and retinal detachment[45].

Delaying vitreous surgery for 5–14 days, rather than performing this operation at the time of initial repair of the wound, permits further diagnostic evaluation and allows the operation to be performed under optimum conditions. Also, during this interval, spontaneous separation of the posterior cortical vitreous from the retina may occur because of vitreous hemorrhage and inflammation. This permits excision of the cortical vitreous with minimal risk. The likelihood of active intraoperative bleeding may also be reduced by delaying posterior vitrectomy several days.

Vitreous surgery may be performed even later if required by secondary complications. The most common indication is an occluded pupil from organization of residual lens material, vitreous gel and inflammatory debris. Other indications include traction and certain rhegmatogenous retinal detachments, as mentioned earlier. Finally, epiretinal membranes causing distortion of the posterior retina and macula occur occasionally and may be an indication for surgical removal.

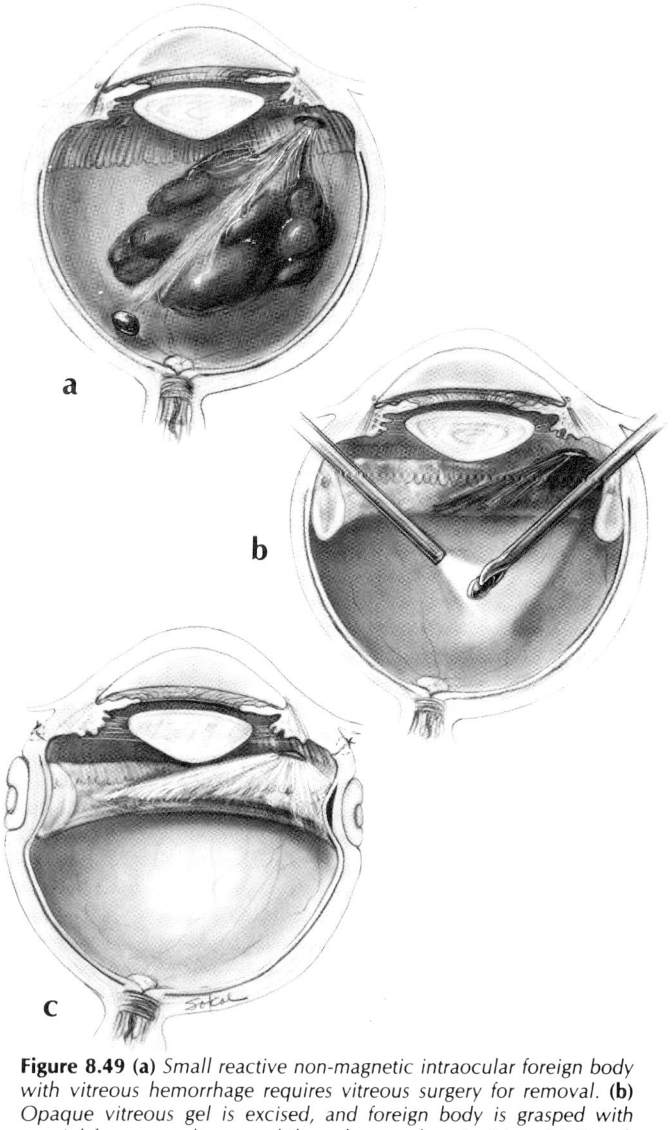

Figure 8.49 **(a)** *Small reactive non-magnetic intraocular foreign body with vitreous hemorrhage requires vitreous surgery for removal.* **(b)** *Opaque vitreous gel is excised, and foreign body is grasped with special forceps and removed through pars plana incision.* **(c)** *Broad, anterior encircling scleral buckle is used to minimize traction effects from remaining anteroperipheral vitreous incarcerated in original injury site and/or surgical incisions*

The comparative results of treating injured eyes by vitreous surgery are difficult to evaluate because several variables are involved, including: (*1*) the amount of initial damage and associated abnormalities; (*2*) the presence and extent of secondary complications; (*3*) differing intervals between the injury and later vitreous surgery; and (*4*) differing mechanical achievements of the operation. Nevertheless experienced vitreous surgeons agree that many eyes can be salvaged that would otherwise be lost because of secondary complications. Nearly normal vision can be achieved in some cases when the macula was not damaged by the original injury. It is estimated that 50 per cent of eyes with an otherwise poor prognosis can be salvaged using vitreous surgery techniques.

Diagnostic vitrectomy

Diagnostic vitrectomy (or vitreous biopsy) is usually reserved for eyes with suspected intraocular fungal infection, possible reticulum cell sarcoma, or severe inflammation after extracapsular cataract extraction and a differential diagnosis of bacterial endophthalmitis or phacoanaphylactic response. The ability to remove intravitreal proliferative tissue and selected membranes from the retinal surface provides biopsy material, permitting clinicopathological correlations, including ultrastructural analysis.

Sufficient tissue is removed to provide an adequate sample for evaluation. The specimen is obtained in a manner to facilitate later analysis – including maintenance of surgical sterility if culture testing is necessary, and avoiding unnecessary dilution by the infusion solution. The specimen is usually collected in a small sterile syringe that is spliced into the aspiration system (*Figure 8.50*). Pieces of tissue, such as epiretinal membranes, can be grasped directly with forceps and removed after dividing all intraocular attachments.

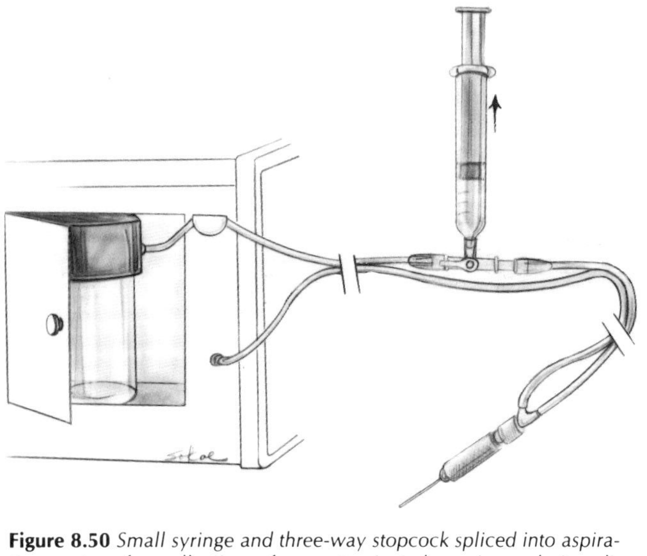

Figure 8.50 *Small syringe and three-way stopcock spliced into aspiration system for collection of uncontaminated specimen during diagnostic vitrectomy. The syringe is operated by the surgical assistant. It provides low levels of suction force, and the biopsy specimen is obtained with minimal dilution*

Anterior segment disorders

Vitrectomy methods now allow treatment of a variety of problems affecting the anterior segment, including: (*1*) an occluded pupillary space; (*2*) complications of vitreous gel in the anterior chamber; (*3*) membranes behind a pseudophakos; (*4*) progressive cystic or sheet-like epithelial invasion of the anterior chamber; (*5*) certain complicated and/or congenital cataracts; and (*6*) total hyphema[46]. A limbal approach is preferred if the surgical objectives are limited to the anterior chamber and/or pupillary-lens plane and if the tissue(s) to be excised are pliable. A pars plana approach is preferred when large amounts of vitreous gel must be excised, when fiberoptic intraocular illumination is needed, and when a posterior entry plane is necessary to minimize corneal damage or to give better access to portions of the anterior segment.

Stiff, non-pliable pupillary membranes cannot be easily aspirated into the cutting port of the vitrectomy probe. Such tissue is first cut into ribbon-like sections using scissors, and then the pliable sections are excised (*Figure 8.51*). When vascularized tissue is encountered, bimanual bipolar diathermy with two instrument tips serving as electrodes is used to control active bleeding (*Figure 8.52*).

When using a limbal approach for anterior segment surgery, we prefer a bimanual operative technique with a

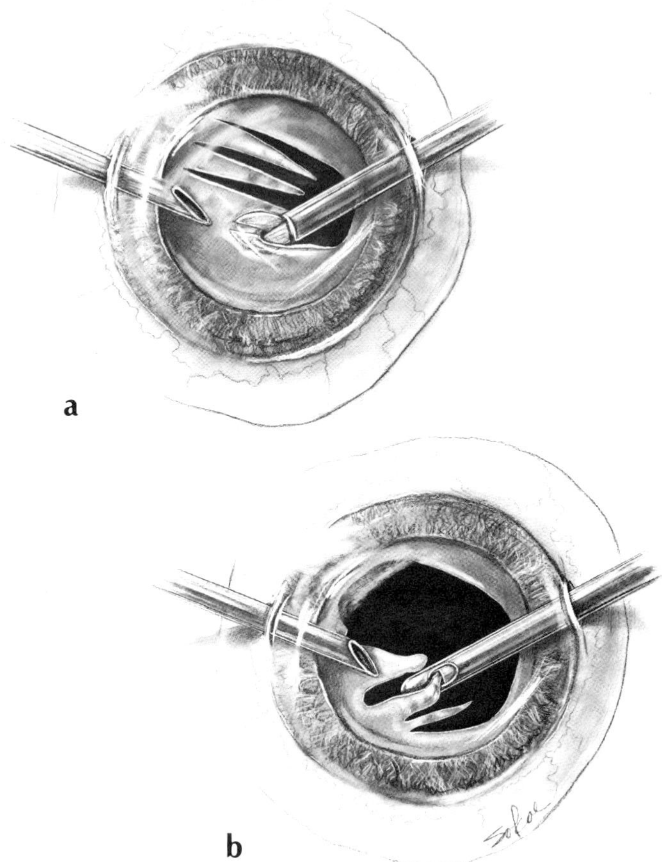

a

b

Figure 8.51 *Excision of fibrotic pupillary membrane composed of lens remnants.* (**a**) *Limbal approach is used, and membrane is cut into ribbon-like sections using right-angle scissors.* (**b**) *The pliable sections are then excised with vitrectomy probe*

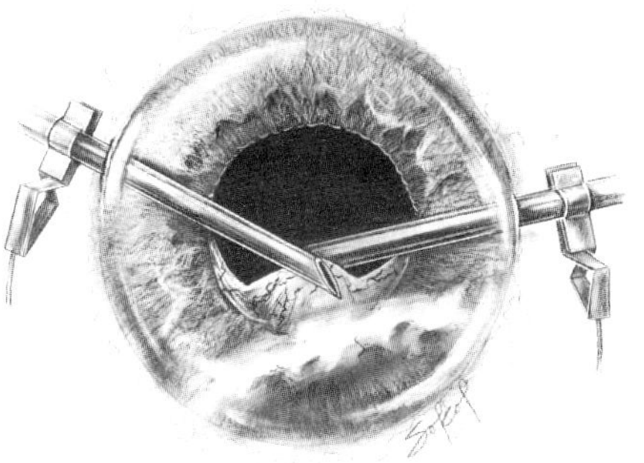

Figure 8.52 *Bimanual bipolar diathermy used to treat vascularized tissue when excising pupillary membrane associated with inferior corneal laceration and adherent leucoma. Instrument tips serve as electrodes, and diathermy current is conducted through vascularized membrane after partial excision. This technique closes abnormal vessels and shrinks fibrotic material farther out of pupillary space*

separate infusion needle. This facilitates rotation of the globe, provides a second instrument to assist in manipulation of intraocular tissues and permits use of bimanual diathermy. The instrument positions can also be exchanged to approach parts of the anterior segment from the opposite direction. Air can be injected into the anterior chamber before withdrawal of the instruments, to prevent incarceration of vitreous gel in the incision sites as the instruments are withdrawn (*Figure 8.53*).

Inadequate pupillary space

Eyes with an inadequate pupillary space include those with: (*1*) fibrotic capsulolenticular membranes (membranous cataract); (*2*) other vascularized membranes occurring after total hyphema or chronic uveitis; (*3*) opacification of the posterior lens capsule after extracapsular cataract extraction; (*4*) an occluded or updrawn pupil in aphakic eyes associated with intraocular inflammation and/or vitreous incarcerated in a cataract wound; and (*5*) eyes with persistent hyperplastic primary vitreous (PHPV) obstructing the pupillary space and/or causing marked shallowing of the anterior chamber. In each of these conditions, iris, lens material and/or other abnormal tissue is excised to create a clear central pupillary space 4–5 mm in size. Excessive excision of iris tissue is avoided to prevent an unnecessary cosmetic abnormality. If the entire iris sphincter muscle is excised, the unopposed dilator fibers cause extreme dilation of the pupil in some eyes.

Results of treating eyes for an inadequate pupil have ranged from nearly uniform success, in eyes with an opaque posterior lens capsule or other thin pupillary membrane, to preservation of the globe but little potential for useful vision in severe PHPV. In eyes with an updrawn pupil improved vision is usually obtained after excision of portions of the iris tissue, and complications are infrequent if excessive traction on the anteroperipheral vitreous is avoided.

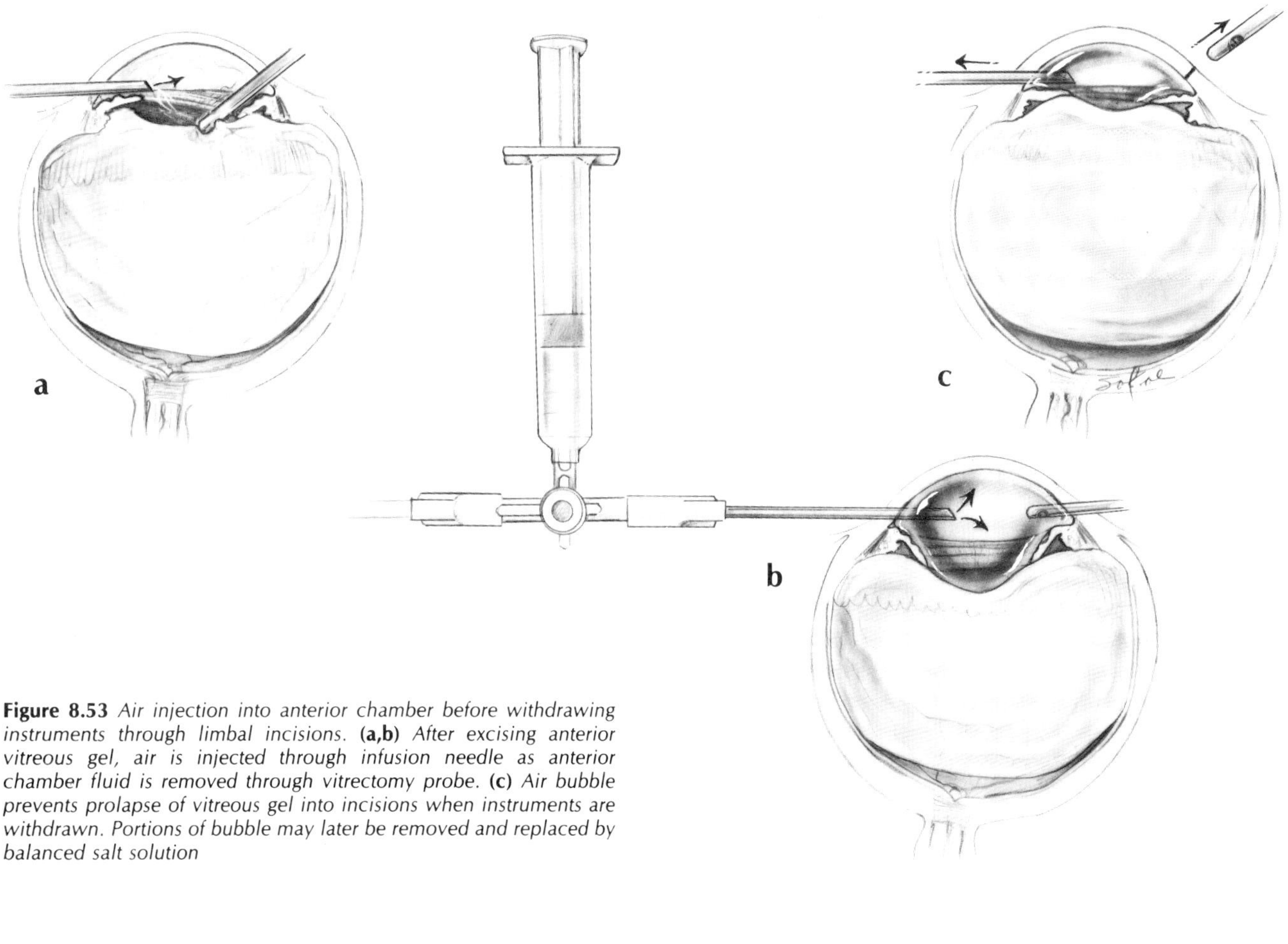

Figure 8.53 *Air injection into anterior chamber before withdrawing instruments through limbal incisions.* **(a,b)** *After excising anterior vitreous gel, air is injected through infusion needle as anterior chamber fluid is removed through vitrectomy probe.* **(c)** *Air bubble prevents prolapse of vitreous gel into incisions when instruments are withdrawn. Portions of bubble may later be removed and replaced by balanced salt solution*

Vitreous complications in the anterior segment

Anterior vitreous complications treated by vitrectomy include: (*1*) vitreocorneal 'touch' with secondary corneal edema; (*2*) aphakic pupillary-block glaucoma; (*3*) vitreous incarceration in a cataract wound, with persistent aphakic cystoid macular edema; and (*4*) the 'vitreous wick' syndrome with externalized vitreous gel. Of these conditions, vitreocorneal touch with early edema of the central cornea is the most widely accepted indication for vitrectomy because of the clinically proven efficacy of vitreous surgery in these cases and the absence of effective alternative therapy (*Figure 8.54*)[47].

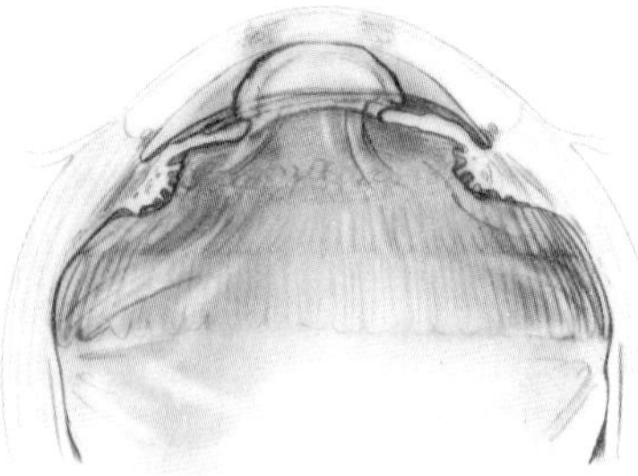

a

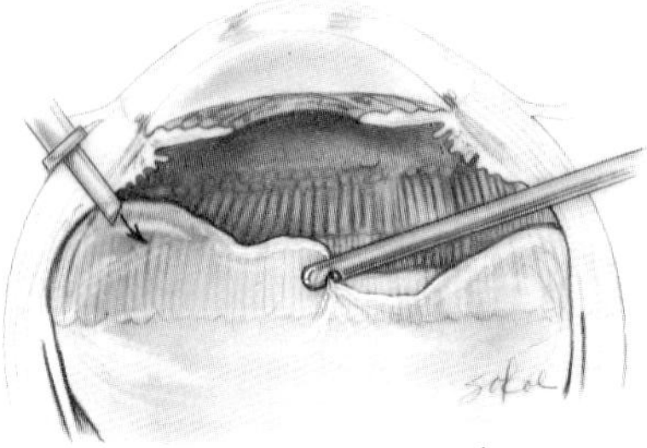

b

Figure 8.54 (a) *Surgical treatment of vitreoretinal touch with central corneal edema due to anterior prolapse of vitreous gel and contact between vitreous and corneal endothelium.* **(b)** *Pars plana approach is preferred to remove vitreous from anterior chamber and excise portions of anteroperipheral vitreous gel to prevent recurrence*

Aphakic pupillary-block glaucoma and the 'vitreous wick' syndrome can be managed by other techniques, although vitreous surgery methods have been helpful in our experience. Treating aphakic pupillary-block glaucoma by vitrectomy relieves the pathogenetic mechanism and prevents recurrence of the pupillary block (*Figure 8.55*). Excision of vitreous gel in the anterior chamber and removal of vitreous from the internal aspect of the fistula is combined with closure of the fistula to treat the 'vitreous wick' syndrome (*Figure 8.56*). The role of vitreous surgery in treating chronic aphakic cystoid macular edema by removing vitreous from the limbal wound and releasing iridovitreal adhesions is unproven, although the initial reported experience is favorable. We prefer a pars plana approach in each of these conditions – except in treatment of the 'vitreous wick' syndrome, in which a limbal approach has proven satisfactory.

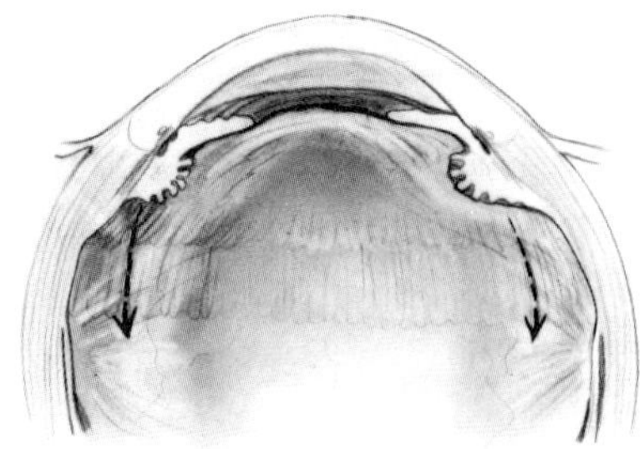

a

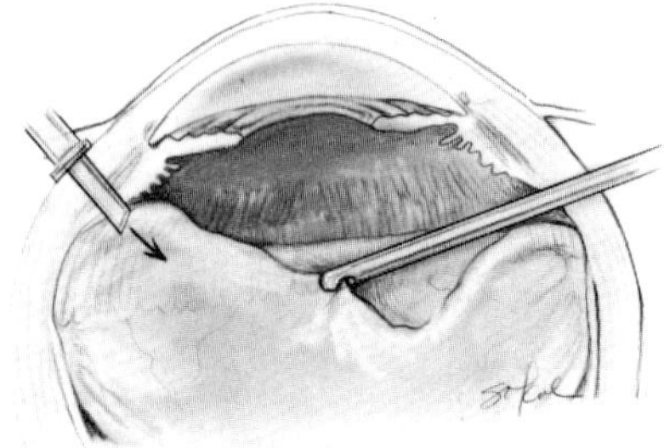

b

Figure 8.55 (a) *Treatment of aphakic pupillary-block glaucoma caused by misdirection of aqueous flow and anterior displacement of vitreous gel causing pupillary block and secondary closure of anterior chamber angle.* **(b)** *Pars plana approach is preferred to excise the anterior vitreous face, thereby relieving the pupillary block, and to remove portions of anterior central vitreous gel to prevent recurrence*

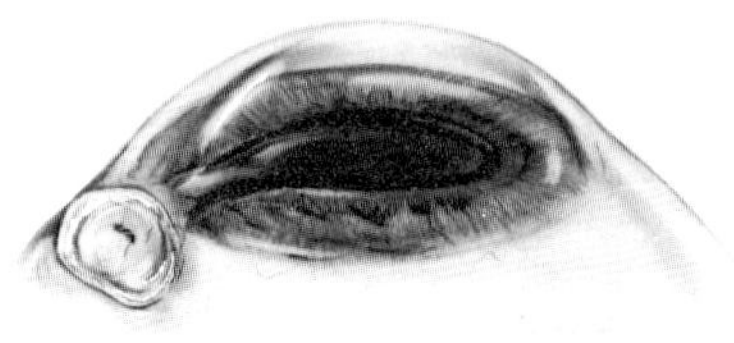

a

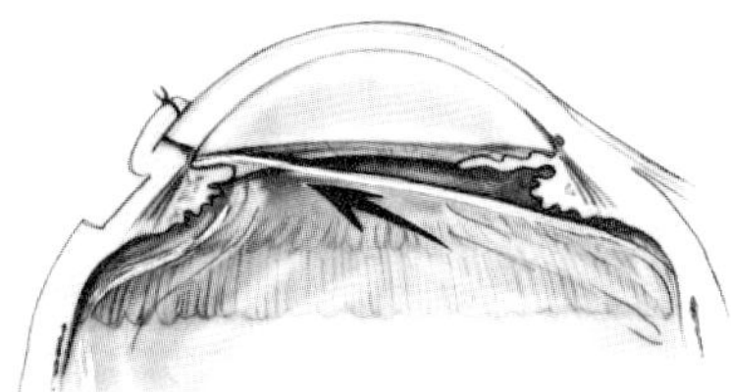

b

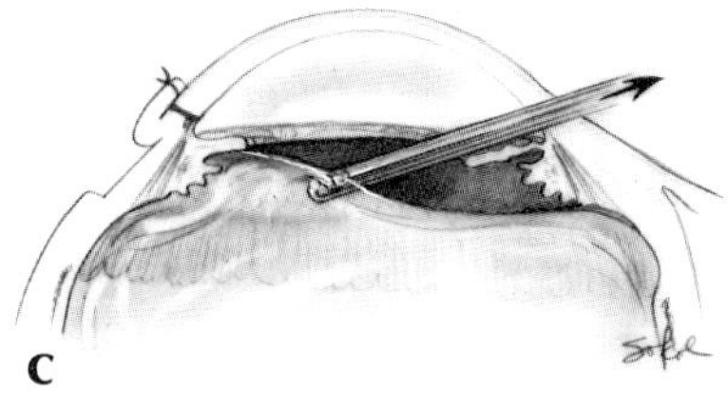

c

Figure 8.56 (a) *'Vitreous wick' syndrome with externalized vitreous gel prolapsed through enlarged suture tract or limbal fistula.* **(b)** *Limbal opening covered by partial-thickness anteriorly hinged scleral flap (or closed with sutures).* **(c)** *Vitreous gel extending to internal aspect of incision is then excised with vitrectomy probe through limbal approach*

Retropseudophakos membranes

Opaque membranes posterior to a pseudophakos can result from inflammation and secondary changes of the anterior vitreous gel and/or opacification of a posterior lens capsule. Vitrectomy probes permit excision of the opaque tissue in the pupillary space. The route of approach and amount of tissue removed depend on the type of intraocular lens and its method of fixation. However, we usually prefer a pars plana approach. An infusion needle can be used in the anterior chamber to maintain a deep chamber and thus prevent contact between the pseudophakos and the cornea (*Figure 8.57*). This is not usually necessary and a pars plana infusion cannula can be used instead.

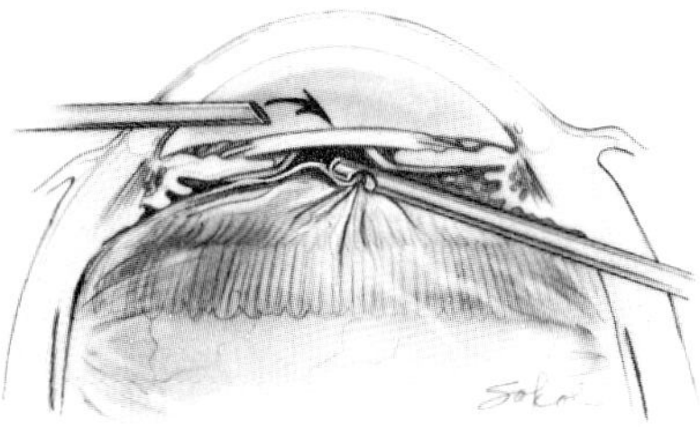

Figure 8.57 *Excision of retropseudophakos membrane using vitrectomy probe through pars plana approach. Infusion is provided through needle introduced through limbus to prevent anterior displacement of IOL. Thin membranes are easily excised, whereas thicker membranes are first fenestrated with a knife or scissors before excision with vitrectomy probe*

Epithelial ingrowth

Epithelial invasion of the anterior chamber can occur as a cyst or as a sheet-like epithelial ingrowth on the posterior corneal surface, the anterior chamber angle, the anterior iris and vitreous surfaces, and posteriorly over the ciliary body. Sheet-like epithelial ingrowth is usually progressive and results in absolute glaucoma from obstruction of the anterior chamber angle.

An epithelial cyst is treated only if it enlarges enough to obstruct the visual axis or to cause other complications that cannot be managed by medical means. Incision of an epithelial cyst is avoided to prevent conversion of the cyst into a sheet-like ingrowth. Instead, the cyst is collapsed by aspirating its contents with a needle introduced through the attachment of the cyst to the eyewall, and the anterior vitreous gel is then excised (*Figure 8.58a,b*). An intraocular air bubble is used to tamponade the cyst against the eyewall and also to provide thermal insulation so that transscleral cryotherapy is effective in devitalizing the epithelial cells of the cyst wall (*Figure 8.58c*).

Sheet-like epithelial ingrowth (*Figure 8.59a*) is treated by first applying photocoagulation to define the extent of iris involvement. Involved iris tissue and vitreous are then excised with the vitrectomy probe (*Figure 8.59b*), and an intraocular air bubble is used to fill the anterior segment (*Figure 8.59c*). The air bubble, acting as a thermal insulator, increases the effect of transscleral and transcorneal cryotherapy in devitalizing the epithelial cells remaining on the posterior corneal surface and in the anterior chamber angle[48].

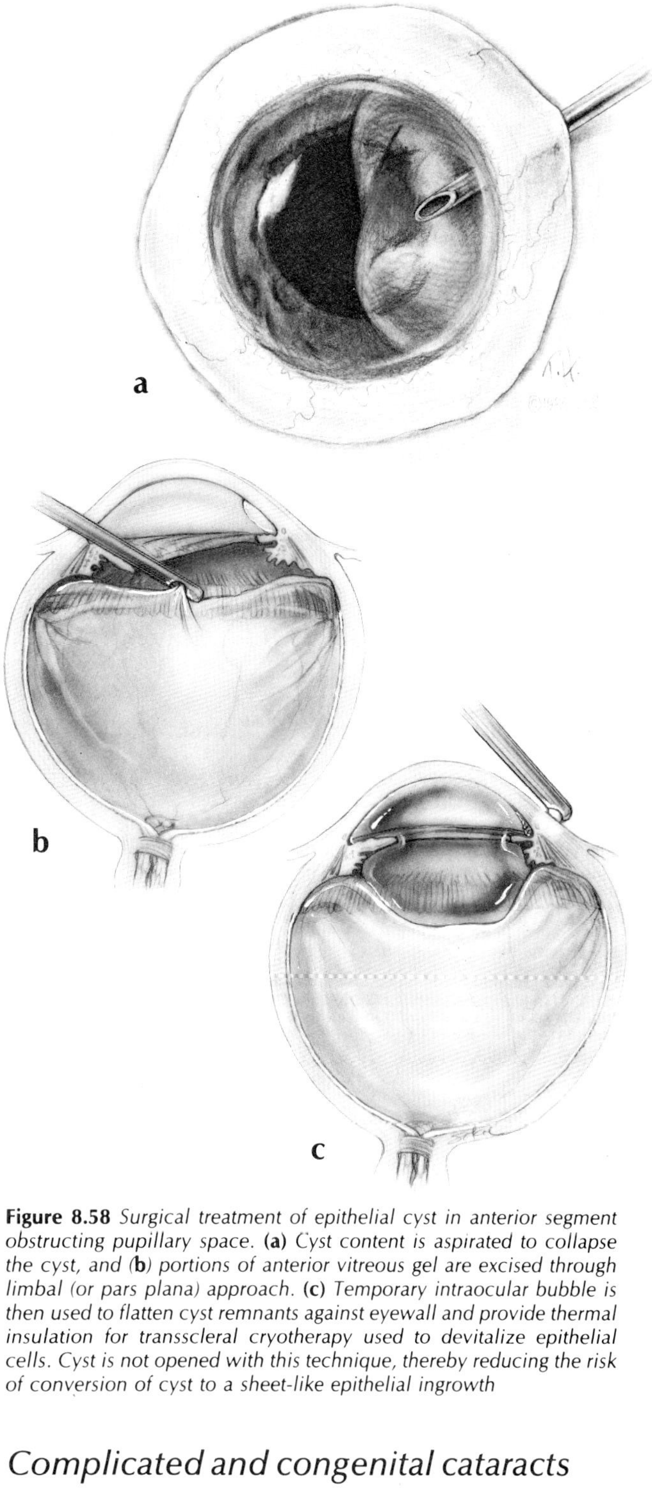

Figure 8.58 *Surgical treatment of epithelial cyst in anterior segment obstructing pupillary space.* **(a)** *Cyst content is aspirated to collapse the cyst, and* **(b)** *portions of anterior vitreous gel are excised through limbal (or pars plana) approach.* **(c)** *Temporary intraocular bubble is then used to flatten cyst remnants against eyewall and provide thermal insulation for transscleral cryotherapy used to devitalize epithelial cells. Cyst is not opened with this technique, thereby reducing the risk of conversion of cyst to a sheet-like epithelial ingrowth*

Complicated and congenital cataracts

Virectomy techniques are useful to remove complicated cataracts, including certain dislocated lenses and others with extensive iridolenticular adhesions and/or prelenticular membranes. A pars plana approach with ultrasonic emulsification is preferable. A dislocated lens is often stabilized by penetration with an infusion needle or illumination pick while it is emulsified with an ultrasonic needle and/or excised with a vitrectomy probe.

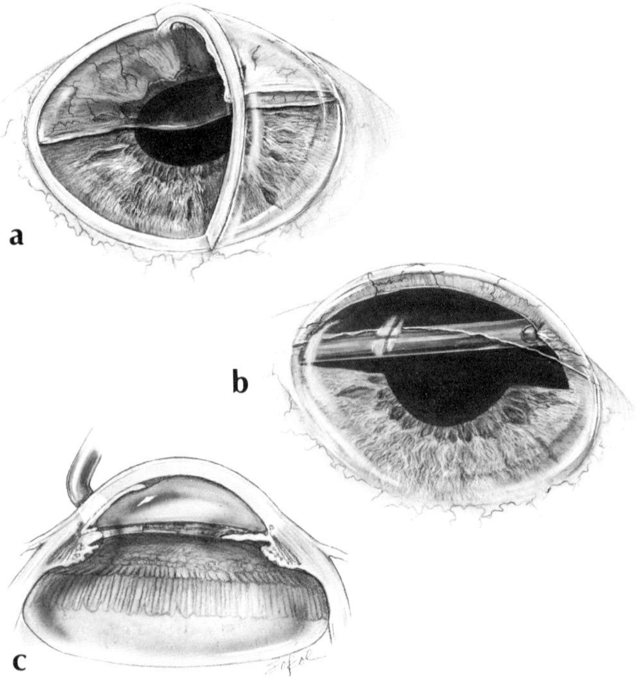

Figure 8.59 **(a)** *Sheet-like epithelial ingrowth involving posterior cornea, iris and anterior vitreous surface.* **(b)** *Vitrectomy instrument, through pars plana approach, is used to excise involved portions of iris and vitreous gel after using photocoagulation to delineate area of iris involvement.* **(c)** *Portions of anterior vitreous are excised, and an air bubble in the anterior segment provides thermal insulation during transcorneal and transscleral cryotherapy to devitalize epithelial cells remaining on posterior corneal surface and in anterior chamber angle*

Congenital and juvenile cataracts are now often removed through a limbal approach, using vitrectomy instruments to aspirate the soft lens material (*Figure 8.60a*) and to excise the posterior lens capsule and portions of the anterior vitreous gel. Wide pupillary dilation is necessary for this technique. We prefer a bimanual technique, so that the pupillary margin can be manipulated with the infusion needle and so that the instrument positions can be transposed to remove easily lens material beneath the iris on the opposite side of the eye (*Figure 8.60b*). Excision of the posterior lens capsule and portions of the anterior vitreous gel (*Figure 8.60c*) seems to reduce the likelihood of secondary membrane formation, which commonly required later discission when previous methods of aspiration were used.

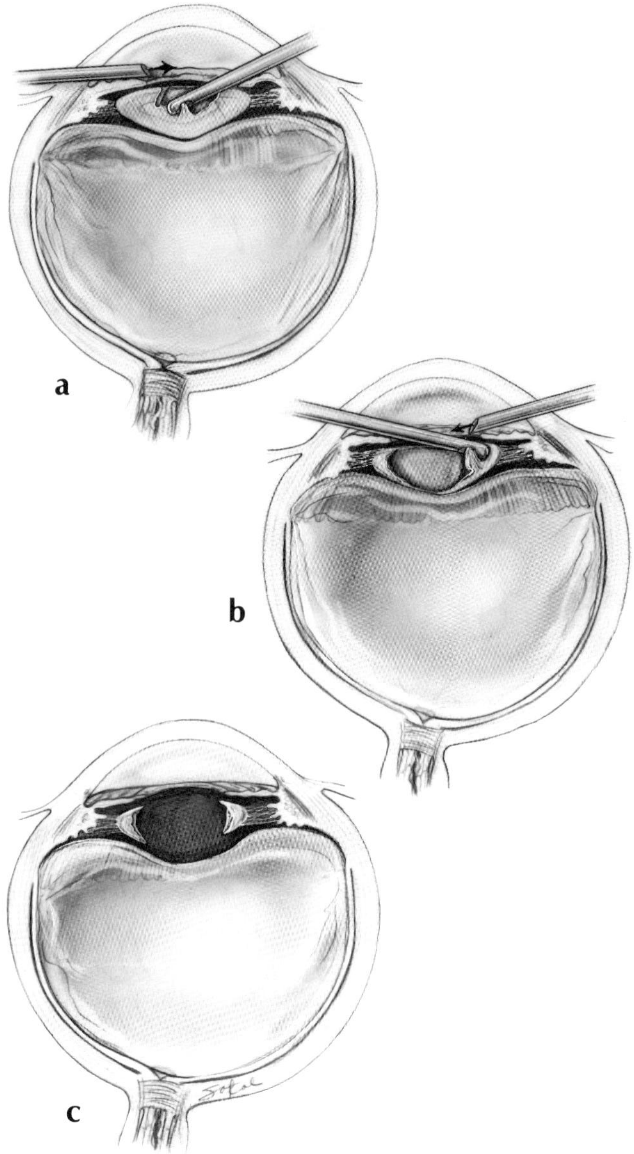

Figure 8.60 *Excision of congenital or juvenile cataract using vitrectomy instruments through limbal approach.* **(a)** *Soft lens material is easily excised with vitrectomy probe.* **(b)** *Positions of probe and infusion needle can be transposed to improve access to lens material under opposite portion of iris.* **(c)** *Posterior capsule and portions of anterior vitreous gel are excised to ensure clear pupillary space without secondary membrane*

Hyphema

Vitrectomy instruments can be used to treat certain eyes with total hyphema when removal of the anterior segment hemorrhage is necessary because of intractable glaucoma or early corneal blood-staining[49] (*see* Chapter 13). Patients with sickle-cell hemoglobinopathy and hyphema require surgical intervention earlier when only mild intraocular pressure elevation is present, to prevent intravascular sickling and ocular ischemic damage. We prefer a bimanual technique with the vitrectomy probe and a separate infusion needle introduced through opposite limbal incisions. A peripheral iridectomy is performed it iris tissue prolapses into the limbal wound when the initial incision is made, because this suggests that pupillary block is also present with increased pressure in the posterior chamber. Loose blood in the anterior chamber is then lavaged from the eye through the vitrectomy probe while the infusion needle maintains normal depth of the anterior chamber. The remaining clot is excised with the vitrectomy probe. However, no effort is made to separate portions of the clot that remain adherent to the iris, in order to avoid further bleeding. The vitrectomy probe is then withdrawn, followed by the infusion needle, to avoid hypotony which can also be associated with further bleeding.

Secondary open-angle glaucoma

Vitrectomy methods are useful to treat eyes with secondary open-angle glaucoma caused by obstruction of the trabecular outflow channels by cells and extracellular debris associated with chronic vitreous hemorrhage or lens material producing a phacolytic or phacoanaphylactic reponse. Blood-induced glaucoma complicating vitreous hemorrhage is more common in aphakic eyes than in phakic eyes. This type of glaucoma is caused by mechanical obstruction of the anterior chamber outflow channels by erythrocytic debris, pigment-laden macrophages (hemolytic glaucoma) or devitalized erythrocytes with rigid plasma membranes that cannot pass through the narrow sinusoidal passages of the trabecular meshwork (ghost-cell glaucoma)[50,51]. A combination of hemolytic macrophages, devitalized erythrocytes and extracellular debris probably accounts for the glaucoma in most eyes with vitreous hemorrhage.

Vitreous surgery through a pars plana approach is used to excise the opaque vitreous gel and remove the reservoir of erythrocytes when blood-induced glaucoma cannot be controlled by medical therapy[52]. However, antiglaucoma therapy with topical medications may be required indefinitely, even after removing the vitreous hemorrhage, because of permanent damage to the filtering meshwork. Similarly, excision of retained lens material, as described later, is used to treat eyes with severe glaucoma caused by obstruction of the trabecular meshwork by inflammatory cells and/or macrophages occurring as a response to extracapsular lens material.

Retained lens material

Extracapsular lens material causing secondary complications can be conveniently removed by vitrectomy methods. Various surgical techniques can be used – depending on the amount, consistency and location of the lens material and the type and severity of secondary complications[53,54]. Remnants of cortical material and lens capsule in the pupillary space are readily removed through a limbal approach using the aspiration and cutting functions of the vitrectomy probe.

Various techniques are needed to deal with extracapsular material dislocated into the vitreous cavity (*Figure 8.61a*). A pars plana approach is used to remove lens material from the vitreous cavity. Portions of the anterior and central vitreous gel are first excised to create a fluid space into which the lens material can be positioned to permit removal without causing excessive vitreoretinal traction when strong suction force is needed. Portions of the posterior cortical vitreous are temporarily left intact when possible. Lens material of soft consistency is removed with the vitrectomy probe using the aspiration and cutting functions (*Figure 8.61b*). A second instrument, such as an infusion needle or fiberoptic illumination probe, can be used to assist in engaging firm lens material in the cutting port.

However, we prefer an ultrasonic needle when lens material is not easily removed through the vitrectomy probe with only moderate suction force. While using only suction force, lens fragments are engaged with the ultrasonic needle and positioned in the fluid space within the vitreous cavity. Then ultrasonic energy is applied. If the lens material is especially firm, the illumination probe may be needed to prevent displacement of the lens fragment away from the needle tip when ultrasonic energy is used (*Figure 8.61c*). As each fragment is removed, smaller particles may fall posteriorly and these, in turn, are retrieved with the needle tip and then emulsified within the fluid-filled central vitreous cavity. Remaining portions of the posterior vitreous surface are later excised with the vitrectomy probe.

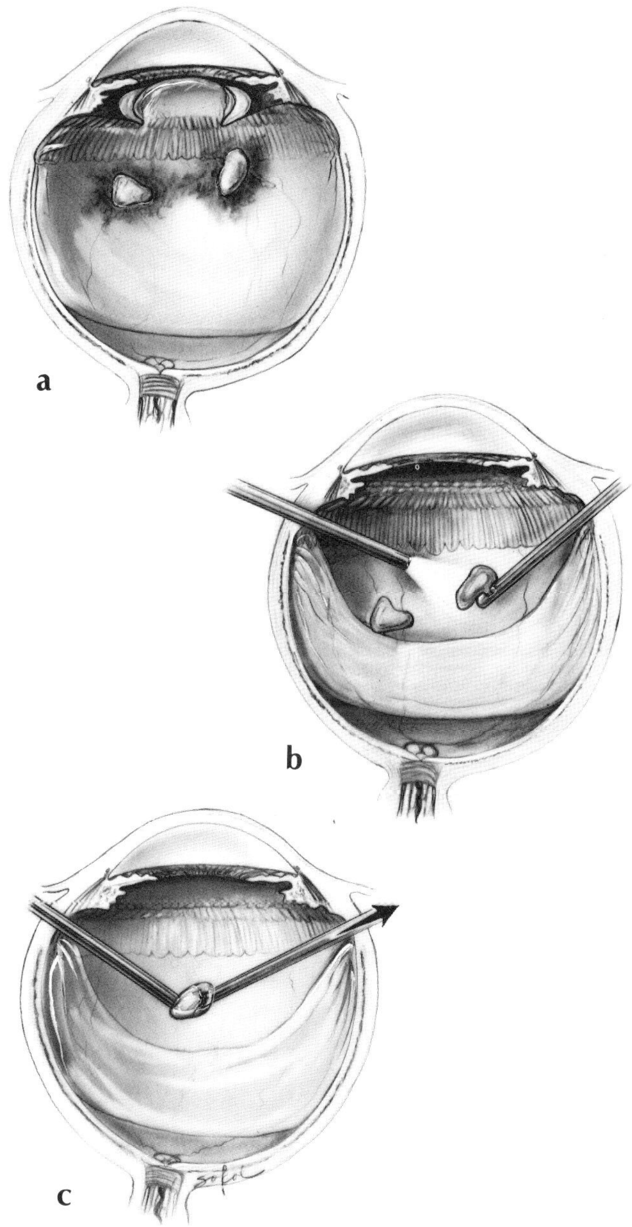

Figure 8.61 **(a)** *Removal of lens remnants from vitreous cavity is necessary when lens material causes severe intraocular inflammation. Pars plana approach is used to excise portions of anterocentral vitreous and provide access to lens remnants.* **(b)** *Soft lens material is removed with vitrectomy probe.* **(c)** *Firm lens material is removed through ultrasonic needle by emulsification, and illumination probe is used to assist in positioning lens material against ultrasonic needle tip*

When an intact lens nucleus of firm consistency is present (*Figure 8.62a*), a limbal extraction technique is preferable. This minimizes the volume of irrigating solution passing through the eye and reduces the possibility of retinal damage due to vitreoretinal traction from strong suction force or direct damage during repeated retrieval of lens fragments from the inner retinal surface. Portions of the vitreous gel are first excised to expose the lens nucleus, and any remaining cortical fibers are stripped from the nucleus and excised with the vitrectomy probe. The lens nucleus is then grasped with the vitrectomy probe and positioned in the anterior chamber through a partially dilated pupil (*Figure 8.62b*). Acetylcholine is injected into the anterior chamber to constrict the pupil and thereby incarcerate the lens nucleus. The vitrectomy instruments are withdrawn, the sclerotomy sites are closed, and the lens nucleus is extracted through a limbal incision (*Figure 8.62c*). When a separate pars plana infusion cannula secured to the sclera is used, this is left in place during removal of the lens nucleus to prevent collapse of the globe. A double Flieringa ring may be sutured to the sclera to assist further in preventing infolding of the sclera when the limbal incision is opened.

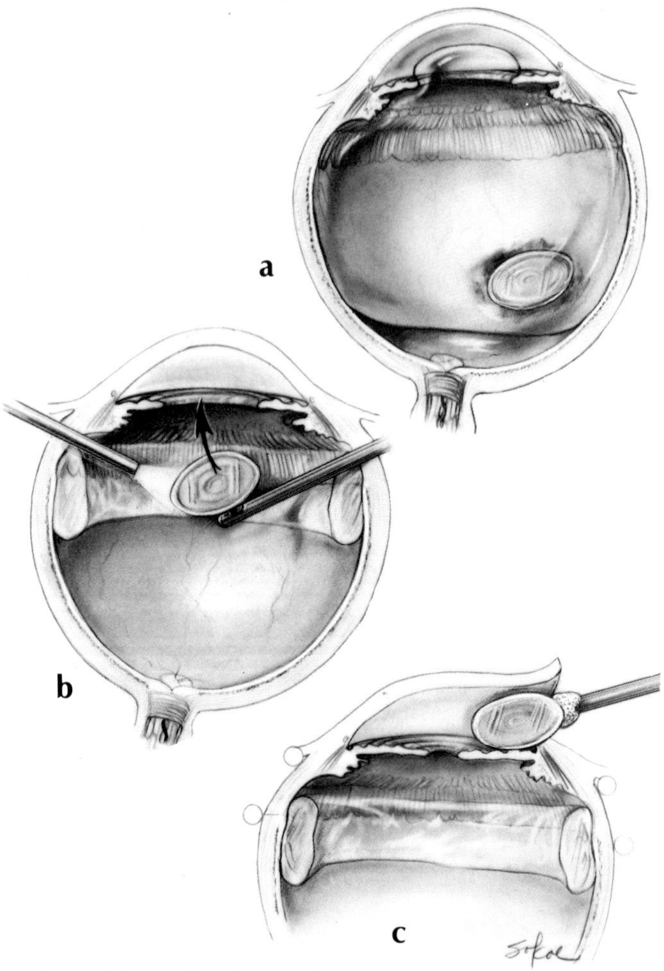

Figure 8.62 **(a)** *Hard lens nucleus in vitreous cavity after trauma or unplanned extracapsular cataract extraction.* **(b)** *Vitreous gel excised through pars plana approach, and lens nucleus grasped with vitrectomy probe and positioned in anterior chamber.* **(c)** *Pupil is constricted with acetylcholine, double Flieringa is ring sutured to sclera, and limbal incision is made to remove lens nucleus with cryoprobe*

Infective endophthalmitis

Vitrectomy techniques now allow treatment of both bacterial and fungal endophthalmitis by direct removal of organisms and inflammatory debris. This provides suitable material for microscopic examination and culture testing, and it seems to have a beneficial effect by reducing retinal and uveal damage caused by bacterial toxins and proteolytic enzymes from the inflammatory cells. Vitreous surgery may also improve penetration of locally and systemically administered antibiotic and antifungal medications.

Vitrectomy is often combined with intracameral antibiotic and steroid therapy and is used to treat selected cases of bacterial endophthalmitis with an otherwise poor prognosis because of an especially virulent pathogen and/or severe or prolonged intraocular inflammation[55]. Vitrectomy is recommended in aphakic eyes when the infected vitreous gel is sufficiently opaque that the retinal vessels cannot be seen by indirect ophthalmoscopy. Other clinical features suggesting that vitrectomy should be performed include: (*1*) extensive intravitreal opacities and/or prominent thickening of the cortical vitreous, retina and choroid as demonstrated by ultrasound examination; (*2*) presence of gram-negative organisms seen on examination of intraocular fluids; (*3*) an untreated infection of longer than 48 hours duration; and (*4*) worsening of the clinical course despite antibiotic therapy.

The vitrectomy is performed as an emergency operation through the pars plana, and as much of the infected vitreous gel is excised as possible. However, no effort is made to separate the posterior vitreous surface from the retina unless a posterior vitreous detachment is already present, because the retina is often friable and retinal breaks and/or hemorrhage may occur as a result of traction on the adjacent vitreous gel. Vitrectomy is often combined with intraocular injection of antibiotics, such as gentamicin 200–400 μg and cefazolin 2.25 mg, and steroids; and high dosage intravenous antibiotic and systemic steroid therapy is used postoperatively. A small syringe spliced into the aspiration line, as described earlier (*see Figure 8.50*), is used to retrieve portions of the excised material for microscopic study and culture testing.

Vitrectomy is recommended to treat presumed fungal endophthalmitis when there is involvement of the vitreous gel and when: (*1*) the organism cannot be isolated from other sources to confirm this presumptive diagnosis; (*2*) there is worsening of the clinical course despite systemic therapy with antifungal medications; and (*3*) when systemic therapy cannot be used because of preexisting renal damage or progressive damage caused by antifungal medications. In addition, mechanical separation of the posterior vitreous surface from the inner retina at the time of vitrectomy may reduce the severity of later epiretinal membrane formation, which commonly occurs after fungal endophthalmitis even though the infective agent is successfully treated with antifungal medications. As much of the involved posterior vitreous gel is excised as possible, and a dilute dose of antifungal medication is often instilled into the vitreous cavity at the end of the operation. Systemic treatment with an antifungal medication is continued postoperatively, when possible, until a full course of the antifungal medication has been given and the infection appears to be cured.

Vitreopapillary and vitreomacular traction

Vitreous traction on the optic nerve and/or macula is common in certain conditions such as proliferative retinopathies, penetrating injuries of the posterior segment and presumed nematode endophthalmitis. This traction may severely distort or displace the macula and peripapillary retinal tissue and may markedly reduce vision. Rarely, direct vitreous traction on the macula or optic nerve also occurs as a separate abnormality. Vitreomacular traction can occur after a partial posterior vitreous separation when the cortical vitreous remains adherent to the macular area, resulting in anteroposterior traction and cystoid macular edema. Vitreous surgery can be used to complete the separation of the posterior vitreous from the retina, and this is followed by reduction in the amount of macular edema. Release of traction on the optic nerve and peripapillary retina also improves vision in selected eyes with disorders such as a proliferative retinopathy or nematode endophthalmitis.

Epiretinal membranes

Cellular membranes growing on the inner retinal surface occur in a variety of disorders, including: (*1*) various proliferative retinopathies; (*2*) massive periretinal proliferation (MPP) complicating rhegmatogenous retinal detachment and as a localized change after otherwise successful retinal reattachment surgery; (*3*) as a secondary change associated with penetrating injuries, intraocular inflammation, vitreous hemorrhage and non-proliferative retinal vascular disorders; and (*4*) as an idiopathic condition, especially during the later decades of life. These membranes can cause moderate or severe visual loss by distortion and displacement of the macula, localized retinal detachment from tangential traction, and retinal vascular leakage with cystoid macular edema.

Non-vascularized membranes can usually be separated from the inner retinal surface, thereby minimizing secondary changes. Portions of the posterior vitreous gel are excised and then the epiretinal tissue is engaged with a vitreoretinal pick and gently separated from the inner retinal surface (*Figure 8.63*). When firm attachments between the membrane and retina are encountered, the epiretinal tissue is amputated at these points using intraocular scissors or the vitrectomy probe. A membrane can usually be separated completely from the macular area, and this results in lessening of the retinal distortion and partial visual improvement (*Figure 8.64*)[56–58].

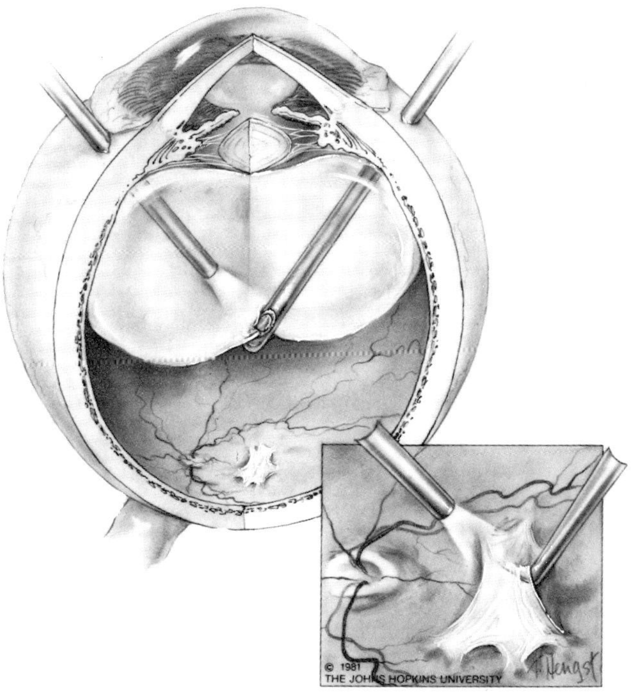

Figure 8.63 *Surgical removal of epiretinal membrane causing macular pucker. Portions of detached posterior vitreous gel are excised, and epiretinal membrane is then dissected from inner retinal surface using vitreoretinal pick*

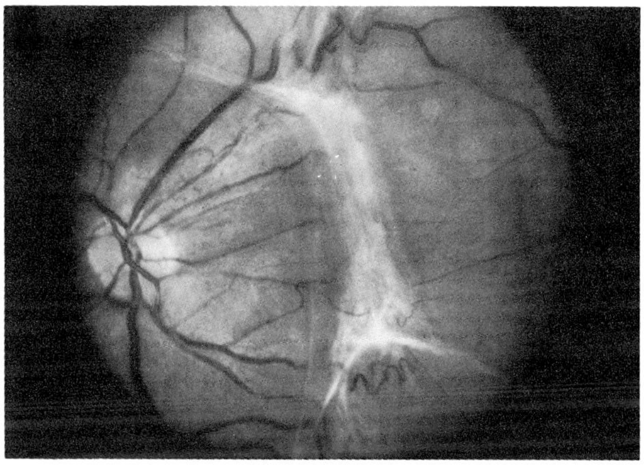

a

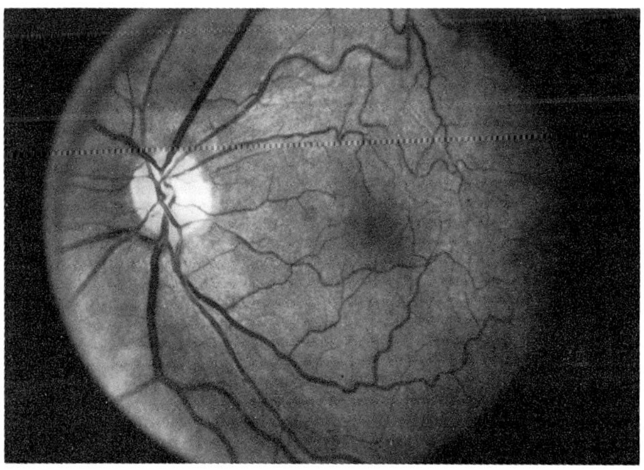

b

Figure 8.64 **(a)** *Preoperative appearance of epiretinal membrane causing macular pucker after otherwise successful retinal reattachment surgery.* **(b)** *Vision improved from 8/200 to 20/25 after removal of abnormal tissue (from Michels, R. G., Gilbert, H. D. American Journal of Ophthalmology 1979; 88:925)*

Postoperative care

Postoperative management begins with certain intraoperative decisions and the selection of postoperative orders to minimize the chance of later ocular and systemic complications. The main ocular concerns are possible infectious endophthalmitis, severe elevation of the intraocular pressure, intraocular hemorrhage and retinal detachment. Infective endophthalmitis is rare postoperatively, and we give gentamicin 20 mg by subconjunctival injection at the end of each operation.

Elevated intraocular pressure may occur postoperatively in any case after vitreous surgery, and this may be especially harmful in eyes with severe intraretinal vascular disease and poor perfusion of the capillary bed. To minimize the possibility of postoperative pressure elevation, before completing the operation a stable situation is achieved regarding the height of any scleral buckle, the composition of any intraocular gas bubble, the amount of blood remaining in the eye and the intraocular pressure itself. If glaucoma was present preoperatively, acetazolamide 500 mg is given intravenously at the end of the operation to reduce aqueous humor secretion during the early postoperative period.

When the operation is performed under general anesthesia, use of nitrous oxide (N_2O) is discontinued about 20 minutes before introduction of any intraocular bubble. This provides time for elimination of the N_2O via the lungs, thereby avoiding the risk of rapid bubble expansion due to systemic N_2O entering the vitreous cavity to equilibrate with any other gases. This also avoids rapid postoperative reduction of the bubble size, which occurs if N_2O is present in the vitreous cavity bubble because it is rapidly cleared from the body through the lungs when the operation is completed.

Immediate postoperative period

Management during the first 3 days after vitreous surgery is directed toward: (*1*) re-establishing the preoperative state of general health; (*2*) diagnosing acute ocular complications, including infective endophthalmitis, elevated intraocular pressure, intraocular bleeding and retinal detachment; (*3*) achieving early corneal reepithelialization if an epithelial defect is present; (*4*) proper use of an intravitreal bubble to seal retinal breaks and avoid lens damage; and (*5*) promoting mobility of the pupil.

To reduce the possibility of elevated intraocular pressure, acetazolamide (250 mg every 6 hours) is routinely given intravenously or by mouth after surgery. This is discontinued if the intraocular pressure is normal or low when it is measured on the first postoperative day. Postoperative elevation of the intraocular pressure occurs sporadically, although it is more likely if the lens is removed and/or if a scleral buckle or intraocular gas bubble is used.

The patient must be specially positioned when an intraocular bubble is used, to permit effective tamponade of any retinal breaks and to avoid pupillary block or corneal damage in aphakic eyes and damage to the lens in phakic eyes. Usually the patient is put in a face-down position. This is especially important if the eye is phakic, to avoid prolonged contact between the gas bubble and the lens (*Figure 8.65*). Posterior subcapsular lens changes may occur after 12–24 hours of contact between the lens and a bubble composed of any inert gas. Initially these lens changes are reversible, but permanent opacification occurs if there is prolonged contact. Therefore, appropriate positioning is begun immediately after the operation.

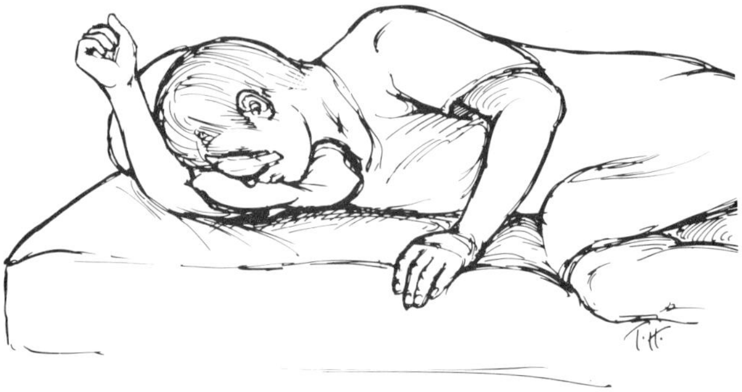

Figure 8.65 *Postoperative face-down position may be achieved by having patient lie on his or her side with the face turned toward the bed sheet. The patient may alternate body position by lying on either side or abdomen. Metal shield covering the eye prevents excessive external pressure on the globe*

Ocular examination is usually performed at the bedside on the first day after surgery and in a fully equipped examination room on the second or third postoperative day. The anterior segment is evaluated with a hand light during bedside examination, the intraocular pressure is measured with a Schiotz tonometer and the fundus is examined by indirect ophthalmoscopy. The eye is usually treated topically with a combined steroid and antibiotic ointment, four times daily.

Management of systemic medical problems is especially important in diabetic patients; postoperative nausea, vomiting and anorexia that may result in dehydration, hyperglycemia and metabolic acidosis are the most common complications. Good control of the blood sugar level by fractional insulin use and prevention of severe dehydration seem to be effective in avoiding serious metabolic disequilibrium. When adequate hydration is combined with antiemetic medications, resumption of normal eating habits and routine insulin usage is usually possible within 24–48 hours. Early mobility of the patient is also attempted, especially in patients over 40 years old.

Intraocular infection is a rare complication after vitrectomy. However, when it occurs the symptoms and physical signs usually appear on the first or second postoperative day. Severe postoperative pain is the most important symptom of infective endophthalmitis. The most important physical feature is a hypopyon. Although a hypopyon may occur with sterile intraocular inflammation, this is rare after vitrectomy.

If infection is suspected, an immediate paracentesis is done to obtain fluid for microscopic study and culture testing. This is performed at the bedside using a 30 gauge needle and tuberculin syringe. The paracentesis is done through the limbus in aphakic eyes, and through the pars plana in phakic eyes. Gentamicin 200 μg is then injected slowly into the vitreous cavity, and sometimes other intravitreal antibiotics are injected such as cefazolin 2.25 mg. All such patients are treated intravenously with broad spectrum antibiotics, and high doses of corticosteroids are given orally in non-diabetic patients. The choice of antibiotics is modified later, depending on the results of culture and antibiotic sensitivity testing. If the signs of infection are especially severe, additional intravitreal antibiotic and steroid injections may be given, including a second dose of gentamicin, more cefazolin, or methicillin 2 mg, and possibly dexamethasone 400 μg.

The intraocular pressure may vary widely during the first 3 days after vitrectomy, and transient elevation of intraocular pressure occurs in about 50 per cent of eyes. This may be due to various causes. There may be transient blood-induced glaucoma caused by residual erythrocytes obstructing the trabecular outflow channels. An intraocular gas bubble can cause increased pressure by pupillary block in aphakic eyes or from postoperative bubble expansion. Glaucoma or subclinical reduction in aqueous humor outflow capacity may have been present before surgery, and the filtration mechanism may be damaged further by the operation. Usually treatment with acetazolamide and topical antiglaucoma medications is successful in lowering the elevated intraocular pressure, and eventually the pressure returns to normal. However, if an expanding intravitreal bubble is present, some of the bubble is promptly removed at the bedside to control the intraocular pressure.

If some of the corneal epithelium was removed during the operation, a semipressure bandage is used postoperatively to encourage corneal re-epithelialization. Dressing changes are performed only once daily until complete re-epithelialization occurs. In cases without an epithelial defect, a single eye pad is used to cover the eye. A metal protective shield is used in all cases to prevent external pressure on the globe.

The fundus is examined daily by indirect ophthalmoscopy. If a rhegmatogenous retinal detachment is seen, prompt repair is recommended. Sometimes blood is layered on the posterior retina at the end of the operation, in which case bilateral eye bandages may be used for several days postoperatively to reduce eye movement. This minimizes early dispersion of blood that would limit visualization. Even so, blood usually becomes dispersed by the third postoperative day.

Pupillary movement is evaluated daily. Normal dilation and constriction are desirable to avoid synechiae between the iris and the lens, or between the iris and remaining peripheral portions of the anterior lens capsule after combined lens removal and vitrectomy. If the pupil is widely dilated on the first postoperative day, pilocarpine is applied. Similarly, if the pupil is small, a short-acting mydriatic is used to produce temporary dilation. When iris motility returns to normal, the pupil is dilated with a short-acting mydriatic only before examination of the fundus.

Intermediate postoperative period

After the third postoperative day the eye is usually relatively stable, and tissue healing occurs in a proper fashion. Discharge from the hospital occurs between the third and sixth postoperative day, when the eye has been stable for about 48 hours. If a corneal epithelial defect persists, a soft contact lens (bandage lens) can be applied to ensure proper healing and preservation of an intact epithelial layer until adherence to the superficial stroma occurs. The eye is treated topically with a combined steroid and antibiotic medication until the vascular injection clears and the eye feels comfortable.

Any remaining portion of an intraocular bubble is absorbed at a predictable rate. Therefore, the patient is instructed at the time of discharge from the hospital regarding the need for special positioning and the length of time this is necessary. Patients are advised against flying if more than 20 per cent of the vitreous cavity is filled with a bubble, to avoid possible complications from rapid bubble expansion when the cabin pressure is reduced.

During the first several weeks after vitreous surgery the retina is repeatedly examined by indirect ophthalmoscopy to detect any progressive retinal detachment. This is especially important when an intraocular bubble becomes small, because unrecognized retinal breaks that were previously flattened against the pigment epithelium by the bubble may cause progressive retinal detachment.

Residual or recurrent blood in the vitreous cavity often obscures proper visualization of the fundus for weeks or months. Such blood becomes dispersed throughout the vitreous cavity by the third postoperative day, despite measures to minimize eye movement. The rate of clearing of vitreal blood depends on the amount of blood present and on whether the crystalline lens has been removed. Postoperative hemorrhage clears more rapidly in aphakic eyes. A diffuse vitreous hemorrhage of moderate severity in an aphakic eye may clear enough within 2 weeks to permit visualization of the fundus. However, clearing takes 6–16 weeks in most phakic eyes with a moderate amount of intravitreal blood. While diffuse vitreous hemorrhage is present, the posterior segment is periodically evaluated by B-scan ultrasonography. This is performed just before discharge from the hospital and again 2–3 weeks after the operation.

Management later than 2 weeks after vitreous surgery depends on the type of condition for which the operation was done and individual features of each case. However, in general, after discharge from the hospital the eye is examined about every 2 weeks during the first 6 postoperative weeks until the eye appears well healed and stable. Thereafter examination is performed every 3–4 weeks for the next 3 months. During this time the primary concerns are possible retinal detachment or rubeosis iridis. Therefore, both the anterior segment and fundus are examined during each visit, and ultrasonography is performed when necessary.

Postoperative rubeosis iridis occurs almost exclusively in eyes with retinal vascular disorders such as diabetic retinopathy. The incidence of this complication is considerably higher in aphakic eyes than phakic eyes. Prompt detection of rubeosis iridis is important because it will regress after further scatter retinal photocoagulation in some eyes and/or after successful treatment of retinal detachment if this is also present.

The anatomical and visual result obtained at 4–6 months after the operation is likely to persist unchanged, although there is a possibility of even later complications such as recurrent intraocular hemorrhage, lens opacification, retinal detachment and rubeosis iridis. When surgery is performed in a hospital at some distance from the patient's home, cooperation from the referring ophthalmologist is of great value to provide timely postoperative evaluation.

Complications

Various complications are associated with vitreous surgery, ranging from mild non-progressive abnormalities that do not affect the vision to severe complications resulting in blindness, discomfort and/or a cosmetically unacceptable appearance. Intraoperative complications are usually caused by mechanical or toxic damage to intraocular tissues. Postoperative complications result from: (*1*) late effects from intraoperative damage; (*2*) progressive changes due to structural alterations caused by the operation; and (*3*) changes in the balance of biologically active substances that, in turn, cause abnormalities such as iris neovascularization. Any ocular tissue can be involved by these complications, either separately or in combination with others. The type, incidence and severity of complications depend on several factors, including: (*1*) the clinical condition for which the operation was performed; (*2*) the complexity of intraocular abnormalities in each case; (*3*) whether or not the objectives of the operation were achieved; and (*4*) whether iatrogenic damage occurred. The overall incidence and severity of complications has been reduced by improved instrumentation and surgical techniques and by better understanding of the factors causing complications.

Corneal complications

Corneal complications usually occur postoperatively, although they are caused by intraoperative mechanical and/or toxic damage. Intraoperative corneal edema only rarely causes enough opacification to interfere with visualization. However, posterior stromal folds occur if the epithelium is removed, and this may be a problem during fluid-gas exchange in aphakic eyes because the combination of posterior corneal folds and air in the anterior chamber markedly reduces visualization.

Postoperative corneal complications are mainly limited to persistent or recurrent epithelial defects and/or stromal and epithelial edema. Troublesome epithelial defects occur almost exclusively in diabetic patients when some of the epithelium was removed intraoperatively. Therefore, removal of the epithelium is avoided whenever possible.

Both the occurrence of inadvertent epithelial defects and aspects of delayed postoperative healing are explained by the abnormal physiological and ultrastructural features of the diabetic cornea. In these eyes there is a loose adhesion between the basal epithelial layer and Bowman's membrane, due to marked thickening of the interposed basement membrane material which is characterized by multiple laminations and contains aberrant anchoring fibrils[59]. Therefore, relatively minor trauma with the operating corneal contact lens can cause an epithelial defect.

An epithelial defect is first covered by reparative sliding of adjacent epithelial cells, and this has been shown to be normal even though the neurotrophic influences of the diabetic cornea are not normal[60]. However, a more important feature is the additional time required to form a new basement membrane layer and to develop anchoring fibrils attached to the superficial stroma. During this time, recurrent epithelial defects can occur. Semipressure bandaging is used postoperatively to encourage healing of an epithelial defect, and this can usually be achieved within 3 days. Topical medications are not used until the epithelial layer is intact.

Corneal edema persisting after the epithelial layer is intact is due to endothelial damage. This may be caused by a combination of factors, including: (*1*) the composition, volume and turbulence of flow of the intraocular irrigating solution; (*2*) mechanical damage to the endothelium by ultrasonic energy, lens fragments or surgical instruments during the operation; (*3*) toxic damage from topically applied phenylephrine used while an epithelial defect is present or from use of intracameral epinephrine (adrenaline) in a high concentration; and perhaps (*4*) mechanical damage from an intraocular bubble. Severe endothelial damage is rare. This occurs most commonly in eyes with pre-existing corneal damage or eyes in which combined pars plana lens removal and vitrectomy is complicated by flattening of the anterior chamber and/or anterior displacement of lens fragments.

Improved irrigating solutions with additional ingredients such as glucose for cell metabolism, calcium and glutathione for cell-membrane stability, and a physiological buffer system have reduced the amount of endothelial damage[61–63]. Also, the volume of irrigating solution used has been reduced by the use of automated devices to produce the suction force. Special techniques, such as segmentation of stiff pupillary membranes with scissors and ultrasonic emulsification of firm lens material, reduce the need for strong suction force which is associated with high volume flow.

Corneal endothelium damage may also occur from toxic effects of other pharmacological agents. Phenylephrine seriously damages the endothelium if applied topically while an epithelial defect is present[64]. Therefore, this drug is not used intraoperatively or postoperatively when a portion of the epithelium has been removed. Epinephrine (adrenaline) can also have a damaging effect on the endothelium when used in the anterior chamber to redilate the pupil. This depends on the concentration of the drug, and therefore only a dilute solution of 1:10 000 or weaker is used in the anterior chamber[65].

The rate of important postoperative corneal complications was high during the early days of vitreous surgery, ranging from 50 per cent in diabetic eyes to nearly 75 per cent if lens removal was combined with vitrectomy[66,67]. The current incidence of these complications is much lower, and permanent corneal opacification is rare. This improved situation is the result of efforts to: (*1*) avoid epithelial defects during the operation; (*2*) encourage rapid postoperative healing of inadvertent epithelial defects; (*3*) avoid direct mechanical damage to the endothelium; (*4*) use only physiological irrigating solutions; and (*5*) prevent toxic effects from topical phenylephrine and intracameral epinephrine (adrenaline) in certain circumstances and in excessive concentrations.

Lens complications

Lens complications include cataract formation and intraocular inflammation or mechanical damage to other tissues from lens remnants. Cataract formation may occur because of direct mechanical damage by the vitrectomy instruments, toxic effects from the irrigating solution and/or prolonged postoperative contact with an intravitreal bubble. Direct contact between the surgical instruments and the lens is rare and is most likely to occur while excising portions of the retrolenticular and/or anteroperipheral vitreous gel (*Figure 8.66a*). Contact is avoided by using caution when working near the lens and by use of retroillumination while excising anteroperipheral vitreous gel using a two-instrument method (*Figure 8.66b*).

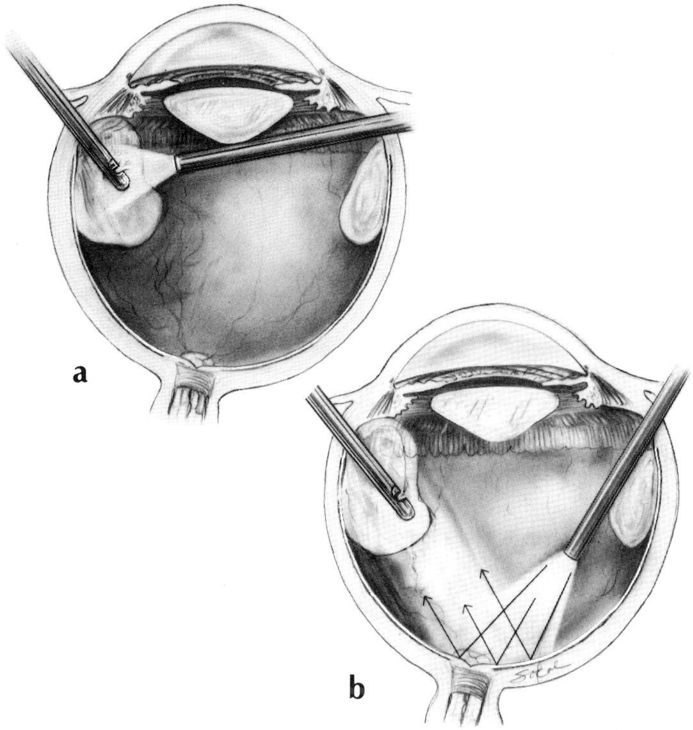

Figure 8.66 (a) *Lens damage by fiberoptic probe during excision of anteroperipheral vitreous on opposite side of the eye.* **(b)** *Lens contact is avoided by using retroillumination with light reflected off posterior pigment epithelium*

The composition of the irrigating solution seems to be an important factor in maintaining lens clarity, especially if the operation is prolonged. Fern-like posterior subcapsular opacities occur intraoperatively in some eyes when a balanced salt solution is used for irrigation, whereas this does not occur if a suitably enriched solution is used, as mentioned earlier[68]. A similar effect was demonstrated when the lens from rhesus monkey eyes was incubated in various irrigating solutions[69].

When an inert intravitreal gas bubble is used, special postoperative positioning is required to avoid prolonged contact between the bubble and the posterior lens capsule (*Figure 8.67*). Fern-like opacities and vacuoles in the posterior lens cortex occur after about 24 hours of contact between the lens and an intravitreal bubble[70]. These changes become irreversible soon thereafter.

Visually significant lens opacities now occur postoperatively in about 20 per cent of eyes undergoing vitrectomy for posterior segment indications when the lens is not removed. The exact incidence of this complication and the cause-and-effect relationship in each case are difficult to analyze because several factors are involved, including: (*1*) the patient's age and health; (*2*) the length of the operation and the type and volume of irrigating solution used; (*3*) the presence of pre-existing lens opacities; (*4*) use of an intravitreal bubble and/or other accessory techniques such as retinal cryotherapy; and (*5*) the occurrence of other complications such as glaucoma, hemorrhage or retinal detachment.

Lens material remaining after incomplete pars plana lens removal can cause serious postoperative complications depending on the amount, location and type of residual material. Cortical material remaining behind the iris becomes quite swollen and opaque, and it may temporarily obstruct the pupil. However, swollen cortical material usually absorbs spontaneously, and the eye is treated with steroids by topical application or subconjunctival depot injection. Retained nuclear material may cause prolonged inflammation and/or secondary mechanical damage to the retina or the cornea if the fragment(s) are freely mobile. Therefore, every effort is made to remove these fragments during the initial operation, using intravitreal ultrasonic emulsification after excising portions of the vitreous gel, and retrieving the fragments as described earlier (*see Figure 8.61*). The same methods can be used during a second operation when necessary.

Premature rupture of the posterior lens capsule and displacement of some lens material into the vitreous cavity occurs in about 25 per cent of eyes undergoing combined pars plana lens removal and vitrectomy. Most often this is cortical material, rupture of the posterior capsule having occurred when the peripheral cortical material was being separated from the equatorial capsule after the lens nucleus had been removed. The soft cortical material is readily removed with the vitrectomy probe or with the ultrasonic needle before the lens material falls further posteriorly, thus reducing the risk of retinal damage associated with retrieval of lens fragments from the posterior part of the vitreous cavity.

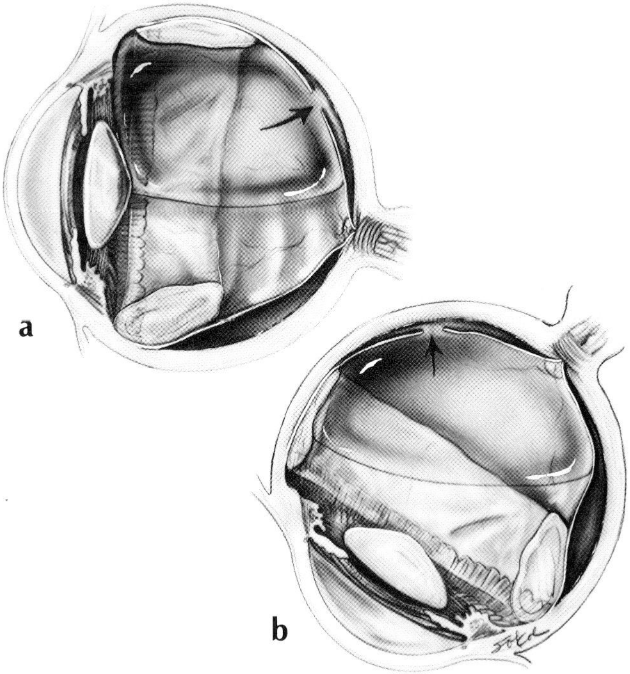

Figure 8.67 (a) *Cataract change caused by prolonged contact between posterior lens surface and intravitreal bubble used to treat posterior retinal break (arrow).* **(b)** *Positioning bubble against retinal break to avoid lens contact treats retinal detachment effectively and prevents secondary cataract*

Sclerotomy complications

Complications related only to the pars plana incision are infrequent. Damage to the adjacent retina can occur if the incision is located too far posterior, if there is excessive traction on the adjacent vitreous base, or if retinal detachment is present and the peripheral retina becomes incarcerated in the wound when the surgical instruments are withdrawn. Fibrovascular ingrowth from the incision occurs postoperatively in some eyes, and can cause traction on the adjacent peripheral retina and perhaps recurrent vitreous hemorrhage[71–74].

Direct retinal damage from preparing the incisions or introducing instruments is rare because the incisions are made 3.5–4 mm posterior to the limbus, near the pars plana ciliaris and safely anterior to the ora serrata and the anterior part of the vitreous base. Bleeding from the pars plana uveal tissue is rare when the incisions are made, although limbal-parallel incisions transect the radially oriented vessels in the pars plana zone.

Incarceration of detached peripheral retina in the pars plana incision can usually be avoided by lowering the intraocular pressure before withdrawing the surgical instruments. However, if this complication occurs or if vitreous gel is incarcerated in the sclerotomy and causes marked traction on the adjacent retina, simultaneous fluid-gas exchange is used to free the tissues. First the incarcerated retina and/or vitreous gel is disengaged from the wound with the vitrectomy probe or a blunt needle (*Figure 8.68a*). Then a bubble is injected (*Figure 8.68b*), and the expanding bubble flattens the peripheral vitreous gel and retina against the eyewall while displacing subretinal fluid posteriorly. This prevents further prolapse of tissue into the incisions when the instruments are again withdrawn (*Figure 8.68c*).

Some fibrous proliferation occurs within every pars plana incision as a part of the normal wound-healing process, and this tissue may grow onto the scaffold of adjacent vitreous fibers incarcerated in the incision. However, clinically significant fibrovascular ingrowth is infrequent in the absence of other complications such as generalized intraocular neovascular proliferation as seen in some diabetic patients with postoperative rubeosis iridis[34]. However, in some eyes neovascular tissue extending from the pars plana incision is visible, and this may cause recurrent vitreous hemorrhage. In such cases, the neovascular tissue extending from the internal aspect of the sclerotomy can be treated with transvitreal coaxial bipolar diathermy or by internal-external bipolar diathermy in suitable aphakic eyes (*Figure 8.69*). Fibrovascular tissue growth can also cause peripheral retinal detachment that may require a scleral buckling operation if traction detachment is progressive or if a rhegmatogenous component occurs.

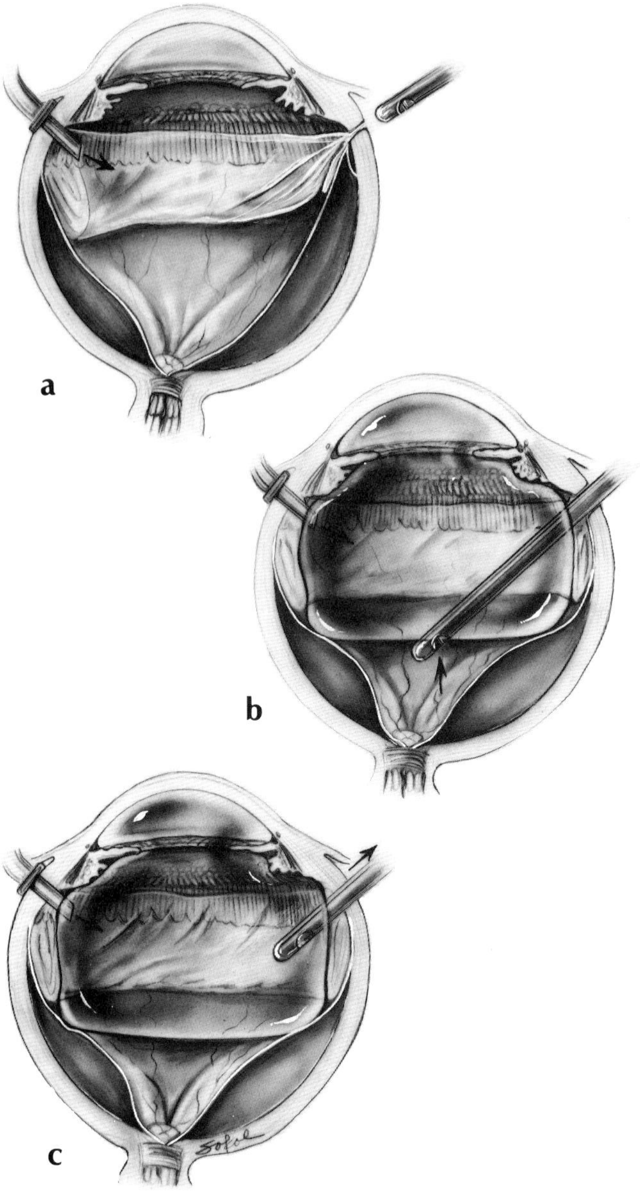

Figure 8.68 *Management of retinal traction caused by vitreous incarcerated in pars plana sclerotomy.* **(a,b)** *Incarcerated tissue is disengaged with vitrectomy probe, and fluid-gas exchange is then performed to displace subretinal fluid posteriorly and flatten peripheral retina and vitreous against the eyewall.* **(c)** *Air bubble prevents recurrence of vitreous or retinal incarceration when instruments are withdrawn*

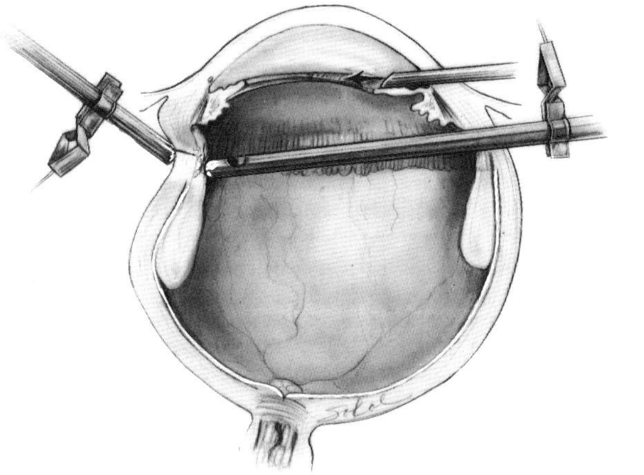

Figure 8.69 *Internal-external bimanual bipolar diathermy used to treat fibrovascular ingrowth at previous pars plana sclerotomy thought to cause recurrent vitreous hemorrhage. Sclera is indented with needle to permit transcorneal visualization, and transvitreal needle or vitrectomy probe is used as internal electrode for direct treatment of vascularized tissue*

Vitreous hemorrhage

Intraoperative bleeding can be a serious complication during vitreous surgery, and recurrent hemorrhages can also occur postoperatively. Intraoperative bleeding is the only major complication that has become more frequent despite improvements in vitreous surgery instrumentation and technique. The increased occurrence of bleeding is probably due to changes in case selection and operative technique. Surgery is now performed in some eyes with severe intraocular neovascularization, and more extensive dissection of this tissue is performed than in the past. Intraoperative bleeding occurs most frequently from the retina and/or from neovascular tissue in the posterior segment. This may occur when vascularized tissue is cut with the vitrectomy instrument or intraocular scissors, or when vitreous sheets and/or proliferative tissue are manipulated, as a result of traction on vitreoretinal attachments.

The possibility of bleeding is reduced by use of scissors to minimize traction on vitreoretinal attachments when adjacent tissue is cut, and by use of diathermy to coagulate abnormal vessels before or immediately after vascularized tissue is cut (*see Figure 8.34*)[19]. Despite these efforts, some bleeding occurs frequently, and clotted blood often remains on the retina at the end of the operation. Residual blood becomes dispersed throughout the vitreous cavity postoperatively, and it may take a long time to clear in phakic eyes.

Some fresh blood remains in the vitreous cavity postoperatively in about 75 per cent of eyes with proliferative diabetic retinopathy, whereas this complication is rare in other conditions when fibrovascular tissue is not cut or manipulated. Postoperative hemorrhage is also common in eyes with proliferative retinopathy; some bleeding occurs in up to 50 per cent of cases. However, this is most common during the initial postoperative period. The amount of early postoperative bleeding tends to be small, and the blood usually clears spontaneously in 4–14 weeks depending on whether the eye is aphakic or phakic.

Later bleeding occurs in about 20 per cent of diabetic patients and is rare in other conditions[34]. The exact origin of later postoperative hemorrhage usually cannot be determined, but possibilities include: (*1*) residual neovascular tissue in the posterior segment; (*2*) fragile retinal or ciliary body vessels damaged by the underlying disease; (*3*) fibrovascular ingrowth from the sclerotomy site(s); and (*4*) abnormal blood vessels on the iris. The latter is probably not a common cause of recurrent bleeding, because this complication seems to occur with equal frequency in phakic and aphakic eyes, and hyphema is rarely present in the involved phakic eyes. However, eyes with abnormal iris vessels seem to have a higher incidence of later vitreous hemorrhage, although the iris changes may only be evidence of more widespread vascular abnormalities.

Photocoagulation is used to treat areas of residual retinal neovascularization in eyes with recurrent vitreous hemorrhage. Non-clotted blood can be removed by later lavage in phakic eyes if spontaneous clearing does not occur. The timing of further surgery depends on several factors, including: (*1*) the status of the fellow eye; (*2*) the visual potential in the eye with recurrent hemorrhage; (*3*) the amount of vitreous blood as judged by clinical and ultrasonic examination; and (*4*) the presence of other complications such as retinal detachment or rubeosis iridis. Lavage of vitreous blood and retinal reattachment surgery are done immediately if progressive detachment is demonstrated by ultrasonography. Eyes with progressive postoperative rubeosis iridis may be treated by lavage of non-clotted blood and intraoperative scatter retinal photocoagulation using a transvitreal fiberoptic probe to cause regression of the anterior segment neovascularization. In other eyes, secondary lavage is performed only if spontaneous clearing does not occur after 3–6 months. If repeated episodes of bleeding occur, lens removal through the pars plana may be performed at the time of vitreous lavage to permit more rapid clearing of any further hemorrhages.

Retinal damage

Retinal tears and detachment are serious and relatively frequent complications of vitreous surgery. Retinal tears can occur from direct damage by the surgical instruments or from traction on areas of vitreoretinal attachment. These tears occur mainly along the posterior margin of the vitreous base or adjacent to areas of posterior vitreoretinal attachment.

Retinal tears from traction along the posterior vitreous base are infrequent when small amounts of suction force are used, and this complication now occurs in only 1–2 per cent of cases[68]. Posterior retinal tears rarely occur from direct damage by the vitrectomy probe or vitreoretinal scissors, although this is more likely when cutting opaque tissue near an area of retinal detachment. Posterior retinal breaks occur most commonly from traction on areas of vitreoretinal attachment when preretinal membranes are cut or epiretinal tissue and/or cortical vitreous is dissected from the retina (*Figure 8.70*). This complication now occurs in about 20 per cent of diabetic eyes with complicated vitreoretinal anatomy. Posterior retinal tears are treated with cryotherapy or photocoagulation, combined with an intraocular bubble if all traction on the area has been relieved. A localized scleral buckle supporting the break is added if anteroposterior or tangential traction persists.

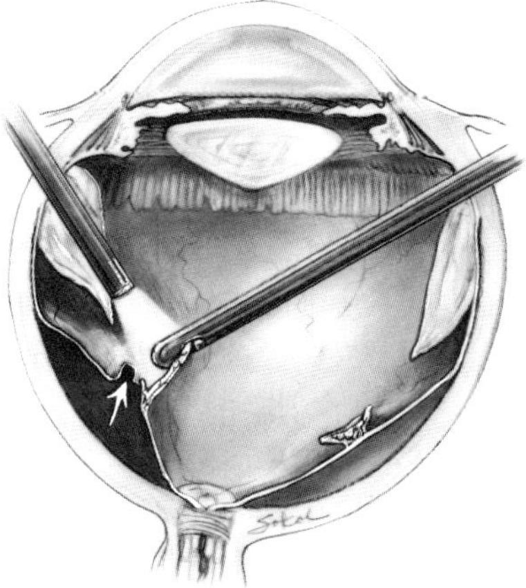

Figure 8.70 *Retinal break (arrow) caused by excessive traction on posterior vitreous surface during vitrectomy for proliferative diabetic retinopathy with pre-existing traction detachment. Retina near posterior areas of fibrovascular proliferation is often thin and atrophic and easily torn by excessive vitreoretinal traction*

Postoperative retinal detachment can result from iatrogenic retinal breaks, from new breaks occurring postoperatively, or from traction by residual vitreous gel and/or epiretinal membranes. New retinal breaks can result from persistent traction by remaining vitreous gel or fibrovascular tissue, or the breaks can occur in other, less involved areas. In the latter case the pathogenesis of the break is unknown. Scleral buckling, together with intraocular gas injection, is used to treat postoperative rhegmatogenous detachments. Often the retinal break is quite small, and careful preoperative evaluation with a contact lens is needed to identify the defect. Further vitreous surgery can also be used to treat persistent traction detachment if a cleavage plane is visible between the contracted membranes and the inner retinal surface.

Rhegmatogenous detachment occurs postoperatively in 5–10 per cent of eyes with diabetic retinopathy, and about one-half of these cases can be successfully treated by further surgery[18,29]. Small areas of postoperative traction detachment are common in these eyes because of tangential traction from remaining epiretinal tissues. However, residual traction detachment is rarely of clinical significance if the original objectives of the operation were achieved. Postoperative retinal detachment is rare in other conditions, except in eyes with previous detachment complicated by massive periretinal proliferation (MPP). In these cases, recurrent detachment occurs in about 50 per cent of eyes because of further epiretinal membrane growth[40].

Rubeosis iridis

Growth of neovascular tissue on the iris (rubeosis iridis) and in the anterior chamber angle is the most frequent postoperative complication causing failure of an otherwise successful vitrectomy procedure. This complication is limited almost entirely to eyes with pre-existing retinal vascular disorders characterized by extensive areas of capillary non-perfusion. The incidence of rubeosis iridis is also considerably higher in aphakic than in phakic eyes. The mechanism causing this complication is unproved, but it is presumed to be an angiogenic substance elaborated by ischemic retinal tissue and capable of producing a neovascular response in adjacent and remote ocular locations.

Rubeosis iridis results in glaucoma from obstruction of the anterior chamber angle by neovascular tissue in some eyes (neovascular glaucoma). This usually occurs 2–12 weeks after the vitrectomy operation. This type of angle-closure glaucoma is especially difficult to treat after extensive obstruction of the anterior chamber angle occurs. Therefore, frequent postoperative observation is necessary to detect early changes, because prompt treatment with scatter retinal photocoagulation causes regression of the anterior segment neovascularization in some eyes (*Figure 8.71*)[26,29]. However, the natural history of iris neovascularization is variable, and not all untreated eyes progress to neovascular glaucoma[75] so that the effect of treatment with scatter retinal photocoagulation is difficult to evaluate. Treatment is nevertheless recommended in suitable cases when neovascular tissue is visible in the anterior chamber angle and before extensive peripheral anterior synechiae develop.

Abnormal iris vessels have been observed in up to 44 per cent of eyes after vitrectomy for complications of proliferative diabetic retinopathy[18,29]. However, this high incidence of vascular abnormalities includes cases of both benign dilation of normal iris vessels (iris hyperemia) and aphakic eyes with total retinal detachment and neovascularization. Diabetic eyes with retinal detachment after vitrectomy are consistently complicated further by rubeosis iridis and neovascular glaucoma or phthisis bulbi[18,29]. Therefore, in some of these eyes the abnormal iris vessels are benign, whereas in others it is a predictable secondary complication superimposed on another blinding condition. Visual loss caused only by rubeosis iridis now occurs in about 10 per cent of cases.

The incidence of rubeosis iridis is also strongly influenced by whether or not the crystalline lens is present, and rubeosis occurs at least twice as often in aphakic as in phakic eyes[27]. Therefore, a clear crystalline lens is preserved whenever possible in eyes with proliferative retinopathies in order to maintain a more physiological optical system and to reduce the risk of postoperative anterior segment neovascularization.

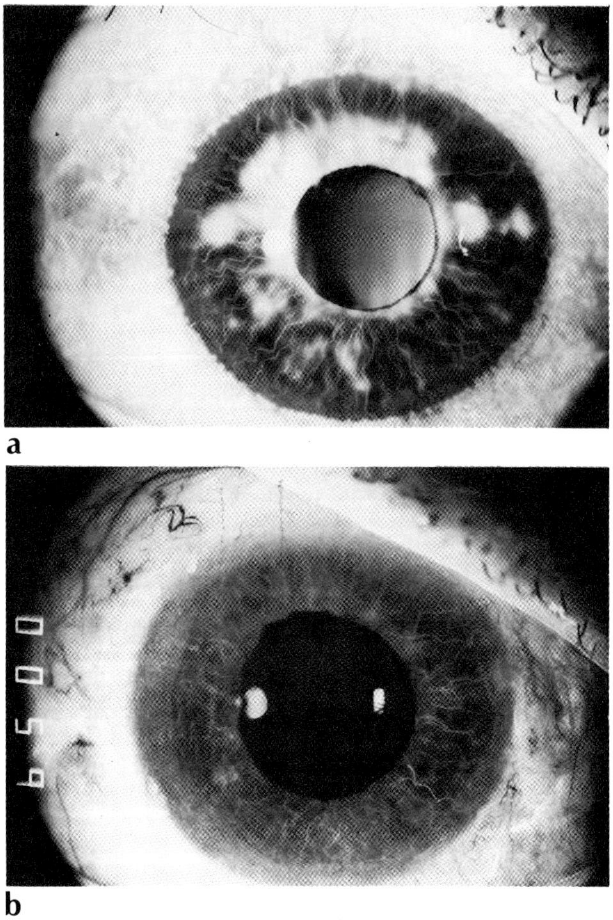

Figure 8.71 *Regression of rubeosis iridis after panretinal scatter photocoagulation in a patient with proliferative diabetic retinopathy.* **(a)** *Iris fluorescein angiogram before photocoagulation demonstrates widespread leakage from abnormal iris vessels.* **(b)** *Angiogram repeated 3 weeks after panretinal scatter photocoagulation shows only minimal residual leakage. Clinically, neovascular tissue regressed and did not recur during 4 years of follow-up (from Michels, R. G. Archives of Ophthalmology 1978; 96:237–246)*

Phthisis bulbi

Phthisis bulbi characterized by hypotony, intraocular scarring, and disorganization and shrinkage of the globe is the final complication in some eyes after vitreous surgery. This occurs most commonly in diabetic patients with retinal detachment and rubeosis iridis, after severe penetrating injuries, and after surgery for retinal detachment complicated by MPP. When the vitreous surgery operation is initially successful, phthisis bulbi rarely occurs. However, phthisis happens sometimes after vitrectomy for infective endophthalmitis with severe enzymatic retinal and uveal damage and in eyes with chronic intraocular hemorrhage and hemosiderosis. It is usually therefore a secondary complication. The incidence is probably 15–20 per cent of all vitreous surgery procedures, but many of these eyes are high-risk cases with a poor prognosis.

Summary

Instrumentation and operative techniques used in modern vitreous surgery have evolved rapidly, and predictable methods are now available to deal with various ocular abnormalities. The indications for vitreous surgery are diverse, ranging from selected pupillary membranes to complex vitreoretinal abnormalities associated with proliferative retinopathies, and other conditions with retinal detachment and non-vascularized epiretinal membranes. Vitrectomy techniques provide an effective method of therapy in some conditions when no treatment was possible previously, and in other conditions these methods are an alternative to conventional means of therapy.

The results obtained with vitreous surgery are also diverse. They range from nearly uniform success in certain eyes with thin pupillary membranes or eyes with vitreous opacities and a complete posterior vitreous separation, to a success rate of less than 50 per cent in eyes with rhegmatogenous detachment and MPP. In general, the success rate is inversely related to the complexity of the intraocular structural abnormalities and the severity of pre-existing retinal damage from the underlying disease process or trauma.

The range and incidence of complications are higher after vitrectomy surgery than after any other ophthalmic surgical procedure, and some complications such as rubeosis iridis are almost unique to this operation when combined with lens removal in certain predisposed eyes. Nevertheless, vitreous surgery has become an indispensable part of therapeutic ophthalmic practice because it provides unique capabilities to treat directly intraocular opacities and structural disorders that are causing severe visual loss.

References

1. Kasner, D. Vitrectomy: A new approach to the management of vitreous. Highlights of Ophthalmology 1969; 11:304–329 (Interview)
2. Kasner, D., Miller, G. R., Taylor, W. H., Sever, R. J., Norton, E. W. D. Surgical treatment of amyloidosis of the vitreous. Transactions of the American Academy of Ophthalmology and Otolaryngology 1968; 72:410–418
3. Machemer, R., Buettner, H., Norton, E. W. D., Parel, J. M. Vitrectomy: A pars plana approach. Transactions of the American Academy of Ophthalmology and Otolaryngology 1971; 75:813–820
4. Machemer, R., Parel, J. M., Buettner, H. A new concept for vitreous surgery. 1. Instrumentation. American Journal of Ophthalmology 1972; 73:1–7
5. Machemer, R. A new concept for vitreous surgery. 7. Two-instrument techniques in pars plana vitrectomy. Archives of Ophthalmology 1974; 92:407–412
6. Machemer, R. Vitrectomy, a pars plana approach. New York: Grune and Stratton, 1975
7. Parel, J. M., Machemer, R., Aumayr, W. A new concept for vitreous surgery. 5. An automated operating microscope. American Journal of Ophthalmology 1974; 77:161–168
8. Charles, S., McCarthy, C., Eichenbaum, D. A chin-operated switch for motorized three-axis microscopic movement. American Journal of Ophthalmology 1975; 80:150–151
9. Parel, J. M., Machemer, R., Aumayr, W. A new concept for vitreous surgery. 4. Improvements in instrumentation and illumination. American Journal of Ophthalmology 1974; 77:6–12
10. O'Malley, C., Heintz, R. M. Sr. Vitrectomy with an alternative instrument system. Annals of Ophthalmology 1975; 7:585–588
11. Benson, W. E., Blankenship, G. W., Machemer, R. Pars plana lens removal with vitrectomy. American Journal of Ophthalmology 1977; 84:150–152
12. Charles, S. Fluid-gas exchange in the vitreous cavity. Ocutome Newsletter 1977; 2(2):1
13. Charles, S., White, J., Dennison, C., Eichenbaum, D., Bimanual, bipolar intraocular diathermy. American Journal of Ophthalmology 1976; 81:101–102
14. Michels, R. G., Stark, W. J. Pars plana vitrectomy technique in anterior segment surgery. Transactions of the American Academy of Ophthalmology and Otolaryngology 1976; 81:382–393
15. Charles, S. Vitreous microsurgery. Baltimore, Maryland: Williams and Wilkins Co., 1981
16. Michels, R. G. Vitreous surgery. St Louis: C. V. Mosby Co., 1981
17. Michels, R. G. Vitrectomy techniques in retinal reattachment surgery. Ophthalmology 1979; 86:556–585
18. Michels, R. G. Vitreous surgery in proliferative diabetic retinopathy. In: Shimizu, K., Oosterhuis, J. A., eds. Concilium Ophthalmologicum XXIII, Kyoto, 1978, Acta pars I. Amsterdam, Oxford: Excerpta Medica, 1979: 420–426
19. Meredith, T. A., Kaplan, H. J., Aaberg, T. M. Pars plana vitrectomy techniques for relief of epiretinal traction by membrane segmentation. American Journal of Ophthalmology 1980; 89:408–413
20. Machemer, R., Aaberg, T. M. Vitrectomy, 2nd ed. New York: Grune and Stratton, 1979
21. Norton, E. W. D. Intraocular gas in the management of selected retinal detachments. Transactions of the American Academy of Ophthalmology and Otolaryngology 1973; 77:85–98
22. Abrams, G. W., Edelhauser, H. F., Aaberg, T. M., Hamilton, L. H. Dynamics of intravitreal sulfur hexafluoride gas. Investigative in Ophthalmology and Visual Science 1974; 13:863–865
23. Aaberg, T. M. Results of 100 consecutive vitrectomy procedures. In: McPherson, A., ed. New and controversial aspects of vitreoretinal surgery. St Louis: C. V. Mosby Co., 1977: 245–249
24. Ryan, S. J., Michels, R. G. Pars plana vitrectomy: indications and results in 100 cases. In: McPherson, A., ed. New and controversial aspects of vitreoretinal surgery. St Louis: C. V. Mosby Co., 1977: 250–256
25. Klöti, R. Indications for vitrectomy and results in 115 cases. In: McPherson, A., ed. New and controversial aspects of vitreoretinal surgery. St Louis: C. V. Mosby Co., 1977: 237–244
26. Little, H. L., Rosenthal, A. R., Dellaporta, A., Jacobson, D. R. The effect of pan-retinal photo-coagulation on rubeosis iridis. American Journal of Ophthalmology 1976; 81:804–809
27. Blankenship, G., Cortez, R., Machemer, R. The lens and pars plana vitrectomy for diabetic retinopathy complications. Archives of Ophthalmology 1979; 97:1263–1267

28. Mandelcorn, M. S., Blankenship, G., Machemer, R. Pars plana vitrectomy for the management of severe diabetic retinopathy. American Journal of Ophthalmology 1976; 81:561–570
29. Michels, R. G. Vitrectomy for complications of diabetic retinopathy. Archives of Ophthalmology 1978; 96:237–246
30. Peyman, G. A., Huamonte, F. U., Goldberg, M. F., Sanders, D. R., Nagpal, K. C., Raichand, M. Four hundred consecutive pars plana vitrectomies with the Vitrophage. Archives of Ophthalmology 1978; 96:45–50
31. Blankenship, G. W. Pars plana vitrectomy for diabetic retinopathy. A report of eight years' experience. Modern Problems in Ophthalmology 1979; 20:376–386
32. Aaberg, T. M. Clinical results in vitrectomy for diabetic traction retinal detachment. American Journal of Ophthalmology 1979; 88:246–253
33. Machemer, R. Pathogenesis of proliferative neovascular retinopathies and the role of vitrectomy: a hypothesis. International Ophthalmology 1978; 1:1–3
34. Rice, T. A., Michels, R. G. Long-term anatomic and functional results of vitrectomy for diabetic retinopathy. American Journal of Ophthalmology 1980; 90:297–303
35. Norton, E. W. D., Aaberg, T. M., Fung, W. E., Curtin, V. T. Giant retinal tears. I. Clinical management with intravitreal air. American Journal of Ophthalmology 1969; 68:1011–1021
36. Machemer, R., Allen, A. W. Retinal tears 180° and greater: management with vitrectomy and intravitreal gas. Archives of Ophthalmology 1976; 94:1340–1346
37. Laqua, H., Machemer, R. Glial cell proliferation in retinal detachment (massive periretinal proliferation). American Journal of Ophthalmology 1975; 80:602–618
38. Laqua, H., Machemer, R. Clinical-pathological correlation in massive periretinal proliferation. American Journal of Ophthalmology 1975; 80:913–929
39. Machemer, R., Laqua, H. Pigment epithelium proliferation in retinal detachment (massive periretinal proliferation). American Journal of Ophthalmology 1975; 80:1–23
40. Machemer, R., Laqua, H. A logical approach to the treatment of massive periretinal proliferation. Ophthalmology 1978; 85:584–593
41. Cleary, P. E., Ryan, S. J. Method of production and natural history of experimental posterior penetrating eye injury in the rhesus monkey. American Journal of Ophthalmology 1979; 88:212–220
42. Cleary, P. E., Ryan, S. J. Histology of wound, vitreous and retina in experimental posterior penetrating eye injury in the rhesus monkey. American Journal of Ophthalmology 1979; 88:221–231
43. Topping, T. M., Abrams, G. W., Machemer, R. Experimental double-perforating injury of the posterior segment in rabbit eyes. The natural history of intraocular proliferation. Archives of Ophthalmology 1979; 97:735–742
44. Abrams, G. W., Topping, T. M., Machemer, R. Vitrectomy for injury. The effect on intraocular proliferation following perforation of the posterior segment of the rabbit eye. Archives of Ophthalmology 1979; 97:743–748
45. Michels, R. G. Vitrectomy methods in penetrating ocular trauma. Ophthalmology 1980; 87:629–645
46. Taylor, H. R., Michels, R. G., Stark, W. J. Vitrectomy methods in anterior segment surgery. Ophthalmic Surgery 1979; 10:25–58
47. Wilkinson, C. P., Rowsey, J. J. Closed vitrectomy for the vitreous touch syndrome. American Journal of Ophthalmology 1980; 90:304–308
48. Stark, W. J., Michels, R. G., Maumenee, A. E., Cupples H. Surgical management of epithelial ingrowth. American Journal of Ophthalmology 1978; 85:772–780
49. McCuen, B. W., Fung, W. E. The role of vitrectomy instrumentation in the treatment of severe traumatic hyphema. American Journal of Ophthalmology 1979; 88:930–934
50. Fenton, R. H., Zimmerman, L. E. Hemolytic glaucoma. An unusual cause of acute open-angle secondary glaucoma. Archives of Ophthalmology 1963; 70:236–239
51. Campbell, D. G., Simmons, R. J., Grant, W. M. Ghost cells as a cause of glaucoma. American Journal of Ophthalmology 1976; 81:441–450
52. Brucker, A. J., Michels, R. G., Green, W. R. Pars plana vitrectomy in the management of blood-induced glaucoma with vitreous hemorrhage. Annals of Ophthalmology 1978; 10:1427–1437
53. Michels, R. G., Shacklett, D. E. Vitrectomy techniques for removal of retained lens material. Archives of Ophthalmology 1977; 95:1767–1773
54. Hutton, W. L., Snyder, W. B., Vaiser, A. Management of surgically dislocated intravitreal lens fragments by pars plana vitrectomy. Ophthalmology 1978; 85:176–189
55. Forster, R. K., Abbott, R. L., Gelender, H. Management of infectious endophthalmitis. Ophthalmology 1980; 87:313–319
56. Machemer, R. Die chirurgische Entfernung von epiretinalen Makulamembranen (macular puckers). Klinische Monatsblätter für Augenheilkunde 1978; 173:36–42
57. Michels, R. G., Gilbert, H. D. Surgical management of macular pucker after retinal reattachment surgery. American Journal of Ophthalmology 1979; 88:925–929
58. Shea, M. The surgical management of macular pucker in rhegmatogenous retinal detachment. Ophthalmology 1980; 87:70–74
59. Kenyon, K. R. Recurrent corneal erosion: pathogenesis and therapy. International Ophthalmology Clinics 1979; 19:169–195
60. Snip, R. C., Thoft, R. A., Tolentino, F. I. Similar epithelial healing rates in the corneas of diabetic and nondiabetic patients. American Journal of Ophthalmology 1980; 90:463–468
61. Edelhauser, H. F., Van Horn, D. L., Hyndiuk, R. A., Schultz, R. O. Intraocular irrigating solutions: their effect on the corneal endothelium. Archives of Ophthalmology 1975; 93:648–657
62. Edelhauser, H. F., van Horn, D. L., Schultz, R. O., Hyndiuk, R. A. Comparative toxicity of intraocular irrigating solutions on the corneal endothelium. American Journal of Ophthalmology 1976; 81:473–481
63. Edelhauser, H. F., Gonnering, R., Van Horn, D. L. Intraocular irrigating solutions: A comparative study of BSS-Plus and lactated Ringer's solution. Archives of Ophthalmology 1978; 96:516–520
64. Edelhauser, H. F., Hine, J. E., Pederson, H., *et al.* The effect of phenylephrine on the cornea. Archives of Ophthalmology 1979; 97:937–947
65. Hull, D. S., Chemotti, M. T., Edelhauser, H. F., Van Horn, D. L., Hyndiuk, R. A. Effect of epinephrine on the corneal endothelium. American Journal of Ophthalmology 1975; 79:245–250
66. Perry, H. D., Foulks, G. N., Throft, R. A., Tolentino, F. I. Corneal complications after closed vitrectomy through the pars plana. Archives of Ophthalmology 1978; 96:1401–1403
67. Brightbill, F. S., Myers, F. L., Bresnick, G. H. Postvitrectomy keratopathy. American Journal of Ophthalmology 1978; 85:651–656
68. Faulborn, J., Conway, B. P., Machemer, R. Surgical complications of pars plana vitreous surgery. Ophthalmology 1978; 85:116–125
69. Christiansen, J. M., Kollarits, C. R., Fukui, H., Fishman, M. L., Michels, R. G., Mikuni, I. Intraocular irrigating solutions and lens clarity. American Journal of Ophthalmology 1976; 82:594–597
70. Fineberg, E., Machemer, R., Sullivan, P., Norton, E. W. D., Hamasaki, D., Anderson, D. Sulfur hexafluoride in owl monkey vitreous cavity. American Journal of Ophthalmology 1975; 79:67–76
71. Tardif, Y. M., Schepens, C. L., Tolentino, F. I. Vitreous surgery. XIV. Complications from sclerotomy in 89 consecutive cases. Archives of Ophthalmology 1977; 95:229–234
72. Tardif, Y. M., Schepens, C. L. Closed vitreous surgery. XV. Fibrovascular ingrowth from the pars plana sclerotomy. Archives of Ophthalmology 1977; 95:235–239
73. Pülhorn, G., Teichmann, K. D., Teichmann, I. Intraocular fibrous proliferation as an incisional complication in pars plana vitrectomy. American Journal of Ophthalmology 1977; 83:810–814
74. Buettner, H., Machemer, R. Histopathologic findings in human eyes after pars plana vitrectomy and lensectomy. Archives of Ophthalmology 1977; 95:2029–2033
75. Madsen, P. H. Rubeosis of the iris and haemorrhagic glaucoma in patients with proliferative diabetic retinopathy. British Journal of Ophthalmology 1971; 55:368–371

9

Retinal surgery

Ronald G. Michels MD
Thomas A. Rice MD
L. Harrell Pierce MD
Robert B. Welch MD
John D. Scott MD

Introduction

Retinal disorders treated by surgical means are mainly limited to retinal detachment and retinal vascular disorders. The latter are usually treated by photocoagulation, and this is considered in Chapter 11. Retinal detachment can be caused by several different mechanisms, and selected cases are treated by vitreous surgery (*see* Chapter 8). However, most cases of retinal detachment are treated by conventional methods to identify and seal retinal breaks.

Pathogenesis of retinal detachment

There are three separate (but sometimes coexisting) types of retinal detachment caused by different mechanisms: (*1*) traction detachment caused by vitreoretinal traction; (*2*) exudative (or secondary) detachment due to leakage of fluid from the choroid into the subretinal space; and (*3*) rhegmatogenous detachment (*Greek*, rhegma: rent, tear, break in continuity) caused by a retinal break and fluid passing from the vitreous cavity through the retinal break into the subretinal space. Each type of detachment can be identified by its distinctive clinical features, and each type is managed differently. This chapter deals mainly with rhegmatogenous retinal detachment which is the most frequent type.

Traction detachment

Traction retinal detachment is due to traction from the vitreous gel and/or from vascularized or non-vascularized epiretinal or intravitreal proliferative tissue elevating the retina above the pigment epithelium. No retinal break is present, and the origin of the subretinal fluid is not known, although it probably comes from the choroid. Traction detachments are usually associated with proliferative retinopathies or previous damage to the vitreous gel as occurs following penetrating injuries or vitreous prolapse during cataract extraction.

Traction retinal detachments often remain unchanged in size, and the condition may be asymptomatic unless the macula becomes involved. Usually the area of retinal elevation surrounds the location of greatest vitreoretinal traction, the surface of the affected retina has a concave configuration, and the detachment does not extend to the adjacent ora serrata. Previously, techniques for scleral buckling and/or scleral shortening were used to treat selected cases. Now, vitreous surgery methods are preferred to deal directly with the pathogenetic mechanism causing retinal detachment (*see* Chapter 8).

Exudative detachment

Extensive exudative retinal detachment is rare and can be confused with rhegmatogenous detachment. Exudative detachments often have turbid subretinal fluid, and no pigmented debris is present in the vitreous gel when examined with a slit lamp. No retinal break is present. A characteristic feature is marked shifting of the subretinal fluid with changes in posture. When the eye is rotated the subretinal fluid shifts and assumes a dependent position so that it no longer extends to the ora serrata in the quadrant where previously the retina had been most elevated. This usually permits differentiation from rhegmatogenous detachment.

Exudative detachments may be associated with ocular disorders such as the Vogt–Koyanagi–Harada syndrome or posterior scleritis. However, often the condition is idiopathic, and most cases undergo spontaneous resolution after several months. The area(s) of leakage from the choroid and pigment epithelium can be identified by fluorescein angioscopy. With this technique fluorescein dye is injected intravenously, and the fundus is examined by indirect ophthalmoscopy using blue light from a cobalt excitation filter. Photocoagulation applied to the leakage sites is followed by slow absorption of the subretinal fluid in some cases. This is performed after rotating the head so that the retina is temporarily flat in the area of leakage when the photocoagulation treatment is applied.

Rhegmatogenous detachment

Rhegmatogenous retinal detachment is the most common type of detachment, and the incidence is estimated to be 1:10 000 people per year. It is usually progressive and results in blindness in the affected eye unless successfully treated by surgical means. The pathogenetic retinal break(s) are typically caused by acute changes in the vitreous gel and vitreoretinal traction. However, chronic vitreoretinal traction can also result in thinning of the underlying retina and eventual formation of atrophic retinal holes.

As a result of aging changes or physical alterations such as cataract extraction, there is a reduction of hyaluronic acid content in the vitreous gel. This may lead to collapse of the gel and detachment (or separation) of the posterior cortical vitreous from the retina (posterior vitreous detachment, vitreous separation) displacing the cortical vitreous anteriorly[1] (*Figure 9.1a*). The amount of separation is usually more extensive superiorly, probably because of the effect of gravity on the vitreous gel during upright posture.

Traction from the partially separated posterior vitreous surface on areas of vitreoretinal attachment results in retinal breaks in 8–15 per cent of eyes[2,3]. The retinal breaks are often flap-shaped (horseshoe tears) (*Figure 9.1b*) or round holes with a free operculum, and they tend to occur in certain predisposed eyes with areas of abnormally strong vitreoretinal attachment. Fluid from the vitreous cavity then seeps through the retinal defect in some eyes and accumulates in the subretinal space, thereby separating the retina from the pigment epithelium (*Figure 9.2*).

The extent and progression of retinal detachment depend on several factors including: (*1*) the size and location of the retinal break(s); (*2*) the amount of the fluid in the space behind the posterior vitreous surface; (*3*) the status of the remaining vitreous gel; and (*4*) factors that directly affect the retinal break(s) such as persistent vitreous traction or intermittent obstruction of the break(s) by the vitreous gel. Usually retinal detachment caused by superior retinal break(s) progresses more rapidly than detachment due to inferior break(s), and in eyes with marked liquefaction and collapse of the vitreous gel, such as aphakic and highly myopic eyes, progress of retinal detachment is usually rapid. Since subretinal fluid tends to accumulate in a dependent position, the configuration of the detachment is of special value in predicting the location of retinal break(s) in eyes with subtotal detachment as described later.

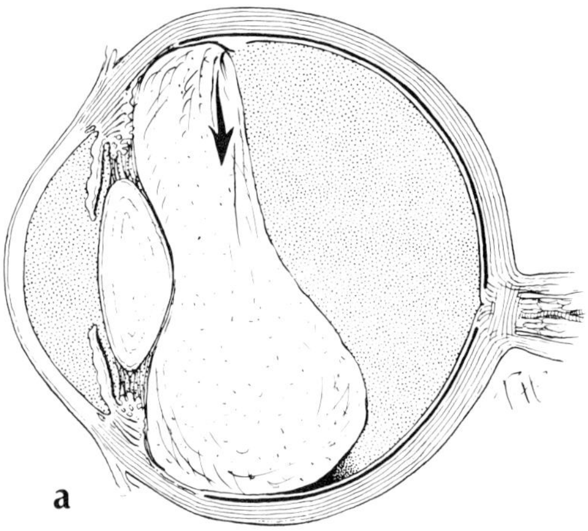

a

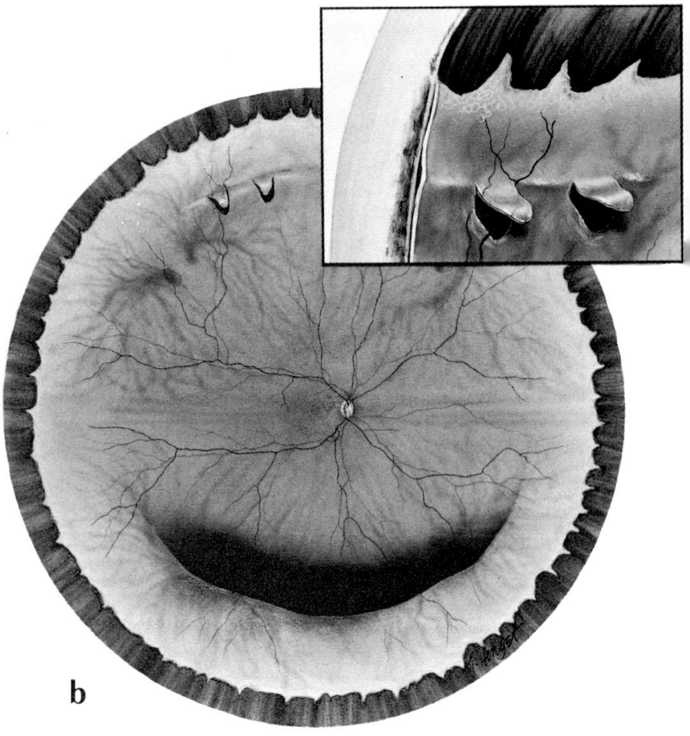

b

Figure 9.1 **(a)** *Anterior collapse of the vitreous gel and traction on areas of persistent peripheral vitreoretinal attachment may cause retinal breaks, especially in the superior quadrants. Blood from the torn retina may accumulate inferiorly beneath the posterior edge of the partially separated vitreous.* **(b)** *The retinal breaks often have a horseshoe-shaped configuration and occur along the circumferential line of vitreoretinal traction. Blood may be present within the vitreous gel or posterior to the gel at the inferior junction of the vitreous and the inner retinal surface*

Retinal detachment occurs more frequently in certain age groups and in eyes with specific predisposing conditions that influence the status of the vitreous gel and/or are associated with abnormal areas of vitreoretinal adhesion. The latter features are genetically determined.

Retinal detachment is most frequent during the sixth decade, with a median patient age of 55 years[4]. This corresponds to the time when ophthalmoscopically visible aging changes occur in the vitreous, including collapse of the gel with posterior vitreous detachment. This is especially frequent in eyes with moderate or high myopia and in aphakic eyes in which the vitreous gel shifts anteriorly after removal of the lens. About 40 per cent of eyes with rhegmatogenous detachment are aphakic. In addition, eyes with abnormally strong vitreoretinal adhesions, such as eyes with lattice degeneration, are more likely to develop retinal break(s) when vitreous collapse and posterior vitreous detachment occur (*Figure 9.3*). Although lattice degeneration is present in only 6 per cent of eyes in the general population it occurs in about 40 per cent of eyes with retinal detachment[4–6].

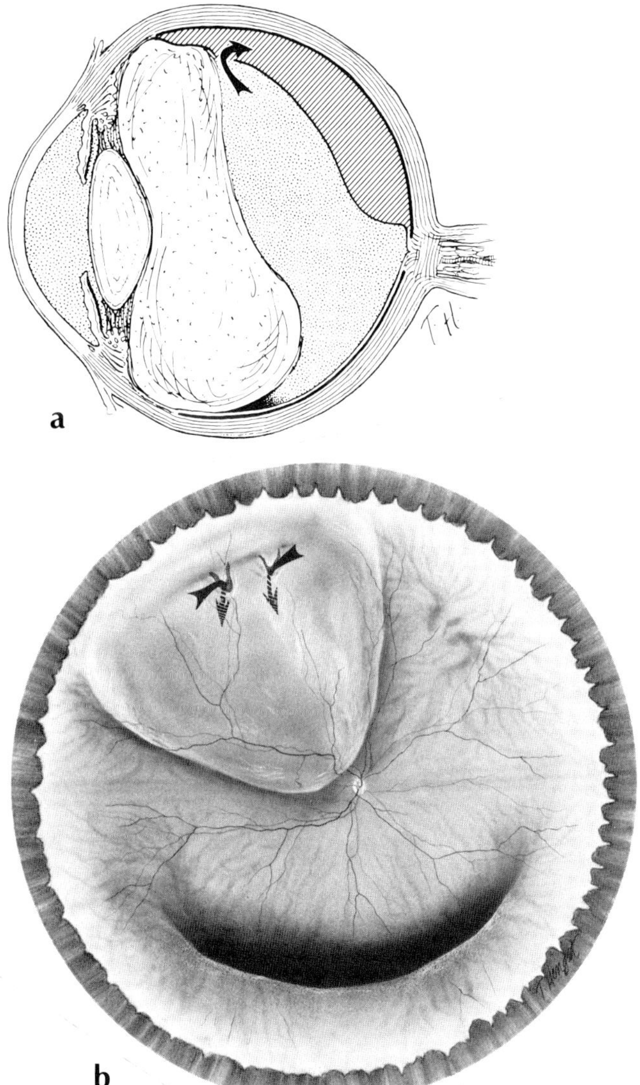

Figure 9.2 *Fluid from the posterior vitreous cavity may pass through the retinal break and accumulate in the subretinal space resulting in separation or detachment of the retina from the pigment epithelium and choroid*

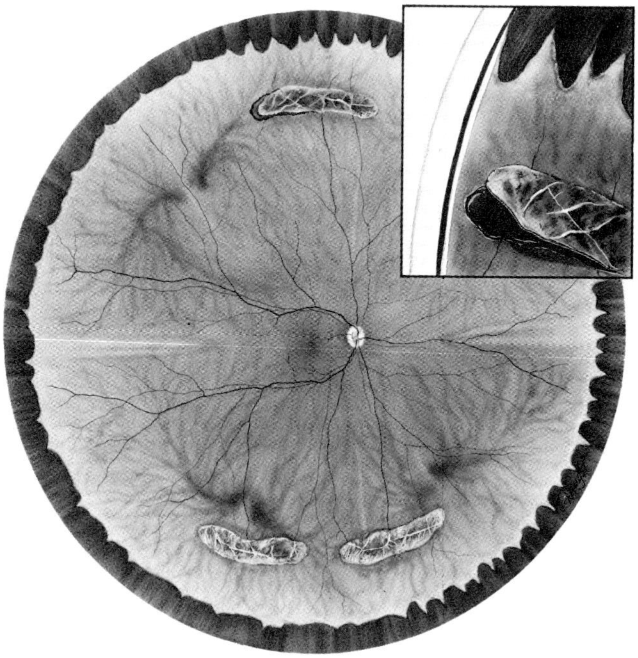

Figure 9.3 *Retinal breaks associated with lattice degeneration. Cortical vitreous is firmly adherent to the peripheral margin of each area of lattice. Atrophic retinal breaks occur within the zone of lattice degeneration and retinal tears occur at the posterior and/or lateral margins (inset)*

History of retinal reattachment surgery

Historically, retinal reattachment surgery evolved through several stages including: (*1*) development of the ophthalmoscope for fundus examination; (*2*) clinical description of retinal separation from the choroid; (*3*) identification of retinal breaks as the cause of retinal detachment and closure of these breaks as the primary objective of surgery; (*4*) refinement of examination and surgical methods to detect and treat retinal breaks and to achieve the mechanical objectives of the operation. Of primary importance was the work between 1919 and 1929 of Jules Gonin[7,8] who both confirmed the suggestion of Leber[9] that retinal breaks due to vitreous traction were the cause of retinal detachment and developed a method for successfully treating retinal detachment by sealing the retinal breaks with thermal cautery (ignipuncture).

During the next 40 years important improvements were made in both the diagnostic methods and the surgical technique. The most important of these improvements were: (*1*) development of the binocular indirect

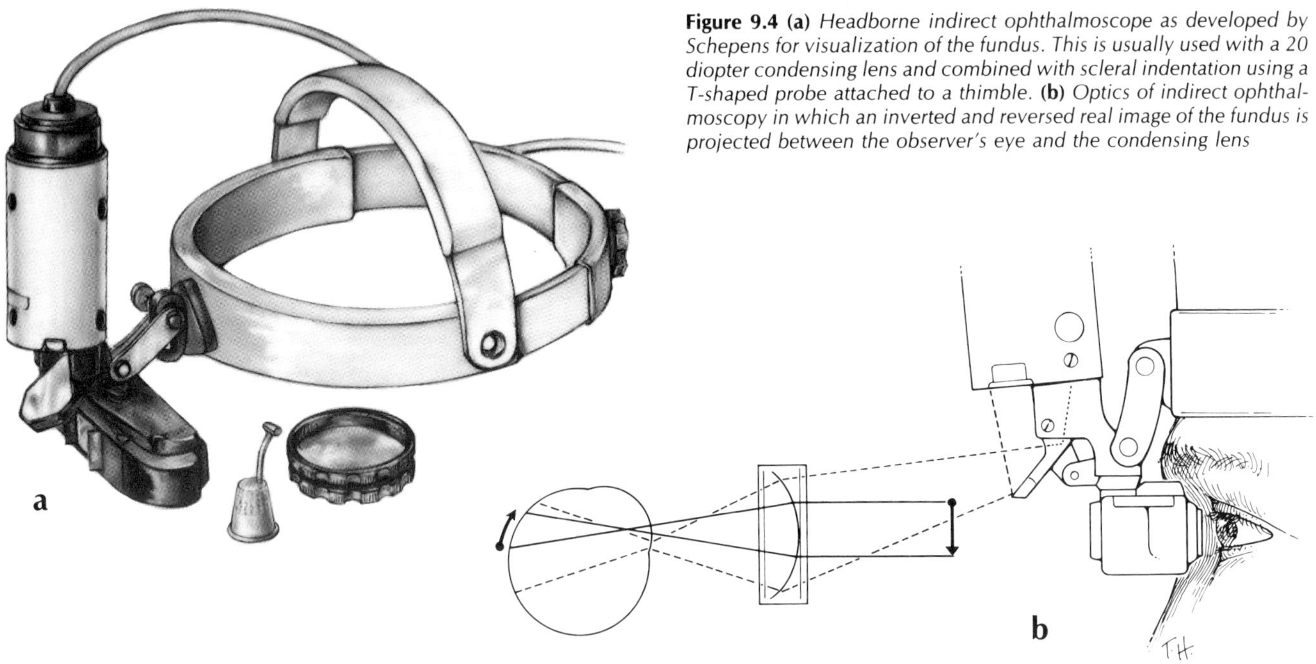

Figure 9.4 (a) *Headborne indirect ophthalmoscope as developed by Schepens for visualization of the fundus. This is usually used with a 20 diopter condensing lens and combined with scleral indentation using a T-shaped probe attached to a thimble.* **(b)** *Optics of indirect ophthalmoscopy in which an inverted and reversed real image of the fundus is projected between the observer's eye and the condensing lens*

ophthalmoscope for fundus examination; (*2*) use of diathermy, photocoagulation and cryotherapy to cause a chorioretinal adhesion; and (*3*) use of scleral buckling as a fundamental part of retinal reattachment surgery.

Schepens[10,11] developed the headborne binocular indirect ophthalmoscope, which provides the best method for examination of the peripheral retina (*Figure 9.4*). He combined indirect ophthalmoscopy with scleral indentation further to improve visualization of the peripheral fundus and to permit kinetic evaluation of the retina and vitreous, which is fundamental to proper preoperative and intraoperative examination (*Figure 9.5*). Goldmann[12] developed a three-mirror fundus contact lens that permits detailed examination of the vitreoretinal anatomy by slit-lamp biomicroscopy (*Figure 9.6*). This is also an important part of modern examination techniques.

Alternative methods for creating a chorioretinal adhesion around retinal breaks soon replaced use of thermal cautery. Diathermy applied through full-thickness sclera was used by Larsson[13] in place of ignipuncture. Weve[14] and Safar[15] applied diathermy with pins that penetrated the sclera into the subretinal space. Although the latter technique is still occasionally useful, diathermy proved to be most effective when used in combination with lamellar scleral dissection[16]. With this method, a partial-thickness scleral bed is made and diathermy is applied to the thin layer of inner scleral tissue. After the scleral bed is closed there is nearly normal scleral strength. Also, when a scleral bed with diathermy is used, larger areas of the choroid can be treated, the effect of the diathermy on the retina and choroid is more predictable, and later scleral necrosis from damage by the diathermy is minimized.

Meyer–Schwickerath[17] developed photocoagulation that is also used to cause a chorioretinal adhesion, and this form of intraocular treatment produces no scleral damage. However, effective use of photocoagulation requires that the edges of each retinal break be near the pigment epithelium. This limits its use in retinal reattachment operations because retinal breaks are usually elevated. Moreover, photocoagulation of retinal breaks in the far periphery is difficult. Therefore, the most important roles of photocoagulation are in prophylactic treatment of acute retinal tears before substantial retinal detachment develops and in postoperative treatment of retinal breaks that do not flatten completely on a scleral buckle.

Cryotherapy to create a chorioretinal adhesion was popularized by Lincoff[18], and this rapidly became the

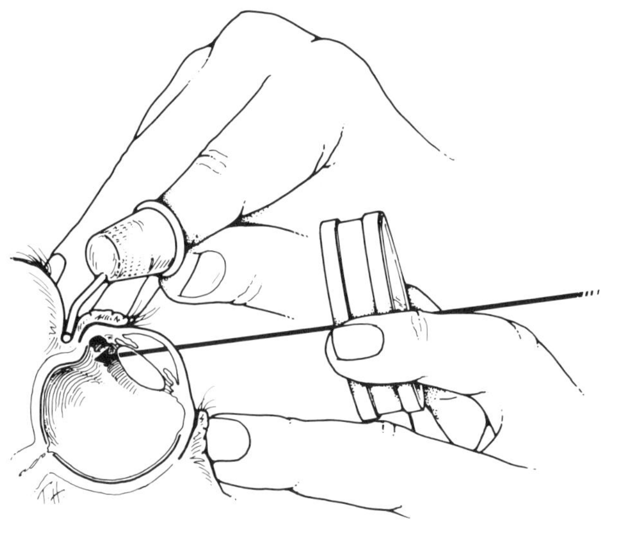

Figure 9.5 *Scleral indentation combined with indirect ophthalmoscopy to improve visualization of the peripheral fundus. The sclera is indented by the thimble depressor placed on the eyelid so that the peripheral retina can be seen*

preferred method of treatment throughout much of the world. Cryotherapy is applied through full-thickness sclera, thereby making treatment simpler and more rapid. This treatment can be applied by the surgeon while he simultaneously monitors the intraocular effect of each freeze by indirect ophthalmoscopy. Cryotherapy causes no long-term scleral damage, and it can conveniently be combined with the methods for scleral buckling.

Of great importance in the evolution of methods to treat retinal detachment was development of scleral buckling techniques. By indenting (buckling) the sclera, the pigment epithelium is positioned close to the retinal break to seal the break and to relieve vitreous traction. Methods were initially tried to shorten the eyewall by resecting partial-thickness or full-thickness strips of sclera and/or imbricating the sclera with sutures.

However, in 1953 Custodis[19] described a scleral buckling technique in which an exoplant of polyviol was sewn to the sclera to indent the eyewall over the retinal break and thereby seal the break. Custodis also demonstrated that it was not necessary to drain subretinal fluid in many cases and that the retina would reattach postoperatively if the break was closed or nearly closed at the end of the operation. Part of this effect is probably due to indenting the sclera, choroid and retina so that the adjacent vitreous gel obstructs the retinal hole from the inside. This is then followed by absorption of the subretinal fluid and flattening of the edges of the retinal break onto the indented and previously treated pigment epithelium, thereby accounting for postoperative flattening of the retinal tear even though subretinal fluid was not drained and the retinal break was not closed by the scleral buckle at the end of the operation. Custodis' observations became the basis for the scleral buckling method.

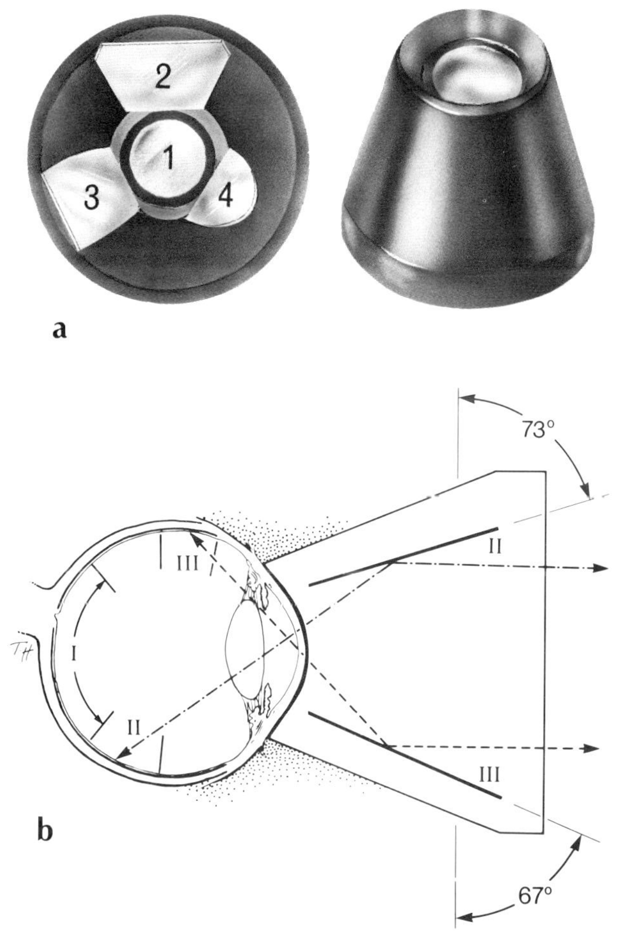

Figure 9.6 **(a)** *Goldmann three-mirror contact lens for a slit-lamp examination. Posterior fundus is examined through central portion (1) and three mirrors are used to examine periphery including equatorial zone (mirror 2), oral zone (mirror 3) and the anterior chamber angle (mirror 4).* **(b)** *Different angulation of the mirrors reflects light so that different zones of posterior segment can be seen*

The techniques of lamellar dissection and implantation of material within the sclera to create a scleral buckle were conveniently combined with diathermy to the scleral bed to make a chorioretinal adhesion. In this way damage to the sclera from the diathermy could be minimized while providing a more predictable reaction in the choroid and pigment epithelium. Schepens[16,20–27] pioneered and refined these techniques and devised implant materials of various sizes and shapes to create buckling effects with different configurations. The buckling effect created by material placed in a lamellar scleral dissection (scleral implant) tends to be permanent, and this lasting effect is enhanced by combining a segmental implant with a band that encircles the globe[28]. The encircling band also serves to relieve vitreoretinal traction in other quadrants. Lamellar dissection and scleral implant techniques for scleral buckling proved to be highly successful, and this is therefore still the preferred method for many surgeons.

Scleral buckling with material sutured to the episcleral surface (episcleral exoplants) was refined by Lincoff[18] who combined scleral buckling with photocoagulation or transscleral cryotherapy. These methods, which were based on the earlier experience of Custodis, used both hard silicone rubber and silicone sponge rubber as exoplant materials[29]. Not only is this technique easier and quicker than lamellar scleral dissection, but the exoplant position and height can be modified as necessary during surgery to achieve the desired result. However, the intraocular height of the buckling effect tends to decrease with time, and there is a higher incidence of late external erosion of the exoplant material than occurs with scleral dissection and intrascleral implants. Nevertheless, use of scleral exoplants combined with transscleral cryotherapy became the most popular method of retinal reattachment surgery because of its ease, rapidity and safety.

The combination of intrascleral implant or episcleral exoplant techniques for scleral buckling with diathermy, photocoagulation or cryotherapy to create a chorioretinal adhesion provides an effective and reliable method for retinal reattachment surgery. The method has been improved over the years by a number of refinements including techniques for safe drainage of subretinal fluid and identification of criteria for selection of cases in which to perform drainage . Use of intraocular air injection to assist in closing retinal breaks was developed along with other techniques for use in special circumstances. Finally, a group of particularly difficult cases, including giant tears, posterior retinal breaks, large and/or multiple retinal tears and detachments complicated by intravitreal and epiretinal membrane formation, was identified, and special methods including vitreous surgery and/or intraocular gas injection were adopted to treat such eyes.

Diagnosis and preoperative evaluation

Patient history

Early diagnosis of retinal tears and/or detachment is important to permit treatment of tears by less invasive techniques before detachment occurs (see p. 283) or to improve the rate of surgical reattachment and the functional result if detachment is already present. Symptoms of vitreous traction and acute retinal tear formation are often characteristic. Collapse of the vitreous gel with posterior vitreous detachment causes condensation of the vitreous fibrils, and the patient often describes a cobweb or multiple translucent lines floating in the visual field. A sudden increase in subjective floaters is the most common symptom of acute posterior vitreous separation. The floaters may be especially severe and appear as dark spots or stringy lines if vitreous hemorrhage accompanies a retinal tear. Patients sometimes experience a dull ache or other discomfort in the involved eye lasting hours or days. Prominent vitreoretinal traction also mechanically stimulates the retina, producing subjective light flashes (photopsia). Light flashes are seen most often in the temporal visual field, but their position occasionally localizes the area of vitreoretinal traction. Photopsia may be more severe if a retinal tear occurs, so that worsening of this symptom may indicate that a retinal break has developed. Light flashes often persist for weeks or months.

When retinal detachment extends posterior to the equator it causes a loss of the corresponding visual field. This is often described as a dark shadow, curtain or cloud in the involved quadrant. Unlike photopsia, loss of a portion of the visual field has important localizing value and indicates the area of retinal detachment and therefore the location of the retinal break(s). For example, peripheral field loss in the superotemporal quadrant suggests an inferonasal retinal break and detachment (*Figure 9.7*). These historical features are especially important in suggesting the location of the retinal hole if the detachment is extensive when the eye is first evaluated. Involvement of the macula is indicated by a marked reduction in visual acuity, although occasionally this visual loss occurs when a highly elevated portion of the superior retina hangs down in front of the macula before it is detached. The duration of macular involvement is important in predicting the likely level of postoperative vision after the retina is reattached.

Other details such as history of previous ocular and systemic disease are important because they may indicate the cause of the retinal detachment or may influence the method of surgery or the final visual result. Medical treatment such as miotic drops and/or systemic steroid therapy is recorded. The previous corrected visual acuity and refractive errors are recorded, including any history of amblyopia or other previous condition that might limit vision. The exact time that visual loss occurred as a result of the detachment is noted.

These pre-existing features may influence the techniques used in surgery. For example, if there is a history of glaucoma it may be necessary to drain subretinal fluid, because it is difficult to obtain an adequately high scleral buckle by other methods in eyes with a low coefficient of outflow. A previous strabismus procedure may make positioning of an episcleral exoplant difficult if a rectus muscle has been recessed behind its usual insertion. The length of time since cataract surgery, and the technique used, determine the wound strength of the previous cataract incision and influence whether additional limbal sutures are needed before beginning the retinal reattachment operation. If previous retinal surgery has been performed, reviewing its details helps to plan the reoperation by anticipating abnormalities such as areas of previous scleral dissection, sclerochoroidal incisions (drainage sites) and temporary disinsertion of extraocular muscles.

Any history of an ocular injury is extremely important including both recent and distant events. These include possible penetrating injuries with or without intraocular foreign bodies, direct contusive injuries to the globe and indirect injuries to the head. Detailed information regarding any injury is recorded because the patient may relate the detachment to the injury for the purpose of obtaining insurance compensation or litigation.

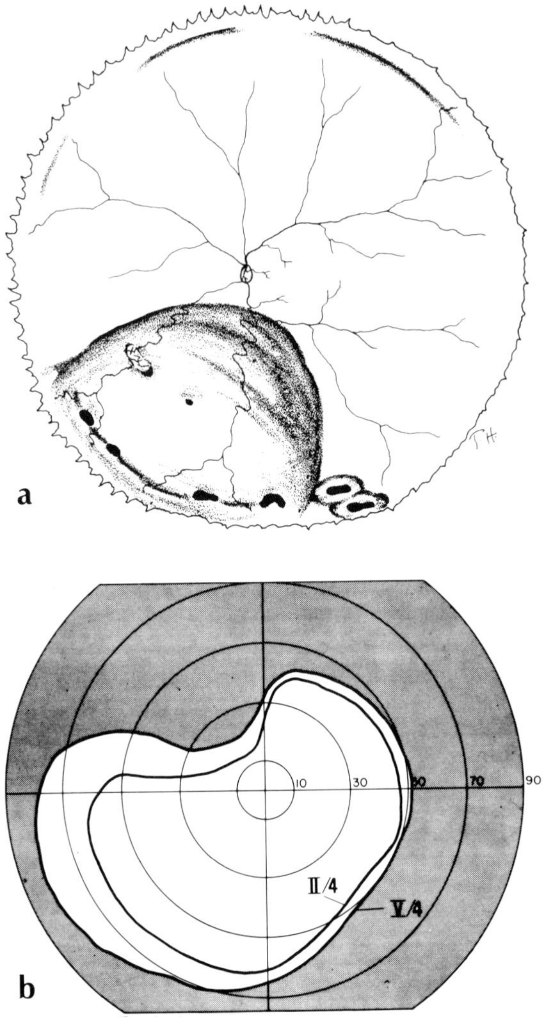

Figure 9.7 *Inferonasal retinal detachment and corresponding visual field defect in superotemporal quadrant. Patient was symptomatic because of field defect described as 'a swollen upper lid'*

Physical examination

Detailed examination of the eye is the most important part of evaluating patients with retinal detachment, with special emphasis placed on studying the vitreoretinal anatomy and physical features of the detachment. However, other aspects of the examination are also important, and these preoperative findings influence the timing and techniques of the operation in various ways. Both eyes are examined in similar fashion.

Visual function

First, the visual function is determined by measuring the best corrected visual acuity in each eye and examining the visual fields. The refractive error is recorded; this is often useful in predicting other features of the physical findings and may also influence intraoperative techniques. For example, if both eyes are emmetropic and preservation of normal vision seems likely in an eye with a peripheral retinal detachment, one may choose not to use an encircling buckle, to avoid causing anisometropic myopia, when a successful result seems likely by other techniques. Eyes with high myopia present special problems. Large and/or multiple retinal tears are more frequent in these cases, and the sclera is often thin, making suture placement difficult. Also, there is a greater risk of choroidal hemorrhage in myopic eyes. Therefore, it may be best to avoid drainage of subretinal fluid or take special precautions when fluid is released in such cases.

The sensory status influences still other features of management. The severity of visual loss in eyes with detachment of the macula is often inversely related to the amount of visual recovery expected after successful reattachment, and it is important to discuss this with the patient preoperatively. The extent of visual field loss usually corresponds to the area of detachment, and this may be helpful in directing ophthalmoscopic examination in eyes with moderately dense lens opacities, small pupils or vitreous hemorrhage that interfere with direct examination of the retina. Demonstration of an absolute scotoma in the visual field suggests the possibility of retinoschisis, with or without rhegmatogenous detachment, rather than retinal detachment alone.

External examination

External examination includes evaluation of the conjunctiva, lid margins and lacrimal drainage apparatus. Any infection is treated before retinal reattachment surgery is performed, especially if scleral buckling or drainage of subretinal fluid is planned. Abnormalities of the lid positions are recorded, and the patient is advised that mild enophthalmos or ptosis may occur postoperatively if an extensive operation is necessary.

The alignment of the eyes in the primary field of gaze and ocular motility are evaluated for evidence of muscle imbalance or restriction of ocular rotations. Abnormalities are more likely after previous retinal reattachment surgery and may become worse if multiple procedures are required. The pupillary responses are evaluated. A relative afferent pupillary defect is frequent in eyes with extensive retinal detachment and does not necessarily imply an abnormality of the optic nerve. Also, the maximum amount of pupillary dilation after use of mydriatic medication is noted to indicate the amount of dilation which can be anticipated during the operation. Finally, examination of the sclera may suggest ectasia or a staphyloma, which could influence the scleral buckling technique chosen if a retinal break is present in that area. Such scleral changes are most common in the superotemporal quadrant and are best detected by elevating the upper lid while the patient rotates the eye inferonasally.

Slit-lamp examination

Slit-lamp examination includes evaluation of the anterior segment and the anterior vitreous gel, and measurement of the intraocular pressure (IOP) by applanation tonometry. Depth of the anterior chamber is recorded because retinal surgery can be complicated by an anterior shift of the lens–iris diaphragm and secondary angle-closure glaucoma. This sometimes occurs in elderly patients when an anterior encircling buckle is used or if more than one vortex vein is cut or compressed. Gonioscopy is performed before pupillary dilation if the anterior chamber is shallow, and a laser iridotomy is considered if the angle seems occludable or if angle closure occurs later after mydriatic drops. If the anterior chamber is unusually deep, such as in eyes with megalocornea, buphthalmos, or in some eyes with myopia, this may facilitate use of anterior chamber paracentesis to soften the eye intraoperatively and to avoid drainage of subretinal fluid. Other iris abnormalities are noted, such as heterochromia, which may suggest a retained iron-containing intraocular foreign body.

Intraocular pressure is measured by applanation tonometry, and a somewhat lower pressure is expected in the eye with detachment. Sometimes involved eyes are hypotonous, in which case choroidal detachment may be present and drainage of the suprachoroidal fluid may be necessary during the operation. If the IOP is near the upper limit of normal or elevated above normal despite extensive retinal detachment, this suggests reduced aqueous outflow and may indicate that it will be difficult to control the IOP intraoperatively or postoperatively.

After the pupil is dilated, the lens, or the anterior vitreous surface in aphakic eyes, is evaluated. Lens opacities may interfere with examination of the fundus, especially during fundus biomicroscopy using a three-mirror contact lens. Rarely, lens opacities are so severe that adequate examination of the fundus is not possible. In these cases, removal of the lens by phacoemulsification without rupture of the posterior lens capsule usually permits adequate examination of the retina, and retinal reattachment surgery can then be performed within 1 week.

The condition of the anterior vitreous surface (anterior hyaloid face) is important in determining whether an anterior chamber paracentesis can be done safely in aphakic eyes. If the anterior vitreous surface is ruptured and loose vitreous fibrils are present in the anterior chamber, paracentesis is not performed. If the anterior vitreous surface is intact and does not bow forward when the pupil is maximally dilated, then a paracentesis can usually be safely done. When a pseudophakos (intraocular lens; IOL) is present in the anterior chamber or iris plane, a paracentesis cannot be done safely (*see* p. 295).

Examination of the anterior vitreous gel is important for other reasons. Pigment debris within the gel is regularly seen in patients with rhegmatogenous detachment, and the absence of pigment suggests another diagnosis, such as retinoschisis or secondary (exudative) detachment[30]. However, in many aphakic eyes pigment debris is present because of the cataract operation, in the absence of retinal breaks or detachment. The amount of pigment debris has no prognostic significance, although the presence of gray clumps of cells within the gel suggests intraocular cellular proliferation which can be a feature of massive periretinal proliferation (MPP) (*Figure 9.8*).

Mobility of the vitreous is evaluated by having the patient rapidly look up and down and then return to the primary position of gaze. Marked reduction in the normal mobility of the vitreous also suggests intravitreal changes as seen in MPP, as does the presence of a visible transvitreal sheet in an equatorial or pre-equatorial plane. When these vitreous changes are present, a high, encircling scleral buckle is used as mentioned later.

The location of the posterior vitreous surface is also recorded. If the posterior vitreous surface has shifted far anteriorly, there is an increased tendency for the fluid behind the vitreous gel to pass through the retinal hole into the subretinal space during drainage of subretinal fluid. Also, in eyes with marked anterior shift of the vitreous gel, aspiration of the fluid from the vitreous cavity behind the gel is possible with a needle and syringe. However, this maneuver is hazardous, especially because the position of the vitreous gel may change when the patient is supine. Fortunately vitreous aspiration is rarely required. Further examination of vitreoretinal features using a three-mirror contact lens may be performed after examination of the fundus by indirect ophthalmoscopy.

Retinal examination

Detailed examination of the retina is of major importance, to study the extent and topography of the retinal detachment, to identify all retinal breaks and to evaluate other features of the posterior segment – including the macula and optic nerve, any areas of abnormal vitreoretinal traction and any epiretinal membranes. Examination is performed with a binocular indirect ophthalmoscope aided by scleral indendation. This is supplemented by direct ophthalmoscopy and fundus biomicroscopy to evaluate the macula, the posterior vitreous gel and the peripheral vitreoretinal interface.

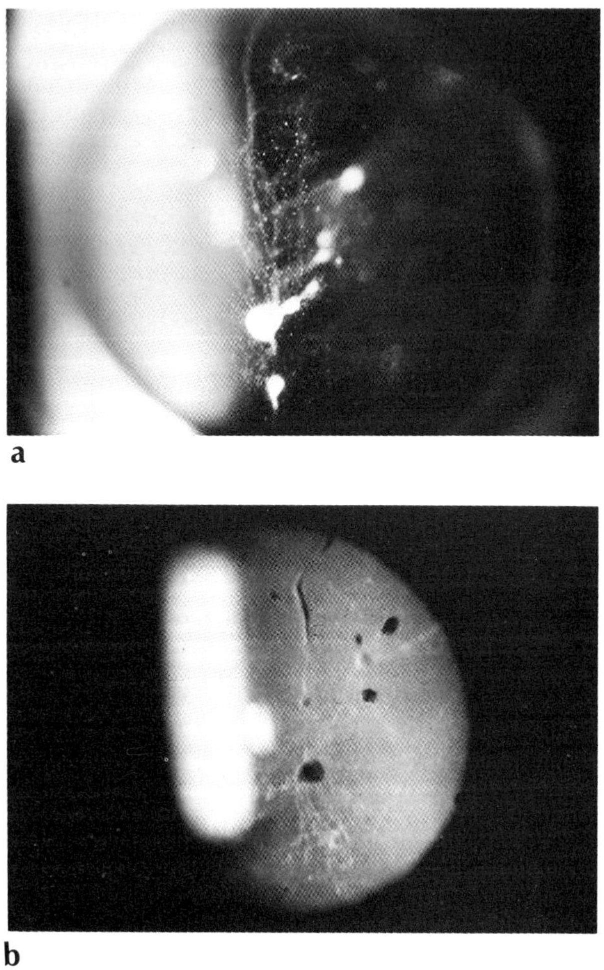

Figure 9.8 *Large clumps of gray-colored debris in vitreous gel of eye with retinal detachment and extensive epiretinal membrane formation. Clumps are composed of macrophages, pigment epithelial cells and fibrous astrocytes indicating cellular proliferation in the vitreous cavity*

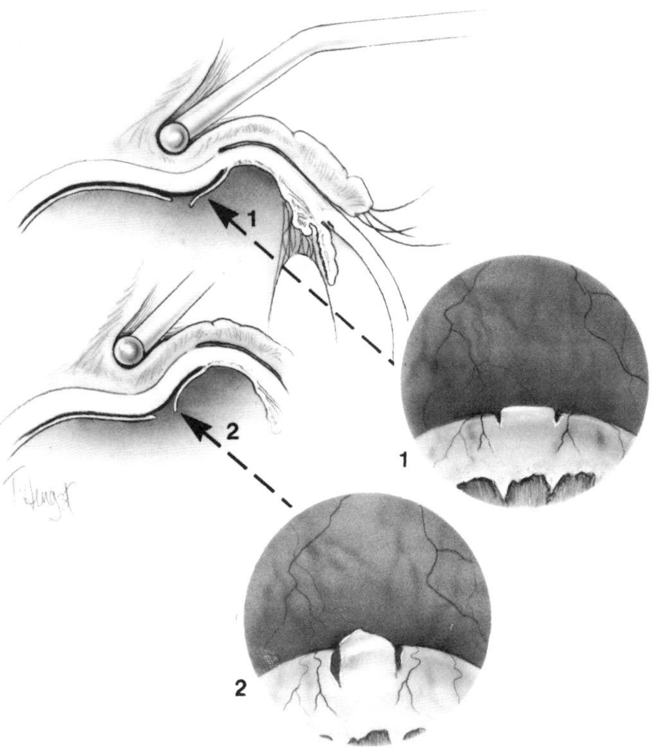

Figure 9.9 *Kinetic examination of peripheral retina combining scleral indentation with indirect ophthalmoscopy. As scleral depressor is moved over the sclera, peripheral retina is seen in oblique view and retinal breaks may be demonstrated*

Indirect ophthalmoscopy allows stereopsis and provides a wide (40°) field of view when a 20 diopter condensing lens is used. This, combined with scleral indentation, allows kinetic examination of the peripheral retina from various angles (*Figure 9.9*). Indirect ophthalmoscopy also permits examination of the peripheral fundus through a small (3–4 mm) pupil, or through opacities such as mild or moderate cataract or mild vitreous hemorrhage. A detailed fundus drawing is prepared using conventional color codes to record the physical findings (*Figure 9.10*), and this is supplemented by written notes as needed. Diagrams representing cross-sections of the vitreoretinal anatomy are made when indicated.

Ophthalmoscopy is performed under optimum conditions in a darkened room with the pupil fully dilated and with the examiner dark-adapted. Examination is done with the patient supine (*Figure 9.11*), and sometimes in a sitting position or with the head hyperextended beyond the end of the examination table. About 20 per cent of patients have marked shifting of subretinal fluid when changing from a sitting to a supine position. This finding may allow selection of an optimum head position during preoperative bedrest and may indicate the need for caution during drainage of subretinal fluid. When an inferior retinal detachment is present, the head is hyperextended beyond

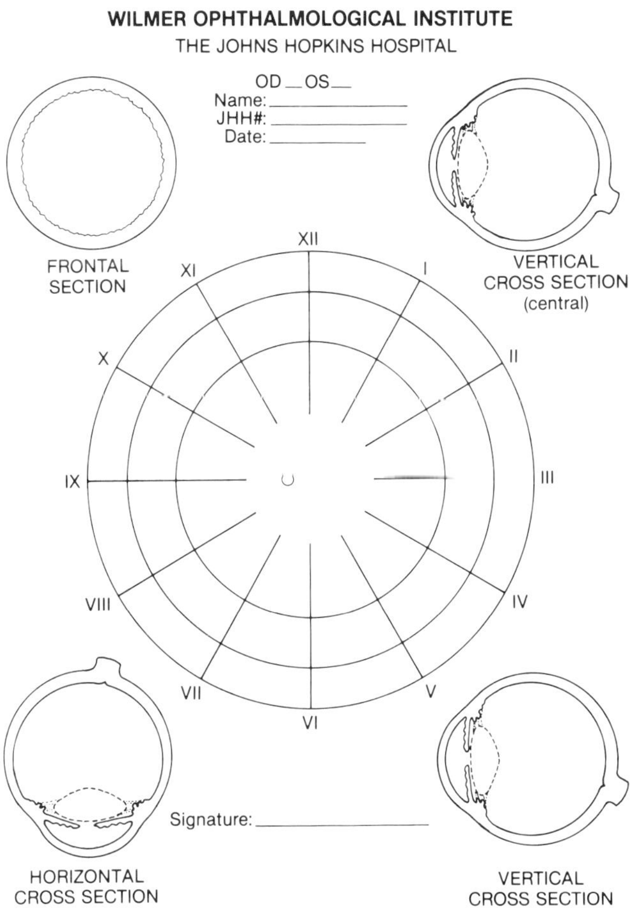

Figure 9.10 *Vitreoretinal drawing chart with space for usual large fundus drawing and cross-section representations of vitreoretinal anatomy*

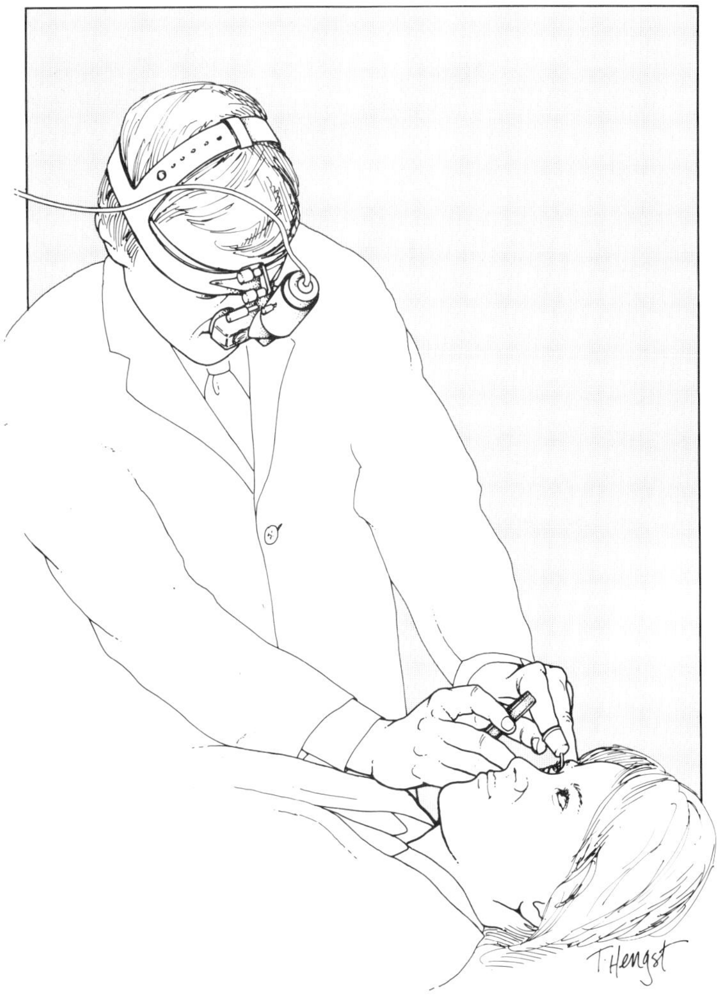

Figure 9.11 *Examination of the fundus by indirect ophthalmoscopy and scleral indentation. Patient is supine on stretcher so examiner can move freely around the head to visualize all meridians of the posterior segment*

the end of the examination table so the superior part of the globe is dependent (*Figure 9.12a*). Superior shifting of the subretinal fluid will demonstrate the true superior extent of the detachment and may show a communication of the subretinal fluid with a superior retinal break (*Figure 9.12b,c*).

The boundaries of the retinal detachment around the optic nerve are recorded first, and it is noted whether the macula is involved. Any retinal breaks or abnormalities posterior to the equator are recorded on the fundus drawing. The entire peripheral retina is then examined by indirect ophthalmoscopy aided by scleral indentation. This is usually begun in the 12 o'clock meridian and proceeds clockwise. The peripheral boundaries of the detachment and shifting of the boundaries with changes in posture are recorded.

All retinal breaks, possible retinal breaks, thin areas of retina, and zones of abnormal vitreoretinal adhesion, including lattice degeneration, are recorded with their circumferential and anteroposterior position carefully noted (*Figure 9.13*). The vortex veins and long posterior

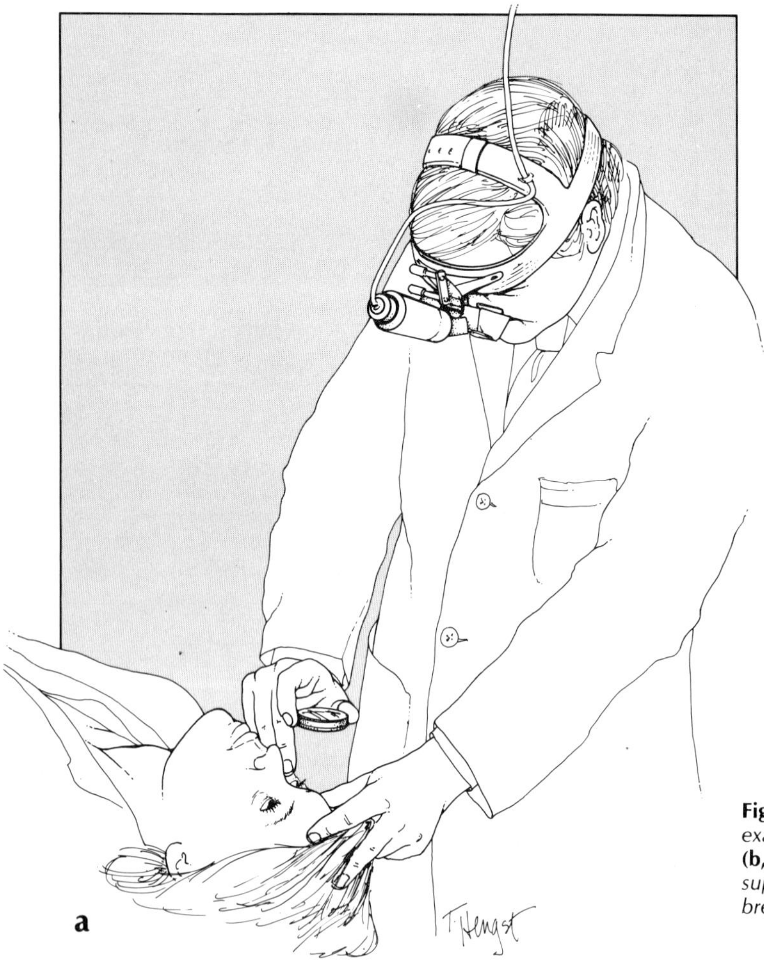

Figure 9.12 (a) *Patient's head hyperextended beyond end of the examination table to aid in evaluation of inferior retinal detachment.* **(b,c)** *As the head is hyperextended, subretinal fluid may extend superiorly and demonstrate communication between superior retinal break and inferior retinal detachment*

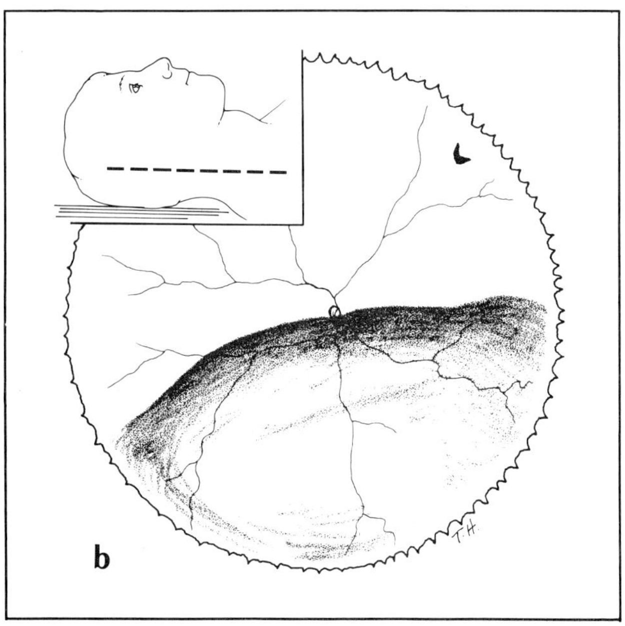

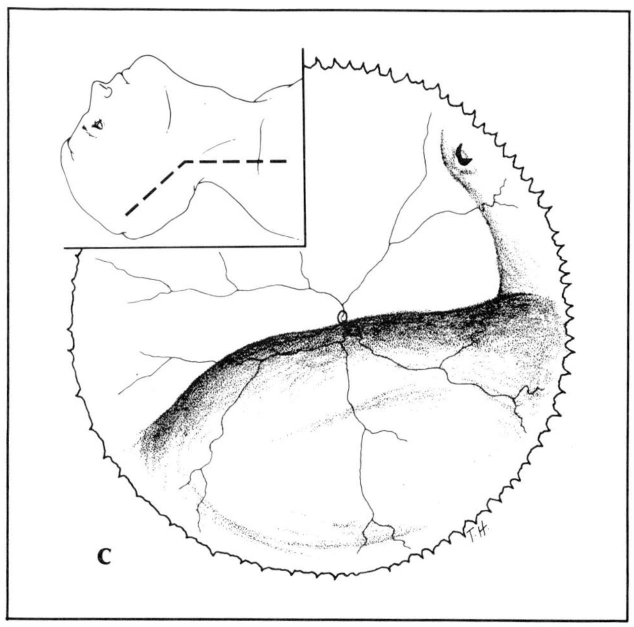

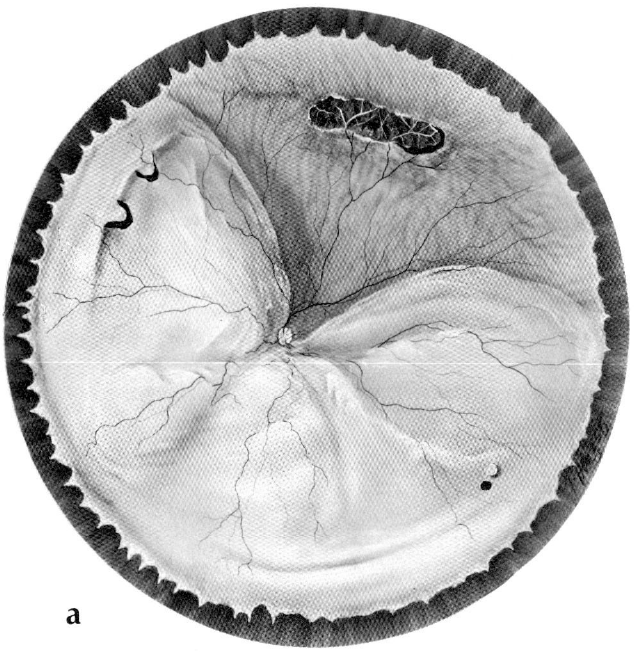

a

Figure 9.13 *Fundus drawing technique.* (a) *Subtotal retinal detachment and distinctive features including horseshoe-shaped retinal breaks, round retinal hole and lattice degeneration in area of attached retina.* (b) *Boundaries of retinal detachment around optic nerve are recorded first. Then peripheral retina is examined in clockwise fashion, recording the boundaries of the detachment, vitreoretinal abnormalities and retinal breaks*

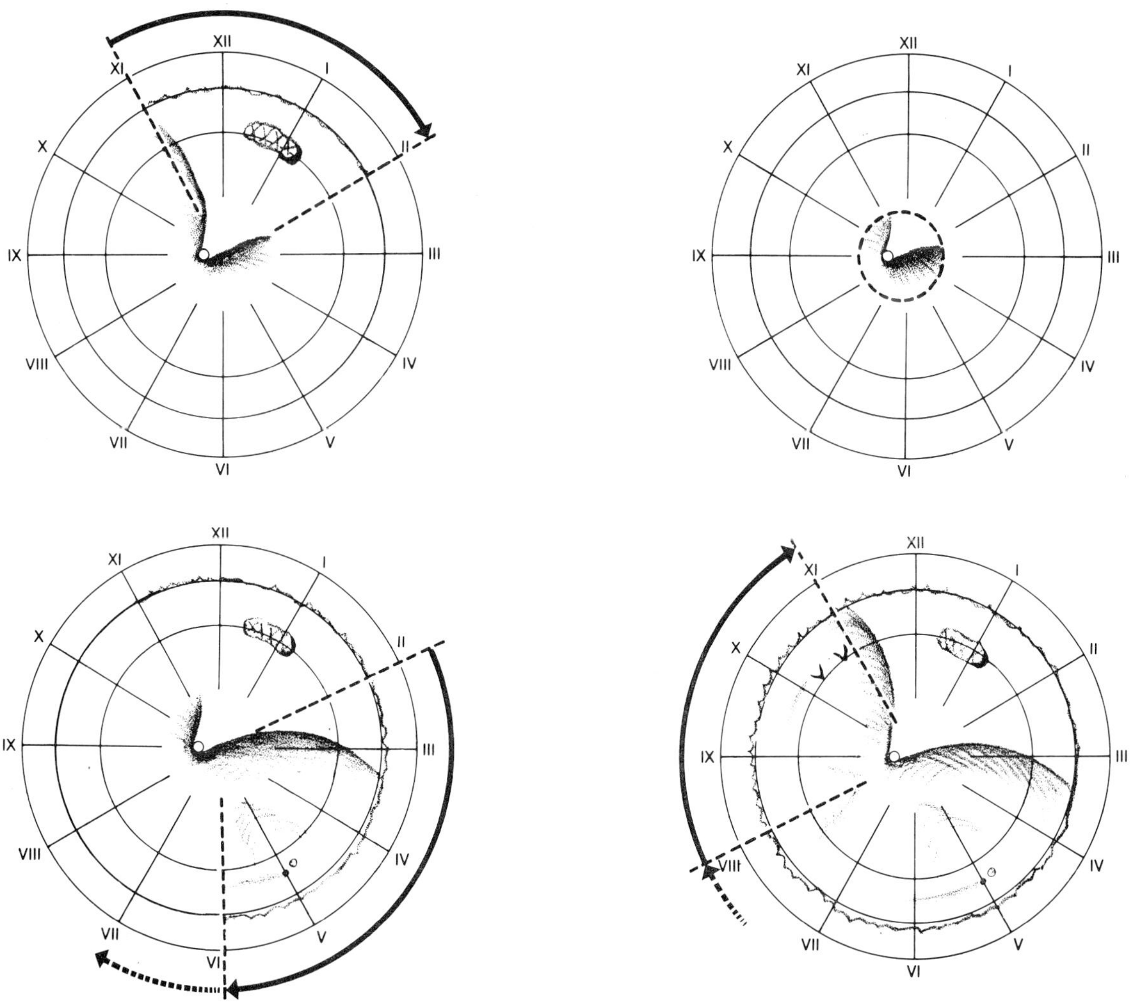

b

ciliary vessels and nerves provide useful reference landmarks to map retinal breaks, as does localizing the retinal breaks by using imaginary locations of the 12 separate clock-hour meridians. The entire retina cannot be represented in an anatomically correct fashion on the usual fundus drawing chart because the circumference of the ora serrata is smaller than the equator, but the opposite is true on the chart (*Figure 9.14*). Abnormalities of the peripheral fundus are usually important and these are carefully recorded.

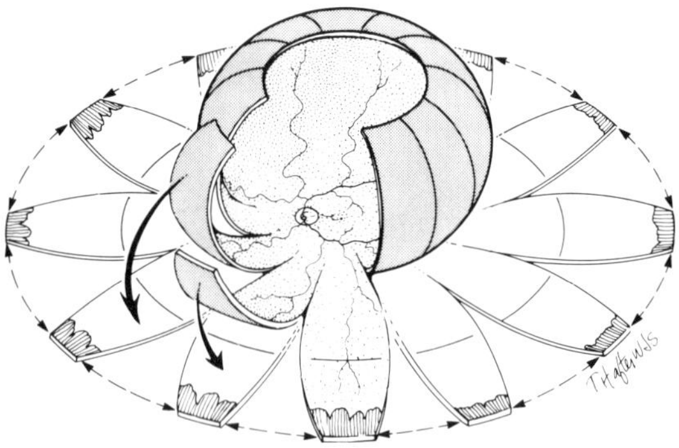

Figure 9.14 *Inconsistency between fundus drawing chart and true posterior segment relations. The equator of the globe has a larger circumference than the ora serrata, whereas the opposite is true on the fundus drawing chart*

Retinal breaks that are difficult to see are carefully localized including their position relative to nearby blood vessels, pigment spots or other physical features, which are added to the fundus drawing to assist in locating the break(s) intraoperatively. However, other than this, the retinal vasculature is not routinely recorded. Other features of the detachment are included on the drawing or written notes are made. These include: (*1*) the height of the detachment; (*2*) the presence of demarcation lines, intraretinal cysts and fixed retinal folds; and (*3*) areas of evident epiretinal membrane formation or retroretinal fibrous proliferation.

Keeping both eyes open during the examination aids the patient in positioning the eyes as requested by the examiner. Examination of the inferior retina requires downgaze, which is more difficult, and the patient is asked to elevate one hand and gaze toward the extended thumb (*Figure 9.15*). The hand position is moved by the examiner to change the ocular position.

After an initial examination of the entire fundus periphery, the examination is sometimes repeated with attention directed to certain areas. Often the patient is better able to cooperate during a second examination because of familiarity with the eye positions required and because the eye has adapted to the bright light of the indirect ophthalmoscope. The fellow eye is examined in the same fashion as the eye with the detachment and a fundus drawing of the fellow eye is made if any abnormality is seen.

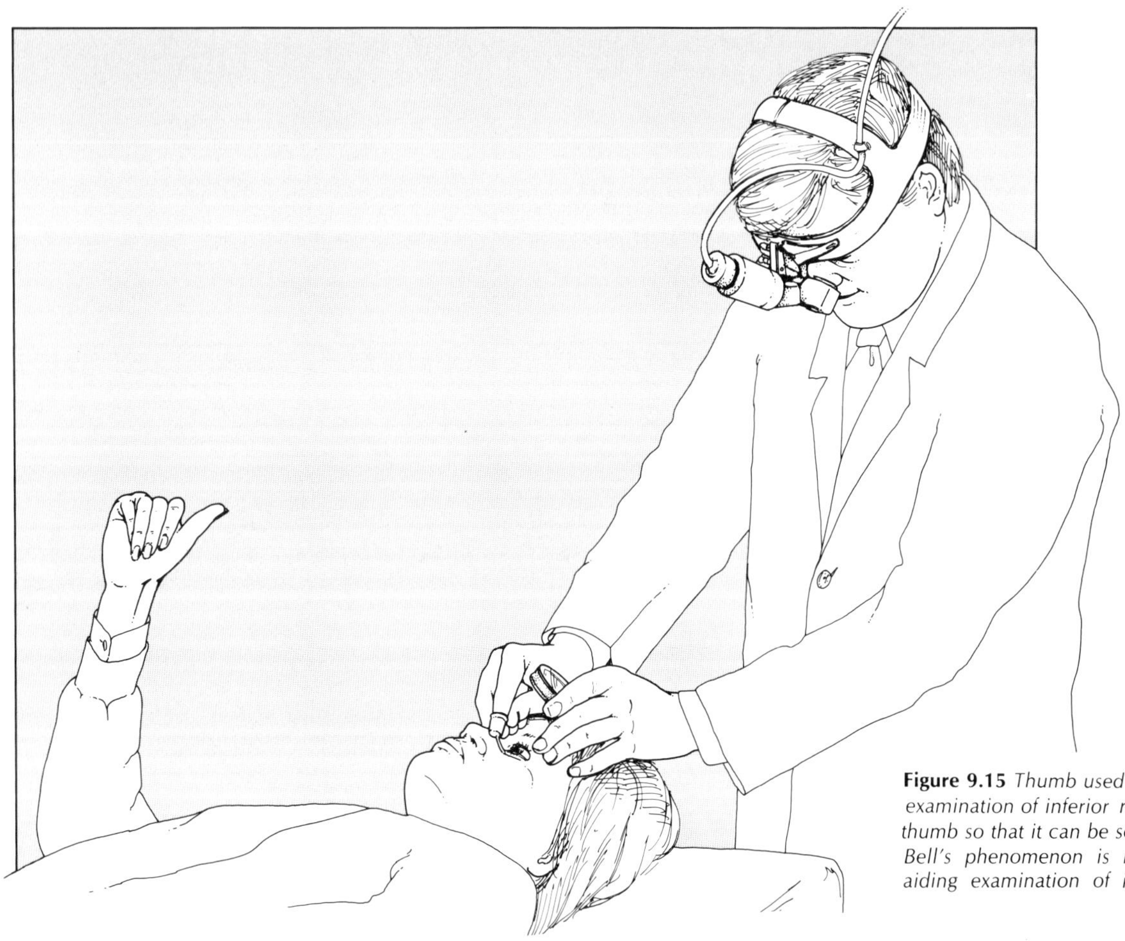

Figure 9.15 *Thumb used to aid patient during examination of inferior retina. By positioning thumb so that it can be seen by the fellow eye, Bell's phenomenon is minimized, thereby aiding examination of inferior fundus*

Locating retinal breaks

The topography of retinal detachment is of considerable value in predicting the location of the retinal break(s)[31]. In cases of rhegmatogenous detachment, retinal break(s) are present within the area of detachment and are usually located near the most superior edge of subtotal detachments that do not involve both superior quadrants. Therefore, if a detachment involves both lower quadrants and extends farther superiorly on one side than the other, retinal break(s) are likely to be present near the most superior edge of the detachment (*Figure 9.16*). When a subtotal detachment involves both superior quadrants, a retinal break is likely to be present near the 12 o'clock meridian on the side with the most extensive detachment (*Figure 9.17*). A retinal break in the 6 o'clock meridian often results in detachment with symmetrical amounts of fluid on both the temporal and nasal sides. Also, detachments due to inferior retinal breaks progress more slowly, and they often show retroretinal fibrosis or pigmentary demarcation lines along the advancing edge of the detachment. Demarcation lines are an important localizing feature in any detachment because they indicate previous boundaries of the detachment and therefore suggest the location of retinal break(s) (*Figure 9.18*). Despite the help of topographical features, it is necessary to examine carefully the entire retina to locate all retinal breaks because each retinal break must be closed to cure the detachment and prevent recurrence.

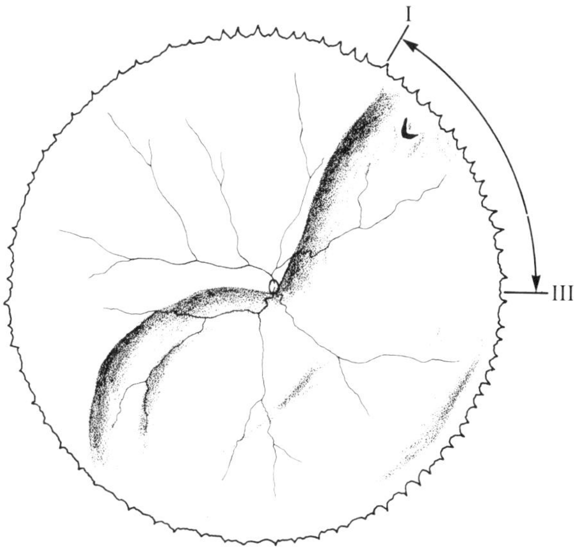

Figure 9.16 *Morphological configuration of subtotal retinal detachment aids in identifying likely location of retinal break(s). Retinal detachment involving both lower quadrants and extending farther superiorly on one side is likely to have retinal break near upper edge of detachment*

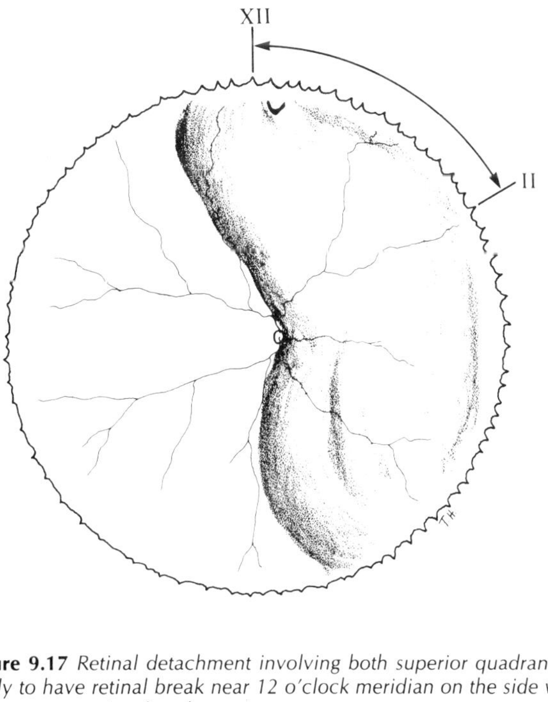

Figure 9.17 *Retinal detachment involving both superior quadrants is likely to have retinal break near 12 o'clock meridian on the side with the most extensive detachment*

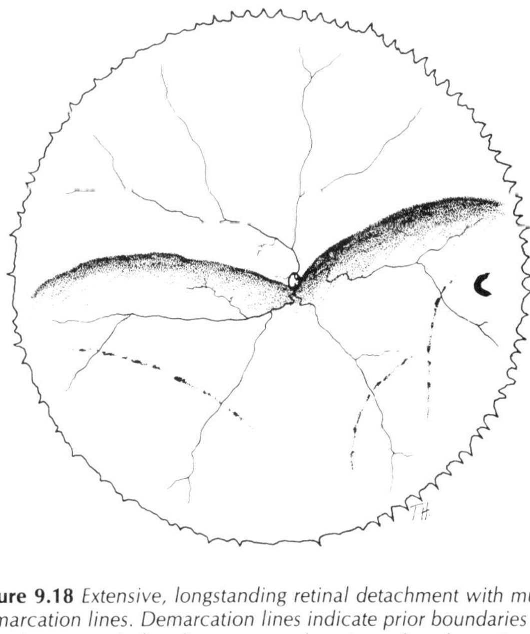

Figure 9.18 *Extensive, longstanding retinal detachment with multiple demarcation lines. Demarcation lines indicate prior boundaries of the detachment and therefore suggest location of pathogenic retinal break(s)*

Fundus biomicroscopy

After examination of the retina by indirect ophthalmoscopy, the macula and optic nervehead are examined by direct ophthalmoscopy and sometimes by fundus biomicroscopy. Any abnormalities are noted on the fundus drawing. The vitreous and vitreoretinal anatomy may then be studied further in certain cases by biomicroscopy with a three-mirror contact lens (*Figure 9.19*). Biomicroscopy allows visualization of the vitreous traction that caused the retinal break. However, its main clinical uses are: (*1*) to study the vitreoretinal anatomy in eyes with transvitreal sheets and/or epiretinal membranes; (*2*) to determine whether areas of thin retina or possible retinal breaks are actually full-thickness retinal defects; and (*3*) to search for small retinal break(s) where the topography of the detachment suggests that a retinal break should be present but where none is seen by indirect ophthalmoscopy. The combination of high magnification provided by the slit lamp and the variable angulation and width of the slit beam is usually sufficient to see subtle retinal break(s). Scleral indentation can also be combined with fundus biomicroscopy, but this is technically difficult. Notations are made on the fundus drawing of the findings of slit-lamp biomicroscopy, and additional cross-section drawings are prepared when necessary.

Formulation and preoperative management

Formulation

After completing the ocular examination, the entire history and constellation of physical findings should provide a logical explanation for the disease process and its manifestations. Any incongruous portions of the history are reviewed, and additional history is elicited if physical findings suggest specific abnormalities such as prior trauma, longstanding retinal detachment, previous macular damage, or still other conditions such as regressed retrolental fibroplasia, old retinal branch-vein obstruction, other proliferative retinopathy or a prior intraocular inflammatory condition.

Portions of the physical examination are repeated when necessary. This may include: (*1*) further examination of the macula if X-linked retinoschisis is suspected; (*2*) gonioscopy if there is evidence of damage from blunt trauma; (*3*) re-evaluation of the anterior vitreous surface in aphakic eyes if anterior chamber paracentesis may be necessary intraoperatively; and (*4*) repeated testing of the visual acuity after prolonged dark adaptation if the amount of visual loss is not explained by the physical findings of

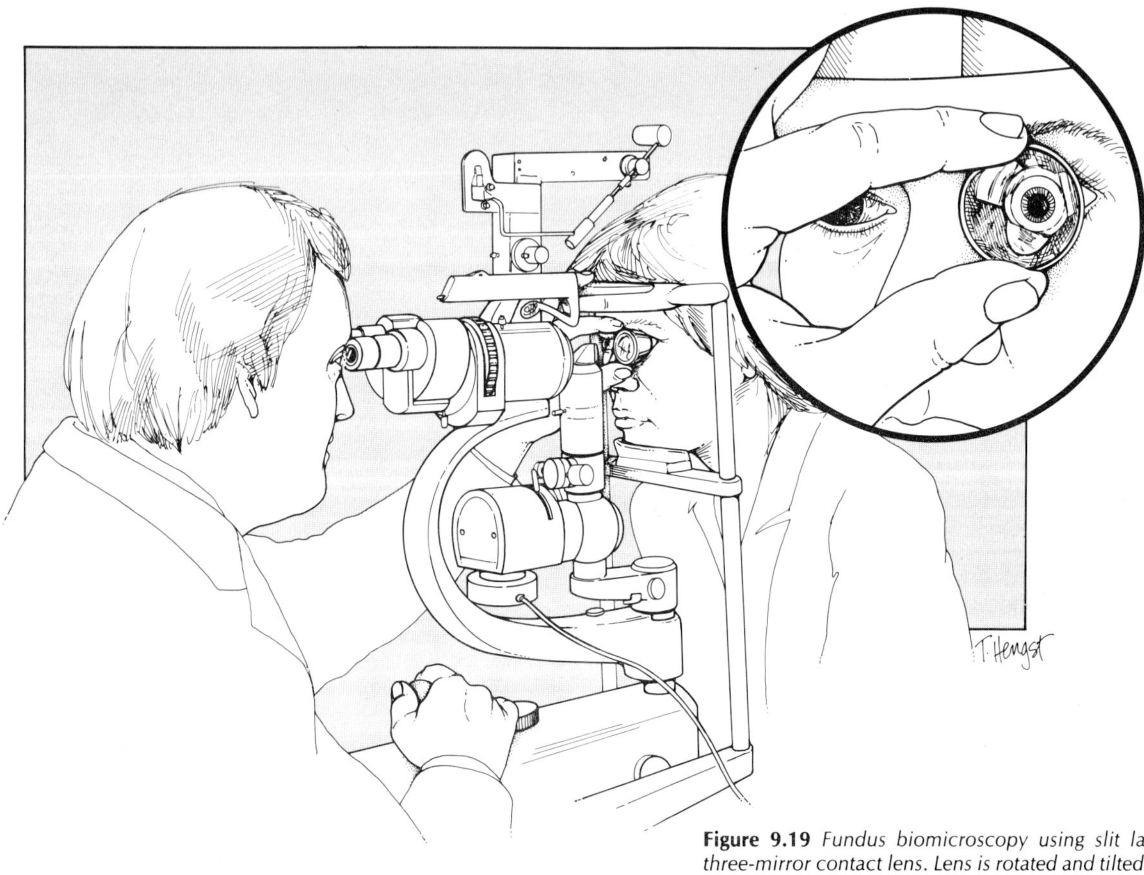

Figure 9.19 *Fundus biomicroscopy using slit lamp and Goldmann three-mirror contact lens. Lens is rotated and tilted to examine different portions of peripheral fundus using each of two posterior segment mirrors*

the detachment. However, when the macula is detached, bleaching of the visual pigments during indirect ophthalmoscopy is not rapidly reversed, and vision may not improve to the level of initial testing until after the retina is reattached.

Fundus examination is repeated at a later time if the previous examination was inadequate or if a retinal break cannot be identified to account for the detachment. In selected cases, additional retinal tests are performed such as quantitative visual field examination, ultrasonography, and/or fluorescein angiography or angioscopy. The latter is useful if a secondary (exudative) detachment is suspected in order to demonstrate leakage of fluorescein dye from the choroid into the subretinal space. Electroretinography is rarely helpful in clinical management of retinal detachment, even though the recording is usually reduced in proportion to the extent of the detachment.

After completion of the evaluation, the diagnosis and recommendations for management are reviewed with the patient and family. Explanation of the disease process is given, although detailed discussion is avoided in most cases to prevent confusion. The patient is told that untreated retinal detachment usually results in permanent blindness in the affected eye, and that no treatment other than retinal reattachment surgery is effective. The variable visual results after successful anatomical reattachment of the retina are reviewed and also the possibility of complications which range from massive choroidal hemorrhage or infection with complete loss of vision to macular pucker or cystoid macular edema which can limit further the postoperative vision despite successful anatomical reattachment. The latter two conditions are especially important to discuss if the macula is not detached preoperatively and the visual acuity is normal. Also, the possibility of prolonged discomfort, diplopia, change in refractive error, cosmetic abnormalities and late complications such as recurrent retinal detachment and extrusion of material used to create a scleral buckle are discussed. The anticipated period of hospital confinement and the postoperative restrictions on activity are reviewed. The patient is given a percentage estimate of the likelihood of an anatomically successful result.

Preoperative management

Preoperative management is directed toward providing optimum conditions for successful reattachment surgery and minimizing the risk of complications. Any preoperative infection of the lid margins or lacrimal drainage system is treated after cultures are taken. In most cases, broad spectrum antibiotic drops are applied preoperatively to decrease the bacterial flora on the conjunctival surfaces. Repeated dilation of the pupil is avoided after completing the fundus examination to minimize fatigue of the dilator muscle of the iris which would limit intraoperative dilation of the pupil. The lashes of the involved eye are cut short.

Bilateral eye bandages are used preoperatively in most cases to limit eye movement. This results in considerable flattening of the retina within 24–48 hours in about 20 per cent of eyes. Flattening of the retina makes it easier to treat and localize the retinal breaks, reduces the need for draining subretinal fluid, shortens the length of the operation and reduces the risk of complications. In some cases, special preoperative head positioning may promote absorption of the subretinal fluid by temporarily occluding the retinal breaks with vitreous gel. Use of bilateral eye bandages also seems to halt the progression of retinal detachment in most eyes. This is especially important if the macula is not yet involved and if surgery must be delayed for a day or longer. Other decisions regarding preoperative management depend on particular features of the case and the patient's general medical condition, which may require further tests or therapy.

Other preoperative decisions must be made, including the choice of anesthesia and use of medications in some cases to lower the IOP before surgery. Usually the duration and complexity of the operation can be anticipated based on the preoperative findings. However, modification of the surgical plan may become necessary because of changing intraoperative conditions.

The choice of anesthesia depends on specific features of the case and also the preferences of the surgeon and the patient. When the operation is expected to take less than 2 hours or when active patient cooperation is desirable, we prefer local anesthesia supplemented by intravenous sedatives and continuous monitoring of the cardiovascular system by an anesthesiologist. For example, in some aphakic eyes with giant retinal tears, vitrectomy is combined with fluid–gas exchange with the patient in a face-down position (*see* Chapter 8). If the patient is awake, he can assist in assuming a face-down position and there is also no risk of displacement of an endotracheal tube during this maneuver. When local anaesthesia is used, we anesthetize the facial nerve, infiltrate the lateral canthal region and give a retrobulbar injection using 4 per cent lidocaine (lignocaine) mixed half-and-half with 0.75 per cent bupivacaine (*Figure 9.20*).

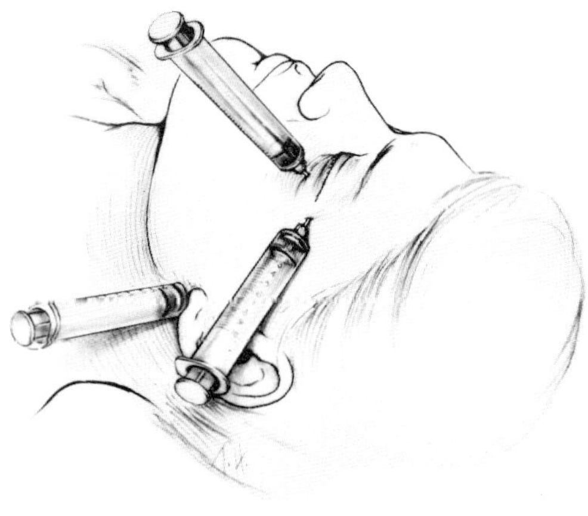

Figure 9.20 *Injections of medications for local anesthesia, including facial nerve block posterior to earlobe, infiltration of lateral canthal area and retrobulbar injection into extraocular muscle cone*

General anesthesia is preferred for children, cases expected to require more than 2 hours, cases with retinal breaks located posterior to the equator and cases undergoing reoperation. In addition, general anesthesia is used if that is the personal preference of the patient and if no medical contraindication is present. The agents and techniques for general anesthesia are chosen by the anesthesiologist.

Medications such as acetazolamide and/or intravenous hyperosmotic agents are sometimes given immediately before the operation to lower the IOP and thereby facilitate scleral buckling when drainage of subretinal fluid is unnecessary or hazardous. Hyperosmotic agents act only for a short period and are given about 1 hour before creation of the scleral buckle. Therefore, these agents may be given just before beginning the operation if a short procedure is anticipated or during the operation in longer cases. Acetazolamide has a longer duration of action and can be given either before the operation or during the procedure. When used, we administer an intravenous dosage of 500 mg of acetazolamide and/or 400 ml of 20 per cent mannitol solution to adult patients in whom there are no medical contraindications. Both medications cause prompt diuresis. Because of the extensive diuresis from mannitol, we prefer not to use it in patients who are under general anesthesia as catheterization of the bladder may be necessary.

Operative methods

Principles of surgery

The objectives of retinal detachment surgery are to close and seal all retinal breaks and to relieve significant vitreous traction on the retina. The latter is achieved by indentation of the globe so as mechanically to support the areas involved by vitreoretinal traction. Every operation is planned to achieve these objectives while dealing with individual features of the case and attempting to minimize the risk of complications.

Alternative techniques for retinal reattachment exist, and various methods are used to deal with different anatomical situations. However, we prefer, when applicable, certain techniques – including cryotherapy to cause a chorioretinal adhesion, an episcleral exoplant for scleral indentation (scleral buckling) and avoiding drainage of subretinal fluid – because they decrease the operating time, reduce the risk of complications and minimize damage to ocular tissues.

Closure of retinal breaks is the most important objective of retinal reattachment surgery. This requires identification and accurate localization of each break during surgery. Retinal breaks are closed by apposing the edges of the torn retina to the underlying pigment epithelium, and the break is sealed by creating a surrounding chorioretinal scar.

The desired chorioretinal scar is usually caused by cryotherapy, although a similar scar can be created with diathermy or photocoagulation. Cryotherapy is preferred because it is easily applied under direct visualization, does not require scleral dissection and causes minimal damage to the sclera. When the retinal break is not highly elevated, both the retina and underlying pigment epithelium are treated with cryotherapy. It is sufficient to treat the pigment epithelium beneath the margins of the retinal break without treating the retina when the overlying retina is highly detached.

Retinal breaks in attached retina are treated with cryotherapy alone, and breaks in detached retina are treated and then brought into apposition with the pigment epithelium by indenting the wall of the eye (scleral buckling), with or without drainage of subretinal fluid. An intravitreal gas bubble can be used to assist in flattening the retina against the pigment epithelium although this is rarely necessary.

Various techniques are used to create a scleral buckle, including suturing silicone rubber to the episcleral surface (episcleral exoplant) and lamellar dissection of the sclera followed by implantation of silicone rubber or other materials within the sclera (scleral implant). We prefer episcleral exoplants for the reasons mentioned, and exoplants are readily combined with cryotherapy. Also, the location and amount of indentation from an exoplant can be easily modified during surgery if necessary.

Sometimes a scleral buckle high enough to close a retinal break(s) can be created without drainage of subretinal fluid, and the subretinal fluid absorbs after the operation. This may be due, in part, to temporary closure of the retinal break by adjacent vitreous gel followed by absorption of the subretinal fluid and settling of the retinal break onto the buckle. In other cases, it is necessary to drain the subretinal fluid to allow flattening of the retinal tear on the scleral buckle. Draining subretinal fluid not only flattens the retina but also decreases the intraocular volume so a higher scleral buckle can be created if necessary. The choice of technique can often be made preoperatively, but final decisions are made intraoperatively based on the anatomical findings and the response to various manipulations.

Surgical exposure

The operative technique requires intraocular visualization by indirect ophthalmoscopy and exposure of the sclera external to the retinal breaks. Therefore, the pupil is widely dilated preoperatively by several applications of mydriatic drops. We use 5 per cent homatropine and 10 per cent phenylephrine, with one drop of each medication given every 15 minutes for a total of six applications beginning 2 hours before the operation. The patient is instructed to keep both eyes closed between drop applications to avoid damage to the corneal epithelium from drying which sometimes occurs after use of topical phenylephrine if the eye remains open. A 0.2 ml subconjunctival injection of mydriatic solution containing 0.4 per cent homatropine, 0.5 per cent phenylephrine and procaine is given preoperatively in selected cases if there is no systemic hypertension. This is used if the pupil does not dilate widely in response to topical medications or if intraoperative pupillary constriction seems likely because: (*1*) a prolonged procedure is anticipated; (*2*) the intraocular pressure is low; or (*3*) vitreous surgery and/or intraocular air injection are to be used. The lids of the involved eye are taped closed after local anesthetic agents have been injected or before induction of general anesthesia to avoid damage to the corneal epithelium while the patient cannot voluntarily keep the eye closed.

The lashes are trimmed if this has not been done earlier. The lid margins and skin surrounding the involved eye are carefully cleaned with a mild soap, the conjunctival surfaces are lavaged with sterile saline, iodine is applied to the lids and skin around the eye, and alcohol is used to remove the iodine. Care is taken to prevent corneal damage from the iodine and alcohol. Iodine and alcohol are used because of their bactericidal effects and also because alcohol dries the skin surface and allows more firm application of an adhesive plastic drape to the lid margins and surrounding skin. Care is taken to ensure adhesion of the drape to the skin near the medial canthus and the nasolabial fold because the plastic drape is especially likely to loosen from these areas during surgery and communication could occur between the surgical field and unprepared portions of the face.

A 360° conjunctival peritomy is performed in most eyes, although sometimes an incision limited to 100–200° is performed if scleral exposure is necessary in only one or two quadrants. The incision can be made at the limbus, although we prefer an incision 2–3 mm posterior to the limbus that allows later closure of the cut conjunctival edges with multiple bites of a running suture (*Figure 9.21a*). A lateral canthotomy is performed to gain additional exposure if the palpebral fissure is narrow or if placement of scleral sutures or drainage of subretinal fluid must be performed posterior to the equator.

Blunt dissection in Tenon's space is carried out (*Figure 9.21b*). Then traction sutures of 4/0 black silk are placed beneath the insertion of each rectus muscle to assist in rotating and manipulating the globe (*Figure 9.21c,d*). Temporary disinsertion of extraocular muscles is rarely necessary, although this is occasionally done to improve visualization if exposure of a posterior portion of the globe is necessary in the meridian of a rectus muscle. The scleral surface is cleaned of its delicate attachment to Tenon's capsule in each quadrant using a cotton-tip applicator. The objective is to expose and clean the sclera in all quadrants where retinal breaks are present and/or where scleral sutures will be placed, scleral dissection performed or where subretinal fluid will be drained. Care is taken to avoid damage to the vortex veins.

Exposure of the sclera may be difficult and time consuming in reoperation for retinal detachment because of scarring and abnormal adhesions from the previous operation. In such cases the episcleral dissection may include exposure and/or removal of previous exoplant or implant material. A decision is made, based on the preoperative findings, as to which portions of the previous buckle must be removed or modified and which portions can be left intact.

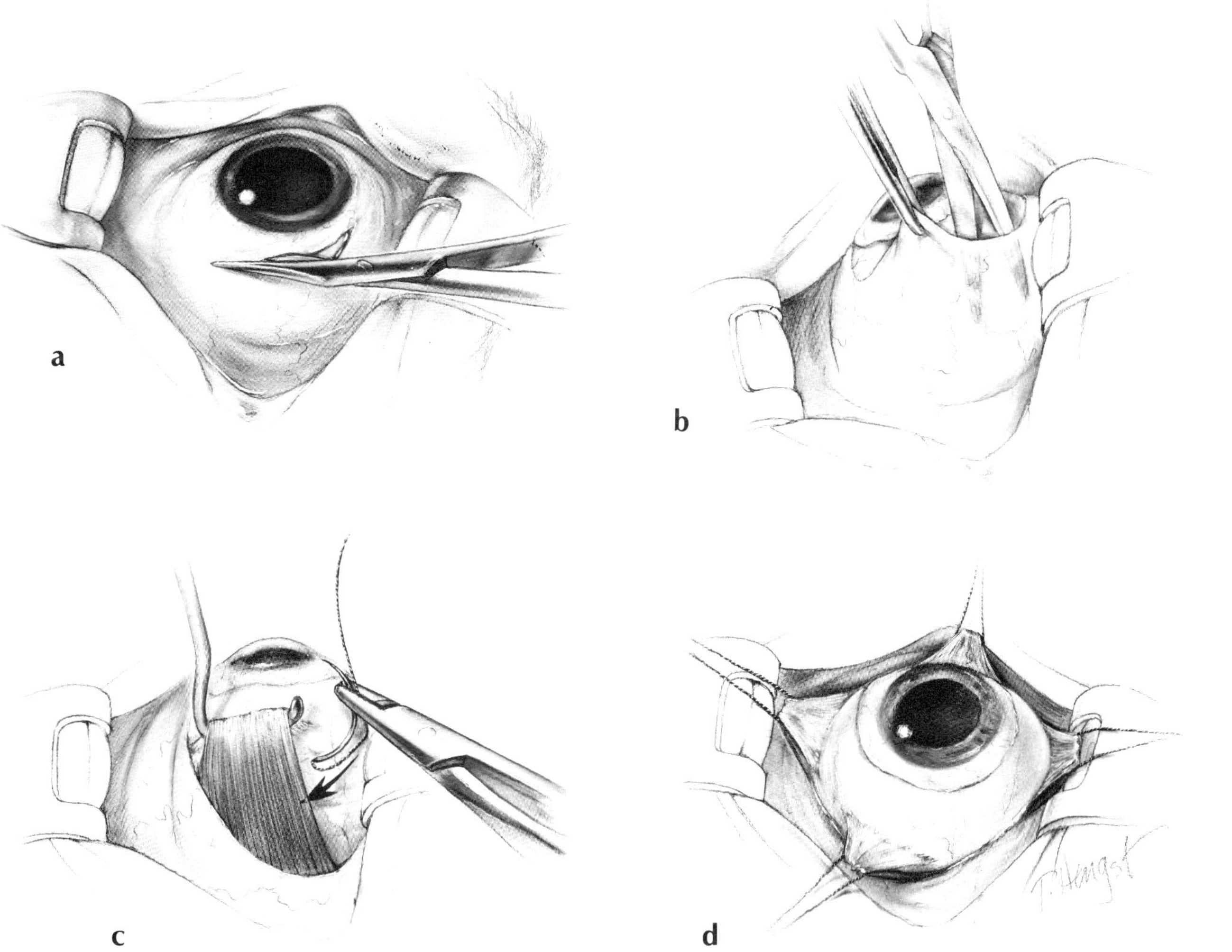

Figure 9.21 *Initial steps in retinal reattachment surgery.* **(a)** *360° conjunctival incision (peritomy) is made near the limbus and* **(b)** *blunt dissection is done with scissors in Tenon's space.* **(c,d)** *4/0 black silk sutures are placed beneath each rectus muscle to permit rotation and stabilization of globe*

Examination and localization of retinal breaks

The entire fundus is examined by indirect ophthalmoscopy including examination of the periphery by scleral indentation. The area of retinal detachment is carefully evaluated – including the extent of the detachment, the amount of elevation, whether the macula is detached or not, and the number and location of retinal breaks. Any changes occurring since the preoperative examination are noted, especially flattening of the detached retina, which may permit closure of the retinal break(s) without drainage of subretinal fluid.

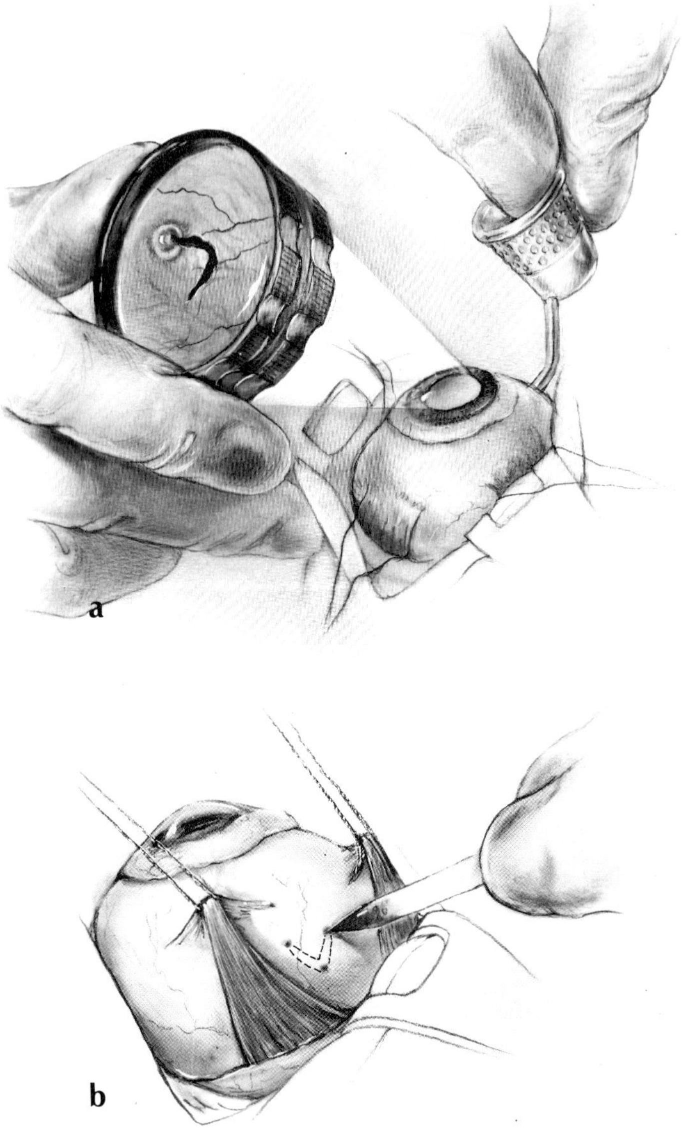

Figure 9.22 (a) *Location of each retinal break is marked on sclera using Gass thimble localizer to leave mark on sclera after pressure is released.* **(b)** *Both anterior horns and posterior edge of large horseshoe-shaped tears are marked with methylene blue applied with a tapered wooden applicator*

Usually the position of each retinal break is then marked on the sclera. The sclera is indented beneath each break to identify its precise location, and the sclera is then marked with dye or diathermy. Small retinal breaks are marked with a single spot, and larger horseshoe-shaped tears are marked with three spots that include the most posterior extent and each of the two anterior horns (*Figure 9.22*). During this time the surgeon decides whether the pigment epithelium can be positioned near the retinal break by scleral indentation alone, and this may determine whether later drainage of subretinal fluid is necessary. When there are multiple anterior retinal breaks and an encircling scleral buckle is used, it may be unnecessary to localize all breaks.

The location of other important areas to be supported by scleral buckling are also marked on the sclera, including areas of prominent vitreoretinal traction such as some zones of lattice degeneration. Thus, the location of each retinal break and each important area of vitreoretinal traction is identified so that a scleral buckle of suitable size and configuration can be prepared. The junctions between attached and detached portions of the retina may also be marked. Using this method when an encircling band is planned allows optimum positioning of the band in each quadrant. The band is often used to support the posterior aspect of zones of prominent vitreoretinal traction, which are often in an equatorial location or pre-equatorial along the posterior margin of the vitreous base. It is unnecessary for an encircling band to follow the largest circumference of the globe, and the band can be located anterior to the equator in all quadrants if it is firmly secured to the sclera.

Treatment of retinal breaks

All retinal breaks are then treated with photocoagulation, diathermy or cryotherapy with the exception of macular holes in eyes with other peripheral holes. Photocoagulation is rarely used intraoperatively, although occasionally posterior retinal breaks are treated with photocoagulation after drainage of subretinal fluid flattens the break against the pigment epithelium. When diathermy is used to treat retinal breaks, it is applied to the scleral bed after lamellar dissection of the sclera as described later. However, most often cryotherapy is used while monitoring the location and effect of each application with indirect ophthalmoscopy.

Each retinal break is surrounded by a 1–2 mm zone of contiguous cryotherapy applications while avoiding refreezing of the same tissue. The probe is moved from one position to the next while monitoring the location of the tip as determined by the indentation seen by indirect ophthalmoscopy (*Figure 9.23*). Each freezing application is terminated as soon as its effect is visible in the pigment epithelium or the overlying retina. If the pigment epithelium freezes, as evidenced by a slight whitening, but the overlying detached retina does not quickly freeze, then the application should be terminated without waiting for the retina to whiten; otherwise a prolonged freeze will occur, producing excessive choroidal damage. Often, indentation caused by the cryoprobe positions the pigment epithelium near the retina, and the freezing effect involves the overlying retina, causing the retina to become

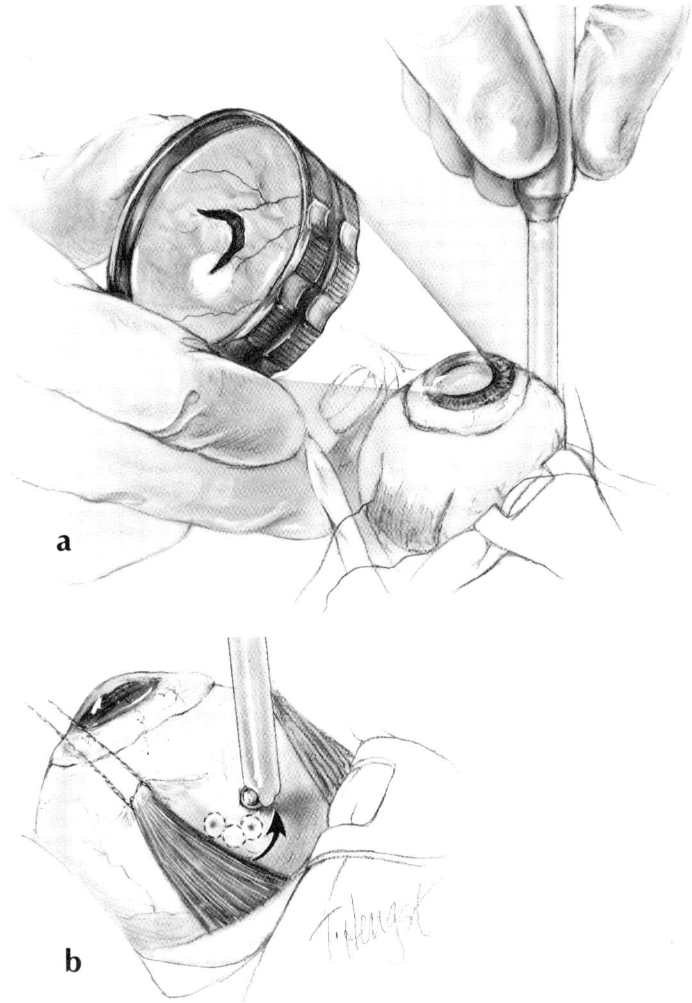

Figure 9.23 *Retinal break(s) are treated with cryotherapy, and probe is moved from one location to next until all margins have been treated*

a distinct white color. When the choroid and pigment epithelium can be positioned sufficiently near the retina so the retina is immediately involved by the freeze, this suggests that scleral buckling alone without drainage of subretinal fluid may be adequate.

Suspicious areas of the retina that may harbor breaks are also treated by cryotherapy, and sometimes it is possible to determine whether or not a retinal break is present by the visible features of the freeze. A retinal break appears dark and is highlighted when the surrounding retina turns white from the cryotherapy. However, spots of blood and pigment sometimes give a similar appearance, and it may be impossible to determine whether a small retinal break is present despite careful observation during cryotherapy. Occasionally pigment is released from the pigment epithelium and passes through the retinal break during cryotherapy. This is clear evidence of a full-thickness retinal defect.

In some eyes it may be impossible to see retinal breaks because they are small, obscured by opacities in the media, or because of other factors. Even though breaks are seen in other locations, there may be portions of the retina that cannot be visualized well enough to rule out the presence of additional retinal breaks. In these cases, cryotherapy can be applied to the areas, within the limits of the detachment, that are most likely to harbor retinal breaks. Cryotherapy is often applied between the ora serrata and the equator throughout the limits of the detachment, where visualization is inadequate and where a retinal break could be present (*Figure 9.24*). This generalized therapy is used only if repeated preoperative and intraoperative examinations fail to identify specific retinal breaks.

Cryotherapy is also applied around areas of abnormal, strong vitreoretinal adhesion, such as zones of lattice degeneration. Contiguous applications are made to cause a chorioretinal adhesion surrounding such areas.

In summary, cryotherapy is used to treat specific retinal breaks, possible retinal breaks and certain areas of abnormal vitreoretinal adhesion and/or traction.

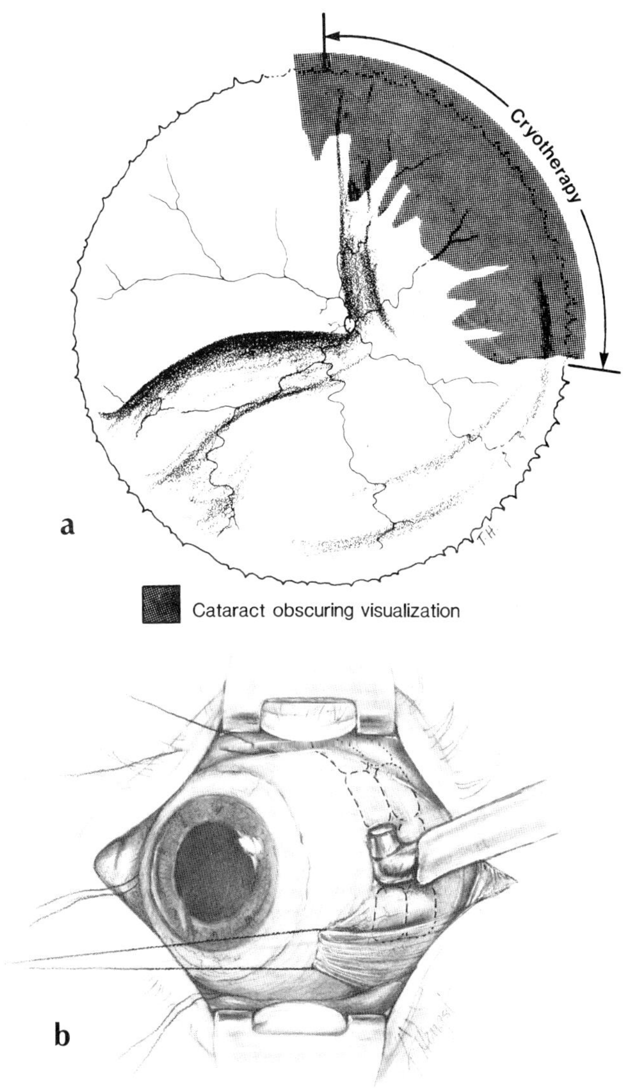

Figure 9.24 **(a)** *Contiguous rows of cryotherapy applied to peripheral retina throughout limits of detachment where retinal break is likely and visualization is limited due to cataract or vitreous hemorrhage.* **(b)** *Treatment is done with flat end of cryoprobe to increase surface area of each application. Each freeze is monitored by indirect ophthalmoscopy and freezing effect can be seen through peripheral opacities even though visualization is not adequate to see retinal break*

Closure of retinal breaks

A scleral buckle is prepared to support all retinal breaks and usually any other areas treated with cryotherapy. The configuration of the scleral buckle depends on the number, size, location and other physical features of the retinal breaks as well as the locations of any zones of abnormal vitreoretinal traction. Various materials can be used to create the scleral buckle, although specially fabricated pieces of silicone rubber are now used almost exclusively. Buckling effects of different widths and heights are determined by the size and shape of the piece of silicone chosen and by how it is secured to the eyewall.

Various kinds of silicone are used, including silicone rubber sponge and solid silicone rubber. These are shaped into bands, grooved pieces, hemispheres, etc. and are constructed in various widths and thicknesses (*Figure 9.25*). We prefer silicone sponge to create separate radially

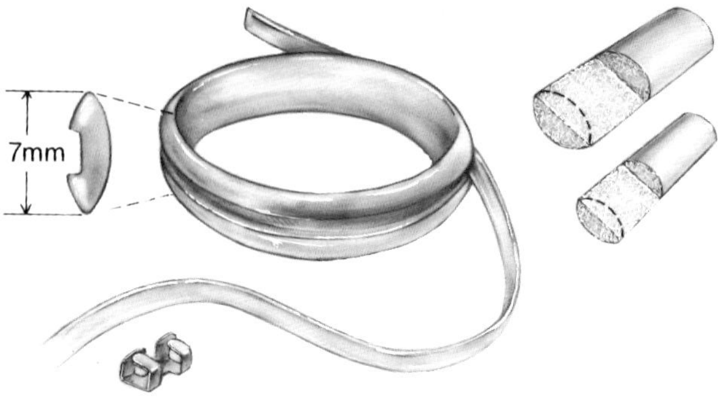

Figure 9.25 *Commonly used pieces of hard silicone rubber and silicone sponge for episcleral exoplant technique. Grooved piece (7.5 mm wide) with convex inner surface is often combined with a narrow (2.5 mm) encircling band that is secured with a double tantalum clip. Pieces of sponge 5 or 7 mm wide are often cut lengthwise, and the convex surface applied to sclera*

oriented scleral buckles, and sponge can be used to encircle the globe if a broad and high scleral buckle is necessary. Solid silicone rubber bands are used to encircle the globe if a narrow buckle is needed, and this can be combined with underlying grooved pieces of solid silicone rubber to create circumferentially oriented buckles of greater width extending partially or entirely around the eye. In most cases, a suitable buckle can be created with various combinations of silicone pieces, using either sponge or solid rubber materials or combinations of the two. The materials chosen depend on the experience and preferences of the surgeon.

Scleral buckles may be radially or circumferentially oriented, or a combination of the two may be used. Radial buckles reduce the amount of radial retinal folding that is sometimes seen with circumferential scleral buckles. Single retinal breaks are often supported on a radially oriented exoplant secured to the sclera by mattress-type sutures. Multiple retinal breaks in different quadrants may be supported by a radially oriented exoplant beneath each break, with or without an encircling silicone-rubber band.

Alternatively, multiple retinal breaks in the same or different quadrants may be supported on a circumferentially oriented scleral buckle that can be extended around the globe to support retinal breaks or areas of vitreoretinal traction in three or more quadrants. A circumferential buckle of 180° or less may be created with only a segmental piece of silicone rubber and sutures, whereas a circumferential buckle of 180° or more is usually created with a piece of grooved silicone combined with an overlying encircling band. An encircling band ensures a permanent buckling effect and it reduces the chance of later exposure of the silicone material as is sometimes seen with localized exoplants. Also, the encircling band creates a narrow buckling effect that is useful to support areas of vitreoretinal traction in other quadrants, and this is commonly used beneath the posterior vitreous base in aphakic eyes.

The width of both radial and circumferentially oriented scleral buckles is selected to support all retinal breaks and areas of surrounding cryotherapy. The elevation of the buckle should be enough to position the treated pigment epithelium near the retinal break and to relieve any vitreous traction. The height chosen for the buckle also depends on whether or not subretinal fluid is drained. After the eye is softened by drainage of subretinal fluid, it is easier to produce a higher buckle. However, a lower buckle height may be all that is needed after the retina has been flattened by release of the subretinal fluid. We prefer using the minimum buckle height necessary to relieve vitreous traction and to close the retinal breaks, although this varies considerably from case to case.

Episcleral exoplants

Silicone rubber material used to create a scleral buckle is usually secured to the sclera by overlying mattress-type sutures. These sutures indent the exoplant and underlying eyewall. The buckle height is determined by the distance between the intrascleral limbs of each mattress suture and by how tight the sutures are tied. A low buckling effect is produced by sutures about 2 mm wider than the silicone exoplant, and a high scleral buckle is produced by sutures 3–4 mm wider than the silicone rubber.

The intrascleral suture limbs are placed parallel to the meridian of the retinal break when a radially oriented buckle is needed (*Figure 9.26*) and parallel to the limbus

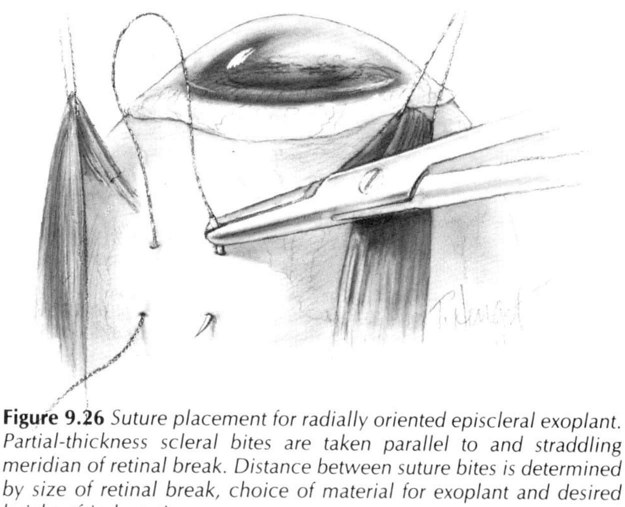

Figure 9.26 *Suture placement for radially oriented episcleral exoplant. Partial-thickness scleral bites are taken parallel to and straddling meridian of retinal break. Distance between suture bites is determined by size of retinal break, choice of material for exoplant and desired height of indentation*

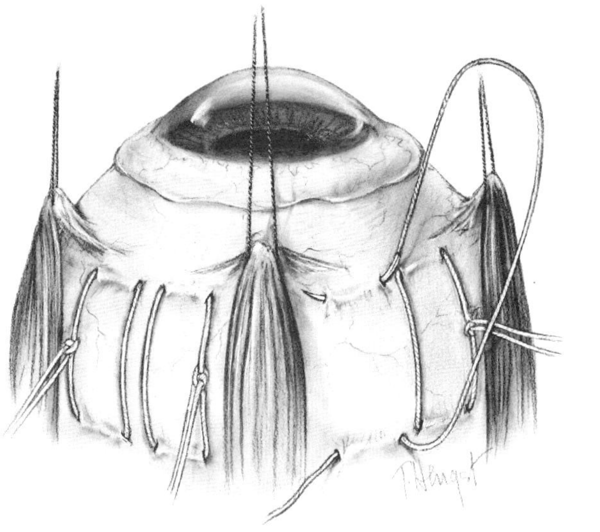

Figure 9.27 *Suture placement for broad circumferentially oriented scleral buckle. Partial-thickness scleral bites are made parallel to the limbus. Two mattress-shaped sutures are placed in each quadrant where buckling effect is needed*

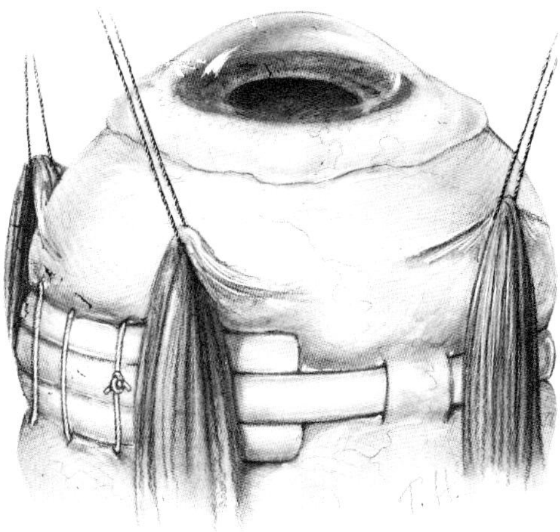

Figure 9.29 *Grooved solid silicone rubber combined with encircling silicone-rubber band to create circumferentially oriented scleral buckle. Indentation is caused by overlying mattress-type scleral sutures plus effect of silicone-rubber band. Band passes through partial-thickness scleral tunnels where the broader grooved exoplant is not used*

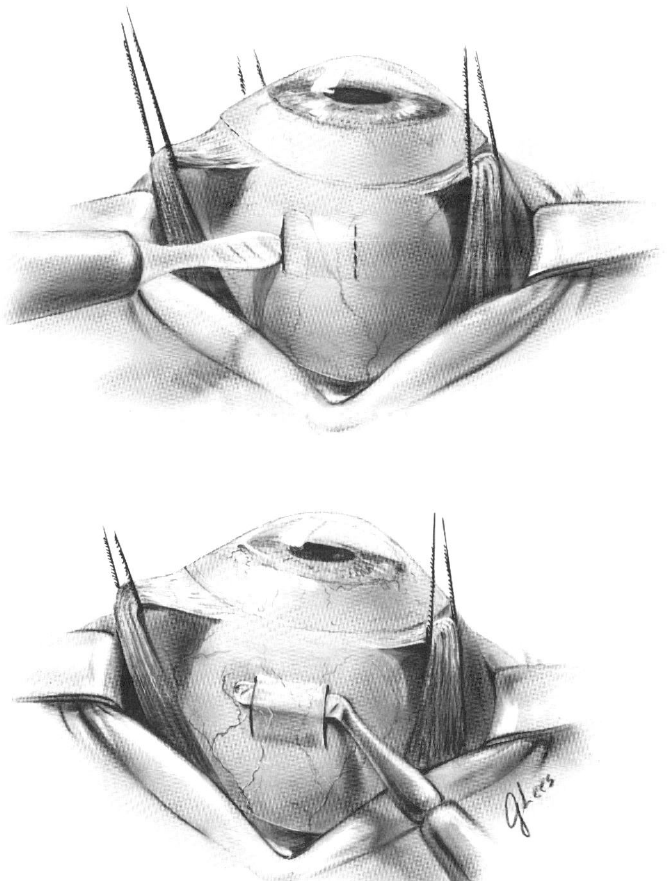

Figure 9.28 *Partial-thickness scleral tunnels used to secure encircling band in the proper anteroposterior location. Radial incisions are made and tunnel created with convex Castroviejo corneal dissector*

for a circumferentially oriented buckle (*Figure 9.27*). When a silicone-rubber band is used, this may be secured to the sclera using partial-thickness scleral tunnels in areas where there is no underlying larger exoplant (*Figures 9.28* and *9.29*). The silicone-rubber material is then positioned beneath the sutures and/or scleral tunnels.

Intrascleral implants

Partial-thickness (lamellar) scleral dissection may be combined with diathermy to treat the choroid and pigment epithelium and with implantation of silicone material within the sclera to create a buckling effect. The bed of the scleral dissection must be large enough so that the buckle supports all edges of each retinal break. A circumferential half-thickness scleral incision is usually made in an anteroposterior location coinciding with the most posterior edge of each retinal break. The dissection is extended anteriorly and posteriorly to create a bed that extends about 3 mm beyond the anterior and posterior edges of the retinal break(s). Grasping the scleral flap with forceps facilitates this dissection, and an effort is made to maintain uniform scleral thickness in the bed of the dissection (*Figure 9.30a,b*). Often a blue color from the choroid is seen through the thin inner scleral fibers.

The scleral dissection is extended circumferentially beyond the meridians where the retinal breaks are present. The dissection may be terminated or brought into a more superficial plane in the region of the long posterior ciliary vessels and nerves. Damage to the intrascleral portion of the vortex veins is to be avoided, and the scleral flap may be notched in these locations to avoid cutting the veins while permitting sufficient posterior placement of the scleral buckle to support all retinal breaks.

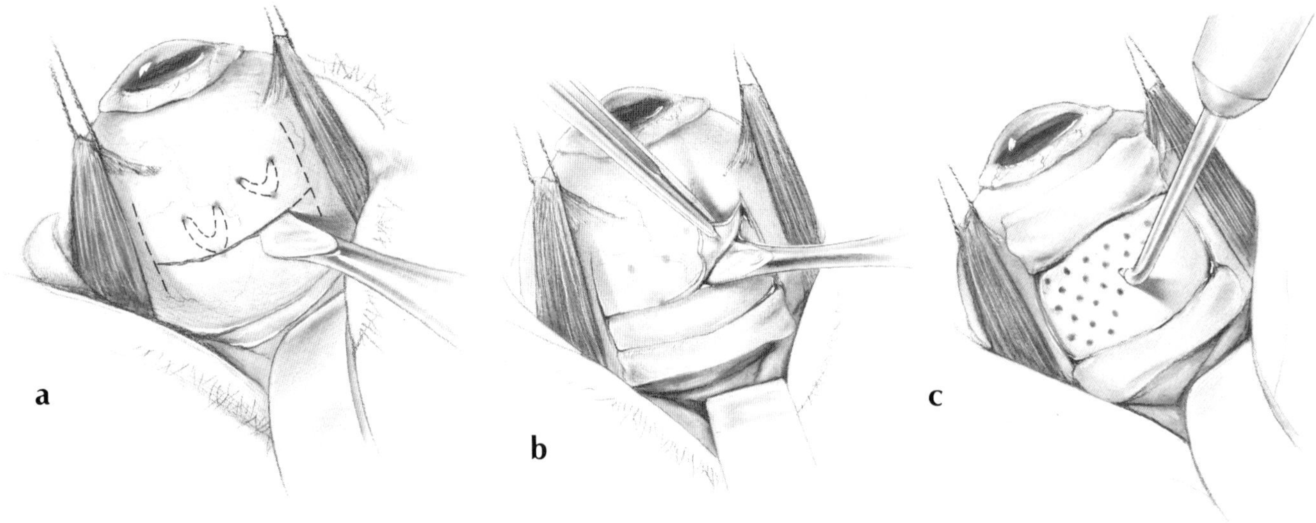

Diathermy is applied in alternating, staggered rows in the bed of the scleral dissection (*Figure 9.30c*). This is done with a blunt electrode, and the energy level is set so that a moderate coagulation effect with slight shrinkage of the underlying sclera is seen after each application which lasts about 1.0 second. Diathermy is applied throughout the entire bed of the scleral dissection so that the pigment epithelium beneath and surrounding each retinal break is treated. Usually the intraocular appearance of the diathermy applications is not monitored by indirect ophthalmoscopy. The intensity of treatment is determined by prior experience, the thickness of the inner scleral bed and the visible external effect.

Silicone-rubber material is placed in the bed of the scleral dissection, and subretinal fluid may be drained in the bed of the dissection by making a horizontally oriented incision and penetrating the choroid with a sharp electrode. The edges of the scleral flaps are then closed with multiple interrupted mattress-type sutures (*Figure 9.30d*). The sutures are tightened, using temporary knots initially, so that the buckle can be examined by indirect ophthalmoscopy to make certain it is of proper height and correctly positioned. Rarely, anterior or posterior extension of the scleral dissection is necessary with additional diathermy. Sometimes additional pieces of silicone rubber are placed in the bed of the scleral dissection to create a higher buckling effect or a different configuration before permanently tying the sutures to close the scleral flaps.

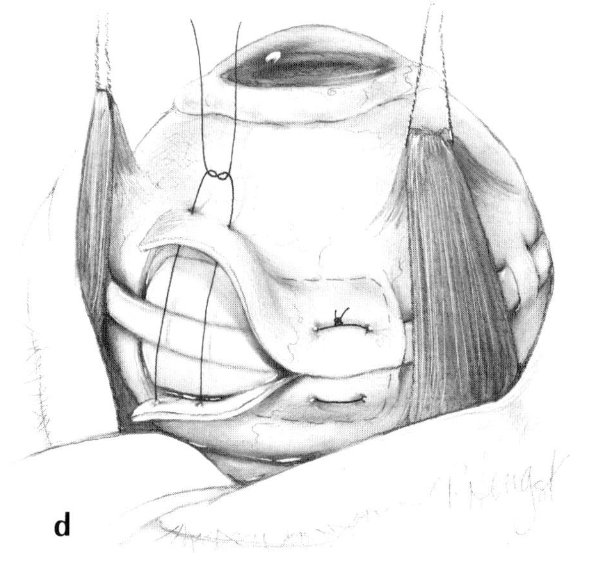

Figure 9.30 *Scleral dissection and diathermy technique for scleral buckling with intrascleral implant.* **(a,b)** *Flaps of partial-thickness sclera are dissected to create bed with adequate margins on all sides of retinal breaks.* **(c)** *Diathermy is applied to scleral bed.* **(d)** *Scleral flaps are sutured to indent intrascleral silicone rubber implant after release of subretinal fluid*

Management of subretinal fluid

After treating the retinal breaks and preparing for the scleral buckle, a final decision is made on whether or not to drain subretinal fluid. The scleral sutures straddling the retinal break(s) may be temporarily tightened, and the fundus is then examined by indirect ophthalmoscopy to determine whether the retinal break(s) are closed or nearly closed by the buckle effect. If the scleral buckle is not in the proper position, the sutures are replaced, and the exoplant repositioned to produce a buckling effect directly beneath the retinal break(s).

Experience is required to determine whether the operation can be terminated at this point without drainage of subretinal fluid. If the edges of the retinal break(s) are mostly supported by the scleral buckle, drainage of subretinal fluid is unnecessary even though the retinal breaks may not be entirely flat on the buckle, and considerable subretinal fluid is present (*Figure 9.31*). However, drainage of subretinal fluid is usually performed in eyes with: (*1*) severe vitreoretinal traction with or without massive periretinal proliferation; (*2*) longstanding retinal detachment with viscous subretinal fluid; (*3*) inferior retinal breaks; and (*4*) multiple retinal breaks unless they are located near the ora serrata in the superior quadrants or unless the amount of subretinal fluid is small. Conversely, drainage of subretinal fluid is often unnecessary in eyes with one or more small retinal breaks located near the ora serrata in the superior quadrants, or in eyes in which nearly all of the subretinal fluid was absorbed preoperatively during the period of bedrest with bilateral bandages.

In eyes where drainage of subretinal fluid may not be necessary, the scleral buckle is elevated to the desired height, and the proximity of the retinal break(s) to the buckle is re-evaluated. In such cases, additional elevation of the buckle can be obtained by softening the eye further. This is done by anterior chamber paracentesis in phakic eyes and in some aphakic eyes that have an intact anterior hyaloid face. This technique is especially effective in phakic eyes with megalocornea or buphthalmos and in certain eyes with high myopia, because a large amount of fluid can often be removed from the limbus without significant shallowing of the anterior chamber due to fluid passing anteriorly from the vitreous cavity.

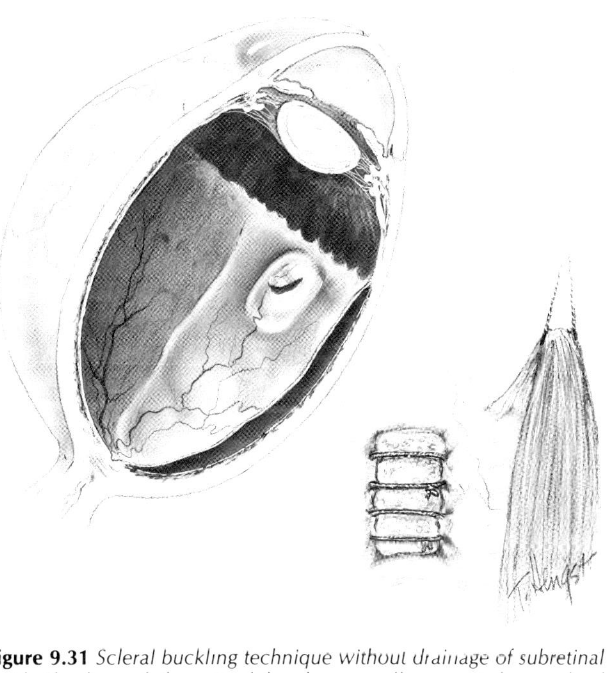

Figure 9.31 *Scleral buckling technique without drainage of subretinal fluid. If edges of the retinal break are well supported on scleral indentation, drainage of subretinal fluid is unnecessary and fluid absorbs quickly during the postoperative period*

An anterior chamber paracentesis is performed with a knife introduced through the peripheral cornea. The tip remains over the iris and does not enter the pupillary space. The blade is tilted to permit release of aqueous humor, and the knife is withdrawn when the anterior chamber becomes shallow (*Figure 9.32*). The amount of fluid that can be removed with this technique is variable, and the anterior chamber deepens again in 5–10 minutes.

Increased height of the scleral buckle can also be achieved without draining subretinal fluid by tightening the scleral sutures one at a time and monitoring the intraocular pressure (IOP) to make sure it is not extremely high before tying the next suture. The IOP is checked by

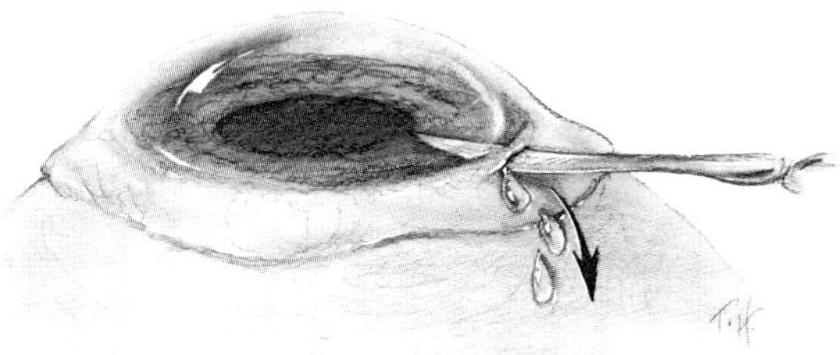

Figure 9.32 *Anterior chamber paracentesis to soften eye during retinal reattachment surgery. A 3 mm Ziegler knife is passed tangentially into anterior chamber with needle tip over iris surface. Blade is tilted to permit outflow of aqueous humor*

indentation tonometry, and the central retinal artery is periodically observed by indirect ophthalmoscopy to make certain it is not closed. If no pulsations of the central retinal artery are present, digital pressure on the globe is used to cause pulsations. In this way one can be certain that the central retinal artery is open rather than flow being already interrupted due to the elevated IOP. If the retinal breaks remain quite elevated over the buckle despite these measures, or if further softening of the globe is required to produce an adequate buckling effect, then subretinal fluid is drained.

A sclerotomy site is chosen for release (drainage) of subretinal fluid in an accessible location where there is sufficient fluid to drain safely. A number of factors are considered in selecting the location for drainage of subretinal fluid, including: (*1*) the configuration of the detachment and the distribution of the subretinal fluid; (*2*) features of vitreoretinal traction; (*3*) the location of the retinal break(s) and the configuration of the proposed buckle; (*4*) vascularity of the choroid; and (*5*) ease of exposure for preparation of the drainage site and for monitoring intraocular changes by indirect ophthalmoscopy during drainage. The most important factor is the height of the detachment, and drainage is usually done where the retina is most highly detached.

A good location for drainage of subretinal fluid is under a zone of peripheral vitreoretinal traction or epiretinal membrane formation because the retina tends to flatten elsewhere first, allowing more complete removal of the subretinal fluid with a lower chance of the retina becoming incarcerated in the wound. The site for drainage is usually selected as far away from the retinal break(s) as possible, to minimize the chance of additional fluid passing from the vitreous cavity through the breaks and into the subretinal space.

Usually a location for drainage of subretinal fluid is selected at the equator or slightly anterior, and the preferred meridians are just superior or inferior to the horizontal rectus muscles. The choroid has smaller vessels in these areas, so there is less chance of serious hemorrhage and external exposure is often better. Draining in a nasal quadrant is advantageous because, if the procedure is complicated by subretinal hemorrhage, the chance of blood accumulating under the macula is reduced. However, this complication is rare, and exposure is often easier if drainage is performed in a temporal quadrant. When an encircling scleral buckle is planned, we prefer to drain so that the sclerotomy site will be supported on the buckle.

However, unless complications occur at the drainage site a separate buckle is not used in this location.

In certain situations it is desirable to perform drainage of subretinal fluid posterior to the scleral buckle. This is sometimes done during reoperations when the previous scleral buckle is only to be modified rather than removed and when the retina is flat over the previous buckle. Also, a posterior drainage site may be used when it is necessary to drain subretinal fluid near a large open retinal break. In such cases the scleral buckle can be elevated as drainage proceeds, so as to close the retinal break and prevent passage of additional fluid through the retinal break into the subretinal space.

The proposed location for release of subretinal fluid is inspected externally to be certain that the sclera is free of episcleral tissue. Ideally the eye is positioned so that while the external opening of the sclerotomy is visible the fundus is also visible with indirect ophthalmoscopy without changing the position of the globe. The sclerotomy site and the fundus are viewed successively by the surgeon or simultaneously by the surgeon and surgical assistant. The lid speculum may be removed if use of separate retractors gives better exposure of a posterior drainage site. However, exogenous pressure on the eye from the lids or instruments is avoided during release of the subretinal fluid to avoid increased intraocular pressure and incarceration of the retina in the drainage site.

The proposed location for drainage is viewed by indirect ophthalmoscopy with the eye in the same position that will be used during actual release of the fluid. This ensures that the subretinal fluid does not shift so that the retina becomes flat at the proposed drainage site. The sclera is indented at the proposed drainage site to assess further the amount of subretinal fluid present. The pattern of the retinal vessels in that area is memorized so that the site can be quickly identified during drainage of the subretinal fluid.

A radial scleral incision about 3.0 mm long is then made to expose a knuckle of the choroid (*Figure 9.33a*), and a mattress-type suture of 6/0 black silk is placed in the lips of the sclerotomy wound at the ends of the incision. The exposed choroidal tissue is treated with surface diathermy (*Figure 9.33b*). This is done until all vessels have been closed as determined by direct visualization while the choroid is transilluminated through the pupil. This is conveniently done by looking at the sclerotomy externally through a condensing lens (indirect ophthalmoscopy lens) that provides increased magnification while the assistant views the fundus in the area of the sclerotomy by indirect ophthalmoscopy to provide the transillumination effect.

The avascular portion of the choroid is then penetrated by a sharp needle or diathermy electrode held nearly tangential to the sclera to avoid retinal damage (*Figure 9.33c,d*). Initially the subretinal fluid is permitted to drain

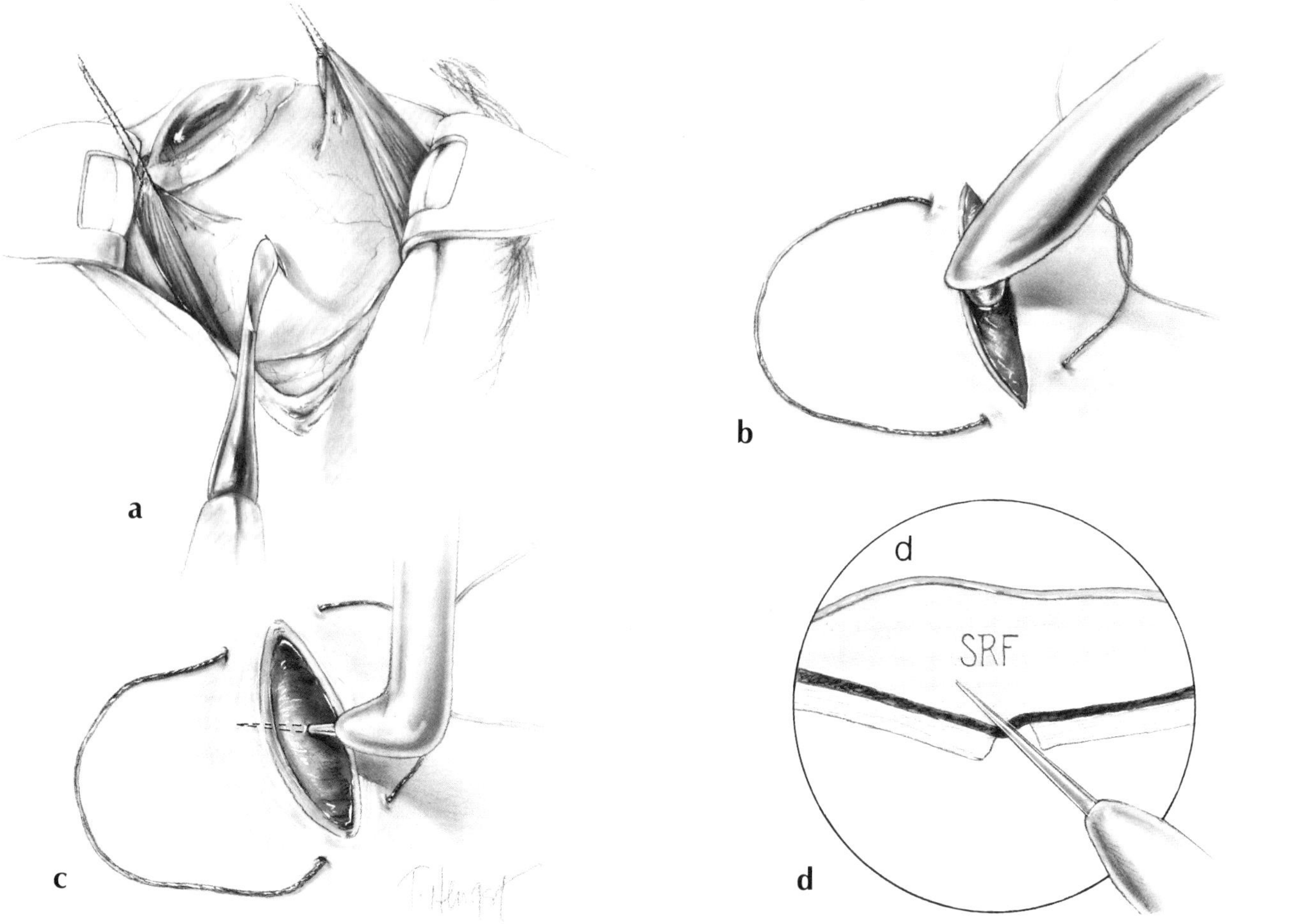

Figure 9.33 *Drainage of subretinal fluid (SRF).* **(a)** *Radial incision (3 mm) is made through sclera to expose the choroid.* **(b)** *A 6/0 silk mattress suture is placed for later wound closure, and diathermy is applied to close vessels in exposed choroid.* **(c,d)** *Choroid is penetrated with sharp electrode passed into the subretinal space and oriented tangentially to reduce chance of retinal damage*

spontaneously without external pressure on the globe. As the globe softens, cotton-tip applicators are placed around the eye between the conjunctiva and sclera to maintain normal intraocular pressure (*Figure 9.34*). These

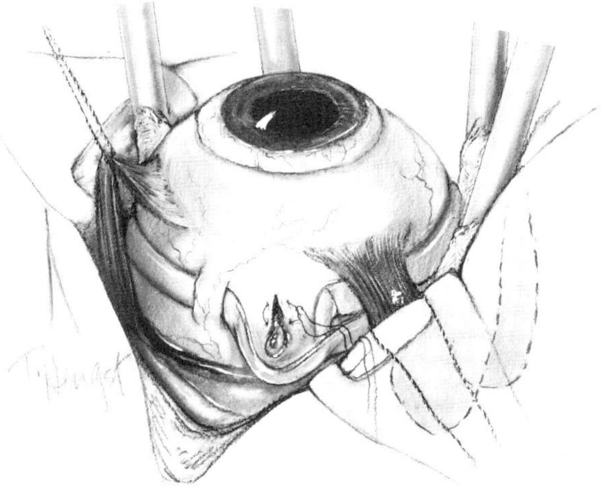

Figure 9.34 *Moistened, cotton-tip applicators placed around the globe to indent sclera and maintain normal intraocular pressure as subretinal fluid drains*

applicators can be placed beneath retinal breaks to indent the sclera and close the breaks, and this minimizes further seepage of vitreous fluid into the subretinal space. Alternatively, scleral sutures on the opposite side of the eye can be tightened over the scleral buckle as the globe softens. Care is taken to avoid excessive elevation of the IOP, which can cause incarceration of the retina at the sclerotomy site when the retina flattens.

Intraocular features of drainage of subretinal fluid are also monitored using indirect ophthalmoscopy. If an open retinal break is present near the drainage site, it can be closed by indenting the sclera with a cotton-tip applicator as drainage proceeds. Often the retina bobbles as it flattens, and this is an indication that drainage is continuing. Also, movement of pigmented debris may be seen in the subretinal space as drainage proceeds. A cotton-tip applicator can be used to displace subretinal fluid from other locations toward the drainage area if the retina remains elevated elsewhere. However, this must be done before the retina is completely flat over the sclerotomy.

As the retina settles near the sclerotomy, the IOP is monitored by digital palpation to be sure that the globe is soft. Sometimes gentle indentation of the sclera just anterior to the sclerotomy aids in draining residual portions of the subretinal fluid. Indentation of the sclerotomy while fluid is draining is avoided because this can prematurely flatten the retina at the sclerotomy and prevent further drainage.

Usually the retina settles evenly throughout the area of detachment as subretinal fluid is drained, even though there may be large amounts of subretinal fluid in opposite quadrants and despite an anterior location of the drainage site. However, in longstanding detachments with viscous subretinal fluid, the retina may settle at the drainage site while a large amount of fluid remains elsewhere. In such cases multiple sclerotomies may be necessary to achieve adequate flattening and closure of all retinal breaks. Also, in many cases a small amount of subretinal fluid remains posteriorly after drainage is completed. This usually absorbs soon postoperatively. The presence of this fluid may be helpful by permitting slower settling of the delicate outer segments of the photoreceptor elements against the pigment epithelium.

The mattress-type suture is immediately tightened to close the sclerotomy when the retina is flat at that location. Then the sclerotomy is indented as the area is viewed by indirect ophthalmoscopy to be certain that retinal incarceration has not occurred. If the retina is incarcerated, with or without an apparent retinal hole, the sclerotomy is treated with cryotherapy and supported on a scleral buckle.

Drainage can be limited to a smaller amount of subretinal fluid and the sclerotomy suture tightened when the eye is soft enough to permit creation of a suitable scleral buckle. However, once the decision to drain fluid has been made, we usually prefer to drain as much of the subretinal fluid as possible, and drainage is permitted to continue until the retina becomes flat at the sclerotomy site. Additional drainage sites can be made if drainage through the initial sclerotomy is inadequate. However, every effort is made to achieve satisfactory drainage through the initial sclerotomy, which has been chosen at the best location with an adequate amount of subretinal fluid.

Adjusting the height of the scleral buckle

Remaining scleral sutures are then tightened to create the scleral buckling effect. Usually these are only temporarily tied so that the buckle height can be adjusted further after examining the retina. If the eye is excessively soft, even after tightening the scleral sutures, saline or air is injected into the vitreous cavity to restore normal intraocular volume and pressure. Saline is used if the retina has settled well and the retinal breaks are flat on the scleral buckle. In other cases air is injected to provide temporary intraocular tamponade. However, visualization of the fundus may be difficult after air injection unless a single bubble is obtained. Therefore, other decisions requiring visualization of the fundus are made before air injection.

Both saline and air are injected through the middle of the pars plana using a 27 or 30 gauge needle (*Figure 9.35*). This is done in an area where the pars plana epithelium

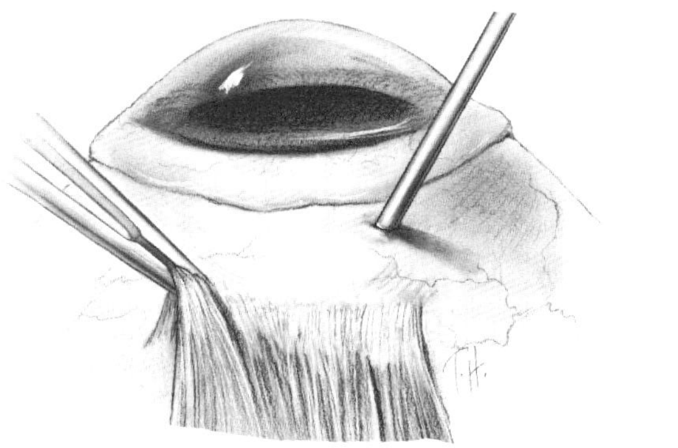

Figure 9.35 *Saline or gas injection to restore normal intraocular volume and tension after excessive drainage of subretinal fluid. Eye is stabilized by grasping rectus muscle, and 27 gauge needle is introduced through mid-pars plana and directed toward center of vitreous cavity*

was not detached preoperatively. If the eye is both phakic and especially soft so that an injection through the pars plana might damage the lens, a partial-thickness circumferentially oriented scleral incision is first made 3 mm posterior to the limbus using a sharp blade. The needle is introduced through this incision while the edge of the incision is grasped with forceps (*Figure 9.36*). This stabilizes the eye, and the partial-depth incision reduces the thickness of sclera that must be penetrated by the needle. Care is taken to avoid damage to the lens, and the needle tip is visualized in the vitreous cavity before injection. Saline is injected slowly while the IOP is monitored, whereas air is injected rapidly to obtain a single large bubble rather than many small bubbles that would interfere with visualization of the fundus. If the needle tip is not placed deeply into the vitreous cavity there is also an increased chance of getting a single large bubble.

The desired height for the scleral buckle will have been chosen previously, and this determines the width of the scleral suture bites if an episcleral exoplant technique is used, or the size and shape of the scleral dissection area if an intrascleral implant is planned. However, the height, position and shape of the buckle may be modified, especially if an episcleral exoplant is used. If the retina flattens well against the pigment epithelium during drainage of subretinal fluid, it may be decided to reduce the height of the buckle unless prominent vitreoretinal traction is also present. If a circumferentially oriented scleral buckle causes excessive radial folding of the retina, this effect can be reduced by lowering the buckle height. The scleral sutures and/or encircling band are loosened, and saline is injected through the pars plana into the vitreous cavity to increase intraocular volume and to restore normal IOP. Conversely, if the edges of the retinal breaks are still elevated above the scleral buckle, the buckle height can be increased further.

Sometimes other modifications in the shape or location of the scleral buckle are necessary, and these are most easily made if an episcleral exoplant is used. Retinal breaks on a circumferential scleral buckle are sometimes involved in radial folds, giving the break a 'fishmouth' appearance. This may result in recurrent detachment if the radial fold extends across the posterior slope of the buckle and communicates with residual subretinal fluid posterior to the buckle. In such cases the height of the scleral buckle may be reduced as mentioned before. If the problem persists, the buckle can be modified by placing an additional radially oriented support under the retinal break (*Figure 9.37*). Alternatively, photocoagulation can be applied to the radial fold intraoperatively, or this can be done postoperatively if persistent leakage occurs from the tear. Photocoagulation usually results in flattening of the fold in 5–15 days.

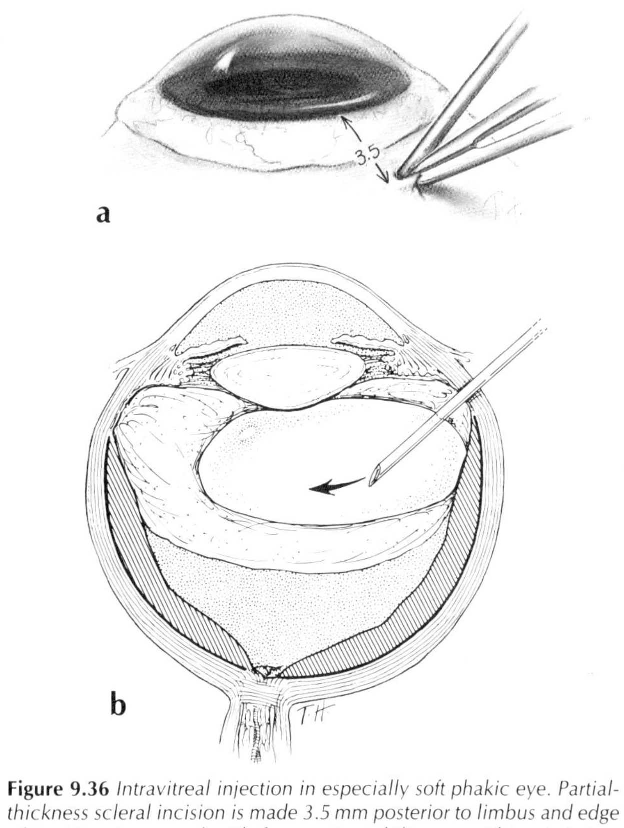

Figure 9.36 *Intravitreal injection in especially soft phakic eye. Partial-thickness scleral incision is made 3.5 mm posterior to limbus and edge of incision is grasped with forceps to stabilize eye. This minimizes force necessary to penetrate remaining sclera and avoids possible lens damage*

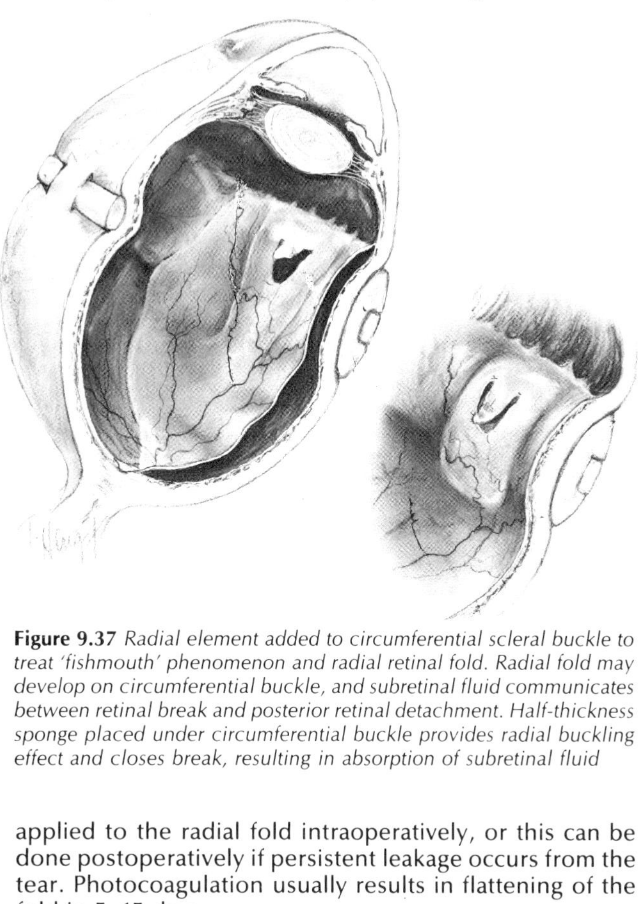

Figure 9.37 *Radial element added to circumferential scleral buckle to treat 'fishmouth' phenomenon and radial retinal fold. Radial fold may develop on circumferential buckle, and subretinal fluid communicates between retinal break and posterior retinal detachment. Half-thickness sponge placed under circumferential buckle provides radial buckling effect and closes break, resulting in absorption of subretinal fluid*

If the scleral buckle is not sufficiently wide or properly located to support all edges of each retinal break, the buckle is moved or modified by adding a piece of silicone rubber as necessary. If retinal breaks remain open and are complicated by immediate reaccumulation of subretinal fluid despite a properly located scleral buckle of desired height, further subretinal fluid can be drained posterior to the previous buckle and then air injected into the vitreous cavity. An intraocular bubble provides tamponade of the retinal breaks and tends to flatten any radial folds (*Figure 9.38*).

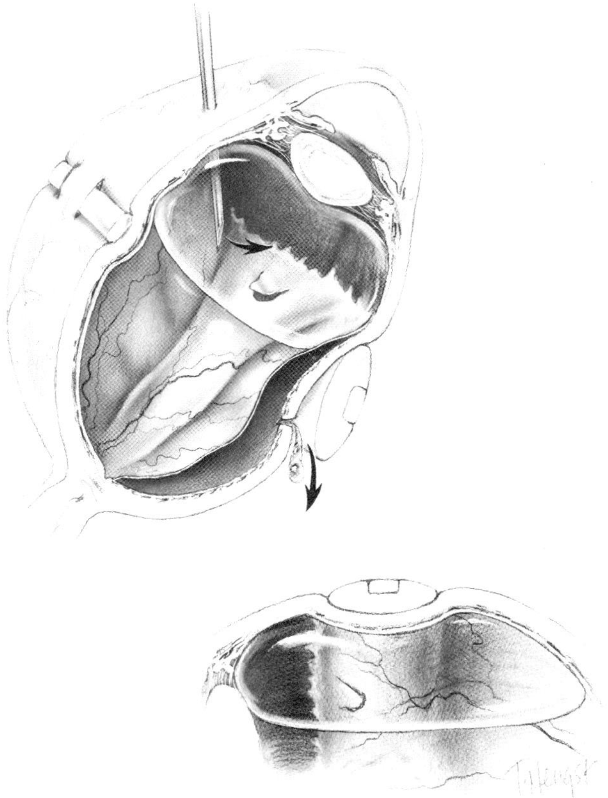

Figure 9.38 *Intravitreal air injection to treat radial retinal folding associated with circumferential scleral buckle. Air is injected into vitreous cavity and patient positioned so that retinal break is flattened against scleral buckle. This results in closure of the break and absorption of subretinal fluid*

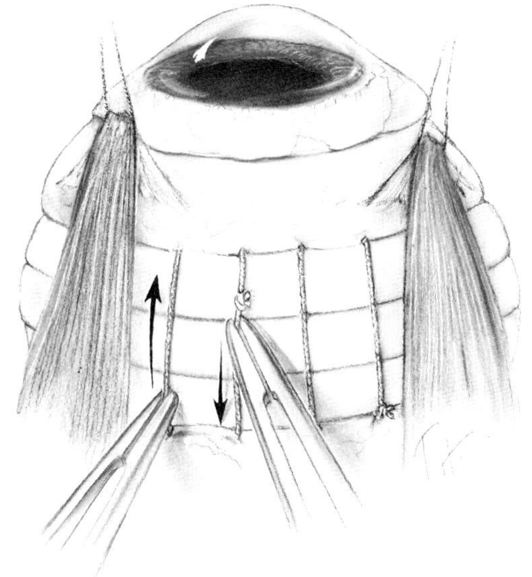

Figure 9.39 *Scleral sutures rotated so that knot is at posterior margin of buckle. This reduces likelihood of erosion of knot through Tenon's capsule and conjunctiva*

Completion of the operation

The completing steps of the operation are made once the retinal breaks have been closed. The scleral sutures are permanently tied, any encircling band is secured and redundant portions of silicone are cut off and discarded. The knots of the scleral sutures are rotated posteriorly (*Figure 9.39*). The IOP is measured by indentation tonometry, and the central retinal artery is examined to be certain that it is patent. If pulsations of the central retinal artery are visible, the IOP can be lowered by performing an anterior chamber paracentesis or administering intravenous acetazolamide or hyperosmotic agents. Moreover, there is usually spontaneous lowering of the IOP after a short interval. The operation is terminated when there is normal flow without pulsations in the central retinal artery and the IOP is less than 25 mmHg.

Tenon's capsule may be sewn to the sclera anterior to the ora serrata in the quadrants where a scleral buckle is present. The conjunctival incision is then closed with a running suture of 6/0 plain catgut. Often the conjunctival opening has been stretched or torn temporally so that a T-shaped closure of the incision is necessary (*Figure 9.40*). Gentamicin is injected beneath the conjunctiva near the bulkiest portion of the scleral buckle. Atropine is applied topically in most cases to maintain partial pupillary dilation so that the fundus can be examined the next day.

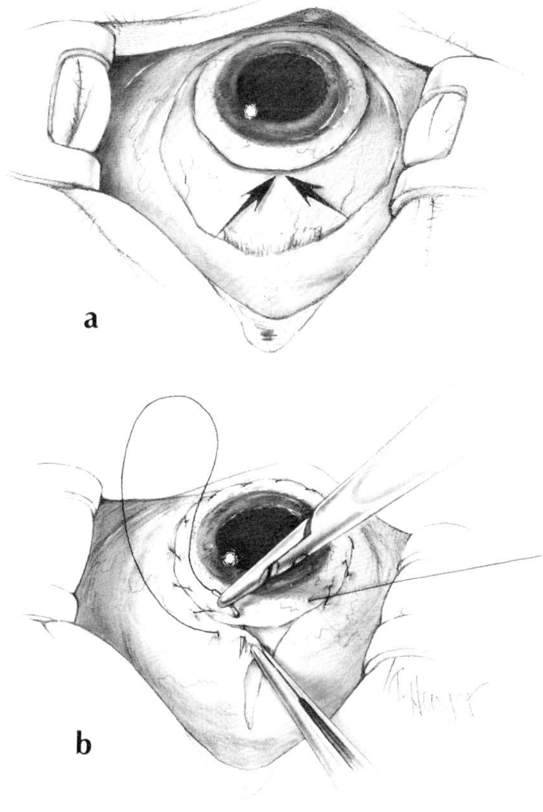

Figure 9.40 *Closure of conjunctival incision after retinal reattachment surgery. Conjunctiva is often torn and/or stretched temporally so 'T' closure of edges is necessary*

Postoperative management

Initial postoperative management is determined at the end of the operation with decisions regarding bandaging one or both eyes, patient activity and positioning, and selection of antibiotics and/or other medications to be used. Only the operated eye is bandaged if the retina is reattached at the end of the operation, if the retinal breaks are located in the superior quadrants and they are well supported by the scleral buckle, or if intravitreal air was used. In cases with inferior retinal breaks or when the edges of the retinal breaks are not flat on the buckle, both eyes are bandaged. Patients are usually restricted to bedrest with bathroom privileges after surgery until postoperative examination demonstrates that the retina is reattached. If a large amount of subretinal fluid remains, head positioning is selected to avoid putting the retinal break(s) in a dependent position.

Systemically administered antibiotics are not routinely used postoperatively, although antibiotics may be ordered when: (*1*) an external infection was treated before the operation; (*2*) there was a break in sterile technique during the procedure; or (*3*) the case was a reoperation and/or the procedure was of excessive length. In such cases, intravenous antibiotics are given of the type and dosage used to treat infective endophthalmitis. This intravenous antibiotic therapy is stopped after 3 or 4 days. Acetazolamide is given during the initial postoperative period if the IOP was elevated before surgery or at any time after creating the scleral buckle. This is given intravenously if the patient is nauseated and cannot take medications by mouth.

The operated eye is examined on the first postoperative day, and the postoperative orders may then be modified. Acetazolamide therapy is discontinued if the IOP is normal. The fellow eye is unbandaged if all subretinal fluid has absorbed and/or if the edges of the retinal break(s) are flat against the pigment epithelium. Unrestricted activity is permitted if the edges of the retinal break(s) are flat against the pigment epithelium and all subretinal fluid has absorbed. A topically applied medication of combined antibiotic and corticosteroid is used four times daily in most cases. One per cent atropine is often used four times daily to maintain pupillary dilation so that the fundus can be examined and because its cycloplegic effect reduces ocular pain.

If subretinal fluid persists postoperatively, the amount and location of the fluid is recorded, noting any change in the distribution of the fluid with change in head position. Bilateral eye bandages are used, and the patient is restricted to bedrest. Eyes with residual or recurrent subretinal fluid are observed frequently to determine whether the amount of fluid is changing and to determine the cause of the fluid. Rarely, an open break is seen that was not discovered previously and which is not supported on the scleral buckle. In such cases, prompt reoperation is recommended to close the additional break.

Usually no new retinal break is seen in eyes with remaining subretinal fluid. One must decide whether this is residual subretinal fluid that will eventually absorb or whether the fluid is from a retinal break that remains open. Usually this can be decided during the first 4–7 postoperative days. During this time the edges of the known retinal breaks usually become flat on the scleral buckle, and visible effects of a surrounding chorioretinal adhesion are evident. If radial folds persist that communicate with a retinal break and extend across the posterior slope of the buckle, these can be treated by photocoagulation using a xenon source or argon laser. This usually requires retrobulbar anesthesia to eliminate pain. The retina whitens, although the whitening may be less on the fold where the retina is most elevated. These folds usually flatten in 5–15 days after such treatment.

With experience, one can also predict whether subretinal fluid is residual or recurrent, based on the appearance of the fundus. Retinal detachment from residual subretinal fluid has a flat appearance and usually does not extend onto the adjacent buckle, even when the eye is rotated so that the adjacent buckle is dependent. Persistent retinal detachment from an open retinal break often has a convex surface and extends onto the adjacent scleral buckle. In eyes with an open retinal break, there may also be folds in the outer part of the retina caused by intraretinal edema. When choroidal detachments are present postoperatively, residual subretinal fluid absorbs slowly. In such cases, remaining fluid may not absorb until the choroidal detachments resolve after about 2 weeks.

Patients with retinal detachment usually remain hospitalized until all retinal break(s) are flat and pigmentary evidence of a chorioretinal adhesion is visible around the break(s). Pigmentary reaction after cryotherapy is usually visible 5 days after surgery, and patients are discharged then if the retina is reattached or if the amount of subretinal fluid is decreasing. Longer hospitalization is recommended if complications are present or if the anatomical success of the operation is uncertain. However, hospitalization longer than 7–10 days is rarely needed to treat eyes with remaining subretinal fluid. By then the edges of visible retinal breaks are usually flat, and it will have become evident whether remaining subretinal fluid is likely to absorb spontaneously. Also, by 7–10 days the media are usually sufficiently clear and the eye sufficiently well healed that detailed examination by fundus biomicroscopy can be performed to search for open retinal breaks.

After hospital discharge, the affected eye is treated with topically applied combined antibiotic and steroid medication for 4–6 weeks. Atropine drops are often prescribed for about 2 weeks. An eye bandage is worn until the eye is comfortable. The patient is permitted to return to normal activity after 1 week of limited activity, but vigorous physical exertion is avoided. The operated eye is reexamined 1–2 weeks after discharge from the hospital, and again 4–6 weeks later if the retina is reattached and the tissues are healing properly. Patients often return to work 4–6 weeks after surgery. Refraction is done 8–12 weeks after the operation to detect refractive errors induced by surgery.

Summary

Preoperative evaluation of eyes with rhegmatogenous retinal detachment, including history taking and physical examination, is organized to ascertain all relevant features of the case before planning the operative procedure. Operative and postoperative management varies from case to case. However, the methods chosen are determined by the basic principles of identifying, closing and sealing all retinal breaks, using techniques that minimize both mechanical damage to the eye and the risk of complications. Successful retinal reattachment surgery requires attention to detail during the procedure, intraoperative achievement of specific mechanical objectives and management of any complications.

We prefer to use episcleral exoplants to support the retinal break(s) and cryotherapy to cause a surrounding chorioretinal adhesion because these techniques are effective and safe compared to other methods. Drainage of subretinal fluid is avoided when possible, although the operation is not terminated until a satisfactory relation between the retinal breaks and the position of the scleral buckle is obtained. Subretinal fluid is drained when necessary to achieve this objective. Postoperatively the fundus is carefully examined to ensure that the retinal breaks are properly closed and any remaining subretinal fluid is absorbing.

Treatment of acute retinal tears

Patients with symptoms of vitreoretinal traction are often seen before significant retinal detachment occurs. Eyes with these symptoms are examined to detect any retinal break(s) so that detachment can be prevented by creating a chorioretinal adhesion around the break(s). Of special importance in examination of such eyes are presence of pigmentary debris in the vitreous gel and/or any evidence of vitreous hemorrhage. Pigmentary debris in phakic eyes is nearly pathognomonic of the presence of a retinal break[30], and retinal breaks are found in 70 per cent of eyes with significant vitreous hemorrhage[2,3,32]. All eyes with symptoms of vitreoretinal traction are carefully examined by indirect ophthalmoscopy with scleral indentation to identify any retinal breaks, and frequent periodic re-examination is performed if pigmentary debris or hemorrhage is present in the vitreous gel and no retinal break is seen.

Acute retinal tears with less than 2 mm of retinal detachment surrounding the edge are usually treated with laser photocoagulation or transscleral cryotherapy without use of a scleral buckle. Laser photocoagulation is preferred for most of these cases. Photocoagulation is especially useful for round holes and for posterior retinal breaks in eyes with clear media. Cryotherapy is preferred for retinal breaks in the far periphery, flap-shaped tears with persistent vitreous traction and those in eyes with a small pupil or opacities in the media that interfere with photocoagulation. In many cases, either treatment method is suitable, and the choice depends on the experience and preference of the surgeon.

Photocoagulation

Laser photocoagulation is applied through a slit-lamp delivery system using a three-mirror contact lens for visualization. Topical anesthesia is usually adequate, although a retrobulbar injection is sometimes necessary if treatment is painful. Topical anesthesia is preferred to avoid the risks of retrobulbar hemorrhage or optic nerve damage associated with retrobulbar injection. Also, when topical anesthesia is used the patient can position his eye to assist the surgeon.

The retinal break or adjacent subretinal fluid is surrounded by two or three rows of confluent photocoagulation applications of moderate intensity producing mild to moderate whitening (*Figure 9.41*). Usually a 500 μm spot

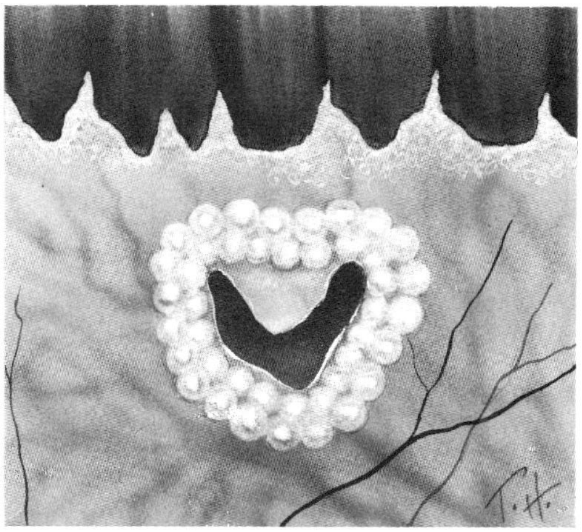

Figure 9.41 *Laser photocoagulation surrounding retinal break. Two contiguous rows of treatment are applied with each application of moderate intensity*

size is used, and each application is 0.1 or 0.2 seconds in duration. If a flap-shaped retinal tear is treated, the photocoagulation may be extended farther anteriorly. This is done to minimize the chance of later retinal detachment if progressive traction on the retinal flap extends the tear anteriorly. When subretinal fluid surrounds the retinal break, the laser treatment is applied to the attached retina around the subretinal fluid. No treatment is applied to the area of detached retina, although this may be treated later if the subretinal fluid absorbs. If the retina anterior to the retinal break and/or localized detachment cannot be easily treated by photocoagulation, simultaneous scleral depression while using the contact lens may allow treatment to the ora serrata; otherwise, remaining anterior portions are treated with cryotherapy.

After laser photocoagulation of acute retinal tears, patients are restricted to limited activity for the next 4–7 days. The rationale for this management is to minimize further vitreoretinal traction from movement of the vitreous gel associated with eye movement and physical activity until a chorioretinal adhesion forms.

Retinal cryotherapy

Cryotherapy is usually applied in transconjunctival fashion, although occasionally a localized conjunctival incision is necessary to permit more-posterior placement of the probe tip. The need for a conjunctival incision can usually be ascertained by attempting to indent the sclera under the retinal break with a sterile cotton-tip applicator placed on the anesthetized conjunctiva.

Before treatment the eye is anesthetized with topical medication and 2 per cent lidocaine (lignocaine; Xylocaine) is injected beneath the conjunctiva in the quadrant(s) where the cryotherapy will be applied. Retrobulbar anesthesia is avoided, even if a conjunctival incision is necessary, so that the patient can rotate his eye as requested by the surgeon. This rotation assists in visualization of the retinal tear(s) and also stabilizes the globe.

The usual cleaning and lavage of the operative field is performed if a conjunctival incision is necessary. The conjunctiva is incised near the fornix in the meridian of the retinal break, and the scissor blades are opened in the episcleral space to create a plane for introduction of the cryoprobe. The posterior edge of the conjunctival incision is grasped with forceps, and the probe tip is introduced into the episcleral space.

Cryotherapy is performed with a probe tip that is insulated except for the surface that is pressed against the sclera. Visualization is provided by indirect ophthalmoscopy. The patient rotates the eye so that the indentation effect caused by the probe tip is easily visualized beneath the retinal break. One must be certain that it is the tip of the probe producing indentation and not the probe shaft because the latter can cause incorrect placement of a posterior freeze.

Cryotherapy is applied as a single continuous row around the tear. When localized retinal detachment surrounds the tear, cryotherapy is applied straddling the junction between the zone of subretinal fluid and the surrounding attached retina. Each application is terminated immediately when the retina turns white, and care is taken to avoid skipping areas or refreezing the same area of the retina. Treatment is begun at a location that can be easily identified, and the probe is moved stepwise around the break (*Figure 9.42*). It is desirable not to remove the probe from the surface of the globe between applications, to minimize the chance of skipping or refreezing an area when the probe is reapplied. A second row of cryotherapy may be applied anterior to flap-shaped tears, to provide a broader zone of chorioretinal adhesion in case further vitreous traction extends the tear anteriorly. If a retinal tear is posterior, the patient is asked to look in the direction opposite the tear to expose more of the posterior sclera in the meridian of the retinal break (*Figure 9.43*). It is unnecessary to hospitalize most patients that have cryotherapy to holes with no associated detachment. These patients are told to avoid strenuous exercise for 1 week.

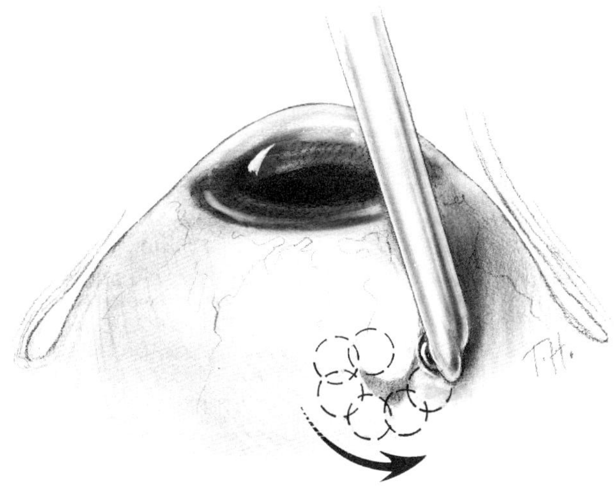

Figure 9.42 *Transconjunctival cryotherapy of retinal break. Probe is moved between freezes in clockwise direction, without removing probe from globe, to apply contiguous treatment without skipping zones or retreating same area. Treatment is applied along peripheral margin of retinal break*

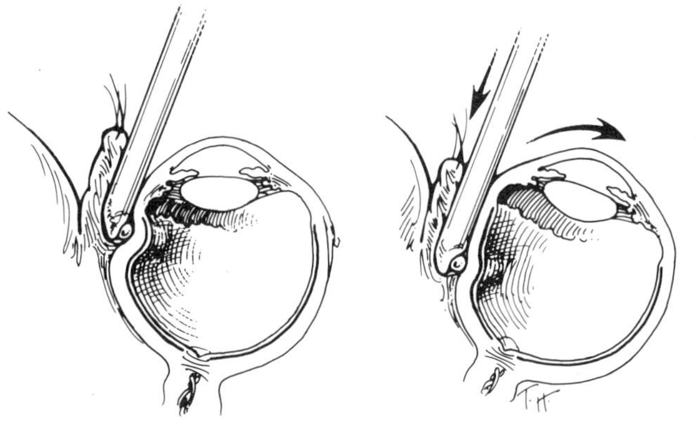

Figure 9.43 *Transconjunctival cryotherapy for posterior retinal break. Patient looks in direction opposite retinal break to permit posterior placement of probe tip*

Patients with both flap-shaped tears and localized surrounding retinal detachment are treated with bedrest and bilateral bandages for at least 48 hours, and limited activity for the next 3 days. If the retinal tear is likely to have occurred less than 5 days previously, the patient may be kept at bedrest until a visible pigmentary reaction is evident. A white color change in the retina is visible 10–20 minutes after cryotherapy is applied, and this clearly indicates the area of treatment. A further change with increased pigmentation at the level of the pigment epithelium occurs on the fifth day.

Post-treatment management

Eyes are re-examined 1 week after treatment if photocoagulation or cryotherapy is performed as an outpatient procedure, and 1 week after discharge following cryotherapy and temporary hospitalization. The eyes are again examined 3 weeks later, when scleral indentation is used. Progressive retinal detachment is treated promptly by retinal reattachment surgery with a scleral buckle. Eyes with an initially successful response are re-examined 3–6 months after cryotherapy and photocoagulation.

Complicated retinal detachments

Certain types of retinal detachments are difficult to treat by conventional scleral buckle techniques. In order of increasing difficulty, these types include: (*1*) highly elevated detachments with multiple large retinal breaks; (*2*) posterior retinal breaks; (*3*) certain giant retinal tears; and (*4*) detachments complicated by epiretinal membrane formation resulting in immobilization of the retina (massive periretinal proliferation; MPP), (massive vitreous retraction; MVR), (proliferative vitreoretinopathy; PVR). Treatment of these detachments requires special techniques, ranging from simple injection of intravitreal air to complex vitreous surgery with dissection of epiretinal membranes. Also there is an increasing frequency of retinal detachment in eyes with an intraocular lens (IOL) and eyes that have previously undergone vitrectomy. These cases present unique problems that require special techniques.

High detachment with large and/or multiple retinal tears

Highly elevated retinal detachments with large and/or multiple tears present difficulties in exact location of the breaks for application of cryotherapy and for proper placement of the scleral buckle. Also, sometimes the retina does not settle well when subretinal fluid is drained, because additional fluid passes through the retinal break(s) into the subretinal space. Therefore, after draining subretinal fluid and elevating the scleral buckle, the edges of the retinal breaks may not be well supported, and fluid may pass from the vitreous cavity through the break and into the posterior subretinal space through radial retinal folds on the buckle.

In some eyes, subretinal fluid is drained and saline is injected into the vitreous cavity before treatment or localization of retinal breaks or preparation for scleral buckling. This is especially useful in aphakic eyes, and saline is injected through the limbus into the anterior chamber to restore normal intraocular volume as subretinal fluid is drained (*Figure 9.44*). Vitreous gel may temporarily tamponade the retinal breaks so that subretinal fluid does not reaccumulate rapidly. This permits exact treatment and localization of the retinal break(s) and use of a low scleral buckle in many eyes. In this manner, a complex anatomic situation can be converted into one that is treatable with simple measures.

If the subretinal fluid reaccumulates rapidly after transscleral drainage then other measures are used. Cryotherapy or diathermy is applied to a broad area beneath and surrounding the retinal break(s). A broad, circumferentially oriented scleral buckle is prepared, and subretinal fluid is drained as far as possible from the retinal breaks (*Figure 9.45a*). If the retina settles well, the scleral buckle is then elevated and later modified as necessary by addition of radial elements beneath retinal breaks associated with radial folds. If the retina does not settle well or if prominent radial folds persist despite modification of the buckle, then air is injected into the vitreous cavity (*Figure 9.45b*).

The desired buckle height is selected and the sutures are temporarily tied before air is injected. If the eye is sufficiently soft, 1.0 ml or more of air is injected into the vitreous cavity through a 27 or 30 gauge needle introduced through the pars plana while the location of the needle tip is monitored by indirect ophthalmoscopy. If the eye is not soft enough to permit injection of an adequate amount of air, additional subretinal fluid is first drained through a second sclerotomy located posterior to the scleral buckle, and then air is injected after closing the scleral incision by tying the preplaced suture.

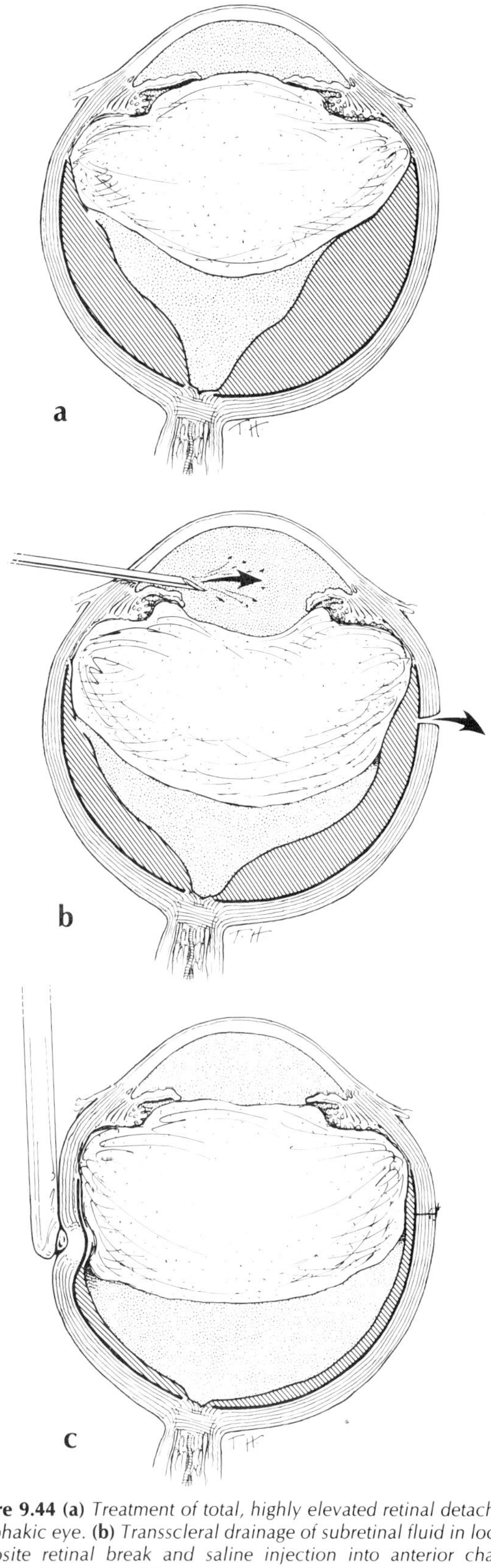

Figure 9.44 **(a)** *Treatment of total, highly elevated retinal detachment in aphakic eye.* **(b)** *Transscleral drainage of subretinal fluid in location opposite retinal break and saline injection into anterior chamber flattens retina. Retinal break is obstructed by vitreous gel.* **(c)** *Proper localization and treatment of retinal breaks can be done including cryotherapy and scleral buckle*

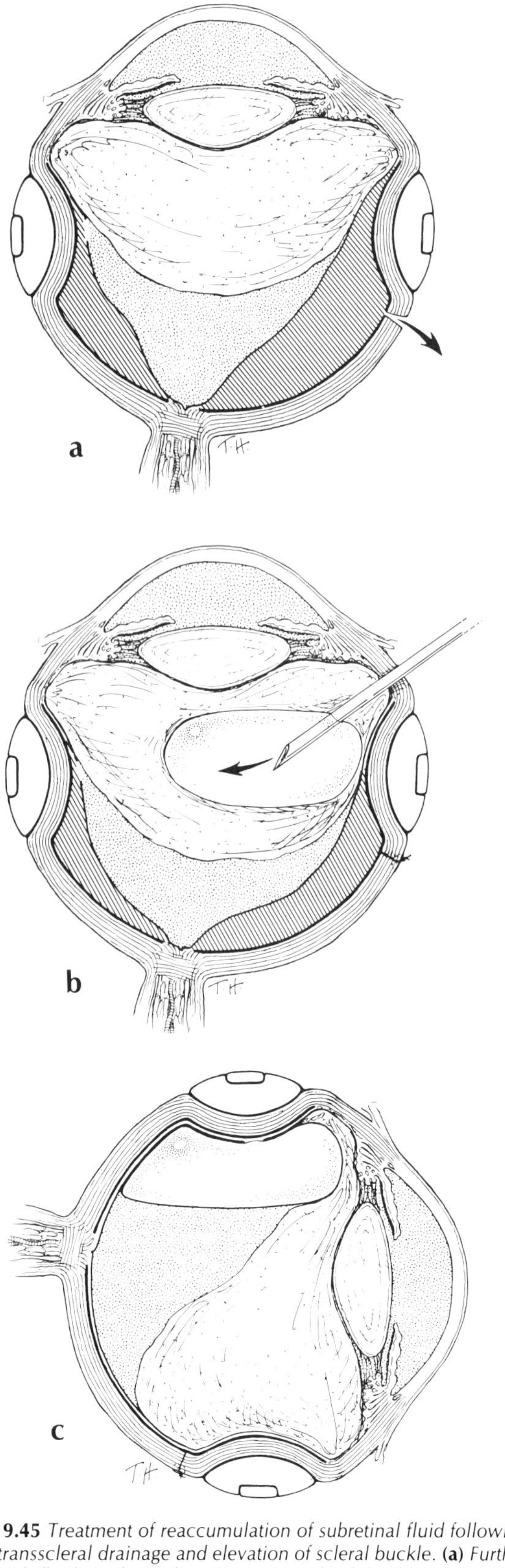

Figure 9.45 *Treatment of reaccumulation of subretinal fluid following initial transscleral drainage and elevation of scleral buckle.* **(a)** *Further subretinal fluid is drained posterior to scleral buckle in location opposite retinal break.* **(b)** *Air is injected to restore normal volume and pressure.* **(c)** *Postoperative positioning is used to seal retinal break by internal tamponade from air bubble*

Postoperatively, the patient's head is positioned so that the air bubble tamponades the retinal break(s) (*Figure 9.45c*). This promotes rapid absorption of the remaining subretinal fluid and flattens any persistent radial folds communicating with the retinal breaks. Photocoagulation can be applied postoperatively if inadequate pigmentation around a break suggests a poor chorioretinal adhesion.

Posterior retinal breaks

There is no precise definition of posterior retinal breaks, but these are usually considered to be breaks located posterior to the equator. Such retinal breaks vary widely in difficulty of management, depending on the number, size, shape, precise location of the breaks, the amount of subretinal fluid and features of vitreous traction. Breaks located near the equator usually are not especially difficult to manage, although proper localization for placement of the scleral buckle may be difficult, and intraocular air may be needed as previously described. Similarly, small posterior breaks located between the equator and the posterior pole and associated with only a limited amount of subretinal fluid are easily treated by cryotherapy or photocoagulation with a localized scleral buckle. In these cases, a 'scleral pocket' technique may be useful to produce a permanent buckle and to prevent possible later migration of the implanted material (*Figure 9.46*).

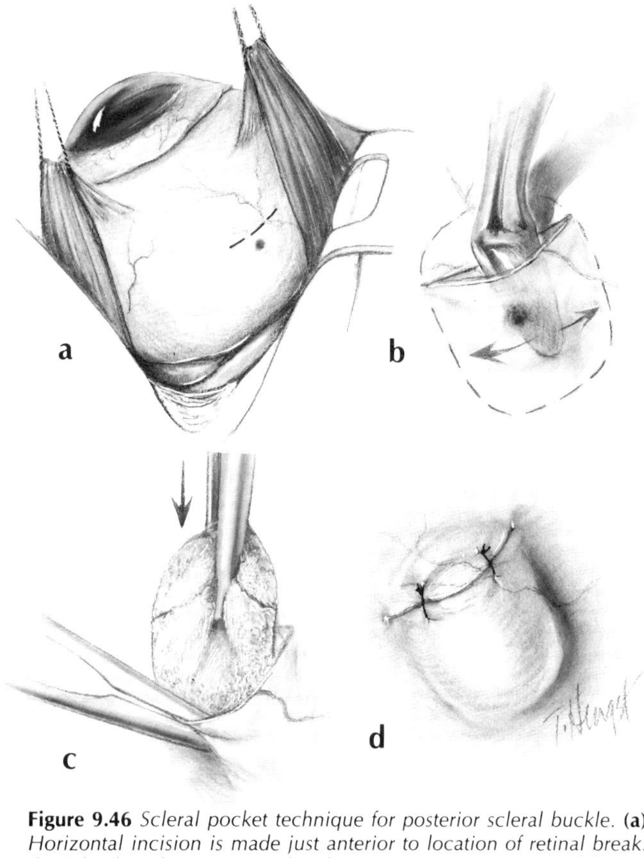

Figure 9.46 *Scleral pocket technique for posterior scleral buckle.* **(a)** *Horizontal incision is made just anterior to location of retinal break.* **(b)** *Scleral pocket is prepared with convex Castroviejo corneal dissector.* **(c,d)** *Half-thickness silicone rubber sponge is placed in scleral pocket and incision closed with sutures. The implanted material cannot migrate and creates low to moderate elevation*

Large posterior retinal breaks, those associated with high retinal detachment or severe vitreoretinal traction such as in proliferative diabetic retinopathy, and breaks located within 20° of the macula present special difficulties. These breaks are more difficult to localize precisely for transscleral treatment and for placement of a scleral buckle. In addition, it may be difficult to get the retina to settle well after drainage of the subretinal fluid. External exposure for far-posterior retinal breaks such as macular and perimacular holes is especially difficult, and there is increased risk of damage to the posterior ciliary vessels and/or damage to the optic nerve if a posterior scleral buckle is used.

Special techniques are used to deal with these eyes. When vitreoretinal traction causes high elevation of posterior retinal breaks, as in some eyes with proliferative diabetic retinopathy, vitreous surgery is used to relieve the traction and remove portions of the fibrovascular tissue (*see* Chapter 8). Then, the retinal break can be treated by ancillary techniques, using methods for transvitreal removal of subretinal fluid, transvitreal application of diathermy, cryotherapy or photocoagulation, and intraocular air for temporary postoperative tamponade of the posterior break. Large posterior retinal breaks may also be treated by vitreous surgery techniques if the edges of the tear do not flatten properly on the scleral buckle after drainage of subretinal fluid and if there is insufficient potential space for injection of a sizable intravitreal bubble.

However, when vitreoretinal traction is absent, most posterior retinal breaks can be treated by intravitreal air injection and temporary face-down positioning followed by photocoagulation or transscleral cryotherapy when the edges of the break become flat against the pigment epithelium. In many cases, space for injection of the air bubble can be obtained by transscleral drainage of the subretinal fluid (*Figure 9.47*). Rarely, direct aspiration of fluid from the preretinal space behind the separated posterior vitreous surface is necessary.

Various techniques have also been used to deal with macular and perimacular holes including: (*1*) permanent or temporary buckling; (*2*) diathermy, cryotherapy, or

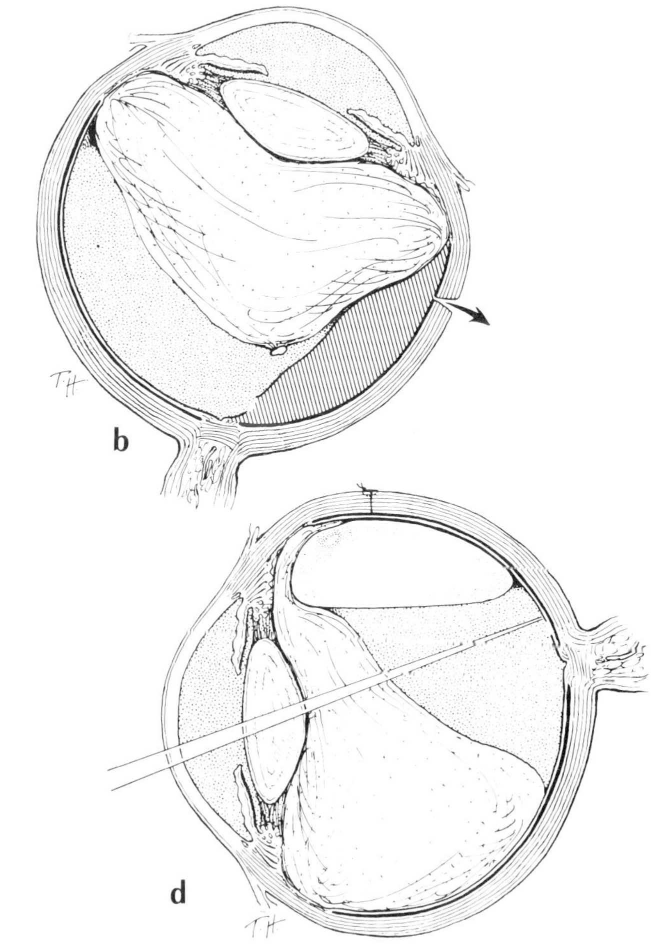

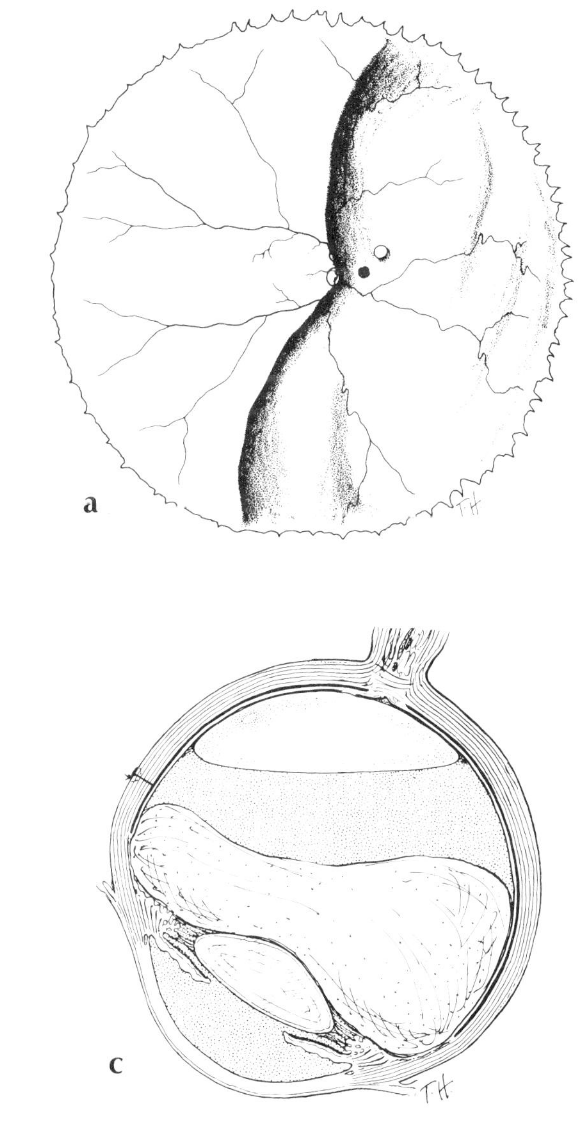

Figure 9.47 *Treatment of nasal rhegmatogenous retinal detachment due to round posterior retinal break near optic nerve.* **(a)** *Complete posterior vitreous detachment is present with operculum on posterior vitreous surface.* **(b,c)** *Transscleral drainage of subretinal fluid is done followed by intravitreal air injection and postoperative facedown positioning to tamponade retinal break by air bubble.* **(d)** *This results in flattening of retina and laser treatment is done to form seal around retinal break*

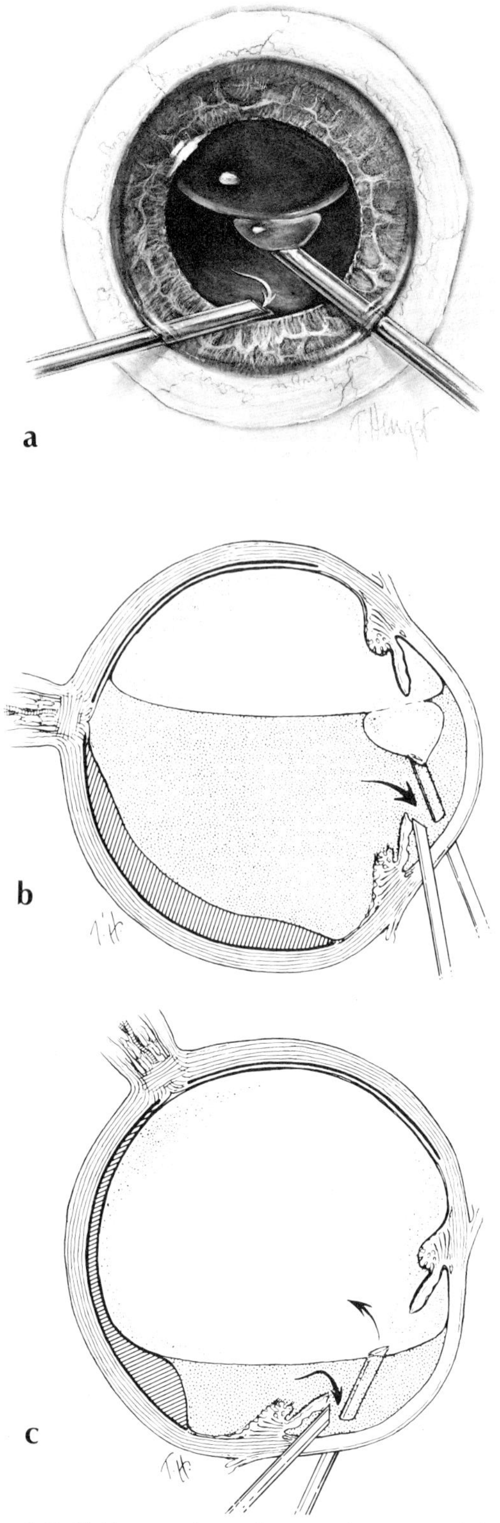

Figure 9.48 *Fluid–gas exchange in a postvitrectomy aphakic eye to supplement or introduce new intraocular bubble postoperatively. Patient is seated upright on operating table and two 27 gauge needles are introduced into anterior chamber.* **(a,b)** *Gas is injected through one needle as intraocular fluid is passively displaced from eye through second needle.* **(c)** *Head is tilted forward until bubble of desired size is obtained and then needles are withdrawn*

photocoagulation combined with intravitreal air injection without a scleral buckle; and (3) vitreous surgery. When there is no vitreous traction on the posterior retina, we prefer transscleral drainage of subretinal fluid followed by intravitreal air injection and laser photocoagulation as mentioned before. Alternatively, transscleral penetrating diathermy can be used directly beneath the retinal break after precise location of the break using indentation with a probe equipped with fiberoptic illumination. A single penetration is made until the electrode is visible in the subretinal space and a grey coagulum forms around the electrode tip. The electrode is then withdrawn, and subretinal fluid may drain through the needle tract. If all subretinal fluid drains and the retina becomes flat, no further treatment is done. If part of the subretinal fluid drains but the retina remains elevated in the region of the hole, a decision is made as to whether additional subretinal fluid can be safely drained through a separate posterior sclerotomy. This is done when possible, and air is injected into the vitreous cavity. If fluid cannot be safely drained, but the eye is sufficiently soft, air is injected into the vitreous cavity. Postoperative face-down positioning is used in these cases to close the retinal break temporarily and thereby promote absorption of residual subretinal fluid.

If a macular or perimacular retinal break is associated with significant traction from the posterior cortical vitreous, or if other methods have failed to seal the break, then vitreous surgery is performed. The vitreous traction is first relieved and the subretinal fluid is then evacuated through the posterior retinal break (*see* Chapter 8) followed by air insufflation into the vitreous cavity. No treatment is done to seal a macular hole in a non-myopic eye if the pigment epithelium appears healthy. Usually, the retina remains reattached postoperatively. If persistent traction, such as tangential traction from epiretinal membranes, prevents flattening of the retinal hole, a segmental scleral buckle is placed under the hole during the original operation or during a second procedure.

If detachment recurs despite these measures, photocoagulation is used to treat the retinal break while a portion of the original air bubble remains in the eye. This is followed by additional face-down positioning. In eyes with abnormal pigment epithelium, such as in eyes with high myopia, the pigment epithelium beneath the retinal break is treated with photocoagulation, cryotherapy, or diathermy applied with a transvitreal probe during the vitreous surgery operation.

When necessary, the intraocular bubble can be supplemented postoperatively in aphakic eyes after vitrectomy by injecting air through the limbus while intraocular fluid is displaced out of the eye through a second needle (*Figure 9.48*). In phakic eyes fluid–gas exchange is performed with a single needle and syringe (Landers, M., Personal communication, 1981). Air is first injected and fluid is then permitted to run out into the syringe. This is repeated several times until a bubble of suitable size is obtained. The air is compressed as it is injected and causes elevation of the intraocular pressure so the fluid enters the syringe without having to pull on the plunger. This is done in small increments of 0.3–0.5 ml to avoid excessive elevation of the intraocular pressure (*Figure 9.49*). The same technique can also be used in aphakic eyes with the patient in a partially face-down position, using a single needle and syringe (*Figure 9.50*).

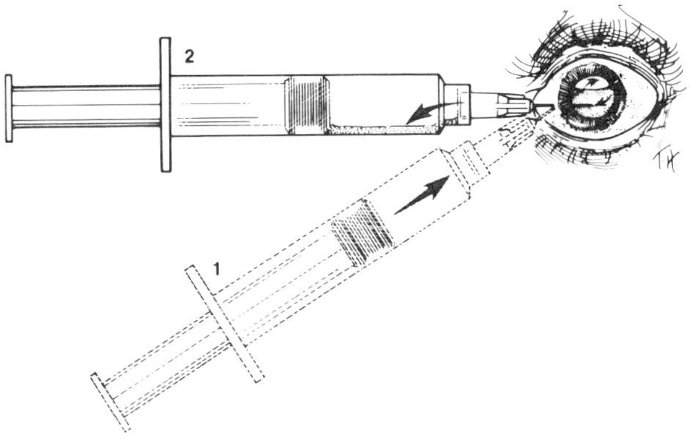

Figure 9.49 *Postvitrectomy sequential fluid–gas exchange in phakic eye. After retrobulbar anesthesia, patient is seated at slit lamp and needle inserted into vitreous cavity through pars plana. Air is first injected and then plunger released so fluid flows out of eye as a result of elevated intraocular pressure. Process is repeated until bubble filling about 60 per cent of vitreous cavity is obtained*

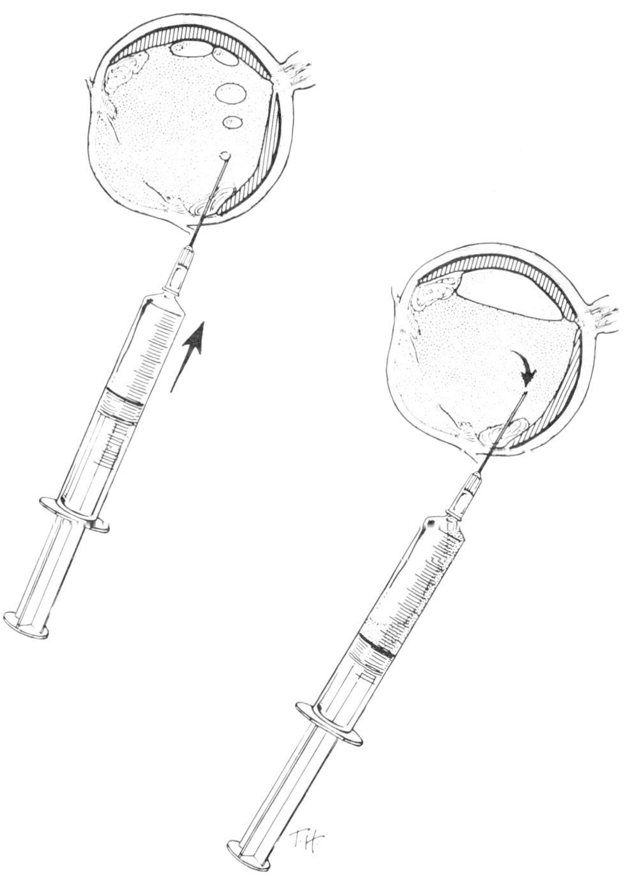

Figure 9.50 *Postvitrectomy sequential fluid–gas exchange in aphakic eye using single needle and syringe. Patient is in partial face-down position and needle introduced through limbus or pars plana. Air is injected and then plunger released for outflow of intraocular fluid due to elevated intraocular pressure. Process is repeated until bubble of desired size is obtained*

Giant retinal tears

Giant retinal tears also present special difficulties in surgical treatment. Giant tears are defined as retinal breaks greater than 90°, and they vary widely in severity depending upon: (*1*) the size and location of the break; (*2*) the position and mobility of the posterior flap of the tear; (*3*) the extent of retinal detachment; and (*4*) features of the vitreous gel. Usually giant tears occur along the posterior margin of the vitreous base because of anterior collapse and contraction of the vitreous gel, or from trauma with avulsion of the vitreous base. The tear extends circumferentially (*Figure 9.51a,b*), but it may also extend posteriorly at one or both ends. When any circumferential retinal tear extends more than one clock hour, there is a tendency for the mobile posterior edge to roll or become inverted (*Figure 9.51c*). This phenomenon is especially common in giant tears, and the amount of folding usually increases as the tear enlarges, although it also depends on the amount of liquefaction of the vitreous gel. If the giant tear results from blunt trauma, and if the gel is not liquefied and collapsed, the amount of subretinal fluid that accumulates may be small and the tear may not become inverted.

Giant tears may be easy to treat if the tear is limited to less than 180° and if the posterior flap is not inverted. These cases can usually be successfully treated with cryotherapy or diathermy and a low, broad scleral buckle throughout the length of the retinal break, together with drainage of subretinal fluid beneath the elevated retinal flap. Elevating the scleral buckle increases the anteroposterior opening of the retinal break and therefore the scleral buckle should extend well posterior to the location of the posterior edge of the retinal tear as originally marked on the sclera. This increased opening of the retinal tear is directly proportional to the height of the scleral buckle and therefore a low, broad buckle is used as mentioned before (*Figure 9.52*). If additional fluid from the vitreous cavity drains through the retinal break when subretinal fluid is released, an air bubble is injected into the vitreous cavity after creating the scleral buckle. In all cases with giant tears an additional zone of chorioretinal adhesion is created along the ora serrata beyond the ends of the tear to prevent recurrent detachment from fluid seepage, because the anterior part of the tear and the adjacent pars plana epithelium remain elevated in some cases.

If the posterior flap of the tear is inverted, and if the tear is 180° or less in length, preoperative rotation and positioning is used to determine whether the inverted flap can be unfolded and positioned near the pigment epithelium. When the flap can be unfolded preoperatively the surgical technique used (as described before) is only cryotherapy or diathermy, a scleral buckle and drainage of subretinal fluid. If the flap does not unfold preoperatively, biomicroscopic examination of the vitreous is performed to determine whether there are mechanical impediments – such as vitreous gel prolapsed between the flap and the pigment epithelium, persistent vitreous traction on the edge of the tear, or epiretinal membrane formation – that prevent unfolding of the flap and require vitreous surgery.

If no mechanical impediments to unfolding the retinal flap are seen, and if the vitreous cavity is filled mainly with fluid, then the eye may be treated with cryotherapy or

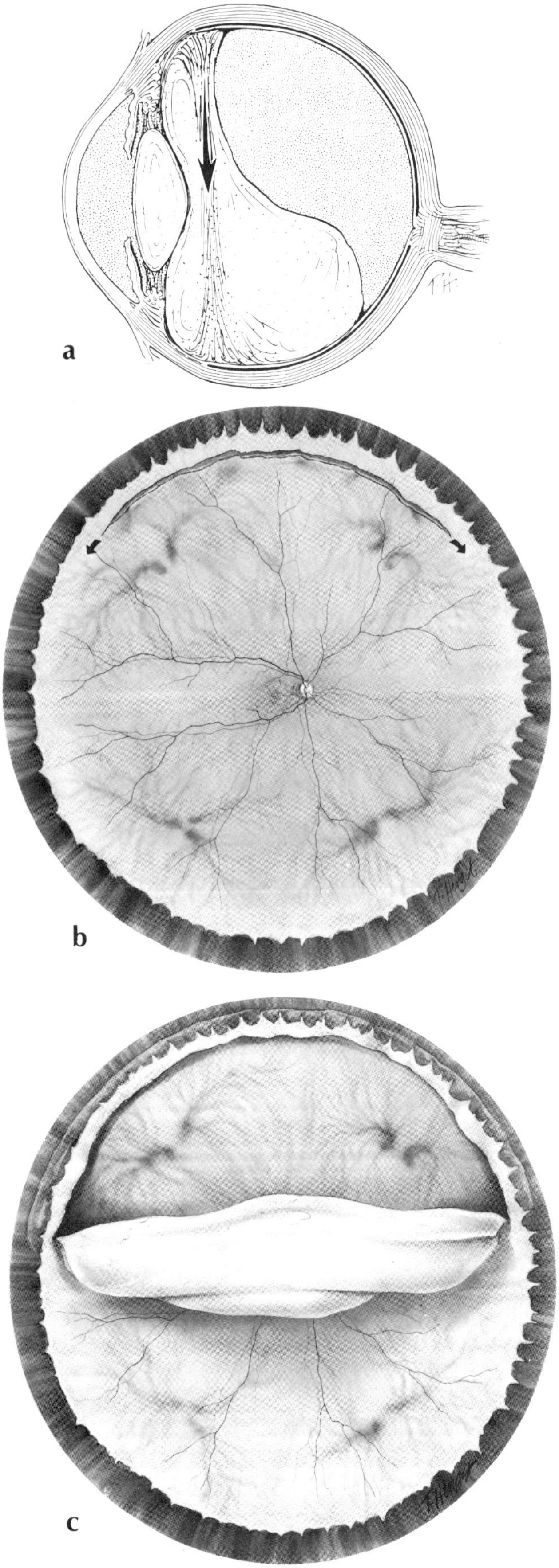

Figure 9.51 *Pathogenesis of giant retinal tears.* **(a,b)** *Vitreous traction along posterior vitreous base results in circumferential retinal tear which may extend in one or both directions.* **(c)** *Mobile posterior flap becomes inverted*

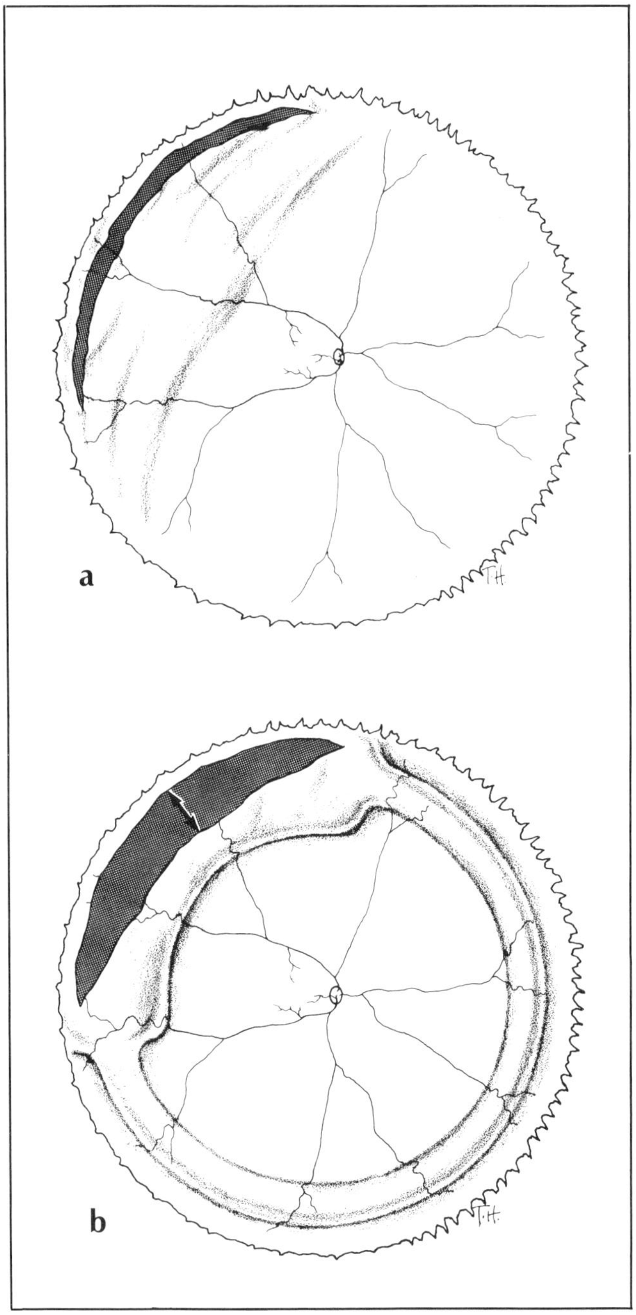

Figure 9.52 *Increased anteroposterior dimension of giant retinal tear after scleral buckling.* **(a)** *Retinal tears without significant folding of posterior edge widen in anteroposterior dimension in response to elevation of scleral buckle.* **(b)** *Therefore buckle must be placed sufficiently posterior to accommodate this change. Low buckle is used to minimize increasing width of retinal break*

diathermy and a scleral buckle, together with an intravitreal bubble to unfold the retinal flap postoperatively. In these cases, drainage of subretinal fluid is performed under areas of detached retina near the edge of the giant retinal tear, with the aim of removing a large amount of intravitreal fluid and still preventing incarceration of vitreous gel in the sclerotomy site (*Figure 9.53*). If enough

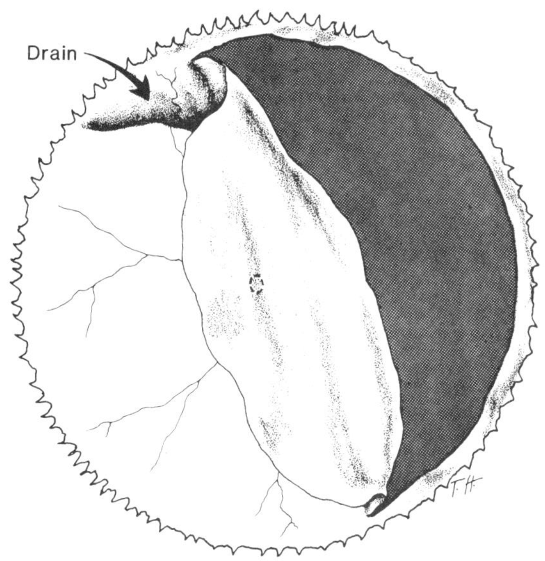

Figure 9.53 *Selection of location for transscleral drainage of subretinal fluid in eye with giant retinal tear. Fluid is drained beneath detached retina in location near retinal break so fluid can pass from vitreous cavity into subretinal space and out through sclerotomy. This permits increased softening of the eye to accommodate elevation of scleral buckle and intravitreal air injection*

intraocular fluid cannot be drained at this location, drainage is repeated anterior to the folded portion of the retinal flap. When the eye is sufficiently soft, the scleral buckle is elevated and at least 1.0 ml of air is injected into the vitreous cavity. Immediate postoperative rotations are used to unfold the retinal flap and position it against the treated pigment epithelium (*Figure 9.54*).

When vitreous gel or other mechanical factors prohibit unfolding of a retinal flap, or when insufficient intraocular fluid can be drained to permit injection of a gas bubble 1.0 ml or larger, vitreous surgery is performed. The posterior two-thirds of the vitreous gel is excised, and any adhesions to the retinal flap or epiretinal membranes immobilizing the flap are released. Then, the flap is unfolded using the vitrectomy instruments. If the flap remains unfolded when the instruments are withdrawn, transscleral drainage of subretinal fluid is performed beneath the flap, the scleral buckle is elevated and air is injected into the vitreous cavity. The patient is then rotated postoperatively to flatten the retinal flap completely against the treated pigment epithelium and buckle.

However, usually the retinal flap becomes inverted again when the instruments are withdrawn (*Figure 9.55a*). In these cases, simultaneous fluid–gas exchange is performed while the patient remains supine. Transscleral drainage of intraocular fluid is not performed. Thirty to 50 per cent of the vitreous cavity is filled with air (*Figure 9.55b*). If the operation is performed under local anesthesia, the patient can be asked to sit upright to determine the actual size of the intraocular bubble. Then, the patient is rotated 360° to determine whether the bubble satisfactorily unfolds the retinal flap (*Figure 9.55c–e*). The same manipulation can be performed postoperatively, but if the flap does not satisfactorily unfold then a further operation is required. If the bubble is excessively large, it may fail to unfold the flap, especially if there is only a small distance between the edge of the flap and the underlying retina. In these cases, the bubble size may be reduced and the rotation repeated.

In eyes with tears greater than 180° and in others in which the flap cannot be properly unfolded with a smaller bubble, fluid–gas exchange is performed with the patient in a face-down position after vitrectomy and removal of the lens (*see* Chapter 8)[33,34]. A 27 gauge needle attached by tubing to a syringe with air is introduced through the limbus or pars plana and directed so that the bubble will rise to the apex of the funnel-shaped detachment or on the side of the eye opposite the giant tear. A second needle is introduced through the limbus into the anterior chamber, and intraocular fluid is displaced out of the eye through this needle as the air bubble expands. The retinal flap is unfolded and flattened against the pigment epithelium by the expanding bubble as the preretinal and subretinal fluid is evacuated. A broad encircling scleral buckle is created by tightening scleral sutures to indent a grooved piece of silicone rubber that has been placed around the eye prior to the fluid–gas exchange. The pigment epithelium is treated with cryotherapy before the vitrectomy.

Patients with an intraocular bubble are rotated frequently during the first 6 hours after the operation to ensure that the retinal flap is smoothly unfolded and properly positioned. As the bubble absorbs, the retinal flap is observed frequently to be certain that a firm chorioretinal adhesion develops. If a portion of the flap becomes elevated, it is immediately treated with laser photocoagulation and the remaining bubble is used to keep the retina flat. When necessary, an additional intraocular bubble is injected. With these techniques, the retinal flap can be satisfactorily unfolded and the tear sealed in most cases. However, there is an increased incidence of later massive periretinal proliferation in eyes with giant retinal tears. Thirty to 50 per cent of such eyes redetach later because of proliferation and contraction of epiretinal membranes.

Massive periretinal proliferation

Massive periretinal proliferation (MPP) is the most common cause of failure of retinal reattachment surgery[35]. This condition was previously named massive vitreous retraction (MVR) or massive preretinal retraction (MPR). However, recent studies indicating the cellular nature of the membranes and demonstrating that both sides of the retina are involved suggest that the name massive periretinal proliferation is more descriptive*. The cause of the process is still unknown, but the pathogenesis includes proliferation of cellular sheets on the posterior surface of the vitreous gel and on both the inner and outer surfaces of the retina[35–39]. The cells are probably of both

* Recently the term proliferative vitreoretinopathy (PVR) has been advocated along with a new classification for this condition[39a]

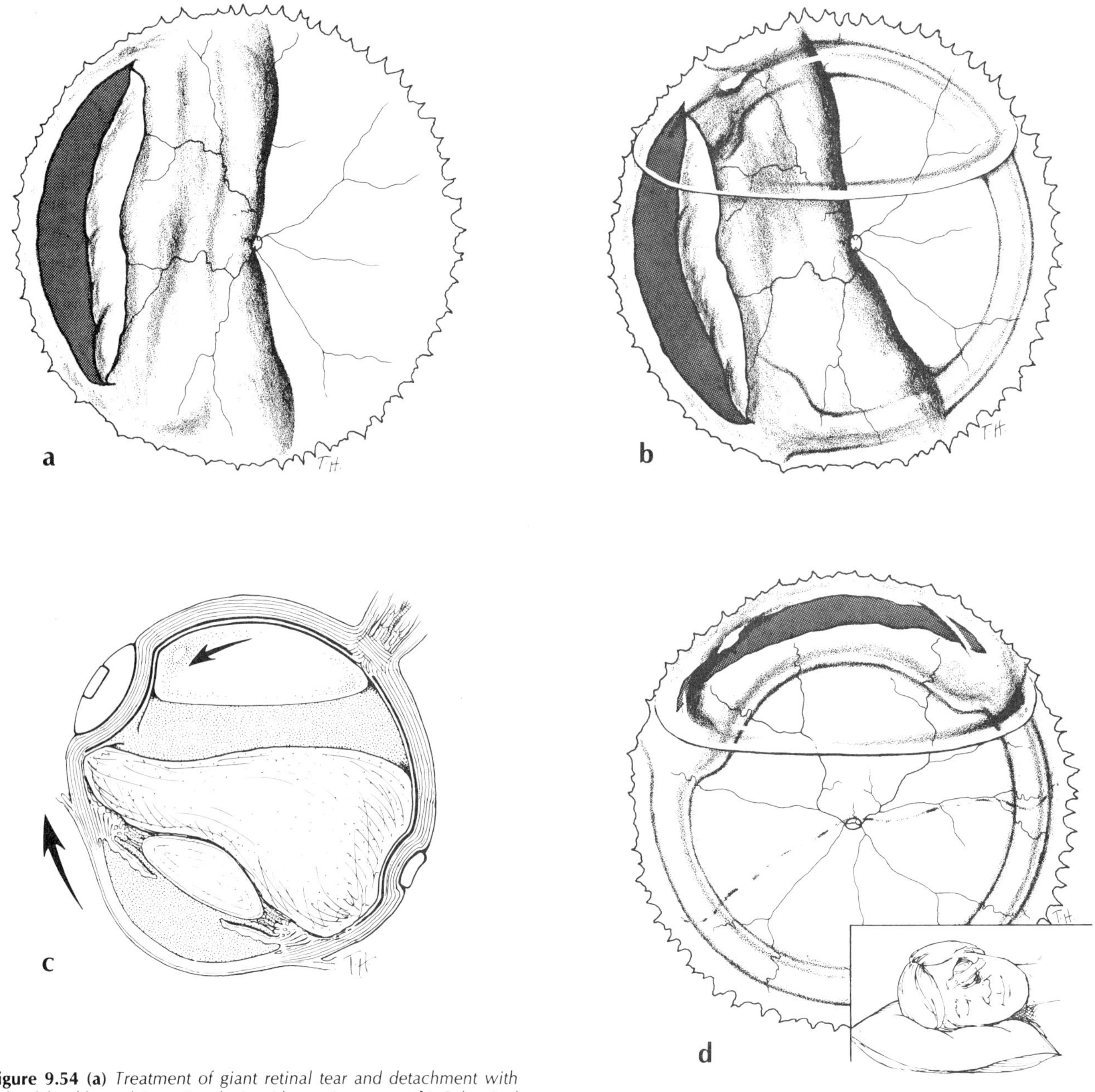

Figure 9.54 (a) *Treatment of giant retinal tear and detachment with scleral buckle and intravitreal air without vitrectomy.* **(b)** *Subretinal fluid is drained to permit elevation of scleral buckle and intravitreal air injection.* **(c,d)** *Patient is then rotated so that retinal flap is unfolded by air bubble and is held against pigment epithelium and scleral buckle*

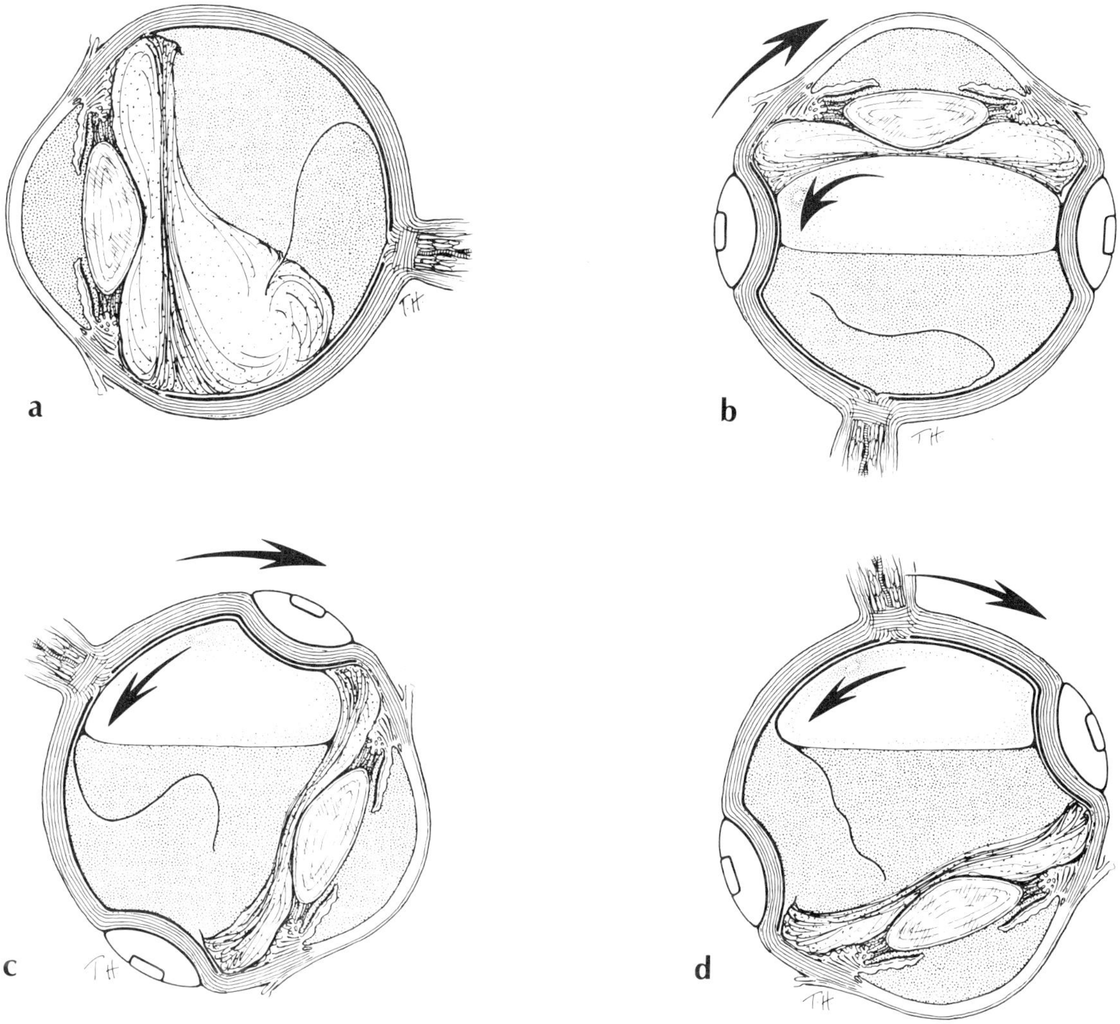

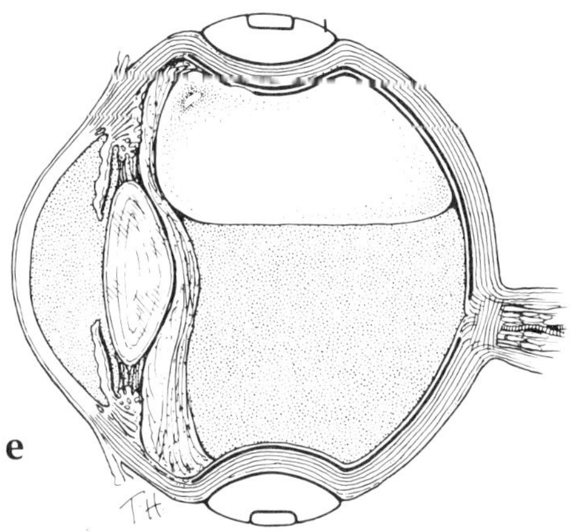

Figure 9.55 (a) *Surgical treatment of giant retinal tear of less than 180° with inverted immobile flap.* **(b)** *After vitrectomy, peripheral retinal cryotherapy and placement of scleral buckle, air bubble is introduced filling 30–50 per cent of vitreous cavity.* **(c–e)** *Patient is then rotated so bubble unfolds retinal flap and positions it against the treated pigment epithelium and scleral buckle*

pigment epithelial and astroglial origin. Contraction of these cellular membranes causes a high, funnel-shaped configuration of the detached retina with numerous retinal folds.

MPP may be present as a continuum of clinical features ranging from only localized retinal folds (starfolds) (*Figure 9.56*) to severe involvement of the entire retinal surface.

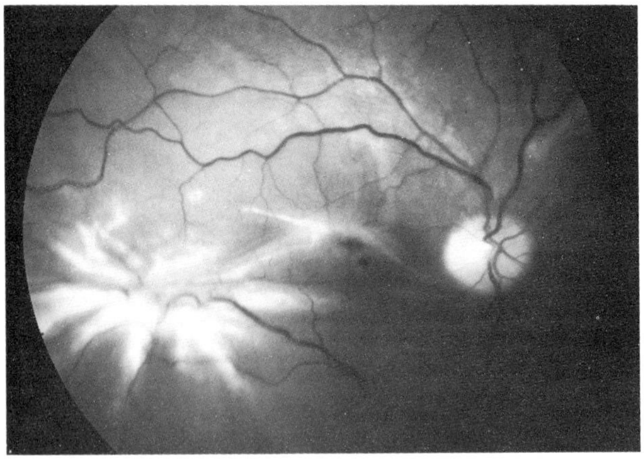

Figure 9.56 *Posterior retinal starfold inferotemporal to macula in eye with extensive rhegmatogenous retinal detachment. Starfold is caused by contraction of localized epiretinal membrane*

Mild stages, in which the retina is still mobile, are treated with conventional scleral buckling techniques. However, a high and broad encircling scleral buckle is often used in these eyes because there may be some progression of this process postoperatively with formation of a transvitreal sheet causing traction on the equatorial or pre-equatorial retina in all quadrants. Retinal breaks are supported on a high scleral buckle because progressive traction tends to elevate and reopen the breaks postoperatively.

Vitreous surgery is used to treat some eyes with MPP when the retina is immobile and/or when marked traction prevents closure of the retinal breaks by scleral buckling techniques alone[40]. Vitrectomy is used to excise all transvitreal membranes and to separate epiretinal membranes causing fixed folds (see Chapter 8). The epiretinal membranes can often be removed in a posterior-to-anterior direction up to the location of the prominent transvitreal sheet. Here a ring of epiretinal tissue is usually encountered that is firmly adherent to the inner retinal surface. In some eyes, this ring can be segmented with scissors to reduce the circumferential traction, although most often this is not possible. Also, in some cases portions of the anterior cortical vitreous can be excised where it extends between the equatorial ring of firm vitreoretinal attachment and the anatomical vitreous base. The equatorial and anterior portion of retina is supported on a broad and high scleral buckle because, typically, sufficient amounts of the cortical vitreous and epiretinal membranes cannot be removed in these areas.

Many factors influence the prognosis for eyes with MPP undergoing vitreous surgery. These factors include: (*1*) the severity of the intraocular proliferative process; (*2*) the anteroposterior location of the transvitreal sheet and ring of epiretinal tissue causing traction on the anterior retina; (*3*) the number and location of retinal breaks; (*4*) the extent to which the abnormal membranes can be removed; and (*5*) the likelihood of recurrent membrane growth postoperatively. Vitreous surgery seems to be most effective if the proliferative process has been present for about 3 months, perhaps because by then the proliferative stage has nearly ended, and therefore the chance of additional postoperative membrane growth is reduced. The prognosis also seems to be better when there are no retinal breaks located posterior to the equator, when the circumferential ring of proliferative tissue is located anterior to the equator and when there is only mild or moderate shrinkage of abnormal membranes in the region of the vitreous base.

In addition to vitrectomy, certain otherwise inoperable eyes with MPP can be treated by intravitreal injection of silicone oil. A large oil bubble is injected into the preretinal space as subretinal fluid is drained through a sclerotomy located beneath the area of most severe epiretinal membrane growth. The silicone bubble fills the preretinal space, and as the bubble enlarges, the retina and the contracted membrane on the inner retinal surface are stretched. The abnormal epiretinal tissue is shorter than the underlying distorted retina. Therefore, as these combined tissues are stretched the epiretinal tissue often ruptures and partially separates from the retina. The silicone oil then tends to pass into the space between the membrane and the retina, and as it expands further it displaces the membrane anteriorly while flattening the retina against the pigment epithelium. The tip of the needle used to inject silicone oil can also be used to assist in separating the epiretinal tissue from the inner retina by lifting and stretching the torn edge of the membrane. The best result is achieved if the membrane can be completely separated from the retina posterior to the equator, so that the posterior retina becomes mobile and is held against the pigment epithelium by the silicone bubble filling the preretinal space.

Injection of silicone oil to treat MPP is usually done with visualization provided by indirect ophthalmoscopy. This observation method provides a wide field of view, considerable depth of focus and stereopsis, so that the complex features of the detached retina, vitreous, preretinal membranes, and the interfaces with the surface of the oil bubble, are well seen. However, precise movement of the needle tip within the vitreous cavity is difficult because of the inverted and reversed image seen through the indirect ophthalmoscope. Movement of the intraocular needle in an anteroposterior direction appears normal, whereas lateral movement appears inverted and reversed. Until the skill and dexterity are acquired to permit good hand–eye coordination, the surgeon guides the intraocular needle tip by moving the extraocular end of the injection apparatus in the intended direction as seen through the indirect ophthalmoscope. Despite the difficulty of hand–eye coordination, these maneuvers can be learned so that the needle tip is properly positioned to inject silicone oil and to cause tangential traction on the partially separated membrane.

In addition to intravitreal injection of silicone oil, all open retinal breaks are closed with a scleral buckle, and an encircling band is used at the equator. If there is marked transvitreal traction on the anterior retina, use of silicone oil can be combined with pars plana vitrectomy to cut the transvitreal sheet. When possible, however, excision of anterior vitreous gel is avoided so as to maintain a physical barrier between the silicone oil bubble and the posterior surface of the lens in phakic eyes. If cataract changes occur later, the opaque lens can be removed by conventional means.

Silicone oil can also be used in aphakic eyes without necessarily causing corneal damage. In such cases, mid- or wide pupillary dilation is maintained so that the surface tension of the silicone oil causes the bubble to remain spherical, thereby avoiding herniation of silicone into the anterior chamber and contact with the corneal endothelium.

Sometimes the intravitreal bubble is not sufficiently large to maintain contact with the entire posterior retina. Moreover, the silicone oil bubble tends to rise because its specific gravity is less than water, and typically the superior retina is flattened against the pigment epithelium whereas subretinal fluid remains or reaccumulates inferiorly. A second operation may be done in these circumstances combining transscleral drainage of the remaining subretinal fluid with further injection of silicone into the preretinal space.

Presence of an intraocular lens

Intraocular lens (IOL) implantation during cataract surgery has become a common practice, and therefore an increasing number of eyes with retinal detachment also have a pseudophakos. The presence of an IOL introduces special problems that depend on (*1*) the type of cataract operation performed; (*2*) the design and location of the intraocular lens; and (*3*) its method of fixation. Intraocular lenses can adversely affect retinal detachment surgery by limiting visualization of the fundus, becoming dislocated into the vitreous cavity or increasing the possibility of traumatic damage to the corneal endothelium during or after retinal surgery.

IOLs are of three general types: (*1*) anterior chamber lenses that rest on the anterior iris surface with haptics in the anterior chamber angle; (*2*) iris plane lenses with haptics anterior and/or posterior to the iris; (*3*) posterior chamber lenses with haptics located in the equatorial recess of the lens capsule or in the peripheral part of the posterior chamber, anterior to the ciliary processes. Usually anterior chamber and posterior chamber IOLs are not secured to the iris. Iris plane lenses may or may not be sutured to the iris tissue. Usually the pupil can be widely dilated in eyes with an anterior chamber or posterior chamber IOL without dislocating the lens. If an iris plane lens is sutured to the iris, the pupil can be dilated without fear of causing complete lens dislocation, although one or more of the haptics may shift to the opposite side of the iris. Therefore, the pupil is only partly dilated in such cases so that the end of the haptic is not visible in the pupil. Pupillary plane lenses that are not sutured to the iris may be totally dislocated posteriorly if wide dilation is used.

Visualization during retinal reattachment surgery may also be limited not only by limited pupillary dilation but by troublesome reflexes from the IOL or from other opacities such as the posterior lens capsule or peripheral lens material remaining after phacoemulsification or other forms of extracapsular extraction. Reflexes from the IOL are most troublesome during preoperative examination of the fundus when performing slit-lamp biomicroscopy with a three-mirror contact lens. Usually the fundus can be adequately examined through an IOL when using the indirect ophthalmoscope if the pupil can be dilated to more than 3.0 mm.

Opacification of the posterior capsule and/or peripheral lens remnants causes various amounts of difficulty, depending on the technique of the original cataract surgery. When modern methods are used to remove the posterior cortical lens fibers and most of the equatorial lens material, visualization by indirect ophthalmoscopy is adequate, although fundus biomicroscopy may be difficult. If peripheral lens material results in a prominent Sommering ring with posterior synechiae and a miotic pupil, then visualization may be severely impaired requiring considerable scleral indentation to examine the peripheral retina. This may be accomplished preoperatively after giving acetazolamide and intravenous hyperosmotic agents. However, often the peripheral fundus cannot be adequately examined until the operation is begun. A broad scleral buckle and extensive cryotherapy to the peripheral retina are used in some cases if portions of the peripheral retina cannot be examined well enough to rule out the possibility of retinal breaks.

The presence of an IOL presents other intraoperative problems because corneal damage may occur if there is contact between the lens and the corneal endothelium. Therefore an anterior chamber paracentesis to soften the globe cannot be performed safely in certain eyes, and special techniques are needed if gas is injected into the vitreous cavity. The greatest chance of corneal damage during paracentesis is in eyes with an anterior chamber IOL if the ends of the lens do not extend well into the anterior chamber angle, and paracentesis is not used in these cases. Paracentesis is also avoided when possible in eyes with an iris plane lens, and care is taken to avoid much shallowing of the anterior chamber when paracentesis seems necessary. Paracentesis can usually be performed without risk in eyes with a posterior chamber lens unless vitreous gel is present in the anterior chamber. In some cases the posterior chamber IOL seems to maintain an unusually deep anterior chamber during paracentesis, thereby permitting removal of an increased amount of intraocular fluid.

Gas injection into the vitreous cavity causes anterior displacement of an IOL when the patient is in a supine position and can cause serious corneal damage. Gas injection can usually be performed in eyes with an anterior chamber lens or a posterior chamber lens without anterior displacement of the IOL. In eyes with an iris plane lens, air may be injected first into the anterior chamber before injection into the vitreous cavity[41]. This is done through a 27 or 30 gauge needle introduced through the limbus. As the air is injected, aqueous humor is permitted to escape along the blade of a Ziegler knife introduced through the opposite clear cornea near the limbus (*Figure 9.57*). With this technique the anterior chamber fluid is replaced by air, and gas can then be safely injected into the vitreous cavity through the pars plana. In eyes with an iris plane IOL, an alternative method with a temporary trans-anterior-chamber suture can be used to restrain the IOL and prevent anterior displacement[42,43]. One such technique uses a 25 or 27 gauge needle to transfix the anterior chamber just in front of the iris plane[43]. A 9/0 or 10/0 nylon suture is threaded through the needle lumen. The process is then repeated to create a mattress-type suture, and the two strands then are tied externally (*Figure*

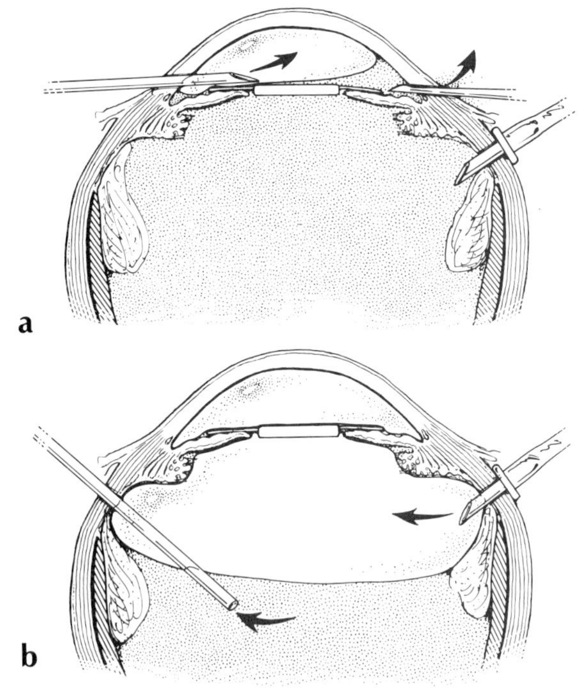

Figure 9.57 *Introduction of air bubble into anterior chamber before posterior segment fluid–gas exchange in an eye with an iris plane IOL.* **(a)** *Air is injected through small needle as knife blade in anterior chamber is tilted to permit egress of aqueous humor.* **(b)** *Air bubble in anterior chamber prevents subsequent anterior displacement of IOL and corneal damage when fluid–gas exchange is performed in vitreous cavity*

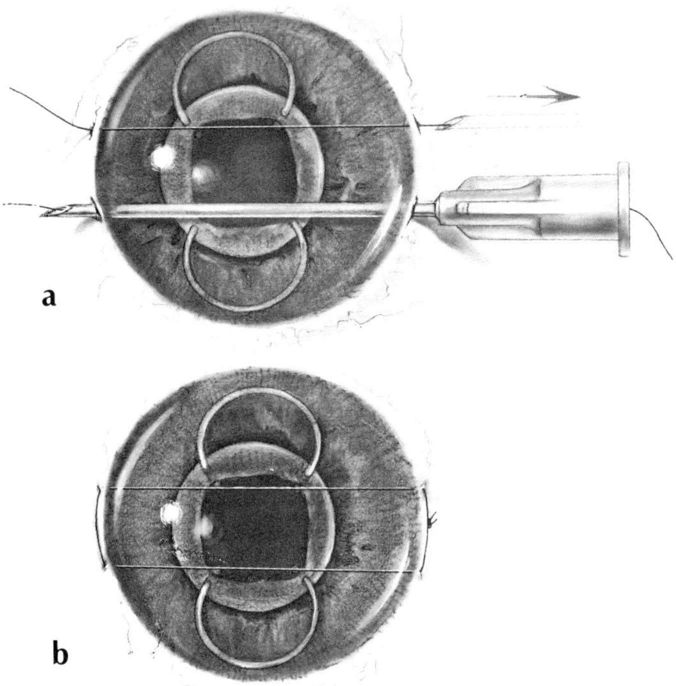

Figure 9.58 *Transcameral suture technique in eye with iris plane IOL before introduction of air bubble into vitreous cavity. One-inch (2.5 cm) 27 gauge needle is used as guide to pass 9/0 monofilament suture across pupillary space in two locations. The suture is tied externally to provide tight restraint that prevents anterior displacement of IOL*

9.58). The suture can be cut and removed after the intravitreal bubble has absorbed.

In summary, an IOL presents difficulties during retinal reattachment surgery by interfering with visualization and by increasing the risk of corneal damage if an anterior chamber paracentesis is performed or if intravitreal gas is used. Anterior chamber and posterior chamber IOLs usually permit wide pupillary dilation and do not interfere with visualization unless there is an opaque posterior capsule or excessive peripheral lens remnants after extracapsular cataract extraction. Iris plane lenses that are not secured to the iris severely limit pupillary dilation, and only mid-dilation is used with iris plane lenses that are fixed to the iris, to avoid dislocation of the haptics. Anterior chamber paracentesis and/or intravitreal gas injection can be safely done when a posterior chamber IOL is present, but these techniques are more dangerous but possible in eyes with an anterior chamber lens. Paracentesis and intravitreal gas injection are even more hazardous in eyes with an iris plane lens. Special measures such as a separate anterior chamber bubble or a transcameral restraining suture are used when intravitreal gas is needed in eyes with an iris plane IOL.

Retinal detachment in eyes after vitrectomy

Retinal detachment sometimes occurs in eyes that have previously undergone vitrectomy. These eyes usually have other abnormalities in addition to retinal detachment, such as proliferative retinopathy or scarring from a prior injury. Usually most of the posterior vitreous gel has been removed, and this introduces certain difficulties, while at the same time providing unique capabilities for treating retinal detachment. When retinal detachment occurs after most of the vitreous gel has been excised and replaced by fluid, open retinal breaks usually result in rapidly progressive retinal detachment. The amount of retinal elevation tends to be low or moderate, however, unless there is also persistent vitreoretinal traction. The retina rarely settles preoperatively in response to bedrest and bilateral eye bandages, perhaps because the retinal break(s) are not occluded by the now-absent vitreous gel.

Retinal detachment following vitrectomy often does not flatten well on a scleral buckle intraoperatively or postoperatively, even after drainage of subretinal fluid. Fluid from the vitreous cavity usually passes through the retinal break(s) into the subretinal space during transscleral drainage of subretinal fluid, so that the retina does not settle against the pigment epithelium. Therefore, an important element in treating these cases is use of an intravitreal gas bubble. Also, transscleral drainage of subretinal fluid may be unnecessary because enough fluid can often be withdrawn from the vitreous cavity to permit elevation of a scleral buckle and/or injection of an intravitreal bubble. The exact surgical technique depends on the features of each eye, such as: (*1*) the number, size and location of the retinal break(s); (*2*) the presence or absence of traction on the retina from remaining vitreous gel or epiretinal membranes; and (*3*) the status of the crystalline lens.

In postvitrectomy phakic eyes, a conventional type of retinal reattachment operation is often performed using cryotherapy and a scleral buckle. An encircling scleral buckle is used in eyes with retinal tears anterior to the equator. A localized episcleral exoplant is used beneath retinal break(s) located posterior to the equator and associated with persistent traction from vitreous gel or epiretinal membranes. Posterior retinal break(s) without evidence of traction may be treated with cryotherapy or photocoagulation without a scleral buckle.

Transscleral drainage of subretinal fluid may be performed in phakic eyes if this is convenient, and the operation is terminated if the retinal break(s) flatten well on the scleral buckle. However, if the retina fails to flatten, or if prominent radial folds are associated with retinal break(s), then intravitreal gas is used. After elevating the scleral buckle, air is injected into the vitreous cavity if the eye is still sufficiently soft (see *Figure 9.45*). In other cases, fluid is first withdrawn from the vitreous cavity and then air is injected. This is done with a 27 gauge needle and two syringes connected by a three-way stopcock. Fluid is first withdrawn, and the stopcock is turned to permit injection of air (*Figure 9.59*). This method of fluid–gas exchange may be used without transscleral drainage of subretinal fluid when a localized scleral buckle is needed and the retina is not highly detached. Enough fluid is withdrawn to permit elevation of the scleral buckle and also injection of an intravitreal bubble.

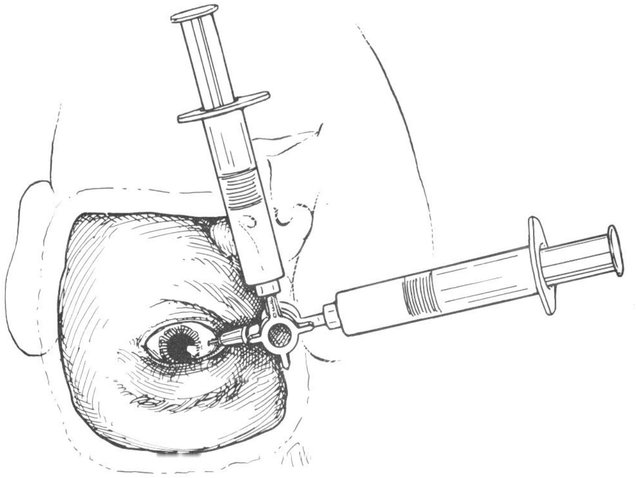

Figure 9.59 *Sequential fluid–gas exchange using two syringes and three-way stopcock in a phakic eye. Needle is introduced through nasal pars plana and stopcock and syringes are supported on bridge of nose. This prevents accidental movement of needle during aspiration of fluid and air injection*

In aphakic eyes a variety of operative techniques may be used. When the retinal breaks are not associated with significant vitreoretinal or epiretinal membrane traction, then an intravitreal bubble can be used without a scleral buckle, and the bubble is combined intraoperatively or postoperatively with use of photocoagulation or cryotherapy. In such cases the location of the retinal break(s) is carefully identified preoperatively in relation to nearby blood vessels, pigment flecks or other landmarks because later identification of the break(s) may be difficult after the retina is reattached and especially while an intravitreal air bubble is present. Peripheral retinal breaks may first be treated with cryotherapy. Fluid–gas exchange is performed through the limbus to replace some of the intravitreal fluid with air (see *Figure 9.48*). The patient is then positioned so that the bubble tamponades the retinal break(s), and usually the subretinal fluid is rapidly absorbed. Untreated anterior retinal breaks are then treated with cryotherapy, and posterior retinal breaks are treated with photocoagulation. Laser photocoagulation is done when the bubble is small enough that treatment can be applied beneath the inferior meniscus of the bubble. The remaining portion of the bubble is then used for further tamponade of the retinal break (*Figure 9.60*).

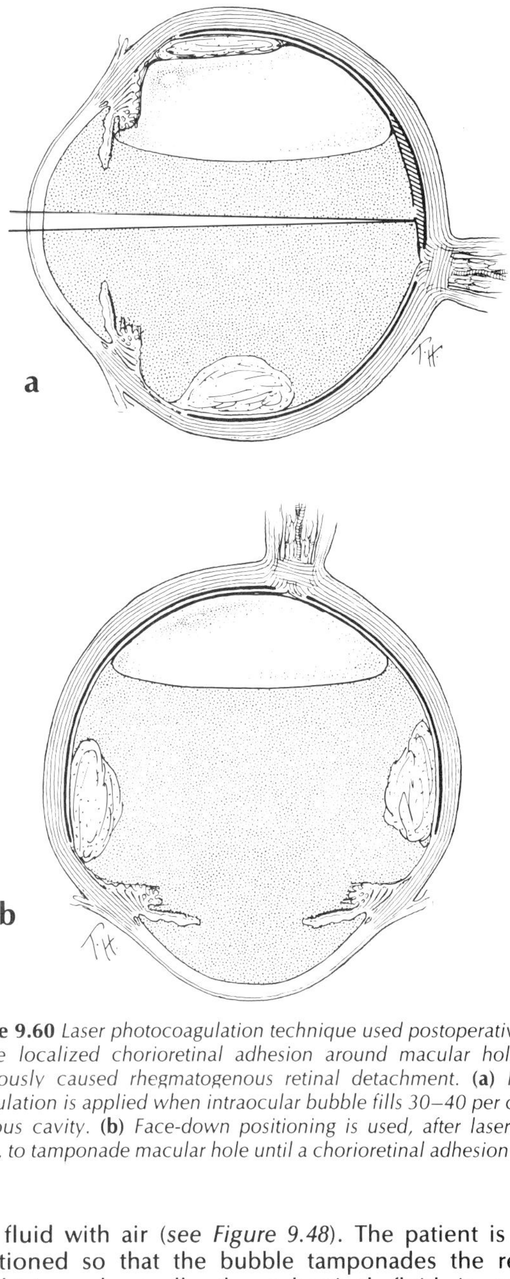

Figure 9.60 *Laser photocoagulation technique used postoperatively to create localized chorioretinal adhesion around macular hole that previously caused rhegmatogenous retinal detachment.* **(a)** *Photocoagulation is applied when intraocular bubble fills 30–40 per cent of vitreous cavity.* **(b)** *Face-down positioning is used, after laser treatment, to tamponade macular hole until a chorioretinal adhesion forms*

In aphakic eyes with a high, total retinal detachment (*Figure 9.61a*) and with anterior retinal breaks, it may be helpful to perform transscleral drainage of subretinal fluid combined with intravitreal air injection to flatten the retina prior to treatment of the retinal breaks and placement of a scleral buckle. Subretinal fluid is drained through a scleral incision located at about the equator in a quadrant opposite the retinal break(s). Air is injected through the limbus or through the pars plana as the eye softens (*Figure 9.61b*).

The globe is rotated so that the intraocular bubble tamponades the retinal break(s) against the pigment epithelium. This permits drainage of remaining subretinal fluid without passage of intravitreal fluid through the retinal break into the subretinal space. Most of the subretinal fluid can usually be drained in this way (*Figure 9.61c*), and additional air is injected to restore normal intraocular volume and pressure. The retinal break is then treated with cryotherapy and supported on a scleral bubble (*Figure 9.61d*).

If the intraocular bubble is small, and if sizable portions of the bubble must be removed to permit elevation of the scleral buckle, then further fluid–gas exchange can be performed with removal of fluid from the preretinal space. A 27 gauge needle is introduced through the limbus for injection of air, and a long 25 or 27 gauge needle is introduced through the pars plana to evacuate the preretinal fluid. The long needle is attached to a handpiece with a central lumen and side port (*see Figure 8.7a*) through which the preretinal fluid is displaced out of the eye. The needle tip is visualized by indirect ophthalmoscopy. Air is injected to enlarge the intraocular bubble and expel preretinal fluid through the other needle (*Figure 9.62*).

The retinal breaks are then treated with cryotherapy, and a scleral buckle is created to support the retinal breaks and other portions of the peripheral retina. Portions of the intraocular bubble are removed through the pars plana using a 30 gauge needle and 1.0 ml syringe to soften the eye. As the eye softens, the scleral sutures are tightened to elevate the scleral buckle.

In summary, retinal detachment in eyes that have previously undergone vitrectomy may be difficult to treat by conventional means because the retina often fails to flatten against the pigment epithelium preoperatively, intraoperatively or postoperatively. Therefore, use of a temporary intraocular gas bubble is helpful to ensure

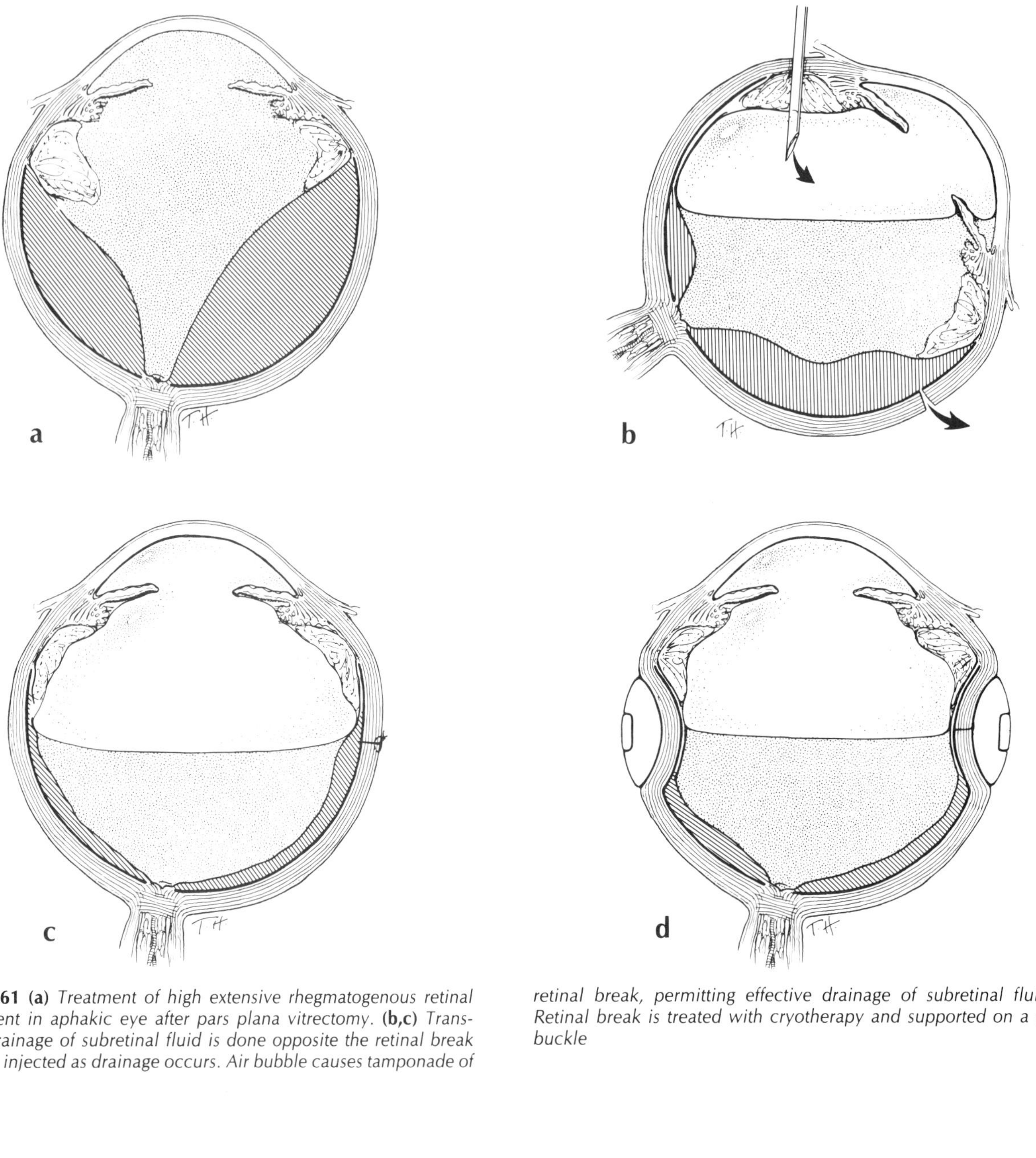

Figure 9.61 **(a)** *Treatment of high extensive rhegmatogenous retinal detachment in aphakic eye after pars plana vitrectomy.* **(b,c)** *Transscleral drainage of subretinal fluid is done opposite the retinal break and air is injected as drainage occurs. Air bubble causes tamponade of retinal break, permitting effective drainage of subretinal fluid.* **(d)** *Retinal break is treated with cryotherapy and supported on a scleral buckle*

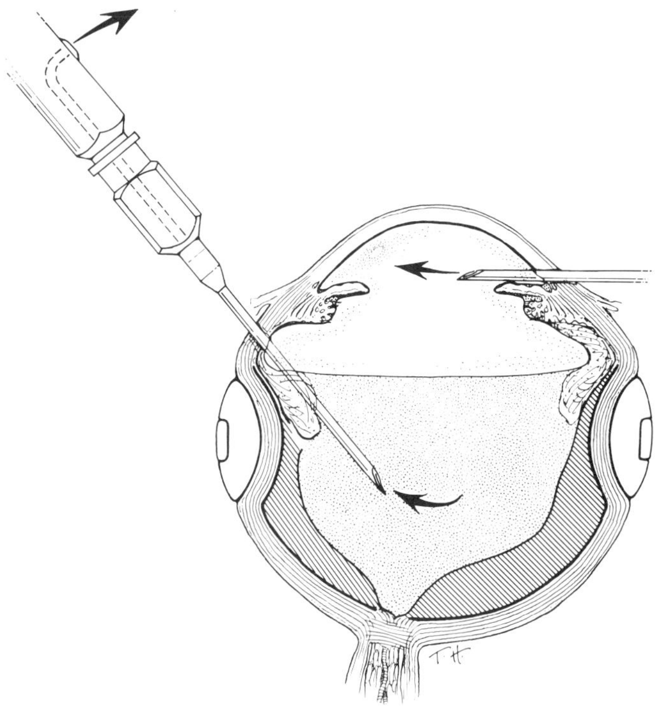

Figure 9.62 *Simultaneous fluid–gas exchange in aphakic vitrectomized eye with extensive rhegmatogenous retinal detachment. After cryotherapy and placement of scleral buckle, air is injected through anterior chamber as intravitreal fluid is displaced out of eye through 27 gauge needle attached to flute handle. Elevated intraocular pressure, caused by expanding air bubble, displaces intravitreal fluid out of eye*

temporary flattening of the retinal break(s) while a surrounding chorioretinal adhesion forms. Various special methods can be used in these eyes, and in some cases these techniques greatly improve the safety of the reoperation procedure and the ease of obtaining a successful result.

Results

Successful retinal reattachment is achieved in slightly more than 90 per cent of eyes with rhegmatogenous detachment, although more than one operation may be required[44–48]. At least 75 per cent of eyes are reattached with a single operation[48]. Most failures ultimately are caused by massive periretinal proliferation.

The likelihood of a successful result also correlates with certain preoperative features. Retinal detachment caused by a retinal dialysis or subtotal detachment due to small anterior retinal breaks can be cured in nearly all cases unless MPP develops later[48–50]. Retinal detachment in aphakic eyes has a less favorable prognosis, perhaps because multiple retinal breaks are often present and there is an increased incidence of occult breaks that cannot be detected during preoperative and intraoperative examination. Also, in aphakic eyes there is an increased incidence of total detachment, thereby removing some topographic features that are helpful in locating the retinal breaks. Similarly, eyes with a pseudophakos have a somewhat lower success rate, perhaps because of greater difficulty in identifying all retinal breaks[51]. Eyes with a poor prognosis are those with giant retinal tears and/or preoperative MPP. Others have observed a lower success rate in eyes with combined preoperative retinal detachment and choroidal detachment, although this has not been our experience[52,53].

Unfortunately, the prognosis for vision is worse than that for reattachment[47,54,55]. When the macula has been involved by the detachment, normal (20/20) postoperative vision is rarely achieved. Even when the macula was not involved preoperatively the final visual acuity is partly reduced in 10 per cent of eyes[47,56,57]. The final level of vision in patients with macular involvement is determined by a number of factors, including the patient's age, duration of macular detachment and amount of elevation of the macular area. For example, if the macula is detached for 1 week or longer, less than 50 per cent of cases achieve final vision of 20/70 or better[55]. Therefore, eyes with retinal detachment threatening the macula are managed as a semi-emergency, to reattach the retina before subretinal fluid damages the macula. Many surgeons believe that prompt reattachment within 48 hours of macular involvement improves further the prognosis for recovery of nearly normal postoperative vision. Thereafter, some permanent visual loss usually results, perhaps due to irreversible damage to the photoreceptors. The final visual acuity rarely improves to better than 20/200 if the macula has been highly detached for more than 4 weeks.

Complications

Various complications are encountered in eyes with retinal detachment. These include pre-existing conditions and intraoperative and postoperative complications. Preexisting conditions include: (*1*) a small immobile pupil, lens opacities or other pupillary opacities obscuring visualization; (*2*) vitreous hemorrhage; (*3*) uveitis with or without choroidal effusion; (*4*) prominent vitreous traction; and (*5*) epiretinal membrane formation with fixed retinal folds. This section emphasizes methods to anticipate and avoid complications.

Pre-existing conditions

Adequate visualization is required for proper identification of all retinal breaks and for monitoring intraocular features of the operation. Usually the fundus can be adequately examined through a 3–4 mm pupil with indirect ophthalmoscopy, although a 30 diopter condensing lens may be required rather than the usual 20 diopter lens. In aphakic eyes with an immobile pupil of 2 mm or less, the pupillary space can be enlarged by excising portions of iris tissue through a limbal approach using a vitrectomy instrument (*Figure 9.63*) or it can be enlarged by photomydriasis. If an opaque posterior lens capsule or other pupillary membrane prohibits proper visualization of the fundus, this tissue is also excised with a vitrectomy instrument. If a markedly cataractous lens is present, this is removed by phacoemulsification in young patients and by planned extracapsular cataract extraction in older patients with a lens nucleus of firm consistency. The posterior lens capsule is preserved in each case, and the limbal incision is closed with multiple sutures. Retinal reattachment surgery can usually be performed within 1 week after phacoemulsification or conventional extracapsular extraction.

Vitreous hemorrhage is frequent in eyes with rhegmatogenous retinal detachment, but the amount of hemorrhage is usually small and does not interfere significantly with examination of the fundus. Eyes with a large amount of vitreous hemorrhage are treated with bilateral eye bandages and bedrest with the head elevated for 24–48 hours. The retina is examined at the bedside to avoid dispersion of blood by eye movement. If retinal breaks can be seen that seem to account for the extent and configuration of the detachment, a conventional scleral buckling operation is performed. Vitrectomy may be performed to remove the opacities if dense hemorrhage is present and extensive retinal detachment is demonstrated by ultrasonography. However, this is rarely necessary other than in eyes with a proliferative retinopathy or after ocular trauma.

Uveitis with discomfort, miosis, vitreous inflammatory debris and even choroidal effusion occurs in some eyes with retinal detachment. The cause of this process is unknown, and usually the intraocular inflammation promptly subsides after the retina is successfully reattached. If the intraocular opacities interfere with visualization of the fundus, or if prominent choroidal effusion is present, the patient is treated preoperatively with topical and systemic corticosteroids. However, the operation is not delayed for long if the media are clear enough to permit identification of all retinal breaks. When choroidal detachments are present, the suprachoroidal fluid is drained at the beginning of the operation by incising the sclera over the area of greatest choroidal elevation. Saline is injected into the vitreous cavity to restore normal intraocular volume before proceeding with the usual steps in the retinal reattachment operation (*Figure 9.64*). If uveitis has caused posterior synechiae that limit dilation of the pupil, subconjunctival injection of a dilating solution containing homatropine, phenylephrine, and procaine is sometimes effective in breaking the adhesions between the iris and the lens.

The most serious preoperative complication is epiretinal membrane formation with fixed retinal folds. This is evidence of active periretinal cellular proliferation that may progress to cause complete immobilization of the retina and an inoperable condition. If the retina is still mobile, and if the retinal breaks can probably be closed by a proper scleral buckle, a conventional retinal reattachment operation is performed using a broad and high encircling buckle as mentioned before. However, if the retina is completely immobile or if a previous scleral buckling operation has failed because of progressive intraocular proliferation, vitrectomy together with revision of the scleral buckle may be advised (see Chapter 8).

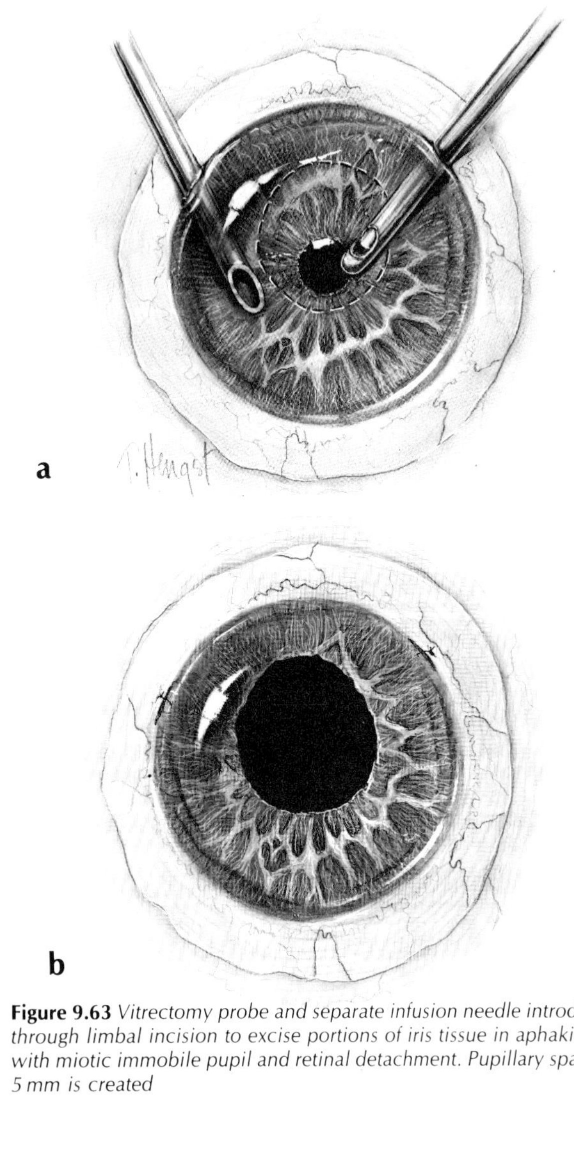

Figure 9.63 *Vitrectomy probe and separate infusion needle introduced through limbal incision to excise portions of iris tissue in aphakic eye with miotic immobile pupil and retinal detachment. Pupillary space of 5 mm is created*

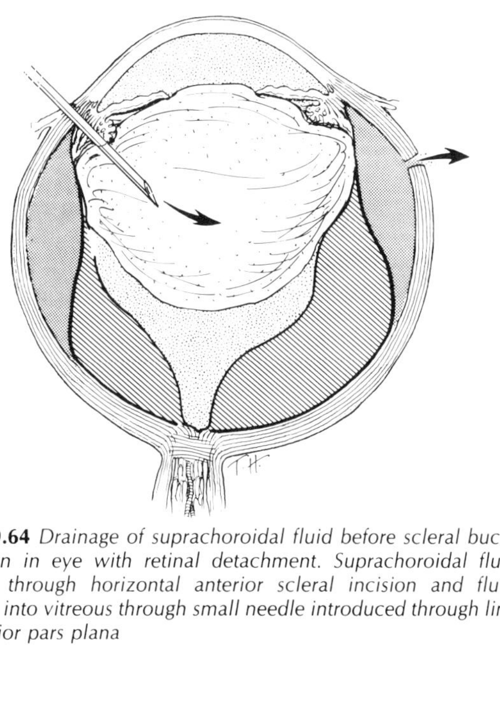

Figure 9.64 *Drainage of suprachoroidal fluid before scleral buckling operation in eye with retinal detachment. Suprachoroidal fluid is drained through horizontal anterior scleral incision and fluid is injected into vitreous through small needle introduced through limbus or anterior pars plana*

Intraoperative complications

Numerous intraoperative complications can occur, including: (1) loss of visualization due to constriction of the pupil or multiple bubbles occurring after intraocular gas injection; (2) scleral rupture during dissection after previous retinal surgery; (3) full-thickness penetration of the sclera during placement of intrascleral sutures for scleral buckling; (4) rupture of an extraocular muscle; (5) choroidal hemorrhage at a drainage site or elsewhere with or without vitreous hemorrhage; (6) incarceration of retina at the drainage site, with or without retinal break formation; (7) failure to close the retinal breaks adequately, for various reasons; (8) closure of the central retinal artery; and (9) migration of pigmentary debris under the macula after cryotherapy.

Loss of visualization

Constriction of the pupil during retinal reattachment surgery is infrequent, although this may occur during reoperations when prolonged dissection of the episcleral tissue is necessary and especially if the eye is somewhat soft. Preoperative subconjunctival injection of a dilating solution seems to help avoid miosis, as does injection of saline into the vitreous cavity if the eye is excessively soft. Intraoperative miosis can sometimes be reversed by topical application of 1 per cent atropine and 10 per cent phenylephrine. The latter is applied to an area of the peripheral cornea using a cotton pledget after creating a local epithelial abrasion. Alternatively, epinephrine in a concentration of 1:10 000 can be injected into the anterior chamber, although this is rarely necessary.

Visualization may also be interrupted if multiple small bubbles (fish eggs) form after injection of air into the vitreous cavity. The chance of this is minimized by rapid injection of the air and by keeping the needle tip in the anterior vitreous cavity within the expanding bubble. Despite these precautions multiple bubbles can still occur, so that final decisions regarding the location and height of the scleral buckle should be made before intravitreal injection of air.

Rupture or penetration of the globe

Scleral rupture during retinal surgery is rare, and it occurs most often during reoperation when a scleral dissection technique was used previously. Therefore, exact knowledge of the previous operation is helpful, and care is taken to identify the proper cleavage plane when cleaning the episcleral surface. When removal of silicone material implanted in an intrascleral dissection plane is necessary, we prefer to place any mattress sutures that are needed and to complete as much of the operation as possible before removal. In removing the silicone, it is exposed in a localized area, any encircling band is cut and the silicone is withdrawn without opening the intrascleral dissection plane further (*Figure 9.65*). If there is leakage of subretinal fluid from the bed, this may flatten the retina. If vitreous fluid leaks, it can sometimes be stopped by placing an

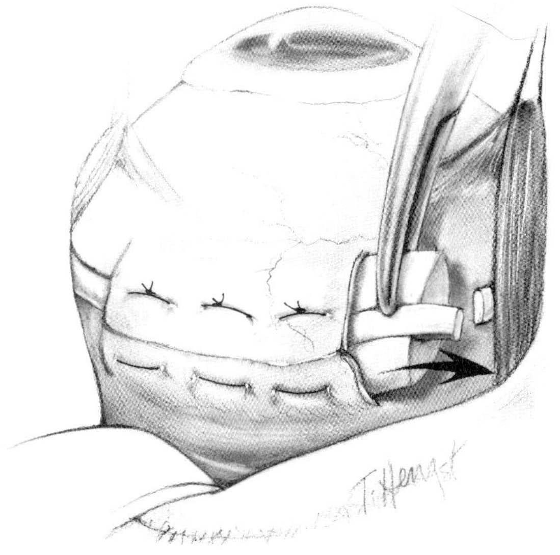

Figure 9.65 *Removal of implanted silicone-rubber material to treat postoperative infection. Small incision is made in scleral bed, encircling element is cut and implanted material is removed without opening scleral dissection further*

external buckle over the leakage site. Sometimes it is necessary to suture the leakage site closed.

Similarly, dissection under the extraocular muscles is done under direct visualization to avoid scleral perforation. When possible, the scissor blades are passed along the external surface of silicone material already present under the muscles.

A more frequent problem is inadvertent full-thickness penetration of the sclera when placing intrascleral sutures for scleral buckling. This is more likely to occur if the sclera is thin. Scleral thinning is often located just posterior to the rectus muscle insertions and sometimes in the superotemporal quadrant. Inadvertent penetration is avoided by use of a spatula needle, by slight elevation of the needle tip as it is passed through the sclera and by constant visualization of the tip. Full-thickness penetration is serious if it occurs where the retina is attached because it can cause a retinal hole, although even here the needle may damage only the choroid and pigment epithelium without passing through the retina.

Any subretinal fluid which drains through a needle tract may be permitted to continue or it may be tamponaded with a cotton-tip applicator, depending on whether all necessary sutures have been placed and whether it is an appropriate time for release of subretinal fluid. If the perforation site is at the posterior location of a suture, the suture is cut at the entry site and the short end is pulled through the intrascleral tract. The suture is then replaced with a slightly more posterior scleral bite if the retina was not damaged. If the retina was damaged, this site is supported on the crest of a scleral buckle, which may require positioning a circumferential buckle further posteriorly, adding a radial element to a circumferential buckle or the use of a broader buckle if the complication occurred during placement of sutures for a radially oriented exoplant. A penetrating suture is not removed if the penetration occurred at the anterior bite of a suture, if the retina was not damaged and if suture material cannot be seen in the tract by indirect ophthalmoscopy. After placing all of the scleral sutures, these areas are routinely examined by indirect ophthalmoscopy to look for evidence of penetration of the sclera, even though there is no apparent drainage of intraocular fluid externally.

Drainage site complications

Complications at the drainage site include premature drainage of subretinal fluid, retinal hole formation, incarceration of retina at the drainage site (with or without retinal hole formation) and choroidal hemorrhage at the drainage site or elsewhere. Accidental penetration of the choroid may occur while preparing the scleral incision, placing a suture in the edges of the scleral incision or during application of diathermy to the choroid. We prefer to use preplaced sutures for later closure of the scleral incision as previously mentioned (see p. 278). Care is taken to avoid elevation of the intraocular pressure as the scleral incision is made and when the suture is placed, because this may prolapse the choroid into the scleral incision and increase the risk of inadvertent penetration. Diathermy, set at low levels, is used to treat the bare choroid, and the tip is constantly moved as the diathermy is applied so the tip does not become adherent to the choroid and rupture it as the tip is pulled away. If premature drainage occurs, all traction on the globe is immediately released to reduce the intraocular pressure and prevent expulsive drainage of subretinal fluid with incarceration of the retina at that site.

A retinal hole may occur from damage by the drainage needle used to penetrate the choroid and the pigment epithelium. This is avoided by selecting a place for drainage where the retina is highly elevated and by penetrating the choroid tangentially. Nevertheless, the needle tip may come near the retina if the choroid is quite elastic and must be considerably indented before penetration occurs. When working with a skilled assistant, we prefer to have the assistant visualize the retina overlying the drainage site as the choroid is penetrated. This is done using indirect ophthalmoscopy, and it is immediately known whether the needle tip damaged the retina.

Drainage of subretinal fluid is monitored both internally and externally as mentioned before, and the safety suture is tightened to close the scleral incision when the retina becomes flat at this location and drainage of subretinal fluid stops. Care is taken to avoid any elevation of the intraocular pressure as the retina begins to flatten near the sclerotomy. The risk of retinal incarceration is greater when a large hole is made in the choroid with a large needle. A thin diathermy electrode or small needle used to penetrate the choroid reduces the chance of retinal incarceration. If retina becomes incarcerated despite these precautions, with or without causing a retinal hole, the area of the sclerotomy is usually treated with cryotherapy and supported on a scleral buckle. Serious postoperative complications are rare unless the retina ruptures with prolapse of vitreous gel which may result in intraocular fibrous proliferation with or without secondary traction retinal detachment.

Hemorrhage from the drainage site is a feared, albeit rare, complication. As previously discussed, the risk of this occurrence may be reduced by the use of diathermy to treat the choroid before penetration. If external bleeding occurs, the fundus is immediately examined. If no blood is seen internally, the bleeding is permitted to stop spontaneously or, if necessary, diathermy is applied. Then the sclerotomy is closed with the scleral suture, and another drainage site is selected. If blood is accumulating internally, the sclerotomy is closed securely by temporarily tying the scleral suture and digital pressure is applied to the globe to increase the intraocular pressure. The area of hemorrhage is examined by indirect ophthalmoscopy until all bleeding stops. Drainage of subretinal fluid may then be attempted in another location.

Choroidal hemorrhage may also occur in a remote location during or after drainage of subretinal fluid. This is most common in highly myopic eyes, and choroidal hemorrhage is often a serious complication that can result in extremely high intraocular pressure with central retinal artery closure or anterior segment ischemia. It can also cause vitreous hemorrhage, recurrent retinal detachment with or without MPP, and loss of vision from other causes. In such cases the sclerotomy is immediately closed, and the scleral sutures are tightened to elevate the scleral buckle. This permits closure of the retinal breaks before the expanding choroidal hemorrhage causes elevation of the intraocular pressure and thereby prevents further indentation of the scleral buckle. Also, tightening the sutures increases the intraocular pressure rapidly, and this may help to tamponade the active bleeding.

Failure to close retinal breaks

Inability to close properly all retinal breaks on the scleral buckle may be a serious problem during retinal reattachment surgery. This may occur because of: (*1*) malposition between the buckle and the retinal breaks; (*2*) vitreous traction; and/or (*3*) radial folds of the retina. Sometimes the size, shape or position of the scleral buckle is not suitable to support all retinal breaks after the retina settles following drainage of subretinal fluid. In such cases the scleral sutures may be replaced and the position of the buckle modified to support all edges of each retinal break, including the anterior margins. This capability is an advantage of the episcleral exoplant technique as compared to scleral dissection with an intrascleral implant. Some experience is needed to judge whether the relationship between each retinal break and the scleral buckle is suitable.

Vitreous traction occasionally prevents adequate closure of retinal breaks. If there is prominent vitreous traction on the flap of a horseshoe tear, a supplemental radially oriented exoplant may be placed beneath the tear. This is combined with an encircling buckle to assist further in relieving vitreous traction. In such cases a larger area anterior to each tear may be treated with cryotherapy to create an extensive chorioretinal adhesion because progressive vitreous traction might cause anterior extension of the tear.

Radial folding of the retina with folds extending from a retinal tear over the posterior aspect of the scleral buckle is a frequent problem, and this is more likely to occur when large horseshoe-shaped tears are present in the superior quadrants and when the retina is highly detached preoperatively. Some retinal folding is seen in many cases, and experience is required to know whether the configuration is likely to persist and cause recurrence of subretinal fluid posterior to the buckle. If the folds are small and narrow, and if the retina is flat on the posterior crest of the buckle for 1 mm or more on both sides of each fold, then no further treatment is needed. If the fold is broad and/or highly elevated, and if it communicates with residual or recurrent subretinal fluid posterior to the buckle, then revision of the buckle or use of intravitreal air is needed.

The encircling buckle may be loosened somewhat if severe radial folding occurs. These folds may be due to excessive tightening of the encircling band. A radially oriented scleral buckle seems to minimize radial folding, and specially designed silicone rubber wedges are available to place beneath such retinal breaks[58]. However, usually a one-half thickness piece of soft silicone sponge smooths out the retinal fold.

When retinal folding occurs because an excessive amount of subretinal fluid was drained, fluid or gas is injected into the vitreous cavity to restore normal intraocular volume and pressure without requiring excessive elevation of an encircling buckle. In such cases, a decision is made – based on the appearance of the worrisome retinal break(s) and the buckle – as to whether the break(s) are likely to settle properly without the use of intraocular tamponade. When a radial buckle is used, saline is usually injected, although further drainage of subretinal fluid and injection of air may be necessary if there is intraoperative reaccumulation of subretinal fluid posterior to the buckle. When a circumferential buckle is used, radial folds are especially likely to persist, and air may be injected to restore the volume in these eyes. Before air injection, the location and height of the scleral buckle is adjusted (as mentioned previously) because visualization may be obscured if the air enters the eye as multiple small bubbles.

Closure of the central retinal artery

Closure of the central retinal artery from excessive elevation of the intraocular pressure is a serious potential complication during retinal reattachment surgery. This is most likely to occur while tightening the scleral sutures if subretinal fluid has not been drained or if only a small amount of fluid can be removed. Therefore, the optic nerve and central retinal artery are observed periodically to be certain that blood flow is not interrupted. The intraocular pressure is also measured periodically by indentation tonometry to correlate the intraocular pressure measurement with the condition of flow in the central retinal artery. If the intraocular pressure is elevated and pulsations in the artery are not visible, gentle digital pressure is applied to the eye until pulsations are induced. This is done to be certain that blood flow is not already interrupted and that the intraocular pressure is lower than the diastolic blood pressure. At the same time the blood pressure is determined, and if found to be low, it may be increased by the anesthesiologist if general anesthesia is being used.

The scleral sutures are tightened one at a time when the intraocular pressure is elevated, and temporary knots are used so they can be immediately loosened if the pressure becomes too high. The technique of tying sutures one at a time and waiting for the intraocular pressure to return to a safe level after each suture is tied is usually effective in eyes with normal outflow of aqueous humor. Anterior chamber paracentesis is also helpful in phakic eyes and in aphakic eyes with an intact anterior hyaloid face or in those with a posterior chamber pseudophakos. Paracentesis permits elevation of the scleral buckle without a marked increase in the intraocular pressure. In some eyes a large amount of aqueous humor can be removed without causing significant shallowing of the anterior chamber, presumably because fluid vitreous passes around the lens or IOL. This reduces further the risk of central retinal artery closure.

If the central retinal artery closes, the intraocular pressure should be lowered immediately by loosening one or more sutures or by performing an anterior chamber paracentesis. However, if these measures fail or if the central retinal artery closes while several sutures remain to be tied, fluid can be aspirated from the vitreous cavity (*Figure 9.66*). This is done with a 1.5 inch (3.8 cm) 25 or 27 gauge needle attached to a 2 ml syringe. The needle tip is

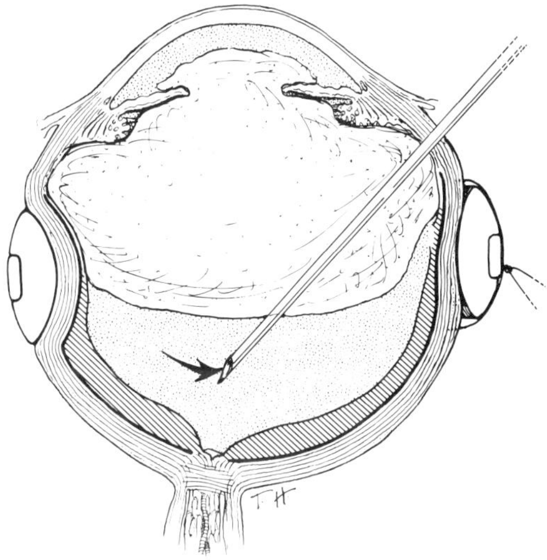

Figure 9.66 *Aspiration of fluid vitreous to soften eye before elevation of scleral buckle in aphakic eye with vitreous in anterior chamber and flat retinal detachment making transscleral drainage of subretinal fluid hazardous. One-inch (2.5 cm) 27 gauge needle is passed through pars plana into fluid space behind posterior vitreous surface. Needle tip is located over optic nerve and fluid aspirated using 1 ml syringe*

passed through the mid-pars plana and positioned directly over the optic nerve posterior to the posterior vitreous surface while the tip is visualized by indirect ophthalmoscopy. The surgeon holds the needle hub and syringe as the assistant gently withdraws the plunger to aspirate fluid. Usually 1–2 ml of vitreous fluid is withdrawn to soften the eye, restore flow in the central retinal artery, and permit tightening of the remaining scleral sutures so as to elevate properly the scleral buckle.

Sometimes there are visible pulsations in the central retinal artery after tightening the last scleral suture. The intraocular pressure is measured by Schiotz tonometry at this time, and the systemic blood pressure is determined. The intraocular pressure is measured periodically as remaining portions of the operation are completed. However, before completing closure of the conjunctival incision, the fundus is again examined to determine whether there is continuous blood flow without pulsations in the central retinal artery. An additional anterior chamber paracentesis may be performed if pulsations persist. Otherwise, an intravenous hyperosmotic agent is given, together with acetazolamide to reduce aqueous humor secretion, and the condition of the central retinal artery is re-examined in the recovery room 20–30 minutes later.

Rupture of extraocular muscles

Serious damage to the extraocular muscles rarely occurs during retinal reattachment surgery, although portions of the insertions of the superior oblique and inferior oblique are deliberateley cut when necessary to provide exposure for localization or treatment of retinal holes or for placement of sutures for scleral buckling. Temporary disinsertion of a rectus muscle is rarely necessary except when retinal breaks are located far posterior in the merdian of the muscle or when treating a macular hole with a scleral buckle. Rarely, a bridle suture ruptures the tendon insertion of a rectus muscle. This is most likely to occur during a reoperation if the muscle was disinserted previously. This is overcome by use of a traction suture attached to the sclera anterior to the muscle insertion, thereby avoiding direct traction on the weakened rectus muscle (*Figure 9.67*). A bridle suture may also rupture the muscle belly.

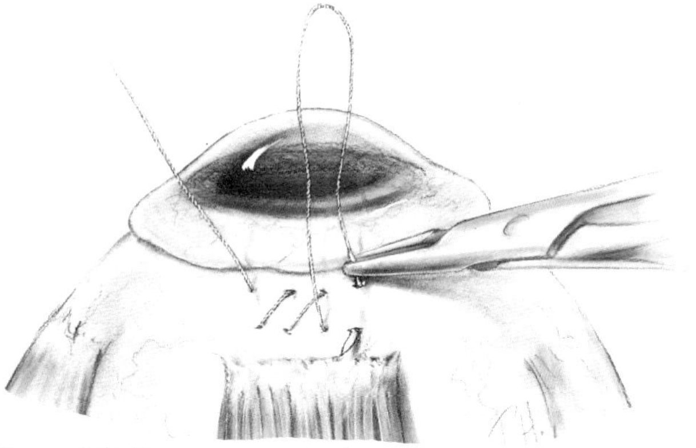

Figure 9.67 *Placement of scleral traction suture anterior to rectus muscle insertion if the muscle was removed previously or is involved with extensive scarring making exposure difficult. Three or four partial-thickness scleral bites are used*

This can occur if the suture loop slips posteriorly beneath the muscle belly rather than beneath the tendon insertion. This complication is avoided by periodically observing the location of the bridle suture loops. If a rupture occurs, the torn edges of the muscle are sutured together with absorbable sutures.

Pigment dispersion under the retina

Cryotherapy applied to the pigment epithelium causes rupture of some cells and dispersion of pigment in the subretinal space. Pigmentary debris may migrate posteriorly and accumulate under the macula (*Figure 9.68*). Some studies suggest that this pigment does not have an important effect on postoperative vision[59]. Nevertheless, it seems unlikely that maximum visual acuity can be achieved if pigmentary debris is present in the center of the macula between the receptor elements and the pigment epithelium. Therefore, pigment dispersion into the macula is avoided when possible.

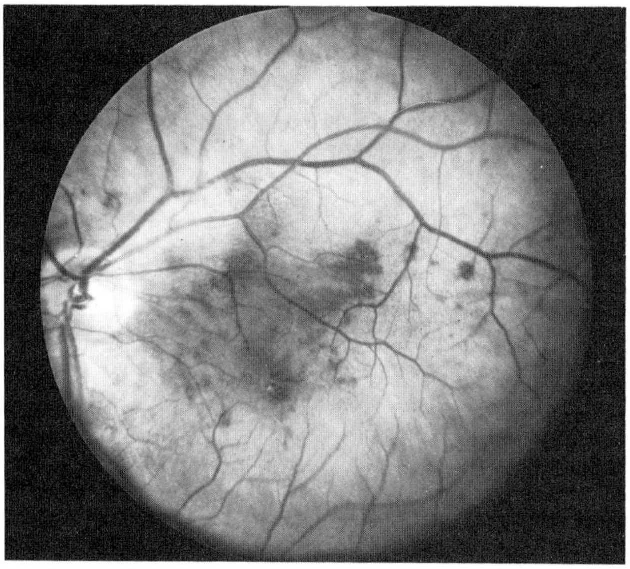

Figure 9.68 *Pigment fallout under macula following cryotherapy in eye with retinal detachment previously involving macula. Pigment released during disruption of pigment epithelial cells may migrate under posterior retina*

In eyes with retinal detachment not involving the macula, cryotherapy is applied as necessary without concern that pigment dispersion may later affect the visual acuity. When the macula is involved, use of cryotherapy is limited to only the retinal breaks to minimize pigment dispersion rather than treating broader areas. Rarely, it is desirable to drain subretinal fluid and inject saline into the vitreous cavity in order to reattach the retina prior to application of cryotherapy. This may be done when large areas of the peripheral fundus are to be treated because of widespread lattice degeneration and yet only a small scleral buckle is needed to close the retinal break(s). When vitreous surgery methods are used, fluid–gas exchange is often performed to replace the intravitreal fluid with air, and this may be combined with drainage of subretinal fluid prior to application of cryotherapy. With this method the peripheral retina is reattached, and cryotherapy applied later is not associated with posterior migration of pigment debris.

Postoperative complications

Numerous complications can occur after retinal reattachment surgery, although the most important are those that result in failure of the retina to reattach, decrease visual acuity despite successful reattachment, or cause discomfort or an unsuitable cosmetic appearance. Postoperative complications may be evident early, during the first 2 weeks after the operation, or they may appear at a later time. Early complications include: (*1*) shallowing of the anterior chamber; (*2*) choroidal detachment; (*3*) residual or recurrent subretinal fluid; and (*4*) anterior segment ischemia. Later complications include: (*1*) recurrent detachment due to new retinal breaks and/or massive periretinal proliferation; (2) macular pucker despite successful reattachment; (3) cystoid macular edema; (4) refractive changes; (5) muscle imbalance and/or cosmetic abnormalities such as enophthalmos and ptosis; (6) ocular pain and (7) exposure or extrusion of the implanted material.

Anterior segment shallowing

Shallowing of the anterior chamber is most commonly seen after retinal reattachment surgery in elderly patients, and it is associated with choroidal detachment and anterior shift of the ciliary body. This is more likely if an encircling buckle is used, if extensive cryotherapy is applied or if the eye becomes very soft during drainage of subretinal fluid. Some surgeons believe that this complication is due to compression or other damage to the vortex veins, causing secondary elevation of the intrachoroidal venous pressure and choroidal effusion. However, choroidal detachment and anterior chamber shallowing can occur when all treatment and surgical manipulations are limited to the region anterior to the equator, and it can occur after only a localized scleral buckle in elderly patients.

Anterior chamber shallowing usually resolves spontaneously in 10–20 days, and it causes no other complication unless it results in angle-closure glaucoma in phakic eyes. Angle closure is most likely to occur if the anterior chamber is shallow preoperatively. The intraocular pressure is routinely measured during the first several postoperative days because of this possibility.

Angle-closure glaucoma is usually not caused by pupillary block but rather by swelling and anterior displacement of the ciliary body[60]. Therefore, treatment of this complication is different from conventional angle-closure glaucoma due to pupillary block. Still, miotic therapy and laser iridotomy or surgical iridectomy may be performed if gonioscopy and slit-lamp examination of the iris surface suggest a true pupillary block mechanism. If a surgical iridectomy is performed, this is combined with drainage of suprachoroidal fluid and injection of saline into the anterior chamber.

Eyes with postoperative angle closure are usually treated with cycloplegic medications, acetazolamide and frequent topical application of steroids. Systemic steroids are used in young, healthy patients. If the intraocular pressure is lowered to 30 mmHg or less with these measures then nothing further is required, and the underlying condition resolves in 1–2 weeks. However, if the anterior chamber is markedly shallow and/or if the intraocular pressure remains elevated above 30 mmHg, we prefer to drain the suprachoroidal fluid promptly. This is combined with injection of saline into the anterior chamber, and frequent postoperative application of topical steroids. If angle closure recurs after these measures, and if more than one vortex vein is compressed by the scleral buckle, then the silicone is removed or modified to relieve compression of the vortex veins.

Choroidal detachment

Choroidal detachment may also occur without shallowing of the anterior chamber, and this is seen postoperatively in about 20 per cent of cases. Although there is probably suprachoroidal fluid in all quadrants, the visible choroidal elevation is often most evident adjacent to the ends of a segmental scleral buckle or on the opposite side of the eye. The choroidal elevation may increase in size during the first 2 or 3 postoperative days. Then it usually remains unchanged for about 10 days before regressing 2 weeks after the operation.

The intraocular pressure is usually low while choroidal detachments are present, and there may also be some increase in the amount of remaining subretinal fluid during the first two postoperative days. Remaining subretinal fluid usually does not resorb while choroidal detachments are present, perhaps due to altered function of the pigment epithelium. The subretinal fluid clears rapidly, however, when the choroidal detachments resolve.

Systemic and/or topical steroids are sometimes used to treat these detachments but there is no evidence that this is effective. Moreover, the choroidal detachments subside spontaneously whether or not steroids are used. Rarely the choroidal detachments are so extensive that elevation on opposite sides of the globe causes contact of the cortical vitreous and peripheral retina centrally ('kissing choroidals'). This can produce adhesions between these tissues and can result in traction retinal detachment or even formation of retinal breaks when the choroidal elevation regresses.

If there is contact between tissues from opposite quadrants, we prefer to drain the suprachoroidal fluid immediately. This is done with a scleral incision over the pars plana to release the fluid, combined with injection of saline into the vitreous cavity to restore intraocular volume. Saline is injected through the limbus in aphakic eyes and through the pars plana in phakic eyes, with the needle introduced through the location of least choroidal elevation and directed into the vitreous cavity.

Choroidal detachments rarely cause separation of a retinal break from the scleral buckle due to distortion of the buckle or due to retinal folds that prevent sealing of the break. If this complication occurs, suprachoroidal fluid may be drained and air injected into the vitreous cavity to ensure closure of the retinal breaks during the early postoperative period.

Residual or recurrent subretinal fluid

The presence of subretinal fluid is a frequent concern in the early postoperative period, and the surgeon must decide whether the fluid will absorb later or whether it is an ominous sign of a more serious underlying problem. When choroidal detachments are present, residual subretinal fluid often does not absorb until the suprachoroidal fluid disappears as mentioned before. In the absence of choroidal detachments, the location and amount of subretinal fluid is recorded, and the eye is examined to identify any open retinal breaks. If breaks are found that were not treated previously and/or supported by the scleral buckle, prompt reoperation is necessary. In other cases, efforts are made to encourage absorption of the subretinal fluid and/or flattening of breaks that remain elevated over a scleral buckle.

Bedrest with bilateral eye bandages is often used in these cases. This seems to encourage settling of the retina and absorption of subretinal fluid, which often occurs between the second and sixth postoperative days. Special head positioning may be helpful, depending on the amount of subretinal fluid and the location of the retinal breaks. The head of the bed is elevated when superior retinal breaks are present, whereas the patient lies flat if there are inferior retinal breaks. The patient may be positioned on one side or the other to displace residual subretinal fluid away from open retinal breaks located over the scleral buckle and to place vitreous gel in contact with the break.

Postoperative photocoagulation and/or air injection into the vitreous cavity is sometimes needed, especially to treat open retinal breaks located over the scleral buckle that are associated with radial retinal folds and that communicate with subretinal fluid posterior to the buckle. Photocoagulation alone is used when sufficient energy can be applied to cause a visible response within the elevated retinal fold, applying treatment along both edges of the fold and on the fold itself. Shrinkage of the fold occurs 3–10 days later. If the fold is so broad or highly elevated that there is no visible response to photocoagulation, air is injected into the vitreous cavity. This may require a reoperation for subretinal fluid drainage, which is performed posterior to the previous scleral buckle. In other cases intravitreal injection can be done at the bedside after softening the eye with hyperosmotic agents, acetazolamide and ocular massage[61].

Anterior segment ischemia

Anterior segment ischemia is a rare but severe complication after retinal reattachment surgery. Because this occurs most commonly in patients with hemoglobin SC, this possibility should be anticipated preoperatively and special precautions taken in such cases[62]. These precautions include partial preoperative exchange transfusion to provide the circulatory system with about 50 per cent hemoglobin A, maintaining low blood viscosity with a hematocrit of about 30 per cent, good intra- and postoperative oxygenation of the patient and the avoidance of elevated IOP. Anterior segment ischemia is also occasionally seen when an extensive operative procedure is performed with cryotherapy applied for 360° and combined with a high and broad scleral buckle extending to the ora serrata in all quadrants. This complication is more likely if two or more of the rectus muscles are temporarily disinserted.

Anterior segment ischemia is recognized on the first or second postoperative day by: (*1*) excessive lid swelling and chemosis; (*2*) corneal edema with folds in the posterior stroma; (*3*) a mid-dilated, nonreactive pupil; (*4*) white flake-like debris in the anterior chamber; and (*5*) progressive lens opacification. In affected eyes, the intraocular pressure may be elevated, low or in the normal range.

Treatment is begun immediately with systemic and local steroids. If an encircling buckle is used, this is loosened. If the intraocular pressure is elevated, a peripheral iridectomy is performed and a sclerotomy performed over the ciliary body to drain any suprachoroidal fluid. Despite these measures, anterior segment ischemia often results in later hypotony or phthisis bulbi, corneal opacity, cataract and poor vision. Fortunately, damage is less severe in some eyes and the process resolves with areas of iris necrosis, mild persistent corneal edema and a mature cataract which can be removed later.

Late recurrent retinal detachment

Late recurrent detachment is usually due to new retinal breaks with or without massive periretinal proliferation. Rarely, prior retinal breaks may reopen due to progressive vitreous traction or changes in the configuration of the scleral buckle. New retinal breaks are also rare, but these may occur during the first 3 months after the retinal surgery due to progressive vitreous traction. However, the most common cause of recurrent detachment after an initially successful result is MPP that occurs between 4 and 12 weeks postoperatively.

MPP is an idiopathic process characterized by intravitreal, epiretinal and subretinal proliferation of nonvascularized cellular membranes, contraction of these cellular membranes and formation of new extracellular collagen. This results in detachment and distortion of the retina and it often causes new retinal tears or reopening of prior tears, leading to a combined traction and rhegmatogenous detachment. These changes range from mild involvement, treatable by revision of the scleral buckle and/or vitreous surgery, to severe conditions that ultimately result in failure despite all efforts. No prophylactic measures are known to avoid MPP. However, if fixed retinal folds or other features of epiretinal membrane formation are evident when the original detachment is seen, then a more extensive operation may be done with use of a broad encircling buckle (*see* p. 291).

Macular pucker

A localized epiretinal membrane covering, distorting or detaching the macula (macular pucker) occurs in 4–8 per cent of eyes after otherwise successful retinal reattachment surgery and accounts for further visual loss (*Figure 9.69a*)[63]. The cause of these membranes is not known, but they are composed of cellular elements derived from both fibrous astrocytes and the retinal pigment epithelium. The cells, in turn, produce new extracellular collagen. Vision is reduced to 20/100 or worse in many eyes with macular pucker. Rarely, these membranes spontaneously separate from the retina, resulting in some visual improvement.

Vitreous surgery can be used to separate the abnormal tissue from the underlying retina (*Figure 9.69b*)[64–66]. Portions of the posterior vitreous surface are excised. Then a vitreoretinal pick is used to engage the epiretinal membrane. The membrane can usually be completely separated from the retina, but areas of firm attachment are sometimes encountered, and the membrane is amputated at these locations using intravitreal scissors or the vitrectomy instrument. Vitreous surgery is considered in eyes with vision reduced to 20/100 or worse by macular pucker.

Visual improvement after removal of an epiretinal membrane causing macular pucker is achieved in about 90 per cent of eyes[65,66]. However, the final vision in technically successful cases usually ranges between 20/40 and 20/100. Therefore, cases are selected for surgery in which vision is already reduced to at least 20/100. Postoperative retinal detachment due to peripheral retinal tears is the most frequent complication of the operation, and this may require revision of the scleral buckle. Progressive nuclear sclerotic lens opacities also occur postoperatively in some phakic eyes.

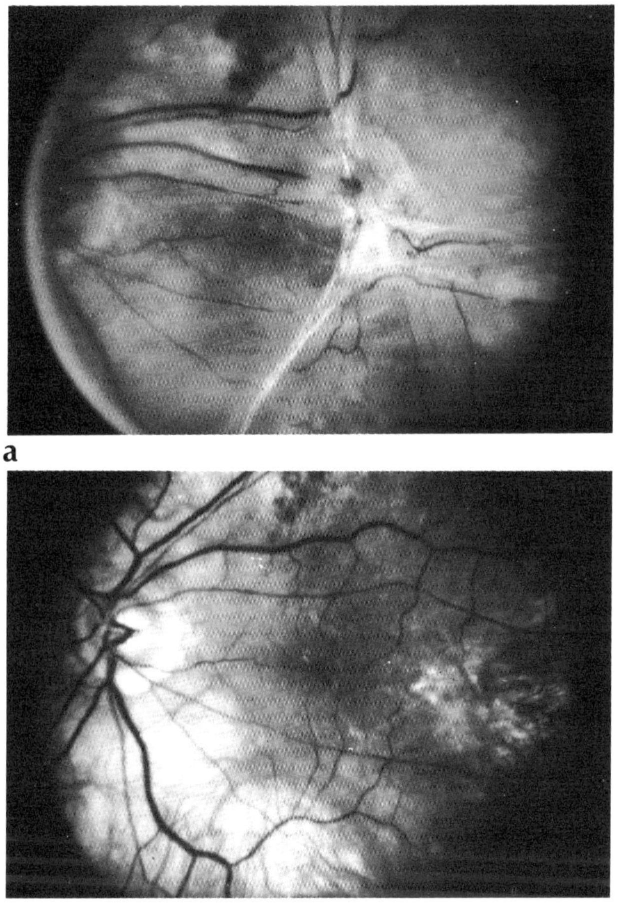

a

b

Figure 9.69 **(a)** *Epiretinal membrane causing macular pucker after otherwise succesful surgery for rhegmatogenous retinal detachment.* **(b)** *Abnormal membrane is removed by vitreous surgery resulting in less distortion of the retina and partial visual improvement*

Cystoid macular edema

Cystoid macular edema occurring after retinal reattachment surgery has only recently been recognized as a postoperative complication. This macular edema occurs in up to 50 per cent of cases, and aphakic eyes are affected more frequently than phakic eyes[67,68]. The etiology of this process is not known, and the features are identical to those of cystoid macular edema seen in some eyes after cataract extraction or associated with ocular inflammatory conditions. Macular involvement is characterized by abnormal leakage from the perifoveal capillary bed, with accumulation of intraretinal extracellular fluid producing a typical cystoid pattern (*Figure 9.70*).

The macular edema clears spontaneously in most cases. However, it can be persistent and reduce vision to 20/200 or worse. No effective treatment is known. Persistent macular edema is most common when extensive cryotherapy has been applied to the peripheral retina, especially if refreezing occurs, causing excessive atrophy of the pigment epithelium and choroid. The possibility of this macular complication is discussed preoperatively with patients in whom the macula is not involved by the retinal detachment and preoperative vision is good.

Refractive changes

Refractive changes are commonly induced by retinal reattachment surgery when a scleral buckling technique is used[69]. The axial length of the eye is increased when an encircling buckle is used, resulting in less hypermetropia or increased myopia. This effect usually changes the refractive power by 1.0–2.5 diopters, although changes of 5 diopters or more may occur if a broad encircling buckle is used. Radial episcleral exoplants often cause changes in astigmatism, but this effect is unpredictable and is influenced by the width and height of the scleral buckle and its location along the anteroposterior dimensions of the globe. Sometimes irregular astigmatism occurs that cannot be corrected with lenses, and this may improve after removal of the silicone implant[70].

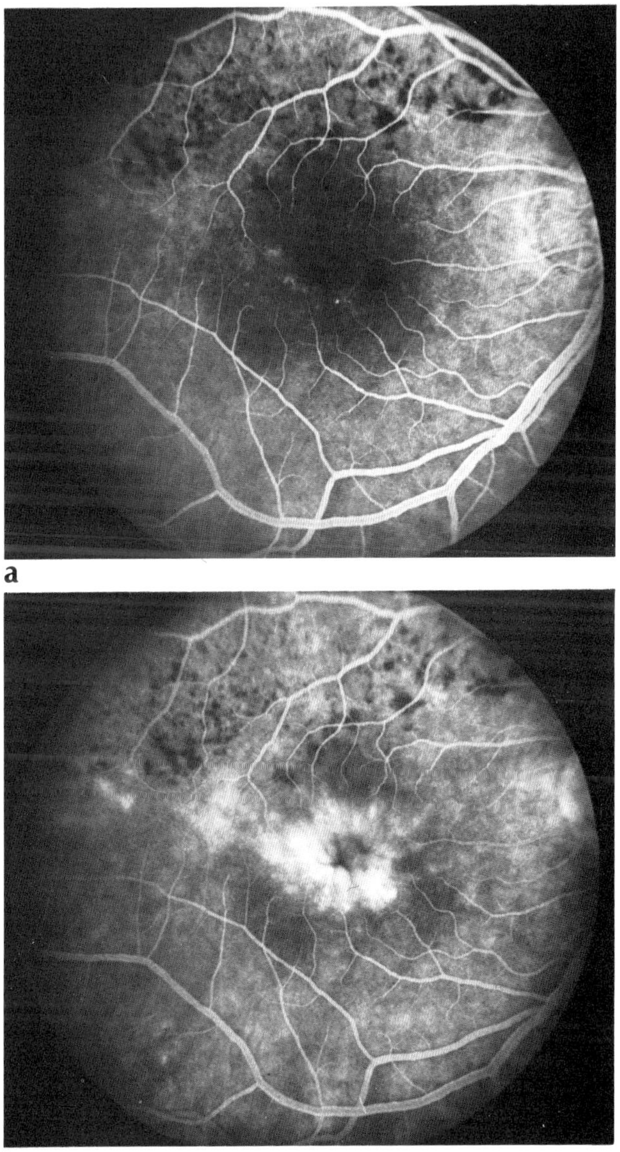

a

b

Figure 9.70 *Cystoid macular edema after otherwise successful retinal reattachment surgery. Fluid leakage occurs from perifoveal capillary bed resulting in accumulation of intraretinal edema. Pigment fallout from prior cryotherapy is seen under superior retina*

The postoperative refractive status may continue to change for 3–6 months after the operation. Therefore, changes in the spectacle prescription are usually not recommended for at least 8–12 weeks postoperatively if the patient is not seriously inconvenienced by imperfect optical correction in the involved eye. Also, during this time there may be improvement in the visual capability of the retina if the macula was involved preoperatively and/or if cystoid macular edema occurred postoperatively. A refraction is often performed 6–8 weeks after the operation, and this is repeated in 2–4 weeks. A lens change is prescribed when two or more successive refractions show no evidence of further change.

Muscle imbalance and/or cosmetic abnormalities

Muscle imbalance and/or changes in the appearance of the eye can occur after retinal surgery. Persistent muscle imbalance causing diplopia is surprisingly infrequent, and this occurs most commonly after two or more operations, perhaps because of an increased amount of episcleral scar tissue. Temporary muscle imbalance is common, and this usually resolves in 6–12 weeks. Persistent muscle imbalance can be treated by prisms or strabismus surgery at a later time if the amount of deviation in the primary position of ocular gaze remains constant.

Ptosis and enophthalmos sometimes occur after extensive surgical procedures. This is probably due to a reduced volume of the globe when a high and broad scleral buckle is used. There may also be atrophy of the orbital fat and/or secondary scarring of the extraocular tissues after extensive surgery. Cosmetic imperfections are most likely if the operation fails to reattach the retina. In such cases a cataract often forms in phakic eyes, and/or the eye may remain quite hypotonous and have further apparent enophthalmos.

Rarely a resection of the levator tendon may be needed to elevate the upper lid as treatment for ptosis. Chronic hyperemia of the conjunctiva and episcleral vessels can be treated by subconjunctival depot steroid injection. If phthisis bulbi develops, a prosthesis can be worn over the shrunken globe to improve the cosmetic appearance.

Ocular pain

Severe persistent pain is rare after retinal reattachment surgery, and chronic pain suggests an infection of the implanted silicone rubber material. However, persistent pain sometimes occurs after use of a high encircling buckle, and rarely it is necessary to cut the encircling band to relieve the pain. When there is both severe pain and excessive injection and swelling of the extraocular tissues during the early postoperative period, but without evidence of an infected exoplant, then an injection of depot steroid under Tenon's capsule is helpful. This is usually combined with frequent use of topically applied steroids.

Chronic pain that complicates an unsuccessful operation can be treated by retrobulbar alcohol injection, and this can also be done in seeing eyes if other measures fail. About 1 ml of 2 per cent lidocaine (Xylocaine) is injected through the lower lid into the retrobulbar muscle cone using a 25 gauge 1.5 inch (3.8 cm) needle. The needle is not removed, but the syringe is exchanged for one containing a 50:50 mixture of absolute ethanol and 2 per cent lidocaine. Two to 3 ml of this mixture are injected, and the syringes are then exchanged again so the needle can be cleared of ethanol by injecting additional lidocaine as the needle is withdrawn.

This technique usually results in prompt resolution of pain, although it is followed by considerable swelling of the orbital tissues and lids. The soft tissue swelling begins to resolve after 3–4 days. The analgesic effect usually lasts at least 3 months and in most cases the effect is permanent. If the first alcohol injection is not successful, this can be repeated about 7 days later. This technique can also be used in seeing eyes without apparent change to the optic nerve, although other measures are first tried to treat the pain.

Infection or exposure of implanted material

Infection or exposure of the implanted silicone material is an infrequent late complication of retinal reattachment surgery, although it occurs in up to 10 per cent of eyes when two or more retinal operations are performed on the same eye[71]. This complication is rarely seen before 6 weeks after surgery, and most cases become evident 4 months or longer after surgery. The involved eye may have mild irritation or severe, unrelenting pain, and the globe is usually tender to palpation. The severity of the pain correlates with the amount of swelling and injection of the extraocular tissues.

A second characteristic feature of an implant infection is chronic purulent discharge. Often a fistula near the conjunctival fornix communicates with the implanted silicone material. Infection involving episcleral exoplants almost never causes infective endophthalmitis, although this sometimes occurs in eyes with an intrascleral implant. Antibiotic therapy is rarely effective, and removal of the implanted silicone material is necessary to cure the infection.

Sometimes the infection can be cured by removing exposed silicone together with any encircling band. This can often be done through the fistula with or without a further local incision. In other cases, the infection persists until all foreign material has been removed, including all sutures used to secure the silicone material to the sclera. Simple removal of the exposed silicone material is usually performed first, however, and this can sometimes be done in the outpatient clinic. If the symptoms persist, a more extensive procedure is necessary to explore each quadrant where silicone material and/or sutures were used and to remove this material.

Retinal detachment can recur after removal of silicone material, especially if the buckle is removed sooner than 4 months after the operation. Before removing silicone material, the retina is examined to locate areas of persistent vitreoretinal traction or other features that might increase the likelihood of reopening a retinal break or causing a new one. Photocoagulation is used preoperatively in some cases to create a firm chorioretinal scar around these areas before the silicone material is removed.

In eyes in which an infected silicone implant is removed and there is a recurrent retinal detachment, systemic antibiotics should be given for at least 10 days before performing another retinal reattachment operation.

Occasionally a portion of the silicone material becomes exposed and yet the eye remains asymptomatic. This usually occurs when the scleral buckle is located anterior to the equator and when the overlying conjunctiva and Tenon's capsule are quite thin. No therapy is recommended in such cases unless features of infection occur later.

Summary

Numerous complications can occur during or after retinal reattachment surgery, and there may be pre-existing conditions that make the operation more difficult or hazardous. The likelihood of most complications can be minimized by proper planning and execution of the operation. However, complications cannot be eliminated entirely. Often a choice must be made that minimizes the possibility of certain complications but increases the risk of others. For example, if subretinal fluid is not drained, the possibility of choroidal hemorrhage or retinal incarceration at the sclerotomy site is avoided, whereas reoperation may be necessary if the retinal break(s) fail to settle on the scleral buckle and the retina remains detached. Similarly, air injected into the vitreous cavity introduces a small risk of intraocular infection or possible damage to the lens or cornea. However, if air is not used to flatten a prominent fold, the operation may fail and further treatment may be needed.

Inadvertent penetration of the sclera with a suture or excessive elevation of the intraocular pressure causing closure of the central retinal artery can usually be avoided, although these complications sometimes occur despite careful measures. However, choroidal hemorrhage in highly myopic eyes at a remote location during drainage of subretinal fluid may occur despite efforts to prevent softening of the globe during drainage.

Complications that are idiopathic and seemingly cannot be prevented include macular pucker and massive periretinal proliferation occurring after a technically uncomplicated and initially successful operation. Postoperative cystoid macular edema or formation of new retinal breaks may also occur without apparent cause. Similarly, infection or exposure of implanted silicone material may occur late after the operation despite observation of strict aseptic technique during the procedure.

The range of complications associated with retinal reattachment surgery is therefore broad, and it includes conditions that subside spontaneously, others that can be successfully treated, and still others for which no treatment is known and that may result in failure. The likelihood of complications can be reduced by anticipating difficult situations, planning the procedure to minimize ocular trauma while achieving the necessary mechanical objectives, and by precise execution of the operation. Careful intraoperative and postoperative observations are needed to detect complications immediately so they can be properly treated. However, despite these efforts it is the nature of retinal detachments and retinal reattachment methods that introduces uncertainty about the anatomical and visual outcome of surgery.

References

1. Heller, M. D., Straatsma, B. R., Foos, R. Y. Detachment of the posterior vitreous in phakic and aphakic eyes. Modern Problems in Ophthalmology 1972; 10:23–36
2. Tasman, W. S. Posterior vitreous detachment and peripheral retinal breaks. Transactions of the American Academy of Ophthalmology and Otolaryngology 1968; 72:217–224
3. Linder, B. Acute posterior vitreous detachment and its retinal complications. Acta Ophthalmologica 1966; Suppl. 87:7–101
4. Ashrafzadeh, M. T., Schepens, C. L., Elzeneiny, I. I., Moura, R., Morse, P., Kraushar, M. F. Aphakia and phakic retinal detachment. I. Preoperative findings. Archives of Ophthalmology 1973; 89:476–483
5. Byer, N. E. Clinical study of lattice degeneration of the retina. Transactions of the American Academy of Ophthalmology and Otolaryngology 1965; 69:1064–1081
6. Byer, N. E. Changes in and prognosis of lattice degeneration of the retina. Transactions of the American Academy of Ophthalmology and Otolaryngology 1974; 78:114–125
7. Gonin, J., ed. Décollement idiopathique: Le processus pathogenique. In: Le décollement de la retine. Lausanne: Librairie Payot and Cie, 1934: 82–117
8. Gonin, J. Treatment of detached retina by searing the retinal tears. Archives of Ophthalmology 1930; 4:621–625
9. Leber, T. Ueber die Entstehung der Netzhautablösung. Bericht über die Vierzehnte Versammlung der Ophthalmologische Gesellschaft Heidelberg 1882; 14: 18–45
10. Schepens, C. L. A new ophthalmoscope demonstration. Transactions of the American Academy of Ophthalmology and Otolaryngology 1947; 51:298–301
11. Schepens, C. L., Bahn, G. C. Examination of the ora serrata: Its importance in retinal detachment. Archives of Ophthalmology 1950; 44:677–690
12. Goldmann, H. Slit-lamp examination of the vitreous and fundus. British Journal of Ophthalmology 1949; 33:242–247
13. Larsson, S. Electro-endothermy in detachment of the retina. Archives of Ophthalmology 1932; 7:661–680
14. Weve, H. Zur Behandlung der Netzhautablösung mittels Diathermie. Abhundlungen aus der Augenheilkunde, Heft 14. Berlin: Karger, 1932
15. Safar, K. Detachment of the retina. Treatment with multiple diathermic puncture and its results. Archives of Ophthalmology 1934; 11:933–941
16. Schepens, C. L., Okamura, I. D., Brockhurst, R. J. The scleral buckling procedures. 1. Surgical techniques and management. Archives of Ophthalmology 1957; 58:797–811
17. Meyer-Schwickerath, G. Light-coagulation: A new method for the treatment and prevention of retinal detachment. XVII. Concilium Ophthalmologicum 1954; 1:404–411
18. Lincoff, H. A., McLean, J. M., Nano, H. Cryosurgical treatment of retinal detachment. Transactions of the American Academy of Ophthalmology and Otolaryngology 1964; 68:412–432
19. Custodis, E. Bedeutet die Plombenaufnähung auf die Sklera einen Fortschritt in der operativen Behandlung der Netzhautzblösung? Bericht der Deutschen Ophthalmologischen Gesellschafft 1953; 58:102–105
20. Schepens, C. L., Okamura, I. D., Brockhurst, R. J. The scleral buckling procedures. II. Technical difficulties of primary operations. Archives of Ophthalmology 1958; 60:84–92
21. Brockhurst, R. J., Schepens, C. L., Okamura, I. D. The scleral buckling procedures. III. Technical difficulties of reoperations. Archives of Ophthalmology 1958; 60:1003–1012
22. Okamura, I. D., Schepens, C. L., Brockhurst, R. J. The scleral buckling procedures. IV. Reoperations following scleral bucklings. Archives of Ophthalmology 1959; 62:445–458
23. Schepens, C. L., Okamura, I. D., Brockhurst, R. J., Regan, C. D. Scleral buckling procedures. V. Synthetic sutures and silicone implants. Archives of Ophthalmology 1960; 64:868–881
24. Regan, C. D. J., Schepens, C. L., Okamura, I. D., Brockhurst, R. J., McMeel, J. W. The scleral buckling procedures. VI. Further

notes on silicone in primary operations. Archives of Ophthalmology 1962; 68:313–328
25. Okamura, I. D., Schepens, C. L., Brockhurst, R. J., Regan, C. D. J., McMeel, J. W. The scleral buckling procedures. VII. Silicone implants in reoperations. Archives of Ophthalmology 1964; 72:297–308
26. Brockhurst, R. J., Schepens, C. L., Okamura, I. D., Regan, C. D. J., McMeel, J. W. Scleral buckling procedures. VIII. Preoperative complications. Archives of Ophthalmology 1965; 74:792–798
27. Okamura, I. D., Schepens, C. L., Brockhurst, R. J., Regan, C. D. J., McMeel, J. W. Scleral buckling procedures. IX. Complications during operation. Archives of Ophthalmology 1966; 75:615–625
28. Schepens, C. L. Scleral buckling with circling element. Transactions of the American Academy of Ophthalmology and Otolaryngology 1964; 68:959–979
29. Lincoff, H. A., Baras, I., McLean, J. Modifications to the Custodis procedure for retinal detachment. Archives of Ophthalmology 1965; 73:160–163
30. Hamilton, A. M., Taylor, W. Significance of pigment granules in the vitreous. British Journal of Ophthalmology 1972; 56:700–702
31. Lincoff, H., Gieser, R. Finding the retinal hole. Archives of Ophthalmology 1971; 85:565–569
32. Jaffe, N. S. Vitreous detachments. In: The vitreous in clinical ophthalmology. St. Louis: C. V. Mosby Co., 1969: 83–98
33. Machemer, R., Allen, A. W. Retinal tears 180° and greater: Management with vitrectomy and intravitreal gas. Archives of Ophthalmology 1976; 94:1340–1346
34. Michels, R. G. Vitreous surgery. St Louis: C. V. Mosby Co., 1981: 250–255
35. Machemer, R., Laqua., H. Pigment epithelium proliferation in retinal detachment (massive periretinal proliferation). American Journal of Ophthalmology 1975; 80:1–23
36. Laqua, H., Machemer, R. Clinical-pathological correlation in massive periretinal proliferation. American Journal of Ophthalmology 1975; 80:913–929
37. Van Horn, D. L., Aaberg, T. M., Machemer, R., Fenzl, R. Glial cell proliferation in human retinal detachment with massive periretinal proliferation. American Journal of Ophthalmology 1977; 84:383–393
38. Machemer, R., Van Horn, D. L., Aaberg, T. M. Pigment epithelial proliferation in human retinal detachment with massive periretinal proliferation. American Journal of Ophthalmology 1978; 85:181–191
39. Kampik, A., Kenyon, K. R., Michels, R. G., Green, W. R. de la Cruz, Z. C. Epiretinal and vitreous membranes. Comparative study of 56 cases. Archives of Ophthalmology 1981; 99:1445–1454
39a The Retina Society Terminology Committee. The classification of retinal detachment with proliferative vitreoretinopathy. Ophthalmology 1983; 90:121
40. Machemer, R., Laqua, H. A logical approach to the treatment of massive periretinal proliferation. Ophthalmology (Rochester) 1978; 85:584–593
41. Diddie K. R., Smith, R. E. Intraocular gas injection in the pseudophakic patient. American Journal of Ophthalmology 1980; 89:659–661
42. Fuller, D. G., Hutton, W. L. Anterior chamber suture in pseudophakic retinal detachments requiring intraocular gas. Archives of Ophthalmology 1980; 98:1101
43. Holekamp, T. L. R. A safe temporary transcameral IOL stay suture. Retina 1981; 1:197–200
44. Burton, T. C. Preoperative factors influencing anatomic success rates following retinal detachment surgery. Transactions of the American Academy of Ophthalmology and Otolaryngology 1977; 83:499–505
45. Griffith, R. D., Ryan, E. A. Hilton, G. F. Primary retinal detachments without apparent breaks. American Journal of Ophthalmology 1976; 81:420–427
46. Norton, E. W. D. Retinal detachment in aphakia. Transactions of the American Ophthalmological Society 1963; 61:770
47. Hilton, G. F., McLean, E. B., Norton, E. W. D. Retinal detachment: a manual prepared for the use of graduates in medicine. 3rd ed. Rochester: American Academy of Ophthalmology, 1979: 113–115
48. Rachal, W. F., Burton, T. C. Changing concepts of failures after retinal detachment surgery. Archives of Ophthalmology 1979; 97:480–483
49. Hagler, W. S. and North, A. W. Retinal dialyses and retinal detachment. Archives of Ophthalmology 1968; 79:376–383
50. Benson, W. E., Morse, P. H. The prognosis of retinal detachment due to lattice degeneration. Annals of Ophthalmology 1978; 10:1197–1200
51. Hilton, G. F., McLean, E. B., Norton, E. W. D. Retinal detachment: a manual prepared for the use of graduates in medicine. 3rd ed. Rochester: American Academy of Ophthalmology, 1979:156
52. Gottlieb, F. Combined choroidal and retinal detachment. Archives of Ophthalmology 1972; 88:481–486
53. Seelenfreund, M. H., Kraushar, M. F., Schepens, C. L., Freilich, D. B. Choroidal detachment associated with primary retinal detachment. Archives of Ophthalmology 1974; 91:254–258
54. Gundry, M. F., Davies, E. W. Recovery of visual acuity after retinal detachment surgery. American Journal of Ophthalmology 1974; 77:310–314
55. Grupposo, S. S. Visual acuity following surgery for retinal detachment. Archives of Ophthalmology 1975; 93:327–330
56. Tani, P. M., Robertson, D. M., Langworthy, A. Rhegmatogenous retinal detachment without macular involvement treated with scleral buckling. American Journal of Ophthalmology 1980; 90:503–508
57. Wilkinson, C. P. Visual results following scleral buckling for retinal detachments sparing the macula. Retina 1981; 1:113
58. Pruett, R. C. The fishmouth phenomenon. II. Wedge scleral buckling. Archives of Ophthalmology 1977; 95:1782–1787
59. Hilton, G. F. Subretinal pigment migration. Effects of cryosurgical retinal reattachment. Archives of Ophthalmology 1974; 91:445–450
60. Perez, R. N., Phelps, C. D., Burton, T. C. Angle-closure glaucoma following scleral buckling operations. Transactions of the American Academy of Ophthalmology and Otolaryngology 1976; 81:247–252
61. O'Connor, P. R. Intravitreous air injection and the Custodis procedure. Ophthalmic Surgery 1976; 7:86–89
62. Ryan, S. J., Goldberg, M. F. Anterior segment ischemia following scleral buckling in sickle cell hemoglobinopathy. American Journal of Ophthalmology 1971; 72:35–50
63. Lobes, L. A., Jr, Burton, T. C. The incidence of macular pucker after retinal detachment surgery. American Journal of Ophthalmology 1978; 85:72–77
64. Machemer, R. Die chirurgische Entfernung von epiretinalen Maculamebranen (macular pucker). Klinische Monatsblätter für Augenheilkunde 1978; 172:36–42
65. Shea, M. The surgical management of macular pucker in rhegmatogenous retinal detachment. Ophthalmology 1980; 87:70–74
66. Michels, R. G. Vitreous surgery for macular pucker. American Journal of Ophthalmology 1981; 92:628–639
67. Meredith, T. A., Reeser, F. H., Topping, T. M., Aaberg, T. M. Cystoid macular edema after retinal detachment surgery. Ophthalmology 1980; 87:1090–1095
68. Lobes, L. A., Jr, Grand, M. G. Incidence of cystoid macular edema following scleral buckling procedure. Archives of Ophthalmology 1980; 98:1230–1232
69. Rubin, M. L. The induction of refractive errors by retinal detachment surgery. Transactions of the American Ophthalmological Society 1975; 73:452–490
70. Burton, T. C. Irregular astigmatism following episcleral buckling procedure with the use of silicone rubber sponges. Archives of Ophthalmology 1973; 90:447–448
71. Flindall, R. J., Norton, E. W. D., Curtin, V. T., Gass, J. D. M. Reduction of extrusion and infection following episcleral silicone implants and cryopexy in retinal detachment surgery. American Journal of Ophthalmology 1971; 71:835–837

10

Photocoagulation

Thomas A. Rice MD

Introduction

Photocoagulation treatment has become widely used during the past two decades and permits successful management of selected eye diseases for which no treatment was previously available. Meyer-Schwickerath[1] began experimental work about 1946 using sunlight as a source of energy to produce chorioretinal scars. In the early 1950s, the Zeiss Optical Company produced a xenon arc photocoagulator with the collaboration of Meyer-Schwickerath. This instrument has been used extensively, although more recently laser photocoagulation instruments have largely replaced xenon instruments.

In 1958 Schlawlow and Townes[2] conceived the possibility of a laser (*L*ight *A*mplification by *S*timulated *E*mission *R*adiation, LASER). Shortly thereafter the first operational laser was constructed. In the early 1960s, the pulsed ruby laser was adapted for use as a retinal photocoagulation instrument by several researchers[3–5]. A continuous-wave blue-green argon laser photocoagulator, which produces light that is absorbed more by blood than is the red light emitted by the ruby laser, was developed by L'Esperance[6] and by Little, Zweng and Peabody[7]. More recently the red krypton laser has been adapted for use in ophthalmology, and histopathological studies of krypton laser burns were first described by L'Esperance[8].

Principles and instrumentation

Generation of light energy

All photocoagulation therapy utilizes thermal damage to the treated intraocular tissue. Visible light emitted by the photocoagulation instrument passes through the transparent media of the eye and is absorbed by opaque tissue and converted to heat. The thermal damage produces anatomical and pathophysiological changes.

The xenon arc photocoagulator produces light radiation by conduction of electrical current through gas. The Zeiss xenon photocoagulation instrument consists of a xenon lamp, an optical beam director, a direct ophthalmoscope to view the fundus and deliver the photocoagulation, and controls for the instrument. A different xenon photocoagulator is also available with both a direct ophthalmoscope and a monocular indirect ophthalmoscope viewing and delivery system. The spectral distribution of light emitted by a xenon instrument includes not only visible wavelengths but also infrared and ultraviolet energy. The output is not continuous and uniform for all wavelengths but shows energy peaks at certain wave lengths. Much of the emitted, harmful ultraviolet radiation is absorbed by the optical system of the instrument. Infrared energy is partially absorbed by the refractive media of the eye, but the amount absorbed by the crystalline lens is insufficient to produce cataracts. Because light emitted from the xenon lamp passes in all directions and is present across the entire visible spectrum, there is a physical limit to the extent to which this type of light can be focused. This prevents production of small photocoagulation burns.

Lasers used for ocular photocoagulation differ from the xenon arc instruments by emitting a much narrower distribution of wavelengths that are more spatially coherent and therefore can be focused to a smaller spot with a higher energy density. A discussion of the physical principles of lasers is beyond the scope of this chapter. The basic requisites for laser emission, however, are production of a population-inversion of atoms at an excited state, followed by stimulation of the excited atoms by a light beam of the necessary wavelength so that an amplified coherent beam is emitted. The ruby laser, which was the first laser used in ophthalmology, was a pulsed system with energy emitted in millisecond pulses. Argon and krypton lasers currently used are gas filled and emit light continuously. Because of this and other properties, gas-filled lasers allow even better focusing than was possible with the ruby laser.

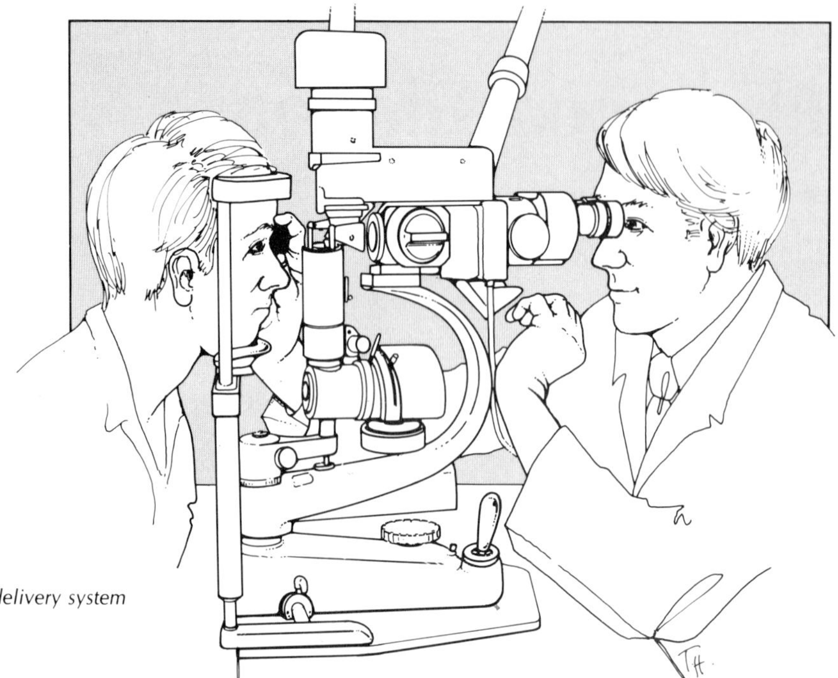

Figure 10.1 *Argon laser with slit-lamp viewing and delivery system*

Most lasers used in ophthalmology do not emit a single wavelength of light, but several wavelengths. These wavelengths are usually close enough together spectrally so that the emitted beam has a characteristic color. Ruby and krypton laser beams have a red color, and the argon laser has a blue-green color because both blue and green wavelengths are produced. Some argon lasers eliminate the blue wavelength, so that the laser emits only the green wavelength.

Argon blue-green, argon green, krypton red, and combinations of these wavelengths in one instrument are commercially available from different manufacturers. Lasers have largely replaced the xenon arc photocoagulator, because the light can be focused to a smaller spot and because selection of certain wavelengths, as discussed below, is advantageous. In addition, lasers generally use a slit-lamp viewing and delivery system through a fundus contact lens (*Figure 10.1*). This allows easier visualization and more accurate placement of burns than is possible with the direct ophthalmoscope delivery system commonly used with xenon photocoagulation instruments. Also, xenon photocoagulation usually causes enough pain to necessitate retrobulbar anesthesia but this is often unnecessary with laser photocoagulation.

Transmission and absorption of light energy

The ocular media transmit almost all light energy between the wavelengths of 400 nm and 900 nm but absorb most of the energy above and below this range. Depending on the wavelength, light energy that reaches the retina, retinal pigment epithelium (RPE), choroid, and intravascular or extravascular blood is absorbed and converted to thermal energy. This produces a burn if the energy is intense enough. Most of the energy from photocoagulation instruments is absorbed by the melanin pigment of the RPE and choroid, because melanin absorbs a significant percentage of almost all wavelengths of light (*Figure 10.2*)[9–11].

Retinal burns from a laser are mostly produced by absorption of energy in the underlying RPE, with conduction of heat anteriorly into the retina. Shorter wavelength light, such as that from a blue-green argon laser (488.0 nm and 514.5 nm), is absorbed by the RPE more readily than that of the longer wavelength, red krypton laser (647.1 nm).

In treating subretinal or choroidal pathology in the macula, a direct burn to the overlying retina can occur if enough energy is absorbed by the intraretinal xanthophyll pigment present in the macula. Xanthophyll absorbs a much higher proportion of shorter than longer wavelength energy. In treating choroidal neovascularization near the fovea, direct foveal damage from absorption of energy by intraretinal xanthophyll can be minimized by using longer wavelength light, such as that from the krypton red laser. Also, as mentioned, some argon lasers

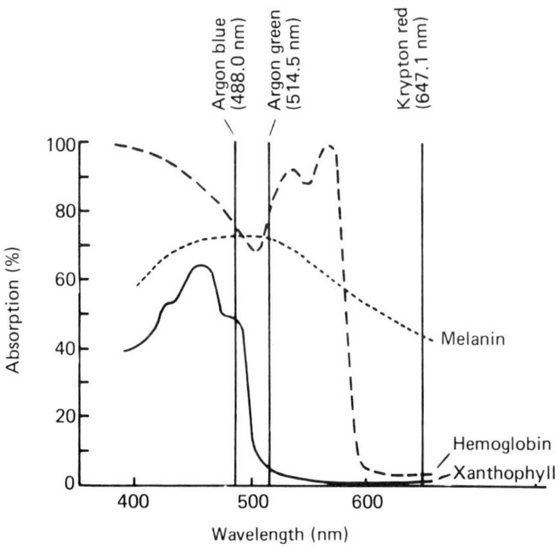

Figure 10.2 *Absorption curves for melanin, hemoglobin and xanthophyll with argon blue, argon green and krypton red wavelengths shown*[9–11]

eliminate the blue component of the laser output so that only the green component is emitted. This is absorbed much less by intraretinal xanthophyll than the blue wavelength and thus minimizes unwanted retinal burns from absorption of energy.

Almost no krypton red laser energy is absorbed by hemoglobin, but both argon blue and argon green energies are highly absorbed. Using the red krypton laser may be advantageous when trying to treat choroidal neovascularization through overlying blood. The red krypton energy is not absorbed by the retinal vessels and therefore these vessels are not directly damaged. Red krypton laser energy penetrates vitreous hemorrhage or a nuclear sclerotic cataract more easily than does the argon blue-green laser, and this allows fundus treatment in some eyes that cannot be treated with the argon laser. In treating retinal neovascularization focally, however, argon blue-green energy is preferable to red krypton energy because the blue-green energy is absorbed by the hemoglobin in the neovascularization. Therefore, the wavelengths produced by some types of lasers offer advantages over other wavelengths in treating certain conditions.

Physiological and pathological effects of photocoagulation

When the retina and deeper tissues are treated with photocoagulation, most of the energy passes through the transparent retina and is absorbed by the RPE, and, to a lesser degree, by the underlying choroidal pigment. Heat is conducted into the overlying outer retina. The initial pathological changes produced are: (*1*) pigmentary dispersion in the RPE; (*2*) damage to the outer retinal layers consisting of pyknotic changes in the nuclei of the outer nuclear layer and edema of the photoreceptors; and (*3*) closure of the choriocapillaries and smaller choroidal vessels[12]. Later the outer retina thins and scars, becoming adherent to the underlying RPE. The inner retina is damaged little when either argon or krypton laser treatment is used, except when argon energy is absorbed by retinal vessels or by intraretinal xanthophyll in the macula[13]. In general, more damage occurs to the inner retina when using xenon photocoagulation than with laser treatment.

The mechanism by which photocoagulation causes the desired effect varies, depending on the disease being treated. In proliferative diabetic retinopathy, for example, scatter photocoagulation (panretinal photocoagulation), consisting of many retinal burns, eliminates retinal neovascularization indirectly, possibly by destroying ischemic retina that liberates a vasoproliferative factor. In contrast, when retinal neovascularization or choroidal neovascularization is treated directly, the blood vessels are obliterated by direct thermal damage. Laser energy can also be used to treat leaks in the retinal vasculature or leaks from the RPE into the subretinal space. Treating the leaking spot creates a local scar and often stops the leakage. Photocoagulation can be used to create a chorioretinal scar around a retinal hole, which seals the retina to the choroid and prevents fluid vitreous from passing into the subretinal space and causing a retinal detachment. There are other uses for photocoagulation as discussed below.

Preoperative evaluation

Preoperative evaluation of patients considered for photocoagulation treatment includes history taking, ocular examination, and often fundus photography and fluorescein angiography. Only after careful evaluation can treatment be recommended, and the risks and treatment alternatives are discussed with the patient.

Ophthalmic history

A complete ophthalmic and medical history is taken to determine the time of onset of the condition, symptoms that might suggest a specific diagnosis, and any underlying systemic disease that is related to the ocular pathology. Details of previous visual acuity, ocular pathology, and previous treatment, including photocoagulation treatment, help in making a diagnosis and in deciding on treatment. A history of disease in the fellow eye may also aid in establishing the diagnosis and prognosis.

Ocular examination

Both eyes are carefully examined, including a best corrected visual acuity, external and pupillary evaluation, tonometry, slit-lamp examination, binocular indirect ophthalmoscopy, and usually fundus biomicroscopy with a slit lamp and fundus contact lens. The best corrected visual acuity is measured before exposing the eyes to bright light, because eyes with retinal disease are slow to recover full visual acuity after exposure to bright light.

Pupillary responses are noted, especially the presence of an afferent pupillary defect, which usually indicates severe retinal or optic nerve damage. The maximum amount of pupillary dilation is noted, because a small pupil can interfere with photocoagulation treatment.

Slit-lamp examination is done to assess pathology of the cornea, iris and lens. Opacities of these tissues may prevent effective photocoagulation. Iris neovascularization and anterior chamber angle neovascularization are also recorded. Iris neovascularization can be present in eyes with retinal vascular disease and may progress to neovascular glaucoma. Scatter retinal photocoagulation may cause regression of iris neovascularization, as discussed below.

The vitreous cavity is carefully examined to observe opacities, vitreoretinal traction and other pathology. The presence of vitreous hemorrhage in diabetic retinopathy often requires modification of treatment, and therapy may be applied over a shorter period in an attempt to prevent further hemorrhage.

Indirect ophthalmoscopy, with its wide-angle stereoscopic view, allows indentification of abnormalities such as retinal elevation, retinal neovascularization and peripheral retinal abnormalities. Biomicroscopy of the fundus with a slit lamp and contact lens affords a more magnified stereoscopic view and is especially useful in detecting shallow retinal elevation, small patches of retinal neovascularization, cystoid macular edema and other subtle abnormalities. The view obtained with a fundus contact lens is superior to that of the Hruby lens. The midperipheral and peripheral retina is examined with the mirrors of a three-mirror fundus contact lens, and the posterior retina can be examined directly through the center of the lens. It is often helpful to use a narrow slit beam from the slit lamp directed from an acute angle to allow better visualization of retinal thickening or to visualize shallow elevations of the retina. Because a viscous solution of methylcellulose is often used with a fundus contact lens, residual methycellulose on the cornea may interfere with later fundus photography. Therefore, contact lens examination is usually deferred until after photography.

Fundus photography and fluorescein angiography

Fundus photography and fundus fluorescein angiography document pathology and often help in making a diagnosis. They are also often necessary before the photocoagulation treatment can be chosen. If all retinal pathology is limited to the macula, stereo 30° photographs of the macula and optic nervehead alone are sufficient. More widespread fundus abnormalities can be photographed with overlapping 30° fields posterior to the equator, and often are photographed as seven stereoscopic pairs (*Figure 10.3*). Wide-angle photography of 60° is used for the

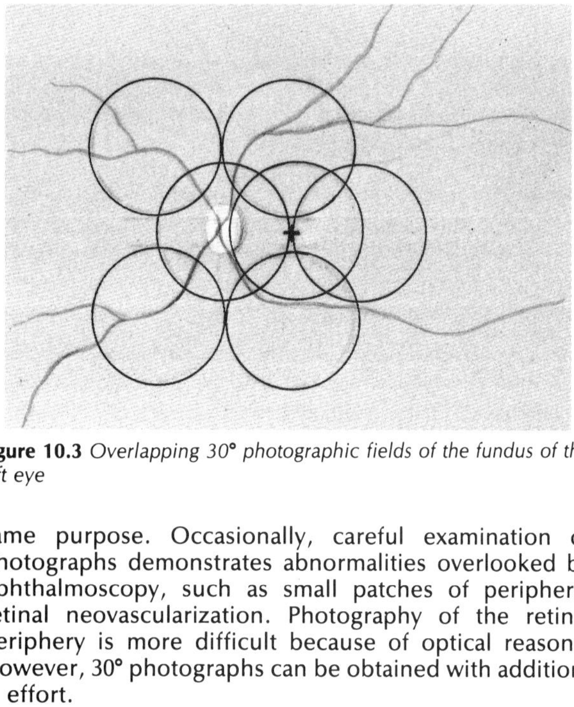

Figure 10.3 *Overlapping 30° photographic fields of the fundus of the left eye*

same purpose. Occasionally, careful examination of photographs demonstrates abnormalities overlooked by ophthalmoscopy, such as small patches of peripheral retinal neovascularization. Photography of the retinal periphery is more difficult because of optical reasons. However, 30° photographs can be obtained with additional effort.

Fundus fluorescein angiography is indispensible in evaluating many eyes considered for photocoagulation treatment. All eyes with choroidal neovascularization or leaks in the RPE must have fluorescein angiography to show the location, pattern and extent of the lesions. Angiography assists in determining whether they can be safely treated and also serves as a guide to placement of photocoagulation. Routine fluorescein angiography, however, is not used to detect peripheral neovascularization in diabetic retinopathy, because most such neovascularization can be found by ophthalmoscopy or can be seen on color fundus photographs.

Fluorescein angiography is performed using a 30° or a wide-angle fundus camera adapted for angiography with the proper exciter and barrier filters. The patient's pupil is maximally dilated, and 5 ml of 10 per cent sodium fluorescein solution is injected during 5–10 seconds into an antecubital or other arm vein. Blood should be aspirated from the vein before injection, to make certain that the needle is in the vein. Inadvertent extravasation of fluorescein into the tissue causes severe pain. Photography is begun 5–10 seconds after beginning the injection, just before fluorescein reaches the eye. One exposure of the main field of interest is made approximately every second for about 25 seconds. Thereafter exposures are made less frequently and sometimes as late as 20 minutes after the injection. When investigating the macula of one eye, a few frames of the macula of the fellow eye should also be taken for comparison, even if ophthalmoscopy has shown no obvious abnormality. This sometimes records subtle pathology in the fellow eye. A variety of areas can be photographed if the pathology is more extensive; this is sometimes termed a 'sweep'. The black-and-white film used in angiography can be developed rapidly and the negatives can be examined the same day if necessary. A positive-transparency contact print can then be made for later use.

Occasionally, fluorescein angioscopy is useful in locating peripheral fundus pathology, such as leaks into the subretinal space from the choroid in eyes with exudative retinal detachment. After fluorescein injection, the fundus is examined with an indirect ophthalmoscope with a cobalt-blue filter over the light source. Fluorescein leakage is identified by its green color.

Angiography should not be done if the patient has had a previous, severe, allergic reaction, such as anaphylaxis. Nausea from injection of fluorescein is not an allergic reaction but a side effect. Nausea can usually be lessened or prevented by pretreating the patient with an oral anti-emetic drug and by injecting the fluorescein more slowly than usual. If there is a history of urticaria from fluorescein injection, but without a more serious allergic reaction, fluorescein angiography should not be performed unless absolutely necessary. If fluorescein angiography in such patients is necessary, pretreatment with an oral antihistamine is used. As always when fluorescein angiography is performed, oxygen, an airway and appropriate medicines must be available to manage the possible but infrequent severe side effects.

Photocoagulation technique

Photocoagulation is used to treat a wide variety of ocular diseases, and different techniques are used depending on the pathology to be treated. Although xenon photocoagulation can be effectively used to treat some conditions, laser photocoagulation can usually treat these same conditions with more ease and accuracy. Some conditions can be treated only with laser photocoagulation. The following discussion of photocoagulation treatment is limited to laser photocoagulation. A further discussion of xenon photocoagulation can be found elsewhere[1,14]. Basic principles of laser photocoagulation treatment will be described first, and then the methods of treatment used in specific conditions will be discussed.

Patient preparation

After a thorough diagnostic evaluation, a decision is made whether to recommend photocoagulation. In some diseases, such as proliferative diabetic retinopathy, the indications for treatment are definite because previous clinical trials have proved the efficacy of treatment. In other conditions, such as diabetic macular edema, preliminary studies suggest that treatment is beneficial, but conclusive data from controlled clinical trials are not yet available. In still other conditions, no clinical trials have been done, but clinical experience suggests that treatment is useful. The potential benefits of treatment are discussed with the patient, and also the possible side effects and complications. If the patient chooses to have photocoagulation treatment after this discussion, written consent is obtained.

Usually it is unnecessary for a patient to be sedated before laser treatment. A careful explanation of the procedure often alleviates fear. It is important that the pupil is maximally dilated to facilitate treatment. Diabetic patients should not miss a meal before treatment which might result in hypoglycemia and an insulin reaction during the treatment session.

Anesthesia

Laser treatment can often be applied after only topical anesthesia, such as is obtained with topical proparacaine (proxymetacaine). Retrobulbar anesthesia is necessary, however, when laser treatment is painful or when it is important that the eye be immobile, for example while treating perifoveal choroidal neovascularization. The burns of scatter (panretinal) laser photocoagulation can usually be applied after topical anesthesia alone, but a retrobulbar anesthetic is given if the treatment is painful. Scatter photocoagulation of the midperipheral retina, especially in the horizontal meridians, is more painful than is more posterior treatment. Some patients tolerate posterior treatment but require a retrobulbar anesthetic for the more peripheral treatment. Others, especially younger patients, cannot tolerate the pain of any treatment without retrobulbar anesthesia. It is not possible accurately to predict which patient will need retrobulbar anesthesia, and so scatter photocoagulation is usually first begun after a topical anesthetic alone, and retrobulbar injection is given if the patient is uncomfortable. Retrobulbar anesthesia is used before subsequent treatment sessions if pain required retrobulbar injection the first time.

If only minimal retinal neovascularization is present, it may be satisfactory to use topical anesthesia and to treat the patient in several sessions, applying less than 500 burns at each sitting. If the patient has considerable retinal neovascularization and only a small amount of treatment can be applied at each session because of pain, it is better to use a retrobulbar anesthetic to allow the treatment to be completed in 2 or 3 treatment sessions over 1 or 2 weeks. This achieves a faster regression of neovascularization and lowers the risk of vitreous hemorrhage or other complications.

As mentioned, eyes with perifoveal choroidal neovascularization that require heavy treatment near the fovea should have a retrobulbar anesthetic to prevent eye movement that might cause inadvertent treatment of the center of the fovea. Other macular conditions, such as diabetic macular edema, can be treated while using a topical anesthetic alone. This type of photocoagulation treatment is not painful, and a small amount of eye movement can be tolerated.

Retrobulbar anesthesia, when required, is given in the conventional fashion. Usually a 2 ml injection of 2 per cent lidocaine (lignocaine) (without epinephrine; adrenaline) is used. We normally use a 25 gauge sharp disposable needle for this injection, but a blunt-tipped 23 gauge needle can be used instead.

For children, general anesthesia may be necessary to permit photocoagulation. Some children as young as 6 years of age, however, can be treated without general anesthesia. If general anesthesia is required, xenon photocoagulation is usually necessary because with the slit-lamp delivery system of the currently available lasers it is not possible to treat patients in a supine position.

General photocoagulation technique

After anesthesia is achieved, the patient is seated at the slit lamp of the laser (*see Figure 10.1*). If a fluorescein angiogram is necessary as a guide for treatment, a suitable frame of the angiogram is projected onto a screen for viewing or placed in a viewer that allows the angiogram to be easily examined. The initial settings on the laser are made, including spot size, burn duration and power. A contact lens is applied to the cornea. A Goldmann three-mirror lens can be used for treatment of the posterior pole or, using the mirrors of the lens, more peripheral treatment can be applied (*Figure 10.4*). It is often difficult to treat the region of the fundus just peripheral to the area seen through the central part of the three-mirror lens. The most posteriorly directed mirror just barely reaches this area, and visualization is improved by having the patient look toward the mirror. With retrobulbar anesthesia such voluntary movement is not possible, but lateral pressure on the eye, applied with the contact lens, moves the eye enough to allow posterior treatment through the mirror.

A Rodenstock lens is an alternative fundus contact lens that can be used for scatter laser photocoagulation. It acts optically in a manner similar to an indirect ophthalmoscope when used with the slit-lamp viewing system of the laser. As compared to a conventional fundus contact lens, the view is inverted, minified and wide-angle (*Figure 10.5*). The wide-angle view makes it easy to identify the macula and keep it in sight while treating the midperipheral retina. This lessens the chance of inadvertently treating the fovea. In addition to being safer in this respect, the Rodenstock lens allows those who are facile in its use to apply scatter photocoagulation more quickly than with a three-mirror lens. A Rodenstock lens is also easier to use when applying treatment through a small pupil. The Rodenstock lens has a magnification effect on the laser

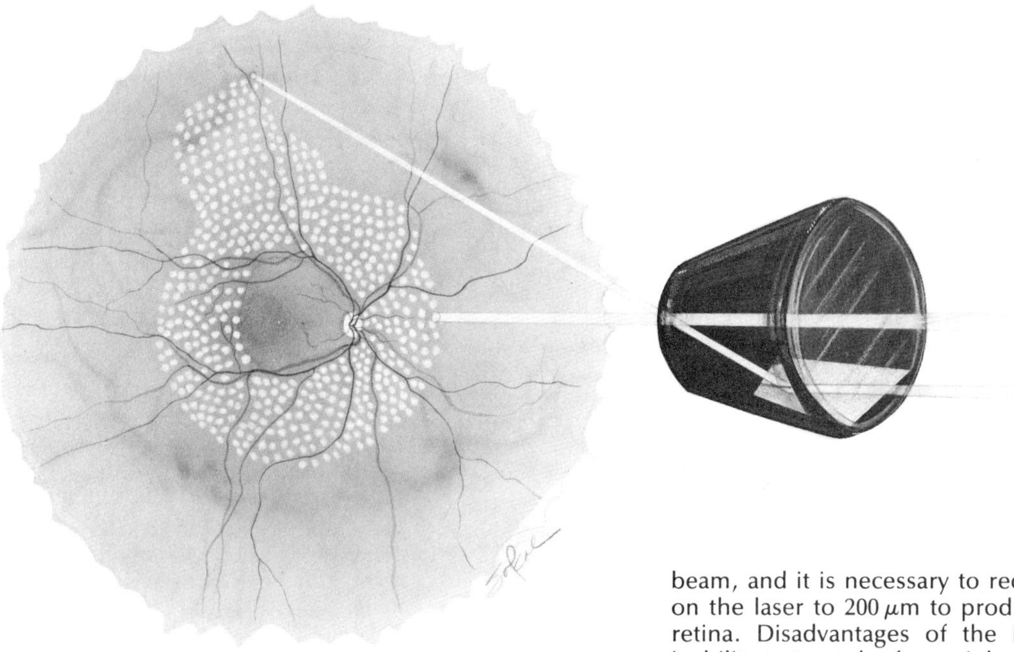

Figure 10.4 *Photocoagulation through three-mirror fundus contact lens. The posterior pole is treated directly through the lens, and the midperipheral retina is treated using the most posteriorly directed mirror (shown)*

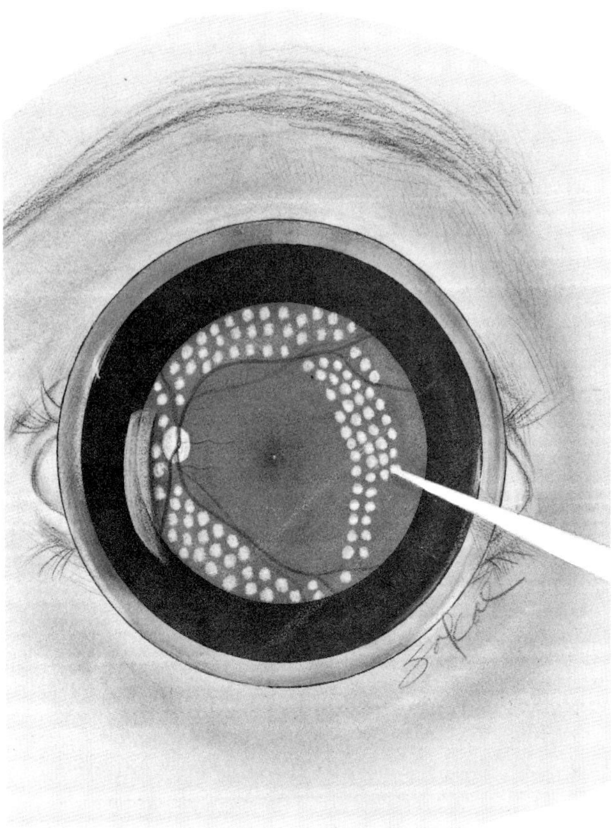

Figure 10.5 *Photocoagulation of a right eye through a Rodenstock lens with an inverted, wide-angle view*

beam, and it is necessary to reduce the spot-size setting on the laser to 200 μm to produce a 500 μm burn in the retina. Disadvantages of the Rodenstock lens include inability to treat the far peripheral retina, distracting light reflexes and decreased optical resolution. Because of the minification of the image and its decreased optical resolution, this lens should not be used to treat subtle macular lesions.

After the fundus contact lens is in place, the retina is viewed using the slit lamp. Lower magnification settings are used for applying scatter retinal photocoagulation, and higher magnification is used to treat macular lesions. The slit beam is adjusted to illuminate the area to be treated and to minimize distracting light reflexes and scattered light. When using a three-mirror contact lens, pressure on the lens can be used further to stabilize the eye or to move the eye slightly, and the ability to move an eye that is paralysed by retrobulbar anesthesia is often useful. When viewing through a mirror a more posterior view is obtained by having the patient look toward the mirror, and a more peripheral view is obtained by having the patient look away from the mirror. The contact lens can be tilted or the slit lamp moved to achieve the same result. Treatment can be applied at the ora serrata by performing simultaneous scleral depression with a thimble depressor such as is used with indirect ophthalmoscopy, or by the use of a depressor ring that is attached to the three-mirror lens.

The appropriate parameters for treatment with the argon laser are chosen. This includes selection of spot size, duration of the burn and the power of the laser burn. For scatter photocoagulation, treatment around peripheral retinal holes and other less exacting treatment, a 500 μm spot size is often used. Choroidal neovascularization in the macula is often treated in part with a 100 μm or 200 μm spot size. Microaneurysms in diabetic macular edema are often treated with 50 μm or 100 μm burns. The smaller the burn size used, the less it spreads and extends into the surrounding retina.

The duration of the burn selected depends on what condition is being treated and on what burn size and wattage have been chosen. For scatter argon laser photocoagulation, a 0.1 second duration is often chosen. A short duration burn such as this spreads less and is less painful. Short duration burns, however, have a greater chance of creating choroidal hemorrhage. For example, if a 500 μm spot size is used at only 0.05 second duration to minimize pain, there is an increased risk of producing a choroidal hemorrhage when adequate power settings are used. A duration of 0.2 second can be used to lessen further the risk of this complication, but this longer duration is more painful.

Microaneurysms and vascular leaks causing diabetic macular edema are often treated with a 0.1 second burn of 50 μm or 100 μm size. Longer duration burns, when treating macular pathology in eyes not immobilized by retrobulbar anesthesia, are risky because inadvertent eye movement may cause accidental damage to the center of the fovea. In treating perifoveal choroidal neovascularization with intense, 100 μm or 200 μm burns, a longer burn duration is desirable to reduce the chance of choroidal hemorrhage. Retrobulbar anesthesia allows the safer use of a 0.2 second or 0.5 second burn in this condition.

The power setting of the burn is the third controllable variable determining the characteristics of the treatment effect. Usually the spot size is chosen first, the burn duration second, and the power setting is chosen last. The power setting is adjusted to achieve the desired burn intensity. The three settings are interrelated, so that a larger spot size or a shorter burn duration requires a higher power setting to get the same effect. It is desirable to start with a low power setting and gradually increase the setting on successive burns until the desired intensity is achieved. This lessens the chance of applying an excessively heavy first burn. As a general rule, in eyes with clear media and a burn duration of 0.1 second, a moderate-intensity, 500 μm burn is achieved at a 500 mW setting with an argon laser. For other spot sizes, this same moderate intensity burn can be achieved by setting the power, in milliwatts, equal to the spot size in microns. For example, a 200 μm moderate intensity burn at 0.1 second duration might be achieved at a power of 200 mW. If the burn duration is shorter, or if the media are hazy, more power will be necessary. Conversely, if the burn duration is longer, less power is required.

Moderate-intensity burns are often used for scatter photocoagulation, treatment of vascular leaks causing macular edema, and treatment around retinal breaks. Heavier burns are used for obliteration of choroidal neovascularization or destruction of tissue in other conditions. Light-to-moderate burns are used in treatment of leaks in central serous retinopathy.

Clinical use of photocoagulation

There are two basic types of photocoagulation treatment. *Scatter* (panretinal) photocoagulation is used to treat proliferative retinopathies such as diabetic retinopathy. *Focal* photocoagulation is sometimes used to treat proliferative retinopathies and is also used: (*1*) to seal retinal vascular and choroidal leaks; (*2*) to destroy choroidal neovascularization; (*3*) to form chorioretinal adhesions; (*4*) to destroy selected intraocular tumors; and (*5*) for other less frequent indications. Scatter photocoagulation for treating proliferative diabetic retinopathy will be described below, although this type of treatment is also used in other conditions. Scatter photocoagulation can be applied in a more localized, 'sector' pattern such as in the area of distribution of a retinal branch vein obstruction to treat secondary optic nervehead neovascularization and retinal neovascularization. A more peripheral pattern of scatter photocoagulation can be used to treat peripheral retinal neovascularization that sometimes occurs in Eales' disease, sickle-cell retinopathy and sarcoidosis. Focal photocoagulation will be described under the individual disease entities.

Photocoagulation treatment of proliferative and preproliferative diabetic retinopathy

Proliferative diabetic retinopathy is the leading cause of adult blindness in the more 'developed' countries. Photocoagulation has been shown to be effective in reducing the incidence of blindness from complications of proliferative diabetic retinopathy. Results of the Diabetic Retinopathy Study (DRS) show that both argon laser and xenon photocoagulation reduce the risk of severe visual loss in eyes with significant proliferative retinopathy[15].

Pathogenesis of proliferative diabetic retinopathy

Eyes with proliferative diabetic retinopathy have widespread areas of retinal capillary non-perfusion as seen by fluorescein angiography (*Figure 10.6*). There is evidence

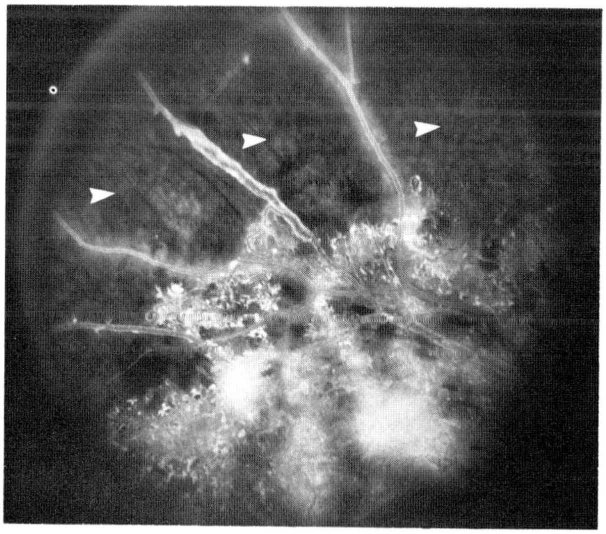

Figure 10.6 *Fluorescein angiogram of an eye with diabetic retinopathy showing extensive areas of capillary non-perfusion (arrows)*

that eyes with extensive retinal capillary non-perfusion liberate a diffusible vasoproliferative factor[16]. This theory suggests that the 'vasoproliferative factor' produces retinal neovascularization at the margin of the non-perfused areas and/or that it diffuses and produces neovascularization at a distance such as at the optic nervehead or the iris (*Figure 10.7*).

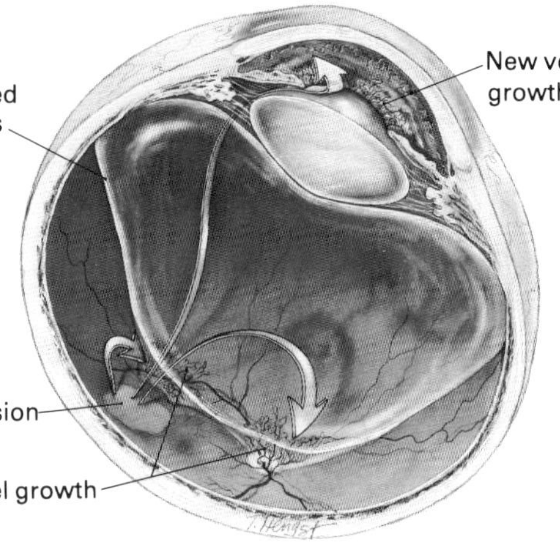

Figure 10.7 *Schematic diagram showing hypothetical vasoproliferative factor diffusing from an area of capillary non-perfusion and producing peripheral neovascularization, optic nervehead neovascularization, and iris and anterior chamber angle neovascularization*

Many abnormalities are present in the blood and microvasculature of diabetics with proliferative retinopathy, and some of these changes undoubtedly produce retinal capillary damage and retinal capillary non-perfusion. It is unclear, however, which abnormalities are important and precisely how they interact to produce damage. For example, diabetics usually have an increased level of hemoglobin A_{1c}. This decreases the erythrocytic oxygen release and can result in hypoxia and damage to retinal capillaries[17]. Increased red-cell aggregation is also present, and this may contribute to vascular occlusion and hypoxia[18]. Platelet aggregation is abnormally increased in patients with diabetic retinopathy and may produce retinal vascular endothelial cell damage[19]. These are but a few of the abnormalities present in diabetics with retinal vascular disease, and other factors may also be important in the pathogenesis of hypoxia, capillary damage and capillary occlusion.

Scatter (or panretinal) photocoagulation of the retina in eyes with proliferative retinopathy is intended to eliminate neovascularization or cause it to regress. One theory is that treatment destroys ischemic non-perfused retina, thus decreasing liberation of 'vasoproliferative factor' and causing regression of neovascularization.

In proliferative diabetic retinopathy the ischemic non-perfused retina is located mostly outside the macula. Scatter photocoagulation treatment is applied to this affected area. Heavy focal photocoagulation to optic nervehead neovascularization and peripheral neovascularization, including attempts to close the 'feeder' arterioles of the neovascularization, has also been used to destroy neovascularization directly. Direct photocoagulation of disc neovascularization is no longer used, however, because scatter photocoagulation alone is usually effective and has fewer complications. Confluent, moderately intense focal photocoagulation of flat peripheral neovascularization, combined with scatter photocoagulation, is still used because it is more effective in eliminating this type of neovascularization than is either type of treatment alone.

Evaluation of eyes with diabetic retinopathy

Diabetic patients without retinopathy should have yearly examinations to be certain they are not developing diabetic retinopathy. If clinically significant background diabetic retinopathy develops, with a moderate number of microaneurysms or intraretinal hemorrhages, the eyes should be re-examined at more frequent intervals. Further progression – with signs of retinal ischemia (including cotton-wool spots, beaded retinal veins and/or intraretinal microvascular abnormalities) – is termed preproliferative retinopathy and may soon be followed by proliferative retinopathy. Eyes with preproliferative retinopathy should be examined about every 4 months.

Indirect ophthalmoscopy allows detection of large amounts of disc or peripheral retinal neovascularization. Lesser amounts may be seen only by careful direct ophthalmoscopy or three-mirror fundus contact lens examination. The most common sites of retinal neovascularization are: (*1*) the optic nervehead or peripapillary retina; (*2*) along the temporal arcades; (*3*) temporal to the macula; and (*4*) other areas posterior to the equator adjacent to areas of capillary non-perfusion. Retinal neovascularization can be 'flat', if the posterior cortical vitreous is not separated from the retinal surface, or 'elevated' and growing along the posterior surface of the detached vitreous cortex. Retinal neovascularization is almost always attached to the posterior cortical vitreous, whether or not the vitreous is separated from the retina. Early neovascularization is composed of blood vessels without accompanying fibrous tissue, but later, extensive fibrous tissue is also present.

Most retinal neovascularization can be detected on careful ophthalmoscopy, but small patches can be missed. If significant background retinopathy or preproliferative changes are present, fundus photographs can be useful to detect these small areas. Overlapping, 30° photographic fields of the fundus posterior to the equator, often taken

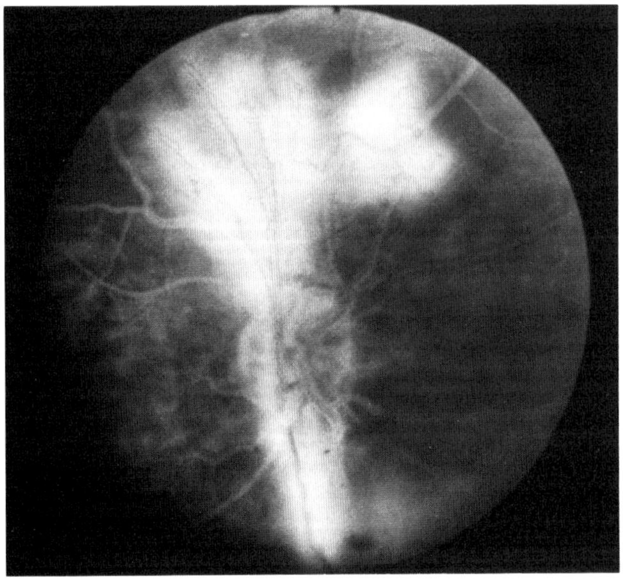

Figure 10.8 *Fluorescein angiogram of an eye with proliferative diabetic retinopathy showing profuse leakage of fluorescein dye from neovascularization*

as seven stereoscopic pairs, are useful for this purpose (*see Figure 10.3*). Fluorescein angiography also helps to detect small areas of neovascularization because neovascular tissue leaks fluorescein dye profusely and therefore is easily identified (*Figure 10.8*). Fluorescein angiography is usually not routinely performed in diabetics solely to detect retinal neovascularization, as this condition can usually be seen by ophthalmoscopy or fundus photography. If a vitreous or preretinal hemorrhage is present and if no neovascularization is visible, a fluorescein angiogram may help locate hidden neovascularization. The retina posterior to the equator is photographed with overlapping fields during angiography to detect leakage from the neovascular tissue.

Indications for photocoagulation

We use scatter photocoagulation in virtually all eyes with optic disc or peripheral retinal neovascularization. Exceptions are eyes with only one or two small patches of flat peripheral neovascularization and those with 'inactive' proliferative retinopathy characterized by atrophic largely avascular fibrous tissue. Eyes with small localized patches of neovascularization can be either left untreated or treated with confluent focal treatment alone. The Diabetic Retinopathy Study (DRS) has shown a statistically beneficial effect of photocoagulation in certain 'high-risk' eyes, including those with: (*1*) moderate or large amounts of disc neovascularization, with or without vitreous hemorrhage; or (*2*) mild disc or peripheral neovascularization with vitreous or preretinal hemorrhage[15]. Although no definite statistical benefit was attributable to photocoagulation in eyes with peripheral neovascularization or mild disc neovascularization, but without vitreous hemorrhage, the DRS found that untreated eyes with these changes progress more quickly to severe grades of retinopathy than treated eyes. Because of this, it is probably reasonable to treat eyes with these earlier proliferative changes. Similarly, eyes with severe preproliferative retinopathy tend to worsen. In cases with bilateral severe preproliferative retinopathy, it seems reasonable to treat one eye with scatter retinal photocoagulation until the results of other studies suggest a better method of management. Alternatively, it is acceptable to follow carefully and frequently these eyes and to apply photocoagulation if they develop definite retinal neovascularization. Untreated eyes with preproliferative retinopathy should be examined about every 4 months to detect development of retinal neovascularization.

Scatter and focal photocoagulation

Photocoagulation for proliferative diabetic retinopathy is usually applied with an argon laser or xenon photocoagulator. Both argon laser and xenon scatter photocoagulation have been determined to be effective in reducing the incidence of blindness, but xenon photocoagulation has more frequent side effects such as loss of peripheral vision. The slit-lamp delivery system used with the argon laser is considerably easier to use than the direct or indirect ophthalmoscope of the xenon instruments.

Argon laser photocoagulation often does not require a retrobulbar anesthetic and allows more accurate, controlled placement of burns. The following discussion of photocoagulation is limited to use of the argon laser. Similar patterns of treatment, however, can be achieved with xenon arc photocoagulation using a 4.5° spot size at a power setting and duration to produce a moderately white burn[14].

Complete scatter photocoagulation is usually not applied in one treatment session because this often would result in complications and excessive pain. Usually treatment is applied in three sessions if done with only topical anesthesia but it may be done in two sessions if retrobulbar anesthesia is needed. A spot size of 500 μm and duration of 0.1 second is used. The power setting is initially set at a low level, such as 300 mW, and adjusted upwards in small steps until it produces a gray-white burn. In eyes with clear media, 500 mW of power often produces the proper intensity of burn, but if the media are hazy the power setting may need to be increased to as much as 2000 mW or more. Occasionally it is also necessary to increase the duration of the burn to 0.2 second to achieve the proper intensity. Heavy chalk-white burns should be avoided, to lessen complications and pain.

The first portion of the treatment is usually applied through the center of the contact lens (not using a mirror) to treat around the posterior pole while avoiding the macula (*see Figure 10.4*). Burns are applied within 500 μm of the nasal, superior and inferior margins of the optic nervehead. Burns are spaced one-half burn width apart, and blood vessels are avoided. Burns are then applied above the superotemporal arcade and below the inferotemporal arcade. If the temporal arcades are farther from the macula than normal, burns are applied inside the arcades but not closer than two disc diameters from the center of the fovea. Treatment is applied temporally to within approximately three disc diameters of the center of the macula. After the posterior pole has been surrounded, treatment is applied more peripherally, by having the patient look in the direction to be treated (*Figure 10.9*). If

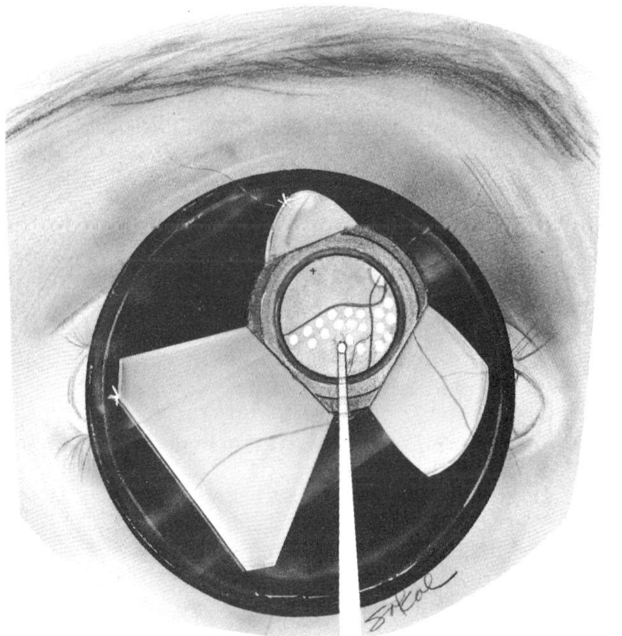

Figure 10.9 *Photocoagulation to inferior portion of posterior retina is accomplished by having the patient look downward and treating directly through the contact lens*

retrobulbar anesthesia has been used, the eye is rotated with pressure on the contact lens while the slit lamp is moved to a different angle.

After as much as possible of the posterior retina has been treated, more peripheral treatment is begun, using the most posteriorly directed mirror of the three-mirror lens. When using this mirror, it may be necessary to rotate the eye to allow sufficiently posterior treatment so that there is no gap of untreated retina between the area treated using the mirror and that treated through the center of the lens. This more posterior treatment can be achieved by having the patient look toward the mirror (*Figure 10.10*).

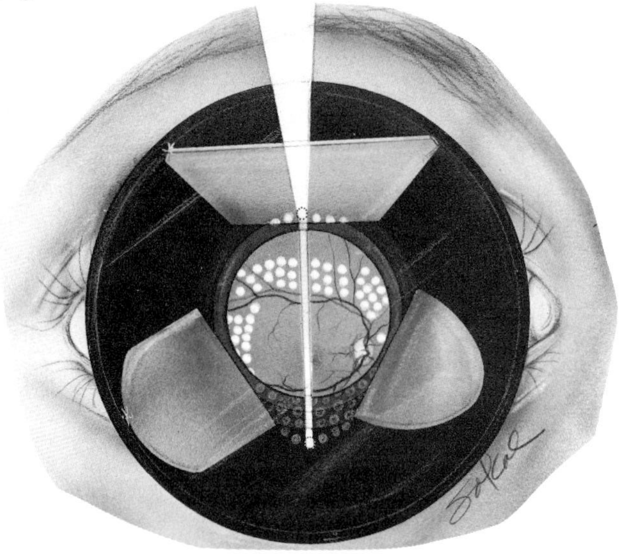

Figure 10.10 *When using a mirror of the three-mirror contact lens more posterior treatment is achieved by having the patient look toward the mirror*

Usually enough additional burns are applied through the posterior mirror to bring the total of 500 μm burns to 600–700 burns for the first treatment session. Treatment should first be done inferiorly if the eye has severe proliferative disease since there is a chance that vitreous hemorrhage could soon occur and interfere with further treatment, and the blood is likely to settle inferiorly (*Figure 10.11*), but in less severely affected eyes other sequences of treatment can be used. If there is significant pain during the first treatment session under topical anesthesia, treatment can be applied in all quadrants posteriorly, leaving the more sensitive peripheral fundus for later treatment with retrobulbar anesthesia.

Treatment is completed in later sessions by extending the application of burns to the equator (just anterior to the vortex vein ampullae) in all quadrants. The total number of 500 μm burns usually needed for 'complete' treatment ranges from 1400 to 2000, depending on various factors. The total number administered is less important than their being spaced one-half burn width apart and the absence of unsuitable gaps in the treatment.

If the eye has severe neovascularization it is advisable to complete the photocoagulation within 1 or 2 weeks because of the chance that vitreous hemorrhage will occur before the neovascularization regresses. If there is only minimal neovascularization the treatment may be completed more slowly over 4–6 weeks.

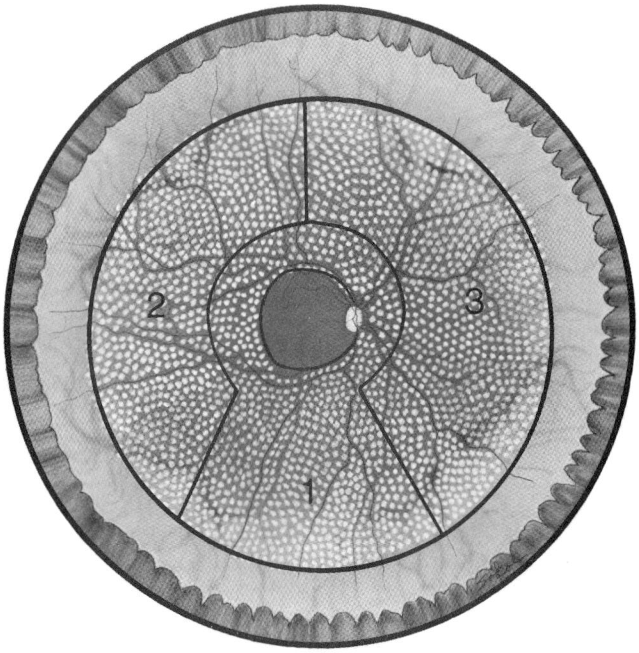

Figure 10.11 *'Complete' scatter photocoagulation applied in three treatment sessions. The first treatment session (1) surrounds the posterior pole and extends to the inferior periphery, so that if vitreous hemorrhage occurs the inferior retina will have been treated. In the second (2) and third (3) treatment sessions, the peripheral treatment is completed*

In addition to applying scatter photocoagulation, areas of flat peripheral neovascularization (*Figure 10.12a*) are treated with moderately intense, confluent 500 μm burns extending 500 μm beyond the margin of the neovascularization (*Figure 10.12b*). Occasionally, if there are only one or two small flat areas of peripheral neovascularization, focal confluent treatment alone can be applied without using scatter photocoagulation, or focal treatment can be used in combination with localized scatter treatment to the zone of capillary non-perfusion peripheral to the neovascularization.

Elevated peripheral neovascularization should not be treated directly, because obtaining an effective burn is difficult, and intense treatment is likely to cause vitreous hemorrhage from the elevated neovascularization or severe damage to the underlying retina and choroid. Areas of traction retinal detachment should not be treated, and treatment should not come within one disc diameter of the elevated retina. There is no clear evidence, however, indicating that photocoagulation itself increases the size of a traction retinal detachment. Eyes that have progressive traction retinal detachment after photocoagulation might have had similar progression occur from contracture of active fibrovascular proliferation, even if photocoagulation had not been done.

After photocoagulation treatment, regression of neovascularization usually begins within a few days or weeks, with a decrease in the vascular component of the fibrovascular tissue (*Figure 10.12c*). The fibrous component persists and can cause more vitreoretinal traction. However, once the vascular component has completely regressed, there is usually no further growth of the fibrous component and little additional traction on the retina. If

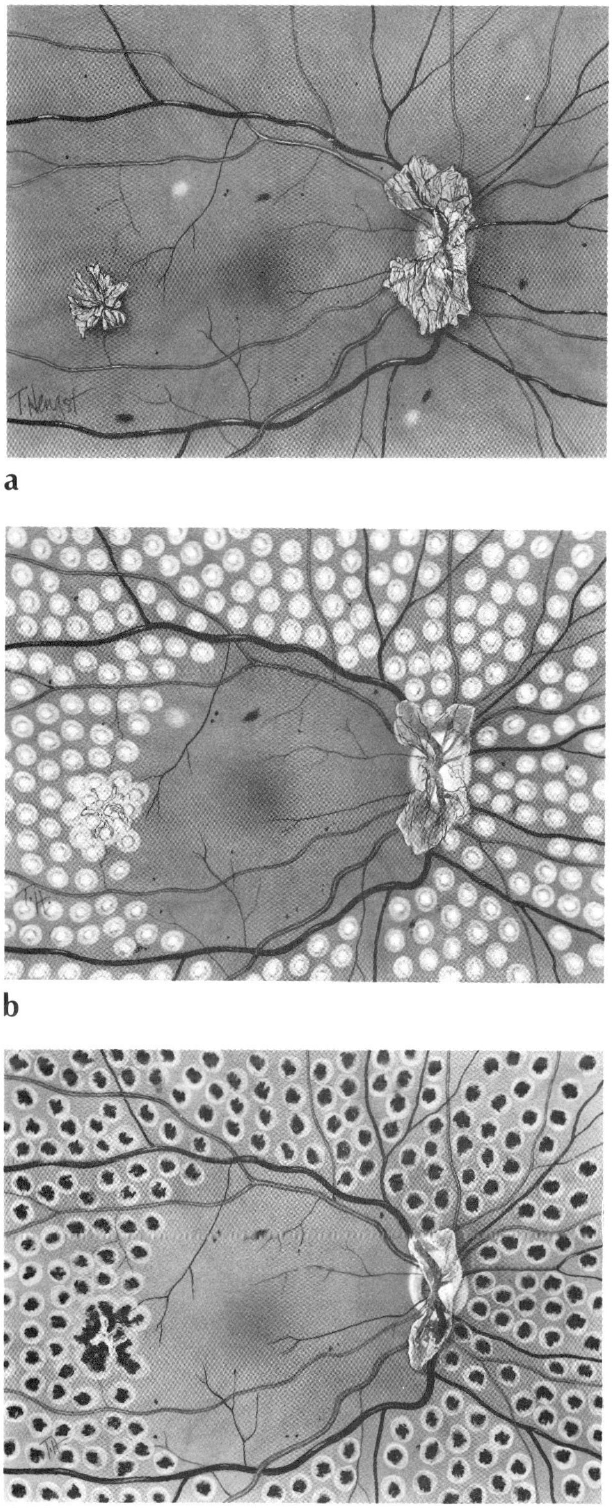

Figure 10.12 *Photocoagulation treatment of optic disc and peripheral neovascularization in diabetic retinopathy.* **(a)** *Optic nervehead and peripheral neovascularization.* **(b)** *Scatter retinal photocoagulation and focal confluent photocoagulation to peripheral neovascularization.* **(c)** *Regression of disc neovascularization and peripheral neovascularization after photocoagulation, with only atrophic fibrous tissue remaining on the optic nervehead*

the eye had only minimal neovascularization, the neovascularization often completely regresses after treatment, but a small amount of neovascularization often remains after treatment if severe neovascularization was present before.

It is advisable to apply additional photocoagulation treatment if significant neovascularization remains a few months after use of complete scatter photocoagulation, even if there has been considerable regression. This is done because vitreous hemorrhage can occur from the residual neovascularization. In eyes that have received extensive scatter photocoagulation and have only a small amount of quiescent neovascularization remaining, further treatment is not done unless there are signs of instability such as vitreous hemorrhage or an increase in neovascularization. If a vitreous or preretinal hemorrhage occurs, supplemental ('fill-in') scatter treatment is used. This is applied as 500 μm burns placed between previous burns. One or two rows are placed closer to the macula and up to the margin of optic nervehead nasally, superiorly and inferiorly, and additional treatment can be applied anterior to previous treatment. The first supplemental treatment may consist of 500–600 additional burns, and later retreatments may raise the total number of burns applied to 3000 or more. Months may pass between retreatment sessions, while one waits for a vitreous hemorrhage to clear enough to allow additional treatment. In some eyes with recurrent severe vitreous hemorrhages that do not clear, it may be best to perform pars plana vitrectomy (*see* Chapter 8).

Results

The DRS has shown that photocoagulation is beneficial in reducing the incidence of severe visual loss in certain stages of proliferative retinopathy[15]. In this study one eye of each patient was randomly assigned to receive either xenon or argon laser photocoagulation. Untreated eyes did significantly worse than treated eyes (*Table 10.1*). For these groups as a whole, xenon photocoagulation was slightly more effective in preventing blindness than argon laser photocoagulation, but the difference in effectiveness was not statistically significant and the complications and side effects of xenon treatment were greater. Another study also demonstrated that xenon and argon laser photocoagulation are beneficial in causing regression of optic disc neovascularization[20].

Table 10.1 Cumulative event-rate of severe visual loss for argon laser or xenon laser treated eyes[15]

Follow-up (years)	*Control* (%)	*Treated* (%)
1	3.6	2.3
2	14.0	6.2
3	21.7	9.0
4	27.8	11.6
5	33.0	13.9
6	36.7	16.6

In the DRS several subgroups of eyes that were graded according to severity of retinopathy also had statistically significant lower rates of blindness with photocoagulation as compared to untreated eyes, and certain 'risk factors' were identified. These risk factors are the presence of: (*1*) vitreous or preretinal hemorrhage; (*2*) any retinal neovascularization; (*3*) optic nervehead neovascularization; and (*4*) moderate or severe retinal neovascularization[21]. Photocoagulation is recommended for eyes with three of more of these factors because they have an especially high risk of progressing to severe visual loss. Evidence also suggests that treatment at earlier stages might be preferable to deferral of treatment until progression occurs. Photocoagulation has not been shown to lower significantly the incidence of blindness in eyes with lesser degrees of retinopathy and yet it did prevent progression to high-risk retinopathy groups for all grades of retinopathy included in the DRS study. Another collaborative clinical trial which is now in progress, The Early Treatment Diabetic Retinopathy Study (ETDRS), will attempt to answer, among other questions, whether it is better to perform treatment at earlier stages of retinopathy or to defer treatment and only treat later if the high-risk factors develop. Until the results of the ETDRS are available, it seems reasonable to apply photocoagulation treatment to all eyes with proliferative retinopathy.

Photocoagulation treatment of central retinal vein occlusion

Photocoagulation can be used in eyes with central retinal vein occlusion to treat retinal neovascularization or iris neovascularization. The pathogenesis of central retinal vein occlusion is probably thrombosis in the vein near its narrowed portion at the lamina cribosa[22]. In some cases, blood dyscrasias (such as macroglobulinemia or polycythemia) or perivasculitis can cause occlusion.

Some eyes with central retinal vein occlusion have severe intraretinal hemorrhages and massive hemorrhagic necrosis of the retina. These eyes, which generally also have extensive capillary non-perfusion (*Figure 10.13*), presumably liberate a 'vasoproliferative factor' such as may occur in proliferative diabetic retinopathy. Although many eyes with central retinal vein occlusion have extensive capillary non-perfusion, most do not develop retinal neovascularization, possibly because there is such severe destruction of the vascular endothelial cells that endothelial proliferation cannot occur and cause neovascularization[23]. It is more common, however, for eyes with severe central retinal vein occlusion and extensive capillary non-perfusion to develop iris neovascularization and neovascular glaucoma, and this occurs in up to 60 per cent of such eyes[24]. Unfortunately, most eyes with a severe central retinal vein occlusion also have marked visual loss because of capillary non-perfusion in the macula and severe cystoid macular edema. Laser treatment is not beneficial in improving vision in those cases.

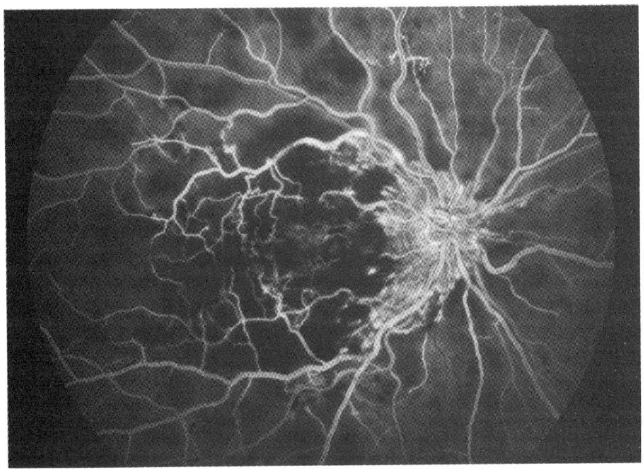

Figure 10.13 *Wide-angle fluorescein angiogram showing extensive retinal capillary non-perfusion in an eye with a central retinal vein occlusion. Capillaries remain only around the optic nervehead*

Evaluation of central retinal vein occlusion

Evaluation is similar to that described for proliferative diabetic retinopathy, but with special emphasis on identifying iris and anterior chamber angle neovascularization. The iris is examined before pupillary dilation, and gonioscopy is performed on all eyes with central retinal vein occlusion. Mild iris and anterior chamber angle neovascularization can progress rapidly over several weeks to cause severe neovascular glaucoma. The optic nerve is examined for neovascularization. Fluorescein angiography is performed to assess the severity of retinal capillary non-perfusion by photographing the midperipheral retina in addition to the posterior pole. If an eye has severe non-perfusion but no retinal or anterior segment neovascularization, the eye is re-examined every 3–4 weeks for the first 3 months after the occlusion because this is when iris neovascularization usually develops. Examination is done at less frequent intervals thereafter for at least 2 years.

It is also important to evaluate young patients with central retinal vein occlusion, or patients with bilateral involvement, for macroglobulinemia, polycythemia and other systemic abnormalities. Medical treatment of these conditions may allow improvement or prevent progression in the affected eye and, in unilateral cases, can prevent involvement of the second eye. Eyes with central retinal vein occlusion also have an increased prevalence of concomitant chronic open-angle glaucoma, and this should be treated.

Indications for photocoagulation

Photocoagulation is not recommended in central retinal vein occlusion to improve visual acuity damaged by capillary non-perfusion in the macula, and treatment is also ineffective in reducing cystoid macular edema[25]. Complete scatter photocoagulation is used, however, if secondary iris or anterior chamber angle neovascularization develops, and photocoagulation is usually effective in causing regression of the neovascularization if initiated at an early enough stage[24–26]. Photocoagulation may even be recommended in the absence of anterior chamber neovascularization if there is severe retinal capillary non-perfusion and therefore a substantial risk of developing neovascular glaucoma. If severe retinal non-perfusion is present and the patient cannot be re-examined frequently, photocoagulation is advisable[24]. Treatment is also recommended if optic nervehead neovascularization develops, to prevent further visual loss from vitreous hemorrhage and to avoid a situation in which vitreous hemorrhage is followed by neovascular glaucoma, but in which scatter retinal photocoagulation then cannot be done because of the vitreous opacity.

Techniques and results

For treatment of central retinal vein occlusion, the method is similar to the scatter laser photocoagulation described for proliferative diabetic retinopathy. When possible, the burns should be applied while avoiding large intraretinal hemorrhages. Krypton laser photocoagulation has the possible advantage of penetrating intraretinal blood better in eyes with extensive intraretinal hemorrhage. However, most clinical experience has been with the argon laser.

Scatter retinal photocoagulation is effective in preventing and also eliminating both optic nervehead and anterior segment neovascularization (*Figure 10.14*). In eyes with neovascular glaucoma when the anterior chamber angle is more than three-quarters closed by peripheral anterior synechiae, scatter photocoagulation will probably not control the intraocular pressure, because the synechiae remain even after the neovascular component disappears.

Photocoagulation treatment of proliferative retinopathy with branch retinal vein occlusion

Branch retinal vein occlusion can reduce vision from macular damage or from complications of secondary retinal neovascularization. In branch vein occlusion, a retinal vein is occluded at an arteriovenous crossing where the vein is compressed by the arteriole. Systemic hypertension, associated with arteriosclerosis, is found in more than 50 per cent of patients with branch retinal vein occlusion[27]. Occasionally, periphlebitis from sarcoidosis or other conditions can also cause branch retinal vein occlusion.

Branch retinal vein occlusion can occur on or near the optic nervehead with involvement of half the fundus if there is occlusion of an inferior or superior division of the central retinal vein before these divisions further divide into nasal and temporal branches. If the occlusion occurs in one of the four main branch veins near the optic nerve, one-quarter of the fundus is affected. The most frequently involved vessel is the superotemporal branch vein. A more distal branch vein occlusion, such as a tertiary

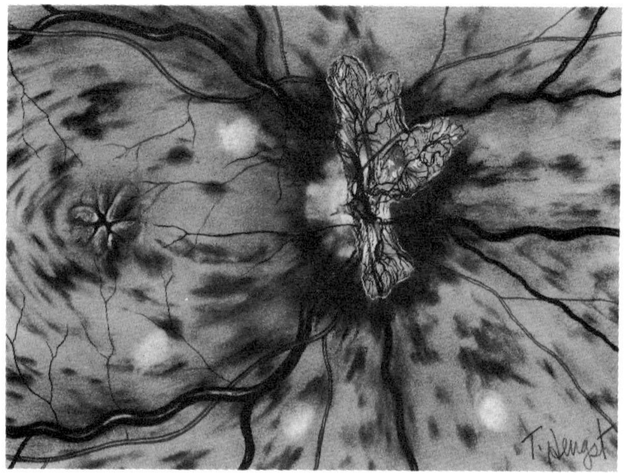
a

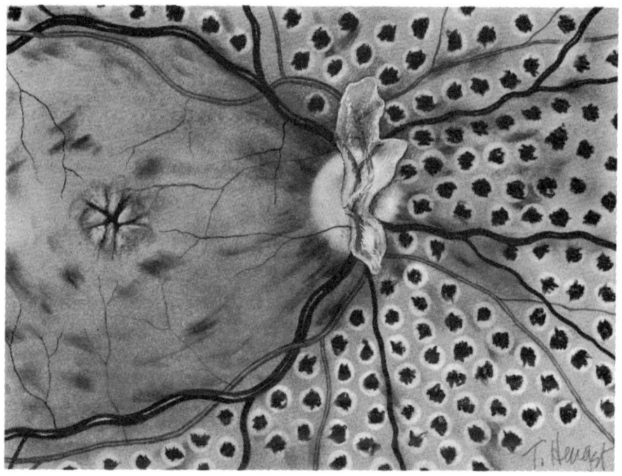
b

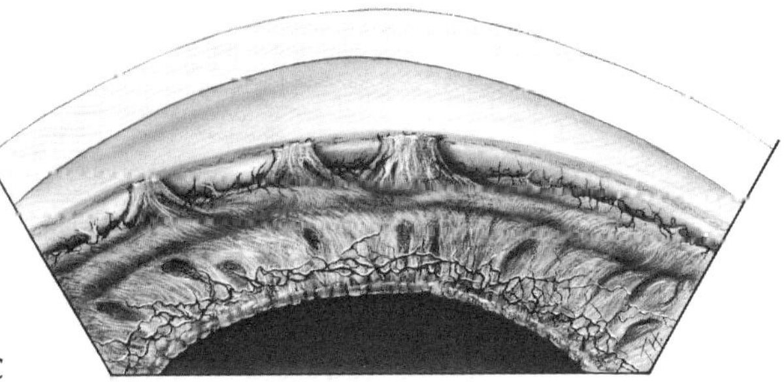
c

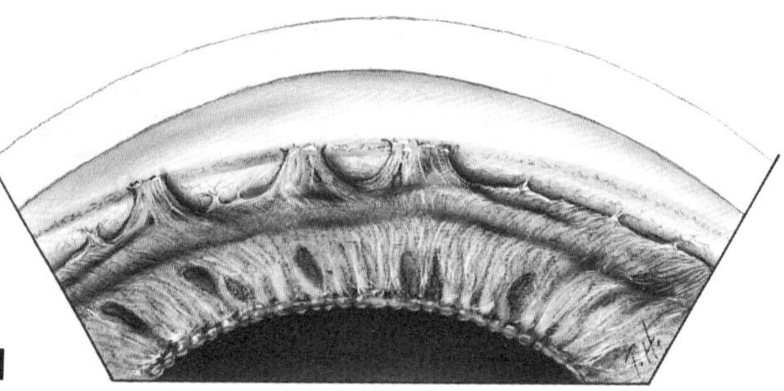
d

Figure 10.14 *Laser treatment of an eye with central retinal vein occlusion.* **(a)** *Optic nervehead neovascularization, intraretinal hemorrhages, cystoid macular edema.* **(b)** *Regression of optic nervehead neovascularization after scatter laser photocoagulation, with persistence of cystoid macular edema.* **(c)** *Iris and anterior chamber angle neovascularization with scattered peripheral anterior synechiae before scatter photocoagulation.* **(d)** *Regression of neovascularization of iris and anterior chamber angle after scatter laser photocoagulation, with persistence of peripheral anterior synechiae* branch vein, involves less of the fundus but this may reduce central vision if the venous drainage of the macula is affected.

A branch retinal vein occlusion can cause capillary non-perfusion with secondary optic nervehead neovascularization, peripheral retinal neovascularization, or both. Optic nervehead neovascularization can occur even if the occlusion is not adjacent to the optic nervehead, but peripheral retinal neovascularization usually occurs only adjacent to an area of capillary non-perfusion at the margin of the involved and uninvolved retina. Rarely, peripheral neovascularization occurs in portions of normal retina not involved by the occlusion[28]. Decreased vision occurs if the venous occlusion involves the macula with capillary non-perfusion or with macular edema.

Evaluation of branch retinal vein occlusion

Special attention is directed toward detecting optic nervehead and peripheral retinal neovascularization. Fundus biomicroscopy allows detection of macular edema, hard exudates and retinal thickening. Fluorescein angiography is helpful to determine: (*1*) the distribution and extent of the involved retina; (*2*) how much of the perifoveal capillary net is affected; (*3*) whether or not significant capillary non-perfusion is present (*Figure 10.15*); and (*4*) the severity of cystoid macular edema.

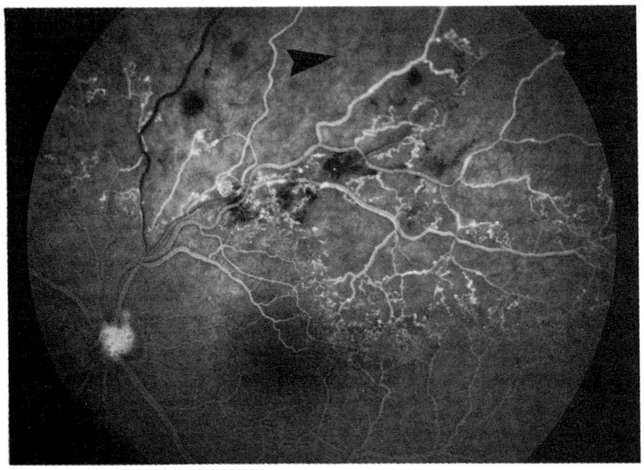

Figure 10.15 *Fluorescein angiogram of an eye with retinal branch vein occlusion showing severe capillary non-perfusion (arrow) and secondary optic nervehead neovascularization that leaks fluorescein dye*

Fluorescein angiography is also useful in differentiating retinal neovascularization from collateral retinal vessels that often occur within a few months after branch retinal vein occlusion. Collateral vessels pass from an involved to an uninvolved area of the retina. These are seen most often: (*1*) across the horizontal raphe temporal to the macula; (*2*) around the arteriovenous obstruction site; (*3*) between involved and uninvolved portions of the venous drainage pattern on the nasal side of the macula; and (*4*) on the optic nervehead. Ophthalmoscopy usually allows differentiation between neovascularization and collateral vessels. When this is difficult, fluorescein angiography helps because neovascularization leaks fluorescein profusely but collaterals do not leak.

Indications for photocoagulation

If optic nervehead neovascularization is present, segmental scatter retinal photocoagulation is applied to the involved area of the retina, sparing the macula itself. This is done to prevent vitreous hemorrhage. Small patches of peripheral neovascularization without preretinal or vitreous hemorrhage can be treated or followed without treatment. If such patches grow or are associated with later hemorrhage, treatment should be done. Indications for treatment of macular edema from branch retinal vein occlusion are described below.

Techniques and results

Treatment technique is similar to that used for proliferative diabetic retinopathy, except that scatter photocoagulation is applied only to that portion of the retina involved by the occlusion. Both ophthalmoscopy and fluorescein angiography are useful in defining the area of retinal involvement. Argon laser scatter photocoagulation with 500 μm burns that are spaced one-half burn width apart is applied to the area of occlusion (*Figure 10.16*), but the macula itself is spared. Confluent 500 μm burns are usually applied to flat areas of peripheral neovascularization, just as is used for proliferative diabetic retinopathy. Elevated peripheral neovascularization is not treated focally. Instead, scatter photocoagulation alone is used.

Treatment usually results in prompt regression of the neovascularization, perhaps even more markedly than is seen with proliferative diabetic retinopathy. A clinical trial is currently in progress to define the exact effects of this treatment in branch retinal vein occlusion[29].

Photocoagulation treatment for other causes of retinal neovascularization

Retinal neovascularization can be seen in other diseases such as sickle-cell anemia, ocular ischemia[30], sarcoidosis, pars planitis, Eales' disease, retrolental fibroplasia and other miscellaneous conditions. In all of these conditions, peripheral neovascularization can be found, although the pattern of neovascularization varies in different diseases. In all diseases, except retrolental fibroplasia, optic nervehead neovascularization can also be present.

Evaluation of miscellaneous causes of retinal neovascularization

It is important to diagnose the cause of retinal neovascularization when it is not due to diabetic retinopathy, central retinal vein occlusion or branch retinal vein occlusion. A thorough ocular examination and a medical evaluation often enable a correct diagnosis to be made.

Photocoagulation treatment of sickle-cell retinopathy

Black patients with sickle-cell retinopathy often have peripheral neovascularization in a 'sea-fan' configuration. Hemoglobin electrophoresis confirms the diagnosis in cases in which the systemic diagnosis has not been made previously. Hemoglobin S-C is the most frequent cause of sickle-cell retinopathy, but S-thalassemia, S-S, S-A and other hemoglobinopathies can cause the retinopathy.

If an eye with sickle-cell retinopathy has significant peripheral neovascularization, or vitreous or preretinal hemorrhage, treatment is indicated. Traditionally, a 'feeder-frond' technique has been used with success, although serious complications can occur with this type of treatment. We prefer peripheral scatter treatment for sickle-cell retinopathy. This is similar to that used for proliferative diabetic retinopathy, except for the distribution of the treatment. Medium-intensity, 500 μm burns spaced one-half burn width apart are applied as far anteriorly as possible beginning one to two disc diameters posterior to the peripheral neovascularization (*Figure 10.17a,b*). A fluorescein angiogram is useful to determine

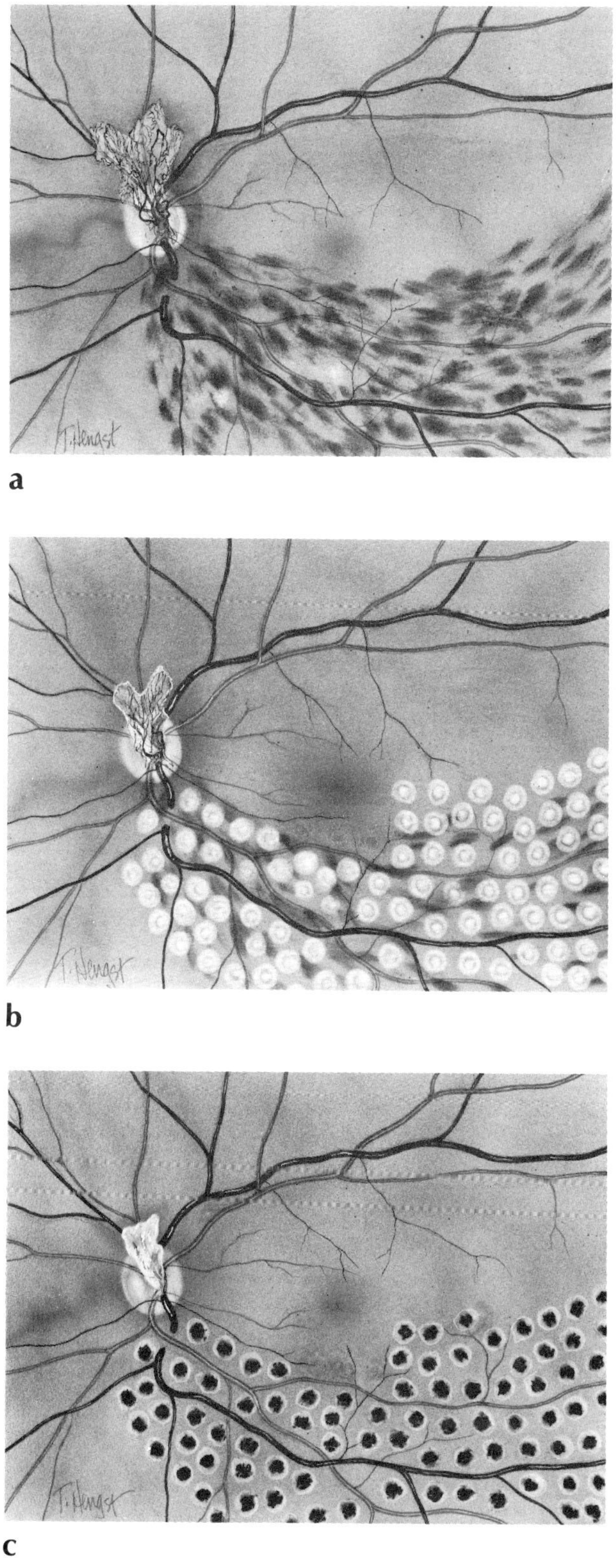

Figure 10.16 *Laser treatment of an eye with branch retinal vein occlusion and optic nervehead neovascularization.* **(a)** *Inferotemporal branch retinal vein occlusion with numerous intraretinal hemorrhages and optic nervehead neovascularization.* **(b)** *Scatter photocoagulation applied to involved segment.* **(c)** *Regression of disc neovascularization after segmental scatter photocoagulation*

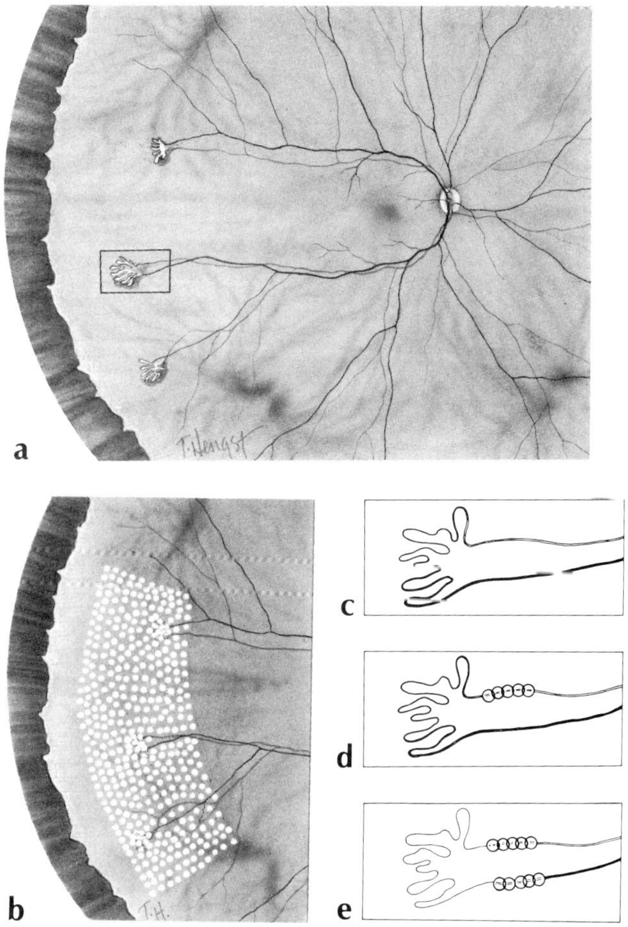

Figure 10.17 *Laser treatment for peripheral neovascularization resulting from sickle-cell retinopathy.* **(a)** *Peripheral neovascularization ('sea-fans').* **(b)** *Peripheral scatter photocoagulation treatment.* **(c)** *Peripheral neovascularization with a feeding arteriole and a draining venule.* **(d)** *Occlusion of feeding arteriole with 500 μm laser burns.* **(e)** *Collecting venule closed with 500 μm laser burns*

the extent of peripheral non-perfusion, all of which should be treated. Confluent 500 μm burns can also be applied to areas of flat peripheral neovascularization. These forms of treatment usually are successful in eliminating peripheral neovascularization[31,32].

Conventional feeder-frond treatment may also be used[33]. Rapid-sequence fluorescein angiography is performed, photographing the transit of fluorescein through the neovascularization. The rapid-sequence photographs identify the arteriole or arterioles feeding the neovascularization. A test photocoagulation burn is applied elsewhere to determine the laser settings needed to produce a burn of moderate intensity. Then 500 μm burns of 0.2–0.5 second at double that baseline power setting are applied to the feeding arterioles to occlude them (*Figure 10.17c,d*). When they are closed and have no blood flow, the draining venules are treated to occlude them as well (*Figure 10.17e*). Angiography is repeated on subsequent visits and, if the vessels reopen, retreatment is applied in a similar fashion, while avoiding excessive power over areas of pigmentation, which absorb the energy more readily.

Both types of treatment, 'feeder-frond' and peripheral scatter treatment, are effective in eliminating peripheral neovascularization[31,32,34]. A clinical trial has indicated that either treatment is better than no treatment[35].

Photocoagulation treatment for other proliferative retinopathies

Several miscellaneous diseases associated with retinal vascular non-perfusion or ischemia develop peripheral retinal or optic nervehead neovascularization, or both. These conditions include Eales' disease, sarcoidosis, retrolental fibroplasia, and the ocular ischemia syndrome. Photocoagulation is often effective in eliminating the retinal neovascularization and preventing secondary complications. These conditions can usually be distinguished from each other by the findings on ophthalmic examination and by medical evaluation. Eales' disease is a diagnosis of exclusion, made in the presence of idiopathic retinal periphlebitis, peripheral retinal capillary non-perfusion and retinal neovascularization. There is often no associated systemic disease, although systemic tuberculosis is found in some patients. The cause of Eales' disease is unknown, but it is probably an immunological disorder with phlebitis that causes vascular occlusion, capillary non-perfusion and secondary retinal neovascularization.

Eyes affected by sarcoidosis often have retinal periphlebitis with peripheral retinal capillary non-perfusion. They usually also show choroiditis, iritis or other ocular signs of inflammation. Characteristic systemic findings of sarcoidosis can be found.

The ocular ischemic syndrome caused by carotid or ophthalmic artery occlusion can show anterior segment ischemia. However, in some eyes there is little anterior segment involvement, and the fundus may have the appearance of diabetic retinopathy with retinal hemorrhages and retinal neovascularization[30]. Fluorescein angiography shows a prolonged dye-transit time and widespread leakage of fluorescein from retinal blood vessels, presumably as a result of ischemia from diminished blood supply to the eye.

Pars planitis is an idiopathic inflammatory disorder characterized by vitreous cells, a 'snowbank' of inflammatory cells over the inferior pars plana, and occasionally vascularization of organized pars plana infiltrate or frank peripheral retinal neovascularization. Neovascularization can lead to secondary complications such as vitreous hemorrhage. Neovascularization in pars planitis probably has similar causes to that in Eales' disease and sarcoidosis: retinal vasculitis and ischemia[36]. Only occasionaly is photocoagulation treatment useful in this condition.

The indication for treatment in these various conditions is optic nervehead neovascularization or significant peripheral neovascularization, especially if there is secondary preretinal or vitreous hemorrhage. Optic nervehead neovascularization is treated just as is diabetic disc neovascularization, with a complete scatter photocoagulation pattern. Extensive peripheral neovascularization can also be treated with complete scatter treatment. Presumably this treatment destroys areas of peripheral retina that are non-perfused or ischemic, just as it does in diabetic retinopathy, which results in elimination of the neovascularization. If the non-perfused ischemic retina is confined mostly to the peripheral retina, scatter photocoagulation may only be necessary in the periphery, extending from near the ora serrata to one or two disc diameters posterior to the peripheral neovascularization. If only one or two small patches of peripheral neovascularization are present, they can be observed periodically without treatment, or they can be treated focally with confluent 500 μm argon laser burns.

Peripheral neovascularization from retrolental fibroplasia in an infant is not usually treatable with photocoagulation because of inability to use a slit-lamp photocoagulator with general anesthesia and difficulty in treating the far-peripheral retina with xenon photocoagulation because of opacities in the media. This disease is usually managed by observation or various types of surgery.

Photocoagulation for retinal vascular leakage

Photocoagulation may be beneficial in treating macular edema resulting from selected types of retinal vascular leakage. In diabetic macular edema, focal leaks can often be identified and treated. Some eyes with diabetic macular edema have a more diffuse type of leakage from all parts of the macular capillaries, and treatment of this is more difficult. Other diseases with macular edema often show this more diffuse type of leakage, such as central retinal vein occlusion, aphakic cystoid macular edema, perifoveal telangiectasis and some other types of cystoid macular edema. Still other eyes have macular edema or macular lipid deposition resulting from a more distant site of peripheral retinal leakage, such as with peripheral Coats' disease and angiomatosis retinae. Argon laser photocoagulation of these different entities is discussed below, with major emphasis on treatment of diabetic macular edema.

Evaluation of diabetic macular edema

Evaluation of macular edema includes measurement of best corrected visual acuity. Day-to-day changes in the refractive error of a diabetic eye can make unrefracted visual acuity measurements inaccurate. This is especially important if the visual acuity is used as a basis for deciding whether photocoagulation should be applied.

The best method for detecting edematous thickening of the retina or small hard exudates is slit-lamp biomicroscopy with a fundus contact lens. In eyes with edematous thickening of the retina, a thin slit beam directed at an angle shows the thickening best (*Figure 10.18*). The normal foveal reflex is also lost if the center of the macula is involved by edema. Cystoid macular edema is usually visible and is best seen by directing the slit beam just to the side of the macula. This highlights the cystoid changes by retroillumination (*Figure 10.18*). A Hruby lens gives a less clear view, but its use may be indicated when fundus photography is to be performed as it avoids the reduction in corneal clarity which occurs after the use of a contact lens. Direct or indirect ophthalmoscopy shows the position and number of hard exudates, the presence of moderate or severe cystoid macular edema, and the loss of the foveal reflex. Visualization of more subtle changes requires biomicroscopy, however.

Fundus photography is useful to document the position and amount of hard exudates, but fluorescein angiography is necessary to evaluate adequately most cases of diabetic macular edema. Fluorescein angiography shows the location of leakage and whether it is focal or diffuse (*Figures 10.19* and *10.20*). Capillary non-perfusion and diffuse leakage from capillary walls can also be seen (*Figure 10.21*). The later phases of the angiogram show the severity of the edema, as indicated by the amount of fluorescein that accumulates in the retina. If cystoid macular edema is present, fluorescein dye accumulates in the macula in a characteristic cystoid pattern (*Figure 10.22*).

Indications for photocoagulation

Several clinical studies suggest that photocoagulation treatment of diabetic macular edema is effective[40–44] However, no prospective controlled clinical trial has yet been completed that properly tests the effect of treatment. Still, certain indications for treatment are widely accepted.

Eyes with circinate deposits of hard exudate are treated if the ring impinges on the center of the macula. Even if the center of the macula is not involved and vision is normal, if the ring of exudate is close to the fovea, treatment is still recommended to prevent worsening of vision as the ring expands. Circinate deposits respond to photocoagulation better than other types of macular edema, probably because usually there are fewer leaks and these are centered within the ring. In eyes with simple ring exudates and one or only a few microaneurysms in the center of the ring, it is not always necessary to perform a fluorescein angiogram before treatment. Circinate exudates that are not close to the center of the macula are not treated. Sometimes leaks in the center of the ring seal spontaneously, and the circinate deposits disappear without photocoagulation treatment.

In eyes with macular edema without circinate deposits, the visual acuity is an important factor in deciding whether to apply photocoagulation or not. Treatment is advised if the visual acuity is reduced to 20/40 or worse from focal leaks, as seen on fluorescein angiography, causing macular edema. Eyes with diffuse leakage from all portions of the capillary wall as seen on fluorescein angiography show equivocal results after photocoagulation.

Photocoagulation is not beneficial in eyes with severe visual loss when fluorescein angiography shows extensive macular capillary non-perfusion. In these eyes ischemia has already permanently damaged the macula. In eyes with macular edema and milder damage to the perifoveal net, photocoagulation is applied if there are also focal leaks.

Technique of treatment

Photocoagulation for diabetic macular edema is applied more easily and safely with a slit-lamp argon laser than with other delivery systems. Treatment is usually done after topical anesthesia since treatment of the posterior pole with small burns is painless. However, sometimes retrobulbar anesthesia is used to achieve akinesia if sudden uncontrolled eye movements increase the chance of accidental damage to the center of the macula.

A three-mirror fundus contact lens is preferred even though only the center part of the lens is used because the larger three-mirror lens is easily held and manipulated to steady the eye. A fluorescein angiogram is used to locate the leakage sites. One method of viewing the angiogram is to project a frame onto a screen behind the patient. This facilitates identification of leaks and allows more accurate treatment, although the use of an angiogram may be unnecessary if there are only a few focal leaks in the center of a circinate pattern of hard exudates. For projection, a frame is chosen in which leaks are visible and in which both the arterioles and venules are filled with fluorescein. The frame should be late enough in the dye passage so that a small amount of leakage extends beyond the hyperfluorescent spots, but it should be early enough so that extensive leakage does not obscure landmarks. Methods other than a projection system are also available that allow viewing of the angiogram while treating the eye.

To treat focal leaks, a choice of burn size, burn duration and power setting must be made. A 100 μm burn at 0.1 second is often chosen to treat solitary microaneurysms. The power setting is adjusted to achieve a darkening of the microaneurysm or a mild whitening of the surrounding retina. The power setting should not be so high, however, that it is associated with significant spread of the burn beyond the treated area. Each leak is treated with a single burn (*Figure 10.23*). If there are several adjacent focal leaks, a larger spot size such as a 200 μm or 500 μm can be used to treat several leakage sites with each burn. These larger coagulation spots are more destructive and should not be used near the center of the macula, nor should a large number of 500 μm spots be used in the papillomacular bundle. In eyes with a circinate pattern of hard exudates the focal leaks in the center of the ring and elsewhere are treated, and the circinate deposits disappear after several months (*Figure 10.24*).

Leaks in the perifoveal capillary net usually are not treated because of the risk of damaging the macula. For

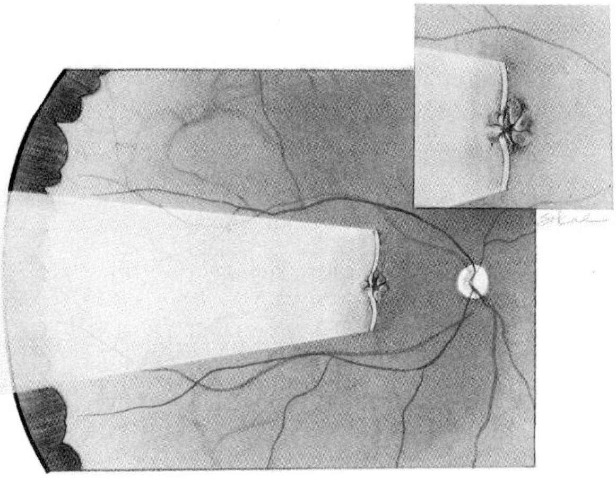

Figure 10.18 *Diabetic cystoid macular edema as seen on slit-lamp fundus biomicroscopy*

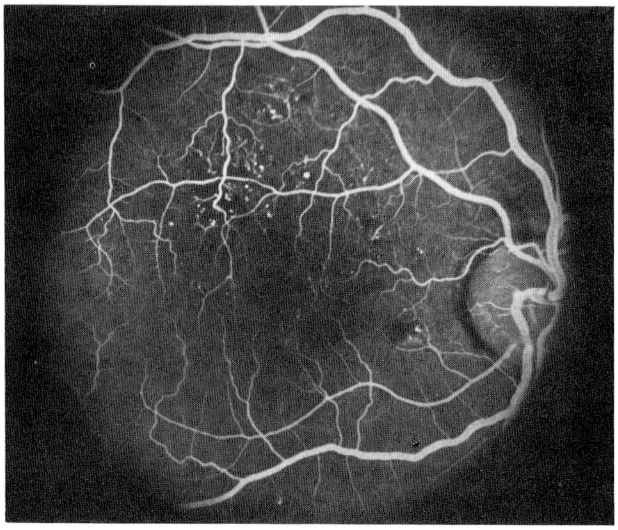

a

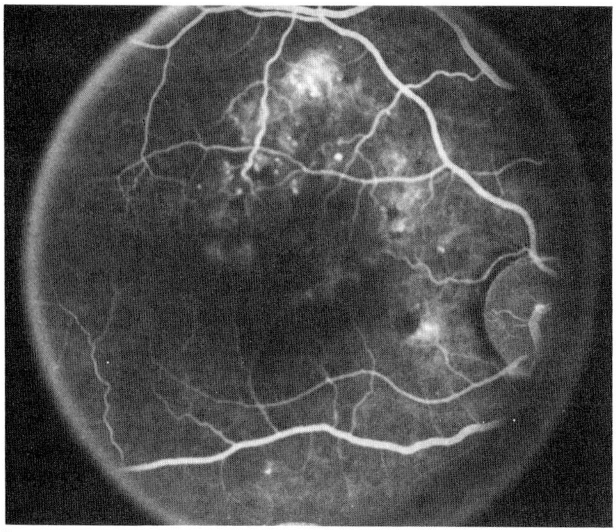

b

Figure 10.19 *Fluorescein angiogram of an eye with diabetic macular edema.* **(a)** *Microaneurysms are visible as hyperfluorescent spots.* **(b)** *Fluorescein leakage from microaneurysms in the later-phase angiogram*

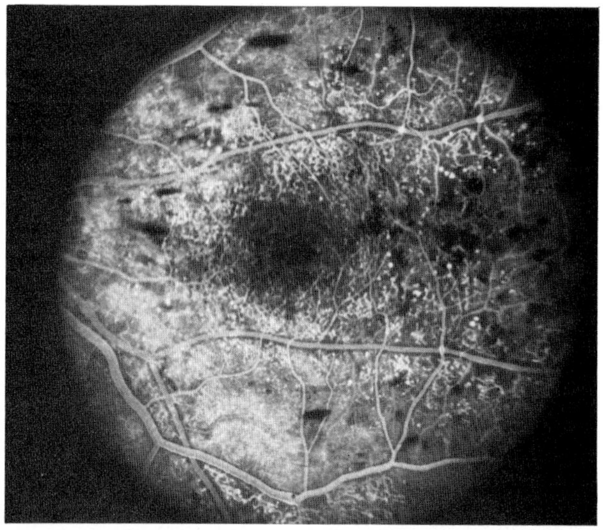

Figure 10.20 *Fluorescein angiogram of an eye with diabetic macular edema, showing a diffuse type of fluorescein leakage from all capillaries*

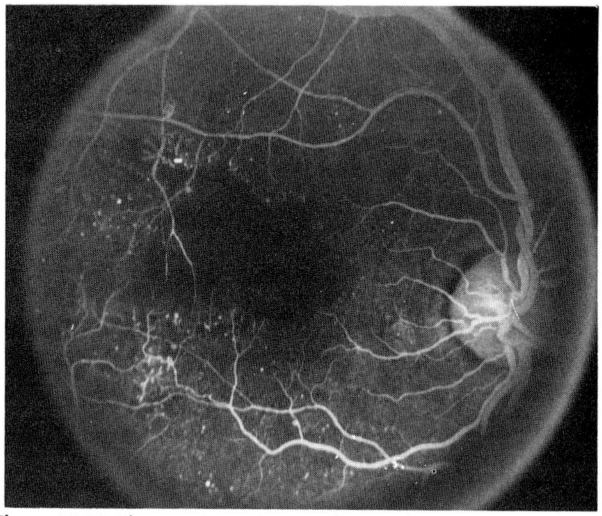

Figure 10.21 *Fluorescein angiogram showing loss of perifoveal capillaries in an eye with diabetic retinopathy*

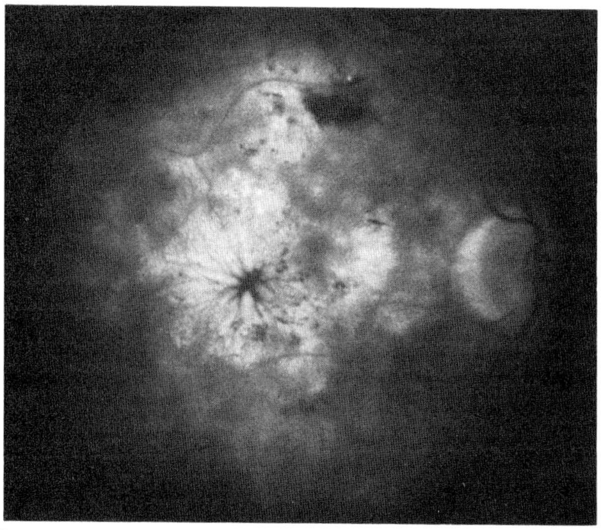

Figure 10.22 *Late-phase fluorescein angiogram showing diabetic cystoid macular edema*

the same reason, leaks that are 300–500 μm from the center of the macula should rarely be treated. If there are a few leaks within 300–500 μm of the center of the macula and multiple leaks farther away that are contributing to the edema, the more distant leaks are treated in the initial

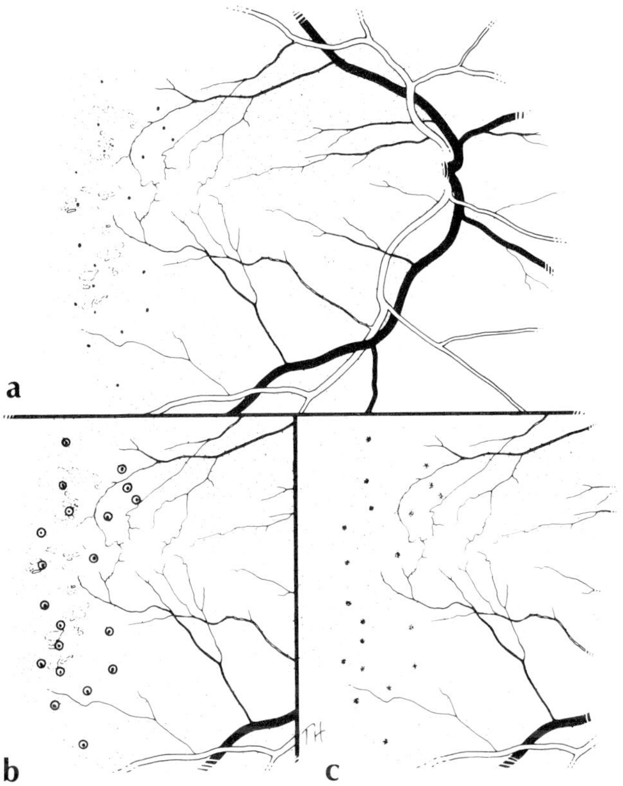

Figure 10.23 *Laser treatment of focal leaks with diabetic macular edema.* **(a)** *Multiple microaneurysms that leak fluid and 'hard' exudate.* **(b)** *Focal laser treatment to leaking microaneurysms.* **(c)** *Resolution of hard exudates and retinal thickening after laser treatment*

session. This less hazardous treatment may have a beneficial effect, and it may be unnecessary to treat the sites nearer the fovea. If fluorescein angiography shows only a few leaks and these are close to the center of the macula, treatment is done with small burns of a 50 μm or 100 μm size and of short duration (0.1 second) to minimize the spread of energy. Extensive treatment of the perifoveal capillary net is not done.

Usually, all hyperfluorescent spots near the macula that leak on fluorescein angiography are treated. However, all leaks are not treated if they are so numerous that treatment would require nearly confluent burns around the macula with damage to the paracentral visual field and the vasculature of the macula. Other patients have a diffuse type of leakage from every capillary, and similar extensive damage would result if all the leaking capillaries were treated. Therefore, eyes with multiple focal leaks or diffuse leakage are not as easily and safely treated as those with fewer focal leaks.

A grid pattern of photocoagulation can be used to treat eyes with numerous focal leaks or diffuse capillary leakage

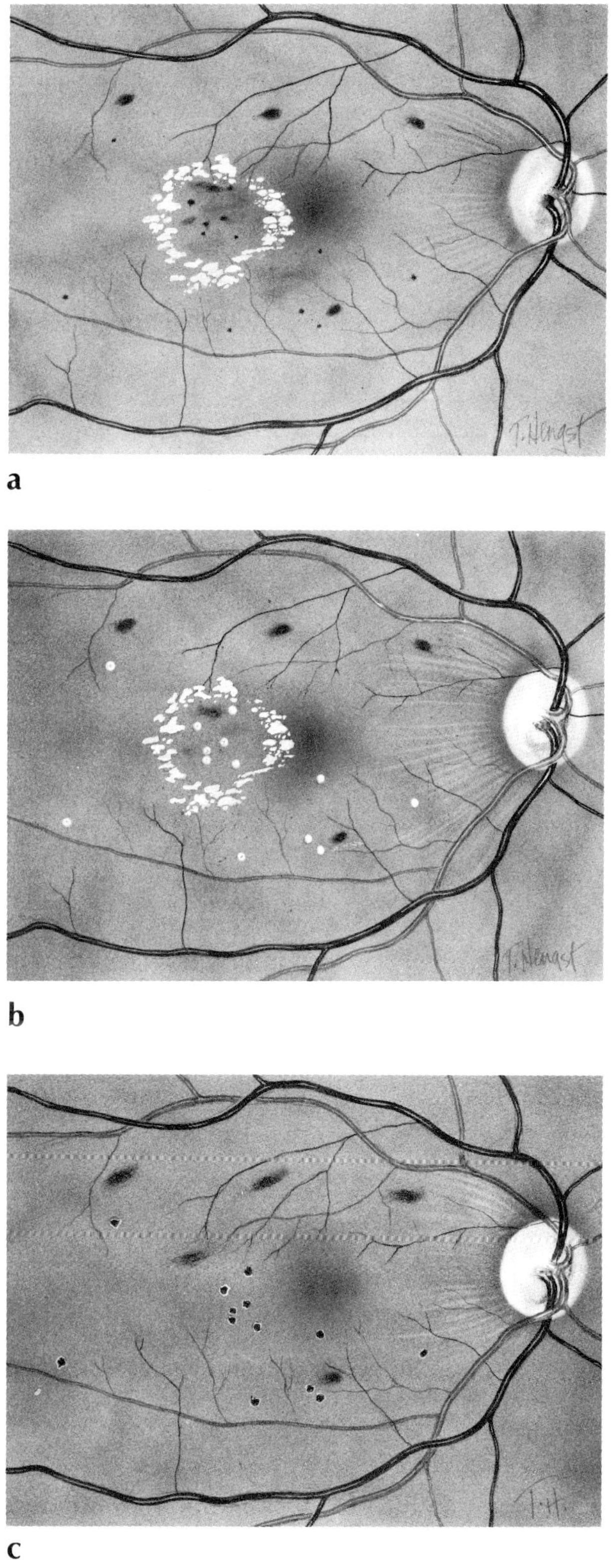

Figure 10.24 *Laser treatment of a circinate pattern of hard exudates in diabetic macular edema.* **(a)** *Circinate pattern with edge of ring impinging on fovea, and focal leakage from microaneurysms in the center of the ring.* **(b)** *Focal laser treatment to leaking microaneurysms in the ring and elsewhere.* **(c)** *Resolution of the ring of hard exudates after laser treatment*

causing macular edema (*Figure 10.25*). About 100–200 burns of 100 μm or 200 μm spot size at lower power intensity and short duration are applied in a grid pattern, spaced one burn width apart. Treatment is applied to the macula but avoiding the fovea by staying 1000 μm away from the center of the macula. Burns in this grid pattern are directed to treat preferentially the sites of worse leakage. No attempt is made to treat all leaks visible on

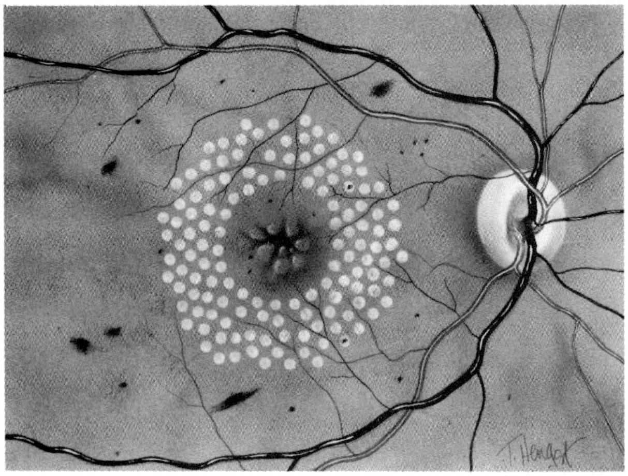

Figure 10.25 *Grid pattern of 200 μm laser burns in an eye with diffuse leakage and diabetic cystoid macular edema*

fluorescein angiography. All areas of non-perfusion in the posterior pole, but outside the fovea, are also treated with a grid pattern. Such treatment, possibly by thinning the retina and disrupting the normal barriers to diffusion, may improve diffusion of edematous fluid from the retina into the choroid and may also allow better oxygenation and diffusion of nutrients from the choroid into the retina.

Retreatment of focal leaks is considered if there is no change in the macular edema as evidenced by a persistence or increase in hard exudates, retinal thickening, or worsening of visual acuity. Fluorescein angiography is repeated to assess the extent and location of leakage. If there are only a few local leaks, additional treatment is applied, even to previously treated leaks that were not successfully closed. However, additional treatment is not done if extensive treatment was used before and there are still extensive focal leaks or diffuse leakage from all capillaries. In this situation, extensive supplemental treatment can be damaging.

Results

Several studies have indicated that argon laser photocoagulation of eyes with diabetic macular edema is beneficial. There have been three main randomized controlled studies on such treatment, and two of these have shown a favorable effect. The first of these, a study of argon laser photocoagulation in 63 patients, found that 27 per cent of treated patients had vision improved by two or more chart lines, 66 per cent remained the same and only 7 per cent worsened[40]. The untreated eyes fared worse: only 10 per cent had improved vision, 27 per cent had the same vision and 63 per cent had worse vision. In this study, focal photocoagulation was applied to microaneurysms and to suspected areas of leakage without the aid of fluorescein angiography. The second controlled study, using argon laser photocoagulation that was applied to specific leaks but also in a grid pattern to the macula, found no statistically significant difference in visual acuity in treated as compared to untreated eyes[41]. The third controlled study, utilizing xenon arc photocoagulation in a variety of treatment patterns, including focal treatment of leaks and use of grid patterns, showed a statistically significant beneficial effect, but the visual acuity of treated eyes averaged only one line better than that of untreated eyes[42].

As mentioned earlier, some types of macular edema seem to respond more favorably to photocoagulation than others. Treatment seems to be beneficial in eyes that have circinate patterns with focal leaks in their centers[43,44]. In another study, argon laser or xenon photocoagulation was used to treat eyes with three different types of fluorescein angiographic findings[45]. Photocoagulation seemed to be beneficial in eyes with focal leaks in which burns were applied to the individual leaks. Eyes with cystoid macular edema were treated using both focal treatment of leaks and a grid pattern of burns, and these eyes responded favorably if the macula had rather good capillary perfusion. Eyes with cystoid macular edema and poor capillary perfusion of the macula, and eyes with extensive areas of non-perfusion, did not respond well to photocoagulation. Another study found that diabetic eyes with poor capillary perfusion in the macula have a poor prognosis and do not have visual improvement after photocoagulation[46].

Although most of the reports and studies on photocoagulation treatment of diabetic macular edema indicate that treatment may be beneficial, the studies are inconclusive. The Early Treatment Diabetic Retinopathy Study (ETDRS), which is currently in progress, is a large controlled, prospective, multicenter clinical trial that will evaluate several types of photocoagulation treatment for diabetic macular edema as well as the use of aspirin treatment. Photocoagulation treatment includes focal treatment of discrete leaks and a 'grid pattern' of treatment for multiple focal leaks and for diffuse leakage. The effect of scatter retinal photocoagulation (as used in the treatment of proliferative retinopathy) on diabetic macular edema will also be assessed.

Photocoagulation treatment of macular edema resulting from branch retinal vein occlusion

Decreased visual acuity can occur if a branch retinal vein occlusion involves the macula. If the occlusion is severe, closure of the perifoveal capillaries severely damages the central vision. If the perifoveal capillaries are involved by the occlusion but are not closed, they can leak fluid and produce macular edema. The amount of damage depends on the severity of the occlusion and the distribution of the occluded vein. About 50 per cent of cases of macular edema improve spontaneously and achieve at least partial visual improvement[47]. The chance for recovery is less if the perifoveal capillary net is involved by the occlusion[48].

In evaluating macular edema resulting from branch vein occlusion, fundus biomicroscopy allows detection of retinal thickening, hard exudates or both. Fluorescein angiography is useful in determining the distribution of the occluded vein, how much of the perifoveal capillary net is affected and whether there is significant capillary non-perfusion. Late leakage of fluorescein into the macula confirms the presence of macular edema, including whether or not cystoid changes are present.

Eyes with poor central vision resulting from extensive capillary non-perfusion are not improved by laser treatment. If non-perfusion involves only a portion of the perifoveal net, good vision may be recovered spontaneously or after photocoagulation treatment. When good perfusion is present but there is leakage from focal leaks, laser treatment to the specific leaking sites is probably indicated. Occasionally a branch vein occlusion does not involve the perifoveal capillaries, but instead fluid and hard exudates diffuse into the foveal region from a more distant site. Photocoagulation in these cases is beneficial in eliminating macular edema, and it improves vision if permanent damage from hard exudates has not occurred.

Photocoagulation treatment of macular edema resulting from branch retinal vein occlusion is similar to that used for treatment of diabetic macular edema, as described above. Focal leaks and microaneurysms are treated with single burns. Areas of diffuse leakage can be treated with a grid pattern of laser burns.

Eyes with extensive involvement of the perifoveal capillary net have a poorer prognosis for improvement after photocoagulation than eyes with lesser amounts of involvement[48]. Because many eyes improve spontaneously, it is difficult to assess the effect of laser treatment. A collaborative clinical trial of laser photocoagulation treatment for branch retinal vein occlusion is currently underway[29].

Photocoagulation treatment of macular edema resulting from other causes

Macular edema with or without cystoid changes can occur as a result of a variety of eye diseases other than diabetic retinopathy or branch retinal vein occlusion. Central retinal vein occlusion often shows severe cystoid macular edema associated with extensive capillary leakage or non-perfusion in the macula. Laser treatment is not beneficial in reducing macular edema or improving vision in this condition.

Aphakic cystoid macular edema and cystoid macular edema resulting from ocular inflammatory disorders are due to diffuse leakage from the perifoveal capillaries. Similar leakage occurs in radiation retinopathy and in ocular ischemia resulting from carotid artery occlusion. Laser photocoagulation is not beneficial in these conditions.

Some adults develop idiopathic juxtafoveal retinal telangiectasis with telangiectatic vessels involving part or all of the perifoveal capillary net. Leakage of fluid into the macula causes retinal thickening, with or without cystoid changes. Some such eyes have only a mild decrease in vision. If progressive visual loss occurs, laser photocoagulation can be applied to the leaking vessels. Multiple treatment sessions may be necessary, a grid pattern of 100–200 μm burns of moderate intensity can be used to treat diffuse leakage[49]. Treatment is beneficial in some cases.

Eyes with idiopathic epiretinal membranes in the macula and macular pucker, resulting from various causes, often have both distortion of the macula and macular edema from diffuse retinal vascular leakage. Such eyes are not improved by photocoagulation, but surgical removal of the epiretinal membranes is beneficial in some cases[50,51].

Macular edema with accumulation of hard exudates can be caused by leakage from extramacular or peripheral retinal vascular lesions. This can occur from macroaneurysms, Coats' disease with peripheral retinal telangiectasis, and angiomatosis retinae. Other conditions with vascular abnormalities such as retrolental fibroplasia may show similar leakage. In children, these conditions often are discovered only after permanent macular damage has occurred as a result of large accumulations of hard exudates.

a

b

c

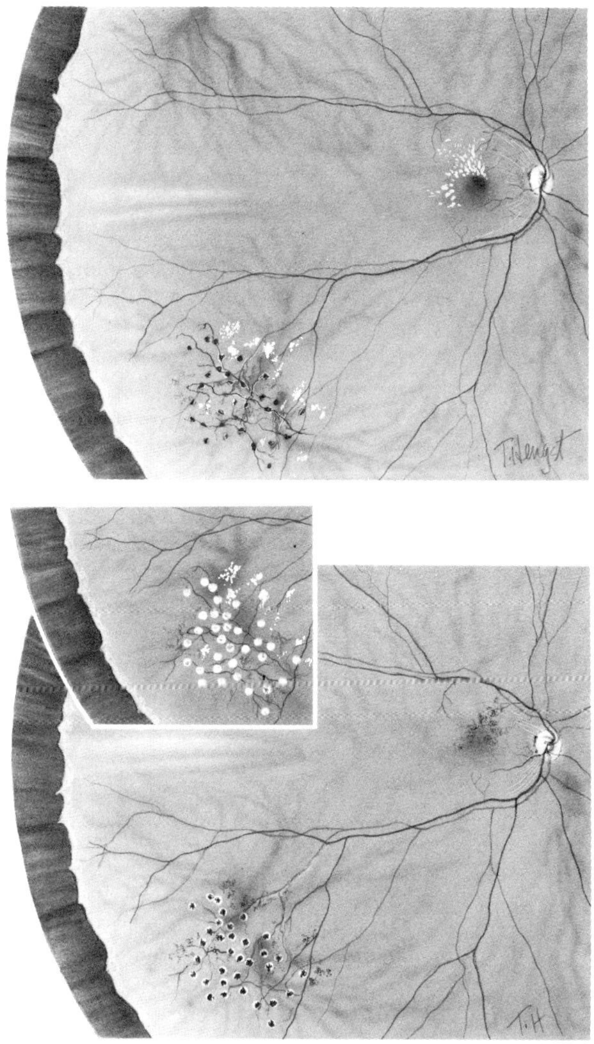

Figure 10.26 *Laser treatment for Coats' disease with macular edema.* **(a)** *Peripheral retinal telangiectasia with hard exudate producing macular edema.* **(b)** *Focal laser treatment to leaking peripheral telangiectasia.* **(c)** *Resolution of macular edema after laser treatment, with residual pigmentary changes in the macula*

Macroaneurysms, usually on one of the major temporal retinal arterioles, can cause vitreous hemorrhage or macular edema. If hard exudates begin to collect in the macula, argon laser treatment can be applied to the macroaneurysm. This causes mild scarring that stops leaking without occluding the arteriole. Light-to-moderate intensity 500 μm burns at 0.2–0.5 second are used.

Laser treatment can also be applied to peripheral retinal vascular abnormalities to stop leakage, and hard exudates gradually clear during several months. Visual recovery occurs if the edema was mild. For peripheral retinal telangiectasis with macular edema, moderate to heavy 200 μm or 500 μm laser burns are applied to the telangiectatic vessels (*Figure 10.26*). Retreatment may be necessary to seal all abnormal vessels. Treatment of angiomatosis retinae is discussed in Chapter 11.

Photocoagulation treatment of localized retinal pigment epithelial leakage

Leakage through the retinal pigment epithelium (RPE), which is normally a barrier against diffusion of fluid from the choroid into the subretinal space, can result in serous detachment of the sensory retina. Central serous retinopathy is the most prevalent disease of this type, but some exudative retinal detachments have demonstrable leaks through the RPE. Choroidal tumors – including metastatic tumors, malignant melanomas, choroidal nevi and choroidal hemangiomas – can also leak and produce serous elevation of the sensory retina. Laser treatment of tumors in some cases allows flattening of the retina and improved visual acuity, and this is discussed in Chapter 11.

Central serous retinopathy

Central serous retinopathy is an idiopathic condition that often occurs unilaterally in men between the ages of 30 and 50 years. Initially it produces metamorphopsia and a mild decrease in central vision. Fundus biomicroscopy shows a circular elevation of the sensory retina involving the macula. This is due to leakage of fluid from the choroid into the subsensory retinal space through a defect in the RPE cell layer (*Figure 10.27*). On fluorescein angiography, the RPE has a small leak, through which fluorescein passes into the subretinal space beneath the

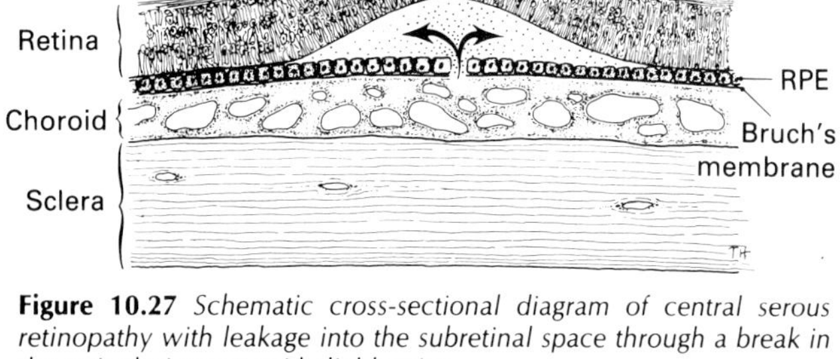

Figure 10.27 *Schematic cross-sectional diagram of central serous retinopathy with leakage into the subretinal space through a break in the retinal pigment epithelial barrier*

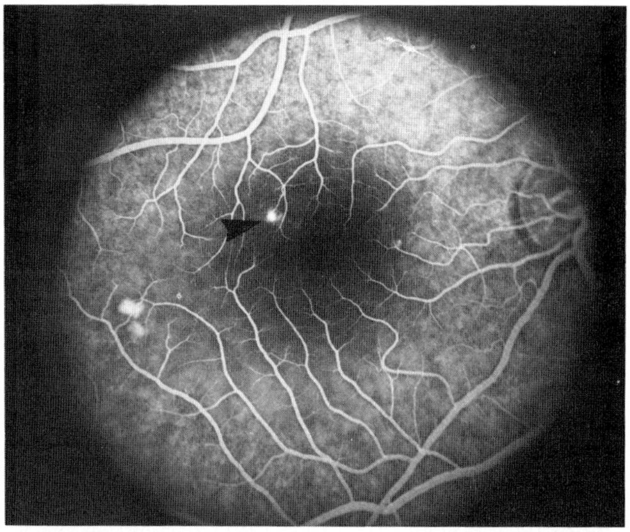

a

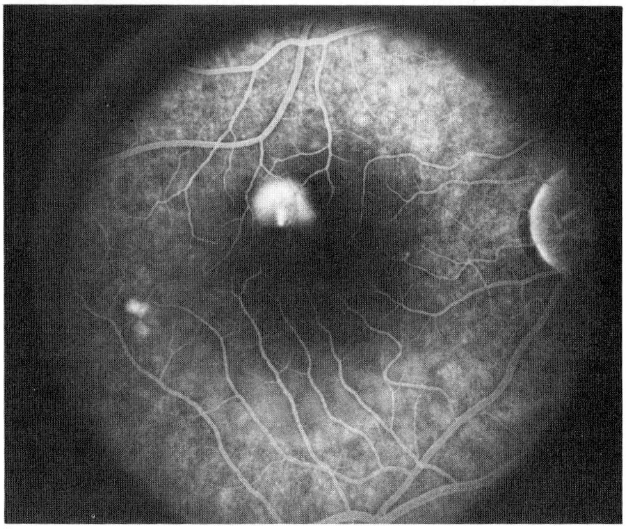

b

Figure 10.28 *Fluorescein angiography showing central serous retinopathy.* **(a)** *Focal hyperfluorescent leak is visible (arrow).* **(b)** *Leakage spreads into the subsensory retinal space in the later phase of the angiogram*

area of sensory retinal elevation (*Figure 10.28*). Sometimes more than one leak is present, and occasionally there are several separate areas of sensory retinal elevation in one or both eyes. The leaks often seal spontaneously, and the retina flattens over several weeks with nearly complete recovery of vision[52]. Sometimes the leak does not close spontaneously. If the serous elevation persists and a fluorescein angiogram shows, after 6 weeks, that the leak is still present, laser photocoagulation can be used to seal the leak. Occasionally, treatment can be applied earlier if there is need for rapid recovery of full visual acuity.

One laser burn applied to each RPE leak is usually enough to close the leak[53]. A mild-to-moderate intensity, 100 μm to 500 μm burn of 0.1 second duration is applied to the leaking site after it has been located by fluorescein angiography (*Figure 10.29*). Occasionally, central serous retinopathy recurs and may require retreatment of a new leak.

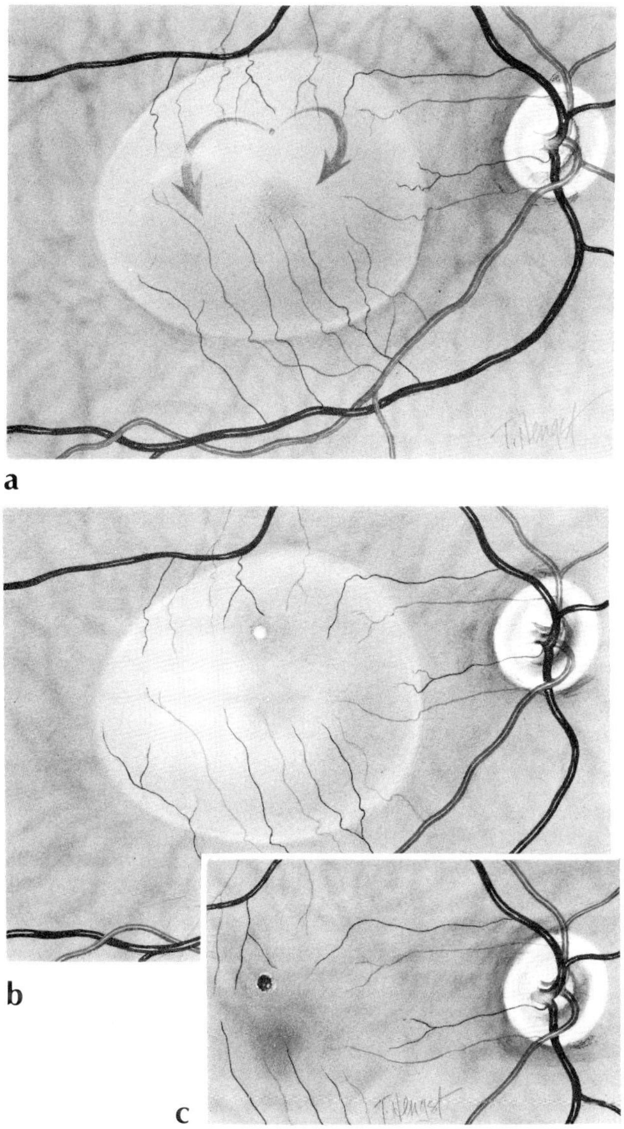

Figure 10.29 *Laser treatment of central serous retinopathy.* **(a)** *Sensory retina elevated, with one focal leak present superior to the fovea.* **(b)** *Laser treatment to focal leak.* **(c)** *Resolution of central serous retinopathy after laser treatment*

Exudative retinal detachment

Exudative retinal detachment can occur: (*1*) as an idiopathic condition; (*2*) associated with systemic disease such as eclampsia of pregnancy of Vogt-Koyanaga-Harada disease; (*3*) with other ocular conditions such as posterior scleritis, uveal effusion syndrome or choroidal detachment; (*4*) with retinal vascular leakage such as in retinal telangiectasia; (*5*) with extensive disciform macular scars; and (*6*) with choroidal tumors such as malignant melanoma, choroidal nevi and choroidal hemangiomas.

Fluorescein angiography can show the location and amount of choroidal leakage. In conditions such as Vogt-Koyanaga-Harada disease and eclampsia of pregnancy, there may be many leaks from the choroid, and laser treatment is not feasible. If leakage is from a more localized area such as a choroidal or retinal tumor, laser treatment can be considered, and this is discussed in Chapter 11. Occasionally, eyes with idiopathic exudative retinal detachment have only one or two leaks from the choroid. These are often large areas of leakage of one or more disc diameters in size, and often they are located in the periphery. It may be necessary to perform fluorescein angioscopy to locate these peripheral leaks.

Laser photocoagulation of such leaks often seals them. The retina then reattaches during several months as the subretinal fluid slowly absorbs. Treatment is applied as moderate-intensity, confluent 500 μm burns to the choroidal leaks. Because the subretinal fluid often shifts in eyes with exudative retinal detachment, it may be possible to tilt the patient's head in such a way as to flatten the retina at the site of leakage and make laser treatment easier. Otherwise, treatment can be applied to the choroid through the detached retina if the subretinal fluid is clear.

Photocoagulation treatment of choroidal neovascularization

Choroidal (subretinal) neovascularization occurs more often from senile macular degeneration (SMD) and the presumed ocular histoplasmosis syndrome (POHS) than from other conditions. It can also occur with angioid streaks, high myopia, choroidal rupture, as an idiopathic condition, and in still other diseases with choroidal or retinal scarring. The pathogenesis is probably related to a break in Bruch's membrane through which choroidal vessels grow into the sub-RPE or subretinal space.

The cause of the break in Bruch's membrane in SMD and idiopathic choroidal neovascularization is unknown. In eyes with angioid streaks occurring in pseudoxanthoma elasticum, the break in Bruch's membrane is a result of a defect in the elastic tissue component of the membrane. Eyes with choroidal rupture have a traumatic break in Bruch's membrane, and a similar break presumably results from stretching of the coats of the eye in high myopia. Scars from many conditions including histoplasmosis presumably cause a focal weakness or defect in Bruch's membrane through which choroidal neovascularization grows.

The abnormal choroidal neovascularization can leak fluid or exudate, and thus elevate the RPE and/or sensory retina (*Figure 10.30a*). Involvement of the macula results in decreased vision and metamorphopsia. Choroidal neovascularization can bleed into the sub-RPE or subsensory retinal space (*Figure 10.30b*). Scarring can eventually occur and create a subretinal fibrovascular disciform scar in the macula, with permanent reduction of vision (*Figure 10.30c*).

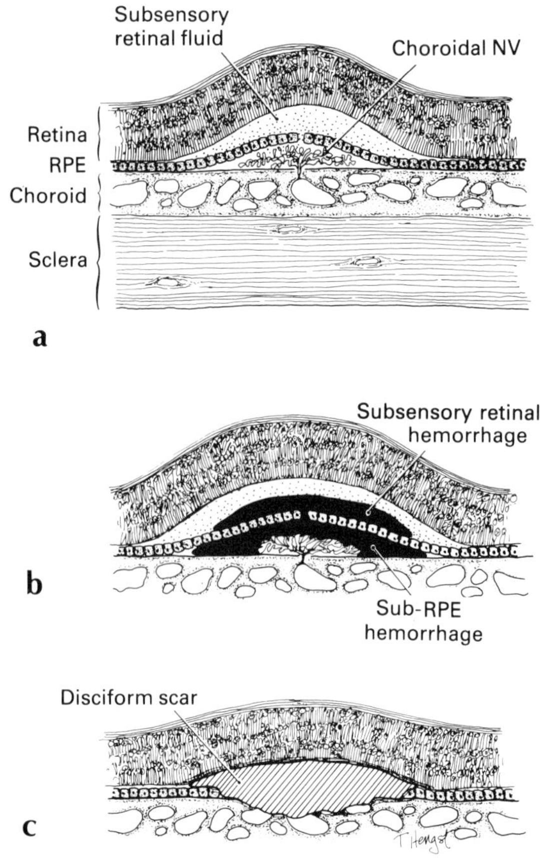

Figure 10.30 *Schematic cross-sectional diagram of exudative senile macular degeneration.* **(a)** *Choroidal neovascularization (NV) causes elevation of the retinal pigment epithelium and the sensory retina.* **(b)** *Hemorrhage from choroidal neovascularization is present in the sub-RPE and the subsensory retinal spaces.* **(c)** *Disciform scar involving the retina and choroid after choroidal neovascularization*

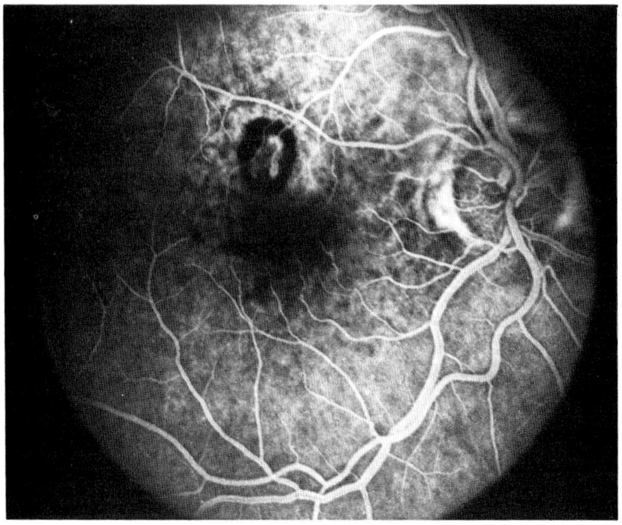

Figure 10.31 *Fluorescein angiogram shows choroidal neovascularization in senile macular degeneration as a hyperfluorescent patch in the superior macula. Surrounding hypofluorescent ring is from sub-RPE blood*

Photocoagulation treatment of senile macular degeneration

In elderly patients SMD is a leading cause of blindness. Patients with SMD and choroidal neovascularization have decreased vision and metamorphopsia if the macula is involved. Fundus biomicroscopy shows elevation of the RPE, elevation of the sensory retina, or both. There may be a visible gray-green area deep to the retina indicating choroidal neovascularization. Subretinal hemorrhage or exudate is virtually pathognomonic of choroidal neovascularization in eyes with drusen and other signs of SMD.

If choroidal neovascularization is suspected, fluorescein angiography is performed. Choroidal neovascularization is manifested as a very hyperfluorescent patch or net of vessels that is visible in the early phase of the angiogram and that leaks profusely in later phases (*Figure 10.31*). The neovascularization may be as small as 50 μm in diameter or larger than one disc diameter in size. It is important to obtain multiple rapid-sequence frames in the angiogram to show not only the choroidal neovascularization but also the position of the overlying retinal perifoveal capillary net. The position of the foveola is at the center of the foveal avascular zone inside the perifoveal capillary net.

Indications for photocoagulation

The indications for treatment of choroidal neovascularization in SMD have recently been more fully defined from results of a randomized clinical trial, the Macular Photocoagulation Study[54]. This study found photocoagulation treatment beneficial for choroidal neovascular membranes located 200–2500 μm from the center of the foveal avascular zone, if the visual acuity was 20/100 or better in the eye. Treatment of choroidal neovascularization closer than 200 μm from the center of the foveal avascular zone has not been shown to be beneficial. Krypton laser photocoagulation can be considered for lesions closer than 200 μm from the center of the foveal avascular because the krypton red wavelength is not absorbed by the intraretinal xanthophyll pigment in the macula and therefore is less damaging to the retina. Krypton laser photocoagulation can be considered as an alternative to argon laser photocoagulation for all types of choroidal neovascularization[55], and its use in treating choroidal neovascularization closer than 200 μm from the center of the fovea is currently being evaluated in the Macular Photocoagulation Study.

Lesions more distant from the fovea, such as peripapillary lesions, probably need not be treated unless elevation of the sensory retina extends into the fovea or the lesion grows further toward the fovea. Choroidal neovascularization with part or all of its margins obscured by hemorrhage is not treated unless it is certain that the neovascularization does not extend closer to the fovea than the recommended safe distance for treatment. Serous detachments of retinal pigment epithelium in SMD are not treated. Although treatment may flatten the RPE detachments, the results of treatment appear to be no better than those of non-treatment[56–60]. Also, such lesions may harbor occult choroidal neovascularization, and partial treatment can stimulate rapid growth of the neovascularization, causing more extensive damage.

Technique of treatment

Argon laser photocoagulation of choroidal neovascularization in SMD is done to obliterate the choroidal neovascularization. Heavy treatment is necessary but this can also damage central vision. Damage to the macula can occur from several causes. Macular xanthophyll pigment and hemoglobin in retinal vessels absorb blue-green argon laser energy, and this directly damages the sensory retina in the treated area. There is also often a lateral 'spreading' or conduction of heat, so that damage extends beyond the area of the laser burn. Treatment is done to allow for this spreading effect, so that the center of the macula is not damaged. When the sensory retina receives an argon laser burn, it becomes white and opaque, and it partially or completely blocks penetration of further burns to the underlying choroidal neovascularization. Therefore it is important to apply heavy burns initially because retreatment of the same area is less likely to penetrate to the choroidal neovascularization.

Photocoagulation should extend 100–125 μm beyond the margin of the choroidal neovascularization, to increase the chance of completely destroying the neovascularization. If blood, pigment or another opacity obscures the margin of the neovascularization, these opacities are treated as if choroidal neovascularization is beneath them, and the treatment should extend 125 μm beyond the margin of the opacity.

Treatment requires retrobulbar anesthesia to paralyze extraocular movements so that there is no eye movement during the long-duration burns. A fluorescein angiogram frame that shows both the choroidal neovascularization and the perifoveal capillary net is projected to show landmarks that are used as a guide to precise placement of the laser burns. The first row of laser burns is applied on the foveal side, extending 100–125 μm beyond the margin of the neovascularization (*Figure 10.32*). If the neovascularization is near the fovea, 200 μm burns of 0.5 or 0.2 second duration are used. For choroidal neovascularization even closer to the fovea, between 200 μm and 350 μm from the center of the foveal avascular zone, 100 μm burns of 0.2 second are used. If the choroidal neovascularization is more distant from the fovea, 500 μm burns of 0.5 second can be used for the row closest to the fovea. The remainder of the choroidal neovascularization is treated with confluent, heavy 500 μm burns of 0.5 second extending 100–125 μm beyond the margin of the choroidal neovascularization.

Follow-up examinations are directed toward detecting recurrence of choroidal neovascularization. The eye should be evaluated 2–3 weeks after treatment, and fluorescein angiography is performed if recurrence is suspected. Recurrences are treated using the same indications and techniques as for fresh choroidal neovascularization. If recurrent choroidal neovascularization extends beneath the fovea, retreatment is not done.

Krypton laser photocoagulation can be used instead of the argon laser to treat choroidal neovascularization from SMD[55,61,62]. The red light of the krypton laser has potential advantages over that of the blue-green argon laser. There is little absorption of red wavelength energy by intraretinal xanthophyll in the macula and little damage to retinal vessels because it is not absorbed by blood. Also, because it is not absorbed by blood, the krypton laser may more easily penetrate blood overlying choroidal neovascularization and allow more effective treatment in such cases. Because of its poor absorption by blood, however, there is a greater chance of causing choroidal hemorrhage with treatment and more difficulty in stopping bleeding if it occurs. The advantages of krypton laser probably outweigh the disadvantages in treating eyes with choroidal neovascularization near the center of the fovea.

Krypton laser photocoagulation can sometimes be used to treat safely choroidal neovascularization that comes almost to the center of the foveal avascular zone. On the foveal side of the choroidal neovascularization, moderately heavy 200 μm burns of 0.2 second duration are used to minimize spreading of the burns. The rest of the lesion is treated with confluent 500 μm burns of 0.5 second, extending 100–125 μm beyond the margin of the neovascularization. If the choroidal neovascularization is closer to the fovea than 100–125 μm, a smaller margin of treatment is used on the foveal side so that treatment does not extend through the center of the fovea.

The power setting on the krypton laser is set to produce whitening equivalent to a medium-intensity argon laser burn. Burns produced with the krypton laser are not as white as those of equal intensity produced with the argon laser because the overlying retina does not absorb much of the energy and does not turn white. Krypton laser burns that are very white are of excessive strength and may produce complications such as choroidal hemorrhage or choroidal vascular occlusion. Because the overlying retina does not whiten and thus does not block retreatment of the same area, it is possible to apply additional krypton laser treatment to the same site.

Recurrences of choroidal neovascularization are treated using the same principles as for the original krypton

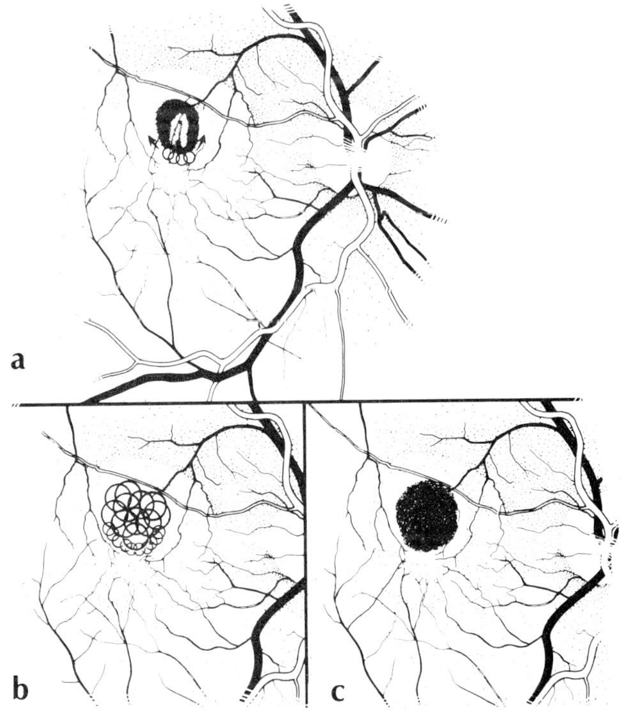

Figure 10.32 *Laser treatment of choroidal neovascularization superior to the fovea in senile macular degeneration.* **(a)** *The border nearest the fovea is treated with 200 μm burns, and* **(b)** *the remainder is treated with 500 μm burns, extending 125 μm beyond the neovascularization.* **(c)** *Choroidal neovascularization obliterated, with residual scar*

treatment. Follow-up examinations of krypton laser treated eyes are done 1–2 weeks after treatment. Fluorescein angiography is routinely performed at this time, and because there is little whitening and opacity of the overlying retina, any recurrent neovascularization is usually visible on the angiogram. This differs from argon laser photocoagulation, in which the whitened retina interferes for several weeks with visualization on repeat angiography.

Results

As mentioned earlier, the results of a randomized clinical trial, the Macular Photocoagulation Study, demonstrate the efficacy of laser treatment for choroidal neovascularization in SMD[54]. Eyes with symptomatic choroidal neovascular membranes at least 200 μm from the center of the foveal avascular zone, with vision of 20/100 or better, were treated with blue-green argon laser photocoagulation. For eyes with 6 months or more follow-up, twice as many of the treated eyes maintained their initial visual acuity or showed improvement; and three times as many untreated eyes experienced a six-line drop in visual acuity (equal to a fourfold increase in the subtended visual angle). After 18 months of follow-up, 60 per cent of untreated eyes versus 25 per cent of treated eyes experienced severe visual loss. Results of the study were highly significant statistically ($P < .001$). At the end of 1 year of follow-up, 73 per cent of untreated eyes versus 35 per cent of treated eyes had an active choroidal neovascular membrane extending under the foveal avascular zone. Furthermore, a natural history study of untreated eyes with SMD and choroidal neovascularization near the fovea showed a poor prognosis for eyes without treatment[63].

A controlled clinical trial has not yet been completed testing the efficacy of krypton red laser treatment for choroidal neovascularization in SMD. The Macular Photocoagulation Study will address this issue also. Until the study results are available, it seems reasonable to consider krypton laser photocoagulation to treat eyes with choroidal neovascularization that is closer than 200 μm to the fovea but not under the center of the fovea.

Eyes with serous or hemorrhagic detachments of the RPE, and eyes with disciform lesions in the fovea do not benefit from photocoagulation treatment. In some cases, it can stimulate further growth of choroidal neovascularization. Photocoagulation treatment of serous detachments of the RPE may also result in atrophy of the RPE itself and damage to central vision. As mentioned, there also appears to be no benefit from photocoagulation to serous RPE detachments in the elderly[59,60].

Photocoagulation treatment of the presumed ocular histoplasmosis syndrome

The presumed ocular histoplasmosis syndrome (POHS) is a frequent cause of loss of vision in the United States. Patients affected may have some or all of the following fundus findings: (*1*) peripheral chorioretinal scars; (*2*) peripapillary atrophy; (*3*) atrophic scars in the macula; and (*4*) choroidal neovascularization in the macula. Patients are presumably infected with ocular histoplasmosis at an earlier age without visual symptoms. Some eyes develop asymptomatic chorioretinal scars, and from some of these scars later choroidal neovascularization develops. Argon laser or krypton laser photocoagulation treatment can be used to treat choroidal neovascularization in the POHS.

The indications and technique for treatment of perifoveal choroidal neovascularization are the same as described for senile macular degeneration. Asymptomatic peripapillary lesions can be followed-up without treatment. However, treatment is applied to the peripapillary choroidal neovascularization if neovascularization extends from the optic nerve toward the fovea, if leakage elevates the sensory retina in the macula, or if choroidal neovascularization comes within one-quarter disc diameter of the fovea (*Figure 10.33*)[64].

Several studies have indicated that photocoagulation treatment in POHS is beneficial[65–68]. However, as yet there has been no controlled clinical trial demonstrating the efficacy of treatment, although it is currently being evaluated in the Macular Photocoagulation Study. Untreated choroidal neovascularization in the POHS does not have as poor a prognosis as it does in SMD[69], and so the potential benefits of treatment are not as clear-cut.*

* Since this chapter was written, the Macular Photocoagulation Study has found a beneficial treatment effect for argon laser photocoagulation of choroidal neovascularization 200–2500 μm from the center of the fovea for the POHS (Macular Photocoagulation Study Group, Argon laser photocoagulation for ocular histoplasmosis: Results of a randomized clinical trial. Archives of Ophthalmology 1983;101:1347)

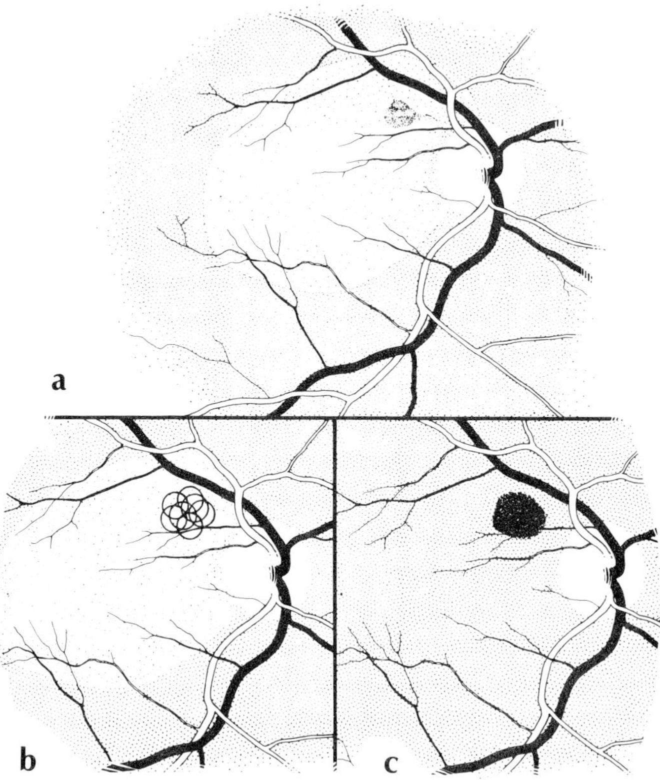

Figure 10.33 *Laser treatment of peripapillary choroidal neovascularization in ocular histoplasmosis.* **(a)** *Peripapillary choroidal neovascularization with an overlying sensory retinal elevation involving the fovea.* **(b)** *Confluent 500 μm burns applied to choroidal neovascularization, extending 125 μm past the neovascular margin.* **(c)** *Scar at site of destroyed choroidal neovascularization, with resolution of the sensory retinal elevation*

Photocoagulation treatment of choroidal neovascularization with angioid streaks

Eyes with angioid streaks have a propensity to develop choroidal neovascularization and macular damage. Angioid streaks may occur in pseudoxanthoma elasticum and less frequently in Paget's disease, sickle-cell hemoglobinopathy, Ehlers-Danlos syndrome, senile elastosis and other conditions. Breaks in Bruch's membrane occur, and choroidal neovascularization may grow through these breaks, causing overlying serous and/or hemorrhagic detachment of the retina with decreased vision. Disciform scars may eventually develop. In pseudoxanthoma elasticum and Paget's disease there is an abnormal calcification of the elastic component of Bruch's membrane, and this probably predisposes to cracks in this membrane. In other conditions, such as sickle-cell disease, iron is deposited in Bruch's membrane, and this may also lead to breaks in the membrane and to angioid streaks.

Prophylactic treatment of angioid streaks is not indicated and may stimulate choroidal neovascular membrane formation[70]. Choroidal neovascularization in the macula can be treated using the guidelines given above for SMD. Results of treatment seem encouraging in some patients[71,72]. The long-term prognosis for such eyes must be considered guarded because of the progressive nature of the disease and the chance of developing additional choroidal neovascularization.

Photocoagulation treatment for other causes of choroidal neovascularization

Choroidal neovascularization may occur in conditions such as high myopia and choroidal rupture, in other conditions that produce chorioretinal scarring, or it can be idiopathic occurring in eyes with no other apparent abnormality. Indications for laser treatment in these conditions are the same as for SMD. Asymptomatic, non-progressive peripapillary lesions probably need not be treated. The results of treatment depend on the location of the choroidal neovascularization and the presence of coexisting damage from the underlying disease.*

Photocoagulation of retinal holes and localized retinal detachments

Laser treatment causes chorioretinal scarring and an adhesion between the treated choroid and retina. Laser treatment can be used to create a chorioretinal adhesion around retinal breaks to reduce the chance of the lesion progressing to a rhegmatogenous retinal detachment. Laser treatment can also be used to cause an adhesion around a localized rhegmatogenous detachment to prevent progression, rather than performing retinal reattachment surgery. The photocoagulation-induced adhesion does not have much strength for the first 5–7 days, and it does not reach full strength for several weeks.

* Since this chapter was written, the Macular Photocoagulation Study has found a probable beneficial treatment effect for argon laser photocoagulation of idiopathic choroidal neovascularization (Macular Photocoagulation Study Group, Argon laser photocoagulation for idiopathic neovascularization: Results of a randomized clinical trial. Archives of Ophthalmology 1983;101:1358)

Indications for photocoagulation

Asymptomatic retinal holes in emmetropic, phakic eyes have a low risk of progressing to rhegmatogenous retinal detachment, probably less than 1 per cent[73,74]. Symptomatic retinal breaks, associated with subjective light flashes or 'floaters', have about a one-third chance of progressing to rhegmatogenous retinal detachment[73,74]. Such high-risk breaks should have photocoagulation treatment to lessen the chance of retinal detachment. Alternatively cryotherapy can be used (*see* Chapter 9). Certain asymptomatic retinal breaks that have a high risk of progressing to retinal detachment can also be treated and these include: (*1*) large tears; (*2*) retinal breaks in highly myopic eyes; (*3*) retinal breaks in aphakic eyes; (*4*) retinal breaks in phakic eyes that are to have cataract surgery; and (*5*) breaks in the fellow eye of a patient who has had retinal detachment in the other eye. Eyes with stable, localized retinal detachment less than one clock-hour in size can also be treated with laser photocoagulation. If the detachment is larger, a retinal reattachment operation should be performed instead. Fellow eyes with lattice degeneration unassociated with retinal breaks, in which the other eye has had a retinal detachment, also possibly should have laser treatment around the lattice degeneration[75].

Technique of treatment

Argon laser burns of a 500 μm size of 0.1 or 0.2 second duration are placed in two or three rows around the retinal hole or localized retinal detachment. Treatment should be of moderate intensity. Treatment is applied to surround a flat retinal break up to the margins of the break (*Figure 10.34*). If a localized retinal detachment is present,

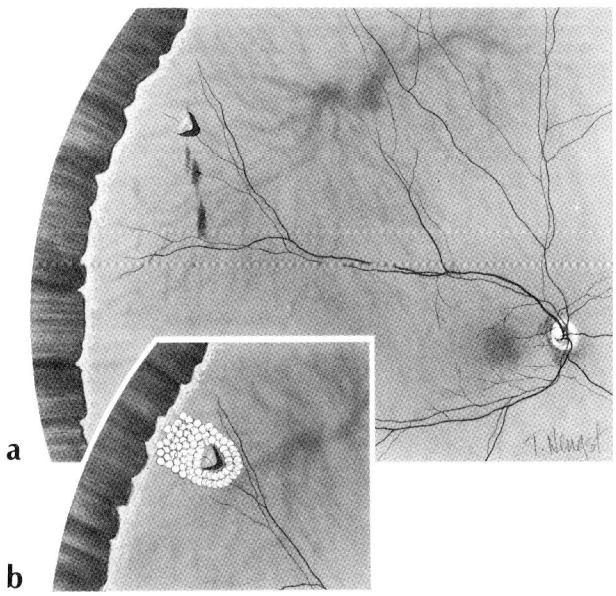

Figure 10.34 *Laser treatment around symptomatic horseshoe retinal break.* **(a)** *Peripheral horseshoe retinal break visible, with no retinal detachment and with small amount of vitreous hemorrhage inferior to the break.* **(b)** *Two rows of confluent 500 μm laser burns placed around the break, with additional treatment extending toward the ora serrata*

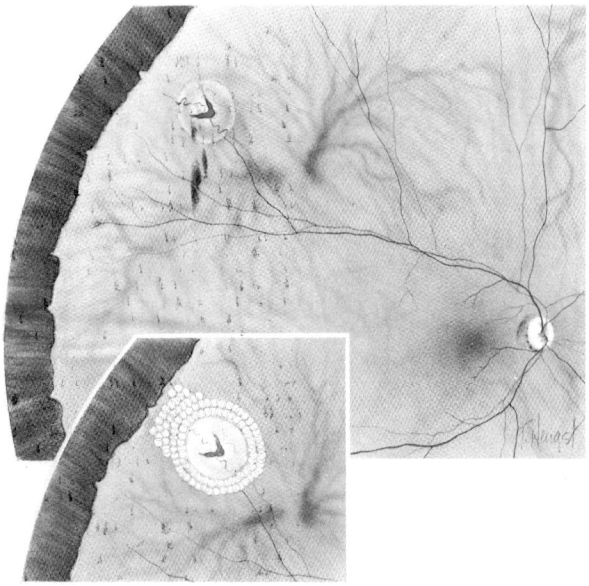

Figure 10.35 *Laser treatment around retinal break with localized retinal detachment.* **(a)** *Horseshoe retinal break with localized detachment and torn retinal vessel with small amount of vitreous hemorrhage.* **(b)** *Two rows of confluent 500 μm laser burns placed around localized detachment, with additional burns placed anteriorly, up to the ora serrata*

treatment of the same type is applied to attached retina up to the margin of the detachment (*Figure 10.35*). In eyes with clear media and with retinal breaks in the equatorial retina, treatment is easily done. If the breaks are nearer the ora serrata, and especially if there are opacities in the ocular media, treatment is more easily done with cryopexy (see Chapter 9). If the media are clear and the breaks are near the ora serrata, treatment can be done with laser photocoagulation by using simultaneous scleral indentation with a thimble scleral depressor or by using a special depressor cone that fits over a three-mirror fundus contact lens (*Figure 10.36*).

Lattice degeneration can be treated, if indicated, by surrounding the lattice degeneration area by two or three rows of burns. If there is a break at the edge of the lattice degeneration, both the break and the area of lattice degeneration can be surrounded (*Figure 10.37*).

Patients are usually not hospitalized after such treatment. They are seen on an outpatient basis at 7–10 days after treatment and again several weeks later, to be certain that there is a good chorioretinal adhesion at the treatment site and that there has been no progression to rhegmatogenous retinal detachment.

Results

Laser treatment is almost always successful in sealing retinal holes so that they do not progress to rhegmatogenous retinal detachment. If a detachment occurs in a treated eye, it is usually from development of a new retinal hole. Treatment around a localized retinal detachment also is usually successful, although occasionally the detachment spreads through the laser treatment.

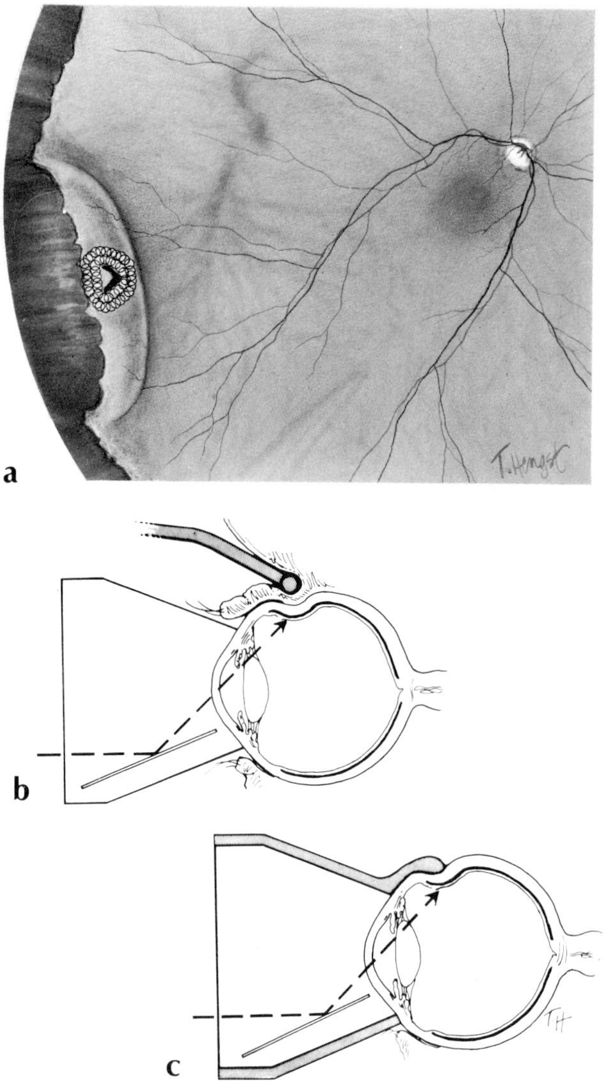

Figure 10.36 *Laser treatment to far peripheral retinal break, using scleral depression for visualization.* **(a)** *Retinal break just posterior to ora serrata. Scleral depression is used, and laser treatment is applied around the break.* **(b)** *Scleral depression and simultaneous laser treatment, using thimble-type scleral depressor.* **(c)** *Laser treatment, using simultaneous scleral depression with depressor cone over three-mirror fundus contact lens*

Photocoagulation treatment in special cases of retinal detachment

Laser treatment is occasionally used to treat selected retinal breaks in conjunction with retinal reattachment surgery and/or vitreous surgery. In eyes with macular holes and retinal detachment, vitreous surgery is often used to relieve vitreoretinal traction and to allow the injection of an intravitreal gas bubble. Postoperative face-down positioning flattens the detachment. This alone, with no treatment of the macular hole, may cure the detachment. Some detachments recur, and it is necessary to treat around the macular hole to form a chorioretinal adhesion. This is more likely to be necessary in an

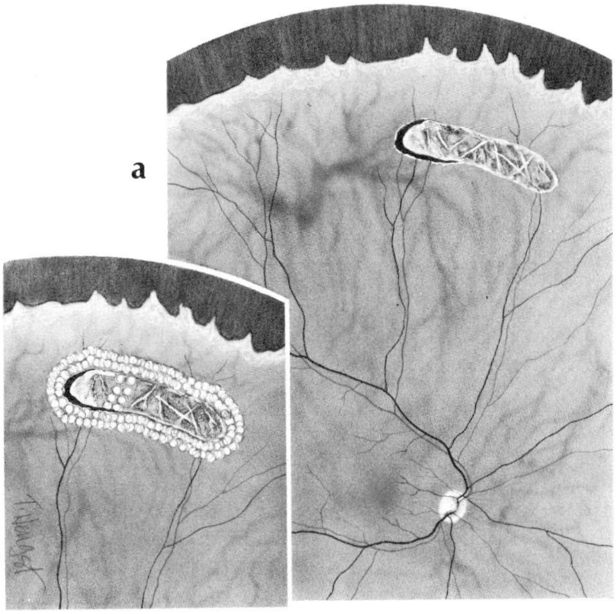

a

b

Figure 10.37 *Laser treatment around lattice degeneration with a retinal break.* **(a)** *Lattice degeneration with a break at one edge.* **(b)** *Two rows of 500 μm laser burns surrounding lattice degeneration, with additional burns surrounding the retinal break*

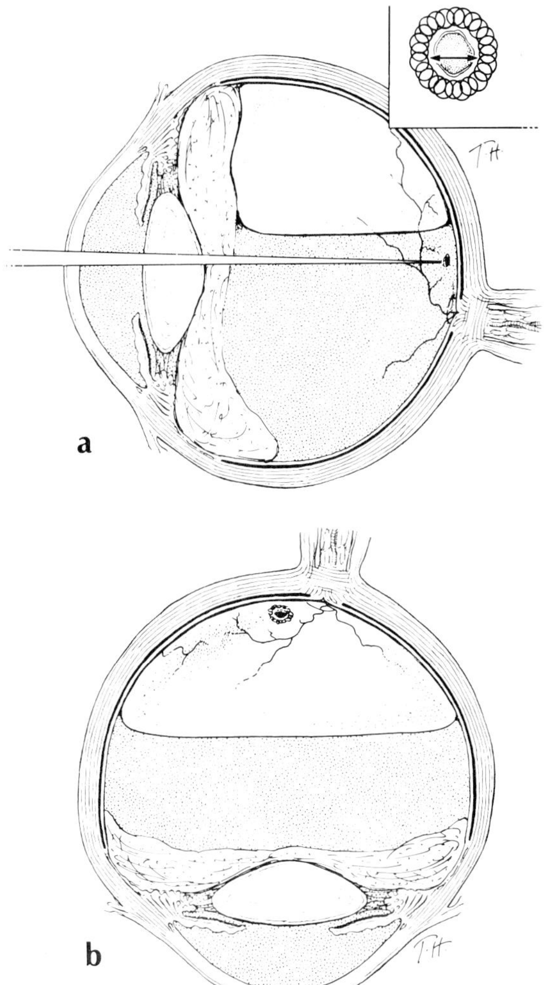

a

b

Figure 10.38 *Laser treatment around a macular hole after vitrectomy.* **(a)** *Retinal detachment caused by macular hole becomes reattached after vitrectomy and placement of an intraocular air bubble. Laser burns of 50 μm spot size are applied around the hole beneath the air bubble.* **(b)** *After laser treatment, patient is positioned face-down to continue to keep the macular hole flat against the choroid*

elongated, myopic eye or in an eye with residual vitreoretinal traction, such as a diabetic eye with a macular hole.

If the detachment recurs after vitrectomy, fluid-air exchange is performed to flatten the macular hole. After the air bubble decreases to less than 50 per cent of the volume of the vitreous cavity, and when the macular hole can be seen with a fundus contact lens beneath the air bubble, laser treatment is applied. One row of 50 μm argon laser burns is applied around the macular hole (*Figure 10.38a*). The patient is again positioned face-down so that the air bubble will keep the macular hole flat until a chorioretinal adhesion forms (*Figure 10.38b*). This type of treatment can be used after vitrectomy, without waiting to see whether redetachment occurs.

An alternative method is to treat the detached macular hole before vitrectomy. Small 50 μm argon blue-green laser burns are applied to the detached retina. The intraretinal xanthophyll in the macula absorbs laser energy, causing a retinal burn and whitening around the macular hole. Energy also penetrates to the underlying choroid. After photocoagulation, a vitrectomy is performed, with placement of an intravitreal air bubble and postoperative face-down positioning. This flattens the retina and the macular hole, allowing reattachment. The advantages of laser treatment around a macular hole are that less extensive damage occurs to the macula than if cryotherapy or other treatment is applied. If intravitreal traction is present that cannot be relieved by vitrectomy, or if the eye is markedly elongated by myopia with marked atrophy of the choroid and RPE, these types of treatment may fail unless posterior scleral buckling is also used.

Laser treatment can be used in other eyes to increase the chance of successful retinal reattachment. Some eyes that have conventional reattachment surgery, with or without vitreous surgery, do not develop an adequate chorioretinal adhesion around a retinal hole, as evidenced by only slight pigmentary change in the underlying choroid. This problem most frequently occurs when cryotherapy only lightly treats the choroid, and the elevated retina is not frozen. Eyes with giant retinal tears treated by vitrectomy in combination with scleral buckling often have an inadequate chorioretinal adhesion. The margin of the giant tears can be treated postoperatively with photocoagulation to increase the strength of the chorioretinal adhesion (*Figure 10.39*). Argon laser photocoagulation of moderate intensity is used, applying 500 μm burns. If it is necessary to treat through an intravitreal air bubble, this can be done in aphakic eyes with a Goldmann lens, and in phakic eyes using a Rodenstock lens.

Occasionally after retinal reattachment surgery a retinal hole remains elevated over a properly positioned scleral buckle, with or without residual detachment posterior to the buckle. Argon laser photocoagulation applied around the hole often results in flattening of the hole and absorption of residual subretinal fluid without the need for

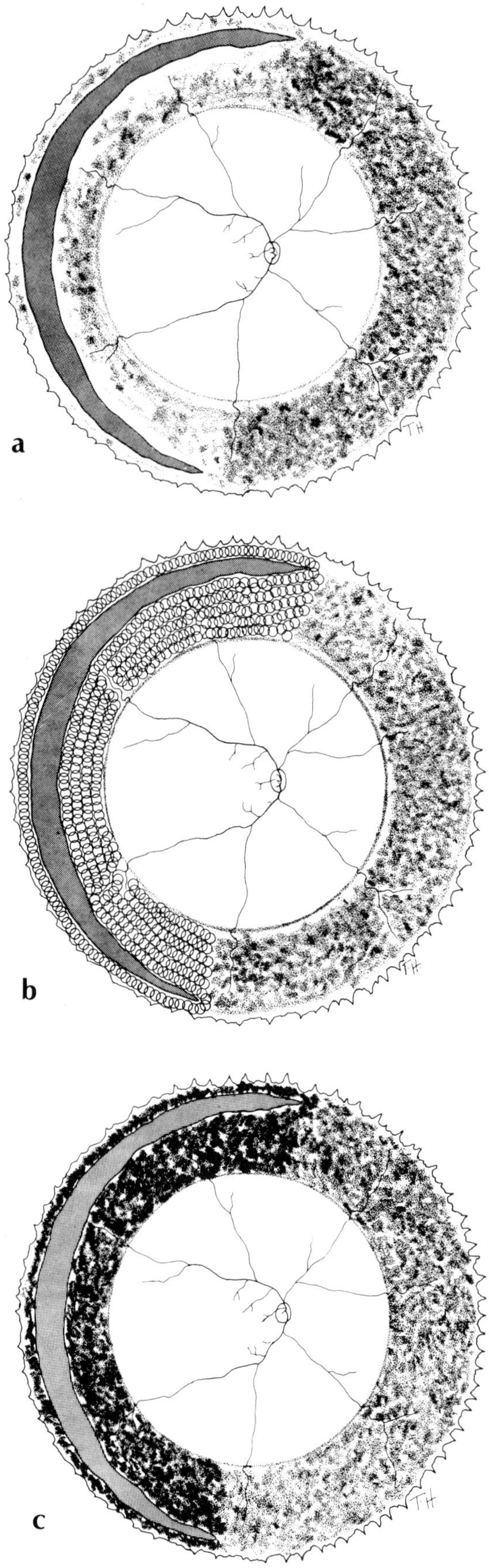

Figure 10.39 *Laser treatment to cause additional chorioretinal adhesion around a giant retinal tear supported on the encircling buckle.* **(a)** *Giant retinal break is flat on buckle, but with poor chorioretinal scarring around break.* **(b)** *Confluent 500 μm laser burns applied around retinal break.* **(c)** *Increased pigmentary change around break, indicating strong chorioretinal adhesion*

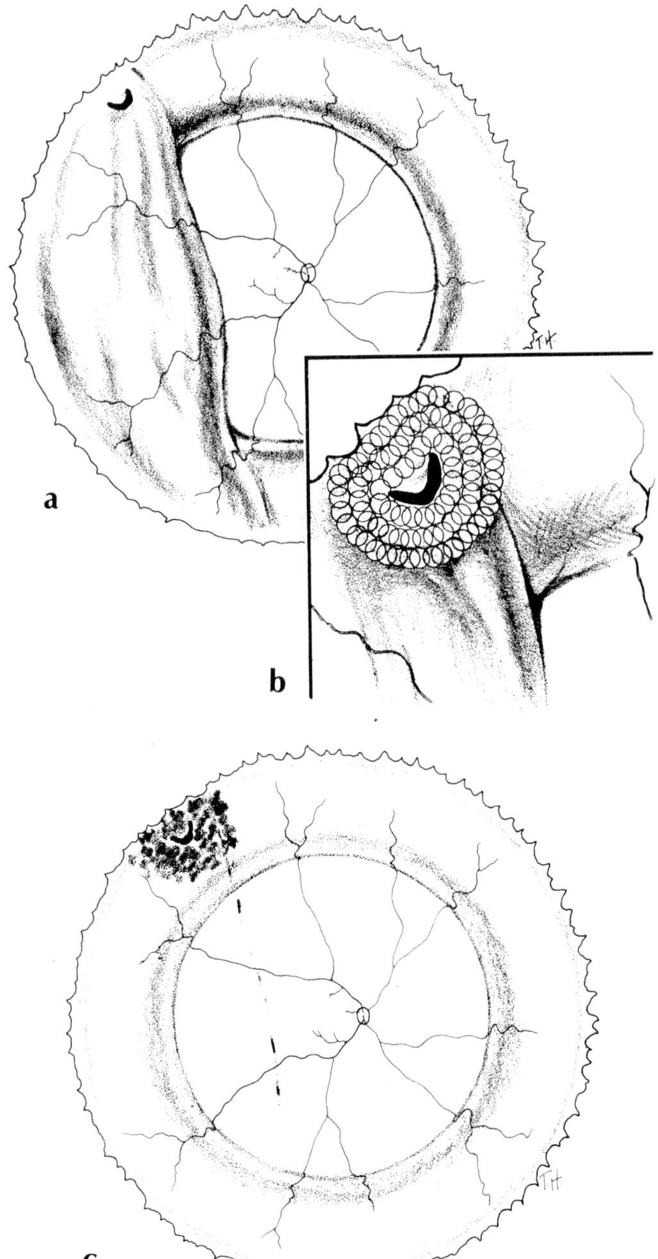

Figure 10.40 *Laser treatment around an elevated retinal hole over a buckle, to seal the hole.* **(a)** *Elevated retinal hole over a scleral buckle with persistent retinal detachment.* **(b)** *Laser burns of a 500 μm spot size applied around shallowly elevated retinal break on the buckle; the break communicates with retinal detachment posterior to the buckle.* **(c)** *After laser treatment, retinal break is flattened and the retinal detachment has resolved*

further surgery (*Figure 10.40*)[76]. This type of treatment possibly causes choroidal swelling that supplements the height of the buckle and seals the hole. Retrobulbar anesthesia is usually required because this treatment must be heavy and is often painful. Laser burns of 500 μm size of 0.2 or 0.5 second duration are applied to the retina and choroid over the buckle in the area of the hole and detachment. The retina turns white where it is flat on the choroid and may even show some whitening where it is shallowly detached. In areas where there is greater retinal elevation, no whitening occurs, and very high power should not be used to try to achieve whitening. Often the retinal hole will flatten on the buckle within a few days after treatment. However, it may take longer for residual subretinal fluid to absorb. The treatment has the best chance of success in eyes in which the hole is only shallowly elevated from the choroid.

Photocoagulation treatment of retinoschisis

Laser treatment has been used in eyes with retinoschisis: (*1*) to block and 'wall-off' retinoschisis that is progressing posteriorly; (*2*) to collapse a retinoschisis cavity; (*3*) to treat flat outer-layer retinal holes; and (*4*) as a test to differentiate retinoschisis from retinal detachment. Laser treatment is seldom needed for any of these reasons. Retinoschisis usually remains localized to the peripheral retina and does not progressively extend posteriorly. If definite signs of progression are present, with potential involvement of the macula, laser treatment can be applied posterior to the retinoschisis to form a chorioretinal adhesion in an effort to prevent the retina from splitting further posteriorly[77]. Some eyes that have this treatment, however, have extension of the schisis through the chorioretinal scar, and occasionally they develop multiple posterior retinal holes in the treated area.

Treatment of the flat outer retinal layer in an attempt to collapse the schisis is probably contraindicated, at least in juvenile retinoschisis. Inner and outer layer holes with retinal detachment can occur as a result of treatment[78]. Treatment of flat outer layer holes, if inner layer retinal holes are also present, is sometimes done because the combination of inner and outer layer holes can lead to rhegmatogenous detachment. Most eyes with only outer layer holes never develop retinal detachment. Therefore treatment of such eyes is probably not indicated.

Laser photocoagulation can be used to differentiate retinoschisis from rhegmatogenous retinal detachment[79]. This is rarely necessary because ophthalmoscopic features usually allow differentiation. Sometimes a shallow chronic retinal detachment with no obvious retinal holes has the appearance of retinoschisis. A laser burn can be used to determine whether schisis is present. A burn is applied in attached retina to select a setting that produces a mild or moderate burn. If the same intensity burn applied to the area of retinal elevation produces a whitening at the level of the RPE, this indicates that an outer layer of retina lies against the retinal pigment epithelium and that the elevation is probably retinoschisis (*Figure 10.41a*)[80]. If no whitening occurs, then the elevation is a retinal detachment (*Figure 10.41b*).

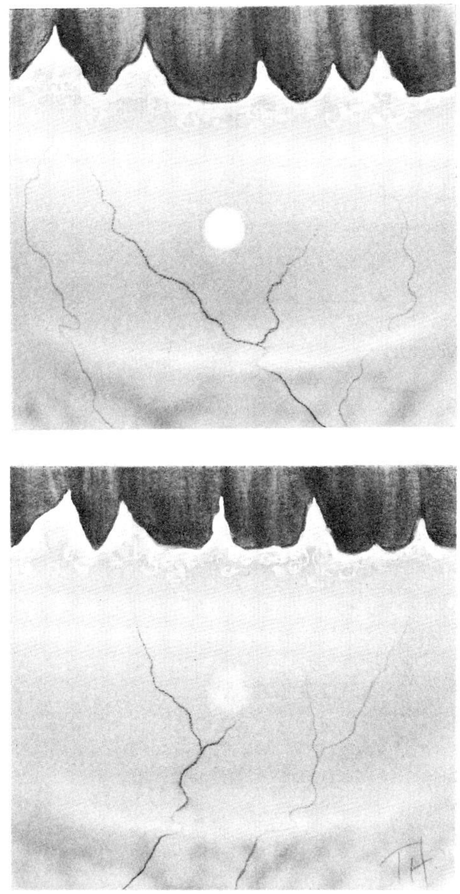

a

b

Figure 10.41 *Laser treatment used to differentiate retinoschisis from retinal detachment.* **(a)** *Laser treatment to retinoschisis produces white burn in attached outer retinal layer.* **(b)** *Same laser treatment to retinal detachment produces minimal or no whitening*

Photocoagulation treatment of the iris and anterior chamber angle

Photocoagulation is used in the treatment of a variety of iris conditions: (*1*) to treat angle-closure glaucoma; (*2*) to treat iris and anterior chamber angle neovascularization; (*3*) to produce photomydriasis; and (*4*) to outline an area of epithelial ingrowth on the iris. Laser iridotomy is discussed in Chapter 7, and laser treatment of epithelial ingrowth on the iris is described in Chapter 8.

Iris neovascularization sometimes occurs in eyes with a retinal vascular disease such as central retinal vein occlusion or diabetic retinopathy, or in carotid occlusive disease with ocular ischemia[30]. It is frequent in diabetic eyes that have had vitrectomy and lens removal[81]. Treatment is unnecessary in eyes with mild, stable iris neovascularization and no anterior chamber angle involvement. If there is progressive iris neovascularization, and especially if anterior chamber angle neovascularization is present, treatment is advisable to prevent progression to neovascular glaucoma.

Iris neovascularization is probably the result of anterior diffusion of a 'vasoproliferative factor' from the damaged retina. Presumably, scatter retinal photocoagulation decreases production of the 'vasoproliferative factor'. Laser treatment is applied in the same way as for treatment of proliferative diabetic retinopathy. If 'complete' retinal scatter treatment can be applied before three-quarters of the anterior chamber angle is closed by peripheral anterior synechiae, neovascular glaucoma usually can be prevented, or the increased pressure can be controlled with antiglaucoma medications[82,83]. Even if the anterior chamber angle has become more extensively closed, so that medically uncontrollable neovascular glaucoma is present, laser treatment may make the neovascularization regress even though the peripheral anterior synechiae persist. Thereafter, filtering surgery may have a better chance of success. Unfortunately, once neovascular glaucoma occurs, scatter retinal photocoagulation often is not possible because of corneal edema due to increased intraocular pressure.

Direct laser photocoagulation to neovascularization in the anterior chamber angle (goniophotocoagulation) has also been used to control this condition[84]. Scatter retinal photocoagulation is more effective, but goniophotocoagulation may be useful in eyes with a clear cornea in which lens or vitreous opacities prevent scatter retinal photocoagulation. Laser burns of a 50 μm or 100 μm size of 0.2 second duration are applied to vessels on the trabecular meshwork to close them. Retreatment may be necessary.

In some eyes with an inadequate or eccentric pupil, laser treatment to the iris can dilate or alter the position of the pupil by causing tissue shrinkage[85]. To dilate a pupil by photomydriasis, one or two rows of 200 μm or 500 μm burns of 0.2 or 0.5 second duration are applied to the iris stroma surrounding the pupil, just inside the pupillary margin. A contact lens may or may not be used. If posterior synechiae are not present, the treatment often dilates the pupil. Treatment can also be used to enlarge an eccentric pupil so that it is located more centrally. Burns are applied to the iris stroma on the side of the pupil where shrinkage is desired.

Ocular care after photocoagulation

It is usually unnecessary to use topical medications after photocoagulation. An eye that has had a retrobulbar anesthetic injection should be patched for 6–12 hours to protect the eye from exposure. Usually there is no pain after mild photocoagulation. In eyes that have more extensive treatment, such as scatter photocoagulation, there may be moderate pain lasting from a few hours to a day or longer. Often mild analgesics such as aspirin or acetaminophen relieve this pain, but occasionally codeine or other narcotics are needed. Aspirin probably should not be used by patients who have active retinal or choroidal neovascularization because aspirin's anticoagulant effect might increase the severity of any hemorrhage. Patients who have severe pain after retinal photocoagulation should be re-examined to be certain they do not have choroidal effusion and angle-closure glaucoma.

Patients who have photocoagulation for retinal or choroidal neovascularization are told not to engage in strenuous physical exertion until subsequent examination shows that the neovascularization has been eliminated or stabilized. Patients who have photocoagulation for other reasons, such as for diabetic macular edema, may resume normal activities immediately.

Complications and side effects of photocoagulation

There are many potential complications and side effects of photocoagulation treatment. Some occur because of incorrect treatment, but others can occur despite proper application of photocoagulation. Some types of treatment are frequently accompanied by side effects or complications. Every attempt should be made to reduce complications by the use of proper technique. In all cases, and especially when side effects are likely to occur despite correct treatment, the patient is told of these effects before treatment.

Complications will be discussed for: (*1*) scatter and focal photocoagulation of proliferative retinopathy; (*2*) vascular feeder-frond photocoagulation of sickle-cell retinopathy; (*3*) focal photocoagulation for macular edema; (*4*) photocoagulation of choroidal neovascularization.

The most frequent proliferative retinopathy treated is proliferative diabetic retinopathy, and the complications that occur in treating this condition are similar to those encountered in scatter retinal photocoagulation of other proliferative retinopathies.

Complications and adverse effects of photocoagulation for proliferative diabetic retinopathy

Peripheral visual field loss

Complications and adverse effects after scatter photocoagulation treatment for proliferative diabetic retinopathy are frequent, but severe complications are rare. The Diabetic Retinopathy Study (DRS) found that the most frequent harmful effect was impairment of the peripheral visual field in eyes treated with xenon photocoagulation. Twenty-five per cent of xenon-treated eyes suffered a modest loss of visual field and an additional 25 per cent had more severe loss[86]. Argon laser treated eyes showed only small visual field losses. Other studies have shown, however, that peripheral visual field loss in argon laser treated eyes is common when sensitive testing methods are chosen[87]. Eyes that require supplemental photocoagulation and that eventually have nearly confluent peripheral chorioretinal scarring, have an even more severe loss of peripheral visual field.

Loss of peripheral field can be minimized by using argon laser photocoagulation instead of xenon photocoagulation, and by avoiding unnecessarily extensive and heavy treatment. In general, however, it is wise to sacrifice the peripheral visual field, if necessary, to obtain regression of retinal neovascularization.

Decreased visual acuity

It is common for eyes to have a transient decrease in visual acuity for several weeks after scatter photocoagulation, presumably from worsening of diabetic macular edema. In most cases the vision returns to the pretreatment level. However, a minority of eyes have a permanent reduction in visual acuity. The DRS estimated that persistent decreases of one to four lines in visual acuity occurred in about 10 per cent of argon-treated eyes and 20 per cent of xenon-treated eyes, and about 2 per cent of xenon-treated eyes had a persistent decrease of five or more lines attributable to treatment[86]. The transient decrease in visual acuity can be lessened by applying photocoagulation in divided sessions, preferably a week or more apart, instead of in one treatment session. If the eye has severe proliferative disease, however, it is best to risk the complication of visual acuity reduction and complete the treatment within 1 or 2 weeks.

Pain

Pain during and after scatter retinal photocoagulation is common. Sensory nerves in the suprachoroidal space are directly affected by photocoagulation burns. The amount of pain from argon laser photocoagulation varies from patient to patient. Some patients feel no pain. Others can tolerate the pain, especially the discomfort associated with the less painful posterior burns. Still others have severe pain with both posterior and anterior burns.

The amount of pain felt during treatment can be reduced by limiting the number of burns applied during each session and by using burns of 0.1 second duration. Burns of longer duration, such as those lasting 0.2 second or 0.5 second are more painful. It is better to use a retrobulbar anesthetic injection rather than to apply inadequate photocoagulation. For example, if a patient has moderate optic nervehead neovascularization and can tolerate only 100 burns in each treatment session, it is best to use a retrobulbar anesthetic so that treatment can be completed sooner. A retrobulbar injection, however, can also result in complications such as penetration of the globe by the needle, retrobulbar hemorrhage or central retinal artery occlusion[88]. Also, when the anesthetic effect wears off, the eye is often painful for a day or longer because of extensive treatment.

Other side effects

There are other, less severe effects of scatter photocoagulation. Some patients note decreased color vision, especially in the perception of blue[89]. Some patients also complain of poorer night vision and poorer dark adaptation[90], and they are easily dazzled by bright light.

Exudative retinal detachment

Exudative retinal detachments can occur after scatter photocoagulation (*Figure 10.42*). They can be localized or extensive and can extend into the macula and cause marked reduction in vision. Localized detachment can occur at the site where peripheral retinal neovascularization is treated with heavy, confluent burns. More extensive detachments usually result from widespread, heavy scatter photocoagulation. The detachments spontaneously resolve in 1 or 2 weeks; and the central vision, if affected, usually recovers. These detachments presumably result from damage to choroidal vessels that cause exudation of fluid which passes through the damaged RPE barrier into the subretinal space[91].

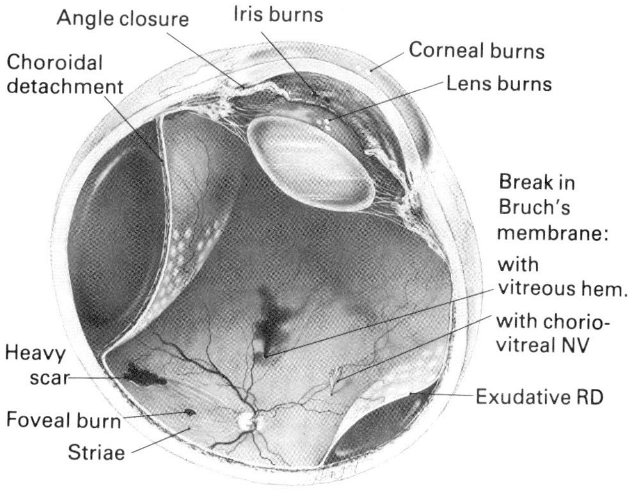

Figure 10.42 *Schematic diagram showing complications that can occur after scatter argon laser photocoagulation*

Choroidal detachment and secondary glaucoma

Choroidal detachments are frequent after extensive photocoagulation. Severe choroidal detachment may cause secondary angle-closure glaucoma due to forward rotation of the ciliary body and the lens-iris diaphragm (see *Figure 10.42*). In one series of eyes that received the entire pattern of scatter photocoagulation in one session, 92 per cent of argon-treated eyes and 100 per cent of xenon-treated eyes developed choroidal detachments[92]. In these cases, transient secondary glaucoma occurred in 15 per cent of argon-treated eyes and 29 per cent of xenon-treated eyes. Some eyes required medical treatment for the glaucoma, and the glaucoma resolved with time.

If a choroidal detachment develops after scatter photocoagulation, usually no treatment is necessary, and the detachment usually resolves spontaneously within 2 weeks. If there is extensive choroidal detachment, additional scatter photocoagulation should not be applied, because it could produce more severe detachment and possible anterior chamber angle closure. Not all anterior chamber angle closure results in glaucoma presumably because the choroidal detachment often reduces aqueous production; but if secondary glaucoma develops, medical therapy with oral acetazolamide, and topical therapy with epinephrine (adrenaline), timolol and possibly pilocarpine are used to control the intraocular pressure until the choroidal detachment resolves and the anterior chamber angle reopens. Extensive choroidal detachments and angle-closure glaucoma are uncommon if photocoagulation is applied in divided sessions a week or more apart. Because of this, and because pain is more severe when complete scatter photocoagulation is applied in a single session, most eyes are treated with at least two sessions. As mentioned, xenon photocoagulation is more likely to produce choroidal detachments than is argon laser photocoagulation, and this may be an additional reason to use laser treatment. Krypton laser scatter photocoagulation also appears more likely to cause choroidal detachments than argon laser treatment[93].

Anterior segment complications

Other anterior segment complications can occur in addition to secondary angle-closure glaucoma (*see Figure 10.42*). Iris burns can produce iris atrophy or posterior synechiae. Corneal burns may occur with very high-power settings, small spot sizes, and long-duration burns. These corneal burns usually clear with time. Burns to the lens capsule can occur under similar circumstances, and these burns do not enlarge to produce a visually significant cataract. Internal ophthalmoplegia after scatter photocoagulation is a frequent complication, resulting from damage to parasympathetic motor fibers in the suprachoroidal space[94].

Breaks in Bruch's membrane, vitreous hemorrhage, and choriovitreal neovascularization

Breaks in Bruch's membrane can occur when retinal photocoagulation is done, and can produce a choroidal or vitreous hemorrhage (*see Figure 10.42*). Usually bleeding is self-limited, but it can usually be immediately stopped by pushing on the eye with the contact lens to increase the intraocular pressure. Then, 500 μm burns of 0.2 or 0.5 second duration with moderately intense power are applied to the bleeding site.

Choriovitreal neovascularization occasionally grows through breaks in Bruch's membrane (*see Figure 10.42*). This is recognized as neovascularization growing into the vitreous cavity from a laser scar where retinal neovascularization had not been present before. The diagnosis is confirmed by rapid-sequence fluorescein angiography that shows the neovascularization filling from the choroidal circulation before the retinal arterioles contain fluorescein dye.

Choriovitreal neovascularization can sometimes be eliminated by heavy focal photocoagulation. However, it is often resistant to any type of treatment, and treatment may result in vitreous hemorrhage. Sometimes choriovitreal neovascularization leads to intractable vitreous hemorrhage; but in a report of 10 diabetic patients with this neovascular complication, only 1 had a vitreous hemorrhage[95]. Because of the risks and difficulties in treating choriovitreal neovascularization, treatment is probably not indicated.

Breaks in Bruch's membrane resulting from photocoagulation treatment can usually be avoided by not using small-size spot burns at short durations and high powers, which tend to 'puncture' Bruch's membrane. Breaks can occur even with 500 μm spot size, however, when excessive power is used. Breaks in Bruch's membrane can also occur when heavy focal treatment is applied, such as: (*1*) when treating to stop blood flow in flat or elevated retinal neovascularization; (*2*) when switching from the posterior portion of the three-mirror contact lens to a mirror without reducing the power setting; or (*3*) when using high power to treat through lens or vitreous opacities and failing to reduce the power when treating a less obscured area. Usually a heavier burn can be anticipated if the reflected light from the aiming beam becomes noticeably brighter. When this is seen, the power setting should be reduced before applying a burn.

Vitreous hemorrhage can occur when applying focal photocoagulation to retinal neovascularization. This complication, along with thermal papillitis and nerve fiber layer visual field defects, was frequent when focal treatment was applied to disc neovascularization[96]. Because of these complications, and because scatter photocoagulation alone seems effective in treating optic nervehead neovascularization, focal treatment of disc neovascularization is no longer recommended. Focal photocoagulation of highly elevated peripheral neovascularization is also dangerous because it may result in vitreous hemorrhage or breaks in Bruch's membrane. Confluent treatment to areas of flat peripheral neovascularization, when combined with scatter photocoagulation, seems more effective than scatter photocoagulation alone, and the combined method rarely results in complications because less power is needed. If bleeding does occur, pressure is applied to the eye with the contact lens to increase the intraocular pressure and heavy 500 μm burns of 0.2 second or 0.5 second are applied to the neovascular bleeding site, just as in treating bleeding from a break in Bruch's membrane.

Accidental treatment of the fovea

A feared complication of scatter photocoagulation is accidental treatment of the fovea. This can occur in a variety of ways. Most commonly it happens when treating through the most posteriorly directed mirror of the three-mirror contact lens. If the eye, contact lens and laser beam are all aligned in a straight-ahead position, the fovea cannot be treated through the mirror. If, however, the eye is markedly rotated toward the posteriorly directed mirror, especially when the mirror is in a nasal position, it is possible to treat the fovea accidentally (*Figure 10.43*).

Accidental treatment of the fovea can be avoided, when using the three-mirror lens, by carefully monitoring the position of the eye. More important, at least one row of photocoagulation burns should be applied temporal to the macula directly through the posterior part of the three-mirror contact lens before applying treatment through a mirror (*Figure 10.44*). This row serves as a marker, so that accidental treatment will not be applied more posteriorly through the mirror.

An alternative method of avoiding a foveal burn is to use a Rodenstock lens instead of a three-mirror contact lens. The Rodenstock contact lens optically acts in a manner similar to an indirect ophthalmoscope when used with a

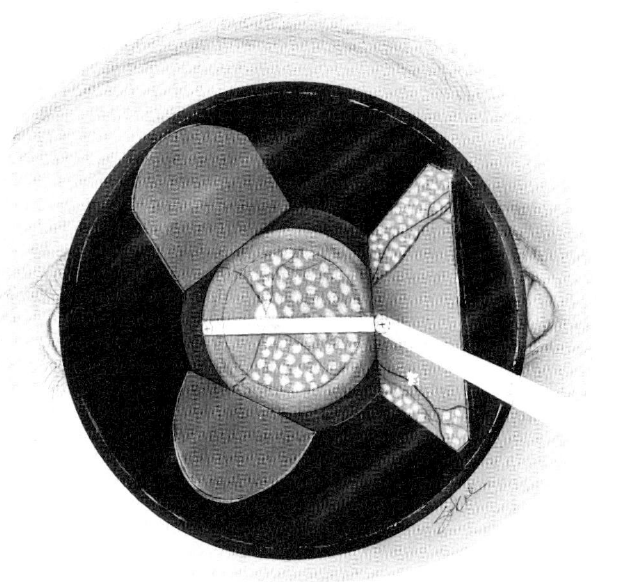

Figure 10.43 *Accidental treatment of the fovea of the right eye when using the most posteriorly directed mirror of the three-mirror contact lens. The eye is rotated nasally toward the mirror*

slit-lamp viewing system. Because of the wide-angle view, it is possible easily to recognize and keep the macula in sight while treating the midperipheral fundus, and there is therefore less chance of treating the fovea accidentally.

The fovea, or the retina near the fovea, can also be treated accidentally when applying the first row of laser burns temporal to the macula directly through the contact lens. This is most likely to occur in a patient who has uncontrolled eye movements. Anything that interferes with the operator's normal clear view, such as opacities in the media or a small pupil, can also increase the chance of accidently damaging the fovea. To be safe, the position

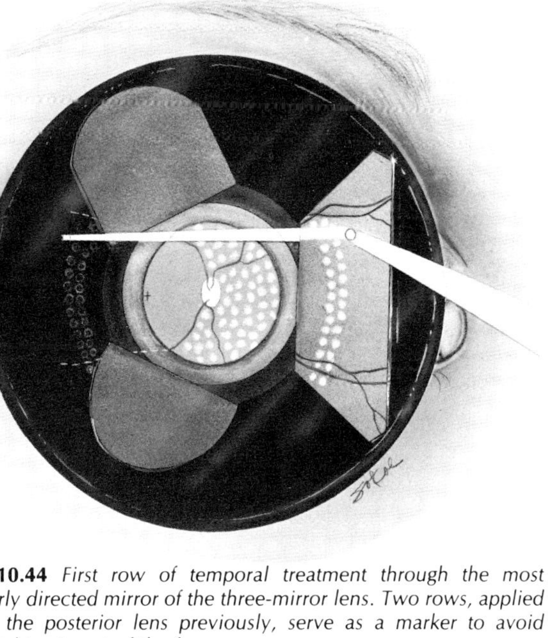

Figure 10.44 *First row of temporal treatment through the most posteriorly directed mirror of the three-mirror lens. Two rows, applied through the posterior lens previously, serve as a marker to avoid accidental treatment of the fovea*

where the row of burns is to be applied should be checked to be certain that the row is approximately two disc-diameters temporal to the fovea. The first burn should not be placed directly temporal to the fovea, because if there is eye movement or if the wrong area was selected, it may hit the fovea (*Figure 10.45*). Instead, it should be placed inferotemporal or superotemporal to

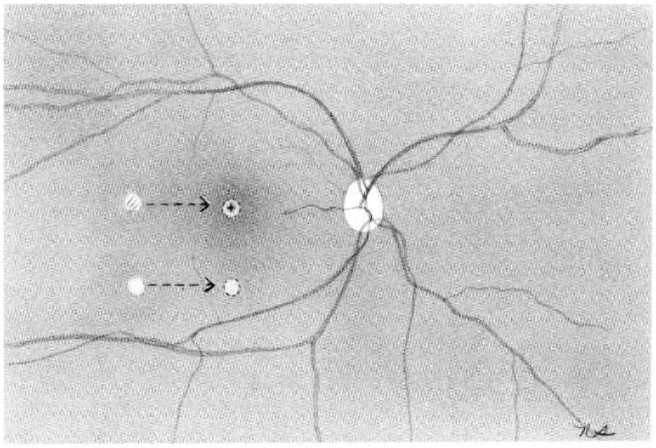

Figure 10.45 *First burn temporal to the macula in scatter photocoagulation should not be applied directly temporal to the fovea (upper arrow) because if it is more nasally placed than intended, it may hit the fovea. Instead the first burn should be applied inferotemporal (lower arrow) or superotemporal to the fovea so that if it is more nasally located than expected, it will miss the fovea*

the macula. The position of this first spot can be checked (with indirect ophthalmoscopy if necessary) and the rest of the row can be safely completed using the first spot as a marker.

The fovea can also be accidentally treated if the physician momentarily forgets which eye is being treated and believes the photocoagulation is being applied to the nasal retina when, instead, the temporal retina is being treated. Occasionally when treatment is being applied through a mirror, the patient or the slit lamp move slightly to the side. Unrecognized movement may cause the laser beam to pass through the center part of the lens rather than onto the mirror, and the fovea may be accidentally treated.

If laser burns are applied to the macula, the central visual acuity will ordinarily not be affected unless the center of the fovea is damaged. Even then, the eye may recover some vision with time. One report cites intentional laser treatment of the fovea in a patient with a malignant melanoma of the choroid in which the eye was to be removed. This eye with foveal damage recovered 20/30 vision the next day[97]. If a severe burn or multiple burns are applied to the center of the fovea, the visual acuity will be severely and permanently affected. Striae through the macula may occur if heavy focal photocoagulation is applied near the fovea. This may produce distortion of central vision but usually only a mild decrease in visual acuity.

Most of the severe complications from scatter photocoagulation can be avoided. Some complications, such as peripheral visual field reduction or decreased visual acuity, occur in a considerable number of patients, and the possibility of these side effects must be accepted if photocoagulation treatment is used.

Complications of vascular feeder-frond photocoagulation treatment of sickle-cell retinopathy

Feeder-frond photocoagulation treatment of sickle-cell retinopathy has a high risk of complications, and we prefer peripheral scatter photocoagulation. If, however, peripheral scatter treatment is ineffective, feeder-frond treatment may be necessary. The main complications are choriovitreal neovascularization[98], retinal holes and detachment[99], vitreous hemorrhage[33], and choroidal ischemia[100].

Choriovitreal neovascularization

Choriovitreal neovascularization can result from a break in Bruch's membrane produced by an excessively heavy burn. Because burns used in direct treatment of sickle-cell peripheral neovascularization are heavy, there is less margin for error than in less heavy treatment used in other conditions. The chance of breaking Bruch's membrane can be lessened by using larger (500 μm), longer duration burns to close the feeding arteriole. If treatment is applied over an area of choroidal pigmentation, the intensity of the burn used should be reduced, because more absorption of energy can be expected from the pigment.

Not all breaks in Bruch's membrane result in choriovitreal neovascularization, but such neovascularization has been reported in up to 19 per cent of treated cases[98]. Chorioretinal neovascularization that does not cause vitreous hemorrhage probably should not be treated because treatment itself can produce vitreous hemorrhage or stimulate further neovascular growth. If the neovascularization continues to grow or results in vitreous hemorrhage, confluent and heavy 500 μm burns of longer duration can be applied. However, this treatment is unsuccessful in most cases.

Retinal holes and detachment

Retinal holes occur in about 9 per cent of eyes with sickle-cell retinopathy when it is treated by the feeder-frond photocoagulation technique[99]. This is probably a result of heavy burns that cause holes in the thin retina and the process may be aggravated by vitreous traction on adjacent peripheral neovascularization. The chance of causing a retinal hole can be lessened by avoiding excessively heavy laser burns. If a hole develops, prophylactic laser treatment or cryopexy around it is used to reduce the chance of retinal detachment. Retinal detachment requires scleral buckling procedures, which are hazardous in patients with sickle-cell disease.

Vitreous hemorrhage

The risk of this complication can be reduced by avoiding excessively heavy burns. Severe persistent hemorrhage may require vitreous surgery.

Complications of focal photocoagulation of the macula

Photocoagulation treatment of retinal vascular leakage causing macular edema or RPE leaks in central serous retinopathy uses medium-power burns applied to the leakage sites. This treatment for macular edema is used most frequently in diabetic retinopathy, but it is also used to treat macular edema from branch retinal vein occlusion, macular telangectasia and other retinal vascular diseases. The complications encountered in treating these conditions are similar, and discussion is limited to complications encountered in treating diabetic macular edema.

Accidental treatment of the fovea

As compared to scatter photocoagulation, accidental treatment of the fovea while treating macular edema is less frequent because in this situation the fovea is usually easily seen and avoided. The fovea can be accidentally treated, however, if there is sudden and unexpected eye movement. This possibility is minimized by instructing the patient to avoid eye movement, and by steadying the eye with pressure on the contact lens. In uncooperative patients it may be necessary to use retrobulbar anesthesia to provide akinesia.

Occasionally the fovea can be accidentally treated if its position is misjudged because it is obscured by diffuse macular edema. In such cases, projection of a frame from the fluorescein angiogram is useful to identify the exact position of the center of the fovea in relation to retinal vessels. Identifying the fovea by asking the patient to fixate on the aiming beam is unreliable if there is massive macular edema, because a relative central scotoma and perifoveal fixation may occur with the edema.

The fovea can also be damaged by spread of energy from laser burns when treating nearby leaks. Spreading of a burn to a size larger than that of the aiming beam can result from several factors including: lateral conduction of energy in the treated tissue; and divergence of the laser beam by induced refractive changes caused by absorption of laser energy by a partially cataractous lens. Lateral conduction of energy can be minimized by using small spot sizes (50 μm or 100 μm), short duration burns (0.1 second) and the minimum power necessary to achieve an adequate burn. Burns should first be tested at a location away from the fovea to assess how much spreading is likely to occur when treating nearer the fovea. It should be remembered that increased spreading can be expected when treating near the fovea because of added absorption of energy by intraretinal xanthophyll. Divergence of the laser beam in a partially cataractous lens can be minimized by using short duration burns and small spot sizes.

To minimize the possibility of foveal damage, heavy burns should not be placed within 300 μm of the center of the fovea; and only under exceptional circumstances should burns be applied to leaks in the innermost capillaries of the perifoveal net. In addition, use of argon green laser photocoagulation, without the argon blue wavelengths, has theoretical advantages for treatment of microaneurysms near the fovea – a microaneurysm absorbs energy from the argon green wavelength but little is absorbed by the intraretinal xanthophyll. There is also less divergence of the beam when treating through nuclear sclerotic lenses with this wavelength.

Paracentral visual field defects

Extensive confluent areas of photocoagulation treatment in the macula may produce large paracentral scotomas, and this should be avoided. Extensive treatment in the papillomacular bundle can damage the nerve fiber layer and produce arcuate field defects affecting central vision. Nerve fiber layer damage is more likely if heavy treatment is applied to intraretinal hemorrhages. These hemorrhages absorb energy, and the inner layers of the retina are damaged. Heavy confluent treatment can also produce retinal striae and cause metamorphopsia or a decrease in visual acuity.

Other complications

Heavy focal burns for macular edema should be avoided, because such treatment can cause breaks in Bruch's membrane or hemorrhages. These complications are less likely to occur during treatment of macular edema as compared to scatter treatment. Subretinal neovascularization in the macula also has been reported as a complication of focal photocoagulation for diabetic macular edema[95].

Complications of photocoagulation treatment of choroidal neovascularization

Treatment of choroidal neovascularization requires heavy burns, usually applied near the fovea. Therefore the risk of adverse side effects and complications is high. The closer the treatment must be applied to the center of the fovea, the greater are the risks. One complication, recurrence of choroidal neovascularization, can be caused by too mild treatment; and others, such as choroidal hemorrhage, can be caused by treatment that is too heavy. In some situations, there is only a fine dividing line between avoiding one complication and producing another.

Recurrence of choroidal neovascularization

Recurrence of choroidal neovascularization can occur if treatment does not extend beyond the margins of the neovascularization, is too light, or does not penetrate blood that is covering part of the neovascularization. Heavy burns of at least 0.2 second, and preferably 0.5 second, duration should be used to ensure adequate treatment. To avoid recurrence as a result of not treating all of the choroidal neovascularization, treatment should extend 100–125 μm beyond the margin of the neovascularization. It may be necessary to treat blood that is covering and hiding a portion of the neovascularization, to ensure adequate treatment. If blood must be treated, then krypton laser photocoagulation may be preferable to penetrate the blood and reach the underlying choroidal neovascularization.

If choroidal neovascularization recurs, it is important to determine this as soon as possible so that retreatment may be given. The eye is examined frequently, especially if there is a high chance of recurrence, and the patient is given an Amsler grid to check for increased distortion or a paracentral scotoma, which may be early signs of recurrence. Fluorescein angiography is performed to detect suspected recurrence. Angiography within a few weeks after argon laser photocoagulation is difficult to interpret, however, because white retinal edema from treatment can block visualization of the underlying tissue and obscure recurrent neovascularization. Krypton laser photocoagulation produces less retinal edema, and angiography is more useful early than after argon laser treatment.

Additional photocoagulation can sometimes be used to obliterate a recurrence of choroidal neovascularization. Treatment is applied just as for new choroidal neovascularization. If the recurrence extends beneath the center of the foveal avascular zone, partial treatment, avoiding the center of the fovea, may eliminate the neovascularization if this closes the vessels feeding the neovascularization.

Foveal damage

If treatment of choroidal neovascularization is applied too close to the fovea, the effect may spread into the fovea. The damage, if mild, may be subtle and may become apparent only months later as RPE atrophy beneath the fovea. Because it is necessary to treat beyond the margin of choroidal neovascularization by at least 100 μm and because the blue component of argon blue-green energy is absorbed by intraretinal xanthophyll, this wavelength is not normally used for treatment of choroidal neovascularization closer than 200 μm to the center of the fovea. If treatment must be applied closer, use of the krypton laser should be considered. It is not yet known how close choroidal neovascularization can be to the center of the fovea and still be safely treated with the krypton laser. Some cases with choroidal neovascularization extending almost to the center of the fovea have been treated, with good recovery of visual acuity.

Paracentral visual field defects

A paracentral scotoma occurs at the site of treatment of choroidal neovascularization, and this is unavoidable. There may be less of a scotoma when using krypton rather than argon laser photocoagulation, because of less retinal damage.

Hemorrhage

Choroidal hemorrhage, which can even spread into the vitreous cavity, can result from the heavy treatment required for choroidal neovascularization. The chance of its occurrence can be lessened by using longer duration burns with a larger spot size, as described earlier. Also, argon laser photocoagulation, because it is absorbed by hemoglobin, probably results in choroidal hemorrhage less frequently than does krypton photocoagulation. If hemorrhage begins, pressure is exerted on the contact lens to raise the intraocular pressure and stop the bleeding. Then, 500 μm burns of 0.5 second duration with a higher power setting are used to treat over the hemorrhage and close the bleeding vessels.

Summary

Photocoagulation has revolutionized the management of many eye diseases. It has clearly lowered the risk of blindness from proliferative diabetic retinopathy and from choroidal neovascularization in senile macular degeneration. Many other conditions also seem to benefit from suitable photocoagulation. To maximize the chance of successful treatment, careful evaluation must be done. Only those cases that meet the proper indications are treated. Careful and properly selected treatment must be applied, and complications must be avoided or managed properly to increase the likelihood of success. If these practices are followed, photocoagulation can be used to prevent loss of vision or to recover vision in many eyes that would otherwise become blind.

References

1. Meyer-Schwickerath, G. Light coagulation, St Louis: The C. V. Mosby Co., 1960
2. Schlawlow, A. L., Townes, C. H. Infrared and optical lasers. Physiological Review 1958; 112:1940
3. Koester, C. J., Snitzer, E., Campbell, C. J., Rittler, M. C. Experimental laser retina coagulator. Journal of the Optical Society of America 1962; 52:607
4. Kapany, N. S., Peppers, N. A., Zweng, H. C., Flocks, M. Retinal photocoagulation by lasers. Nature 1963; 199:146–149
5. Zaret, M. M., Ripps, H., Siegel, I. M., Breinin, G. M. Laser photocoagulation of the eye. Archives of Ophthalmology 1963; 69:97–104
6. L'Esperance, F. A., Jr. An ophthalmic argon laser photocoagulation system: design, construction, and laboratory investigations. Transactions of the American Ophthalmological Society 1968; 66:827–904
7. Little, H. L., Zweng, H. C., Peabody, R. R. Argon laser slit-lamp retinal photocoagulator. Transactions of the American Academy of Ophthalmology and Otolaryngology 1970; 74:85–97
8. L'Esperance, F. A., Jr. The ocular histopathologic effect of krypton and argon laser radiation. American Journal of Ophthalmology 1969; 68:263–273
9. Yannuzzi, L. A., Shakin, J. L. Krypton red laser photocoagulation of the ocular fundus. Retina 1982; 2:1
10. Francois, J., Cambie, E. Retinal photocoagulation (xenon arc and lasers). Annals of Ophthalmology 1971; 3:1201
11. Wald, G. Human vision and the spectrum. Science 1945; 101:653–658
12. Marshall, J., Hamilton, A. M., Bird, A. C. Histopathology of ruby and argon laser lesions in monkey and human retina: A comparative study. British Journal of Ophthalmology 1975; 59:610–630
13. Marshall, J., Bird, A. C. A comparative histopathological study of argon and krypton laser irradiations of the human retina. British Journal of Ophthalmology 1979; 63:657–658
14. Arribas, N. P., Johnston, G. P., Okun, E. Photocoagulation in diabetic retinopathy. International Ophthalmology Clinics 1976; 16:59–77
15. The Diabetic Retinopathy Study Research Group: Photocoagulation treatment of proliferative diabetic retinopathy: Clinical application of Diabetic Retinopathy Study (DRS) findings, DRS report number 8. Ophthalmology 1981; 88:583–600
16. Glaser, B. M., D'Amore, P. A., Michels, R. G., Brunson, S. K., Fenselau, A. H., Rice, T., Patz, A. The demonstration of angiogenic activity from ocular tissues. Ophthalmology 1980; 87:440–446
17. Schanzlin, D. J., Jay, W. M., Fritz, K. J., Tripathi, R. C., Gonen, B.: Hemoglobin A_1 and diabetic retinopathy. American Journal of Ophthalmology 1979; 88:1032–1038
18. Little, H. L., Sacks, A., Vassiliadis, A., Greer, R. Current concepts of pathogenesis of diabetic retinopathy: A dysproteinemia. Transactions of the American Ophthalmological Society 1977; 75:397–426
19. Dobbie, J. G., Kwaan, H. C., Colwell, J., Suwanwela, N. Role of platelets in the pathogenesis of diabetic retinopathy. Archives of Ophthalmology 1974; 91:107–109
20. The Diabetic Retinopathy Study Research Group: Four risk factors for severe visual loss in diabetic retinopathy. The third report from The Diabetic Retinopathy Study. Archives of Ophthalmology 1979; 97:654–655
21. Yassur, Y., Pickle, L. W., Fine, S. L., Singerman, L., Orth, D. H., Patz, A.: Optic disc neovascularization in diabetic retinopathy: II. Natural history and results of photocoagulation treatment. British Journal of Ophthalmology 1980; 64:77–86
22. Green, W. R., Chan, C. C., Hutchins, G. M., Terry, J. M. Central retinal vein occlusion: A prospective histopathologic study of 29 eyes in 28 cases. Retina 1981; 1:27
23. Chan, C. C., Little, H. L. Infrequency of retinal neovascularization following central retinal vein occlusion. Ophthalmology 1979; 86:256–263
24. Magargal, L. E., Brown, G. C., Augsburger, J. J., Parrish, R. K. Neovascular glaucoma following central retinal vein obstruction. Ophthalmology 1981; 88:1095–1101
25. Laatikainen, L., Kohner, E. M., Khoury, D., Blach, R. K. Panretinal photocoagulation in central retinal vein occlusion: A randomised controlled clinical study. British Journal of Ophthalmology 1977; 61:741–753
26. Laatikainen, L. Preliminary report on effect of retinal panphotocoagulation on rubeosis iridis and neovascular glaucoma. British Journal of Ophthalmology 1977; 61:278–284
27. Blankenship, G. W., Okun, E. Retinal tributary vein occlusion: History and management by photocoagulation. Archives of Ophthalmology 1973; 89:363–368
28. Finkelstein, D., Clarkson, J., Diddie, K., Hillis, A., *et al.* Branch vein occlusion: retinal neovascularization outside the involved segment. Ophthalmology 1982; 89:1357–1361
29. Branch Vein Occlusion Study Group: Letter to the editor: Branch vein occlusion study. Investigative Ophthalmology and Visual Science 1979; 18:1097
30. Brown, G. C., Magargal, L. E., Simeone, F. A., Goldberg, R. E., Federman, J. L., Benson, W. E. Arterial obstruction and ocular neovascularization. Ophthalmology 1982; 89:139–146
31. Hanscom, T. A. Indirect treatment of peripheral retinal neovascularization. American Journal of Ophthalmology 1982; 93: 88–91
32. Rednam, K. R., Jampol, L. M., Goldberg, M. F. Scatter retinal photocoagulation for proliferative sickle cell retinopathy. American Journal of Ophthalmology 1982; 93:594–599
33. Goldberg, M. F., Acacio, I. Argon laser photocoagulation of proliferative sickle retinopathy. Archives of Ophthalmology 1973; 90:35–44
34. Goldbaum, M. H., Goldberg, M. F., Nagpal, K., Asdourian, G. K., Galinos, S. O. Proliferative sickle retinopathy. In L'Esperance, F. A., Jr, ed. Current diagnosis and management of chorioretinal diseases. St Louis: C. V. Mosby, 1977: 132–145
35. Condon, P. I., Serjeant, G. R. Photocoagulation in proliferative sickle retinopathy: Results of a 5-year study. British Journal of Ophthalmology 1980; 64:832–840
36. Pederson, J. E., Kenyon, K. R., Green, W. R., Maumenee, A. E. Pathology of pars planitis. American Journal of Ophthalmology 1978; 86:762–774

37. Wise, G. N. Retinal microaneurysms. Archives of Ophthalmology 1957; 57:151–156
38. Kearns, M., Hamilton, A. M., Kohner, E. M. Excessive permeability in diabetic maculopathy. British Journal of Ophthalmology 1979; 63:489–497
39. Peyman, G. A., Spitznas, M., Straatsma, B. R. Chorioretinal diffusion of peroxidase before and after photocoagulation. Investigative Ophthalmology 1971; 10:489–495
40. Patz, A., Schatz, H., Berkow, J. W., Gittelsohn, A. M., Ticho, U. Macular edema – an overlooked complication of diabetic retinopathy. Transactions of the American Academy of Ophthalmology and Otolaryngology 1973; 77:34–42
41. Blankenship, G. W. Diabetic macular edema and argon laser photocoagulation: A prospective randomized study. Ophthalmology 1979; 86:69–78
42. Cheng, H. Multicentre trial of xenon-arc photocoagulation in the treatment of diabetic retinopathy: A randomized controlled study. Interim report. Transactions of the Ophthalmological Society of the United Kingdom 1975; 95:351–357
43. Spalter, H. F. Photocoagulation of circinate maculopathy in diabetic retinopathy. American Journal of Opthalmology 1971; 71:Suppl.:242–250
44. Reeser, F., Fleischman, J., Williams, G. A., Goldman, A. Efficacy of argon laser photocoagulation in the treatment of circinate diabetic retinopathy. American Journal of Ophthalmology 1981; 92:762–767
45. Whitelocke, R. A. F., Kearns, M., Blach, R. K., Hamilton, A. M. The diabetic maculopathies. Transactions of the Ophthalmological Society of the United Kingdom 1979; 99:314–320
46. Ticho, U., Patz, A. The role of capillary perfusion in the management of diabetic macular edema. American Journal of Ophthalmology 1973; 76:880–886
47. Michels, R. G., Gass, J. D. M. The natural course of retinal branch vein obstruction. Transactions of the American Academy of Ophthalmology and Otolaryngology 1974; 78:166–177
48. Clemett, R. S., Kohner, E. M., Hamilton, A. M. The visual prognosis in retinal branch vein occlusion. Transactions of the Ophthalmological Society of the United Kingdom 1973; 93: 523–535
49. Gass, J. D., Oyakawa, R. T. Idiopathic juxtafoveolar retinal telangectasis. Archives of Ophthalmology 1982; 100:769–780
50. Michels, R. G. Surgical management of epiretinal membranes. Transactions of the Ophthalmological Society UK 1979; 99:54
51. Michels, R. G. A clinical and histopathological study of epiretinal membranes affecting the macula and removed by vitreous surgery. Transactions of the American Ophthalmological Society 1982; 80:580
52. Klein, M. L., Van Buskirk, E. M., Friedman, E., Gragoudas, E., Chandra, S. Experience with nontreatment of central serous choroidopathy. Archives of Ophthalmology 1974; 91:247–250
53. Watzke, R. C., Burton, T. C., Woolson, R. F. Direct and indirect laser photocoagulation of central serous choroidopathy. American Journal of Ophthalmology 1979; 88:914–918
54. Macular Photocoagulation Study Group. Argon laser photocoagulation for senile macular degeneration: Results of a randomized clinical trial. Archives of Ophthalmology 1982; 100:912
55. Bird, A. C., Grey, R. H. Photocoagulation of disciform macular lesions with krypton laser. British Journal of Ophthalmology 1979; 63:669–673
56. Gass, J. D. M. Photocoagulation of macular lesions. Transactions of the American Academy of Ophthalmology and Otolaryngology 1971; 75:580–608
57. Gass, J. D. M. Drusen and disciform macular detachment and degeneration. Transactions of the American Ophthalmological Society 1972; 70:409–436
58. Bird, A. C. Recent advances in the treatment of senile disciform macular degeneration by photocoagulation. British Journal of Ophthalmology 1974; 58:367–376
59. Braunstein, R. A., Gass, J. D. M. Serous detachments of the retinal pigment epithelium in patients with senile macular disease. American Journal of Ophthalmology 1979; 88: 652–660
60. The Moorfields Macular Study Group. Retinal pigment epithelial detachments in the elderly: A controlled trial of argon laser photocoagulation. British Journal of Ophthalmology 1982; 66:1–16
61. Singerman, L. J. Red krypton laser therapy of macular and retinal vascular diseases. Retina 1982; 2:15
62. Yannuzzi, L. A. Krypton red laser photocoagulation for subretinal neovascularization. Retina 1982; 2:29
63. Bressler, S. B., Bressler, N. M., Fine, S. L., Hillis, A., Murphy, R. P., Olk, R. J., Patz, A. Natural course of choroidal neovascular membranes within the foveal avascular zone in senile macular degeneration. American Journal of Ophthalmology 1982; 93:157–163
64. Cantrill, H. L., Burgess, D. Peripapillary neovascular membranes in presumed ocular histoplasmosis. American Journal of Ophthalmology 1980; 89:192–203
65. Okun, E. Photocoagulation treatment of presumed histoplasmic choroidopathy. Transactions of the American Ophthalmological Society 1972; 70:467–489
66. Maumenee, A. E., Ryan, S. J. Photocoagulation of disciform macular lesions in the ocular histoplasmosis syndrome. American Journal of Ophthalmology 1973; 75:13–16
67. Schlaegel, T. F., Jr. Histoplasmic choroiditis. Annals of Ophthalmology 1974; 6:237–252
68. Gitter, K. A., Cohen, G. Photocoagulation of active and inactive lesions of presumed ocular histoplasmosis. American Journal of Ophthalmology 1975; 79:428–436
69. Klein, M. L., Fine, S. L., Knox, D. L., Patz, A. Follow-up study in eyes with choroidal neovascularization caused by presumed ocular histoplasmosis. American Journal of Ophthalmology 1977; 83:830–835
70. Wilkinson, C. P. Stimulation of subretinal neovascularization. American Journal of Ophthalmology 1976; 81:104–106
71. Deutman, A. F., Kovacs, B. Argon laser treatment in complications of angioid streaks. American Journal of Ophthalmology 1979; 88:12–17
72. Singerman, L. J., Hatem, G. Laser treatment of choroidal neovascular membranes in angioid streaks. Retina 1981; 1:75
73. Byer, N. E. Prognosis of asymptomatic retinal breaks. Archives of Ophthalmology 1974; 92:208–210
74. Davis, M. D. Natural history of retinal breaks without detachment. Archives of Ophthalmology 1974; 92:183–194
75. McPherson, A., O'Malley, R., Beltangady, S. S. Management of the fellow eyes of patients with rhegmatogenous retinal detachment. Ophthalmology 1981; 88:922–934
76. Curtin, V. T., Norton, E. W. D., Gass, J. D. M. Photocoagulation: Its use in the prevention of reoperation after scleral buckling operations. Transactions of the American Academy of Ophthalmology and Otolaryngology 1967; 71:432–441
77. Okun, E., Cibis, P. A. The role of photocoagulation in the management of retinoschisis. Archives of Ophthalmology 1964; 72:309–314
78. Brockhurst, R. J. Photocoagulation in congenital retinoschisis. Archives of Ophthalmology 1970; 84:158–165
79. Landers, M. B. III, Robinson, C. H. Photocoagulation in the diagnosis of senile retinoschisis. American Journal of Ophthalmology 1977; 84:18–23
80. Hagler, W. S., Woldoff, H. S. Retinal detachment in relation to senile retinoschisis. Transactions of the American Academy of Ophthalmology and Otolaryngology 1973; 77:99–113
81. Blankenship, G., Cortez, R., Machemer, R. The lens and pars plana vitrectomy for diabetic retinopathy complications. Archives of Ophthalmology 1979; 97:1263–1267
82. Little, H. L., Rosenthal, A. R., Dellaporta, A., Jacobson, D. R. The effect of pan-retinal photocoagulation on rubeosis iridis. American Journal of Ophthalmology 1976; 81:804–809
83. Murphy, R. P., Egbert, P. R. Regression of iris neovascularization following panretinal photocoagulation. Archives of Ophthalmology 1979; 97:700–702
84. Simmons, R. J., Dueker, D. K., Kimbrough, R. L., Aiello, L. M. Goniophotocoagulation for neovascular glaucoma. Transactions of the American Academy of Ophthalmology and Otolaryngology 1977; 83:80–89

85. James, W. A. Jr, deRoetth, A., Jr, Forbes, M., L'Esperance, F. A. Jr. Argon laser photomydriasis. American Journal of Ophthalmology 1976; 81:62–70
86. The Diabetic Retinopathy Study Research Group. Photocoagulation treatment of proliferative diabetic retinopathy: The second report of diabetic retinopathy study findings. Ophthalmology 1978; 85:82–106
87. Frank, R. N. Visual fields and electroretinography following extensive photocoagulation. Archives of Ophthalmology 1975; 93:591–598
88. Klein, M. L., Jampol, L. M., Condon, P. I., Rice, T. A., Serjeant, G. R. Central retinal artery occlusion without retrobulbar hemorrhage after retrobulbar anesthesia. American Journal of Ophthalmology 1982; 93:573–577
89. Birch-Cox, J. Defective colour vision in diabetic retinopathy before and after laser photocoagulation. Modern Problems in Ophthalmology 1978; 19:326–329
90. Pender, P. M., Benson, W. E., Compton, H., Cox, G. B. The effects of panretinal photocoagulation on dark adaptation in diabetics with proliferative retinopathy. Ophthalmology 1981; 88:635–638
91. Peyman, G. A., Bok, D. Peroxidase diffusion in the normal and laser-coagulated primate retina. Investigative Ophthalmology 1972; 11:35–45
92. Huamonte, F. U., Peyman, G. A., Goldberg, M. F., Locketz, A. Immediate fundus complications after retinal scatter photocoagulation: I. Clinical picture and pathogenesis. Ophthalmic Surgery 1976; 7:88–99
93. Schulenburg, W. E., Hamilton, A. M., Blach, R. K. A comparative study of argon laser and krypton laser in the treatment of diabetic optic disc neovascularization. British Journal of Ophthalmology 1979; 63:412–417
94. Rogell, G. D. Internal ophthalmoplegia after argon laser panretinal photocoagulation. Archives of Ophthalmology 1979; 97:904–905
95. Benson, W. E., Townsend, R. E., Pheasant, T. R. Choriovitreal and subretinal proliferations: Complications of photocoagulation. Ophthalmology 1979; 86:283–289
96. Goldberg, M. F., Herbst, R. W. Acute complications of argon laser photocoagulation: Epipapillary and peripapillary neovascularization. Archives of Ophthalmology 1973; 89:311–318
97. Weinstein, G. W., Rylander, H. G. Photocoagulation of the fovea. Transactions of the American Ophthalmological Society 1978; 76:278–293
98. Dizon-Moore, R. V., Jampol, L. M., Goldberg, M. F. Chorioretinal and choriovitreal neovascularization. Their presence after photocoagulation of proliferative sickle cell retinopathy. Archives of Ophthalmology 1981; 99:842–849
99. Jampol, L. M., Goldberg, M. F. Retinal breaks after photocoagulation of proliferative sickle cell retinopathy. Archives of Ophthalmology 1980; 98:676–679
100. Goldbaum, M. H., Galinos, S. O., Apple, D. *et al.* Acute choroidal ischemia as a complication of photocoagulation. Archives of Ophthalmology 1976; 94:1025–1035

11

Management of intraocular tumors*

Jerry A. Shields MD

Introduction

Several important advances have been made in recent years in the diagnosis and management of intraocular tumors. As a result, clinicians have become more skilled in recognizing tumors and pseudotumors of the uveal tract, retina and optic disc. This improved diagnostic accuracy has resulted in prompt appropriate management of these conditions. This chapter reviews current diagnostic methods and therapeutic alternatives in the surgical and non-surgical management of intraocular tumors[1,2].

Diagnostic methods

In contrast to tumors of the skin and other tissues, most intraocular tumors are more difficult to biopsy and diagnosis often must usually be made on the basis of clinical features and special tests without pathological study of a tissue specimen. Therefore, diagnostic errors sometimes occur whereby malignant tumors are misdiagnosed as benign lesions, or benign lesions are misinterpreted as being malignant[3]. To minimize the chance of such a diagnostic error, a systematic complete ophthalmic evaluation is performed in each case and combined with selected ancillary diagnostic studies[4]. This section considers the general principles of clinical evaluation and reviews the most important diagnostic tests.

* Text material, in part, and all photographs extracted from: Shields J. A. Diagnosis and management of intraocular tumors. St Louis: C. V. Mosby, 1983. Additional text material from: Shields, J. A. Surgical and nonsurgical management of intraocular tumors. In: Spaeth, G. L., ed. Ophthalmic surgery. Philadelphia: W. B. Saunders, 1982

History

A detailed history is taken in each case of possible intraocular tumor. It is good policy to take the thorough history *before* examining the patient, and then to review relevant parts of the history in relation to the findings of physical examination and ancillary tests. Depending on the particular situation, one should also inquire about the birth history, medical history and family history.

The birth history is often important in the evaluation of children with suspected intraocular tumors. For example, retinoblastoma is usually not detected until several months after birth, whereas lesions that can simulate retinoblastoma, such as persistent hyperplastic primary vitreous and retinal dysplasia, are often detected at birth or soon thereafter. A history of prematurity and postnatal oxygen therapy in an infant who later developed a white pupillary reflex should suggest retinopathy of prematurity (retrolental fibroplasia, RLF) rather than retinoblastoma[5,6].

The past medical history can also provide clues as to the diagnosis. An amelanotic choroidal mass in a patient with a history of previous surgery for a malignancy elsewhere, particularly breast carcinoma, should suggest the possibility of a metastatic tumor to the eye[7]. The prior excision of a skin melanoma in a patient with a pigmented fundus lesion should suggest a possible metastatic melanoma to the choroid. Recent anorexia or weight loss may indicate that an intraocular mass is a metastatic tumor and part of a widely disseminated process. A history of diabetes mellitus or hypertension in a patient with a dark fundus mass should suggest intraocular hemorrhage or retinal detachment.

A careful ocular history frequently provides information that is helpful in the differential diagnosis. Previous ocular trauma may predispose to retinal detachment, intraocular hemorrhage or proliferation of the retinal pigment epithelium (RPE), all of which can be mistaken for an intraocular malignancy. A history of recent intraocular surgery on the eye with a dark peripheral fundus mass suggests the likelihood of a choroidal detachment. A history of high myopia in a patient with retinal elevation suggests the possibility of a rhegmatogenous retinal detachment.

The family history frequently provides other diagnostic information. Patients with retinoblastoma, retinal angiomatosis or retinal astrocytoma may have a family history of the same condition. Patients with a uveal melanoma or choroidal hemangioma are not likely to have a positive family history. In addition to the family history, it can be helpful to perform a general physical and ocular examination on other family members. Evidence of neurofibromatosis, tuberous sclerosis or regressed retinoblastoma in a family member can aid in establishing the correct diagnosis.

Medical evaluation

Medical evaluation, including attention to the patient's age, race, physical examination and laboratory tests may provide important diagnostic information. A pigmented fundus lesion in a black patient is likely to be a benign process such as a melanocytoma or hyperplasia of the RPE rather than a malignant melanoma, because melanomas are extremely rare in blacks. A thorough physical examination may detect a primary tumor elsewhere which has metastasized to the eye, whereas metastatic spread from an untreated primary eye malignancy is rare. In patients with a possible fundus hamartoma, the skin should be checked carefully for café au lait spots (*Figure 11.1*), angiomas or sebaceous adenomas (*Figure 11.2*) to aid in diagnosis of a specific type of phacomatosis.

Laboratory studies are helpful in some cases. A blood count, bone marrow aspiration, cerebrospinal fluid examination or lymph node biopsy may establish the diagnosis of leukemia or histiocytic lymphoma in a patient with a diffuse fundus mass, vitreous hemorrhage or vitreous cells. A chest X-ray can detect a primary lung tumor with

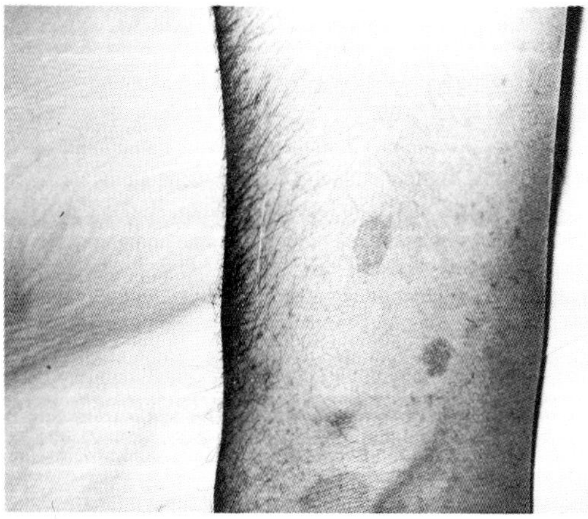

Figure 11.1 *Cutaneous café au lait spots on forearm of patient with neurofibromatosis*

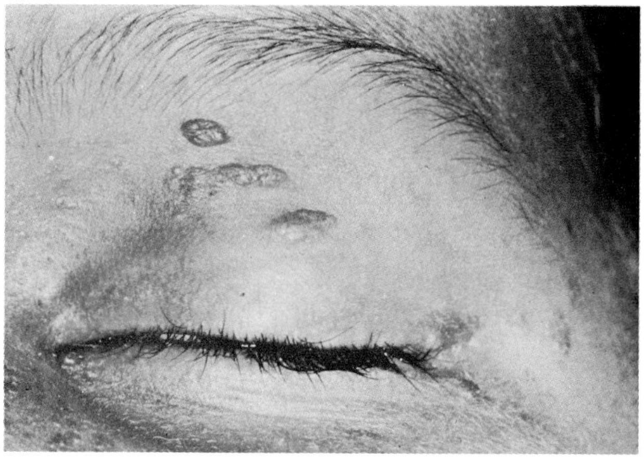

Figure 11.2 *Sebaceous adenoma on eyelid of patient with tuberous sclerosis*

metastasis to the eye. A chest X-ray may also show evidence of sarcoidosis, which may cause an intraocular granuloma appearing as a pseudotumor. Plasma carcinoembryonic antigen (CEA) levels are sometimes helpful in determining the nature of an intraocular tumor, as well as suggesting the presence of systemic involvement[1].

Ocular examination

Evaluation of the fellow eye

The fellow eye is carefully examined *prior* to examining the symptomatic eye. This is helpful to detect clues as to the correct diagnosis and/or to identify pathological changes which could alter management of the involved eye. Tumors such as retinoblastoma, metastatic carcinoma to the uvea, retinal capillary hemangioma and astrocytoma can be bilateral, whereas uveal melanomas and choroidal hemangiomas are almost always unilateral.

Certain lesions that can simulate an intraocular neoplasm can be bilateral, thus providing a clue to the correct diagnosis. Central exudative hemorrhagic chorioretinopathy (disciform macular degeneration) due to any one of several causes can ophthalmoscopically resemble a melanoma. This condition can be bilateral, and the findings in the fellow eye should suggest the correct diagnosis. Similarly, drusen in the macular area of the fellow eye of an elderly patient should suggest disciform degeneration rather than melanoma as the cause of a posterior pole lesion. Bullous retinoschisis can sometimes simulate a melanoma but is also usually bilateral and symmetrical.

External examination

External examination may reveal signs associated with an intraocular tumor and thus provide diagnostic clues, even before slit-lamp biomicroscopy and ophthalmoscopy are performed. For example, strabismus or heterochromia

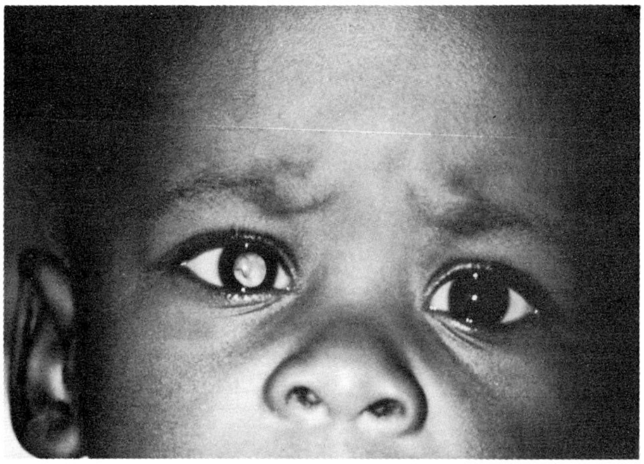

Figure 11.3 *Esotropia and right leukocoria in patient with retinoblastoma. The esotropia preceded the leukocoria by several weeks*

may be initial signs of retinoblastoma (*Figure 11.3*). Acquired hyperchromic heterochromia may be the presenting manifestation of a diffuse iris melanoma or the iris-nevus syndrome. An afferent pupillary defect (Marcus-Gunn pupil) can be associated with a benign tumor of the optic disc such as a melanocytoma, or with invasion of the optic nerve by a malignant tumor such as retinoblastoma or malignant melanoma (*Figure 11.4*). A large choroidal melanoma may also be associated with an afferent pupillary defect, even though the optic disc is not involved.

Signs of episcleral inflammation may be associated with a benign pseudotumor such as nodular posterior scleritis or with a necrotic melanoma of the posterior uvea. Large dilated blood vessels in the ciliary region often suggest a melanoma of the ciliary body or peripheral choroid in the same quadrant (*Figure 11.5*). A subconjunctival pigmented lesion in the ciliary region may be either a staphyloma of the sclera or extrascleral extension of a uveal melanoma, and differentiation can be made by transillumination as described later. There are many other external ocular findings that are helpful in evaluation of an intraocular tumor.

Biomicroscopy

Slit-lamp biomicroscopy provides excellent visualization of lesions located in the anterior segment. Some anterior segment lesions may be difficult to diagnose by external examination alone, and can be studied in more detail using the magnification and optical sectioning provided by the slit lamp. Biomicroscopy is the best method to evaluate the size, extent and clinical characteristics of iris tumors and pseudotumors and subtle changes in pupillary function. Lens opacities in a child with a white pupillary reflex suggest a congenital cataract or persistent hyperplastic primary vitreous rather than retinoblastoma, because the latter is usually associated with a clear lens. Gonioscopy combined with slit-lamp biomicroscopy is the best method to visualize tumors in the anterior chamber angle. The site, extent and involvement of adjacent structures by peripheral iris lesions can be seen. Anterior extension of ciliary body tumors into the region of the iris root can also be detected.

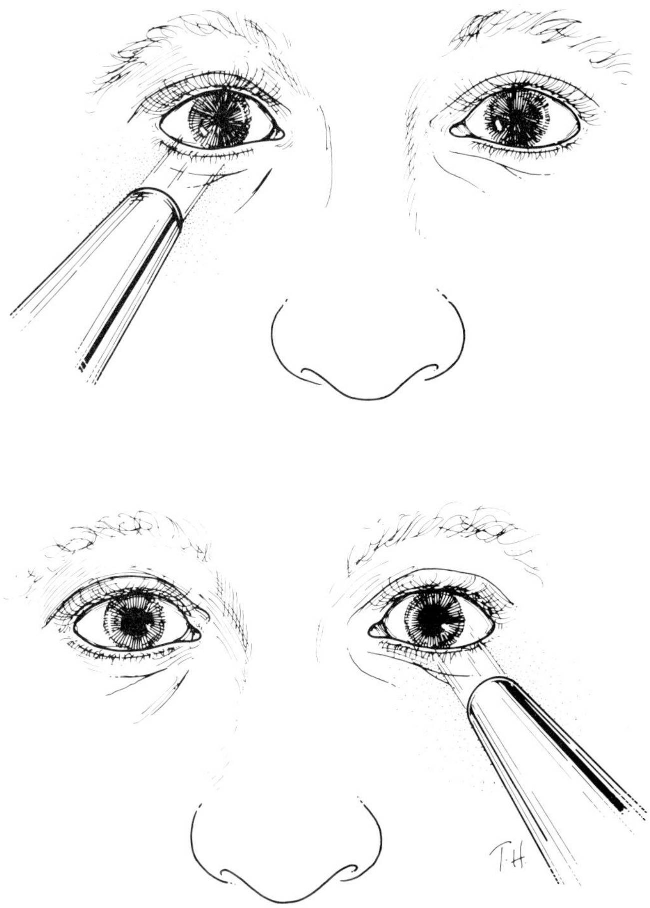

Figure 11.4 *Left afferent pupillary defect (Marcus-Gunn pupil). When light is shined in right eye, both pupils constrict* **(top)**; but when light is shined in the left eye, both pupils dilate, demonstrating defect in the afferent portion of the pupillary reflex mechanism in the left eye **(bottom)**

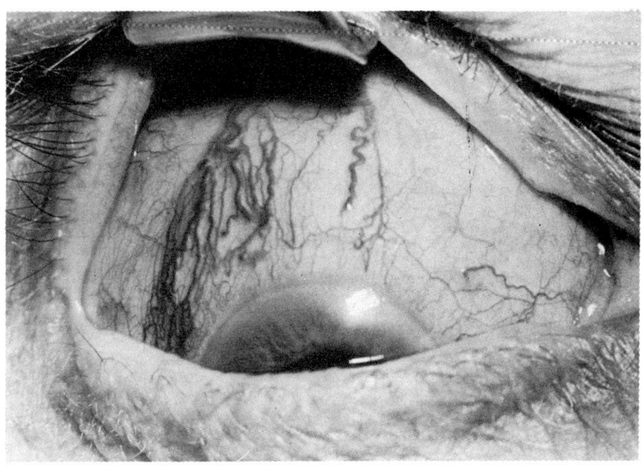

Figure 11.5 *Dilated episcleral vessels overlying location of malignant melanoma of the ciliary body*

Ophthalmoscopy

Ophthalmoscopy is the most important part of examination of tumors in the posterior segment. Both binocular indirect ophthalmoscopy and direct ophthalmoscopy are used, although indirect ophthalmoscopy has important advantages in tumor diagnosis. Indirect ophthalmoscopy provides stereopsis, bright illumination and a wide field of view. Therefore, the extent of a lesion can be easily determined and its relation to adjacent structures can be seen. Elevated tumors can be differentiated from flat or depressed lesions. Indirect ophthalmoscopy also permits visualization of the peripheral fundus and the pars plana region, and can be combined with scleral indentation to detect peripheral lesions overlooked by direct ophthalmoscopy. Indirect ophthalmoscopy permits visualization through moderately hazy media, such as with partial cataract or vitreous opacities.

The stereopsis and wide field of view provided by indirect ophthalmoscopy facilitate detection and evaluation of shifting subretinal fluid. Shifting fluid after movement of the patient's head is characteristic of non-rhegmatogenous retinal detachments, such as those seen with choroidal tumors or choroidal effusions. If the subretinal fluid does not shift, it suggests a rhegmatogenous cause for the retinal detachment rather than its being associated with a choroidal tumor.

Visual fields

Visual field examination is useful in some cases, but it has definite limitations in evaluation of intraocular tumors. Although malignant lesions of the posterior fundus are more likely to produce field defects, some benign lesions also produce a scotoma. Occasionally, a small malignant lesion does not produce an appreciable field defect, and therefore visual field testing alone cannot differentiate between malignant and benign lesions.

Special tests

Transillumination

Transillumination is an important part of evaluation of certain intraocular tumors. Both pigmented tumors and blood block the transmission of light and cast a shadow, whereas non-pigmented lesions and serous fluid permit transmission of light. Transillumination is best performed with a high-intensity fiberoptic probe. There are several ways to perform this test, including transpupillary, transscleral, indirect ophthalmoscopy and slit-lamp techniques. Different methods are used depending on the size, shape and location of the lesion and the type of information needed.

The transpupillary technique of transillumination is performed by placing the light source in the conjunctival cul-de-sac with the light beam directed toward the sclera, and then observing the light transmitted through the pupil. In the normal eye, a distinct red reflex is seen through the pupil regardless of the quadrant in which the light is placed. In an eye with a pigmented tumor or blood, this red pupillary reflex is diminished or absent when the light source is placed on the sclera over the lesion.

The transscleral technique is performed by placing the light source in the conjunctival cul-de-sac or directly on the sclera, in the quadrant opposite the tumor. Rather than observing the pupil, the examiner observes the sclera in the quadrant where the tumor is present (*Figure 11.6*).

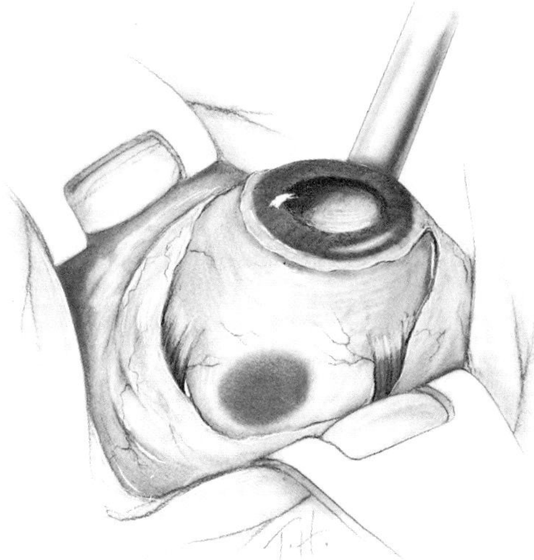

Figure 11.6 *Transscleral transillumination technique used to outline tumor before ^{32}P test. Fiberoptic light probe is placed against sclera in quadrant opposite the tumor, and shadow caused by pigmented tumor outlines its size and location*

This method is useful in localizing and measuring the base of pigmented tumors. It is used when performing the radioactive phosphorus uptake test (^{32}P test) to permit precise placement of the counting probe. We use it routinely to determine the size and extent of ciliary body and choroidal melanomas at the time of treatment by iridocyclectomy, episcleral plaque radiotherapy or eyewall resection.

The indirect ophthalmoscopy method permits the examiner to visualize directly the transillumination characteristics of the lesion. It is performed either in the office or during surgery by placing the light source on the globe directly over the base of the lesion and observing the tumor by indirect ophthalmoscopy through the dilated pupil. When the tumor is in focus, the light of the ophthalmoscope is turned off and the lesion is illuminated only by the transscleral light. The light is seen to be decreased or absent in areas of pigmentation or blood, and the lesion appears dark and surrounded by a red glow (*Figure 11.7*). In cases of serous detachment of the choroid, choroidal hemangioma and other non-pigmented lesions the light is not blocked, and the lesion is brightly illuminated.

The slit-lamp method is used mainly for evaluating anterior segment lesions. It is performed by focusing the slit-lamp beam on the lesion and then placing the fiberoptic probe against the sclera in the quadrant of the lesion. The light of the slit lamp is turned off, and the lesion is visualized by retroillumination. This method is helpful in differentiating between epithelial cysts of the iris or ciliary body and solid pigmented tumors which may have a similar appearance on routine biomicroscopy[8].

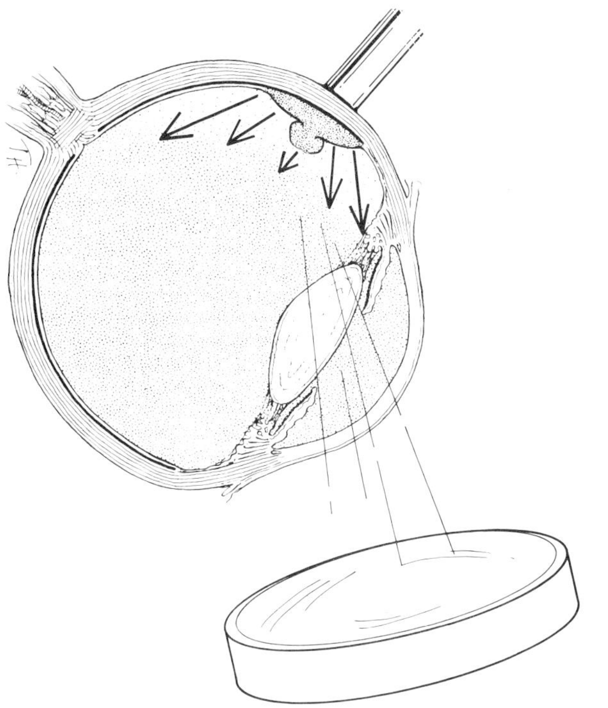

Figure 11.7 *Transillumination technique using indirect ophthalmoscopy. Fiberoptic light source is placed on globe over base of lesion. Pigmented lesion blocks the light, whereas light passes more readily through the surrounding tissues as the fundus is examined by indirect ophthalmoscopy*

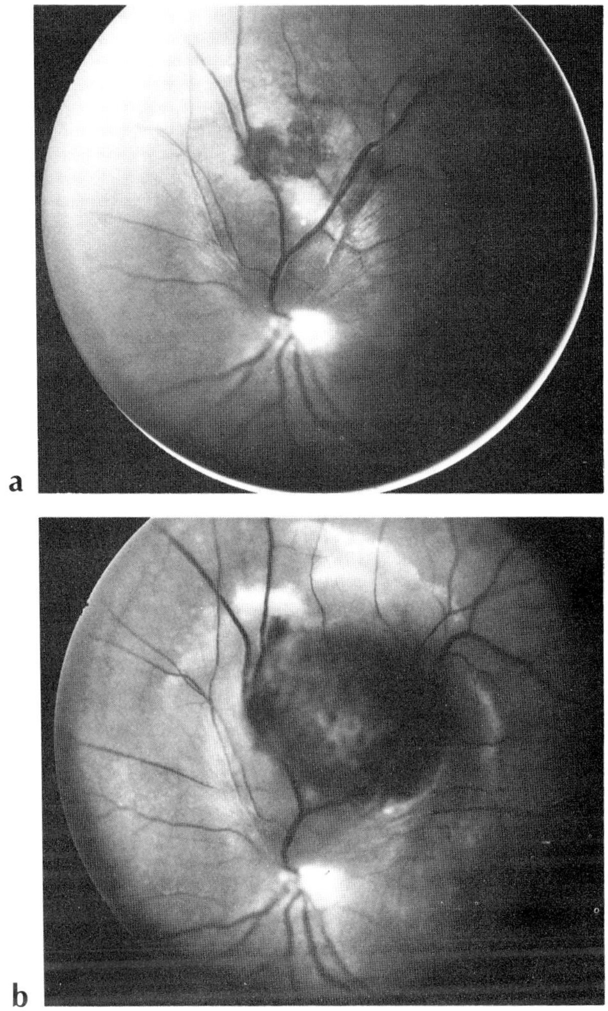

Figure 11.8 *Photographs documenting growth of a small choroidal melanoma.* **(a)** *Initial appearance of lesion superior to optic nervehead.* **(b)** *Same lesion 4 months later, showing marked enlargement*

Slit-lamp and fundus photography

Anterior segment and fundus photography permit better evaluation of certain intraocular lesions and provide a means whereby lesions can be observed and changes precisely compared over a period of time. In evaluation of certain types of tumors, periodic photographs are used for follow-up of the lesion and in determining whether it is growing. This assists in selecting the type of therapy needed (*Figure 11.8*). Photographs allow evaluation in greater detail than does ophthalmoscopy, and stereophotographs are especially useful. Several physicians can study the lesion simultaneously and discuss their findings, and the photographs can be mailed to consultants for diagnostic and therapeutic opinions, thus lessening costly travel for the patient.

Wide-angle fundus photography has become important in ocular oncology. Cameras are available that provide 45° and 60° fields, and with the special 'Equator-Plus' camera a view of the fundus of up to 148° is possible[9]. Therefore, larger lesions can be included in one photographic field (*Figure 11.9*). This is helpful for documenting the overall size of the lesion and in comparing the edges of the lesion to nearby landmarks. Wide-angle photography is especially useful for documenting regression of choroidal melanomas after episcleral plaque radiotherapy.

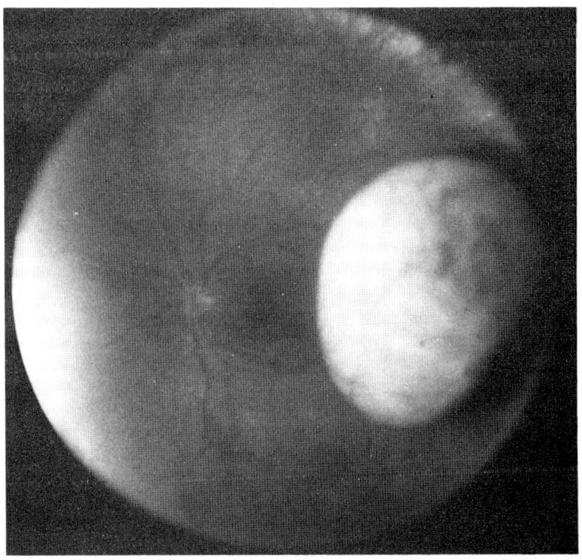

Figure 11.9 *Wide-angle 'Equator-Plus' photograph of a large amelanotic melanoma of the choroid*

Fluorescein angiography and angioscopy

Fluorescein studies often provide helpful information in the evaluation of intraocular tumors. Fluorescein angiography with photographic documentation is preferred when possible to permit detailed study of the lesion, but this can be combined with fluorescein angioscopy using the indirect ophthalmoscope for immediate study of the late-stage staining pattern and/or to study eyes with hazy media. With fluorescein studies one can determine the degree of pigmentation and vascularity of the lesion and study pathological changes such as vascular

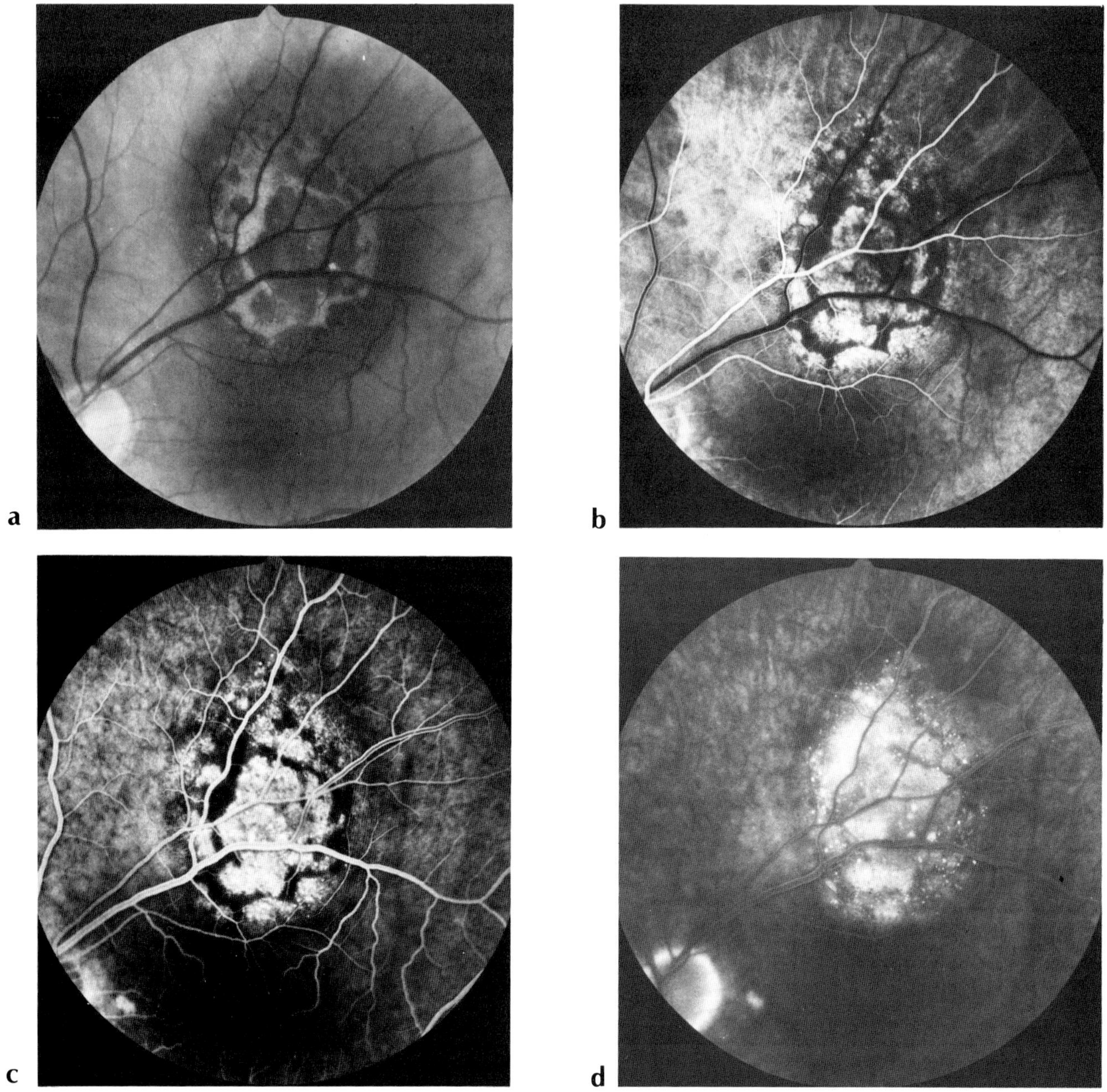

Figure 11.10 *Typical fluorescein angiographic features of small choroidal melanoma.* **(a)** *Tumor located above macula in left eye. Note geographic orange pigment on surface.* **(b)** *Late arterial and early arteriovenous phase showing mottled hyperfluorescence of tumor. Areas of geographic orange pigment remain hypofluorescent.* **(c)** *Venous phase showing increased hyperfluorescence of main portion of tumor and pinpoint areas of hyperfluorescence around margin of tumor. Orange pigment remains hypofluorescent.* **(d)** *Late phase showing diffuse hyperfluorescence and leakage from pinpoint foci of hyperfluorescence. Areas of geographic orange pigment remain hypofluorescent*

leakage. Fluorescein studies demonstrate whether vascular tumors are derived from the retinal or choroidal circulation.

Changes that occur in the tissues adjacent to ocular tumors can also be studied by fluorescein angiography. Multiple leakage spots in the RPE overlying a pigmented choroidal mass is suggestive of a malignant melanoma. Accumulation of subretinal fluid or cystic retinopathy may also be detected with fluorescein studies. Certain retinal or choroidal tumors show rather typical fluorescein patterns. These tumors include malignant melanoma (*Figure 11.10*), cavernous hemangioma of the choroid (*Figure 11.11*), metastatic carcinoma (*Figure 11.12*), retinoblastoma (*Figure 11.13*) and retinal capillary hemangioma (*Figure 11.14*). However, fluorescein angiography is only an ancillary test and cannot be used alone to make a definitive diagnosis.

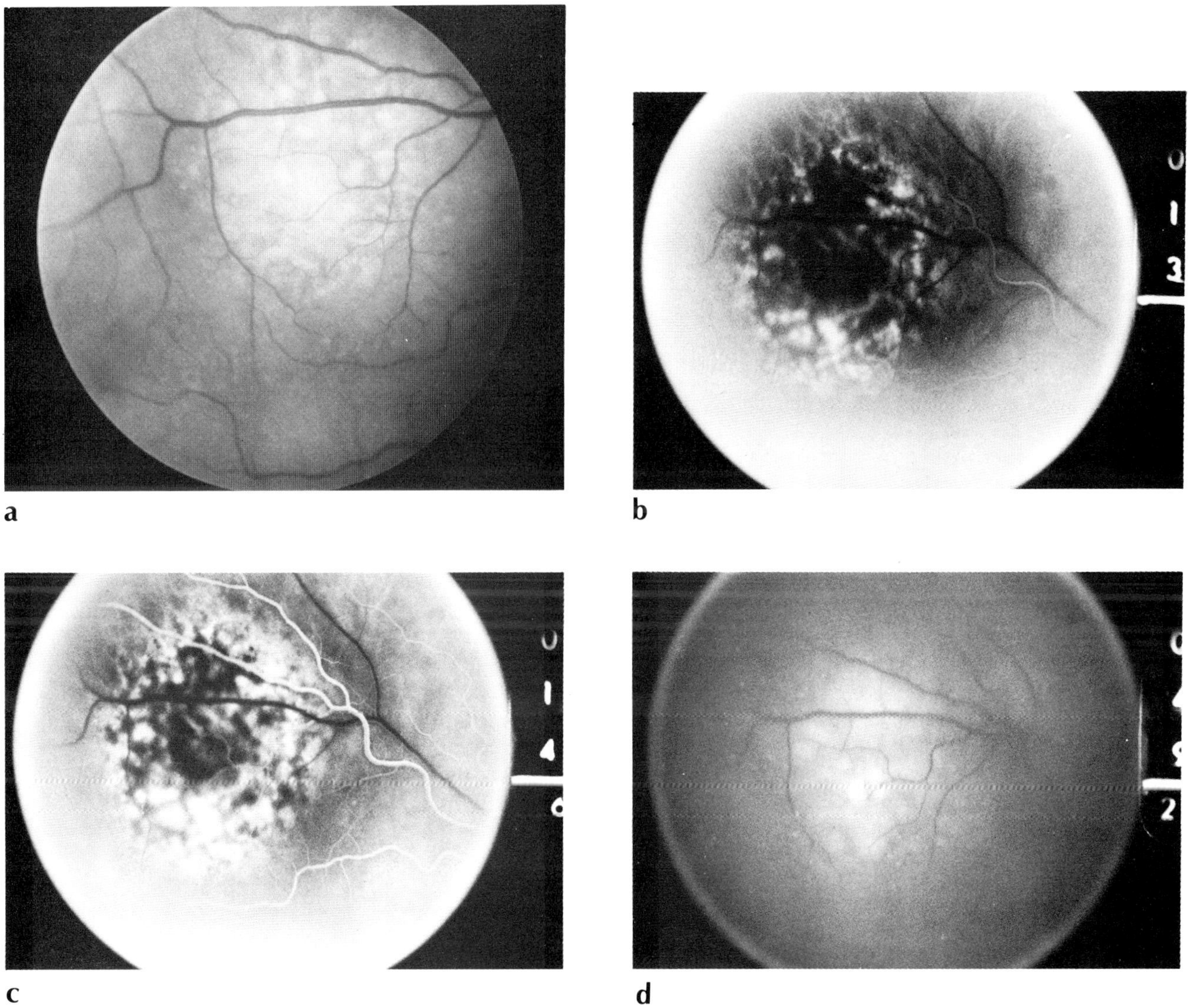

Figure 11.11 *Fluorescein angiography of choroidal hemangioma.* **(a)** *Pre-injection photograph showing amelanotic tumor temporal to macula in right eye.* **(b)** *Early arterial phase showing filling of large choroidal vessels within tumor.* **(c)** *Arterial phase showing more intense hyperfluorescence of vessels within tumor and early leakage from tumor vessels.* **(d)** *Late phase showing diffuse hyperfluorescence of the choroidal tumor. Hyperfluorescent areas in center of tumor represent fluorescein within cystoid spaces in overlying retina*

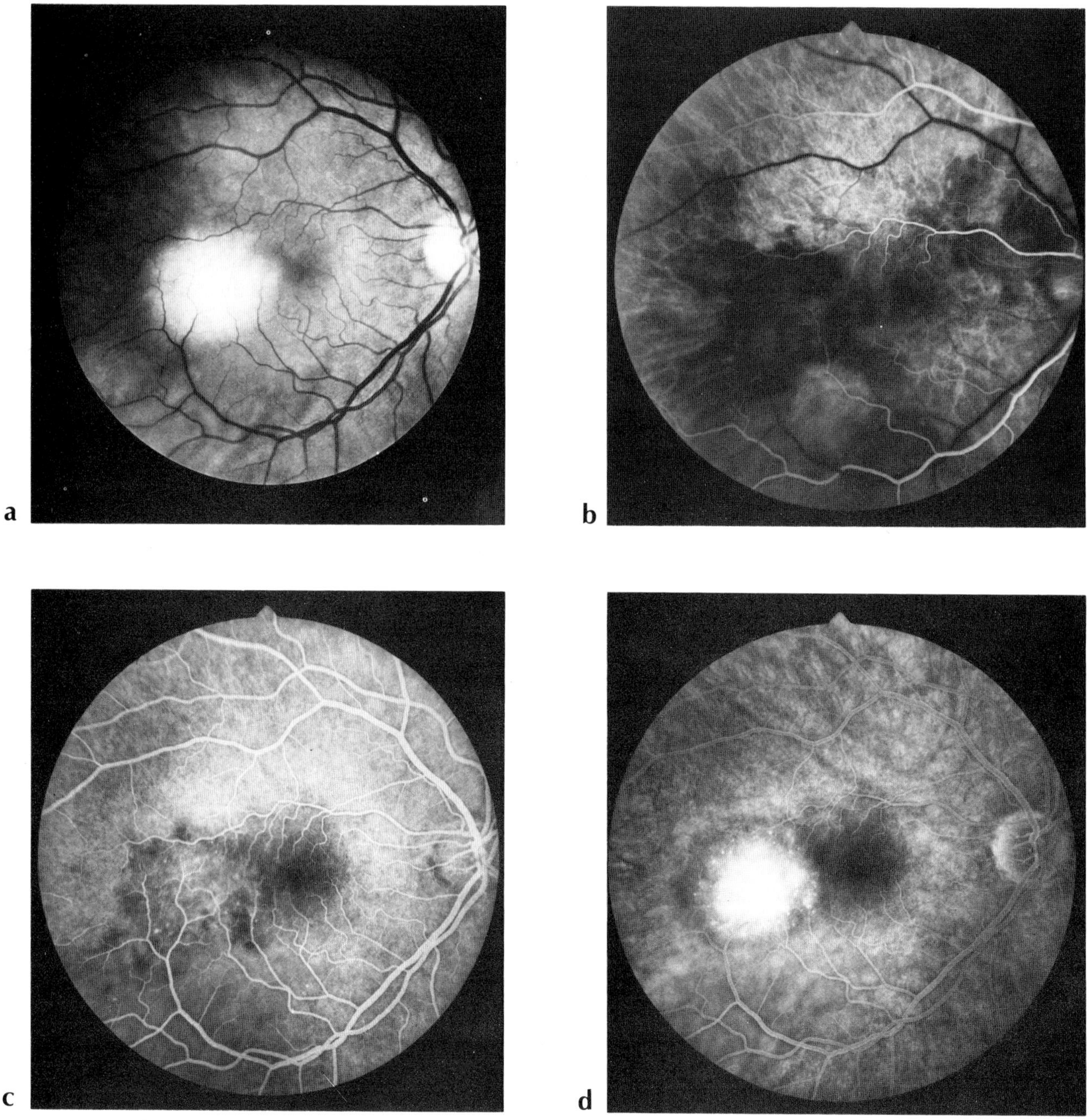

Figure 11.12 *Fluorescein angiography of metastatic tumor to choroid.* **(a)** *Pre-injection photograph showing amelanotic tumor temporal to center of macula.* **(b)** *Arterial phase showing hypofluorescence of metastatic tumor.* **(c)** *Late venous phase showing progressive fluorescence of the tumor. Note the pinpoint foci of hyperfluorescence within the mass.* **(d)** *Late phase showing intense staining of entire tumor. Pinpoint foci of hyperfluorescence are more intense*

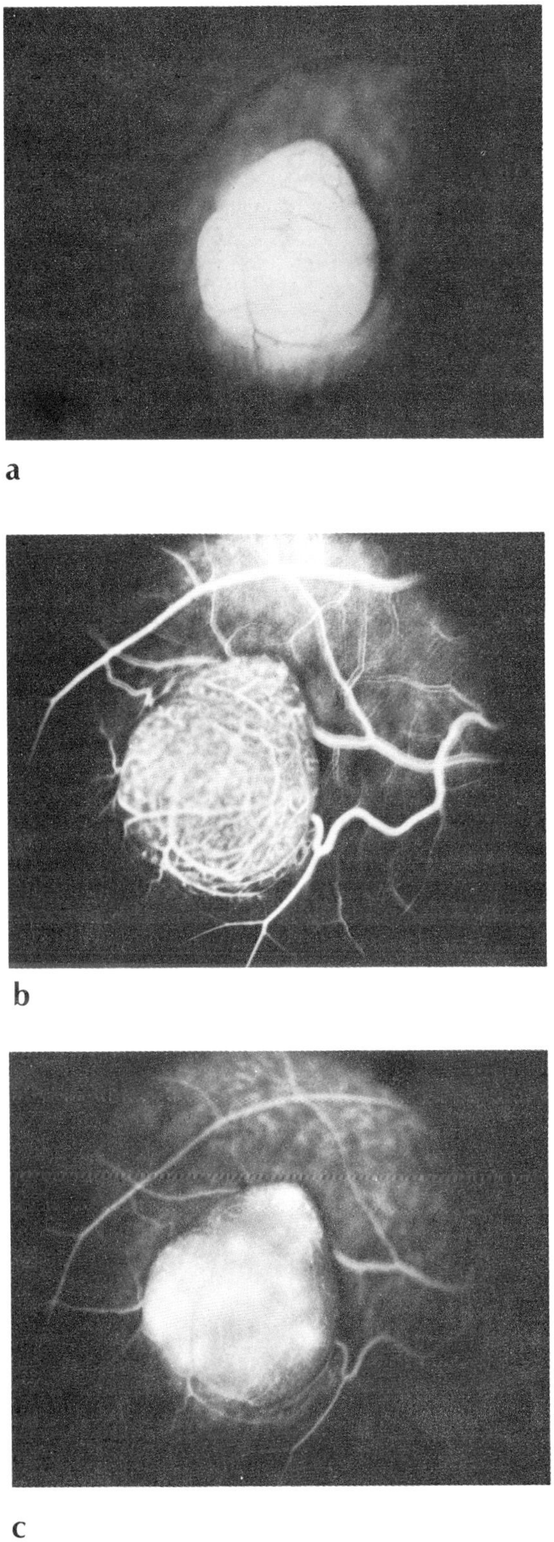

Figure 11.13 *Fluorescein angiography of retinoblastoma.* **(a)** *Pre-injection appearance of small retinoblastoma located temporal to macular area in right eye.* **(b)** *Early venous phase showing numerous vascular channels within tumor.* **(c)** *Late phase showing diffuse hyperfluorescence of the entire tumor.*

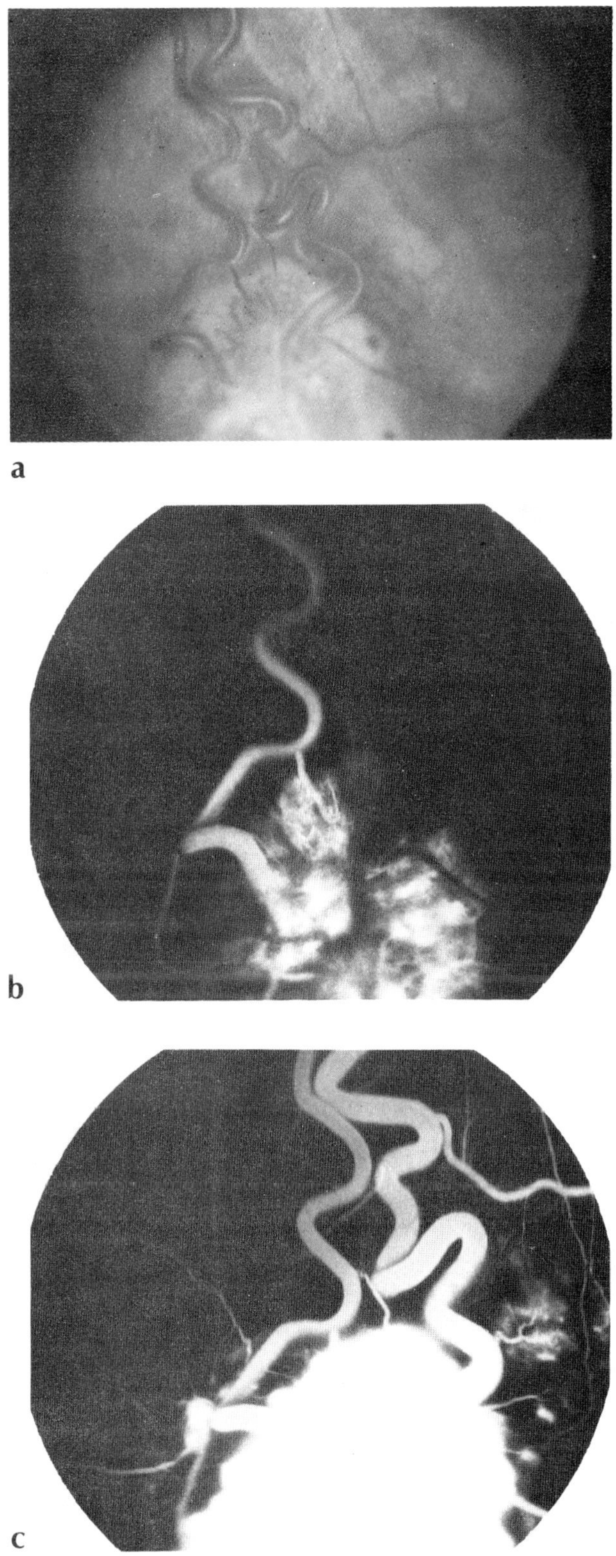

Figure 11.14 *Fluorescein angiography of retinal capillary hemangioma (von Hippel's tumor).* **(a)** *Pre-injection appearance of inferior tumor with dilated feeder vessels.* **(b)** *Arterial phase showing immediate filling of capillaries in the mass from dilated feeder arteriole.* **(c)** *Venous phase showing strong hyperfluorescence of the tumor and fluorescein in both feeder arteriole and draining vein*

Ultrasonography

Since its introduction into ophthalmology, ultrasonography has been used to help in differentiating between intraocular tumors and related lesions. The physics of A-scan and B-scan ultrasonography and their application in ocular tumor diagnosis have been described[10]. Ultrasonography is especially useful in detecting tumors in eyes with opaque media[11], but it is also helpful in the differential diagnosis of tumors that can be directly visualized. Typical, although not pathognomonic, ultrasound patterns are seen with some tumors such as choroidal melanoma (*Figure 11.15*), retinoblastoma (*Figure 11.16*) and choroidal osteoma (*Figure 11.17*). A characteristic pattern may also be seen in eyes with an encapsulated intraocular foreign body simulating an intraocular tumor. The height of a pigmented choroidal lesion, as measured by ultrasound, is probably of most importance in differentiating between a malignant melanoma and a choroidal nevus.

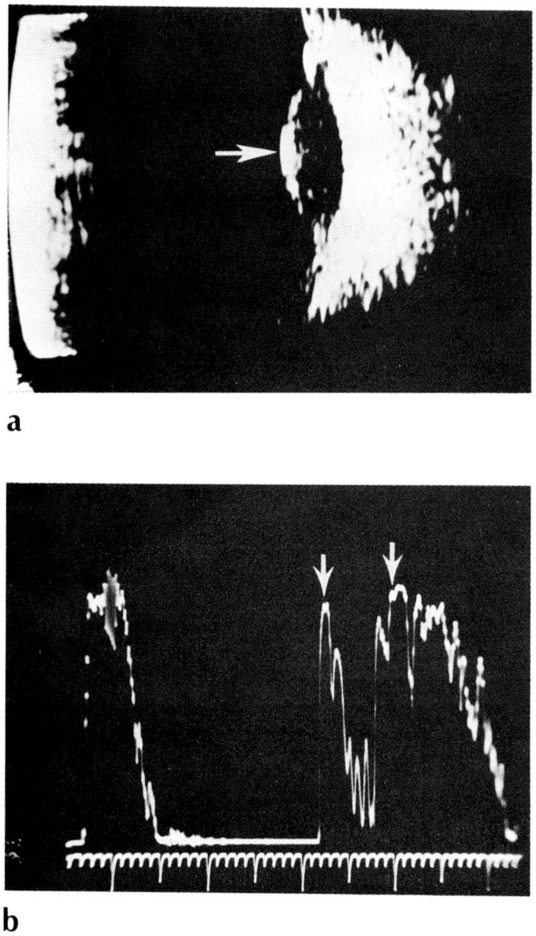

Figure 11.15 *Ultrasonography of medium-size malignant melanoma of choroid.* **(a)** *B-scan ultrasonogram showing dome-shaped tumor (arrow) with low internal sonographic reflectivity and underlying choroidal excavation.* **(b)** *A-scan ultrasonogram of same tumor. First arrow indicates retina and anterior surface of tumor, and second arrow indicates sclera. Note low-to-medium reflectivity within the mass*

Radioactive phosphorus uptake test (^{32}P test)

The ^{32}P test was introduced into ophthalmology in 1952 as an aid in differentiating between benign and malignant intraocular tumors[12]. It is based on the principle that malignant cells incorporate and utilize phosphorus to a greater degree than do normal tissue cells. Therefore, if ^{32}P is administered to a patient with a malignant tumor, the ^{32}P should be more concentrated in the mass. The β-radiation emitted by the isotope can be quantitated by placing a counting probe near the suspected tumor and comparing this to the background radiation emitted from normal tissues in other parts of the eye.

The test is performed by administering 500 μCi of radioactive phosphorus either orally or intravenously. If the lesion is located in the ciliary body region, it is precisely localized by transillumination, and four to six measurements are taken by placing a counting probe

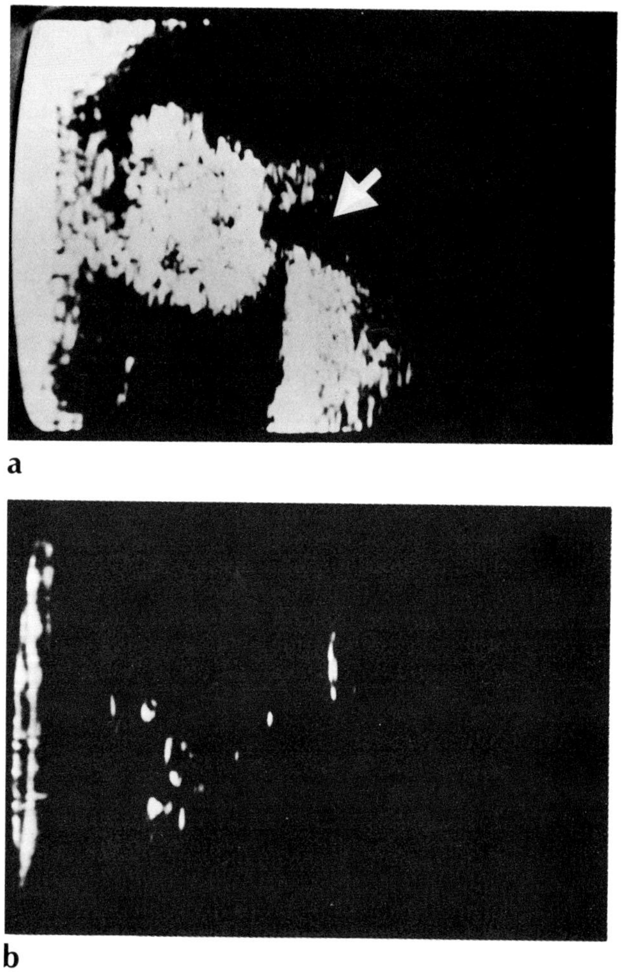

Figure 11.16 *Ultrasonography of a large nodular retinoblastoma. Cornea is to left and orbit to right.* **(a)** *B-scan ultrasonogram at 80 decibels, showing acoustic shadowing of eye wall and retrobulbar tissue posterior to tumor (arrow).* **(b)** *Ultrasonogram at 50 decibels, showing highly reflective echoes within mass that are suggestive of calcification*

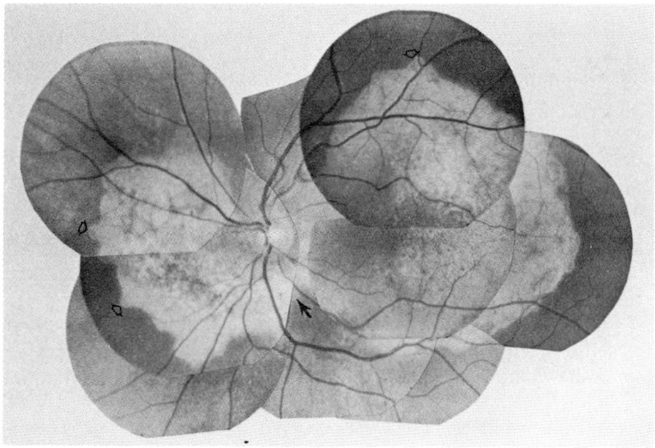

a

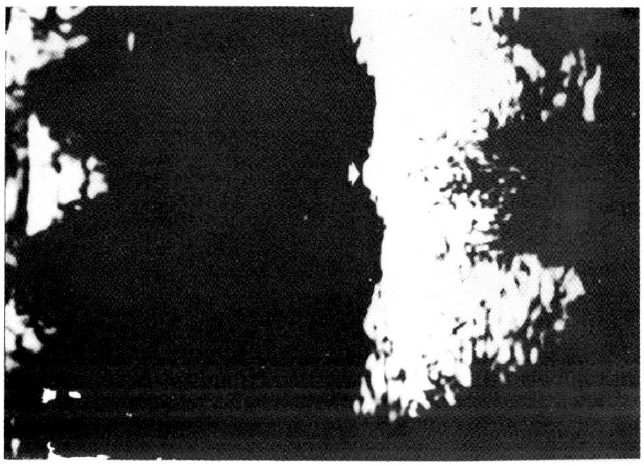

b

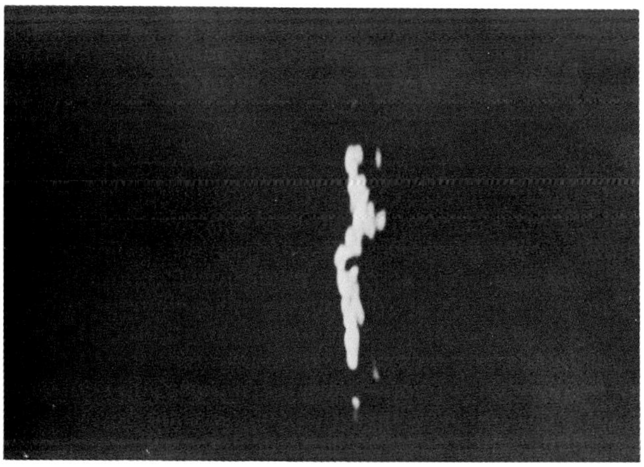

c

Figure 11.17 *Ultrasonography of peripapillary choroidal osteoma.* **(a)** *Montage of clinical photographs showing extensive tumor surrounding optic disc (solid arrow). Open arrows indicate pseudopods which are characteristic of margins of this type of tumor.* **(b)** *B-scan ultrasonogram at 80 decibels, showing solid tumor (arrow) with high internal reflectivity. Cornea is to the left and sclera to the right. Note shadowing in orbit which gives appearance of enlarged optic nerve.* **(c)** *Ultrasonogram at 50 decibels showing persistent echoes from highly reflective calcified plaque after adjacent soft tissue echoes have disappeared*

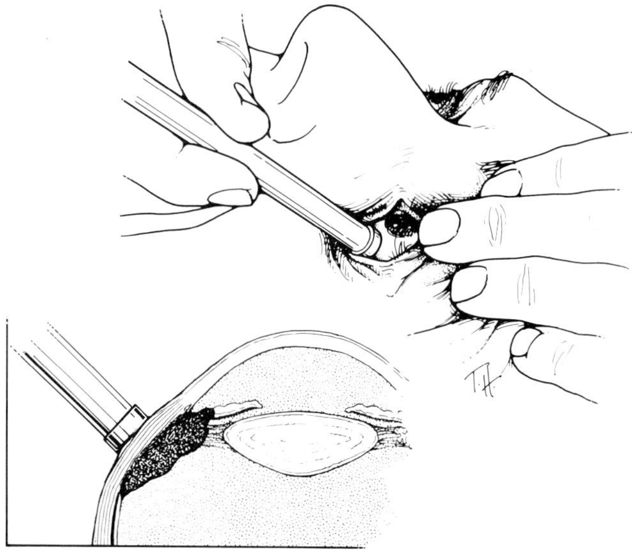

Figure 11.18 *Technique of transconjunctival ^{32}P test for tumor of the ciliary body. Probe is placed on the sclera directly over the lesion*

exactly over the lesion (*Figure 11.18*) 1 hour, 24 hours and 48 hours after administration of the ^{32}P. The opposite quadrant of the same eye is usually used for the same number of control readings. An initial 1-hour uptake of 30 per cent or greater over the lesion as compared to the control area, with an increasing value at 48 hours, is considered a positive test suggesting a malignant tumor. The percentage of uptake is calculated using the formula

$$\frac{L - C}{C} \times 100 = \text{percentage uptake},$$

where L is the average of the readings over the lesion and C is the average of readings over the control area[13].

If the tumor is in the posterior segment, a conjunctival peritomy under anesthesia is necessary to expose the sclera in the area of the lesion[14]. This is usually done 48 hours after administration of the radoactive phosphorus. The lesion is localized by transillumination, and a curved probe is used to take counts over the tumor (*Figure 11.19*). Control readings are made in the opposite quadrant of the same eye. With this technique, a positive test suggestive of a malignant tumor is considered to be a 50 per cent greater uptake over the lesion as compared to the control area[15]. Some workers use 60 per cent as a positive test, and others consider any increased uptake of between 50 and 100 per cent as a 'gray zone' between a positive and a negative result.

Between February 1971 and October 1976, 500 ^{32}P tests were performed for ocular tumors by the Oncology Service at the Wills Eye Hospital, Philadelphia. With the exception of iris tumors, for which the test is not reliable, it was 95–98 per cent accurate in differentiating benign from malignant intraocular lesions[16]. Although this procedure has been criticized by some investigators who believe that it is rarely necessary, the ^{32}P test has proved helpful in making the correct diagnosis in some difficult cases. It should be performed by someone with experience in retinal detachment surgery who is accustomed to using indirect ophthalmoscopy, scleral depression, transillumination and other means to assist in localizing the tumor.

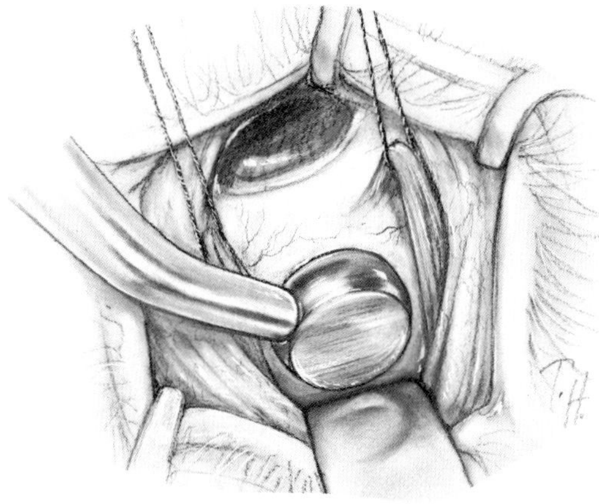

Figure 11.19 *Surgical ^{32}P test for possible choroidal melanoma. After incising conjunctiva and placing traction sutures under adjacent rectus muscles, counting probe is applied to sclera overlying choroidal mass*

The ^{32}P test is more difficult in eyes with opaque media. In such cases, ultrasonography and transillumination are used to localize the lesion, and the ^{32}P test is then used to aid further in the diagnosis. The combined use of these procedures provides important capabilities in the diagnosis of malignant melanoma when the fundus cannot be visualized[11,17].

There are no major complications of the ^{32}P test. Some clinicians have speculated that it may predispose certain patients to leukemia, but this has not been substantiated, and it seems unlikely. We believe that this test is the most reliable ancillary procedure (other than performing a biopsy) now available for differentiating between benign and malignant lesions. It is only a diagnostic adjunct, however, and occasional false positive or false negative results will occur. We now reserve the ^{32}P test for cases in which some means of therapy will be employed if the test result is positive, suggesting a malignant lesion.

Radiology

Radiological examination is useful in the evaluation of suspected orbital tumors, but it has a limited role in the diagnosis of intraocular tumors, for which it is used primarily to detect intraocular calcium in cases of suspected retinoblastoma. Recently, X-ray examination has been found useful in the diagnosis of choroidal osteomas, and it can be of great value in eyes with encapsulated intraocular foreign bodies simulating a neoplasm. X-rays of the chest, skull and other structures are helpful in the overall evaluation of patients with possible malignant intraocular tumors or metastatic lesions to the eye.

Computerized tomography

The recent introduction of computerized tomography (CT scan) has helped considerably in the diagnosis of central nervous system and orbital tumors (*see* Chapter 12). For intraocular tumors, CT scan is valuable in the diagnosis of retinoblastoma and choroidal osteoma and in detecting extraocular extension of malignant tumors. Some investigators believe that it will have an even greater diagnostic role in the future.

Intraocular biopsy

The use of intraocular biopsy establishing the exact diagnosis of an intraocular tumor is usually not justified, because the diagnosis can usually be made with a high degree of accuracy using non-invasive methods. However, in some cases biopsy of intraocular tissue may be necessary. This can be done by vitrectomy to remove intravitreal cells in eyes with possible reticulum cell sarcoma[18]. The author has also used other intraocular biopsy methods in cases in which the diagnosis was especially difficult. First, we used a scleral trapdoor incision to obtain a wedge biopsy with a technique similar to that used for iridocyclectomy. More recently, we have successfully used a fine needle for transocular aspiration biopsy[19]. Our technique is a modification of a previously reported method[20].

The technique of transocular needle biopsy varies with the location of the tumor. If the lesion is on the iris, a 25 gauge needle is passed across the anterior chamber from the limbus on the opposite side. If the lesion is located in the ciliary body, choroid or retina, the approach also depends on whether or not the lens is present. In phakic eyes, the needle is passed through the pars plana on the side of the eye opposite the tumor (*Figure 11.20a*). In aphakic eyes the needle can be inserted either through the pars plana or at the limbus and passed through the pupil to reach the tumor (*Figure 11.20b*). Originally we performed the biopsy under direct visualization using the binocular indirect ophthalmoscope. More recently we have used the operating microscope with a contact lens.

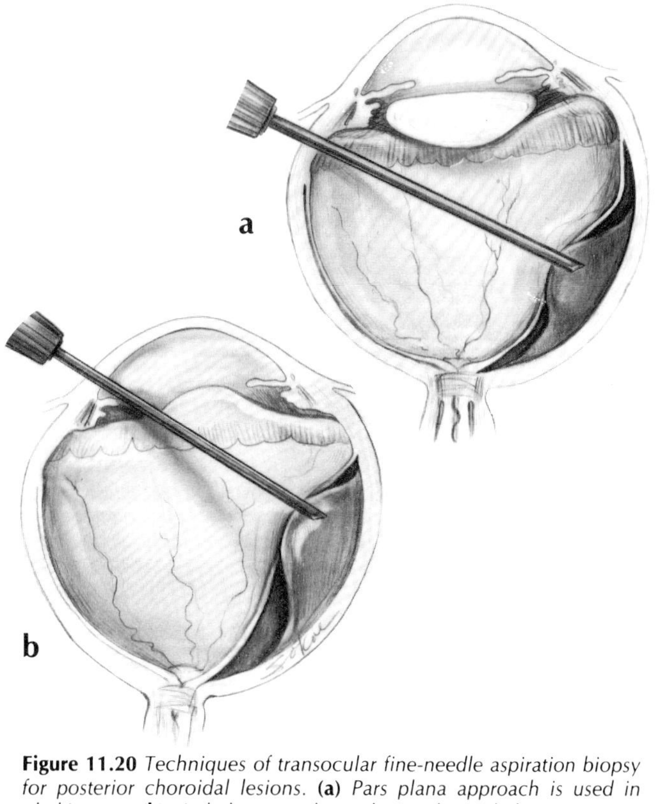

Figure 11.20 *Techniques of transocular fine-needle aspiration biopsy for posterior choroidal lesions.* **(a)** *Pars plana approach is used in phakic eyes.* **(b)** *Limbal approach can be used in aphakic eyes*

For biopsy, the tumor is penetrated with the needle, and a small amount of tissue is aspirated for routine cytological analysis. In cases with opaque media, ultrasonography can be used to guide the needle to the tumor. The indications and technique of intraocular fine-needle aspiration biopsy have been reported[19]. We currently reserve this test for cases in which the diagnosis is uncertain and when a therapeutic decision will be made based on the cytological findings. Fine-needle aspiration biopsy has been helpful in differentiating metastatic tumors from amelanotic melanomas and in the diagnosis of medulloepithelioma and lymphoid tumors. The full evaluation of this biopsy method and its limitations and possible complications must await additional clinical experience.

Additional ophthalmic consultation

Because of inherent difficulties in the diagnosis of intraocular tumors, we recommend that the patient be examined by more than one experienced ophthalmologist before a therapeutic decision is made. If the observers agree about the diagnosis, and if the ancillary diagnostic tests support their clinical impression, then necessary therapy should be begun. This careful approach minimizes the chance of an erroneous diagnosis and/or misdirected therapy.

Therapeutic alternatives

Intraocular tumors present special therapeutic problems. Since the treatment of intraocular tumors varies greatly according to the type of tumor, it is important first to establish the correct diagnosis, using the aforementioned methods. Important factors in making a therapeutic decision include: (*1*) the type of tumor and whether it is benign or malignant; (*2*) the location of the lesion; (*3*) the age and health of the patient; and (*4*) the condition of the fellow eye. In general, benign tumors are managed more conservatively than malignant lesions. Tumors located near the fovea or optic disc and causing visual loss are often managed differently from similar, but asymptomatic, tumors located in the peripheral fundus. Treatment is often different for elderly or chronically ill patients or for patients with the tumor in their only useful eye.

Newly developed methods of treatment have improved the management of certain intraocular tumors. Previously, enucleation of the involved eye was the generally accepted management of malignant tumors. There was no satisfactory treatment for benign tumors, and these sometimes caused significant visual loss from secondary complications. Improved therapeutic methods, such as irradiation, photocoagulation and cryotherapy, and better surgical techniques, combined with improved understanding of the biological behavior of various types of tumor, now provide a variety of reasonable therapeutic alternatives. Depending on the overall clinical situation, a particular tumor may now be managed by simple observation, photocoagulation, radiotherapy, cryotherapy, diathermy, local resection, enucleation, exenteration, chemotherapy or immunotherapy, or by a combination of these methods.

Observation

There are several situations in which simple periodic observation of an intraocular tumor is the preferred management. Benign lesions, for example, have little or no tendency to grow, and they usually require no therapy unless secondary complications occur. However, in some cases lesions that are presumably benign require careful periodic observation to be certain that they do not subsequently show malignant behavior, thereby indicating a need to change the diagnosis.

Benign conditions that do not require treatment include congenital hypertrophy of the RPE (*Figure 11.21*), melanocytoma of the optic nervehead (*Figure 11.22*) and retinal astrocytomas (*Figure 11.23*). Choroidal nevi (*Figure 11.24*) rarely require therapy unless they are associated with leakage through the RPE and symptomatic serous retinal detachment. Other benign tumors are more likely to

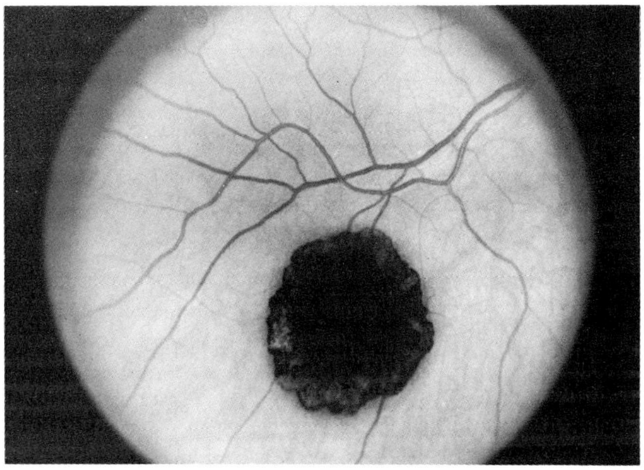

Figure 11.21 *Congenital hypertrophy of the RPE. This lesion is flat and has a sharp margin. It is benign and non-progressive and is managed by observation*

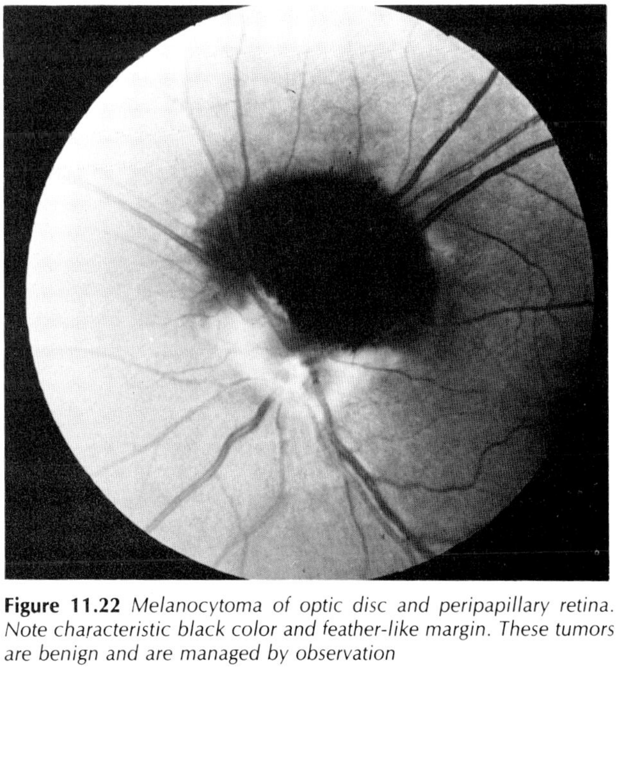

Figure 11.22 *Melanocytoma of optic disc and peripapillary retina. Note characteristic black color and feather-like margin. These tumors are benign and are managed by observation*

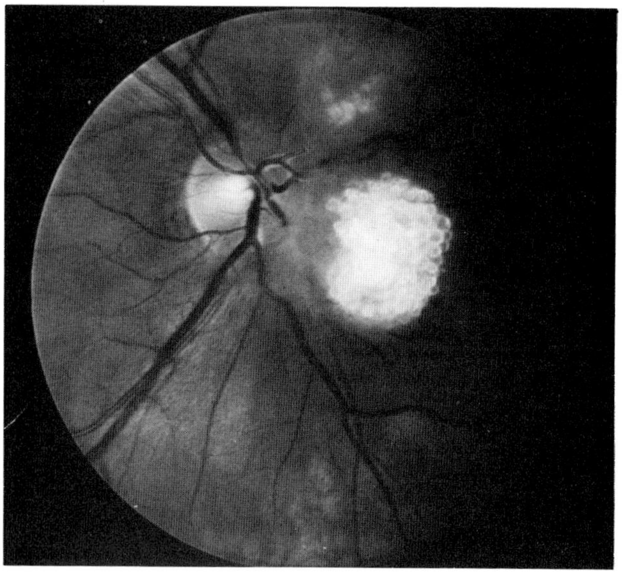

Figure 11.23 *Astrocytoma near optic disc in patient with tuberous sclerosis. These tumors are stationary or only slowly progressive and rarely require treatment*

require treatment because of visual symptoms or to prevent serious secondary complications. Such tumors include capillary hemangiomas of the retina and cavernous hemangiomas of the choroid.

Some form of treatment other than simple observation is usually necessary for malignant intraocular tumors. In recent years, however, we have become increasingly aware that certain small, presumably malignant lesions such as small choroidal melanomas, show little or no potential to cause local tissue damage or to metastasize. Therefore, an increasing number of authorities are advocating only periodic observation of suspected nevi and small to medium-sized melanomas for evidence of change before initiating treatment.

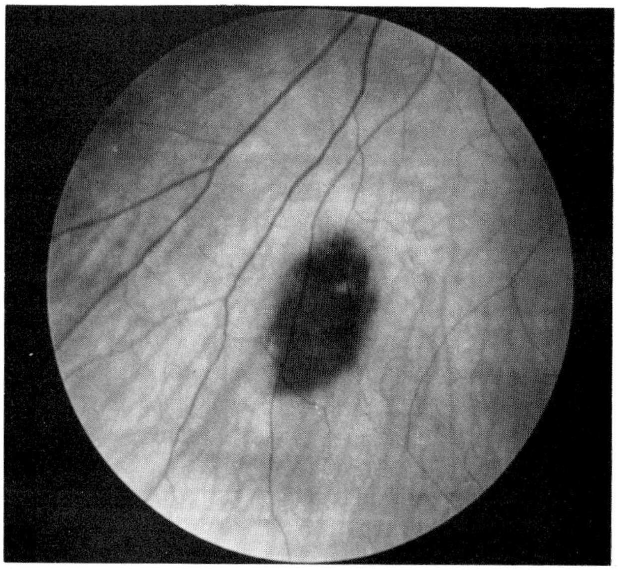

Figure 11.24 *Typical small choroidal nevus. These lesions are flat or only slightly elevated and are managed by observation*

If periodic observation is selected to manage a possibly malignant tumor, careful recording of baseline findings is necessary so that later changes can be detected. Detailed fundus drawings, photography, fluorescein angiography and ultrasonography may be useful. The ^{32}P test, which often involves a surgical procedure, should not be performed if periodic observation alone has already been selected. However, the ^{32}P test may provide useful information in cases in which differentiation between a benign and a malignant tumor is difficult and for diagnostic documentation in cases of choroidal melanoma being considered for treatment.

Photocoagulation (xenon arc and laser)

Light energy has been used for more than 30 years to treat selected intraocular tumors. The principle of therapy is that light energy is absorbed by pigment and thereby converted to heat energy. When there is enough heat to raise the temperature of the tissue sufficiently, protein is coagulated, producing a thermal effect or burn (photocoagulation)[21].

For photocoagulation to be effective, it is necessary to have both a light source and pigment to absorb the light energy. Light sources for ophthalmic use include the xenon arc tube and various types of lasers (*L*ight *A*mplification by *S*timulated *E*mission of *R*adiation, LASER). The RPE and the uveal pigment are well suited for absorption of light. Lesions that may be treated by photocoagulation include selected choroidal melanomas, retinoblastoma, retinal capillary hemangioma and choroidal hemangioma.

Choroidal melanoma

Both xenon arc photocoagulation and the argon laser have been used to treat selected choroidal melanomas. Levels of circulating antibodies produced in response to malignant melanoma increase after photocoagulation with either type of light source[22]. The significance of this finding is unclear.

Our current indications for considering photocoagulation in the management of choroidal melanoma are as follows: (*1*) the clinical diagnosis should seem clear – based on indirect ophthalmoscopy, fluorescein angiography and ultrasonography; (*2*) the lesion should show growth as documented by serial fundus photographs, or there should be strong evidence of prior growth seen on initial examination; and (*3*) the lesion should not exceed 10 mm in diameter or 3 mm in thickness as measured by A-scan ultrasonography[1,17].

There is controversy as to whether photocoagulation should be used for lesions located within 1.0 mm of the optic disc or foveola, or for lesions that have produced extensive retinal detachment. Photocoagulation is probably justified in selected cases of these types, but the prognosis for retention or recovery of good visual acuity is guarded.

Photocoagulation is done through a widely dilated pupil. Retrobulbar anesthesia is usually necessary when xenon photocoagulation is used, but topical anesthesia is often adequate when treatment is done with the argon laser. A Goldmann fundus contact lens or Rodenstock Panfundoscope lens is used with the laser.

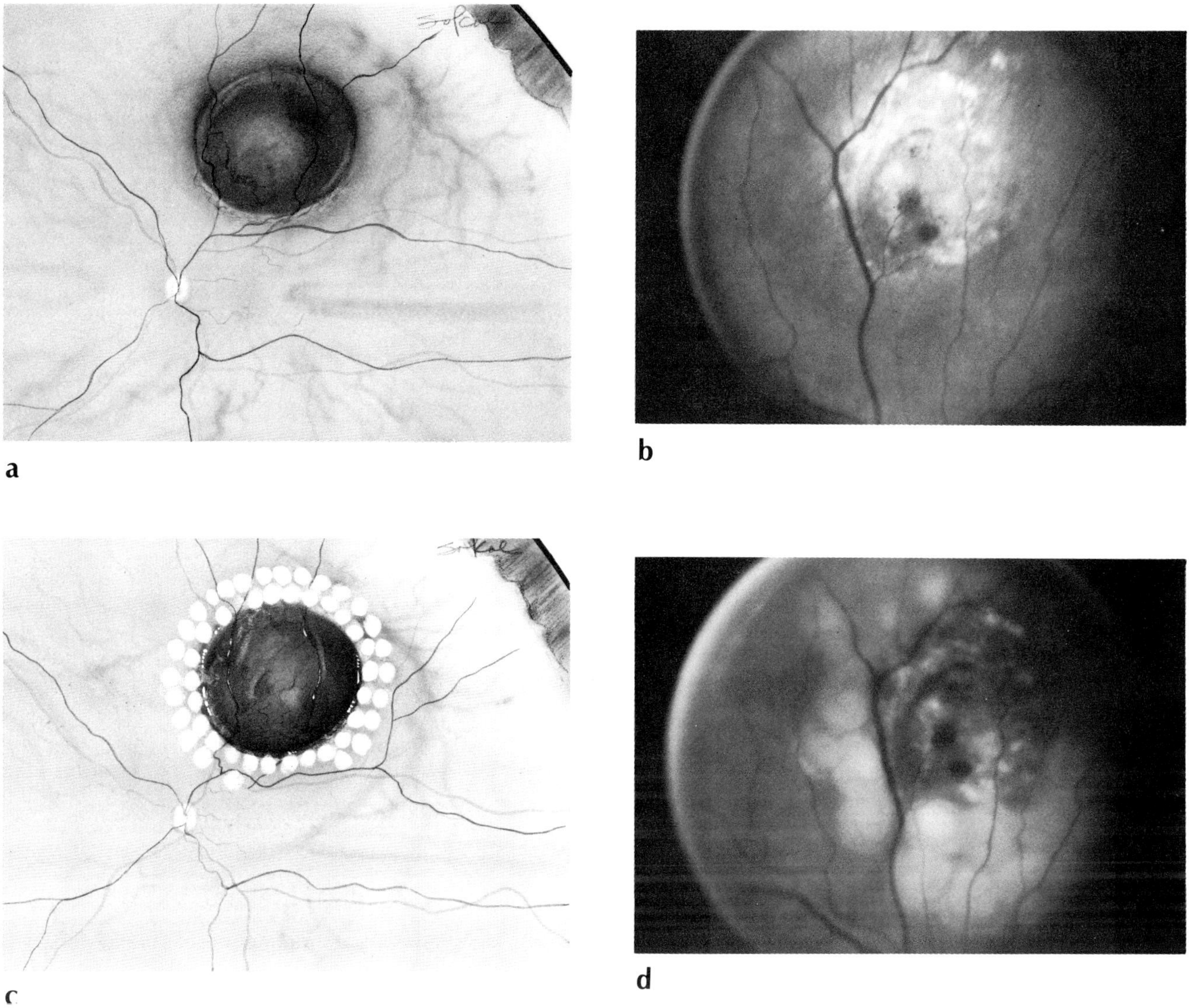

a b c d

Figure 11.25 *Photocoagulation of choroidal melanoma.* **(a,b)** *Tumor located superior to the optic disc in the left eye, with documented growth and positive* ^{32}P *test.* **(c,d)** *Technique of first photocoagulation session. Photocoagulation burns surround margins of tumor. This is repeated during second treatment session.*

Photocoagulation for a choroidal melanoma is done in multiple sessions. During the first session, two rows of treatment are applied in normal retina around the margins of the tumor to cause atrophy of the choroidal vessels (*Figure 11.25a–d*). With the argon laser, a spot size of 500 μm is used with duration of 0.5–1.0 second, and a power setting of 500–1000 mW. The intensity of the visible coagulation effect varies with the degree of pigmentation of the fundus. The same area surrounding the tumor is treated again 3 weeks later, using similar instrument settings.

A third treatment session, again using similar instrument settings, is done to cover the surface of the tumor about 3 weeks after the second treatment (*Figure 11.25e*). Subsequent treatment sessions, given every 3–4 weeks, repeat the photocoagulation covering the surface of the tumor. Four to 10 treatment sessions are usually necessary to produce a circular area of scar tissue through which the yellow sclera is clearly visible. A small flat area of pigmentation often remains in the center of this scar (*Figure 11.25f,g*). This central area of pigmentation is studied by fluorescein angiography, and when it is hypofluorescent, no further treatment is necessary. The residual central pigmentation eventually disappears in some cases.

Complications of photocoagulation for choroidal melanoma can include iris damage, hemorrhage, cystoid macular edema, retinal branch vessel obstruction, preretinal fibrosis, choriovitreal fibroneovascularization and traction retinal detachment. Damage to the iris can occur at the time of photocoagulation, especially if the pupil is not widely dilated, and this can result in focal or sector iris atrophy. An irregular pupil can result from damage to the sphincter or dilator muscles. Bleeding from photocoagulation can occur on the surface of the tumor or in the retina or vitreous. It occurs most often at the time of photocoagulation and usually resorbs within a few weeks.

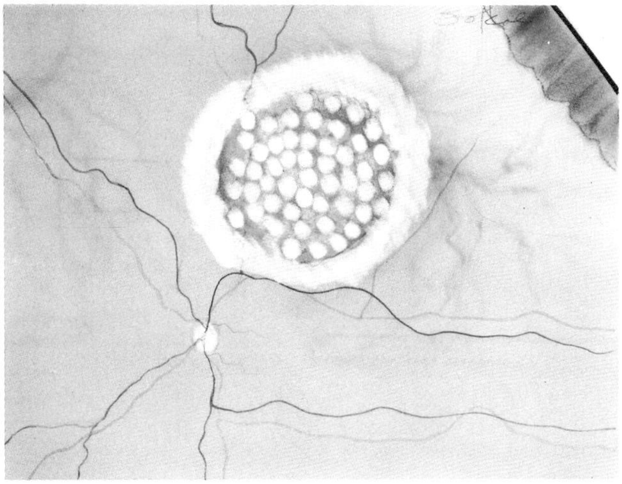

e

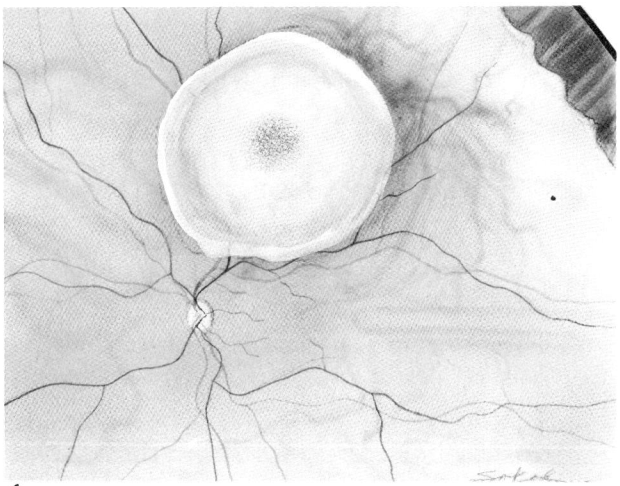

f

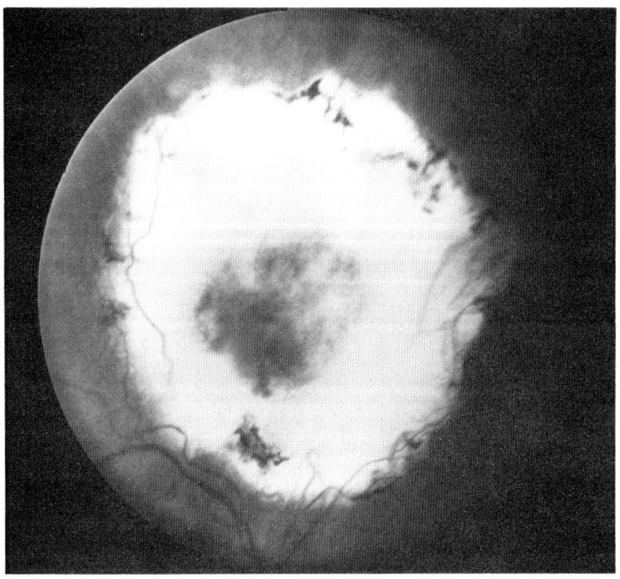

g

Figure 11.25 *(contd)* **(e)** *Photocoagulation is applied over anterior surface of tumor during third session and repeated several times at later sessions.* **(f,g)** *Final result with yellowish scar corresponding to prior margins of tumor, and flat central pigmentation*

Cystoid macular edema can develop after photocoagulation, especially if the xenon arc is used. The edema may result from vitreous traction or from inflammation causing increased permeability of the perifoveal capillaries. Although the cystoid maculopathy may partially resolve in time, it can cause permanent visual reduction.

Obstruction of a branch retinal artery or vein can occur during or after photocoagulation, especially if a large vessel passes over the tumor. Obstruction of a large retinal vein can lead to retinal or optic nervehead neovascularization. Heavy treatment, particularly with xenon photocoagulation, can lead to epiretinal membrane formation and result in macular pucker. If Bruch's membrane is disrupted by photocoagulation, choriovitreal neovascularization can occur. This may lead to vitreoretinal traction and subsequent retinal detachment.

Retinoblastoma

Photocoagulation is the treatment of choice for selected small retinoblastomas[23,24]. Xenon arc photocoagulation is used most commonly, because the currently available unit can be easily transported to the operating room. Photocoagulation can be used either as the primary treatment or as supplementary treatment in cases initially treated with irradiation or cryotherapy. When used properly, photocoagulation has fewer complications than irradiation.

Photocoagulation is indicated for small retinoblastomas confined to the sensory retina that do not involve the optic disc or the fovea (*Figure 11.26a,b*). It is usually performed under general anesthesia because of the patient's young age. Photocoagulation alone is usually contraindicated if there is ophthalmoscopic evidence of vitreous seeding, choroidal invasion or involvement of the fovea, optic disc or pars plana. Photocoagulation would not eliminate tumor cells in the vitreous, it probably would not destroy tumor cells in the choroid, and it might cause dissemination of the tumor in such cases. Photocoagulation would of course result in marked visual loss if used on the optic disc or fovea. External beam irradiation is preferred in such cases.

One or two rows of confluent photocoagulation burns are placed around the tumor, using enough power to whiten the surrounding retina and close the retinal vessels that supply the tumor (*Figures 11.26c,d*). The treatment should be heavy enough to obliterate these retinal vessels but not so heavy that it disrupts Bruch's membrane. Within a few weeks, the tumor regresses to become a depressed scar (*Figure 11.26e,f*). It may be necessary to apply a second and third treatment in some cases, waiting 3–4 weeks between sessions. Tumors located in the peripheral fundus can often be treated, using scleral indentation to assist if necessary.

Major complications from photocoagulation for retinoblastoma are uncommon but may occur if treatment is excessively strong. Vitreoretinal traction may lead to macular pucker or even retinal detachment. If Bruch's membrane is ruptured, choriovitreal neovascularization may occur. Minor complications such as small retinal or vitreous hemorrhages at the time of treatment usually do not cause serious problems.

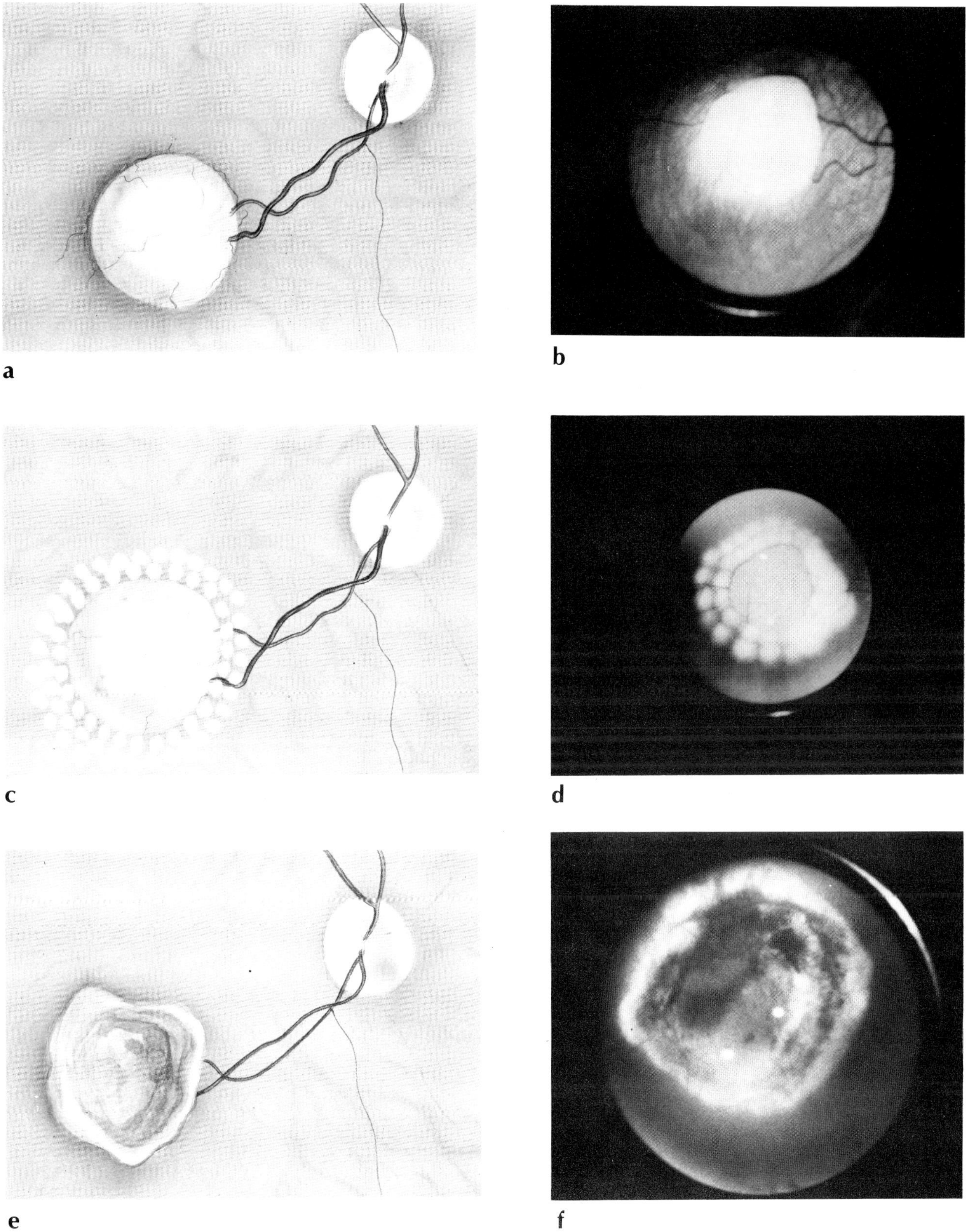

Figure 11.26 *Photocoagulation of small retinoblastoma.* **(a,b)** *Pretreatment appearance of intraretinal tumor inferotemporal to macula in right eye.* **(c,d)** *Photocoagulation technique with two rows of treatment around tumor. Tumor is not treated directly.* **(e,f)** *Final result, with depressed chorioretinal scar and no evidence of viable tumor*

Retinal capillary hemangioma

Retinal capillary hemangioma (von Hippel's tumor) is a non-malignant lesion that can lead to progressive exudative retinal detachment, macular exudation and profound visual loss. This tumor can be treated in some cases with either argon laser or xenon photocoagulation[25]. Photocoagulation can usually be done successfully if the hemangioma is less than 5 mm in diameter and has produced little or no retinal detachment. Because of the potential of these lesions to cause visual loss, most small angiomas are treated whether or not they have already caused secondary complications, unless they are located in the macula or over the optic nervehead.

There is some controversy as to the best technique for treating a retinal capillary hemangioma by photocoagulation. Small lesions less than 2 mm in diameter can be ablated by heavy treatment to the entire tumor (*Figure 11.27*). If the tumor is larger than 3 mm in diameter, photocoagulation should be used first to surround the tumor and close the feeder vessels (*Figure 11.28*). It is important that the feeding arteriole be closed first. The draining vein is closed during a later session. During subsequent sessions the margins of the tumor are treated directly, and the feeder vessels are re-treated until the lesion is atrophic. The macular exudate gradually resolves after the angioma has been destroyed.

The complications of photocoagulation for retinal capillary hemangioma can include hemorrhage, retinal detachment and vitreoretinal traction. Hemorrhage can occur

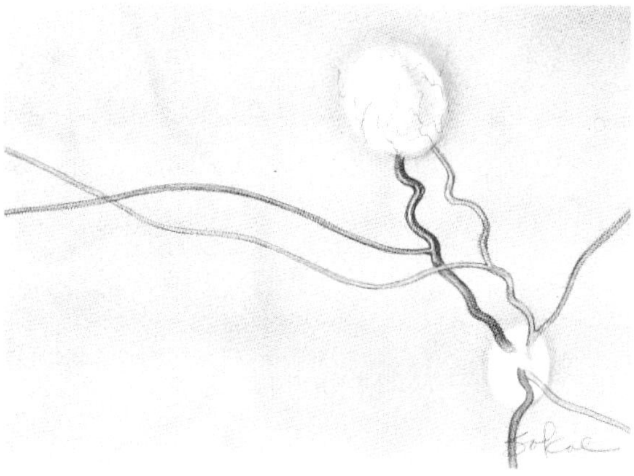

a

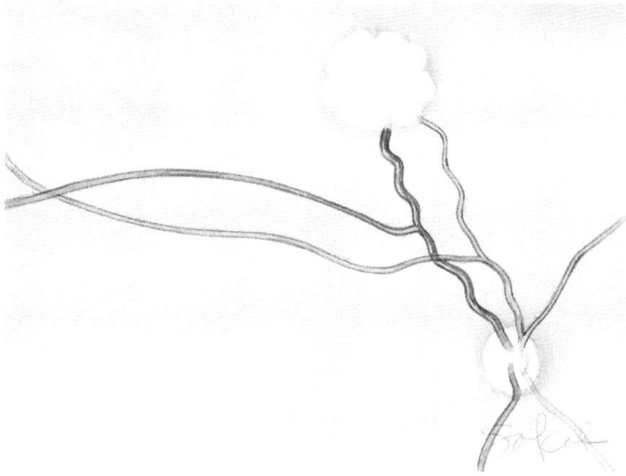

b

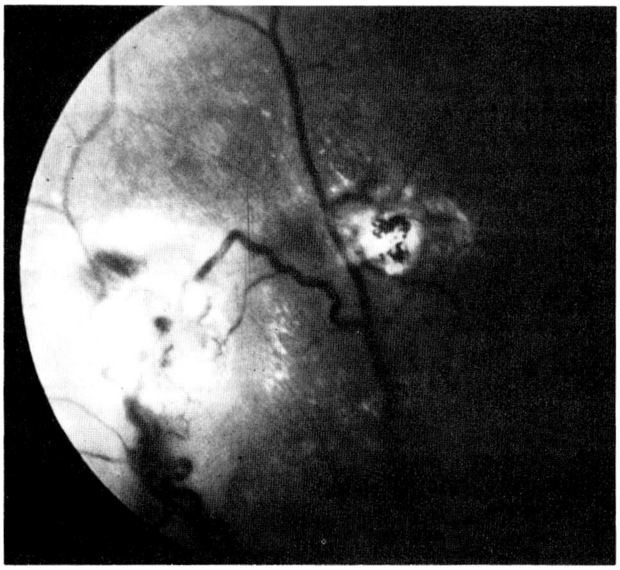

c

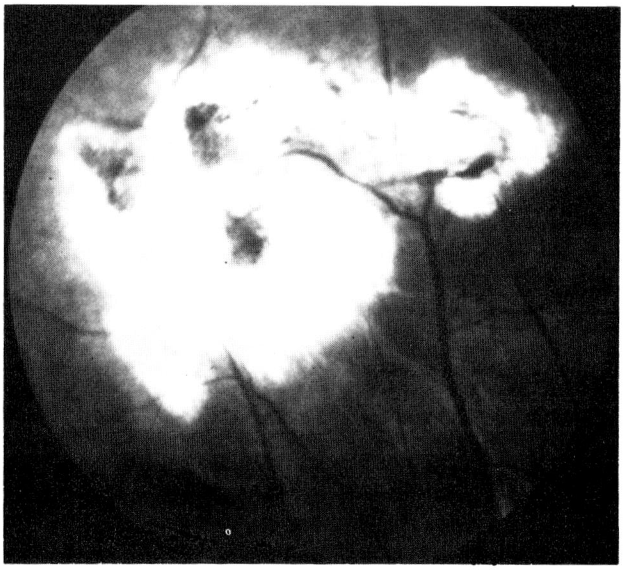

d

Figure 11.27 *Photocoagulation of small capillary hemangioma of retina.* **(a)** *Pretreatment appearance of angioma..* **(b)** *Angioma is treated with intense laser burns over the entire tumor. This usually causes complete destruction of small lesions.* **(c)** *Two capillary hemangiomas prior to treatment. Right tumor is smaller and left tumor is larger.* **(d)** *Appearance after photocoagulation, with complete destruction of both tumors (patient of Dr William H. Annesley, Jr)* from direct treatment to the tumor or from closure of the draining vein before the feeding artery. Transient, exudative retinal detachment can occur after photocoagulation, and this usually resolves spontaneously in a few weeks. Vitreoretinal traction is uncommon after argon laser treatment, but it occurs more frequently when xenon arc photocoagulation is used.

a

b

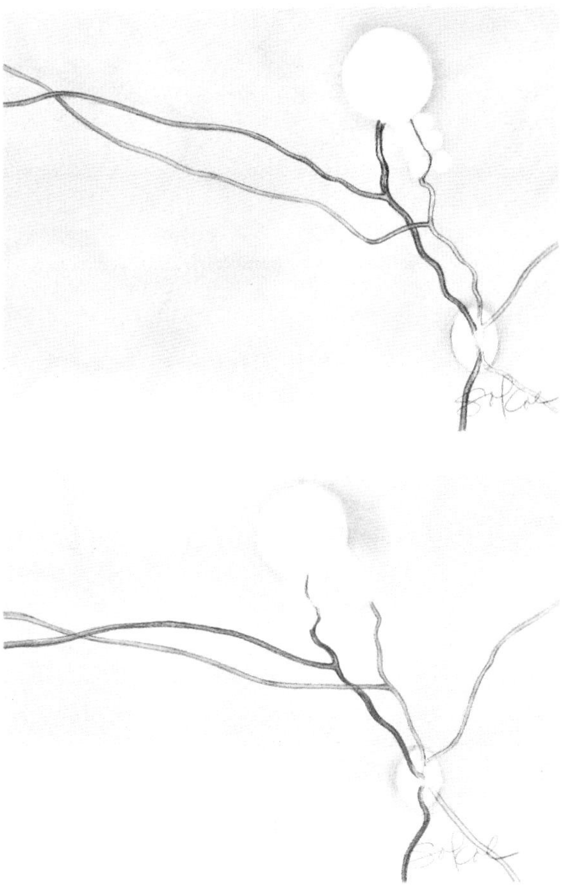

Figure 11.28 *Photocoagulation of larger retinal capillary hemangioma.* **(a)** *First, feeding arteriole is treated to stop blood flow to the tumor, but draining vein is not treated.* **(b)** *Three weeks later feeding arteriole is scarred and tumor is beginning to shrink. Draining vein is then treated with photocoagulation along its margins*

Choroidal hemangioma

Choroidal hemangiomas are benign vascular tumors that can cause marked cystoid edema in the overlying retina and may cause visual loss from serous detachment of the macula. Photocoagulation may help to resolve this detachment and improve vision[26].

Asymptomatic choroidal hemangiomas are not treated, but photocoagulation is recommended if a secondary retinal detachment threatens or involves the macula (*Figure 11.29a,b*).

The photocoagulation technique for choroidal hemangioma differs from that used for choroidal melanoma or retinoblastoma. Argon laser or xenon photocoagulation is applied lightly over the entire surface of the tumor to create a chorioretinal adhesion between the sensory retina and the RPE (*Figure 11.29c,d*). This prevents further accumulation of subretinal fluid and encourages resorption of the fluid already present. Treatment should be just intense enought to create a distinct burn on the surface of the tumor. This is usually done with a spot size of 200 μm of 0.2–0.5 second duration and a power setting of 200–500 mW, depending on the degree of fundus pigmentation and the amount of subretinal fluid over the tumor. It may be necessary to repeat the treatment on two or three occasions, at 3–4 week intervals.

Complications of photocoagulation for a choroidal hemangioma are similar to those of photocoagulation for other tumors. If treatment is too heavy over the surface of the tumor and causes rupture of Bruch's membrane, choroidal neovascularization with secondary exudation can occur. Because choroidal hemangiomas are often located near the fovea, contraction of the internal limiting membrane of the retina surrounding the area of photocoagulation can cause visual distortion (metamorphopsia).

Radiotherapy

Although irradiation may sometimes damage normal intraocular tissues, certain types of intraocular tumors can be successfully treated with radiotherapy[27,28]. These tumors include selected malignant melanomas, retinoblastomas, and metastatic tumors to the uveal tract. The two methods of radiotherapy used to treat intraocular tumors are external-beam irradiation and local application of a radioactive scleral plaque.

There are several methods of treating intraocular tumors with external-beam irradiation. Orthovoltage can be used to deliver radiation to the entire eye, and this is used mainly for diffuse neoplastic processes. Supravoltage, with use of a betatron or linear accelerator, has the advantage of a sharp beam and more precise focus. This is applicable to treatment of isolated or solitary tumors. More recently, other methods such as helium-ion irradiation and proton-beam irradiation using a Bragg peak have been used[29]. These newer techniques await further clinical evaluation.

Radioactive plaques applied to the sclera are especially suitable for treating malignant melanomas of the posterior uvea and retinoblastomas. Radon seeds, gold seeds in radon rings, and other devices have been used, but most ophthalmic oncologists now prefer cobalt-60 applicators. These plaques consist of a series of radioactive cobalt rings within a platinum envelope and are manufactured in several shapes and sizes.

Malignant melanoma

Because most melanomas are relatively radioresistant, a scleral plaque rather than external-beam irradiation is usually recommended for treatment of posterior uveal melanomas. This method provides greater radiation to the base of the tumor and less radiation to uninvolved portions of the eye. The indications for treating a choroidal

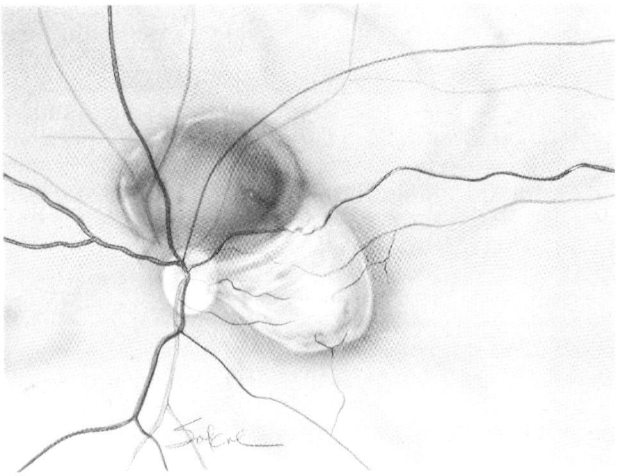

a

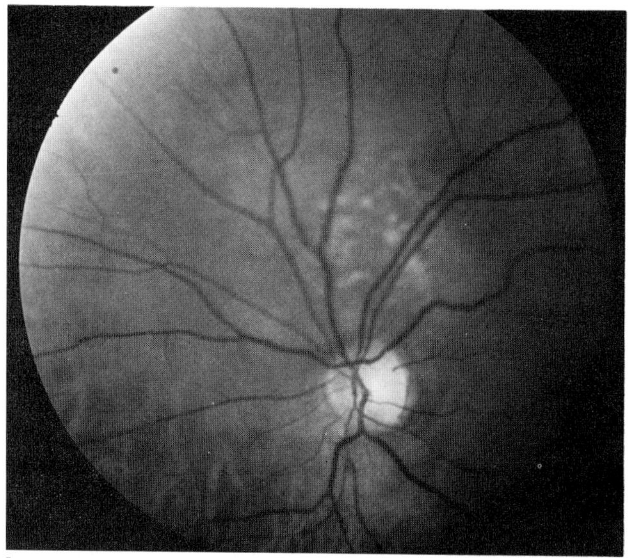

b

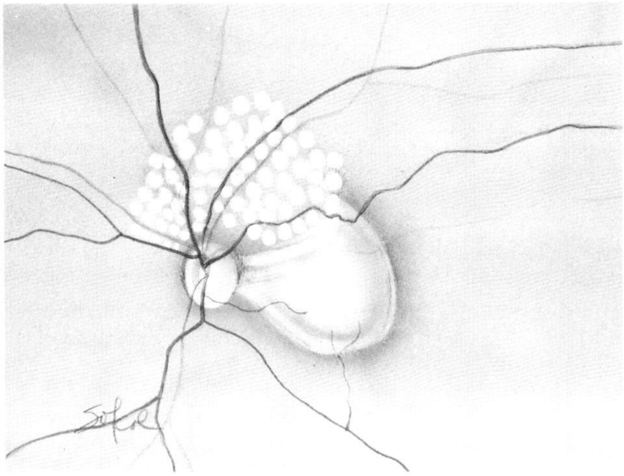

c

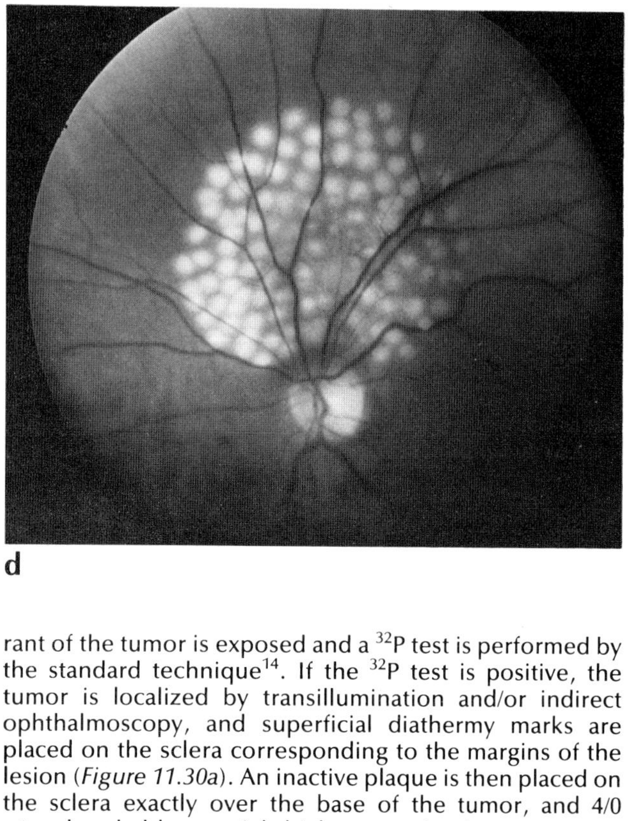

d

Figure 11.29 *Photocoagulation of choroidal hemangioma with secondary serous detachment of retina.* **(a,b)** *Tumor superior to disc, with subretinal fluid extending into macula.* **(c,d)** *Photocoagulation burns are placed over surface of tumor, extending just outside its margins. Subretinal fluid often resorbs in 2–3 weeks*

melanoma with cobalt plaque radiotherapy are still controversial. Our present indications, at the Oncology Service of the Wills Eye Hospital, Philadelphia, include tumors with evidence of growth and of a size greater than 6 × 6 mm diameter and 3 mm elevation but with a greatest diameter of less than 15 mm and an elevation of less than 8 mm. Also, vision should be useful or salvageable in the involved eye. Larger tumors are sometimes treated with a cobalt plaque if the tumor is in the patient's only useful eye.

A-scan ultrasonography is done preoperatively to determine the maximum thickness of the tumor. Calculations are made to determine the time necessary to deliver either a maximum of 8000 rad to the apex of the melanoma or a maximum of 40 000 rad to the base of the tumor. Depending on the strength of the cobalt plaque and the thickness of the tumor, this generally takes 6–12 days.

Insertion of the cobalt plaque can be done under local or general anesthesia. A peritomy is performed, the quadrant of the tumor is exposed and a ^{32}P test is performed by the standard technique[14]. If the ^{32}P test is positive, the tumor is localized by transillumination and/or indirect ophthalmoscopy, and superficial diathermy marks are placed on the sclera corresponding to the margins of the lesion (*Figure 11.30a*). An inactive plaque is then placed on the sclera exactly over the base of the tumor, and 4/0 non-absorbable partial-thickness scleral sutures are aligned with the holes in the plaque (*Figure 11.30b*). When the scleral sutures are in place, the inactive plaque is removed and replaced by the active cobalt plaque (*Figure 11.30c*). The sutures are then tied and cut, and the location of the plaque is rechecked. The conjunctiva is closed with interrupted 6/0 plain catgut sutures. Postoperatively, the patient is kept in a room separate from other patients.

When the calculated dose has been delivered to the tumor, the patient is taken back to the operating room for removal of the plaque. Under local anesthesia, the peritomy is reopened, the sutures holding the plaque are cut,

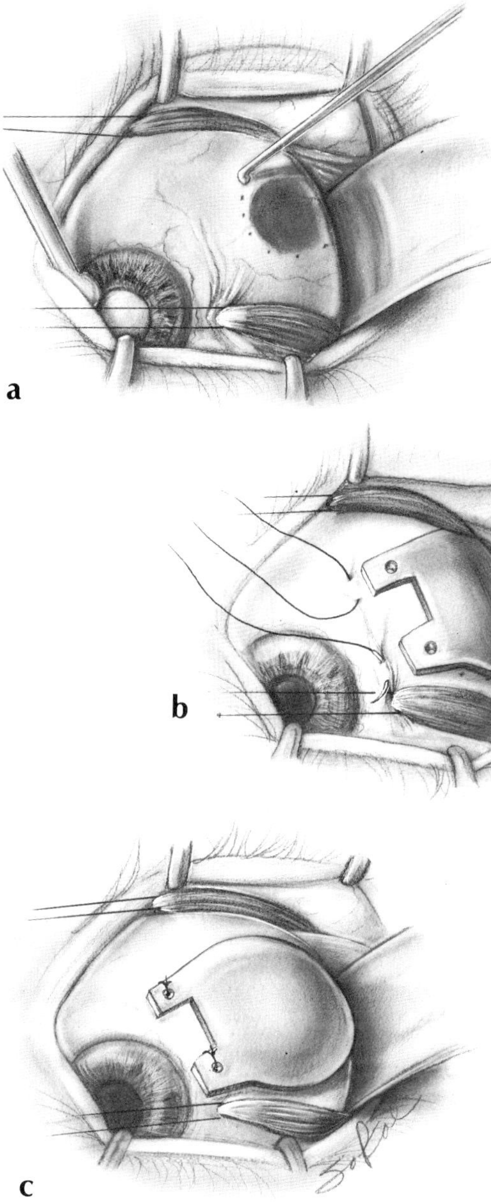

Figure 11.30 *Application of radioactive cobalt-60 plaque to sclera to treat choroidal malignant melanoma.* **(a)** *Tumor is localized by transillumination, and diathermy marks are placed around margin.* **(b)** *Inactive plaque is first positioned over tumor while aligning scleral sutures.* **(c)** *After removal of inactive plaque, cobalt plaque is tied into position*

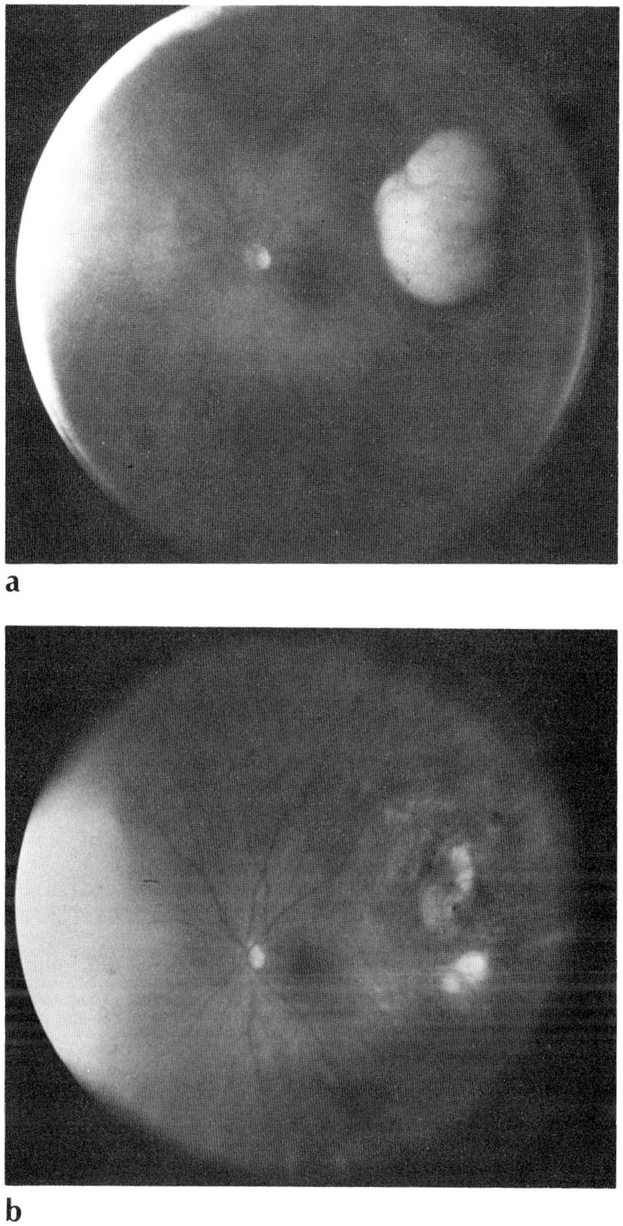

Figure 11.31 *Successful cobalt plaque therapy of mushroom-shaped choroidal melanoma.* **(a)** *Preoperative appearance, with 'Equator-Plus' camera view showing dome-shaped tumor temporal to macula in left eye.* **(b)** *Appearance 18 months later. Tumor has decreased from 7 mm to 1 mm thickness and seems inactive*

and the plaque is removed. The conjunctiva is closed with 6/0 plain catgut sutures, and the patient is discharged from the hospital the next day.

The treated eye is re-examined every 3–4 months. The rate of decrease in the size of the tumor is variable. However, when the melanoma is sensitive to irradiation, it usually becomes markedly smaller by 6–12 months after treatment (*Figure 11.31*).

The most serious complications from scleral plaque treatment are radiation retinopathy and cataract. Radiation retinopathy is characterized by obliteration of retinal capillaries, telangiectasia, exudates and superficial retinal hemorrhages. When radiation retinopathy involves the optic disc or macula, marked visual loss can result. Radiation retinopathy may become apparent between 6 and 24 months after treatment. Cataracts occur most commonly after cobalt plaque therapy of ciliary body melanomas, and they are uncommon after treatment of posterior choroidal melanomas. Such cataracts can be removed by conventional means if necessary.

Retinoblastoma

Retinoblastomas are more radiosensitive than posterior uveal melanoma. This tumor can be treated with either external-beam irradiation or scleral plaque irradiation.

External-beam irradiation is required when it is necessary to treat the entire globe with radiotherapy because of large or multiple tumors or vitreous seeding, or to prevent occurrence of new tumors. This is most frequently needed for treatment of the second eye if there is severe bilateral involvement, and the eye with the more advanced tumor is enucleated. External-beam irradiation is the treatment of choice for large tumors filling more than one-third of the globe, multiple tumors (*Figure 11.32*), or when there is extensive vitreous seeding by tumor cells. Bilateral external-beam irradiation is used if there are moderately advanced tumors in both eyes with sparing of half the retina; after enucleation if tumor is found histologically to extend along the optic nerve to the line of surgical transection; and when there is orbital recurrence of the tumor.

The method of external-beam irradiation most commonly used for retinoblastoma in the United States is via either an anterior or a temporal portal, with a linear accelerator emitting γ-rays. Previously, 7000–8000 rad were recommended, but now 3500–4000 rad delivered in divided doses over a 3 week period is the treatment of choice. The anterior portal technique involves a greater risk of causing radiation-induced cataract, but it provides irradiation to the ora serrata region. The temporal portal approach is less likely to cause cataract, but parts of the anterior retina, especially on the nasal side, may go untreated.

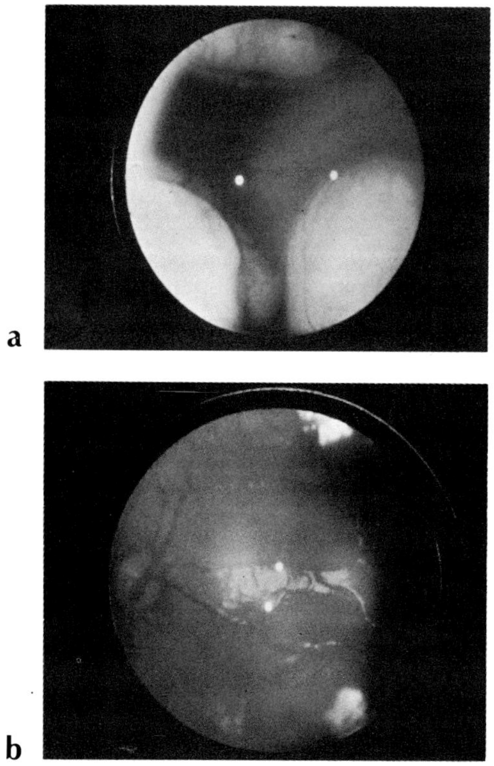

Figure 11.32 *External-beam irradiation for retinoblastoma.* **(a)** *Pretreatment appearance of three medium-size tumors in posterior pole as seen through indirect ophthalmoscope.* **(b)** *Appearance 4 weeks after 3500 rad of external-beam irradiation. Optic nerve is near left edge of lens. There has been marked regression of the tumors, and two show typical calcification*

After successful radiation treatment, a retinoblastoma usually appears as a shrunken white retinal mass. There may be pigmentary alterations and scar tissue around the regressed tumor. Three patterns of tumor regression after irradiation have been described. Type I is characterized by a white calcified mass that resembles cottage cheese. Type II has a pink translucent appearance that resembles fish flesh. Type III is a combination of Types I and II.

The main ocular complications of external beam irradiation for retinoblastoma are radiation retinopathy and cataract. Radiation retinopathy, as described earlier, is characterized by loss of small retinal vessels, secondary telangiectasia, and retinal edema and exudate. This may lead to retinal neovascularization and vitreous hemorrhage 6 months to several years after treatment. In some cases, the normal retinal vessels seem especially sensitive to irradiation, and extensive obliteration of the retinal vessels occurs. Other complications can include a dry eye, a sunken orbit with atrophy of the temporal fossa, and optic atrophy.

Perhaps the most important long-term complication of external irradiation is radiation-induced tumors. Radiation-induced orbital sarcomas, usually in the field of radiation, are the most common, but other malignancies such as lymphomas and leukemias have also occurred. The incidence of these tumors has decreased greatly since the radiation dose was reduced from 8000 to 3500 rad[30]. Recently, occurrence of new tumors distant from the area of irradiation has been noted, and neoplasms have also been recognized in patients who had no irradiation[31]. It is likely that patients with bilateral retinoblastoma have a greater statistical chance of developing other malignancies later in life, regardless of the type of treatment.

An alternative method of irradiation for retinoblastoma is application of a scleral plaque, most commonly a cobalt-60 plaque[24]. These plaques are used to treat retinoblastomas that are 6–15 mm in diameter and that are located at least 3 mm from the optic disc or macula. This treatment method can be used in unilateral cases or when treating the second eye in bilateral cases. Recurrent or residual tumors that have not been controlled by external beam irradiation, photocoagulation or cryotherapy can also be treated with a scleral plaque.

Relative contraindications to use of a cobalt plaque include tumors larger than 15 mm in diameter and those with extensive vitreous seeding. This technique should not be used for tumors touching or overlying the optic disc or tumors that involve the macula.

The surgical technique includes precise localization of the tumor by indirect ophthalmoscopy and scleral depression with a diathermy tip. The sclera is lightly marked with diathermy surrounding the margins of the tumors. An inactive plaque is then sutured over the base of the tumor and later replaced by the active plaque, using the technique previously described for treating malignant melanomas.

Retinoblastomas are treated with 3000–4000 rad delivered to the apex of the tumor. Most of these tumors show a dramatic response to irradiation (*Figure 11.33*). Shrinkage occurs within 3 weeks after removal of the plaque. The regression patterns are similar to those seen after external-beam irradiation.

The complications of cobalt plaque therapy, such as cataract and radiation retinopathy, are the same as can occur after external-beam irradiation. Although it is rare, scleral necrosis may occur many months later at the site of the plaque. It is uncertain whether radiation-induced sarcomas can occur after cobalt plaque therapy.

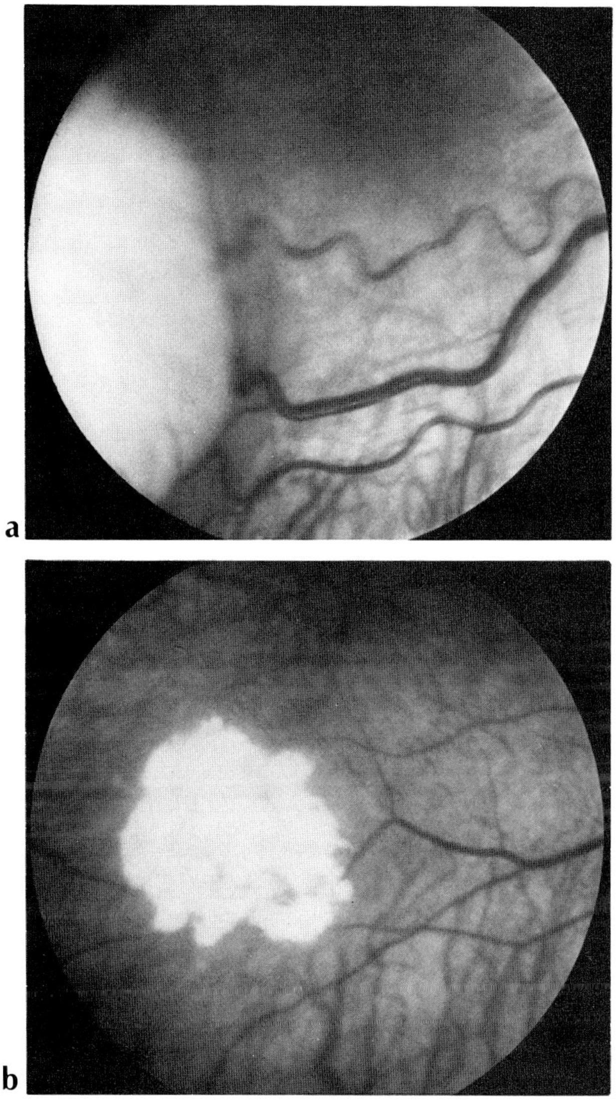

Figure 11.33 *Cobalt plaque therapy of retinoblastoma.* **(a)** *Moderate-size retinoblastoma temporal to macula in patient's only remaining eye.* **(b)** *Appearance 3 weeks after cobalt plaque radiotherapy. Note marked regression of tumor and residual calcification*

Metastatic tumors to the uvea

Chemotherapy is the basic treatment for metastatic tumors to the uvea, and about 50 per cent of these metastatic tumors are either asymptomatic or can be controlled systemically with chemotherapy alone[7]. In some cases this may be combined with ocular irradiation, and irradiation is used for tumors causing visual loss either because the tumor is located beneath the macula or because of secondary retinal detachment that involves the posterior pole.

Metastatic tumors to the uvea are also treated with external-beam irradiation to the whole eye, usually through a lateral portal approach. About 3000–4000 rad are delivered in divided doses over a 3 week period. Visual improvement after such treatment is often dramatic. A successfully irradiated metastatic choroidal tumor appears flat and creamy yellow in color, with overlying clumps of golden brown pigment (*Figure 11.34*).

The complications of irradiation for metastatic tumors are the same as those described previously for other ocular tumors. In our experience, however, there have been fewer complications after treatment of metastatic tumors than after treatment of choroidal melanoma or retinoblastoma. Perhaps this is because many patients with metastatic tumor do not survive long enough to develop the late complications of radiation therapy.

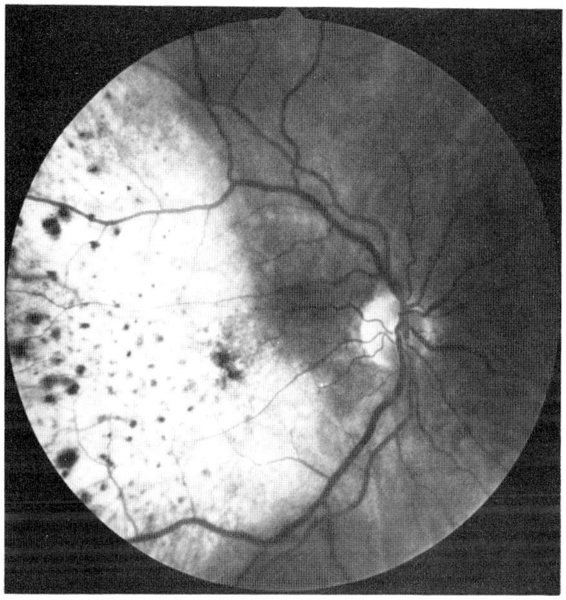

Figure 11.34 *Regression of metastatic tumor to macular area of right eye following radiotherapy. Visual acuity improved from 20/200 to 20/30. Note typical leopard-skin pigmentary changes on surface of flat amelanotic lesion*

Cryotherapy

Cryotherapy is of value in the management of selected intraocular tumors. It has been used successfully to treat retinal capillary hemangiomas and retinoblastoma and is occasionally used for small peripheral choroidal melanomas.

Retinal capillary hemangioma

Cryotherapy is the treatment of choice in cases of retinal capillary hemangioma in which the tumor is more than 5 mm in diameter and is producing secondary retinal detachment and/or exudation. Smaller retinal capillary hemangiomas in the peripheral fundus that cannot be photocoagulated can be treated with cryotherapy. Lesions in the peripheral fundus can be treated in transconjunctival fashion, but those located more posteriorly may require a conjunctival incision to reach the tumor.

The cryotherapy technique uses the cryoprobe as a scleral depressor, and the tumor is frozen while being observed by indirect ophthalmoscopy. (*Figure 11.35*). If the tumor is less than 3 mm in diameter it may be possible to freeze it completely with one application. However, if the tumor is greater than 3 mm in diameter, two or more applications may be necessary to treat the entire lesion. When treating larger angiomas, the cryoprobe is positioned straddling the margin of the tumor and adjacent normal retina. In each application, the freeze is applied until an ophthalmoscopically visible iceball envelops the tumor. The tumor is allowed to thaw for a few seconds and is then refrozen. This cycle is repeated three times.

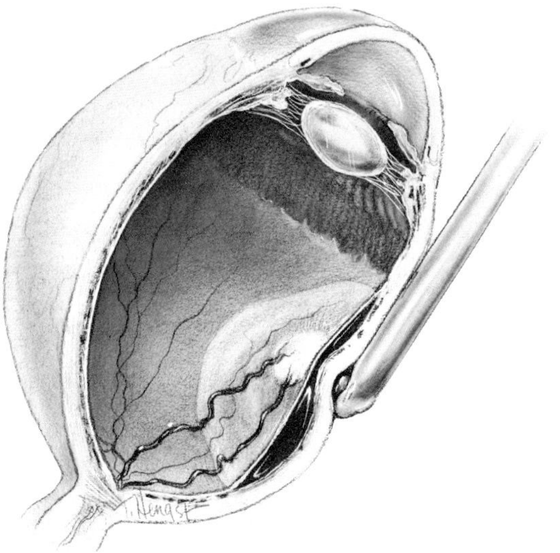

Figure 11.35 *Transscleral cryotherapy for retinal capillary hemangioma with secondary exudative retinal detachment. Cryoprobe is used to indent sclera and iceball envelopes angioma. The lesion is frozen three times*

The lesion is re-examined after 3 weeks, and treatment may be repeated then. The goal of treatment is to improve vision by causing absorption of subretinal fluid and clearing of lipid exudates, and not necessarily to destroy the tumor completely. Even if the tumor is still perfused, further treatment is withheld if macular exudation is resolving (*Figure 11.36*).

The main complications of cryotherapy for retinal capillary hemangioma are hemorrhage and retinal detachment. Hemorrhage can occur suddenly at the time of cryotherapy, and progressive exudative retinal detachment (ablatio fugax) can occur several hours after treatment. In most cases the hemorrhage or retinal detachment resolves spontaneously after several weeks.

Retinoblastoma

Cryotherapy is an effective method of destroying small retinoblastomas[23,24]. It may be used as the primary treatment or combined with other methods. Cryotherapy has the advantage of preserving Bruch's membrane and also the internal limiting membrane of the retina, and these structures may be natural barriers to the spread of tumor cells into the choroid or vitreous. Cryotherapy can also destroy small tumors in the choroid and in the vitreous near the surface of the main tumor.

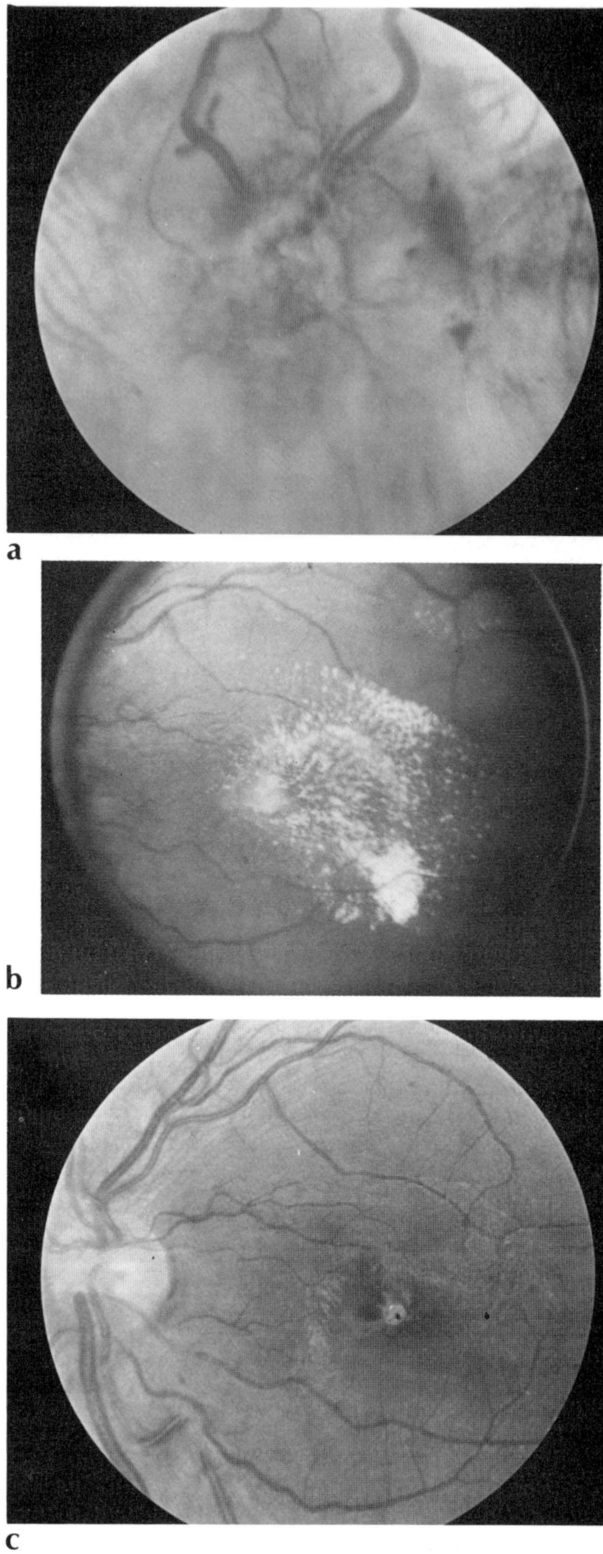

Figure 11.36 *Cryotherapy of retinal capillary hemangioma.* **(a)** *Appearance of lesion after several cryotherapy sessions showing shrinkage of the tumor but only slight change in feeder vessels.* **(b)** *Macular area with lipid deposits prior to treatment. Visual acuity was 20/200.* **(c)** *Macular area several months after cryotherapy of peripheral tumor. Macular exudation resolved, and visual acuity improved to 20/30. Tiny fibrotic nodule remains*

Cryotherapy is the primary treatment for small peripheral retinoblastomas located near the ora serrata. It is also used to treat residual or recurrent retinoblastoma in the peripheral fundus after incomplete eradication with external-beam irradiation. Recurrences are usually near the ora serrata inferiorly, probably because of incomplete irradiation of the anterior retina when a lateral portal is used.

Cryotherapy for retinoblastoma is administered by the triple freeze-thaw technique, as described above for treating retinal capillary hemangiomas. The cryoprobe is used as a scleral depressor, and the tumor is elevated on the probe tip (*Figure 11.37a*). Freezing is applied until the surrounding retina turns white and ice crystals appear in the overlying vitreous (*Figure 11.37b*). After freezing for 10–15 seconds, the tumor is allowed to thaw. It is then immediately refrozen, and the cycle is repeated. Three successive freeze-thaw applications are used. It may be necessary to repeat the treatment in 3–4 weeks if there is still ophthalmoscopic evidence of viable tumor. The tumor is considered to be eradicated when only a flat scar remains (*Figure 11.37c*).

The complications of cryotherapy for retinoblastoma are the same as those for treating retinal capillary hemangioma, although extensive exudative retinal detachment is rare. Local vitreous hemorrhage can occur at the time of treatment, but this usually resolves within several days or a few weeks.

Diathermy

Before the development of photocoagulation and cryotherapy methods, diathermy was used to treat selected cases of choroidal melanoma, retinal angioma and certain other tumors. Since it involves considerable damage to the sclera, it is rarely used today, especially for malignant tumors. Diathermy is still useful, however, to treat retinal capillary hemangiomas associated with extensive exudative retinal detachment. In such cases, a scleral buckling procedure with penetrating diathermy to the angioma can be effective[25].

Iridectomy

Iridectomy is surgical excision of a portion of the iris. Melanomas of the iris, if removed, are most commonly excised with a sector iridectomy, removing a portion of the iris from the pupillary margin to the iris root. Sector iridectomy is not commonly indicated for other iris tumors.

Most melanomas of the iris are relatively benign, slow-growing or non-growing tumors that pose no major threat to the patient's eye or life. If a suspected iris tumor demonstrates unequivocal growth, however, an iridectomy is justified. Iridectomy may also be indicated for biopsy of a diffuse iris tumor with secondary glaucoma, to determine whether the diffuse lesion is a nevus or a melanoma before making a therapeutic decision. Rarely, it may be necessary to perform an iridectomy for a suspected metastatic tumor to the iris when no tissue diagnosis of metastatic disease has been established systemically. However, in these rare cases it may also be possible to aspirate aqueous humor from near the surface of the lesion to gather cells for cytological study rather than excising the lesion.

Local anesthesia is usually sufficient for iridectomy. This may dilate the pupil somewhat, but it does not interfere with the surgical procedure. General anesthesia is used

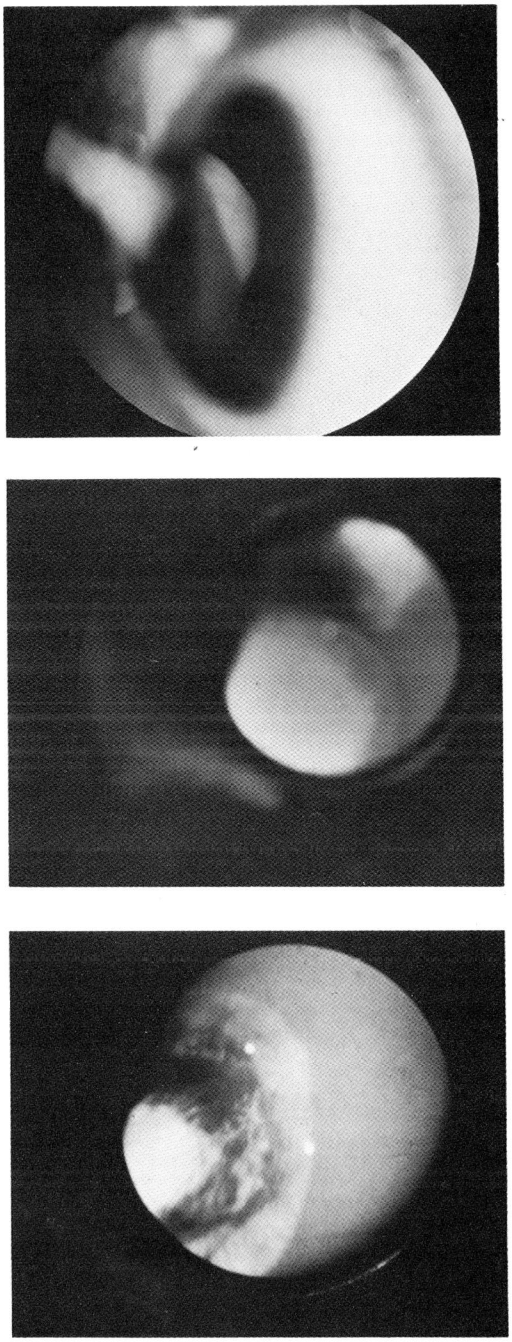

a

b

c

Figure 11.37 *Cryotherapy of retinoblastoma.* **(a)** *Small retinoblastoma near ora serrata as seen on tip of scleral depresser.* **(b)** *Cryotherapy of retinoblastoma, showing iceball extending transsclerally to incorporate intraocular tumor.* **(c)** *Appearance of lesion several weeks later. Retinoblastoma has regressed, leaving flat pigmented scar* when the patient is young. Acetazolamide and/or osmotic agents are used to lower the intraocular pressure before surgery.

The operating microscope is used because high magnification gives better visualization of the tumor and the operative field. A corneoscleral limbal incision for 180° is made in the area of the tumor. This incision may be larger or smaller than 180°, depending on the anticipated size of the iridectomy. However, it is better to have an incision that is too large than one that is too small.

Preplaced sutures may be used. The cornea is retracted with a suture through the corneal margin. The iris is elevated to avoid damage to the lens, and radial incisions are made in the iris on either side of the tumor (*Figure 11.38a*). The iris root is gently torn free or cut with the iridectomy scissors, and the specimen is removed (*Figure 11.38b*). Wet-Field diathermy is used to stop any bleeding from the anterior chamber angle. The preplaced corneoscleral sutures are tied, and additional sutures are added to obtain watertight closure. Removal of the tumor by this method leaves a keyhole-shaped pupil (*Figure 11.38c*).

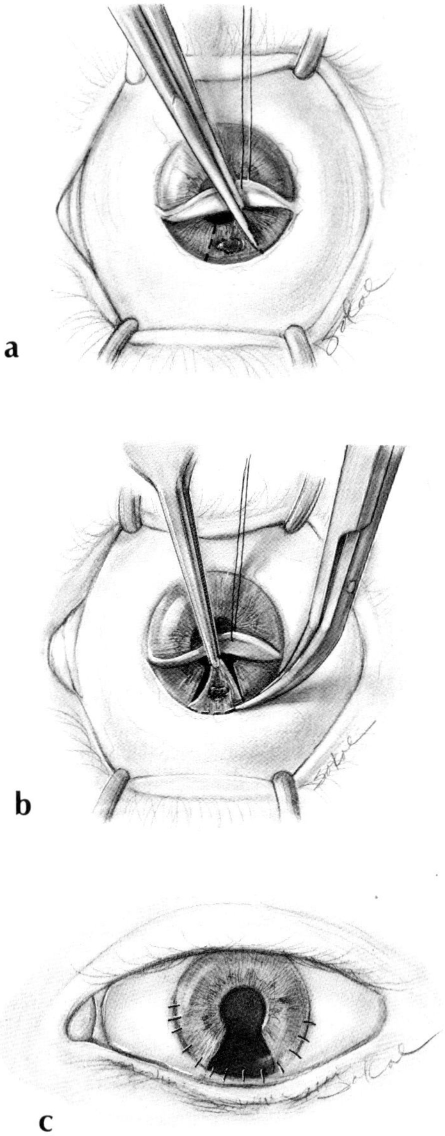

Figure 11.38 *Iridectomy for growing iris tumor.* **(a)** *Limbal incision is made and cornea is retracted. Radial incisions are made in iris on either side of tumor.* **(b)** *Base of iris is cut with the scissors.* **(c)** *Final appearance, with 'keyhole' pupil*

The specimen is kept flat and is allowed to dry for a few minutes on a thin piece of cardboard. It is then placed in 10 per cent formaldehyde. This method prevents rolling or folding of the specimen and facilitates proper orientation for pathological study.

Postoperatively, the eye is treated with a topical cycloplegic medication and a corticosteroid-antibiotic combination. The eye is examined daily, including measurement of the intraocular pressure, and the patient is discharged from the hospital on the second or third day. The eye is examined 1 week later and then monthly for a period of 3 months. The topical medications are discontinued after 1–2 weeks. Re-evaluation is done every 6 months to 1 year, including gonioscopy to look for recurrence of the tumor in the anterior chamber angle.

The complications of iridectomy can include hyphema, iridodialysis, cyclodialysis and, rarely, vitreous loss. A postoperative hyphema usually resolves in a few days. Iridodialysis rarely causes problems unless it is extensive. Cyclodialysis with persistent hypotony can be treated by argon laser photocoagulation applied through a gonioprism, to cause scarring in the anterior chamber angle and to close the cleft. Vitreous loss usually occurs only if the lens is subluxed.

Iridocyclectomy

Iridocyclectomy is the surgical removal of part of the iris and ciliary body. The major indication for this procedure is a melanoma of the iris and ciliary body. The tumor should involve no more than 4 clock-hours as measured along the limbus. Treatment of tumors larger than 4 clock-hours by iridocyclectomy has given such poor visual results that enucleation or scleral plaque radiotherapy is preferred.

Either local or general anesthesia can be used for iridocyclectomy, but we prefer general anesthesia because the operation can be prolonged. Because the chance of vitreous loss is significant, preoperative osmotic agents are used routinely. Preoperative pressure on the eye to reduce the vitreous volume is *not* indicated, because of the possibility of forcing tumor cells out of the eye.

There are several techniques for iridocyclectomy. We prefer a fornix-based conjunctival flap to expose the sclera, and localization of the tumor by transillumination. An anteriorly hinged square or rectangular scleral flap of four-fifths scleral depth is prepared with a 2 mm margin around the tumor (*Figure 11.39a,b*). This flap is dissected forward to the limbus, and diathermy is applied to the remaining inner scleral fibers surrounding the tumor. The anterior chamber is then entered at the limbus, and radial incisions can be made in the iris by the method described previously. Instead of cutting the iris at its root, however, the radial incisions are extended posteriorly to excise the inner wall of the sclera and the underlying ciliary body around the tumor. Alternatively, the deep scleral flap can be prepared first, diathermy applied around the tumor,

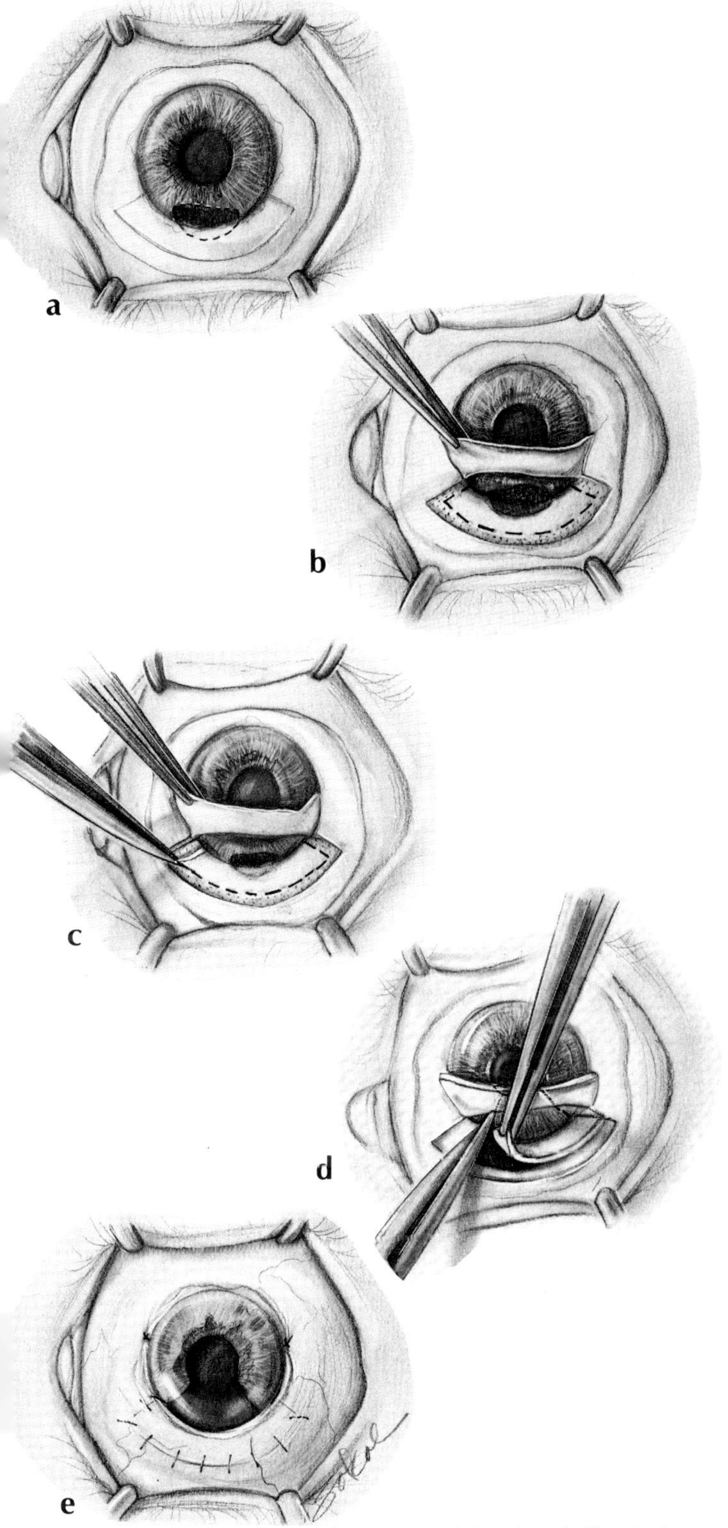

Figure 11.39 *Iridocyclectomy for tumor involving iris and ciliary body.* **(a)** *Flieringa ring is sutured to sclera (not shown), tumor is localized with transillumination, conjunctiva is reflected and scleral flap outlined. Dotted line shows margin of tumor.* **(b,c)** *Scleral flap is pulled forward, and second smaller scleral incision is made 2 mm outside the tumor margin. Diathermy is placed around margin of tumor to prevent hemorrhage or retinal detachment.* **(d)** *Tumor is then resected and sector iridectomy is done along dotted lines.* **(e)** *Final appearance, showing sector iridectomy with sutures used to close scleral flap*

and the ciliary body and iris then excised in a posteroanterior direction (*Figure 11.39c,d*). The iris and ciliary body containing the tumor and the attached inner scleral fibers are removed in one piece. The scleral flap is then closed with interrupted or running sutures (*Figure 11.39e*). The specimen is handled as described previously for iridectomy specimens.

The complications of iridocyclectomy include those that can occur after iridectomy, such as hyphema, iridodialysis and vitreous loss. Also, because of the more posterior incision, iridocyclectomy is more likely to be complicated by subluxation of the lens and vitreous hemorrhage. If the tumor extends to the ora serrata, iridocyclectomy can result in a retinal dialysis and detachment.

Sclerochorioretinal resection

Sclerochorioretinal resection, or full-thickness eye-wall resection, is a technique sometimes used to remove melanomas of the peripheral choroid[17,32]. Some authorities believe that sclerochorioretinal resection is never indicated and that peripheral choroidal melanomas that show signs of growth should be managed by irradiation or enucleation. The author has found it useful, however, in selected cases. The melanoma should be located in the peripheral choroid and should show evidence of growth. The findings of fluorescein angiography, ultrasonography and the ^{32}P test should all be compatible with the diagnosis of malignant melanoma. The tumor should not exceed 8 mm in diameter and 6 mm in thickness. There should be minimal retinal detachment, and the vitreous should be clear, to permit preoperative photocoagulation.

Sclerochorioretinal resection requires preparatory photocoagulation or cryotherapy to produce a chorioretinal adhesion for 2–3 mm around the tumor. It may take two to four treatment sessions to achieve a satisfactory result. Later, at the time of surgery, a specially designed eye basket is used to stabilize the globe, and the ring of the basket is sutured to the sclera surrounding the margins of the tumor.

Alternating partial-thickness incisions and diathermy are used to penetrate the sclera almost to the choroid, around the tumor. A piece of sclera from a donor eye is cut to fit the defect where the eye wall will be removed. The choroid is then incised, and the full-thickness eye wall specimen is removed, including the sclera, the choroidal tumor and the overlying retina (*Figure 11.40a,b*). A vitrectomy is performed through the defect, using a standard vitrectomy probe (*Figure 11.40c*). The scleral graft is then sutured into the defect with non-absorbable 4/0 or 5/0 sutures (*Figure 11.40d*). Postoperative ophthalmoscopy permits a clear view of the scleral graft and the surrounding photocoagulation.

There are many potential complications of sclerochorioretinal resection for choroidal melanomas. Because preoperative photocoagulation is necessary, all of the complications of photocoagulation can also occur. If xenon photocoagulation is used, there is a high incidence of cystoid macular edema. Operative complications can include vitreous hemorrhage and retinal detachment. They are most likely to occur when cutting through the area of previous photocoagulation. Postoperative complications can include cataract, vitreoretinal fibrosis, traction retinal detachment and anterior segment ischemia.

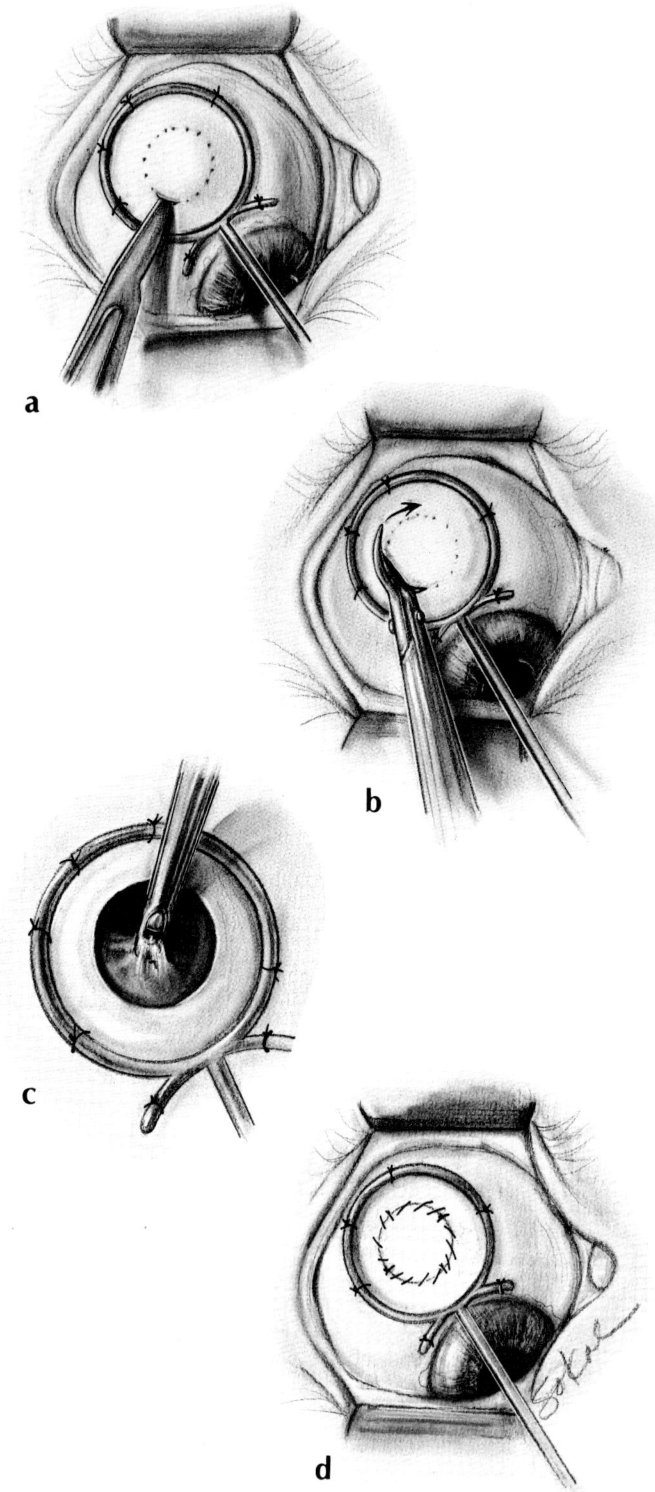

Figure 11.40 *Sclerochorioretinal resection (full-thickness eye-wall resection)*[32] *for peripheral choroidal melanoma.* **(a)** *Eye basket is sutured to sclera, and margins of tumor are outlined with diathermy. Scleral incision is made through diathermy marks within zone of previous photocoagulation surrounding tumor.* **(b)** *Scissors can be used to cut out full-thickness eye wall including the sclera, choroid containing the tumor, and adjacent retina.* **(c)** *Vitrectomy is performed through the scleral opening.* **(d)** *Sclera from eye-bank tissue is sutured in place with running stitch to close defect*

Enucleation

Enucleation (removal of the eye) is sometimes necessary when managing an intraocular tumor. The two intraocular malignant tumors most commonly managed by enucleation are retinoblastoma and malignant melanoma of the uvea. The subject of standard enucleation is discussed and illustrated in Chapter 3. Only additional points related specifically to intraocular tumors are presented here.

Retinoblastoma

Enucleation of the involved eye has been the traditional method of treating severe cases of retinoblastoma. Early enucleation after the clinical diagnosis is probably the main reason for improvement in the survival rate with this tumor during the last 50 years. Enucleation is recommended for all unilateral cases in which the tumor fills most of the globe and in which there is little hope of salvaging useful vision. If half the retina is free of tumor, other methods of treatment may be considered, provided the parents are informed about the possibility of metastasis and the complications of treatment.

In bilateral cases, the eye with the most advanced tumor is usually enucleated, and the less involved eye is managed with irradiation or other methods. However, if the eye with the most advanced disease has sparing of more than half the retina, an attempt may be made to salvage both eyes with treatment other than enucleation.

If both eyes have far-advanced tumors and there is no hope of any vision, bilateral enucleation is advised. Bilateral irradiation and careful follow-up may be an acceptable alternative in such cases, if the parents are fully informed and choose radiotherapy in preference to bilateral enucleation.

The technique of enucleation for retinoblastoma is only slightly different from the standard enucleation technique performed by most ophthalmic surgeons. Because retinoblastoma is a loosely cohesive malignant tumor, special care is taken to ensure gentle handling of the tissues; and because it may invade the optic nerve, as long a section of optic nerve as possible is removed with the eye.

Using general anesthesia, a peritomy is performed at the limbus for 360°, and the connective tissue between the rectus muscles is separated with enucleation scissors. The four rectus muscles are gently hooked, clamped and cut. The stump of the medial rectus muscle on the globe should be long enough to be grasped with a hemostat for traction when the optic nerve is sectioned.

The oblique muscles are then gently hooked, clamped and cut. All four quadrants are checked to make sure there are no adhesions between the sclera and the orbital tissues. A hemostat is used to grasp the stump of the medial rectus muscle, and the globe is pulled forward. Enucleation scissors are placed adjacent to the sclera nasally and are directed as far as possible into the orbit posteriorly. During firm traction on the medial rectus stump, the optic nerve is cut and the globe removed.

Gauze is placed in the socket until hemostasis is achieved. A 14 mm or 16 mm silicone sphere implant is then placed in the socket, and Tenon's capsule is closed over the implant with 4/0 chromic catgut mattress sutures.

A second layer of more superficial Tenon's fascia is closed with interrupted 4/0 chromic catgut sutures. The conjunctiva is then closed with a horizontal running 6/0 plain catgut suture. A plastic conformer is placed between the conjunctiva and eyelids, antibiotic ointment is applied and a pressure patch is used for 36–48 hours. A temporary prosthesis is fitted in 3–5 weeks.

There are few major complications of enucleation for retinoblastoma when performed carefully. Hemorrhage at the time of surgery may be controlled with orbital compression. Postoperative ecchymosis of the eyelids subsides spontaneously. Patients receiving chemotherapy may develop recurrent infections of the eye socket, but this is easily managed with appropriate antibiotic therapy. Long-term complications such as a sunken orbit are managed by adjustments of the prosthesis or by reconstructive plastic surgery.

Malignant melanoma

Enucleation has long been considered the treatment of choice for most choroidal melanomas, but this method of treatment has recently been challenged by some authorities[33]. We believe, however, that there are specific indications for enucleation of an eye with a uveal melanoma. The technique of enucleation has also been challenged, and recently a freezing 'no-touch' technique has been advocated[34]. We use this technique for most cases of malignant melanoma and for some cases of retinoblastoma.

Indications for enucleation in cases of uveal melanoma include: (*1*) a diffuse iris melanoma that is causing severe secondary glaucoma and is too large to resect surgically; (*2*) a ciliary body or choroidal melanoma that has produced significant visual loss and is too large to treat with irradiation or resection; and (*3*) any posterior uveal melanoma that has produced a total retinal detachment, dense cataract and secondary glaucoma.

We use a modification of the 'no-touch' enucleation technique. The conjunctiva is opened at the limbus for 360°, and the subconjunctival connective tissues are gently dissected in the four quadrants, using spring-action scissors. The rectus muscles are identified without hooking them and are cut at their insertions. A retractor is then placed between the sclera and Tenon's capsule in the quadrant of the tumor. A special cryo-ring is inserted between the retractor and the globe (*Figure 11.41a*). The cryo-ring is then activated to freeze the tumor and to attach the globe firmly to the probe (*Figure 11.41b*). When a satisfactory iceball has formed, the enucleation scissors are inserted, the optic nerve is cut, and the eye is elevated by pulling upward with the cryo-ring (*Figure 11.41c*). The oblique muscles and other tissue attachments are cut, and the eye is removed. After hemostasis has been achieved, an 18 mm silicone sphere is inserted into the socket, and the tissues are sutured closed as previously described for enucleation for retinoblastoma.

The technique of enucleation may sometimes be modified further. If invasion of the optic nerve is suspected clinically, it is desirable to obtain a long section of optic nerve. After cutting the rectus and oblique muscles, traction sutures are placed on the rectus muscle stumps to elevate the globe further before cutting the optic nerve.

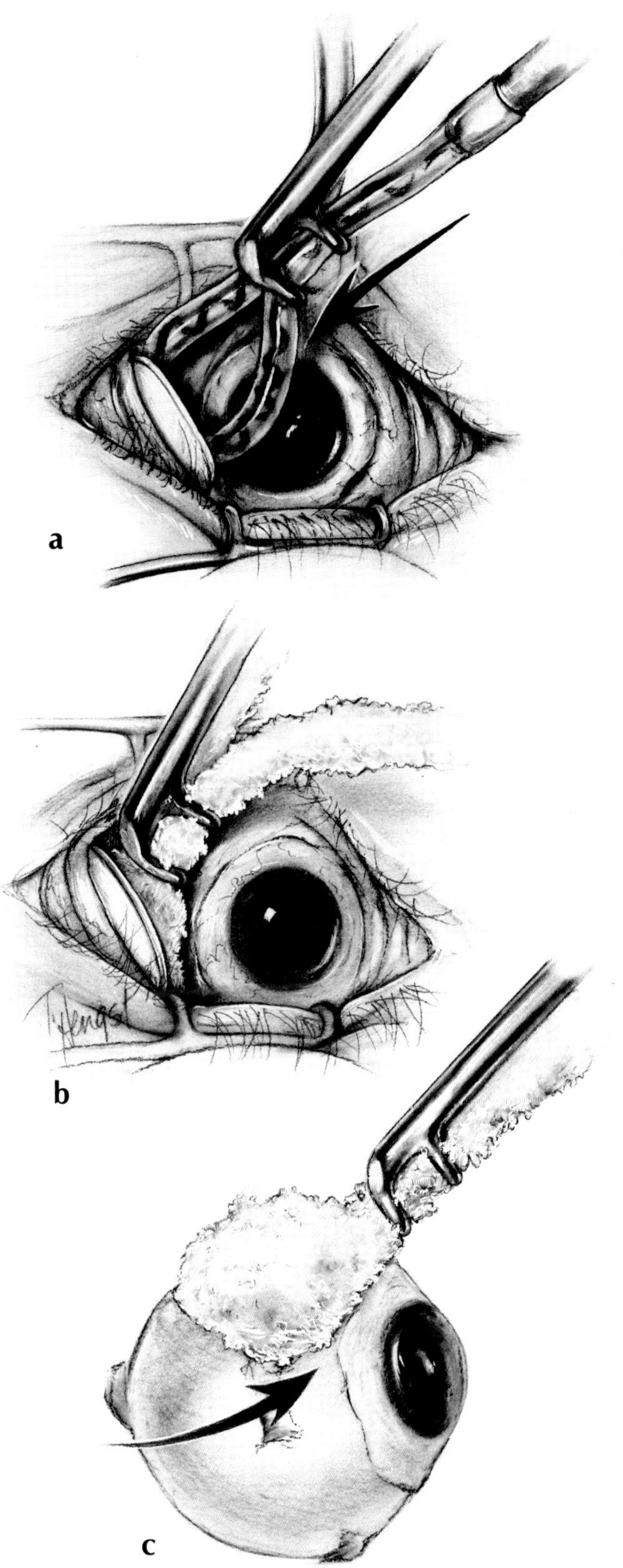

Figure 11.41 *Enucleation of choroidal melanoma using freezing 'no-touch' technique.* **(a)** *Cryo-ring is introduced between retractor and sclera after peritomy is done. The ring is positioned over base of tumor.* **(b)** *Liquid nitrogen, passed through tubing, freezes sclera and underlying tumor.* **(c)** *Optic nerve is cut and eye is removed. Large iceball incorporates sclera and underlying tumor*

This facilitates obtaining a long section of nerve. If there is gross evidence of extraocular extension of a melanoma or retinoblastoma, it is desirable to remove Tenon's capsule or other adjacent tissues with the globe.

Exenteration

Although orbital exenteration is commonly used for certain primary malignant tumors of the orbit, its role in management of intraocular tumors remains controversial. Since it is now uncommon for patients with uveal melanoma or retinoblastoma to present with extensive extrascleral involvement, exenteration is not often performed for these conditions. Some authors, however, advocate exenteration as the treatment of choice in eyes with malignant melanoma that has any degree of extrascleral extension[35]. The technique of orbital exenteration is discussed in Chapter 12.

Chemotherapy and immunotherapy

Chemotherapy and immunotherapy have not proved to be beneficial in preventing or controlling metastasis from malignant intraocular tumors. Such therapy seems reasonable, however, in patients thought to be at high risk of developing metastasis. Chemotherapy is often used in cases of retinoblastoma, patients with tumors metastatic to the eye, and patients with leukemic or lymphomatous intraocular involvement. Immunotherapy is sometimes used in patients with uveal melanomas, but its effectiveness is not yet established. Chemotherapy and immunotherapy should be given by a physician experienced in their use.

Summary

The diagnosis and treatment of intraocular tumors is a rapidly changing field. This chapter has discussed the surgical and non-surgical methods now used in the diagnosis and management of benign and malignant intraocular tumors.

Diagnostic methods include thorough systemic and ophthalmic examinations and ancillary studies such as transillumination, fluorescein angiography, ultrasonography, radioactive phosphorus uptake test, radiology, computerized tomography and fine-needle aspiration biopsy with cytological analysis.

Current methods of management include simple periodic observation, photocoagulation, radiotherapy, cryotherapy, diathermy, local surgical resection, enucleation, exenteration, chemotherapy and immunotherapy. The method of management selected varies depending on whether the tumor is benign or malignant, the type of tumor, the status of the opposite eye and the patient's visual acuity, age and general health. The indications for each method of management have been discussed in relation to the type of tumor and these other related findings.

Acknowledgement

Research for this chapter was supported, in part, by the Retina Research and Development Foundation, Philadelphia; The Pennsylvania Lions Sight Conservation and Eye Research Foundation, Inc.; the Ocular Oncology Fund, Wills Eye Hospital; and the Research Department, Wills Eye Hospital.

References

1. Shields, J. A. The diagnosis and management of intraocular tumours. St Louis: C. V. Mosby, 1983
2. Shields, J. A. Surgical and nonsurgical management of intraocular tumors. In: Spaeth, G. L., ed. Ophthalmic surgery. Philadelphia: W. B. Saunders, 1982: 721–741
3. Shields, J. A. Lesions simulating malignant melanoma of the posterior uvea. Archives of Ophthalmology 1973; 89:466–471
4. Shields, J. A., McDonald, P. R. Improvements in the diagnosis of posterior uveal melanomas. Archives of Ophthalmology 1974; 91:259–264
5. Shields, J. A., Stephens, R. F., Sarin, L. K. The differential diagnosis of leukocoria. In Harley, R. D., ed. Pediatric ophthalmology, 2nd ed. Philadelphia: W. B. Saunders, 1982
6. Tasman, W., Shields, J. A. Disorders of the peripheral fundus. Hagerstown, MD: Harper & Row, 1980; 117–128
7. Stephens, R. F., Shields, J. A. Diagnosis and management of cancer metastatic to the uvea. A study of 70 cases. Ophthalmology 1979; 86:1336–1349
8. Shields, J. A. Primary cysts of the iris. Transactions of the American Ophthalmological Society 1981; 79:771–809
9. Ducrey, N., Pomerantzeff, O., Schepens, C. L., Delori, F. C., Schneider, J. Clinical trials with the Equator-Plus camera. American Journal of Ophthalmology 1977; 84:840–846
10. Coleman, D. J. Reliability of ocular tumor diagnosis with ultrasound. Transactions of the American Academy of Ophthalmology and Otolaryngology 1973; 77:677–686
11. Shields, J. A., McDonald, P. R., Leonard, B. C., Canny, C. L. B. The diagnosis of uveal malignant melanomas in eyes with opaque media. American Journal of Ophthalmology 1977; 83:95–105
12. Thomas, C. I., Krohmer, J. S., Storaasli, J. P. Detection of intraocular tumors with radioactive phosphorus: preliminary report with special reference to differentiation of cause of retinal separation. Archives of Ophthalmology 1952; 47:276–286
13. Hagler, W. S., Jarrett, W. H., Humphrey, W. T. The radioactive phosphorus uptake test in diagnosis of uveal melanoma. Archives of Ophthalmology 1970; 83:548–557
14. Shields, J. A., Sarin, L. K., Federman, J. L., Mensheha-Manhart, O., Carmichael, P. L. Surgical approach to the ^{32}P test for posterior uveal melanomas. Ophthalmic Surgery 1974; 5(3): 13–19
15. Shields, J. A., Hagler, W. S., Federman, J. L., Jarrett, W. H., Carmicheal, P. L. The significance of the ^{32}P uptake test in the diagnosis of posterior uveal melanomas. Transactions of the American Academy of Ophthalmology and Otolaryngology 1975; 79:297–306
16. Shields, J. A. Accuracy and limitations of the ^{32}P test in the diagnosis of ocular tumors. An analysis of 500 cases. Ophthalmology 1978; 85:950–966
17. Shields, J. A. Current approaches to the diagnosis and management of choroidal melanomas. Survey of Ophthalmology 1977; 21:443–463
18. Michels, R. G., Knox, D. L., Erozan, Y. S., Green, W. R. Intraocular reticulum cell sarcoma: Diagnosis by pars plana vitrectomy. Archives of Ophthalmology 1975; 93:1331–1335
19. Augsburger, J. A., Shields, J. A. Fine needle aspiration biopsy in the diagnosis of intraocular tumours. Indications, instrumentation and techniques. Ophthalmic Surgery (in press)

20. Jakobiec, F. A., Coleman, D. J., Chattock, A., Smith, M. Ultrasonically guided needle biopsy and cytologic diagnosis of solid intraocular tumors. Ophthalmology 1979; 86:1662–1678
21. Zweng, H. C., Little, H. I., Peabody, R. R. Laser photocoagulation and retinal angiography. St Louis: C. V. Mosby, 1969:15
22. Federman, J. L., Felberg, N. T., Shields, J. A. Effect of local treatment on antibody levels in malignant melanoma of the choroid. Transactions of the Ophthalmological Society of the United Kingdom 1977; 97:436–439
23. Shields, J. A. Modern techniques in the management of retinoblastoma. Transactions of the Pacific Coast Oto-Ophthalmological Society 1979; 60:235–243
24. Shields, J. A., Augsburger, J. J. Current approaches to the diagnosis and management of retinoblastoma. Survey of Ophthalmology 1981; 25:347–372
25. Annesley, W. H., Leonard, B. C., Shields, J. A., Tasman, W. S. Fifteen year review of treated cases of retinal angiomatosis. Transactions of the American Academy of Ophthalmology and Otolaryngology 1977; 83:446–453
26. Sanborn, G. E., Augsburger, J. J., Shields, J. A. Treatment of circumscribed choroidal hemangiomas. Ophthalmology 1982; 89:1374–1380
27. Grant, G. D., Shields, J. A., Brady, L. W. The radiotherapy of ocular diseases. In Brady, L. W., Perez, C. A., eds. Basics and clinical practice of radiation oncology. New York: John Wiley & Sons (in press)
28. Brady, L. W., Shields, J. A., Augsburger, J. J., Day, J. L. Malignant intraocular tumors. Cancer 1982; 49:578–585
29. Gragoudas, E. S., Goitein, M., Verhey, L., Munzenreider, J., Urie, M., Suit, H., Koehler, A. Proton beam irradiation of uveal melanomas. Archives of Ophthalmology 1982; 100:928–934
30. Cassady, J. R., Sagerman, R. H., Tretter, P., Ellsworth, R. M. Radiation therapy in retinoblastoma. Radiology 1969; 93: 405–409
31. Abramson, D. H., Ronner, H. J., Ellsworth, R. M. Second tumors in nonirradiated bilateral retinoblastoma. American Journal of Ophthalmology 1979; 87:624–627
32. Peyman, G. A., Ericson, E. S., Axelrod, A. J., May, D. R. Full-thickness eye wall resection in primates: an experimental approach to treatment of choroidal melanoma. Archives of Ophthalmology 1973; 89:410–412
33. Zimmerman, L. E., McLean, I. W., Foster, W. D. Does enucleation of the eye containing a malignant melanoma prevent or accelerate the dissemination of tumour cells? British Journal of Ophthalmology 1978; 62:420–425
34. Wilson, R. S., Fraunfelder, F. T. 'No-touch' cryosurgical enucleation: a minimal trauma technique for eyes harboring intraocular malignancy. Ophthalmology 1978; 85:1170–1175
35. Shammas, H. F., Blodi, F. C. Orbital extension of choroidal and ciliary body melanomas. Archives of Ophthalmology 1977; 95:2002–2005

12

Surgery of the orbit

Neil R. Miller MD
W. Jackson Iliff MD

Introduction

In 1774, Thomas Hope of Scotland reported the successful removal of a longstanding, inferior orbital tumor with preservation of the eye and ultimate relief of proptosis. Although Hope credited his teacher, St Yves, with having first performed a similar, successful procedure, this report marked the beginning of the concept of orbital surgery. Subsequent discoveries and improvements in technique have gradually led to the emergence of orbital surgery as a distinct ophthalmological entity. Major advances have occurred in diagnosis (computed tomography, ultrasonography), surgery (anesthesia, operating microscope, bipolar cautery, cryoprobe) and postoperative treatment (antibiotics, corticosteroids).

In order to perform a competent orbital evaluation, to determine the appropriate management and to perform successful surgery if indicated, the orbital surgeon must have a solid knowledge of normal orbital anatomy, of the disease processes that can involve the orbit, of the procedures available to aid diagnosis of orbital disease, and of the surgical techniques and approaches best suited to specific orbital diseases. We will discuss many of these issues, concentrating primarily on surgical techniques. A complete discussion of all aspects of orbital disease is beyond the scope of this chapter. The interested reader is encouraged to pursue the subject, using the texts of Henderson[1], Jones and Jakobiec[2], and Korhel, Stewart and Chavis[3].

Indications for surgery

Following a complete evaluation of the patient with orbital disease, a decision must be made either to: (*1*) follow-up the patient without giving treatment; (*2*) begin non-surgical therapy; or (*3*) perform surgery. When there is evidence of a mass within the confines of the orbit, it is generally advisable to obtain a specimen for pathological diagnosis whenever possible. The decision to perform surgery is usually based on a complete clinical evaluation including appropriate diagnostic studies. In addition to considerations directly related to the orbital disease process, the physician must also consider such variables as the patient's age and general health. Based on this evaluation, the physician can elect to perform a biopsy (either incisional or excisional), total excision, drainage, decompression or repair-reconstruction. In situations where there is some controversy regarding the appropriate management of an orbital process (e.g. thyroid ophthalmopathy, optic nerve glioma, lacrimal gland carcinoma, blow-out fracture), the physician must consider all options and discuss these extensively with the patient.

Although in most instances a careful preoperative evaluation will determine the surgical approach to be used, the surgical procedure may be modified when the lesion is actually encountered and its nature becomes apparent. The preoperative evaluation of a patient with presumed orbital disease will usually not provide the orbital surgeon with a precise diagnosis, but it will provide knowledge regarding several important characteristics. If a lesion is present, the evaluation should determine its location, extent and biological activity.

Preoperative evaluation

Ophthalmic history

The examination of a patient with orbital disease must be methodical and comprehensive. The initial step in any evaluation is a complete history, which should focus on the patient's symptoms and signs and their progression or stability over time. Although a history of proptosis is important, it may be neither the chief complaint nor the first sign. Frequently, patients with orbital disorders complain of decreased visual acuity, diplopia, ptosis, tearing, redness or pain. The precise order of symptoms and the rapidity with which they have developed are often important clues to the underlying diagnosis. The examiner should not confine himself to a review of ocular symptoms and signs. A complete review of the patient's general health and a concise past medical history may be crucial to the diagnosis of orbital disease which may represent but a single manifestation of a systemic process. The examiner should spend enough time taking a history so that he can reconstruct precisely the events that have led to the patient presenting for examination.

Examination

After the history has been obtained, a complete examination should be performed, including measurement of the best corrected visual acuity at distance and near, visual field testing, pupillary examination, slit-lamp examination, intraocular pressure measurements and ophthalmoscopic examination. A careful external examination is also imperative. Changes in the texture and color of the soft tissues of the eyelid may be helpful in differential diagnosis. The presence of swelling, edema, and redness of these tissues may suggest the appropriate diagnosis. Proptosis should be noted and measured. Such measurements are made with the Hertel exophthalmometer or similar instrument. The examiner should also determine the exact position of the eye, since the eye may not only protrude but may also be displaced vertically or horizontally. The presence or absence of pulsation should be noted, and auscultation should be performed to determine whether a bruit is present. After the external examination, careful palpation of the orbit and its accessible surrounding bony walls is essential. Anterior tumors are palpated and their extent partially determined. Abnormalities in the orbital bone are also noted. When a lesion is discovered on palpation, it should be determined whether the lesion is hard or soft, well-circumscribed or diffuse, movable or fixed, tender or non-tender.

Diagnostic tests

Once it has been determined that orbital disease is present, further diagnostic studies are performed. Plain skull X-rays may help in assessing the integrity of the bony orbit and the presence of soft-tissue masses, and polytomography may further characterize bony lesions. However, the primary diagnostic tests for orbital disease are computed tomographic (CT) scanning and ultrasonography[4–7].

The availability of CT scanning for the past decade has revolutionized orbital diagnosis. Using thin-section scanning techniques, appropriate positioning, and intravenous contrast enhancement when necessary, virtually all orbital lesions, whether involving soft tissue or bone, can be identified. We believe that all CT scanning involving the orbital structures should be performed using both axial and coronal (direct or reconstructed) views. Although many orbital lesions can be identified using only axial CT views, CT scanning of the orbit is not complete unless direct or reconstructed coronal views are also obtained (*Figure 12.1*). Only with a combination of axial and coronal views can the precise location and extent of an orbital lesion be determined. Thin (5–8 mm) 'slices' should be obtained, and window width and level should be modified depending on the nature of the lesion. We do not routinely use intravenous contrast enhancement in patients with orbital disease unless: (*1*) no lesion is seen by non-contrast scanning; (*2*) a vascular lesion (e.g. orbital varix) is suspected; or (*3*) it is important to know whether the lesion is vascular, to assess the surgical approach. Used in this manner, the CT scan allows the location and extent of the orbital lesion to be determined and may also give some indication of the lesion's biological characteristics. It is the most useful diagnostic study presently available for orbital disease.

Diagnostic ultrasonography, using the A-scan and B-scan modes, can be helpful in locating lesions directly behind the globe and in giving a clue as to their nature. In general, CT scanning is more useful in determining the location and extent of the lesion, while ultrasonography is more likely to indicate the cause. The use of these two techniques together provides a tremendous amount of information about the nature of an orbital process. Because of the improvement in CT scanning and ultrasonographic techniques, neuroradiological studies such as positive contrast orbitography, orbital venography and arteriography, that were previously thought to be important in orbital diagnosis, are rarely used today.

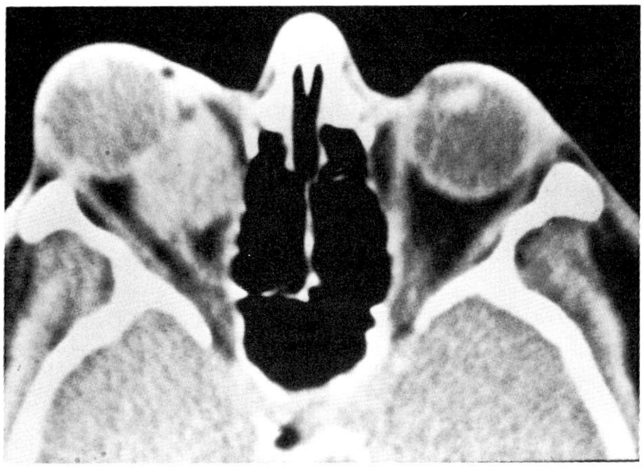

a

Figure 12.1 *Computed tomographic (CT) scans show the location, characteristics and, occasionally, the etiology of orbital lesions. Axial and coronal views are both important.* **(a)** *Axial view of a well-circumscribed mass in the central space of the right orbit. The precise location of the mass with respect to the optic nerve is unclear.* **(b)** *The coronal views in the same case shows the optic nerve lateral to the mass. The tumor should therefore be removed through a medial approach.* **(c)** *Axial view of the orbits of a patient with bilateral proptosis seems to show bilateral apical orbital masses.* **(d)** *Direct coronal views of the orbits in the same patient, however, show generalized enlargement of the extraocular muscles without evidence of any discrete masses. The abnormalities seen are compatible with thyroid eye disease. Note the encroachment of the extraocular muscles on the optic nerves.* **(e,f)** *Axial and coronal views of a patient with a left orbital lesion. Using both views, it can be determined that the lesion is well-circumscribed, of low density and located in the peripheral (extraperiosteal) space. It is associated with expansion and thinning of the surrounding bone, without destruction. The lesion proved to be a dermoid cyst*

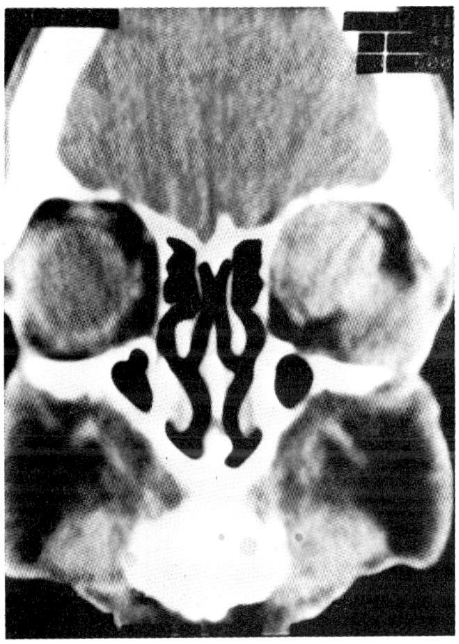

b

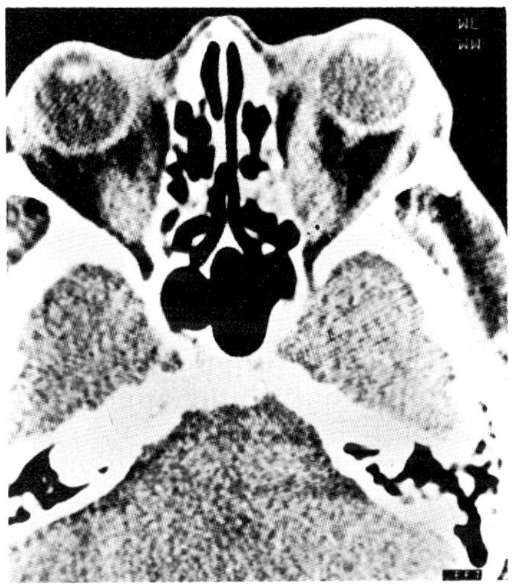

c

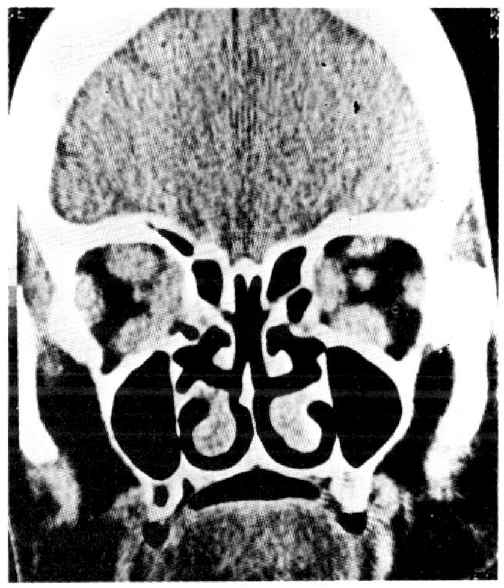

d

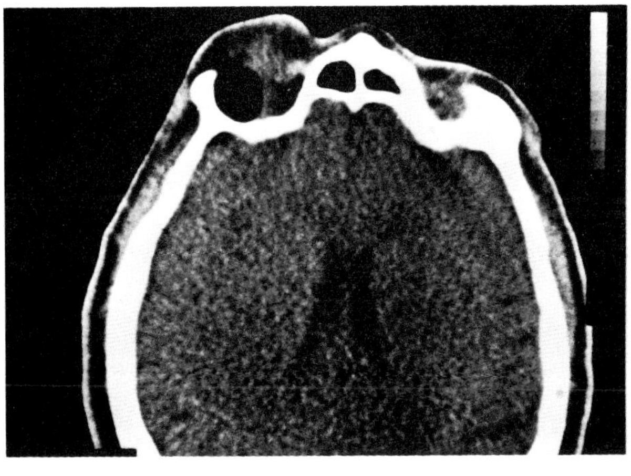

e

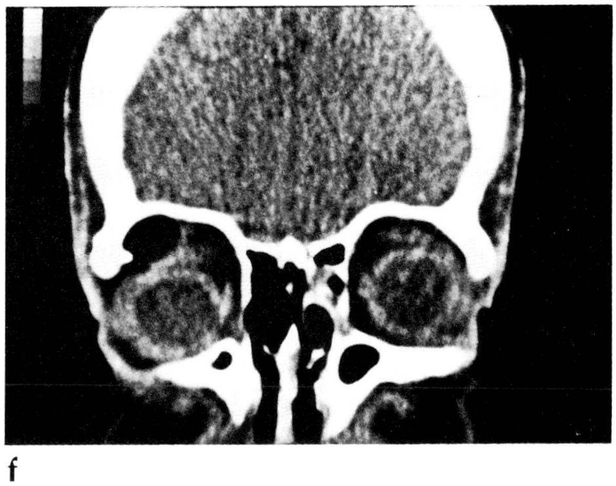

f

Surgical principles and techniques

Orbital anatomy

Successful orbital surgery depends not only on knowing the location, extent and biological activity of a lesion, but also on the surgeon's knowledge of normal orbital anatomy. Whitnall compared the orbit to a pear, with its anterior orbital aperture corresponding to the base of the pear and the optic canal to its stalk. The height, width and depth of a normal adult orbit each measure about 40 mm, and the orbital volume is about 29 ml. The bony walls of the orbit comprises seven individual bones: the frontal bone, the maxilla, the zygoma, the greater and lesser wings of the sphenoid, and the ethmoid, the lacrimal and the palatine (*Figures 12.2* and *12.3*). The superior wall, or roof of the orbit, is formed anteriorly by the frontal bone and posteriorly by the greater and lesser wings of the sphenoid. The roof is thin throughout its extent, and the periorbita easily peels away from its undersurface. The supraorbital notch (which is sometimes a true foramen) is located at the junction of the medial one-third and lateral two-thirds of the orbital rim. The supraorbital vessels and nerve leave the orbit through this structure (*Figure 12.4*). Damage to the supraorbital nerve causes hypesthesia and occasionally dysesthesia in the supraorbital region. Adjacent and medial to the supraorbital notch is the trochlea, through which the tendon of the superior oblique muscle passes.

The lateral wall of the orbit is formed anteriorly by the junction of the frontal and zygomatic bones, and posteriorly by the junction of these bones with the greater wing of the sphenoid. The anterior rim of the lateral wall is sturdy compared to the midportion of the wall. It can only be removed using a sharp saw or chisel. The lateral wall becomes thinner as it passes posteriorly to its junction with the forward and lateral extension of the greater wing

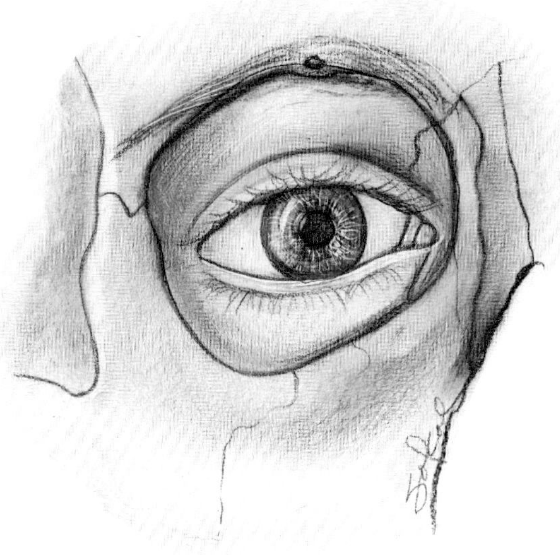

Figure 12.2 *The anatomy of the bony orbital rim with the position of the eyelids and eybrow superimposed*

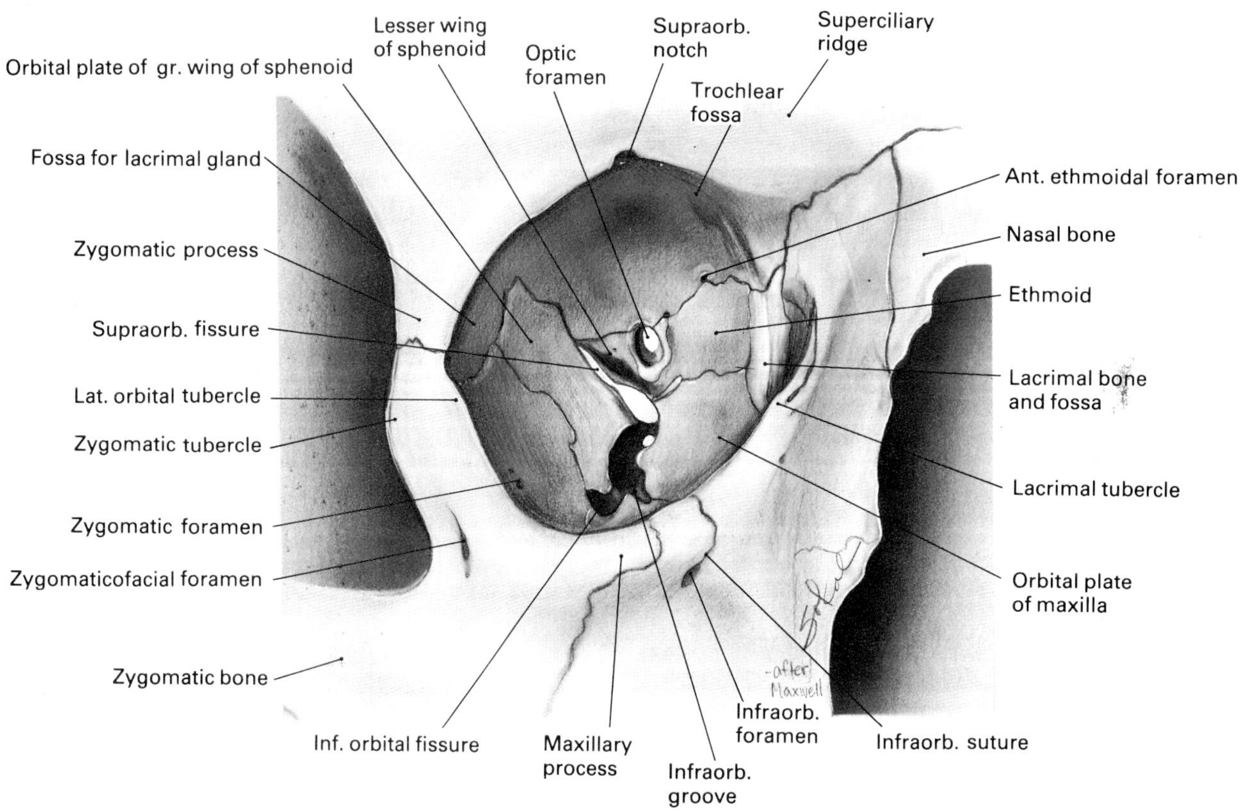

Figure 12.3 *The anatomy of the bony orbit. The skull has been positioned to show all major features of the bony orbit*

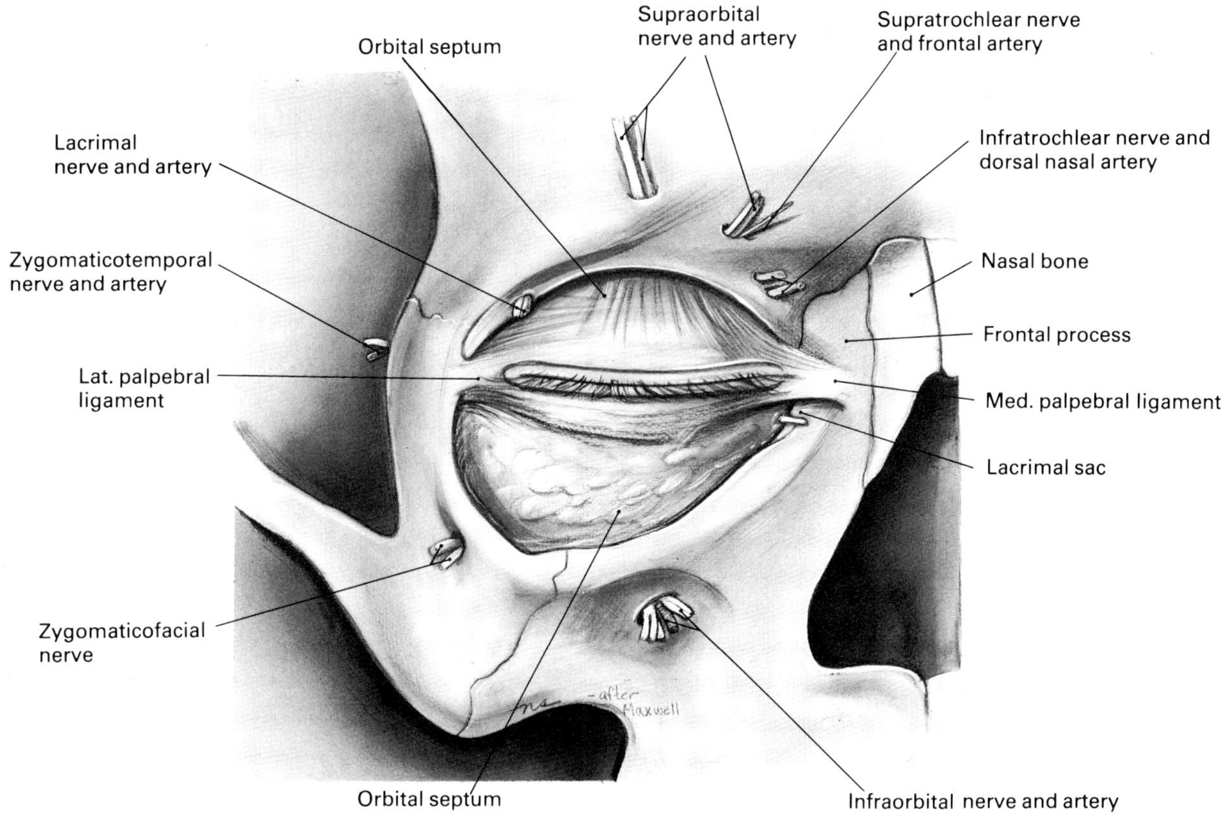

Figure 12.4 *The anatomy of the bony orbit showing the location of the major vessels and nerves as they emerge from the bone*

of the sphenoid. Through the lateral orbital wall pass small zygomatico-orbital branches of the middle temporal artery. Although these always bleed after removal of the wall, the bleeding is easily controlled with cautery or bone wax.

The inferior wall or floor of the orbit is formed by the junction of the maxilla and zygomatic bones. It is both the floor of the orbit and the roof of the maxillary sinus. Running within the orbital floor is the infraorbital groove (or foramen) which contains the infraorbital nerve and artery.

The medial wall of the orbit is the thinnest of the four walls. It is formed by the medial parts of the maxilla and frontal bone and their junctions with the ethmoid, lacrimal and palatine bones. Two foramina in the ethmoid bone transmit arteries (the anterior and posterior ethmoidal arteries) that are important anatomical landmarks and also potential hazards encountered during surgery. The posterior ethmoidal artery is located a few millimeters anterior to the beginning of the optic canal.

Within the orbit, normal structures, and lesions that disturb these structures, can be defined as lying in specific 'spaces' (*Figure 12.5*). The surgical approach to each space is different. The orbital contents are separated from the bony orbital walls by the bony periosteum which, in the orbit, is called the 'periorbita'. The periorbita is often a barrier which limts spread of lesions that originate in the orbital bones. The potential space between periorbita and bone is called the extraperiosteal or subperiosteal space. Henderson[1] has also called this the 'peripheral' space. It is limited anteriorly by the fusion of periorbita with the periosteum and orbital septum along the rim of the orbit, and posteriorly by its junction with the dural sheath of the optic nerve.

The space between the rectus muscles and periorbita is termed the 'middle space'. This space is occupied mainly by fat, although superiorly it also contains the levator palpebrae superioris muscle. Anteriorly, it is limited by the orbital septum. The middle space is the largest of the orbital spaces.

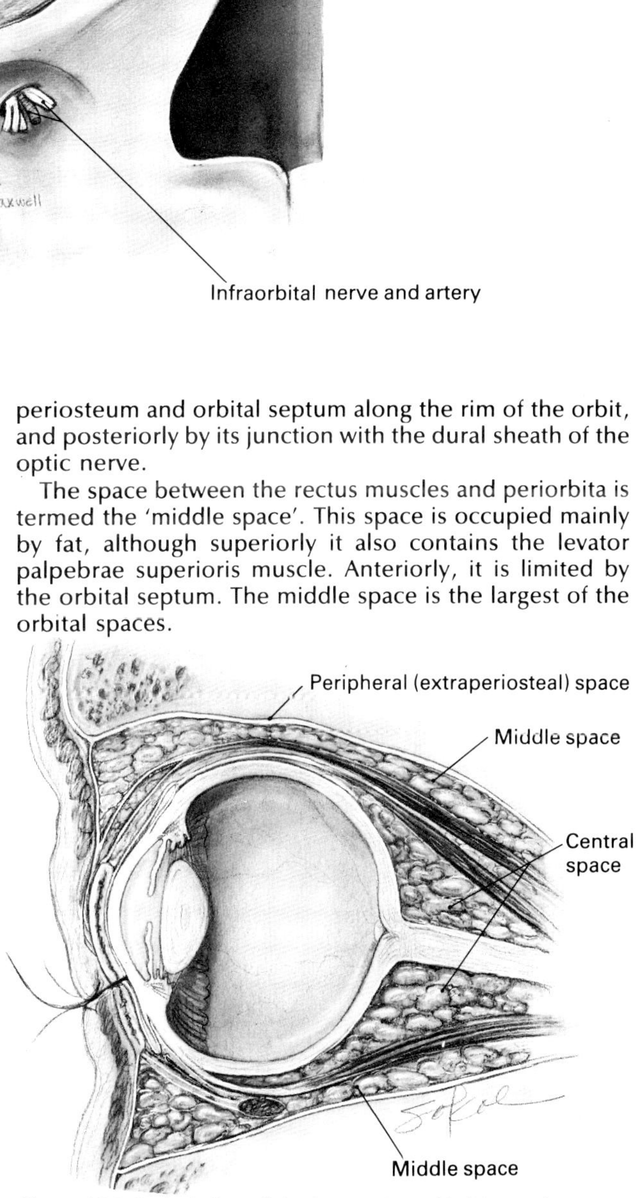

Figure 12.5 *Sagittal view of the three major orbital 'spaces'*

The 'inner' or 'central' surgical space is located between the optic nerve and the rectus muscles. It is cone-shaped, and lesions within the region are often said to be within the 'muscle cone'. The back surface of the eye forms its anterior boundary, while the extraocular muscles and intramuscular septa compose its walls, and the optic nerve runs through the middle of the space.

The lacrimal gland fills the entire anterior portion of the superotemporal orbital region. Posteriorly, the tip of the gland extends almost to the zygomatic-sphenoidal suture, so that when a surgeon enters the superior orbital quadrant from a lateral approach, the lacrimal gland must be pushed forward or retracted to one side to gain better access and visibility into the posterior orbit. Anteriorly, the gland is divided into superior (orbital) and inferior (palpebral) lobes by the lateral sweep of the aponeurosis of the levator muscle. The smaller, inferior lacrimal lobe actually lies outside the orbit, but it is connected to the main lobe by an isthmus of tissue.

Anesthesia and preparation for surgery

When the surgeon discusses surgery with the patient, he or she already has an idea of the location, extent and type of lesion that might be encountered. The physician's plan is carefully explained to the patient, including the possibility of a change in the plan of surgery, depending on the exact nature of the lesion that is encountered. Possible complications of surgery are carefully discussed; these include general complications (bleeding, infection, diplopia, failure to achieve the desired result, visual loss, death) and also complications that depend on the location of the lesion and planned incision (dry eye, supraorbital or infraorbital anesthesia, hypesthesia, dysesthesia). An informed consent form is signed by the patient, the responsible physician and a witness.

Patients undergoing general anesthesia should have a complete physical examination, a complete differential blood count, a chest X-ray and an electrocardiogram before surgery. If the patient has any medical illnesses, further blood studies (e.g. electrolytes) and consultations (e.g. cardiac, pulmonary) may be obtained. Patients undergoing orbital surgery who may need a blood transfusion should have their blood typed and crossmatched, especially when the lesion is posterior or likely to be vascular. Patients taking anticoagulants, such as sodium warfarin (Coumadin), or inhibitors of platelet aggregation, such as aspirin, should have these drugs stopped (if possible) at least 1 week prior to surgery, to reduce the chance of excessive intraoperative or postoperative bleeding.

Most orbital surgery is performed under general anesthesia; however, when the lesion is anterior, or a simple biopsy is contemplated, local anesthesia with infiltration of surrounding tissue with a 50-50 mixture of 2 per cent lidocaine (lignocaine; Xylocaine) and 0.75 per cent bupivacaine can be used.

Instrumentation

The instruments needed for orbital surgery vary depending on whether orbital bone must be removed. If not, the surgeon needs a basic set consisting of fine dissecting instruments, fine malleable retractors, a suction device, a cryoprobe and cautery, including a bipolar cautery. An operating microscope may be needed. When the operating microscope is not used, magnifying loupes are usually used, along with an operating headlight. If orbital bone needs to be removed, the surgeon needs an oscillating saw and possibly a pneumatic drill. Bone wax should be available to stop the mild bleeding that always occurs when any of the orbital walls are cut.

Incisions and surgical approaches

Surgical approaches to the orbit can be made through a variety of incisions, depending on the location and extent of the lesion (*Figure 12.6*). When the lesion is anterior and

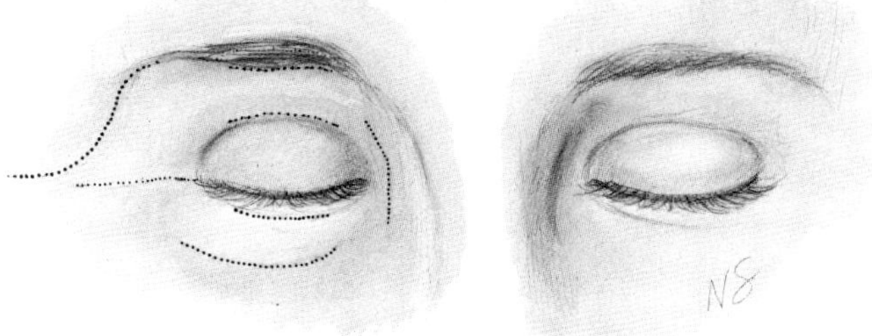

Figure 12.6 *Diagram of the various incisions (dashed lines) that may be used to approach orbital lesions*

can be palpated, a transcutaneous approach – either extraperiosteal or transseptal (*Figure 12.7*) – is usually used. When a palpable lesion is thought to reside in the 'peripheral space' (between periorbita and bone), an extraperiosteal approach is used. The approach to nonpalpable orbital lesions is determined by whether they are located within the peripheral, middle or central orbital spaces.

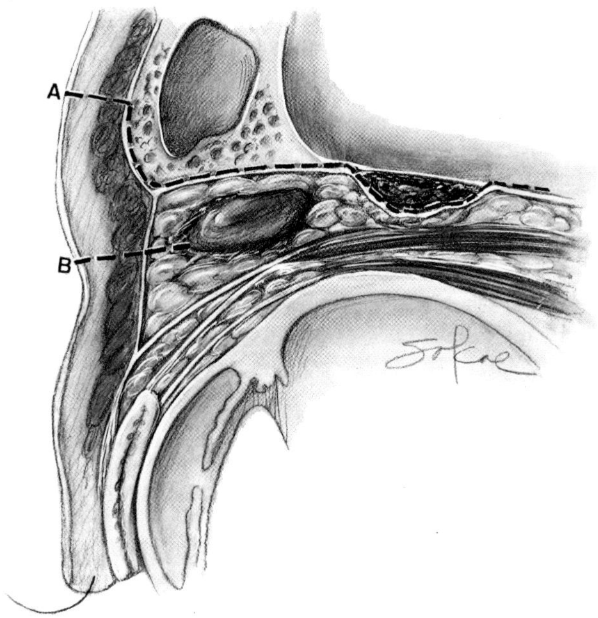

Figure 12.7 *The anatomy of lesions that can occur in the superior peripheral (extraperiosteal) and middle spaces, including the surgical routes for removal (dashed lines).* **(a)** *Surgical route for removal of an extraperiosteal lesion.* **(b)** *Surgical route for removal of a lesion in the superior middle space*

Extraperiosteal approach

For an extraperiosteal approach, a skin incision is positioned outside and parallel to the bony orbital rim. The position and length of the skin incision depend on the site and size of the lesion. For superior orbital lesions, we prefer to place the incision just beneath the eyebrow. This site avoids the heavy bleeding that is often associated with incisions made within the brow, but it is still partially hidden cosmetically by the brow itself. For infraorbital lesions or 'blow-out' fractures of the orbital floor, an incision can be made just beneath the cilia of the lower lid and carried subcutaneously down to the inferior orbital rim, or an incision can be made directly over the inferior rim itself.

Before making the skin incision, its intended position is marked with a dye such as brilliant green or methylene blue. If local anesthesia is used, a 50-50 mixture of 2 per cent lidocaine (lignocaine) and 0.75 per cent bupivacaine may be used. When general anesthesia is used, a small volume of 1 per cent lidocaine (lignocaine) with 1:10 000 epinephrine (adrenaline) can be injected in the region of the operative site to reduce bleeding.

The skin incision is carried through subcutaneous tissue and orbicularis oculi muscle, which is split in the direction of its fibers. Hemostasis is obtained with use of hemostats or with cautery. We find that there is less bleeding if the initial incision is carried just to subcutaneous tissue and the remainder of the incision is extended to periosteum using a cutting cautery. Either traction sutures of 4/0 silk or skin rakes are used to open the incision. When the periosteum is encountered just outside the orbital rim, it is incised sharply and dissected off the bone with a periosteal elevator. Both the Freer and Cottle elevators are useful periosteal elevators. With a superiorly located incision near the brow, care must be taken to identify the supraorbital vessels and nerve. The vessels are ligated or cauterized. If possible, the supraorbital nerve is spared and is traumatized as little as possible. If the incision is carried laterally, care must be taken to prevent injury to the lacrimal gland and laceration of branches of the lacrimal artery and nerve. Medially, care must be taken to preserve the integrity of the superior oblique tendon and trochlea by carefully separating the periorbita in this area from the bone. If an inferior incision has been made, the infraorbital nerve should be identified and care taken to avoid injury to it.

Once inside the bony orbital margin, the 'peripheral' (extraperiosteal or subperiosteal) space is easily entered and the dissection is carried as far posteriorly as necessary. Medially, one must identify the anterior and posterior ethmoidal arteries and ligate or cauterize them when necessary. Laterally, the zygomatico-orbital branches of the middle temporal artery will be encountered.

Once the extraperiosteal lesion is reached, biopsy, excision, drainage or decompression is carried out as necessary. When extraperiosteal lesions involve not only the orbit but also the paranasal sinuses or the intracranial cavity (which is often the case), the orbital surgeon should operate using a team approach in conjunction with a neurosurgeon, otolaryngologist, or both. This is especially true for patients with suspected encephaloceles, mucoceles, or tumors arising from the sinuses.

In dealing with entirely extraperiosteal lesions, care should be taken to keep the periorbita intact, since this structure serves as a barrier protecting the orbital contents. Once the lesion has been biopsied or removed, the wound is closed in layers. If hemostasis is complete, no drain is needed; otherwise a soft rubber drain such as a Penrose drain, is used. Periosteal closure at the orbital margin is performed with absorbable sutures such as 4/0 or 5/0 chromic or plain catgut. Muscle layers are reapproximated with similar sutures. The skin is then closed using interrupted 8/0 fine silk sutures, or running cutaneous or subcuticular sutures of 6/0 nylon or polypropylene. A light dressing is then applied.

Transseptal approach

For anterior lesions that are palpable and thought to be located either subcutaneously or within the 'middle' space between the periorbita and extraocular muscles, we prefer a transseptal approach (*Figure 12.8* and *see Figure 12.7*). An incision is made directly over the lesion. In some instances, gentle pressure on the globe may cause the lesion to protrude slightly and thus permit more precise localization (*Figure 12.8a*). The skin incision is usually made to conform with the natural creases of the eyelids, so that it will be hidden in those creases. The skin incision

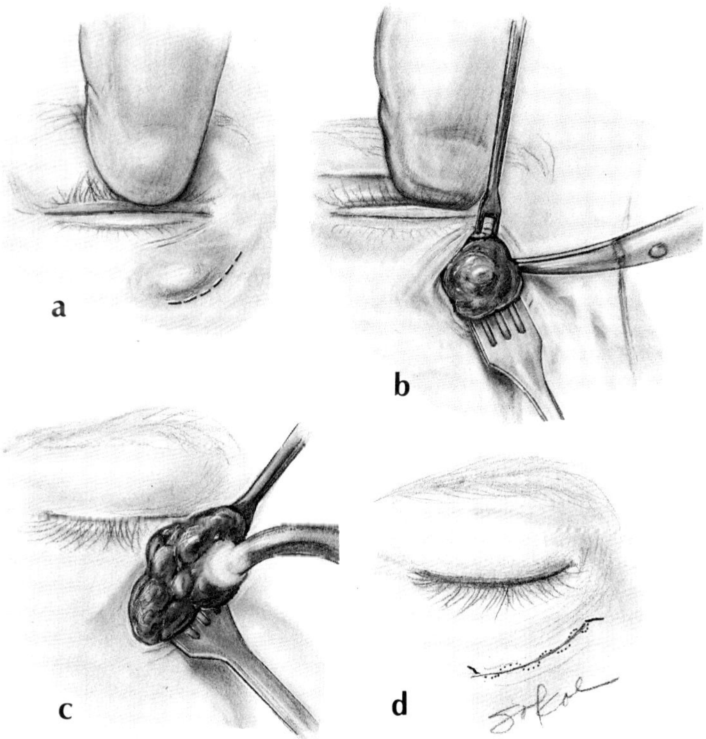

Figure 12.8 *Transcutaneous, transseptal removal of an anterior, inferior orbital mass.* **(a)** *The location and extent of the mass can best be appreciated by placing gentle pressure on the globe which pushes the mass forward.* **(b)** *A skin incision is made along a skin fold overlying the lesion. Using careful blunt dissection, the mass is exposed and separated from surrounding tissue.* **(c)** *A cryoprobe is used to exert gentle traction on the mass, while blunt and sharp dissection are used to free the posterior aspects of the mass from surrounding tissue.* **(d)** *After removal of the mass and control of bleeding, the orbital septum (if opened) has been closed, and the skin incision is closed using a subcuticular suture*

is carried down to the lesion using meticulous blunt and sharp dissection (*Figure 12.8b*). Bipolar cautery is essential in maintaining hemostasis. Once the lesion has been identified, it is either biopsied or removed. If it is biopsied, the tissue should not be crushed because this may interfere with later pathological examination. Crush injury can be avoided by outlining the area to be biopsied with bipolar cautery. An incision is then made into the lesion using a fine scalpel blade. The piece of tissue is grasped at one corner with a pair of fine forceps and held while the remainder of the tissue is excised. If the entire lesion is to be removed, careful dissection is carried out to free it of all attachments to normal orbital structures. Traction on the lesion is best performed using a standard cryoprobe (*Figure 12.8c*) to avoid crush injury to the tissue while manipulating the lesion. Such traction is usually required to allow careful separation of the posterior part of the lesion from surrounding normal tissue. Once the lesion has been removed, careful attention is again paid to hemostasis. The surgical field is irrigated with warm saline until all bleeding stops. If bleeding persists, closure is delayed until a bleeding site is found and cauterized, or a drain is placed in the wound. Avitene (microfibrillar collagen hemostat) can be used to stop diffuse bleeding, but we prefer not to use this in the orbit because it can cause significant scarring. If an inflammatory lesion has been biopsied, we usually irrigate the area with dexamethasone, and occasionally we inject the remainder of the lesion with depot-type steroids.

The subcutaneous tissue is closed using interrupted 4/0 or 5/0 chromic or catgut suture, and the skin incision is closed using either subcuticular or superficial running or interrupted 7/0 suture (*Figure 12.8d*). A non-adherent sterile dressing is then placed over the incision, with an overlying pressure dressing.

Lateral orbitotomy

Lesions in the lateral-central or middle orbital spaces are usually approached through a lateral orbitotomy that involves temporary or permanent removal of a portion of the lateral orbital wall (*Figure 12.9*). The patient is positioned with the head slightly elevated and rotated away from the operative side. The cornea is protected either by closing the lids with a temporary traction suture, or by a protective scleral contact lens or ointment (*Figure 12.9a*). We have also sutured a small piece of Gelfoam over the cornea to protect it during surgery.

The site of the skin incision is marked. The skin incision may be a modification of the Burke incision, extending from the lateral canthal region posteriorly for approximately 4 cm (*Figure 12.9a*), or it may be a curvilinear incision that is begun just beneath the inferior cilia of the lateral third of the eyebrow and is carried inferiorly and posteriorly along the superior and lateral bony orbital rim (see *Figure 12.14a*). The section is carried down through the subcutaneous tissues and orbicularis oculi muscle to the level of the external orbital periosteum anteriorly and the fascia of the temporalis muscle posteriorly (*Figure 12.9a*). As previously noted, the subcutaneous portion of the incision may be made with either a scalpel or cutting cautery. Hemostasis is initially achieved by pressure on the superior and inferior margins of the skin incision and with hemostats. Cautery is then applied as necessary. Traction sutures may be positioned in the upper and lower flaps through the subcutaneous and muscularis tissue, or a self-retaining retractor may be used.

After the periosteum has been exposed, it is incised about 2 mm behind and parallel to the lateral bony margin (*Figure 12.9b*). The incision is carried superiorly as far as the proposed bony excision and may extend as far as the supraorbital foramen. It is carried inferiorly past the superior aspect of the zygomatic arch. The periosteal incision is then carried posteriorly along the zygomatic arch and along the upper part of the temporalis muscle. The periosteum is stripped from the external aspect of the lateral orbital wall. The periosteum and temporalis muscle are reflected posteriorly from the zygomatic process of the frontal bone and the frontal process of the zygomatic bone. This exposes the fossa of the temporalis muscle and the bone of the lateral orbital wall. Initially, it is usually easier to dissect the temporalis muscle using a sharp scalpel or cautery. Once the dissection is begun, a periosteal elevator can be used. Brisk venous bleeding is usually encountered in the bed of the temporalis muscle. This can be controlled by pressure or with bipolar cautery.

After the periosteum and temporalis muscle have been separated from the external portion of the lateral orbital wall, the periorbita is lifted away from the inner portion of the wall (*Figure 12.9c*). The periorbita is loosely adherent in this area and can be easily separated from bone as far posteriorly as the orbital apex. A broad malleable retractor is then positioned in the orbit along the lateral wall between the bone and periorbita. This protects the orbital soft-tissue contents during removal of the lateral wall. If the wall is to be replaced at the end of surgery, drill holes are made with a pneumatic drill on either side of the intended upper and lower edges of the bony incisions. The bone incisions can then be made with an oscillating saw (*Figure 12.9d*). The lower cut is placed along the upper margin of the zygomatic arch. The upper cut is positioned above the frontozygomatic suture. During the bone cutting, malleable retractors over gauze pads or neurosurgical cottonoid pads are used to retract the temporalis muscle and associated soft tissue. The saw blade is gently irrigated with saline to cool it and prevent heat necrosis of bone, and suction is used to prevent scattering of bony fragments. Once superior and inferior cuts have been made, the lateral wall fragment is grasped with bone rongeurs and gently rocked until it fractures posteriorly and can be removed (*Figure 12.9e*). If it is to be replaced, it is temporarily placed in warm, lactated Ringer's solution. Further posterior bony resection may be performed using rongeurs or a pneumatic drill with a diamond burr. Malleable retractors are placed on either side of the bone to prevent injury either to the periorbita and soft tissue contents of the orbit or to the temporalis muscle and fascia. Bone wax may be used to control bleeding, usually originating from the zygomatico-orbital vessels and from the bone itself. The bony opening can be enlarged posteriorly, superiorly and inferiorly to the thick bone that protects the middle cranial fossa. Further retraction of the temporalis muscle can be accomplished using either traction sutures or hand-held or self-retaining retractors.

The intact periorbita is now visualized. The periorbita is incised in an anteroposterior direction below the level of the inferior part of the lacrimal gland, at approximately the level of the upper border of the lateral rectus muscle. A

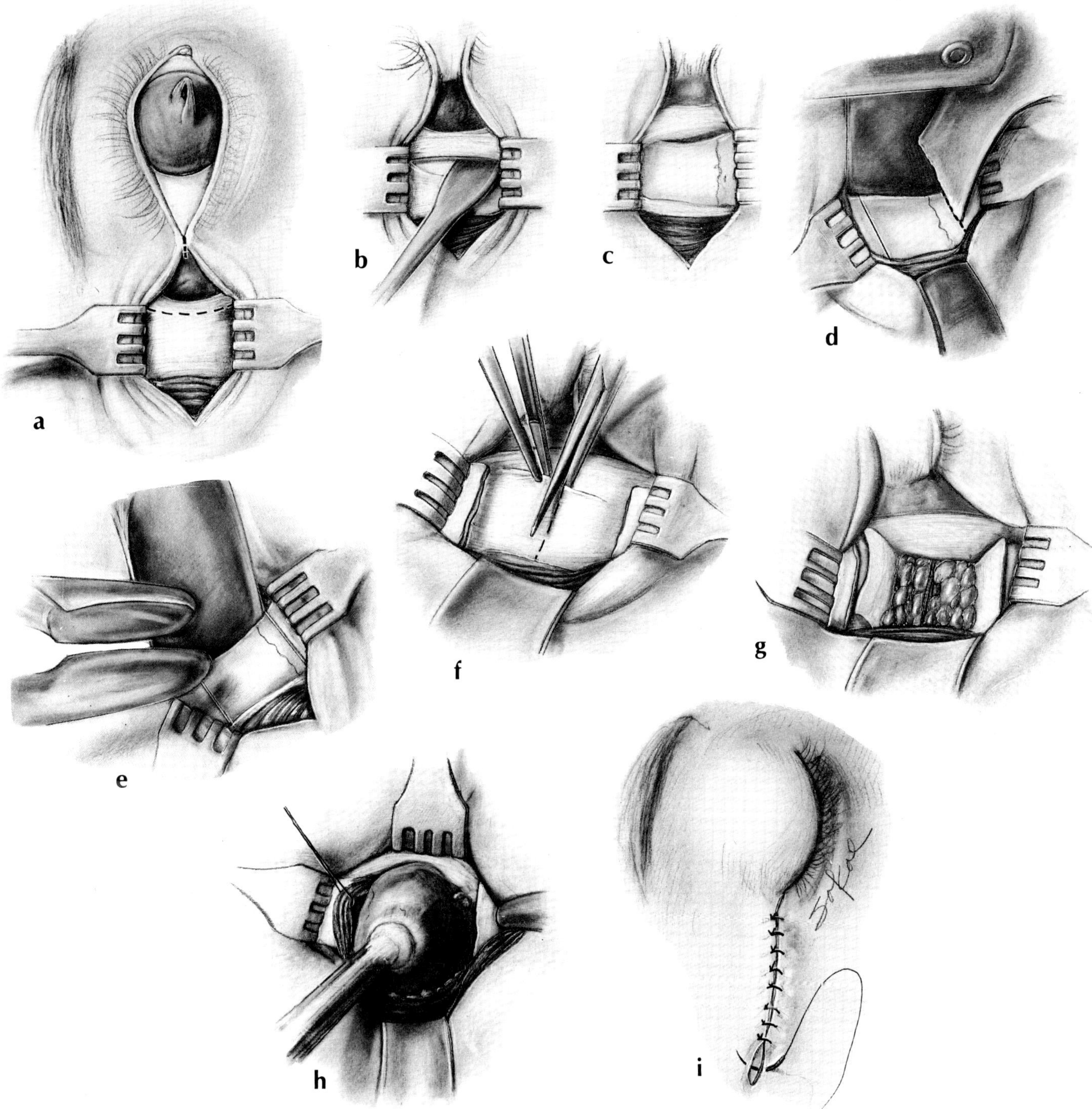

Figure 12.9 *Lateral orbitotomy.* **(a)** *The cornea of the right eye has been covered with a contact lens, and a linear (Burke) incision has been made and carried down to the lateral orbital wall. The thick dashed line shows the area where a sharp scissors will be used to separate the lateral portions of the upper and lower lids at the lateral canthus, thus providing an adequate surgical opening. The thin dashed line shows the location where the periosteum of the lateral orbital wall will be incised.* **(b)** *The upper and lower lids have been separated, and an incision has been made in the periosteum of the lateral orbital wall. The periosteum is being separated from the bone using a Freer elevator.* **(c)** *The periosteum has now been removed from the lateral bony wall externally and internally. The fascia of the temporalis muscle has also been separated from the orbital wall.* **(d)** *An oscillating saw is used to make linear incisions in the lateral bony wall. Note that retractors are used to protect the orbital contents and also the skin and subcutaneous tissue.* **(e)** *Bone rongeurs are used to remove a large piece of bone from the lateral orbital wall. The bony opening may be enlarged by using rongeurs superiorly, inferiorly and posteriorly.* **(f)** *A T-shaped incision is carefully made in the periorbita using sharp scissors.* **(g)** *With the periorbita open, orbital fat protrudes, and the lateral rectus muscle can be identified and looped with a traction suture, umbilical tape or a fine Penrose drain.* **(h)** *A well-circumscribed orbital mass is identified and separated from surrounding tissue using blunt dissection. The mass is removed from the orbit using a cryoprobe. Note that the lateral rectus has not been removed from the globe but is looped away from the lesion.* **(i)** *The periorbita, periosteum and subcutaneous tissue incisions are closed in separate layers. The skin incision is closed using an interrupted suture technique*

vertical (superoinferior) incision in the periorbita is also made anteriorly, producing a T-shaped incision (*Figure 12.9f*). Relaxing incisions in the posterior-most exposed periorbita can also be made if necessary, producing an I-shaped incision. The orbital contents are carefully palpated, determining the position of any mass. The lateral rectus muscle is located by opening the perimuscular fascial sheaths with blunt dissection (*Figure 12.9g*). It is looped with umbilical tape or a fine Penrose drain to allow traction. The lateral rectus need not usually be disinserted from the globe to allow entry into the central orbital space.

Intraorbital dissection is performed using either the operating microscope or operating loupes with a fiberoptic headlight. Intraorbital structures should be identified by careful dissection and divided only under direct visualization, with application of bipolar cautery to stop bleeding when necessary. If the mass is to be removed, a cryoprobe is applied to the mass to facilitate removal (*Figure 12.9h*). Following biopsy or removal of an intraorbital mass, the periorbita is closed using 4/0 or 5/0 chromic or plain catgut. If hemostasis is complete, no drain is placed. If the lateral orbital wall bone fragment is to be replaced, it is placed in position and fixed using 3/0 stainless steel wire. The wire is placed in the previously drilled holes and twisted to proper tightness to ensure satisfactory alignment. The ends of the wire are cut long enough to allow them to be bent into the drill holes on the external surface of the bony surgical rim. Usually we do not advocate replacement of bone, since we believe that the patient's postoperative appearance is not substantially altered by the exclusion of this bone.

The temporalis muscle is repositioned in the temporalis fossa, and the periosteum and anterior temporalis fascia are reapproximated with buried interrupted sutures of 4/0 or 5/0 chromic catgut. Traction sutures are removed, and muscle and subcutaneous tissues are reapproximated with multiple interrupted sutures of catgut. A running subcuticular or cutaneous suture of 6/0 nylon or polypropylene, or interrupted 8/0 silk, is then used to close the skin incision (*Figure 12.9i*). The incision is dressed with a non-adherent sterile dressing with an overlying mild pressure patch. If a drain is used, one end is positioned in the fossa of the temporalis muscle, and the other end is passed subcutaneously and brought out inferior to the lateral aspect of the main incision through a separate stab wound. The drain is removed in 24–48 hours. Skin sutures are removed in 5–7 days.

In patients undergoing orbital decompression for thyroid eye disease, a lateral orbital approach is performed in the manner described above until the bone is removed. The amount of bone removed is variable. Bone rongeurs are used to extend the bony decompression inferiorly to include the orbital floor, up to and beyond the infraorbital nerve (which should always be preserved). One of us (WJI) prefers this approach. The other (NRM) prefers to extend the bony removal just to the lateral border of the infraorbital nerve. Further removal of bone from the medial orbital floor is accomplished through a Caldwell-Luc incision. Through this incision, it is possible to remove an extensive amount of bone from the orbital floor and medial orbital wall inferior to the anterior and posterior ethmoidal arteries (*Figure 12.10*). At this stage, a large segment of temporalis muscle is removed from its position opposite the bony opening (*Figure 12.11a,b*). If this is not done, the temporalis muscle will act as a barrier and will prevent decompression. We prefer to use a cutting cautery to remove the portion of muscle and minimize bleeding. A window of lateral periorbita is then carefully dissected away from the underlying orbital fat and removed (*Figure 12.11c*). The size of the window may vary, but it should be at least 20 × 20 mm. Removal of the periorbita allows fat to protrude from the orbit, producing decompression. If a Caldwell-Luc incision has also been performed, several slits are made in the inferior periorbita to allow fat to protrude inferiorly and produce further decompression. The skin incision is closed as previously described; and, if a Caldwell-Luc incision has been made, the mucous membrane incision is closed using running 3/0 catgut suture.

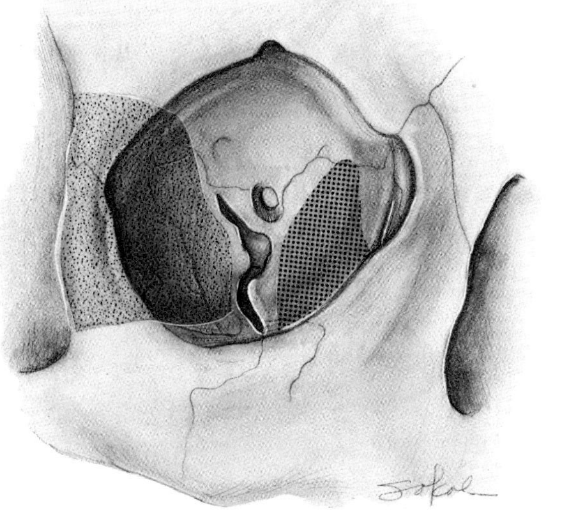

Figure 12.10 *The bony orbit showing the areas of bone removal during orbital decompression for thyroid eye disease. Fine stippled region is removed from a lateral approach. Dense stippled region is removed through a Caldwell-Luc approach*

Transconjunctival approach

Lesions located in the medial-middle or central orbital spaces are best biopsied or removed through a transconjunctival approach, often after a lateral orbitotomy has been performed to provide adequate room for lateral rotation of the globe (*Figure 12.12a*). The lateral orbitotomy is closed after the transconjunctival procedure is completed. A wire speculum is used to retract the eyelids, and a 240° limbal peritomy is performed nasally (from 11 to 7 o'clock for the right eye). The superior and inferior rectus muscles are looped with traction sutures to rotate the eye laterally (*Figure 12.12b*). The medial rectus muscle is identified. For extraconal lesions (in the middle orbital space), the medial rectus need not be removed from the globe, although a traction suture can be looped around it to aid in lateral rotation. Using fine malleable retractors, neurosurgical cottonoid pads and gentle blunt dissection, the lesion can be identified and biopsied or removed. When the lesion is within the central space, the medial

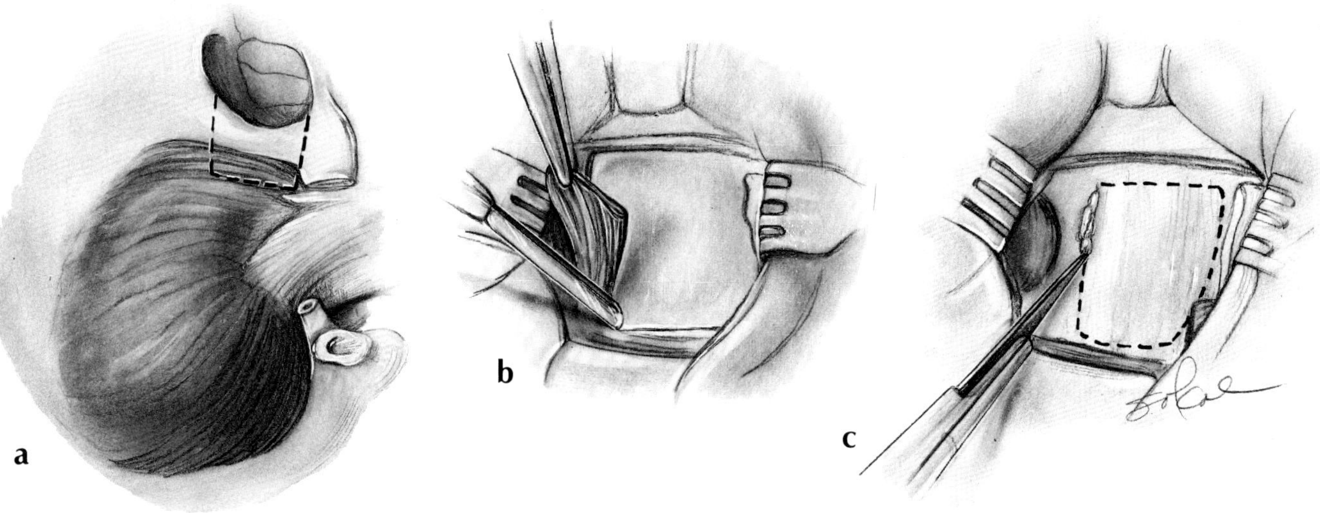

Figure 12.11 *Special considerations in orbital decompression for thyroid eye disease.* **(a)** *The extent of the initial lateral wall excision is outlined (dashed line). Note the relationship of the temporalis muscle to the excision site.* **(b)** *A portion of temporalis muscle is removed opposite and posterior to the bony excision site using a cutting cautery to minimize bleeding.* **(c)** *A window of periorbita is carefully removed from the lateral orbit to allow protrusion of fat in order to produce partial orbital decompression*

rectus is temporarily disinserted from the globe as if a muscle recession were to be performed (*Figure 12.12c*). A traction suture can then be placed through its stump on the globe to improve lateral rotation of the globe. With gentle traction on the rectus sutures, blunt dissection can be used to displace orbital fat and visualize the lesion (*Figures 12.12d,e*). After biopsy or removal of the lesion, the medial rectus is reattached to its original insertion on the globe, and the conjunctiva is closed using 8/0 running or interrupted collagen suture (*Figure 12.12f–h*). The lateral orbitotomy site is closed as described above. The lids are closed, and the eyelids are covered by a non-adherent sterile dressing with an overlying standard oval eye pad, and a light dressing is applied.

In the surgery of orbital masses, a decision must be made whether to perform an incisional biopsy, excisional biopsy or total removal. Lesions that are well-circumscribed can generally be completely removed irrespective of whether they are in the peripheral, middle or inner (central) orbital space. The most common well-circumscribed lesions are dermoid cysts and hemangiomas. With such lesions, adequate visualization, careful blunt dissection, gentle traction on the lesion using the cryoprobe and use of the bipolar cautery usually allow a safe, total removal. On the other hand, most inflammatory orbital lesions and metastatic tumors (including carcinomas and lymphoreticular lesions) cannot – and need not – be totally removed. In some instances, the lesions are obviously diffuse. In other cases, the lesions are surrounded by a 'pseudocapsule' of surrounding tissue that is microscopically invaded by tumor cells. Attempts at total removal of these lesions can result in extensive damage to normal orbital structures, without achieving total removal. Of course, if the main portion of the mass is easily removable, this should be done. As a minimum, an adequate biopsy should be obtained in all cases so that the tissue can be identified and definite treatment begun with chemotherapy, radiotherapy, or both.

Surgical management of specific orbital lesions

Orbital floor (blow-out) fractures

Diplopia from orbital floor (blow-out) fractures can occur as a result of several causes, including: (*1*) hematoma and swelling involving the inferior rectus and inferior oblique muscles; (*2*) damage to the inferior branches of the oculomotor nerve; or (*3*) entrapment of orbital tissue in the fracture site. Thus, unless there is profound enophthalmos on initial examination, we prefer to follow-up the patient for at least 2 weeks without surgery, performing serial quantitative measurements of the degree of diplopia, extent of ductions and amount of enophthalmos. In most cases, diplopia spontaneously resolves, there is no significant enophthalmos and orbital exploration is unnecessary. In other cases, residual diplopia can be corrected with simple surgery on the vertical and/or horizontal extraocular muscles.

If surgery is necessary to repair an orbital floor fracture, a transcutaneous, extraperiosteal approach is used to expose the fracture site (*Figure 12.13a–c*). The intact periorbita is carefully elevated from normal bone until the fracture site is located (*Figure 12.13d,e*). Periorbita is then elevated around the incarcerated tissue (*Figure 12.13f*). The entrapped tissue is released by inserting a narrow spatula through the bony defect and using it to pry the prolapsed tissue back into the orbit (*Figure 12.13g,h*). This is a better method than pulling up on the muscle and fascia using tissue forceps in a hand-over-hand fashion, as is often attempted. In some instances, it may be necessary to remove additional bone from around the defect to allow release of the tissue. A Caldwell-Luc approach may be necessary to release tissue by allowing the tissue to be pushed upward from below, while maintaining traction on the tissue from above.

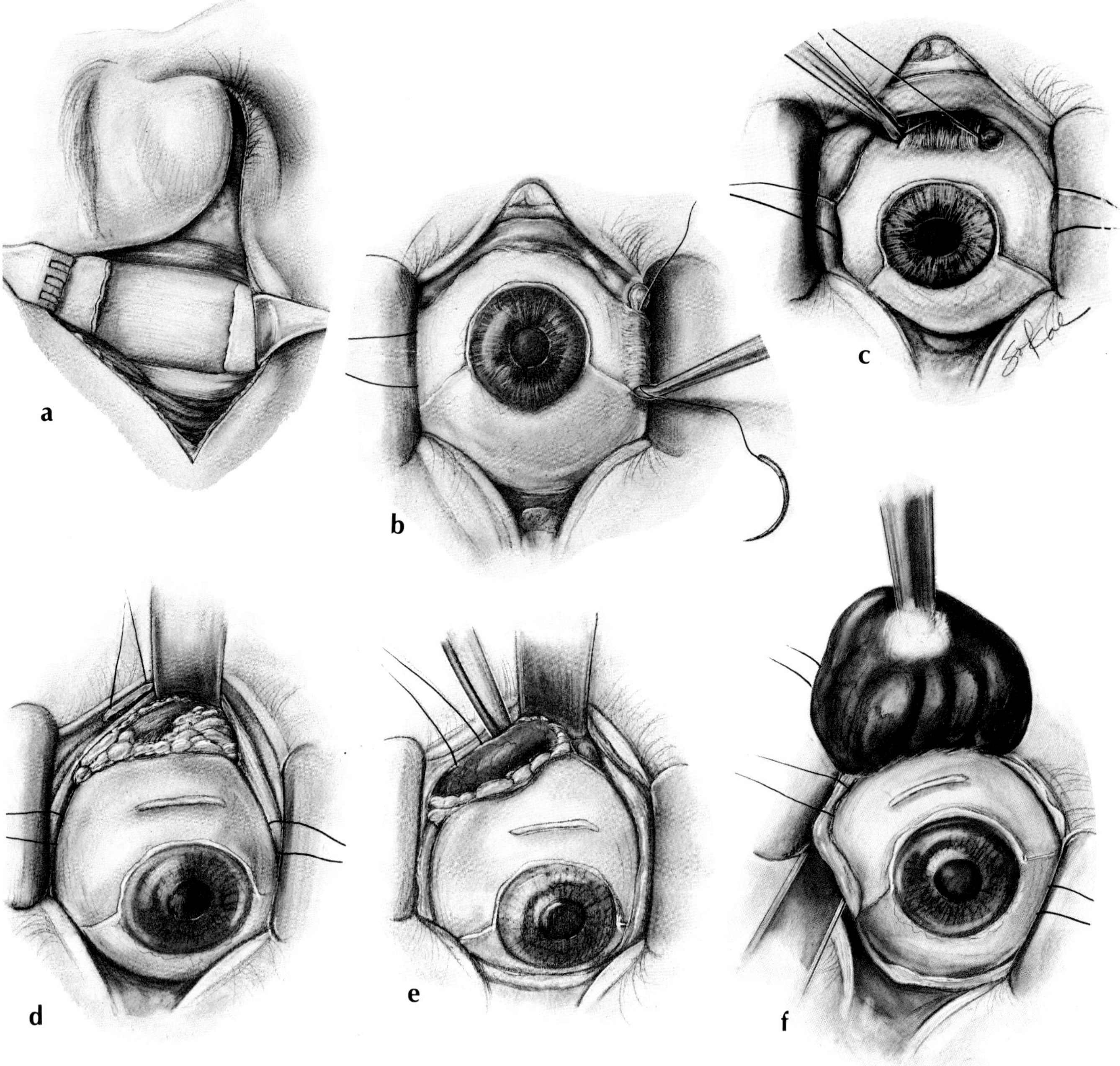

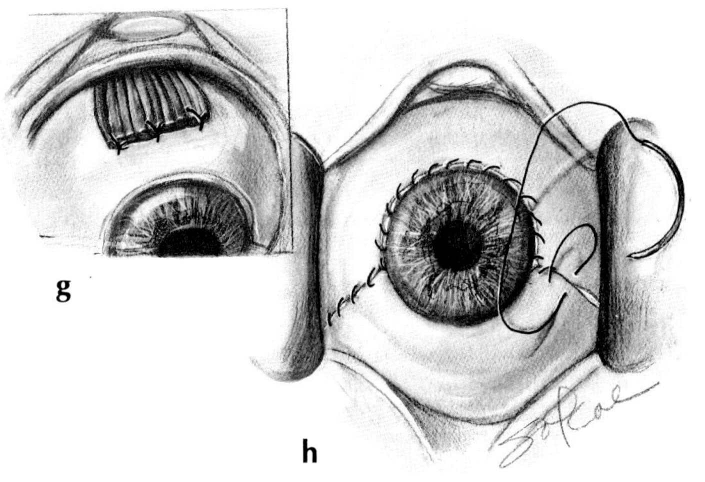

Figure 12.12 *Transconjunctival approach to medial orbital lesions.* **(a)** *A routine lateral orbitotomy is made to allow lateral rotation of the eye.* **(b)** *A peritomy has been performed from 11 to 7 o'clock to expose the superior, medial and inferior rectus muscles and allow access into the medial, middle orbital space. The superior and inferior rectus muscles are isolated and looped with traction sutures to provide lateral eye rotation.* **(c)** *The eye is rotated laterally, and the medial rectus is isolated and disinserted from the globe.* **(d)** *Careful retraction and blunt dissection of orbital tissue are then performed until the lesion is identified.* **(e)** *Blunt dissection is used to free the lesion from surrounding tissue.* **(f)** *The mass is grasped with a cryoprobe and delivered intact from the orbit.* **(g)** *After establishment of hemostasis, the medial rectus is reattached to the globe in its normal location.* **(h)** *The conjunctiva is resutured to the globe using a running collagen suture*

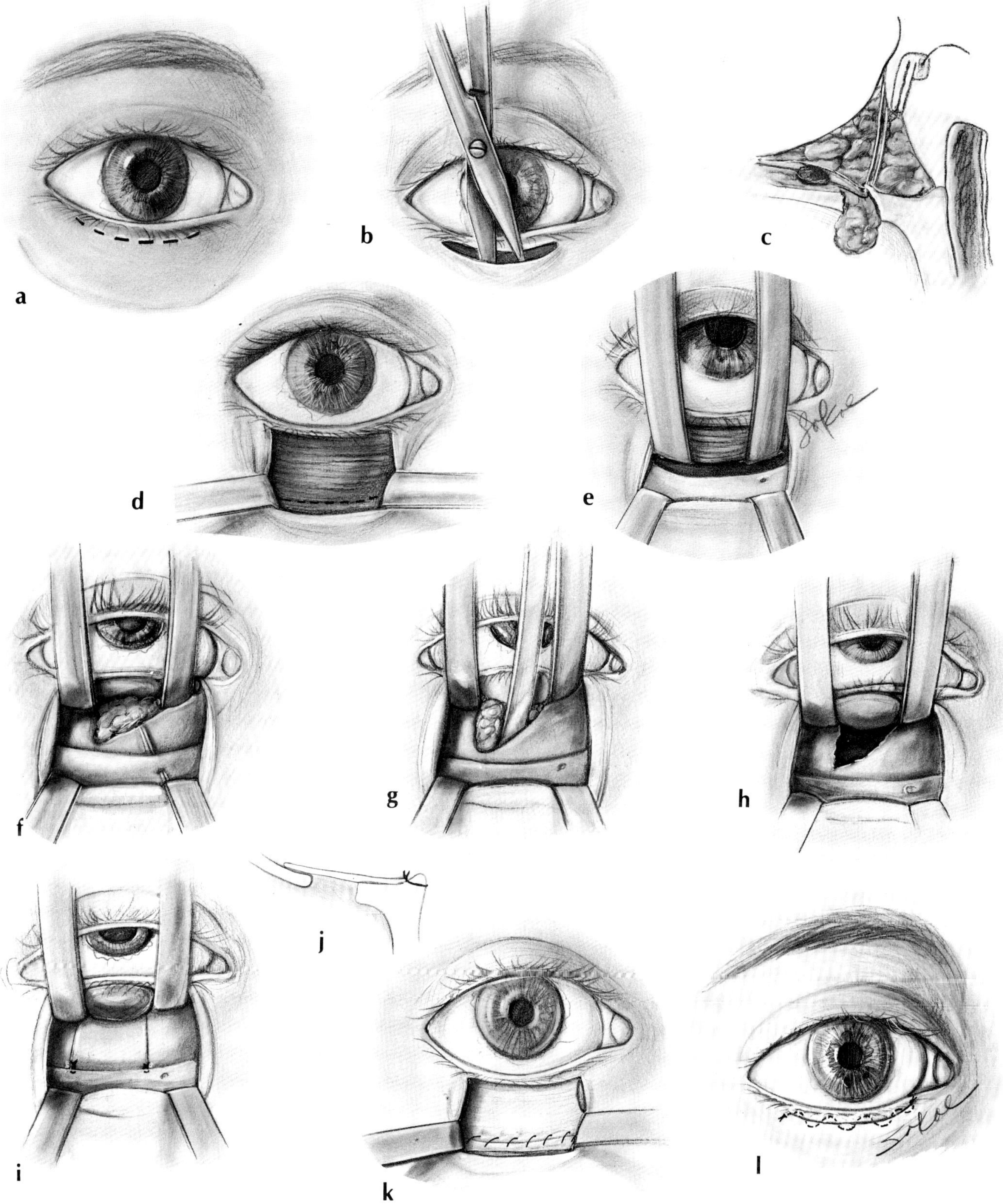

Figure 12.13 *Approach to orbital floor fractures.* **(a)** *An incision is made in the skin just beneath the cilia of the lower lid.* **(b)** *The incision is carried down through orbicularis oculi muscle and then continued inferiorly to the level of the inferior orbital rim* (**c,** *side view).* **(d)** *Malleable ribbon retractors are used to spread the skin and subcutaneous tissue, while an incision is made in the periorbita along the inferior orbital rim.* **(e)** *The periorbita is stripped from the floor of the orbit until* **(f)** *the fracture site is exposed.* **(g,h)** *A small ribbon retractor is inserted into the defect to allow manipulation and freeing of trapped tissue.* **(i)** *A Supramid implant is placed over the fracture site and anchored in place* (**j,** *side view).* **(k,l)** *The periorbital and skin incisions are closed separately*

Once orbital tissue has been removed from the fracture site, any loose bone is carefully removed with a small sphenoidal punch, taking care not to damage the infraorbital nerve. The size of the bony defect is noted, and a piece of Supramid is fashioned to cover the defect. The Supramid should never be longer than 2.5 cm in the anteroposterior dimension; otherwise, it may encroach on the optic nerve. However, the implant should be wide enough so that intact bone medial and lateral to the bony defect can support it. The Supramid is positioned inside the anterior orbital rim or beneath the anterior edge of the bony defect to prevent it from becoming displaced forward. The implant should also be sutured to the orbital rim to prevent it from migrating in any direction (*Figure 12.13i,j*). The operative site is then irrigated with antibiotic solution, and the wound is closed in layers as described above (*Figure 12.13k,l*).

Lacrimal gland lesions

Lesions involving the lacrimal gland require special management. The lacrimal gland may harbor inflammatory lesions as well as benign and malignant lymphoid and epithelial cell tumors. Of these tumors, it is crucial to diagnosis correctly and manage mixed-cell tumors. Failure to excise such lesions completely results in eventual recurrence, often with malignant change and spread beyond the limits of surgical excision. A benign mixed-cell tumor of the lacrimal gland is suspected in any patient (usually aged 30–50 years) with a history of painless eyelid or superotemporal orbital swelling and proptosis of longer than 12 months' duration. In such cases, neuroradiological studies may show only an ill-defined mass involving the lacrimal gland without evidence of bony change in the lacrimal fossa, or there may be some evidence of expansion without destruction of the lacrimal fossa. These findings differ from those in patients with lacrimal gland carcinomas, who usually present with a short history of pain, proptosis, swelling and neuroradiological evidence of bony destruction of the lacrimal fossa. In patients suspected of harboring a benign mixed-cell tumor of the lacrimal gland, the surgical approach is through a lateral orbitotomy as described above (*Figure 12.14*). An S-shaped skin incision is always used, because it provides more exposure than the linear modification of the Burke incision.

Many believe that biopsy of a benign mixed-cell tumor results in eventual growth and spread; and this may be true if a biopsy *only* is performed, the incision closed and

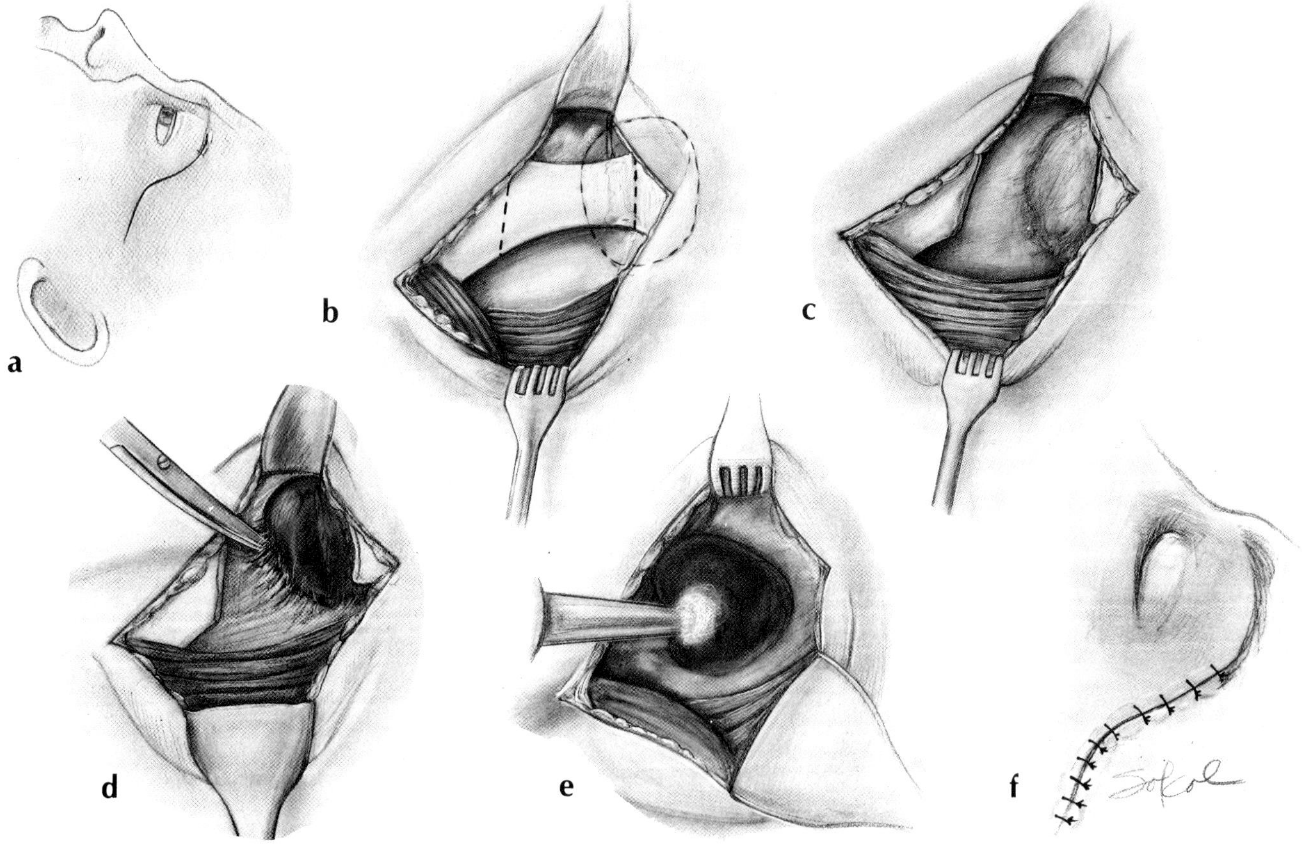

Figure 12.14 *Lateral orbitotomy for lacrimal gland lesions.* **(a)** *An S-shaped incision is used to provide access to the lesion. This incision may be used for any lateral orbitotomy.* **(b)** *The incision has been carried down to the lateral bony wall, and the periosteum (and periorbita) have been separated from the bone. Fine dashed lines outline the location of the lacrimal gland. Dense dashed lines mark sites of bone incision.* **(c)** *A portion of the lateral bony wall has been removed using an oscillating saw and bone rongeurs. The lacrimal gland can be identified beneath its periosteal covering.* **(d)** *Blunt dissection is used to separate the lesion (or gland) from surrounding tissue.* **(e)** *A cryoprobe is used to remove the mass from the orbit.* **(f)** *The perorbita (if not removed), periosteum and subcutaneous tissue incision sites are closed separately, and the skin is closed using interrupted suture*

definitive therapy delayed until permanent histological sections are obtained that disclose the true nature of the lesion. We believe that it is safe and prudent to perform a biopsy and frozen-section study of any lacrimal gland mass. If the diagnosis on frozen section is a benign mixed-cell tumor, removal of the entire tumor, surrounding lacrimal gland and adjacent tissue including periorbita is performed. Removal of adjacent lacrimal gland is important for two reasons: the tumor may be multicentric; and the 'capsule' is, in fact, a pseudocapsule, often permeated by tumor cells. Thus, contiguous tissue may already be seeded with tumor cells at the time of surgery. We are not aware of any cases in which a benign mixed-cell tumor has recurred after frozen-section biopsy followed by complete, *en bloc* removal during a single procedure. For these reasons, we use this approach. If, however, the lesion is found on frozen section to be inflammatory or malignant, we usually elect not to remove the entire mass and lacrimal gland but to terminate the surgery and manage the lesion non-surgically.

Although a transseptal approach to lacrimal gland lesions suspected of being malignant is probably safer than an extraperiosteal approach (since the latter results in loss of the periorbita as a potential barrier to seeding of the extraperiosteal space with malignant cells), we believe that an extraperiosteal approach should be used for lacrimal gland lesions not associated with pain or inflammation, since the likelihood of benign mixed tumor is so high in these cases. We would rather risk spread of an already malignant neoplasm by biopsy through an extraperiosteal approach than risk converting a potentially curable benign mixed-cell tumor into a malignancy by incomplete removal through a transseptal approach.

Orbital abscesses

Prompt surgical treatment of orbital abscesses is essential. Because many abscesses originate from paranasal sinus infections, an ophthalmologist and an otolaryngologist should operate as a team. This approach allows the abscess to be drained and the involved sinuses to be treated appropriately. The possibility of the existence of an orbital or paranasal foreign body as the cause of orbital inflammation should always be considered. If a foreign body is present, it must be completely removed. It is also important to achieve *adequate* surgical exposure in treating orbital abscesses. Simple drainage of an abscess and involved sinuses usually is insufficient to halt the inflammatory process. The involved sinuses should be opened, completely drained and obliterated by the otolaryngologist.

Paranasal sinus mucoceles

A similar team approach, operating with an otolaryngologist, may be used in managing paranasal sinus mucoceles. Mucoceles should be drained and the involved sinus obliterated. Some mucoceles, especially if they are in an older patient and the sinus involvement is minor, can be adequately managed by complete removal of the mucous membrane lining the involved sinus, followed by establishment of an adequate passage for drainage from the sinus into the nose. However, such lesions can be treated more extensively by complete obliteration of the involved sinus by removing the sinus mucous membrane with a pneumatic drill, followed either by collapsing the sinus or packing of the sinus with adipose tissue taken from an abdominal incision.

With large mucoceles, the possibility of intracranial extension should be considered. For this reason, the posterior bony limits of the sinus must be delineated preoperatively, to determine whether neurosurgical assistance will be needed.

Optic nerve gliomas

The surgical treatment of orbital optic nerve gliomas and optic nerves sheath meningiomas remains controversial. These lesions can be completely removed only by removing the optic nerve as well. Because these lesions usually grow slowly, many orbital surgeons believe that removal should not be attempted until virtually all vision is lost. If severe loss of vision has occurred, a combined ophthalmological-neurosurgical approach is used to attempt to remove the *entire* lesion, including the intracanalicular and intracranial extension.

Exenteration of the orbit

Orbital exenteration is performed for malignant neoplasms that are confined to the orbit and unresponsive to chemotherapy and/or radiotherapy. In this procedure, the entire orbital contents, including the periorbita, are surgically removed. The boundary of the orbital incision is usually the orbital rim (*see Figure 12.2*), although the eyelids are occasionally preserved. Elevation of the periorbita, using a periosteal elevator, is carried around the entire orbit posteriorly to the apex. The remaining tissue is cut away using a sharp scalpel, sharp scissors or an exenteration knife. The remaining apical orbital tissue is cauterized extensively to destroy the tissue and stop bleeding. Malignant lacrimal gland tumors that are thought to have bony involvement usually require extensive removal of orbital bone. Following exenteration with bone excision, reconstruction usually involves rotation of a skin flap to cover the exposed intracranial dura and to fill the orbital cavity. When bone has not been removed, the orbital cavity may be covered with a split-thickness skin graft obtained from the thigh or abdomen. The socket can then be filled with gauze or a loose dressing to keep the graft in place and to allow healing. We prefer to eliminate the skin graft and simply allow the orbit to heal by primary epithelialization and granulation of the socket. This technique requires frequent, careful attention to the granulating socket during its healing stage, but it will eventually heal with non-keratinizing epithelium.

The decision to exenterate an orbit should never be made on the basis of frozen-section tissue study alone. Only permanently fixed histopathological sections should be used to diagnose a malignant lesion that requires orbital exenteration.

Postoperative care

In general, pressure dressings are applied after orbital surgery only when a drain has been placed. If pressure dressings are used routinely without a drain, postoperative hemorrhage or swelling may occlude the vascular supply of the optic nerve and/or globe. Postoperative systemic corticosteroids are used when an inflammatory lesion is removed or if a dermoid cyst ruptures during removal. When systemic corticosteroids are used, systemic antibiotics are also given prophylactically for about 10 days. When the orbital lesion is thought to be infectious, appropriate antibiotic coverage is used; however, postoperative antibiotics are not used routinely.

In the immediate postoperative period, the patient is not confined to bed but is encouraged to ambulate. The dressing is removed after 24 hours, at which time the vision is assessed. If a drain has been placed, it is removed at this time, and warm compresses are applied continually to the orbital region for the remainder of the hospitalization. The patient is usually discharged on the second or third postoperative day.

Complications

Complications of orbital surgery can occur intraoperatively, in the immediate postoperative period or later in the course of recovery. Intraoperative complications include hemorrhage, inadvertent breaching of the confines of the lesion, inadvertent damage to normal orbital structures, and inadvertent entry into adjacent sinuses or the intracranial cavity.

When severe hemorrhage occurs during orbital surgery, it is a potential catastrophe, and every effort must be made to find its source and stop it. To this end, exposure, magnification and illumination are essential. Careful manipulation of orbital tissues using fine malleable retractors and suction is often sufficient to expose the bleeding site and allow cautery using a bipolar system. If an operating microscope has not been used, it may be brought into place to provide further magnification and illumination to aid in identification and cauterization of the bleeding site.

In cases of inadvertent rupture of a dermoid cyst, careful attention should be paid first to removing the entire cyst. The contents should be aspirated and the area irrigated vigorously with both saline and dexamethasone because the cyst contents are highly irritating. If the cyst is filled with hair fragments, the operating microscope is used when possible to remove the scattered fragments. Postoperatively, the patient should be placed on systemic corticosteroids.

Inadvertent entry into the paranasal sinuses or intracranial cavity may require otolaryngological or neurosurgical intervention. If the mucosa of the sinuses or the intracranial dura has not been breached, no major manipulation need be performed. However, if a sinus is entered, it may be best to exenterate the sinus by removing all of its mucosa and establishing a drainage site into the nose. The patient should also be placed on systemic antibiotics. If the dura has been lacerated, it must be carefully sutured closed, and systemic antibiotics are begun to prevent meningitis or meningoencephalitis.

Immediate postoperative complications are usually a result of hemorrhage or infection. Proper hemostasis during surgery and appropriate orbital drainage when necessary will significantly reduce the risk of an extensive accumulation of blood or tissue fluid. Nevertheless, the complaint of severe orbital pain in the initial postoperative period must be evaluated immediately because it may signify orbital hemorrhage or infection, which can result in permanent visual loss. When orbital hemorrhage is severe and accompanied by visual loss, prompt orbital decompression must be attempted. Accumulated blood is released, either by opening the operative site or by more extensive decompression procedures. Although CT scanning or ultrasonography may accurately show the location of a hemorrhage, decompression should not be delayed in order to obtain these studies. Accumulation of pus within the orbit must also be promptly relieved. The abscess is opened, the material removed and cultured, and a drain placed. The site can be irrigated with antibiotic solution, and the patient is placed on intravenous systemic antibiotics that are chosen to treat appropriately the responsible organism.

Although in the immediate postoperative period there is often periorbital edema, ecchymosis, ptosis, extraocular muscle imbalance and cutaneous hypesthesia, these findings usually resolve rapidly. Some patients, however, have persistent diplopia after surgery. This can result from damage by the previous orbital lesion or from secondary scar formation involving the extraocular muscles after surgery. If the muscle imbalance is mild, diplopia can usually be managed with prisms. If it is too great to be treated with prisms, extraocular muscle surgery is performed as soon as the motility disturbance has stabilized.

Summary

The ophthalmologist's approach to orbital disease should be – as Krohel, Stewart and Chavis[3] have suggested – a *practical* one. It must include a complete preoperative evaluation, an appropriate surgical approach with meticulous surgical technique and logical intraoperative decision-making, and careful postoperative management.

References

1. Henderson, J. W. Orbital tumors. Philadelphia: W. B. Saunders, 1973
2. Jones, I. S., Jakobiec, F. A., eds. Diseases of the orbit. Hagerstown, Maryland: Harper and Row, 1979
3. Krohel, G. B., Stewart, W. B., Chavis, R. M. Orbital disease: A practical approach. New York: Grune and Stratton, 1981
4. Alper, M. G. Computed tomography in planning and evaluating orbital surgery. Ophthalmology 1980; 87:418–431
5. Dallow, R. L. Reliability of orbital diagnostic tests: Ultrasonography, computerized tomography and radiography. Ophthalmology 1978; 85:1218–1228
6. Dallow, R. L., Momose, K. J., Weber, A. L., Wray, S. H. Comparison of ultrasonography, computerized tomography (EMI scan) and radiographic techniques in evaluation of exophthalmos. Transactions of the American Academy of Ophthalmology and Otolaryngology 1976; 81:305–322
7. Grove, A. S., Jr. Ocular computed tomography. Boston: Little, Brown and Company, 1982

13

Surgery for ocular injuries

Lawrence W. Hirst MD
Thomas A. Rice MD

Introduction

Ocular injuries vary greatly and can affect one or more parts of the eye. Some injuries require surgery and others are managed without surgery. The surgical management of ocular trauma has markedly improved with the advent of microsurgical techniques, vitreous surgery, and the use of new diagnostic tools such as ultrasonography. We will discuss the general principles of management of ocular injuries including a stepwise approach for dealing with complex injuries.

Indications and rationale for surgery

Ocular injuries can damage the eye and cause loss of vision by a number of mechanisms. The injury itself can directly damage the eye by penetration or rupture of the globe, contusion damage, or both. Chemical and burn injuries can also produce severe ocular damage. Later inflammation, infection or growth of scar tissue can produce further damage. The goal of surgery for ocular trauma is to restore the eye to a stable, functional state and to minimize the chance of later complications.

Ocular injuries resulting from a blow to the eye can be divided into those in which the globe suffers a contusion injury but remains intact, and those in which penetration or rupture of the globe occurs. Surgery is more frequently necessary for injuries in which the globe is lacerated or ruptured.

In eyes with a contusion injury alone, severe damage affecting vision can result from hyphema, angle-recession glaucoma, cyclodialysis and hypotony, cataract, lens dislocation, vitreous hemorrhage, retinal dialysis or retinal breaks, retinal detachment, contusion retinopathy, traumatic macular hole, choroidal rupture, choroidal hemorrhage, combined retinal and choroidal rupture, and other damage. Surgery may be required to treat some of these contusion injuries such as: (*1*) hyphema with uncontrolled secondary glaucoma or corneal blood-staining; (*2*) medically uncontrolled angle-recession glaucoma; (*3*) lens dislocation into the anterior chamber with uncontrolled secondary glaucoma or corneolenticular touch; (*4*) non-resolving vitreous hemorrhage; (*5*) retinal breaks or dialysis; (*6*) retinal detachment; and (*7*) combined retinal and choroidal rupture. Of these entities, surgery for angle-recession glaucoma, non-resolving vitreous hemorrhage, and retinal breaks and detachments are described in other chapters. The surgical treatment of hyphema is directed at removing the anterior chamber blood without damaging intraocular tissues. A dislocated lens in the anterior chamber is removed using cataract extraction techniques. Surgery for other contusion injuries is directed at restoring as much as possible the normal anatomy of the eye.

Injuries in which the globe is ruptured or penetrated are often more complex because such eyes can have damage to several ocular structures and often have complicated retinal detachments that are difficult to repair. Furthermore, if hemorrhage or opacities are present, it may be impossible to visualize and accurately assess the full extent of injury. Secondary complications can develop including: (*1*) endophthalmitis; (*2*) intraocular inflammation; (*3*) growth of scar tissue with secondary damage such as retinal detachment; and (*4*) ocular damage from retained intraocular foreign bodies. Therapy is directed not only toward repairing the primary injury but also toward preventing these secondary complications.

In managing the primary injury, any rupture or laceration that is accessible and not self-sealing must be closed. Closure restores the ocular integrity, preventing loss, or additional loss, of intraocular tissue, and it lessens the risk of endophthalmitis. In closing wounds, prolapsed nonviable tissue is excised, but viable tissue that can be salvaged is reposited into a normal position. Meticulous wound closure is required with the goal of removing incarcerated tissues from wounds and achieving permanent watertight closure.

Secondary complications in a ruptured or lacerated globe should be prevented when possible or treated to minimize further damage. Antibiotics are used to prevent or treat endophthalmitis. Vitreous surgery may also be necessary in the management of endophthalmitis. Ocular inflammation can often be managed medically with corticosteroids and cycloplegic drops, but occasionally severe inflammation, such as lens-induced uveitis or phacoanaphylaxis, may require vitrectomy. If an eye contains a reactive foreign body, surgery is necessary to remove it in order to prevent damage to the eye from its toxic components.

A severe secondary effect of penetrating ocular injury is growth of vascularized or non-vascularized scar tissue into the eye. Contraction of such scar tissue can cause retinal detachment, cyclitic membranes with phthisis bulbi, and other severe damage. Experimental studies show that penetrating ocular injuries involving the vitreous often lead to fibrous ingrowth into the vitreous cavity. In one study, monkey eyes with a wound of the pars plana and blood in the vitreous gel developed intraocular inflammation, cyclitic membranes, epiretinal membranes and traction retinal detachments[1]. Another study demonstrated that lensectomy and vitrectomy in such eyes 1 or 14 days after injury prevented cyclitic membranes and traction retinal detachment by removing the vitreous scaffold on which the fibrous tissue proliferates, but the same surgery was ineffective 70 days after injury[2]. In an experimental rabbit model of double-perforating posterior segment injury, fibrous tissue grew along the tract of a previous penetrating injury[3]. Vitrectomy immediately after injury prevented development of transvitreal fibrous tissue, and vitrectomy at 2 weeks removed the transvitreal tissue and it did not recur[4]. Similar pathological findings are seen in human eyes. Rhegmatogenous retinal detachment often results from penetrating injuries, either from a retinal hole created by the penetration itself or from a retinal break resulting from vitreous traction. Such detachments are often difficult to repair surgically[5]; however, vitreous surgery can be used to prevent or remove vitreous traction bands and to facilitate management of complex retinal detachments.

Surgery is indicated in all penetrating injuries, except for small self-sealing wounds with no other significant ocular damage. The type of surgery chosen depends on the extent of the injury and the capabilities of the surgeon. Simple injuries may require only wound closure. More complex injuries may require vitreous or retinal reattachment surgery, usually as a reoperation after primary wound closure. In severe cases, several operations may be necessary to deal with persistent or new complications. We will describe a stepwise approach used to deal with complex injuries.

Preoperative evaluation

History

Although the extent of trauma is often self-evident, it is helpful to know the type of agent which inflicted the injury and the manner in which it involved the eye. If a patient has been hammering metal on metal without protective glasses, intraocular foreign bodies are immediately suspected. A history of eye injury in a child running with a pencil suggests a penetrating injury. It is useful to determine what agent caused the injury and, if possible, to examine a specimen of this agent. In the case of chemicals, this can help establish the prognosis and management. A specimen of a piece of metal that might be in the eye can be checked to see if it is magnetic.

The length of time since the injury is of critical importance in assessing the clinical picture. The presence of a heavy cellular reaction and fibrin in the anterior chamber immediately after injury does not necessarily indicate infection, while the same findings 24–48 hours after injury suggest endophthalmitis. Similarly, with chemical burns, the opacification seen with an alkali burn 3 or 4 days after the injury frequently allows definitive classification and grading of the severity of the injury[6] while corneal opacification seen immediately after the injury can be misleading in assessing the severity of damage.

The clinical picture can also be altered by prior treatment, administered either as first aid or as an attempt at definitive treatment. The use of topical antibiotics can alter the conjunctiva flora so that bacterial cultures are difficult to interpret. The use of eye ointments in eyes with penetrating injury can itself explain the appearance of foreign material in the wound. In chemical injuries, topical anesthetic may have been instilled and can give the impression of total corneal anesthesia, or vigorous irrigation may have denuded the corneal epithelium so that a more extensive corneal injury is mimicked.

A history of ocular pathology preceding injury influences the management and prognosis of the injury. For example, the presence of previous amblyopia tempers the prognosis for visual recovery. Knowledge of a previous cataract extraction may prevent an unnecessarily extensive vitreous examination for a dislocated lens, and previous herpes simplex keratitis may explain some of the corneal nebula seen in a mild chemical burn.

The general health of the patient should be evaluated to decide if special precautions are necessary in administering general anesthesia, the usual type of anesthesia used for patients with significant eye injuries requiring surgery. A history of a bleeding diathesis, frequent aspirin use, or anticoagulant therapy may lead one to prepare for more intraoperative bleeding than usual or possibly to administer medication before surgery to prevent excessive bleeding. The use of systemic medication can alter the planned therapy or surgical approach, and known allergies to antibiotics can modify therapy designed to prevent endophthalmitis.

Ocular examination

The measurement of best corrected vision, either with glasses or with a pinhole, should not be overlooked in the initial assessment of significant eye trauma. If vision is severely limited, it should still be carefully assessed to determine if light perception and good light projection are present. The level of vision is of prognostic importance, but for medicolegal reasons it is also desirable to obtain a recorded visual acuity in each eye. The frustration and anger of the patient who fails to recover good final vision after trauma is blunted if the patient understands at the onset that trauma alone has severely reduced vision. This understanding makes discussion of therapy and the prognosis clearer.

The examination should be undertaken with minimal administration of topical medications until the integrity of the globe is ascertained. If there is a lid laceration, lid swelling, or previous ointment applications, careful separation of the lids using two Desmarres retractors may be required. This minimizes pressure on the eye that might cause extrusion of intraocular contents if the globe is not intact. If finger retraction is possible, it is done using pressure against the orbital rim, again to avoid pressure on a ruptured or lacerated globe. Hand-light examination of the lids and the eye often shows penetration sites and the extent of injury. In the case of chemical injury, careful inspection under the surface of the upper lid and in the superior and inferior fornices is mandatory. Presence of particulate matter at these sites requires further irrigation and removal. Pupillary light reaction should be noted, especially the presence of an afferent pupillary defect, which usually indicates severe posterior segment injury. Slit-lamp examination is done unless the patient is incapable of sitting at the instrument because of other injury. Careful examination is done to detect anterior segment penetration sites, anterior chamber inflammation or hemorrhage, abnormalities in the depth of the anterior chamber, irregularity of the iris or pupil margin, and damage or dislocation of the lens. If the eye appears intact, then careful measurement of applanation or pneumatonometry intraocular pressure can be attempted. If the anterior segment appears normal and the patient is not suspected of having significant central nervous system injury, then the pupils are dilated. Careful slit-lamp examination of the lens and vitreous is performed. Vitreous and fundus examination with indirect ophthalmoscopy may show posterior segment injury.

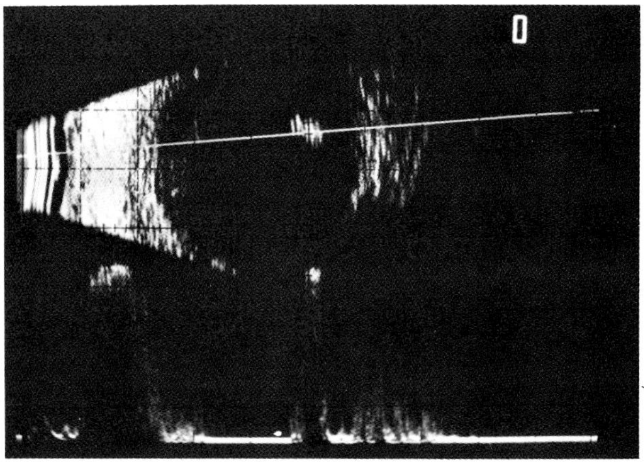

Figure 13.1 *A- and B-scan ultrasonography showing metallic foreign body in the vitreous cavity*

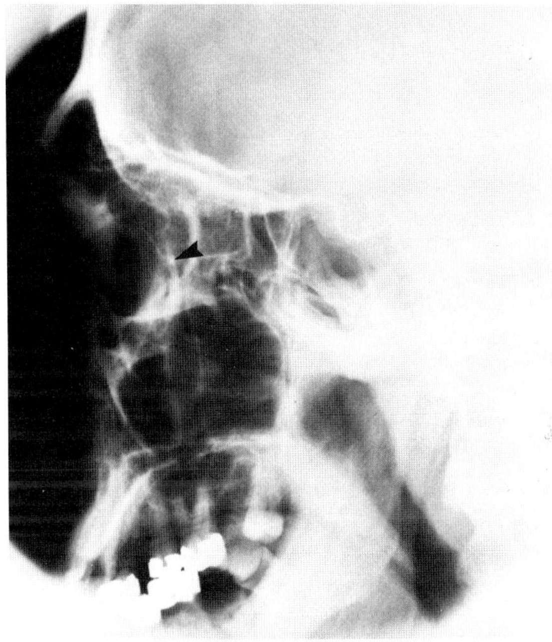

Figure 13.2 *Lateral skull X-ray showing small posterior intraocular foreign body (arrow)*

Diagnostic tests

In significant anterior segment trauma where an edematous cornea, hyphema, cataractous lens, vitreous hemorrhage or other opacity prevents posterior segment examination, gentle B-scan ultrasound examination may be performed. Ultrasonography is useful in determining the presence of vitreous hemorrhage, posterior vitreous detachment, retinal detachment, choroidal detachment and the location of foreign bodies (*Figure 13.1*). Eyes with open wounds should not have ultrasonography if it might cause prolapse of intraocular tissue.

Suspected penetration of the globe by a foreign body requires X-ray examination of the globe and orbit after ocular examination. Plain X-ray films are taken to determine whether a foreign body is present (*Figure 13.2*). If the type of penetrating material is known or a specimen is available, this can help the radiologist obtain optimally exposed X-ray films. Special X-ray localization methods such as the Sweet's localization can be helpful in determining the position of a foreign body. Often X-ray localization, however, does not distinguish between an intraocular foreign body embedded in the posterior eye wall and a foreign body that has passed through the eye and is lodged just behind the posterior sclera. Improved CT scan X-rays with axial and coronal views are superior to conventional X-ray examinations and X-ray localization techniques (*Figure 13.3a,b*).

If possible, photography is used to document the injury for medicolegal reasons.

Examination of the eye under anesthesia is indicated in infants when severe pain or swelling prevents adequate examination or when penetration or rupture of the eye is suspected but not confirmed by clinical examination. This

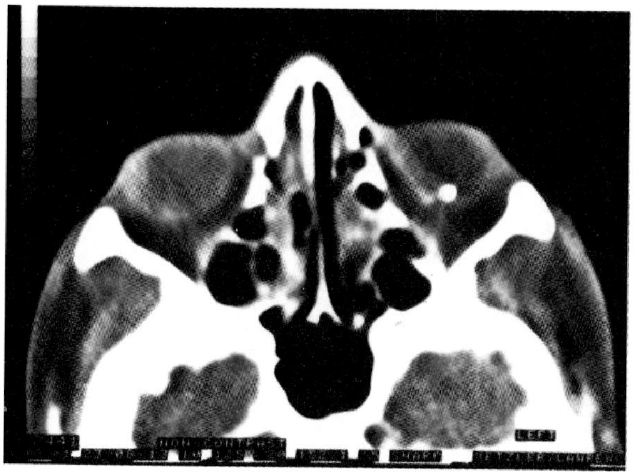

a

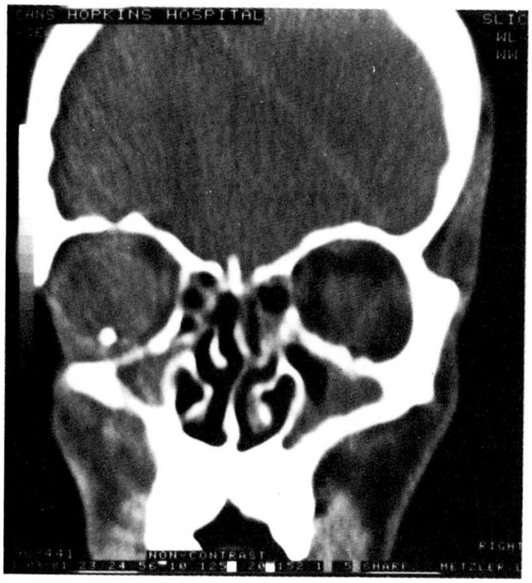

b

Figure 13.3 *CT scan X-ray, showing metallic foreign body in the vitreous cavity.* **(a)** *Horizontal section.* **(b)** *Coronal section*

is particularly so in eyes with conjunctival and Tenon's lacerations or in eyes with subconjunctival hemorrhage after blunt trauma in which a laceration or rupture is suspected but not seen. In these cases surgical exploration may also be required.

Preoperative management

After acute penetrating injury, the eye should be protected with a shield which rests on the frontal and maxillary bones and does not push on the eye. An underlying eye patch should not be used if it exerts pressure on the eye. Patching of the uninjured eye may be useful in limiting movement of the injured eye. Bilateral patching is preceded by an explanation to the patient, so that the anxiety produced by covering the seeing eye is not excessive and counterproductive. Every effort is made to avoid elevation of intraocular pressure and expulsion of intraocular contents through the perforation site by preventing vomiting, coughing and straining. For the same reason, it may be preferable to transport the patient in a sitting position rather than in a supine position. Although topical application of an anesthetic agent may be required for adequate examination of the injured eye, all other topical medications should be avoided. If the patient is not adequately immunized for tetanus, tetanus toxoid should be given, although tetanus infection following ocular penetrating injury alone has not been reported.

The immediate care of the chemically burned eye differs from that of other types of trauma. With chemical burns, immediate irrigation of the eye is crucial and the testing of visual acuity and other examinations of the eye are postponed until adequate ocular irrigation is completed. Irrigation is usually done even if there is a history of previous irrigation elsewhere because it is often difficult to assess whether the previous irrigation was adequate. Copious irrigation with sterile saline is given with a cystoscopy set or other high-flow delivery system to the front of the eye and fornices until all particulate matter is gone and until the pH of the ocular surface has returned to normal. This usually requires a minimum of 10–15 minutes' irrigation, but under certain circumstances it can require up to one or 2 hours' irrigation. Non-soluble particulate matter such as lime may require removal with a cotton swab. After adequate irrigation, the eye is examined carefully. The use of EDTA or other agents in alkali burn or immediate anterior chamber paracentesis is advocated by some, but there is little scientific evidence supporting the use of these treatments. Eye patching to aid in corneal and conjunctival re-epithelialization is used only if any coexisting lid burn has been treated. Coexisting facial burns and burns of the respiratory tract must be treated simultaneously. Patients with eye injuries are frequently in severe pain and narcotic analgesic agents may be required.

Preoperative antibiotics

In eyes with penetrating injury and no overt infection, broad-spectrum intravenous antibiotics are begun immediately to prevent infection. Conjunctival cultures can be taken prior to their use. If an eye has suspected or definite endophthalmitis, antibiotics should be temporarily deferred until proper cultures are obtained. If surgery is to be performed on an infected eye in 1 or 2 hours, cultures can be taken in the operating room and intravenous antibiotics started then. If surgery is delayed longer, then, depending on the type of injury, an attempt should be made to obtain adequate cultures before surgery and begin antibiotics earlier. Broad-spectrum antibiotic coverage for both Gram-positive and Gram-negative bacteria, including anaerobic bacteria, is used. For example, intravenous nafcillin or methicillin is used for prevention of infection from Gram-positive bacteria, intravenous gentamicin for Gram-negative and Gram-positive bacteria, and intravenous penicillin for anaerobic bacteria and Gram-positive bacteria.

Patient explanation

Prior to preoperative sedation of the patient, informed consent is obtained for surgery. The patient should clearly understand that the exact details of the surgery cannot always be predicted and sometimes must be modified intraoperatively. Therefore, the signed consent form should allow for repair of any injury encountered so that retinal reattachment, vitrectomy, lensectomy and other procedures can be done. If the eye is felt to be injured beyond any realistic hope of repair, permission should be obtained for possible enucleation, with the proviso that should operative findings suggest a chance of salvage the enucleation will not be done. A clear statement is made that additional surgery may be necessary, and no guarantee is given that a good visual result will be obtained. Among other complications, that of sympathetic ophthalmia is mentioned.

Choice of anesthesia

In eyes with open wounds, local retrobulbar anesthesia is contraindicated because injection can cause intraocular tissues to be extruded. Preoperative sedation and analgesia are usually chosen in consultation with the anesthesiologist. The type of general anesthesia is left to the choice of the anesthesiologist. The anesthesiologist is told not to allow the patient to become too 'light' and 'buck'. In open eyes, succinylcholine is not used because it causes contraction of extraocular muscles and can cause extrusion of intraocular tissues. Instead, if necessary, a muscle-paralyzing agent which causes no muscle contraction such as tubocurare is used.

Operative technique

The goals of surgery on an injured eye are to: (*1*) restore ocular integrity; (*2*) reestablish as normal an anatomy as possible; (*3*) remove opacities of the ocular media; (*4*) remove certain intraocular foreign bodies; and (*5*) prevent ocular infection, inflammation and scarring. These goals can often be achieved in a variety of ways. Depending on the available surgical capabilities, partial initial repair, such as closure of wounds, can be done followed by later more extensive surgery. In other situations, extensive and definitive repair is attempted at the first surgery. For penetrating injuries or a ruptured globe, the aims of surgery are accomplished in a stepwise fashion. The order of repair when possible is usually: (*1*) closure of corneal and scleral wounds; (*2*) removal of opacities such as hyphema, cataracts and vitreous hemorrhage; (*3*) removal of displaced or incarcerated tissue such as vitreous or iris in a corneal wound, or a dislocated lens; (*4*) prevention and control of intraocular bleeding with coagulation treatment and reestablishment of normal intraocular pressure; (*5*) prevention of vitreous traction bands by removal of vitreous injured by penetrating injury; (*6*) removal of intraocular foreign bodies; (*7*) repair or prevention of retinal detachment; and (*8*) prevention or treatment of infection. Of course, not all these steps will be required or possible in every eye.

Preparation of the operative field

After induction of general anesthesia, the operative field is carefully prepared and irrigated if appropriate. An adhesive plastic drape is placed over the eye. The lashes, if not trimmed previously, are draped with the plastic to keep them outside the operative field. A lid speculum is inserted under each lid so as to avoid pressure on the eye and to avoid introducing the speculum into any perforation. The lid speculum is adjusted to lift the lids from the eye. If this is impossible, lid sutures may be required.

Closure of open anterior segment ocular wounds

Closure of all wounds is usually performed first. We will describe how different types of wounds are closed beginning with more anterior corneal wounds and ending with posterior wounds.

Small corneal laceration with no incarceration of tissue, a formed anterior chamber and no evidence of intraocular damage

Occasionally, small 1–2 mm shelved, corneal lacerations may spontaneously seal (*Figure 13.4a,b*) and further sealing and protection can be achieved with an extended-wear soft contact lens (*Figure 13.4c*). Although this may reduce

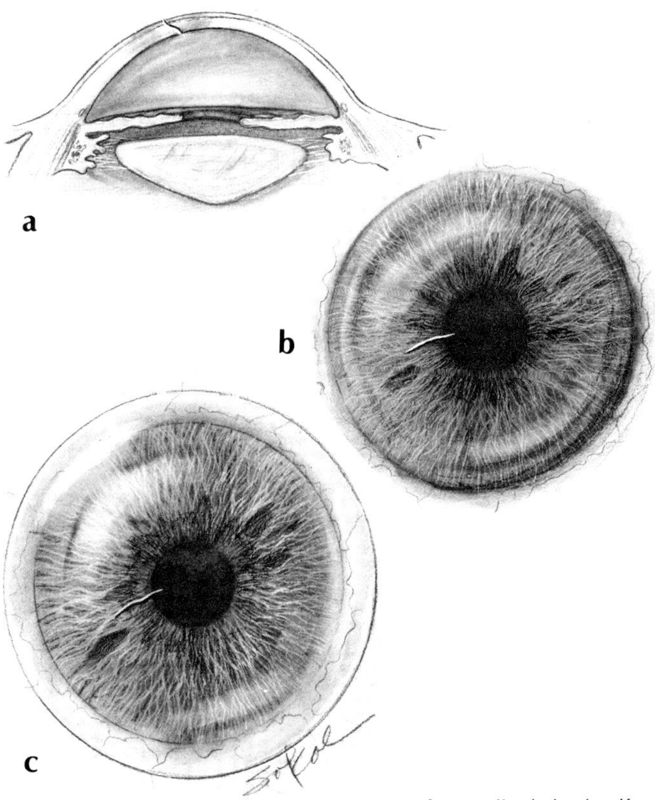

Figure 13.4 *Self-sealing corneal wound.* **(a,b)** *Small, shelved self-sealing corneal wound with anterior chamber formed.* **(c)** *Extended-wear soft contact lens further protects self-sealing corneal wound*

the amount of corneal scarring by avoiding suture scars, treatment without the use of sutures is usually restricted to a self-sealing puncture wound with a formed anterior chamber and no incarceration of intraocular tissue. Frequently such puncture wounds are accompanied by wounds to the lens or other intraocular structures and then other surgical steps may be required. If this is the case, especially if there is doubt as to the adequacy of a self-sealing closure, it is best to suture the wound (*Figure 13.5a,b*). Using an operating microscope at high magnification, a 10/0 nylon interrupted suture is placed with a deep bite in the cornea and with equal bites on each side of the wound (*Figure 13.5c*). One or two sutures may adequately close a small perforation. To obtain the best healing, it is important to aim for deep suture bites, but loss of the anterior chamber during suturing should be avoided. To avoid losing the anterior chamber, careful traction is applied to the edge of the wound into which the needle first passes (*Figure 13.6a,b*), followed by pressure against the opposite wound edge; finally, the procedure is reversed as the needle is passed across the laceration line into the opposite edge (*Figure 13.6c*). The suture is tied so that no tension lines radiate from the suture penetration sites. If the knot has been tied squarely, a super-sharp blade or razor blade can be used to cut the ends of the suture flush with the knot (*Figure 13.6d*). Tying forceps, with the jaws of the forceps perpendicular to the surface of the cornea, are used to bury the knot in the cornea (*Figure 13.6e*), and this is followed by a small amount of reverse traction to allow the tags of suture to line up in the suture tract (*Figure 13.6f,g*). If loose corneal epithelial tags are present at the edge of the wound, they are removed, after two or three approximating sutures are placed, to avoid carrying epithelial cells into the wound or anterior chamber with the sutures.

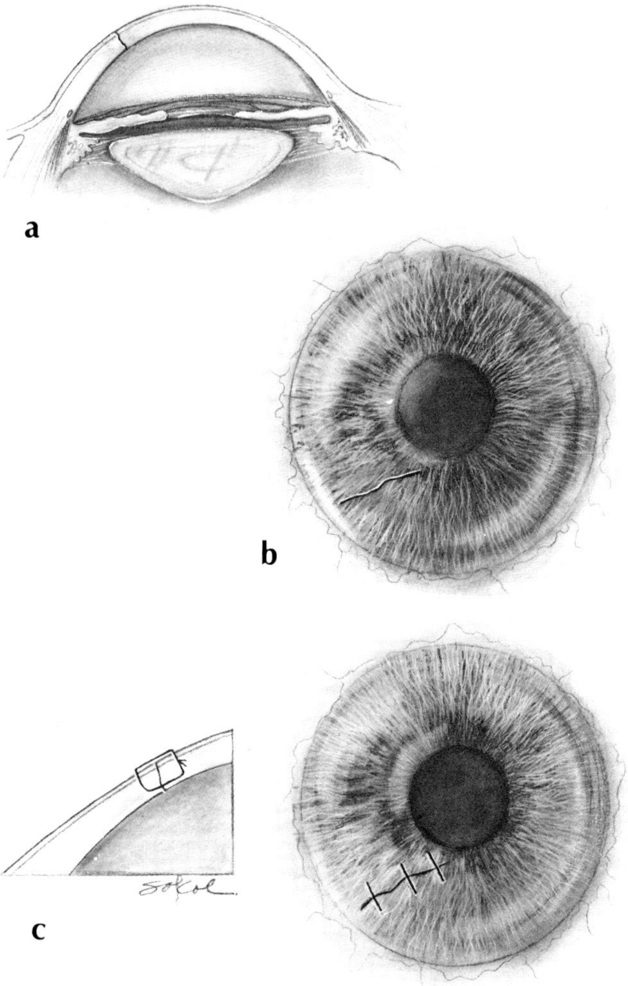

Figure 13.5 *Closure of medium-sized self-sealing corneal wound.* **(a,b)** *Unsutured corneal wound sealed with formed anterior chamber.* **(c)** *Wound closed with deep, interrupted 10/0 nylon sutures with knots buried*

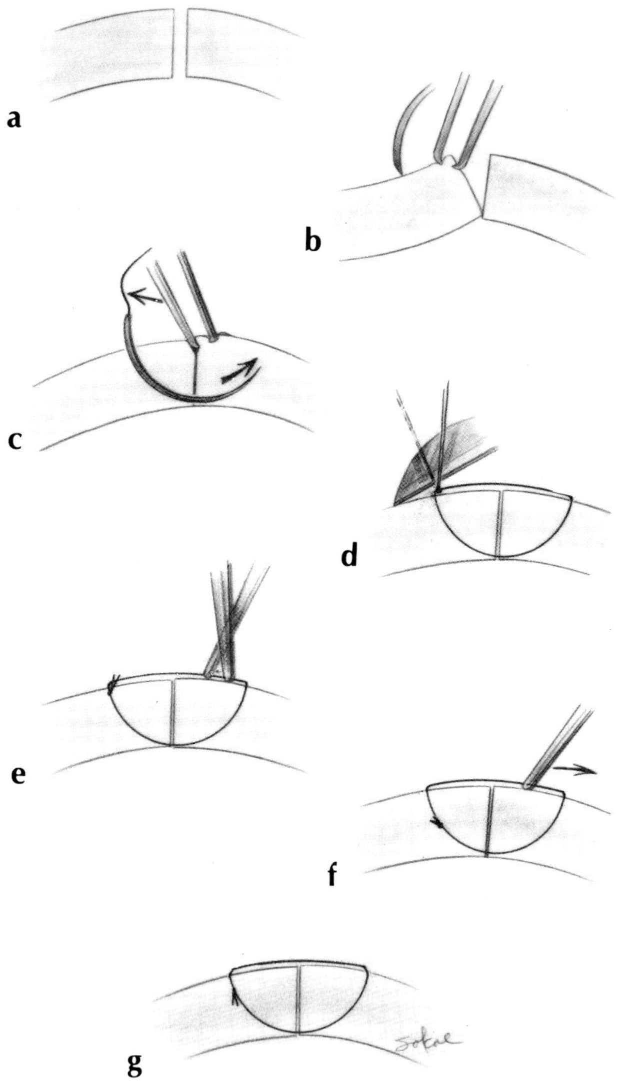

Figure 13.6 *Technique of surgical closure of a corneal wound.* **(a)** *Vertical corneal wound.* **(b)** *Fine-toothed forceps grasping tip of proximal wound and 10/0 nylon needle placed perpendicular to this edge.* **(c)** *Passage of needle in an arc through the depths of wound, using counterpressure to hold the distal edge against the proximal edge to maintain the integrity of wound and prevent loss of the anterior chamber.* **(d)** *Cutting suture flush with knot using a super-sharp blade.* **(e)** *Tying forceps bury knot into the proximal corneal tissue.* **(f,g)** *Reverse maneuver brings ends of suture to lie parallel with suture line just below surface of the cornea*

Corneoscleral laceration with formed anterior chamber and no tissue incarceration

For this type of injury (*Figure 13.7a,b*) the same suturing technique is used as described above, except that the first 10/0 suture is placed at the limbus to approximate it accurately (*Figure 13.7c*). The corneal laceration is closed, placing each successive suture to halve the wound (*Figure 13.7d*). A limbal peritomy is then performed, exposing the sclera for 3–4 mm on either side of the laceration (*Figure 13.7e*). The sclera is exposed and cleaned with Vannas scissors (*Figure 13.7f*). It is essential to expose and repair the full extent of the scleral wound. If the scleral wound has no gaping, it may be sutured with 10/0 nylon sutures (*Figure 13.7g*). If tension is required to close the scleral wound, stronger 8/0 or 9/0 nylon sutures are used. The knots are not easily buried in the sclera and are instead cut flush and covered by conjunctiva, which is closed with interrupted 6/0 collagen sutures (*Figure 13.7h*).

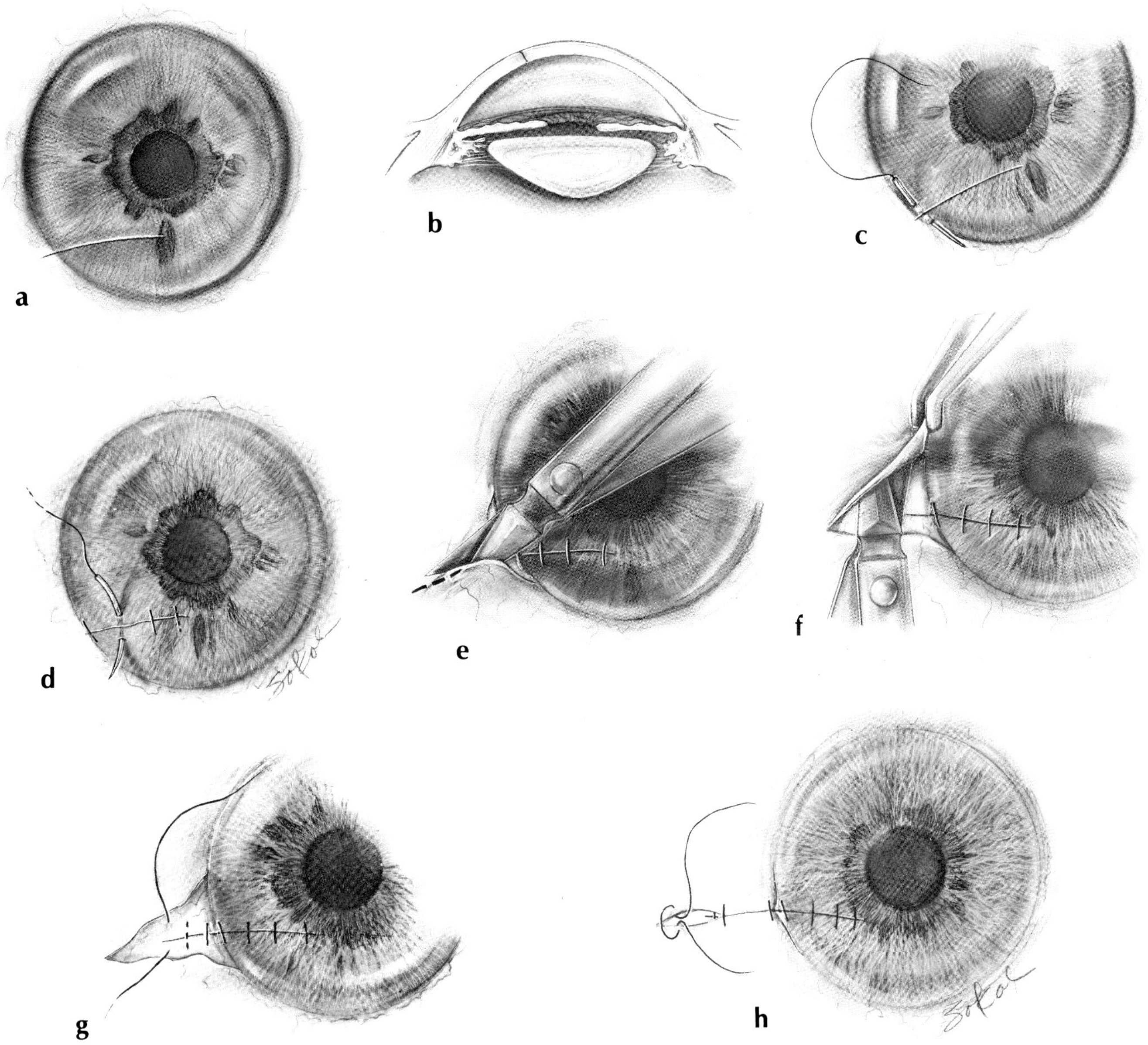

Figure 13.7 *Corneoscleral laceration and formed anterior chamber.* **(a,b)** *Anterior and cross-sectional view.* **(c)** *Placement of 10/0 nylon interrupted suture at limbus.* **(d)** *Closure of corneal wound with 10/0 nylon* **(e,f)** *Conjunctival peritomy and exposure of the sclera, undermining the conjunctiva on either side of the scleral wound.* **(g)** *Closure of scleral wound with 10/0 nylon sutures.* **(h)** *Conjunctiva closed with 6/0 collagen sutures*

Corneal or corneoscleral laceration with no tissue incarceration but the anterior chamber not formed

In these wounds (*Figure 13.8a*), one surgical goal is to avoid incarceration of intraocular tissue in the corneo-scleral wound as it is closed. Tissue that can be incarcerated consists mainly of iris in corneal wounds and ciliary body in the anterior scleral wounds. With a flat anterior chamber, the initial corneal sutures are placed shallowly and examined at high magnification to make certain they do not extend to the posterior lips of the wound (*Figure 13.7b*). When sufficient sutures have been placed to close the wound, the anterior chamber will frequently re-form spontaneously (*Figure 13.8c*). When this occurs, and there is separation of the intraocular structures from the cornea, further suturing is performed with deep sutures to approximate the inner corneal wound (*Figure 13.8d*). The initial, shallow sutures can then be removed. After closure, spontaneous re-formation of the anterior chamber will frequently be sufficient to repressurize the eye and allow assessment of whether or not the wound is watertight. If the eye is soft, a Ziegler-knife puncture is made into the anterior chamber through the limbus, and the anterior chamber is re-formed with balanced salt solution injected through a 30 gauge cannula. The integrity of the wound is assessed by drying the corneal surface with a cellulose sponge and watching for leakage from the laceration. If in doubt, application of sterile 2 per cent fluorescein solution while observing the wound under blue illumination from the operating microscope will allow detection of minor wound leakage (Seidel test).

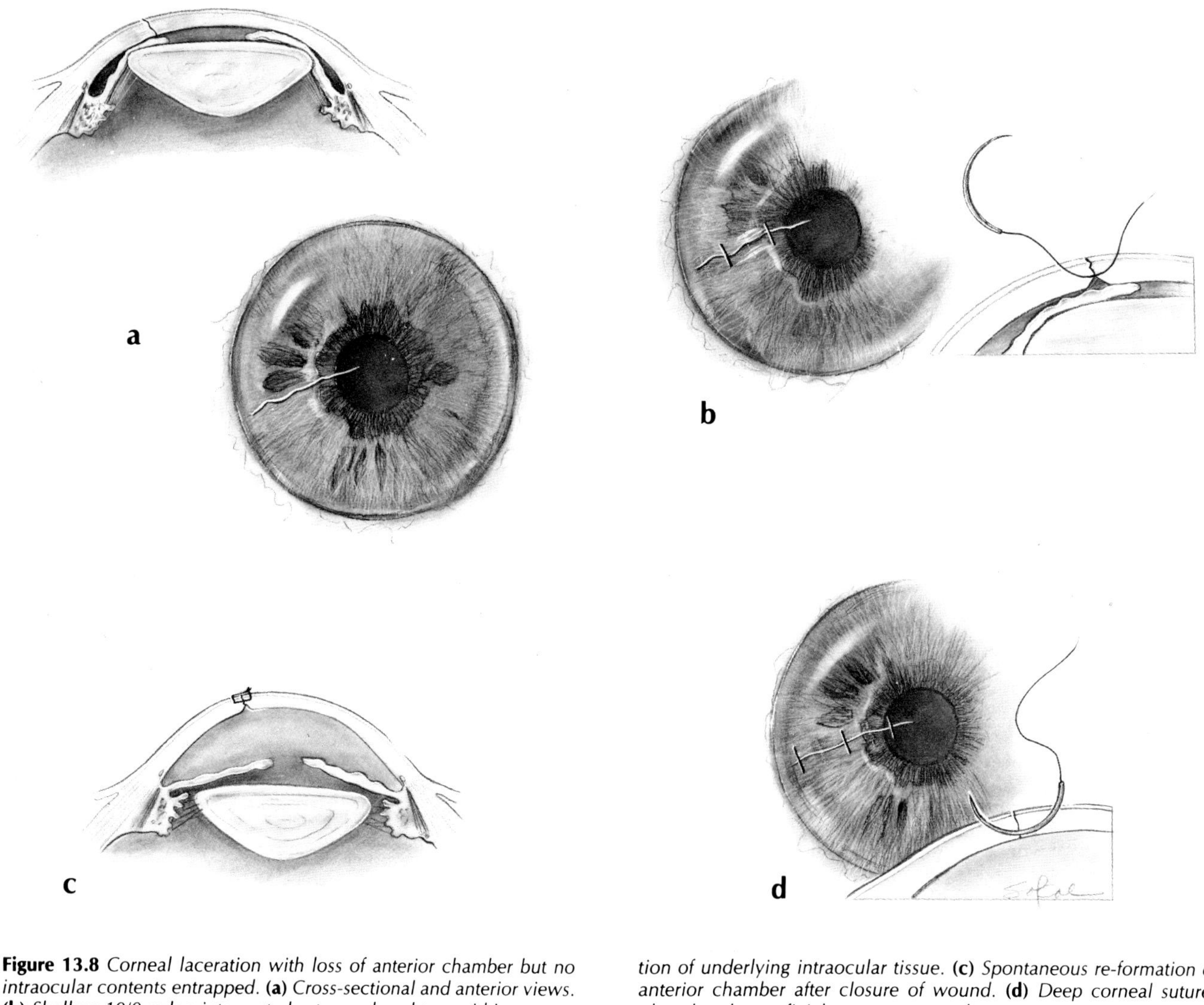

Figure 13.8 *Corneal laceration with loss of anterior chamber but no intraocular contents entrapped.* **(a)** *Cross-sectional and anterior views.* **(b)** *Shallow 10/0 nylon interrupted sutures placed to avoid incarceration of underlying intraocular tissue.* **(c)** *Spontaneous re-formation of anterior chamber after closure of wound.* **(d)** *Deep corneal sutures placed and superficial sutures removed*

Corneal laceration with incarcerated tissue with no lens or vitreous involvement

The management of iris incarceration in a corneal laceration depends on the extent of the incarceration and prolapse, the duration it has been prolapsed, and the length of the laceration. A small corneal laceration with only a peak of iris incarcerated in the posterior wound is usually easily managed (*Figure 13.9a–c*). A superficial corneal suture is placed to close the anterior lips of the wound without suturing the iris into the posterior wound (*Figure 13.9d*). A Ziegler-knife puncture is made through the limbus into the anterior chamber and, if there is no lens damage or need for posterior segment surgery, acetylcholine solution is injected to form the anterior chamber and to constrict the pupil (*Figure 13.9d*). This alone may pull the iris from the wound (*Figure 13.9e*). If further surgery or ophthalmoscopy of the posterior segment is necessary, topical or subconjunctival dilating solution is administered instead of acetylcholine. Although it takes longer to act than acetylcholine, it will also often pull the iris free of the wound. If these methods of disengaging the iris are unsuccessful, a fine Barraquer

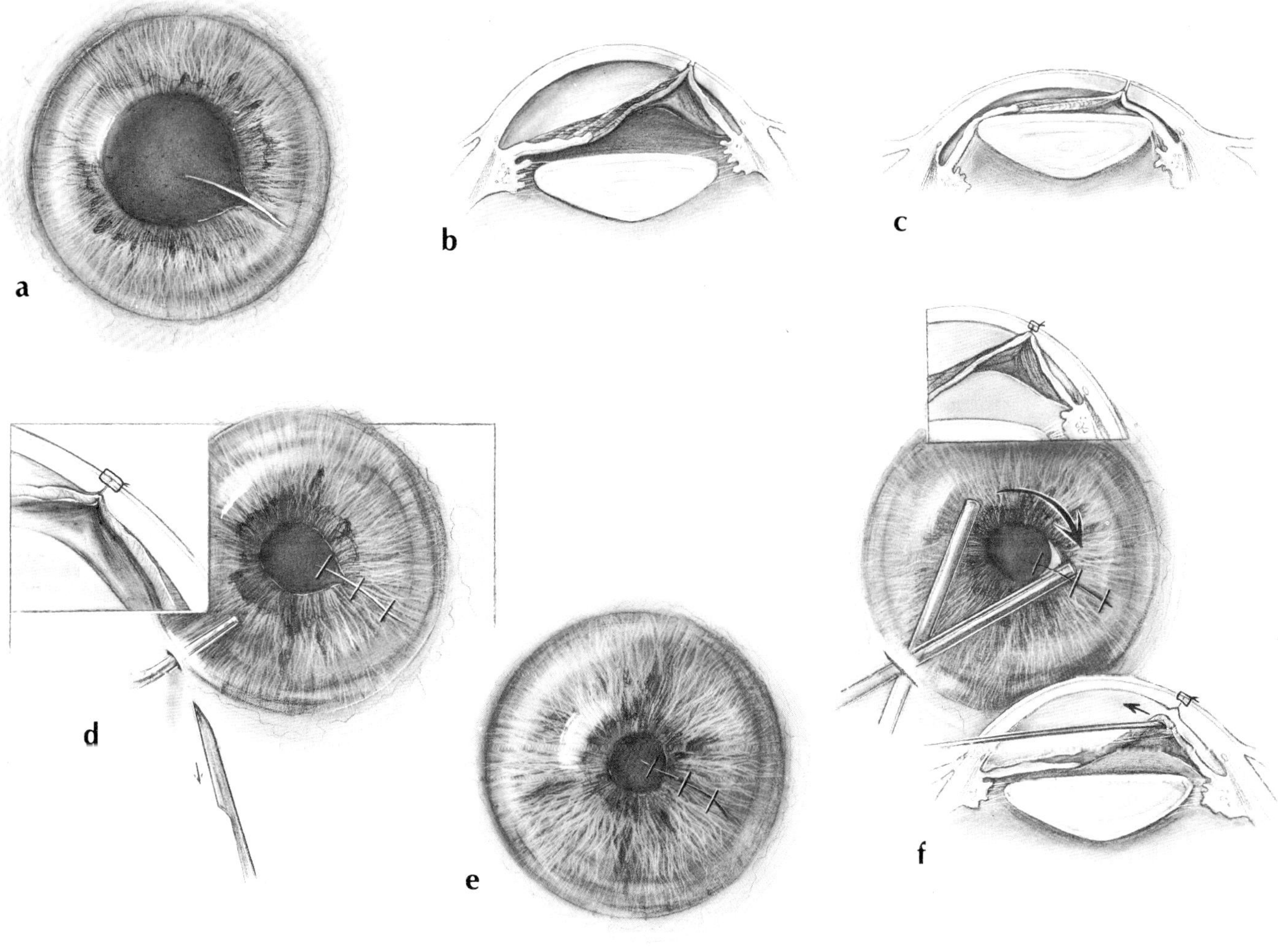

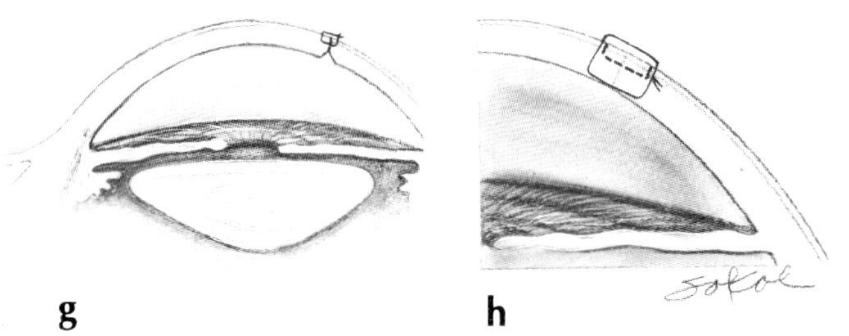

Figure 13.9 **(a)** *Corneal laceration with iris entrapment.* **(b)** *Anterior chamber formed, with iris trapped in the posterior lips of wound.* **(c)** *Anterior chamber flat, with iris caught in posterior lips of wound.* **(d)** *Superficial 10/0 nylon sutures are placed, avoiding incarceration of iris in posterior lips of wound, and the anterior chamber is re-formed with acetylcholine solution injected through a Ziegler-knife puncture at limbus.* **(e)** *Pharmacological retraction of iris from the posterior lips of wound, regaining a miotic, regular pupil.* **(f)** *Fine Barraquer sweep used to sweep iris from posterior lips of wound.* **(g)** *Iris free from wound and anterior chamber formed.* **(h)** *Deep corneal sutures placed and superficial sutures removed*

iris sweep passed through a Zeigler-knife puncture at the limbus is used to sweep the iris from the posterior wound (*Figure 13.9f*). Deep corneal sutures replace superficial sutures after the iris is free of the corneal wound (*Figure 13.9g,h*).

When there is extensive prolapse of iris through a small corneal laceration (*Figure 13.10a*), it is frequently preferable to excise the prolapsed portion of iris, especially if the iris appears non-viable, rather than to attempt to open the wound and allow retraction of the prolapsed iris. After excision of the prolapsed iris (*Figure 13.10b,c*), a corneal suture is placed so that it is superficial to iris remaining in the wound (*Figure 13.10d*). A 30 gauge cannula can be introduced through the corneal laceration and injected acetylcholine solution may flush the iris from the wound; or the instillation of acetylcholine solution may cause the iris to contract enough to pull it free from the wound (*Figure 13.10e–g*). Deeper corneal sutures are then placed to close the wound if the iris is free of the wound. If the iris cannot be freed from the wound, some of the cut edge is reposited into the anterior chamber. After the wound is partially cleared of iris, sutures are placed in that portion of the wound, and an attempt is made to re-form the anterior chamber through the unsutured wound. This maneuver is repeated until more and more iris is reposited into the anterior chamber. Eventually, only a small portion of iris is caught in the unclosed part of the wound with the remainder of the wound held together with superficial sutures. At this stage, with a partially or totally formed anterior chamber, a Ziegler-knife puncture is made through the limbus into the anterior chamber, and a 30 gauge cannula is used to inject acetylcholine solution to cause retraction of the iris (*Figure 13.10h*). If the iris remains incarcerated, a Barraquer sweep is used to sweep the iris from the wound and the wound is closed with deep corneal sutures, replacing the superficial sutures (*Figure 13.10i*).

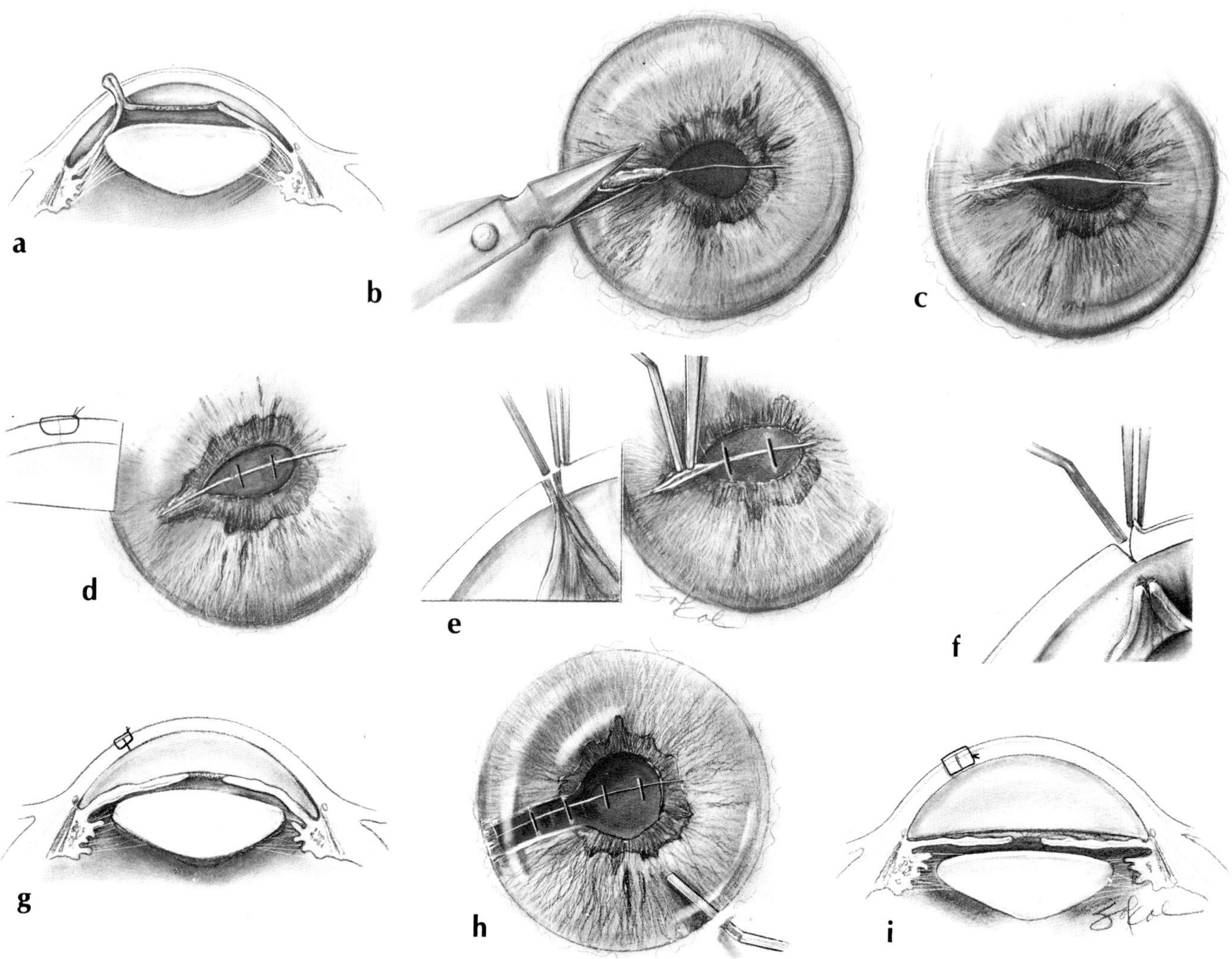

Figure 13.10 *Corneal laceration with extensive prolapse of iris through the wound.* **(a)** *Cross-sectional view.* **(b)** *Iris excised flush with corneal surface using Vannas scissors.* **(c)** *Iris remains incarcerated in posterior lips of wound.* **(d)** *Superficial 10/0 nylon corneal sutures placed in the parts of the wound in which iris is not entrapped.* **(e–g)** *Acetylcholine solution injected into the wound with a 30 gauge cannula to flush trapped iris free of the wound.* **(h)** *After the wound has been closed with superficial sutures, additional acetylcholine solution can be injected through a limbal puncture to free any remaining iris incarcerated and/or to re-form the anterior chamber.* **(i)** *Superficial corneal sutures are replaced with deeper sutures*

Limbal or anterior scleral incarceration of tissue

If tissue is incarcerated in a corneoscleral laceration (*Figure 13.11a*), a peripheral or sector iridectomy is often required to free the iris from the corneal portion of the wound (*Figure 13.11b*). A limbal suture of 10/0 nylon is placed (*Figure 13.11c*) and the corneal wound is closed (*Figure 13.11d*). The anterior scleral wound is closed after exposing it by a limbal peritomy. Sometimes we close the anterior scleral wounds before closing the cornea, because if it is necessary to inject fluid into the anterior chamber to close the corneal wound, there is no chance of the injection forcing ciliary body or vitreous out through the sclera. Ciliary body prolapsed through the anterior sclera can often be reposited and the sclera sutured closed. Every attempt is made not to excise ciliary body tissue because it usually bleeds if cut. If ciliary tissue cannot be reposited, inspection should first be done to make certain there is no external pressure on the eye preventing it. If not, light, Wet-Field cautery to the ciliary body surface may cause enough tissue contraction to allow scleral closure without removing ciliary body. If these techniques fail to reposit the ciliary body or if it has been lacerated with vitreous prolapse, the ciliary tissue is excised (*Figure 13.11e*), applying cautery either before or after cutting. Prolapsed vitreous is excised with scissors, lifting it with cellulose sponges. As little vitreous is removed as possible to minimize vitreous traction on the peripheral retina. The sclera is closed with 8/0 or 9/0 nylon sutures (*Figure 13.11f*). Treatment of more posterior scleral wounds behind the extraocular muscle insertions will be described later in this chapter.

Corneoscleral laceration with lens damage

In cases of extensive anterior segment injury with lens damage and opacification, we prefer not only to close the wound but also to remove the lens and other opacities at the initial surgery. This may allow visualization of the posterior segment so that vitreous or retinal detachment surgery can be performed either at this first operation or more easily at a later surgery.

Before removing the damaged lens, the corneal (*Figure 13.12a,b*) and any scleral wound are closed. Treatment of the iris incarceration is the same as described above (*see Figure 13.10*). Every attempt is made to re-form the anterior chamber, and dilating solution such as 1:10 000 epinephrine (adrenaline; made by diluting 1:1000 epinephrine without preservatives) is used if pupillary dilation is necessary (*Figure 13.12c*). The use of sodium hyaluronate in the anterior chamber may keep it formed, and the sodium hyaluronate can be aspirated and removed later. After wound closure and pupillary dilation

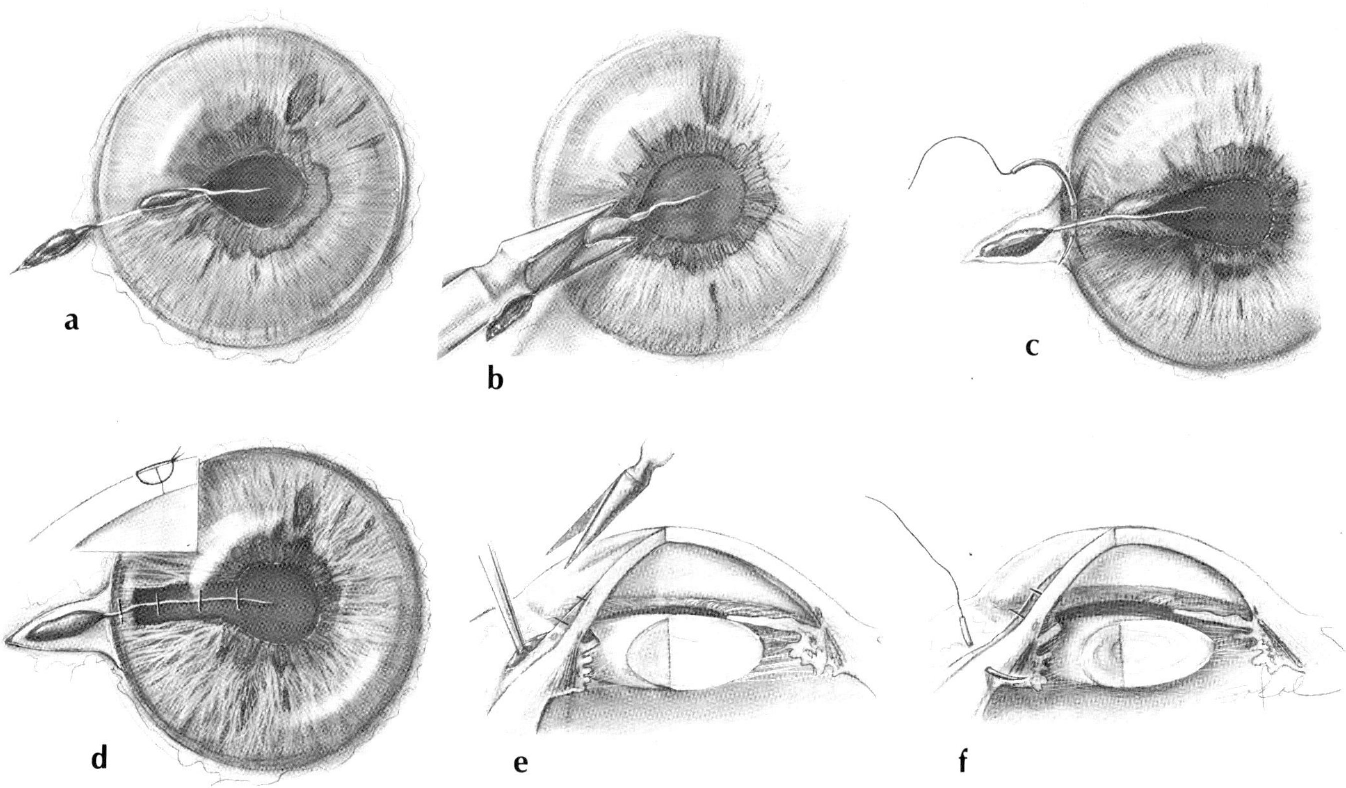

Figure 13.11 *Corneoscleral laceration with iris and ciliary body prolapsed through wound.* **(a)** *Anterior view.* **(b)** *Prolapsed iris excised with Vannas scissors.* **(c)** *Exposure of scleral extent of wound and placement of superficial, limbal 10/0 nylon suture.* **(d)** *Corneal wound closed.* **(e)** *Prolapsed ciliary body is excised if it cannot be reposited.* **(f)** *Sclera sutured with 8/0 or 9/0 nylon*

(*Figure 13.12d,e*), a limbal entry site is made (*Figure 13.12f*). If the posterior lens capsule is intact, an irrigation/aspiration instrument, such as the Cavitron unit, may be used to remove the lens. To minimize postoperative inflammation, as much cortical lens material should be removed as possible. If the posterior capsule is intact, every effort is made not to cut or tear it. If the posterior capsule is broken or its integrity cannot be determined, a vitrectomy cutting instrument can be used instead to remove a soft lens (*Figure 13.12g,h*). This allows removal of anterior vitreous along with lens material, if necessary, to prevent its incarceration in the anterior wound. The limbal wound is then closed (*Figure 13.12i*).

In an eye with lens damage with the posterior lens capsule disrupted, a pars plana lensectomy and anterior vitrectomy can be considered after wound closure. This approach usually allows more complete removal of the lens and easier removal of tissue incarcerated in the previously closed wounds. A pars plana approach can be used if there is no evidence of retinal or choroidal detachment and the lens and anterior segment opacities are not so severe as to prevent visualization of the instruments inserted through the pars plana. With this approach, infusion can be performed through a needle or infusion cannula inserted through the limbus into the anterior chamber or by a pars plana infusion cannula if its tip can be visualized to confirm that it is in the vitreous cavity. These techniques will be described more fully below.

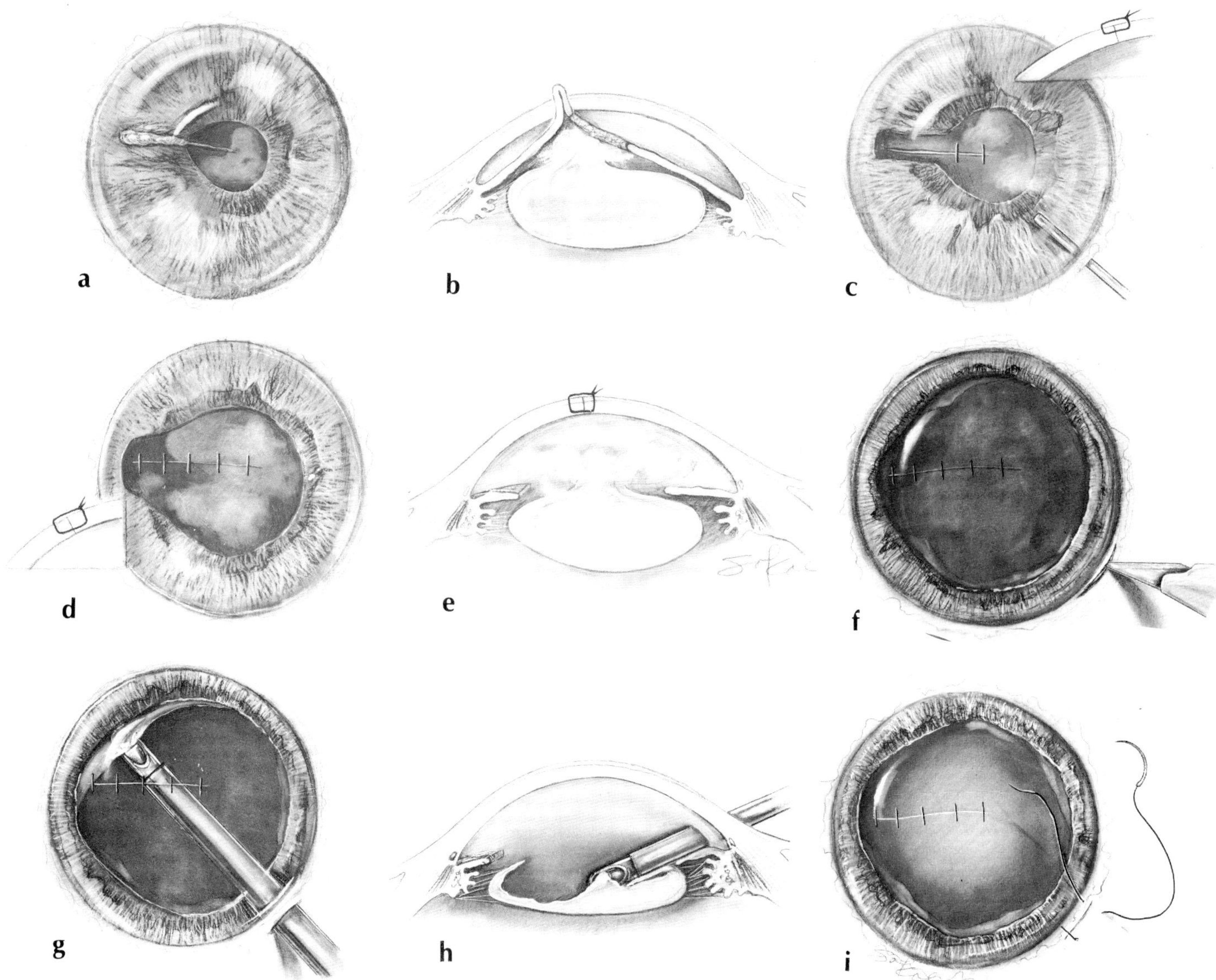

Figure 13.12 *Corneal laceration with iris prolapse, lens rupture and shallow anterior chamber.* **(a)** *Anterior view.* **(b)** *Cross-sectional view.* **(c)** *Corneal wound closed with superficial 10/0 nylon sutures after incarcerated iris removed using techniques shown in Figure 13.10 and Figure 13.11.* **(d,e)** *Deep corneal sutures placed with a formed anterior chamber, iris free of the wound, and lens material in the anterior chamber.* **(f)** *Limbal incision with sharp blade after dilation of pupil with 1:10 000 epinephrine solution.* **(g,h)** *Use of Ocutome vitrectomy instrument with overlying infusion sleeve to remove lens nucleus and cortex (ultrasonic fragmentation may be required).* **(i)** *Limbal wound closed*

Management of other problems associated with perforating injuries of the anterior segment

Iris tears

Iris tears or defects that can produce photophobia, polyopia or glare usually should not be repaired at the time of corneoscleral wound closure. Attempted repair can cause further incarceration of tissue, repeated flattening of the anterior chamber, or lens damage. Primary repair should be attempted only if the lens has been removed and the iris can be easily sutured. Later surgical repair of an iris injury may occasionally be considered.

Intraoperative bleeding

Bleeding from exposed vascularized tissues such as iris or ciliary body is controlled with bipolar Wet-Field cautery. To avoid excessive damage, the initial cautery setting should be low and should be increased gradually to get the correct intensity cautery. If internal bleeding occurs during wound closure, the closure should be completed and the eye re-formed with balanced salt solution in the hope that a normotensive eye will stop further bleeding. Small intraocular hemorrhages frequently clear spontaneously. If bleeding continues even though the eye is closed and normotensive, the intraocular pressure can be increased further with an anterior chamber injection through the limbus, and this usually stops bleeding. An elevated pressure of 40–50 mmHg should not be maintained for more than 10–15 minutes. If bleeding persists and a bleeding point can be seen on the iris or in the anterior chamber angle, two-instrument bipolar diathermy can be used to try to stop bleeding. A 27 gauge or 30 gauge needle is attached to one of the two bipolar cautery leads and the other is attached to a 30 gauge cannula. The needles and cannula are inserted through the limbus and the bleeding site is treated directly (*Figure 13.13*). If bleeding occurs from the anterior chamber angle, internal-external bipolar diathermy is used with one instrument or needle tip in the anterior chamber angle at the bleeding site and the other instrument tip placed externally on the limbus. If the bleeding point is not seen and a significant amount of blood accumulates in the eye, a vitrectomy instrument is introduced through the limbus, or the pars plana in an aphakic eye, to remove clotted blood and replace it with balanced salt solution at an increased intraocular pressure. This may stop bleeding or allow visualization and diathermy treatment of a bleeding point.

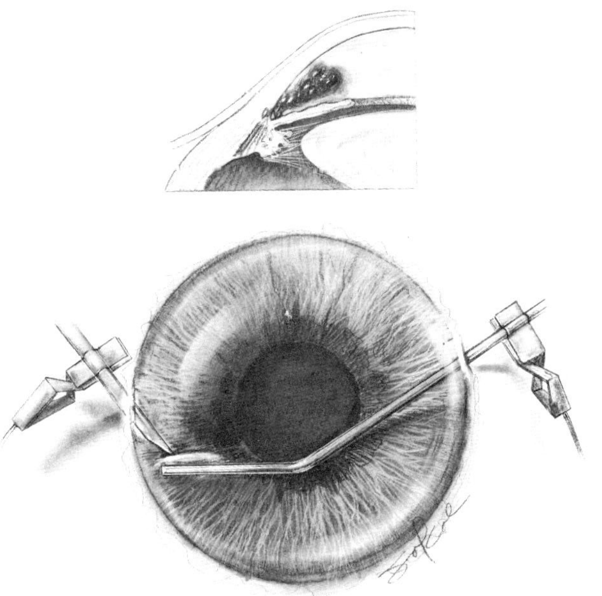

Figure 13.13 *Bimanual bipolar diathermy used to coagulate bleeding peripheral iris vessels. Bipolar clamps attach to a sharp 30 gauge needle and a 30 gauge cannula*

Corneal tissue loss

In stellate or fragmented corneal wounds, enough corneal tissue can be lost so that direct closure of the wound is impossible. In other cases, apposition of the sutured wound edges creates such distortion of the cornea and globe that the anterior chamber cannot be re-formed. In these cases, some form of corneal patching is required. Fresh donor corneal material is preferred as a patch, but stored corneal tissue can be used if fresh material is unavailable. The goal of a patch closure is to re-establish ocular integrity so that later reconstructive surgery can be performed. When a patch graft is insufficient to close the wound and the visual axis of the cornea is involved (*Figure 13.14a*) tissue glue can be used to close the wound. The limbs of the stellate wound are closed with corneal sutures (*Figure 13.14b*). Through the remaining central corneal defect a 30 gauge cannula is used to introduce air or sodium hyaluronate into the anterior chamber beneath the perforation. Isobutyl 2-cyanoacrylate tissue adhesive is then applied to the perforation site with an iris spatula (*Figure 13.14d*)[7]. With re-formation of the anterior chamber (*Figure 13.14e*) further surgery may be deferred. If the central cornea is extensively damaged, a keratoplasty can be performed on the intact, sutured globe (*Figure 13.15a–c*).

Leaking corneal or corneoscleral wound

In some cases where tissue loss is minimal or absent but in which sutures inadequately appose the wounds and the wound leaks, a small amount of tissue adhesive can be applied to the leaking point. An extended-wear soft contact lens is placed over the dried tissue adhesive. The contact lens and adhesive can be removed 2–4 weeks after surgery and the suture line then remains watertight.

Anterior segment foreign bodies

Shelving or partial-thickness corneal lacerations with foreign bodies embedded deep in the wound are difficult to manage. Attempted removal may open a deep penetrating

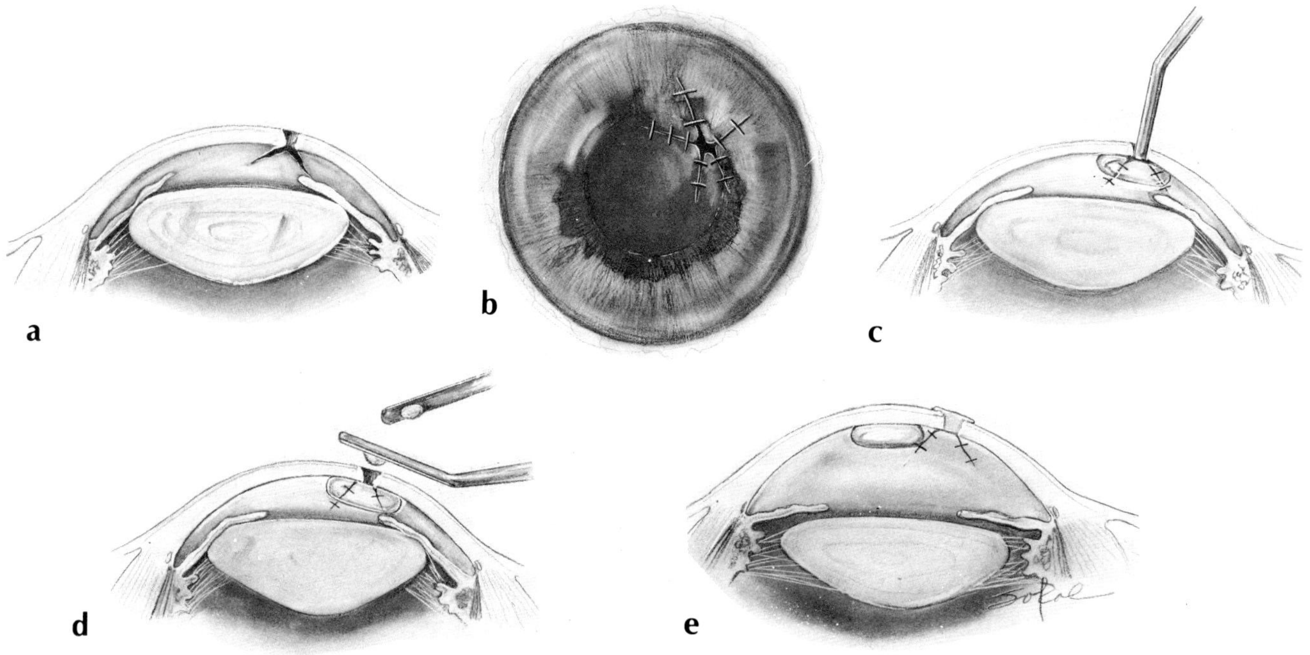

Figure 13.14 *Stellate corneal wound with central corneal tissue loss.* **(a)** *Cross-sectional view.* **(b)** *Closure of limbs of stellate wound using 10/0 nylon sutures.* **(c)** *Small air bubble is placed in anterior chamber through central corneal perforation with a 30 gauge cannula.* **(d)** *Isobutyl 2-cyanoacrylate tissue adhesive on the end of an iris spatula is applied over dry corneal central perforation site.* **(e)** *Firm, adherent plug of dry glue closes the stellate wound*

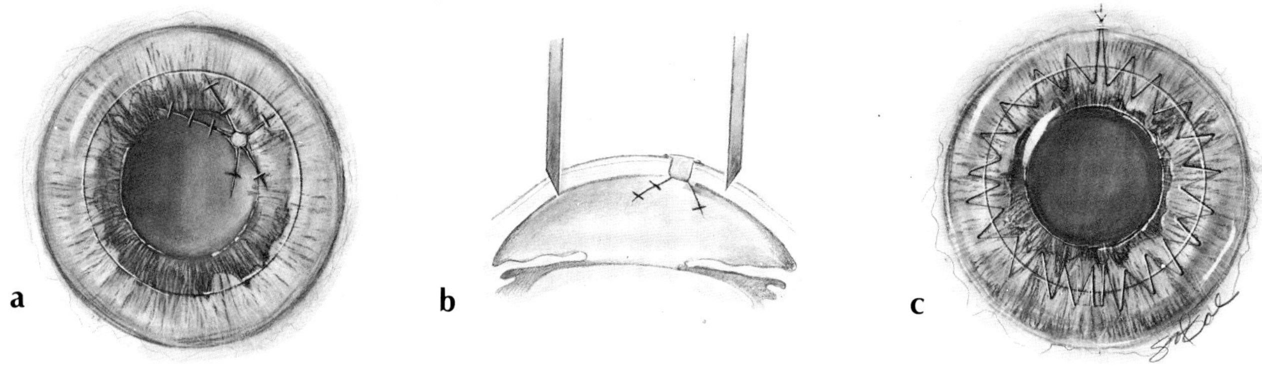

Figure 13.15 *Keratoplasty to repair extensively damaged cornea.* **(a)** *Closed stellate corneal wound with central tissue loss. Trephine mark encloses entire corneal wound.* **(b)** *Corneal trephine removes damaged central cornea.* **(c)** *Donor graft sutured into place*

wound or cause further damage to the surrounding cornea. Small glass, plastic and even metallic foreign bodies can sometimes be left in the cornea without serious problems. Vegetable material, ferrous metals and foreign bodies in the visual axis should usually be removed. Irrigation alone may free the foreign body. The lips of the wound are held apart, and a 30 gauge cannula is inserted to irrigate. Ferrous metals are often magnetic and readily removed with a magnet. Forceps also can be used to remove a foreign body. If removal attempts fail, it is better to wait and see how the cornea responds after surgery rather than undertaking more aggressive and damaging attempts at removal. A residual foreign body may eventually require removal by a lamellar cornea transplant requiring substantial loss of corneal tissue.

Corneal foreign bodies that project into the anterior chamber, usually sharp pieces of glass or metal, are difficult to remove safely. Often the anterior chamber is formed with the foreign body plugging the corneal perforation (*Figure 13.16a*). If the foreign body projects above the corneal surface, and a good grip on this foreign body with toothed forceps is possible, it can be removed. If, however, the foreign body is embedded below the corneal surface with the deep portion projecting into the anterior chamber, attempts at removal are dangerous. Premature loss and flattening of the anterior chamber may impale the sharp tip of the foreign body into the iris or lens. To avoid flattening of the anterior chamber, a 30 gauge cannula is inserted through the limbus and fluid is infused (*Figure 13.16b*). Microforceps are placed through a second limbal incision opposite the infusion site (*Figure 13.16c*). The forceps are used to grasp the tip of the foreign body in the anterior chamber and remove it through the limbus, avoiding damage to the lens and iris (*Figure 13.16c,d*). If necessary, the limbal incision is enlarged to permit easy removal.

Foreign bodies floating in the anterior chamber or in the anterior chamber angle need not always be removed. Indications for removal are: persistent inflammation, risk of siderosis, mobility with corneal endothelial damage, and corneal edema. If the foreign body is visible and free-floating, it may be possible to manipulate the globe to move the foreign body into the superior angle. The limbus is incised over the foreign body. The foreign body is removed with a magnet, fine forceps, or by flushing it out with solution from a 30 gauge cannula. If the foreign body will not move to the superior angle, a similar approach can be used in another portion of the angle.

Intralenticular foreign bodies need not be removed unless they cause a progressive cataract or ocular siderosis[8]. An intracapsular cataract extraction can be used in some cases to remove the foreign body and lens together. If this is inappropriate, an extracapsular cataract extraction can be done. If the posterior capsule is intact, irrigation and aspiration are used to remove the lens followed by the foreign body. If the foreign body is too large for aspiration, microforceps can be introduced into the anterior chamber and the foreign body removed after lens removal. A pars plana vitrectomy may be necessary to remove the lens and foreign body if the posterior lens capsule is broken.

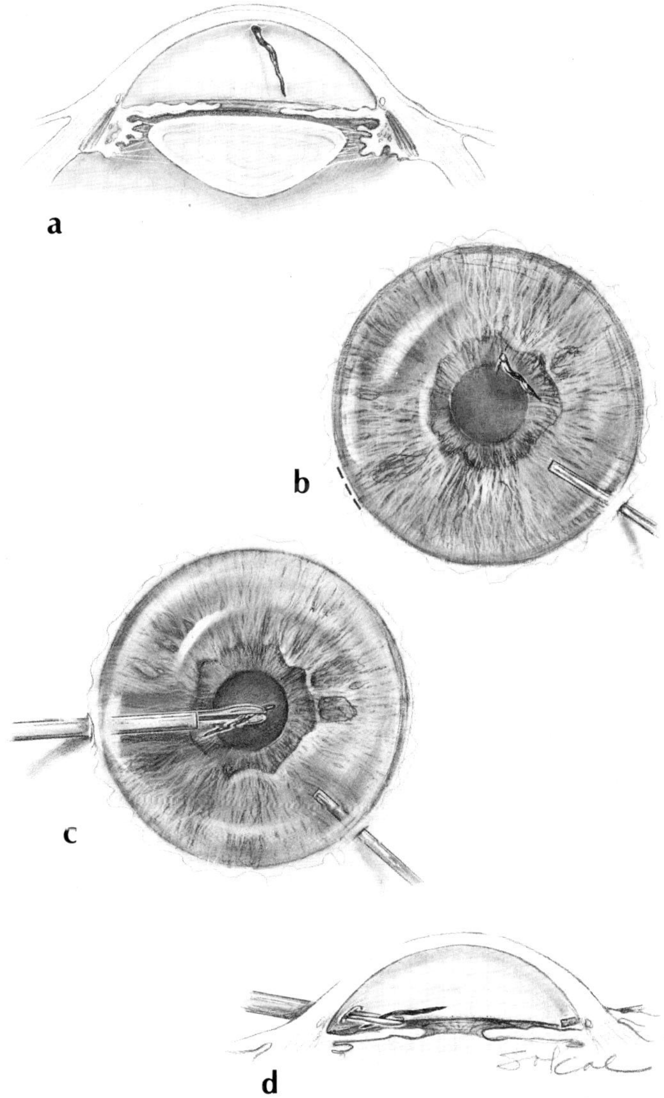

Figure 13.16 **(a)** *Perforating corneal foreign body with sharp tip of foreign body protruding into the anterior chamber.* **(b)** *Irrigation through 30 gauge cannula or 30 gauge needle maintains anterior chamber.* **(c)** *Sutherland microforceps are introduced through a separate limbal stab incision, and foreign body is pulled into the anterior chamber.* **(d)** *Removal of the foreign body from the anterior chamber through the limbal incision. Separate infusion prevents collapse of the anterior chamber*

Management of anterior segment contusion and chemical injuries

Discussion here will be limited to those anterior segment injuries not discussed in other chapters or earlier in this chapter.

Hyphema

Most eyes with acute hyphema are managed with bedrest to prevent further bleeding, and pain and elevated intraocular pressure are managed medically. A systemic evaluation is obtained if a bleeding diatheses is suspected. Surgery is performed to evacuate the hyphema if: (*1*) medical treatment does not control the intraocular pressure; (*2*) there is uncontrolled pain; (*3*) there is early corneal blood-staining or corneal edema; or (*4*) there is a significant decrease in vision or light perception.

For an eye with hyphema in which antiglaucoma medication does not control the intraocular pressure at a level below 40 mmHg, evacuation of the hyphema should be considered. In these patients, it is important to perform coagulation studies to detect preventable causes of rebleeding. In black patients a sickle-cell preparation or hemoglobin electrophoresis is performed to diagnose sickle-cell disease because sickled red blood cells plug the trabecular meshwork and produce intractable glaucoma[9].

The timing of surgery depends on several factors, including the degree of elevation of intraocular pressure, the amount of blood-staining, the severity of pain, the duration of total hyphema, and the presence of retinal detachment on preoperative ultrasound examination. In an eye with an elevated intraocular pressure, preoperative intraocular pressure reduction is attempted with medical therapy including intravenous mannitol if necessary. General anesthesia is normally used for surgery.

We prefer a closed-eye aspiration of the hyphema with a small vitrectomy instrument[10–12] using a limbal approach and a separate limbal infusion cannula. A 20 gauge infusion cannula is first passed through a limbal incision into the anterior chamber and a vitrectomy instrument is introduced through the limbus into the anterior chamber opposite the infusion needle (*Figure 13.17a,b*). The infusion cannula can be directed posteriorly toward the area of excision of clot to try to keep the iris out of the vitrectomy instrument (*Figure 13.17c*). Gentle suction is applied first to blood or clot lying over the midperipheral iris (*Figure 13.17d*). Suction is stopped immediately if the anterior chamber begins to collapse. If the blood or clot can be removed by suction alone without cutting, this is safer. Blood or clot in the peripheral anterior chamber is removed (*Figure 13.17e*). Clot that is weakly adherent to the anterior chamber angle (which is frequently the site of the original and recurrent bleeding) is removed by gentle suction. Firmly adherent clot should be left behind because removal may cause new bleeding. The more central clot is then cut away (*Figure 13.17f*). If the lens is visible, it may be safe to aspirate blood or clot from the lens surface (*Figure 13.17f*). If gentle suction does not remove a clot from the iris surface, the vitrectomy instrument is used to cut and remove the clot.

If rebleeding occurs, cutting and suction are stopped and the infusion bottle is raised to increase intraocular pressure until bleeding stops. Bleeding sites can be treated with bipolar diathermy (see *Figure 13.13*).

If an intumscent cataract is found after the anterior chamber is free of blood, lens removal should be performed, especially if retinal detachment is present. The vitrectomy instrument removes the anterior lens capsule and then the cataract. An attempt is made to maintain an intact posterior lens capsule as a barrier to prevent blood from any rebleeding from passing into the vitreous cavity.

At the end of surgery every effort is made to avoid hypotony and rebleeding during instrument removal. Gentle infusion is continued as the vitrectomy instrument is removed. If iris prolapses, a small peripheral iridotomy is performed in the prolapsed iris after gentle bipolar cautery to the area (*Figure 13.17f*). The iris is reposited and the vitrectomy instrument entry site is closed with interrupted 10/0 nylon sutures. The infusion cannula is then removed and gentle pressure placed over the area with a cotton-tipped applicator until a watertight seal is obtained. Interrupted 10/0 nylon sutures are used to close the infusion site.

Postoperative complications include increased intraocular pressure, rebleeding and inflammation. Antiglaucoma medicines usually control elevated intraocular pressure, and topical steroid and cycloplegic drops may reduce postoperative inflammation and pain.

All black patients with hyphemas should have laboratory testing as described to look for sickle-cell disease or sickle-cell trait[9]. If either of these conditions is found, the patient is examined frequently despite what might appear to be an insignificant hyphema. Sickled red blood cells effectively plug the trabecular meshwork and raise intraocular pressure, and patients with sickle-cell disease or

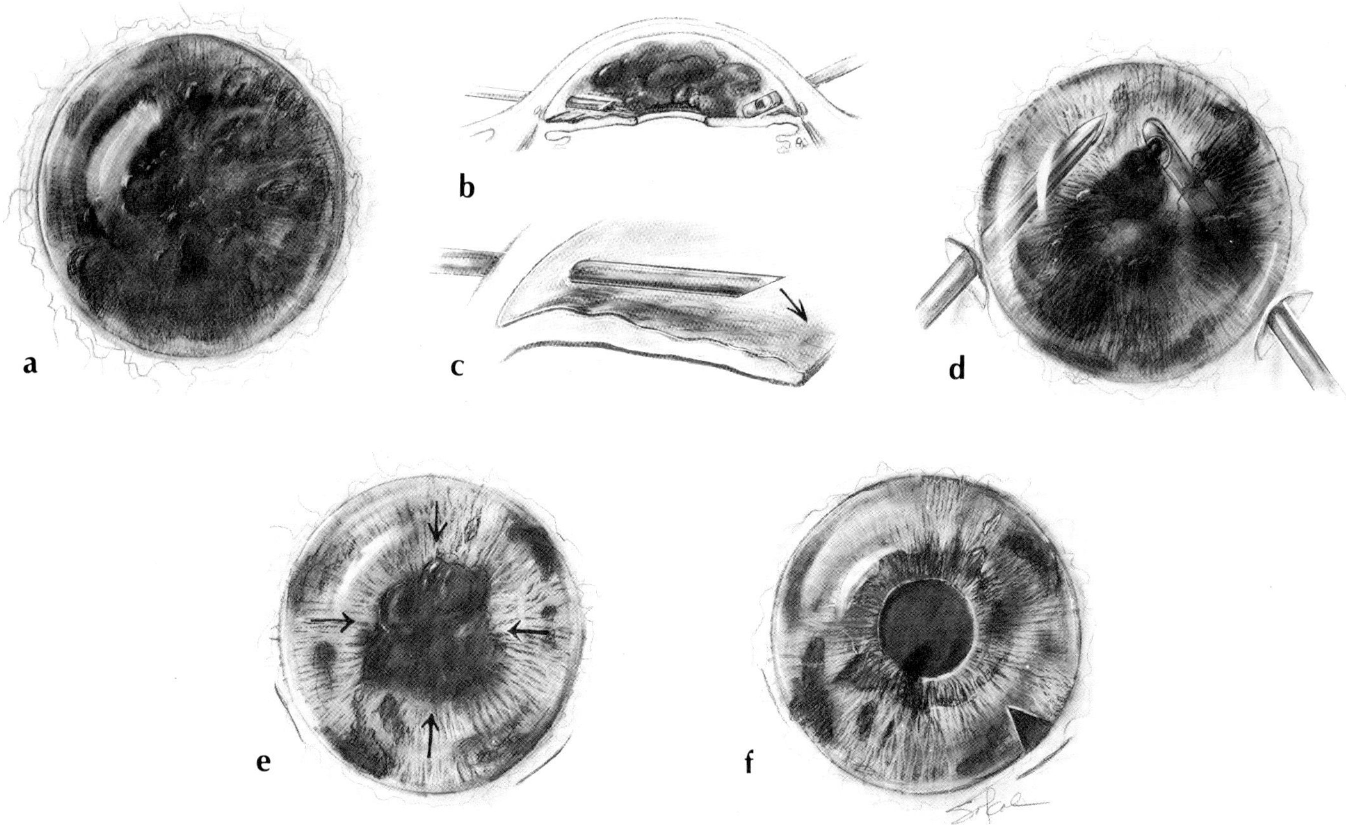

Figure 13.17 *Removal of large hyphema with vitrectomy instrument.* **(a)** *Anterior view of hyphema.* **(b)** *Ocutome and 20 gauge infusion needle introduced into the peripheral anterior chamber through limbal incisions.* **(c)** *Bevel-down position of irrigation needle keeps iris away from Ocutome and needle.* **(d)** *Midperipheral clot is removed first, and irrigation needle is manipulated to keep it near the Ocutome tip so that intraocular structures are more easily visible.* **(e)** *Peripheral clot is removed, leaving some clot in anterior chamber angle.* **(f)** *After removal of central clot, residual anterior chamber angle clot still remains. Peripheral iridectomy has been performed*

trait are more susceptible to optic nerve damage from increased intraocular pressure[13]. Such patients should be initially examined every 2–4 hours, and intraocular pressure and vision should be measured until they are stable. Pressure in the middle to high 20s for more than 24 hours should be treated by paracentesis in the operating room under the operating microscope. Decreasing vision despite a static hyphema should also initiate paracentesis.

Even dense corneal blood-staining from hyphema will usually resolve with time, although it may take several years. In young patients in whom occlusion amblyopia is a threat, in patients whose other eye has lost vision, or in eyes with retinal detachment, penetrating keratoplasty can be considered for treatment of corneal blood-staining. A temporary keratoprosthesis can be used if simultaneous vitreous surgery is performed.

Glaucoma surgery in eyes with medically uncontrolled, elevated intraocular pressure after resolution of hyphema is discussed in Chapter 7.

Dislocated lenses

The indications for removal of a dislocated lens after blunt trauma are (*1*) dislocation into anterior chamber with recurrent corneal edema and decreased vision; (*2*) episodes of pupillary-block glaucoma; and (*3*) lens dislocation with lens-induced inflammation. The management of anteriorly and posteriorly dislocated lenses is dealt with in Chapter 8.

Chemical trauma

There is no proof that surgical treatment is useful in acute chemical burns. Emergency treatment consists of vigorous irrigation, removal of particular matter from the fornices and conjunctival surfaces, and protection of the ocular surface with lubrication, patching and soft contact lens application. Paracentesis has been suggested in the treatment of acute alkali burns[14], but the benefit of this treatment is unproved. Surgery can be considered in the long-term rehabilitation of the severely chemically burned eye. Protection of the cornea with a tarsorrhaphy or a conjunctival flap may be required. Maintenance of satisfactory lid-ocular apposition may require symblepheron lysis, mucosal grafting, and entropion and trichiasis procedures. Uncontrolled secondary glaucoma may require glaucoma surgery. In carefully selected cases, penetrating keratoplasty with or without cataract extraction can permit visual rehabilitation of some chemically injured eyes. Before keratoplasty, factors that are detrimental to the maintenance of a clear graft should be treated. These include dry eyes, poor lid-ocular surface apposition, poor lid closure, corneal vascularization, corneal anesthesia, persistent corneal epithelial defects and persistent elevation of intraocular pressure. Persistent epithelial breakdown can be treated with conjunctival transplantation from the normal eye. Corneal 'melting' in severe aklaki burns is currently being treated with ascorbic acid or citric acid, and such treatment appears promising[15,16].

Treatment of posterior segment injuries

Posterior segment injuries can result from ocular contusion or from laceration or rupture of the globe. Contusion injuries such as choroidal rupture or traumatic retinopathy can cause severe loss of vision but are not managed surgically. Surgical management of non-resolving vitreous hemorrhage, retinal breaks and retinal detachment from contusion injury are discussed in Chapters 8 and 9. Discussion here will be limited to management of eyewall ruptures or lacerating or penetrating injury causing posterior segment damage. Usually, scleral ruptures from a direct blow to the eye have a poor prognosis because of loss of intraocular contents, traction on the retina by vitreous extending to the wound, retinal detachment, choroidal rupture or hemorrhage, and contusion injury to the ciliary body and retina. Lacerations involving the posterior segment can also be severe, depending on the extent of injury. Lacerations not extending posterior to the equator and those with minimal loss of intraocular contents have a better prognosis. Lacerations involving only the anterior segment, however, can be associated with severe posterior damage if the penetrating object extends far enough posteriorly to damage the retina. Even an anterior laceration with vitreous loss can cause enough vitreous traction to produce severe retinal detachment.

All scleral ruptures and almost all penetrating injuries require surgery. Surgery may entail only simple closure of a wound or complex vitreous and retinal reattachment surgery. Depending on the capabilities of the surgeon, more complex injuries can be managed by primary closure and later reoperation with vitreous and retinal reattachment surgery, or vitreoretinal surgery can be performed at the initial operation if this type of surgery is indicated and possible.

There is little controversy over the fact that vitreoretinal surgery has allowed salvage of some injured eyes that would otherwise have been lost. On the other hand, many injuries are so severe that, for example, there is no chance of reattaching the retina or there is so much macular damage that good vision is unattainable. Many eyes are filled with hemorrhage, and some eyes require surgery to clear the blood and other opacities before the full extent of the injury is evident. If the laceration or rupture extends posterior to the equator of the eye, the prognosis is poor. If an eye has had severe loss of intraocular contents, the chance of saving the eye is also poor, although exceptions occur. Ultrasonography also has improved the management of traumatic injuries because it allows diagnosis of preoperative vitreous traction bands, choroidal detachment, retinal detachment, intraocular foreign bodies, and other abnormalities in eyes with opaque media.

In eyes that have simple repair of laceration or rupture first, and later require vitreous surgery, there is controversy about the proper timing of the second operation. It is clear as mentioned earlier that surgery before 2 weeks is better than later surgery, because progressive intraocular fibrosis after 2 weeks often causes irreparable damage. It is also desirable to determine by 2 weeks' time whether the eye needs to be enucleated, because enucleation before 2 weeks lessens the chance of developing sympathetic ophthalmia[17]. Some surgeons feel surgery is best delayed for 7–10 days to lessen the chance of bleeding and to allow the posterior vitreous to detach so that it is more easily removed[18]. Others feel that early vitrectomy offers the best chance for repair and prevention of fibrocellular membranes and should be done immediately or within 3 days of the injury[19]. In certain cases it is desirable to perform surgery before, rather than after, posterior vitreous separation, because the intact, attached vitreous may tamponade posterior retinal breaks and prevent retinal detachment.

In the following discussion, surgery will be described as though it is performed in one operation. It can actually be separated into two operations: a primary wound closure, and later, more extensive surgery performed before 2 weeks. The surgery required for successful repair is performed in a stepwise fashion consisting of wound closure, followed, if necessary, by: (*1*) lens removal; (*2*) vitrectomy; (*3*) repair of retinal detachment; and (*4*) removal of a foreign body.

Repair of scleral wounds

Scleral wounds can be caused either by direct laceration or by blunt injury with scleral rupture. Both are repaired in a similar fashion. Wounds that do not pass posterior to the extraocular muscle insertions (which are good external landmarks of the ora serrata) have a better prognosis than more posterior wounds directly involving the retina. Wounds anterior to the ora serrata can nevertheless be associated with vitreous loss, vitreous traction and severe retinal detachment. Wounds or ruptures directly involving the retina, especially if they extend posterior to the equator, have an even worse prognosis. Almost all scleral wounds are sutured closed except for very small anterior self-sealing wounds (such as those caused by a small penetrating foreign body) and very posterior exit wounds that are hazardous to close because of the high risk of extrusion of intraocular contents during the required surgical exposure.

If a corneal wound is also present, this is usually closed first and then the scleral wound is closed, working from the anterior to the posterior part of the wound. The exception, as described earlier in this chapter, is that of corneoscleral wounds with involvement of only the sclera anterior to the extraocular muscle insertions. In these cases, it is best to close the scleral wound first, to prevent prolapse of vitreous, and then definitively close the corneal wound. An eye with a scleral wound posterior to the extraocular muscle insertions, however, requires more manipulation of the eye to expose the wound, and it is best to close the corneal wound first to prevent extrusion of contents through this wound. Because closing the corneal wound first, with an open scleral wound, does not allow proper re-formation and sweeping of the anterior chamber, it may be necessary to revise the corneal closure after the scleral wound is closed.

For very small scleral wounds, suturing can be done with absorbable 7/0 polyglycolate suture. In general, however, non-absorbable suture material is used to obtain a watertight wound that has less chance of leaking or coming apart if reoperation is necessary. This is especially important if vitrectomy might be used later, because it is more difficult to close a wound leak at reoperation. We prefer closely spaced, monofilament nylon sutures of a 7/0, 8/0 or 9/0 size, depending on the suture strength required. Sutures of 5/0 braided nylon or 6/0 silk can also be used. Whenever exposure permits, an operating microscope is used to aid scleral wound closure.

Every attempt is made to reposit exposed, viable uveal tissue back into the eye. Cutting of the heavily vascularized uveal tissue is avoided because it can result in bleeding and can inadvertently remove apposed retina. If it is necessary to remove choroidal tissue, the choroid should be treated with diathermy first to prevent bleeding. Prolapsed vitreous is cut flush with the wound and the wound is closed. No attempt is made to use cellulose sponges to remove more vitreous, because this only results in greater vitreous traction and the vitreous gel still remains incarcerated in the closed wound.

Some injured eyes have an obvious scleral laceration or rupture visible externally or on ophthalmoscopy. In other eyes, such wounds may not be visible and are only suspected because the eye has significant subconjunctival hemorrhage, hypotony or signs of severe posterior segment injury on ultrasonography. In eyes in which a wound is suspected but not confirmed, exploratory surgery is performed to search for a wound and to repair it if found.

Scleral lacerations or ruptures extending behind the extraocular muscle insertions are associated with retinal breaks unless there is only a superficial scleral laceration. Every attempt is made to prevent or minimize loss of choroid, retina and vitreous while repairing any such wound by not exerting excessive pressure and traction on the eye. Associated retinal breaks must be treated to prevent or repair retinal detachment.

External repair of scleral wounds extending behind the extraocular muscle insertions

The scleral wound is exposed by performing a conjunctival peritomy, usually beginning at the limbus in the quadrant of the wound (*Figure 13.18a,b*). Under microscopic visualization, if possible, the wound is closed with interrupted non-absorbable sutures such as 8/0 nylon sutures (*Figure 13.18c,d*). Every effort is made to avoid removing intraocular tissue. If there is mild prolapse of choroid, the suture needle can be passed completely through each lip of the scleral wound separately to avoid puncturing the choroid. When the suture is tied, this may help force the choroid back into the eye. The closely spaced interrupted sutures are cut close to the knots, although a suture can temporarily be left long so that it can be grasped with forceps to rotate the eye and expose more of the wound (*Figure 13.18e*). A stay suture, such as a 4/0 silk suture, is placed beneath the rectus muscle insertion in the area of the laceration (*Figure 13.18f*). The stay suture provides further traction and additional exposure, along with the use of a retractor (*Figure 13.18g*). The scleral wound is closed to its posterior end (*Figure 13.18h*). The conjunctival peritomy is extended, the other rectus muscles are isolated on stay sutures, and the sclera is examined elsewhere for other wounds (*Figure 13.18i*).

If the retina is ophthalmoscopically visible and attached, with the retina incarcerated in the internal aspect of the

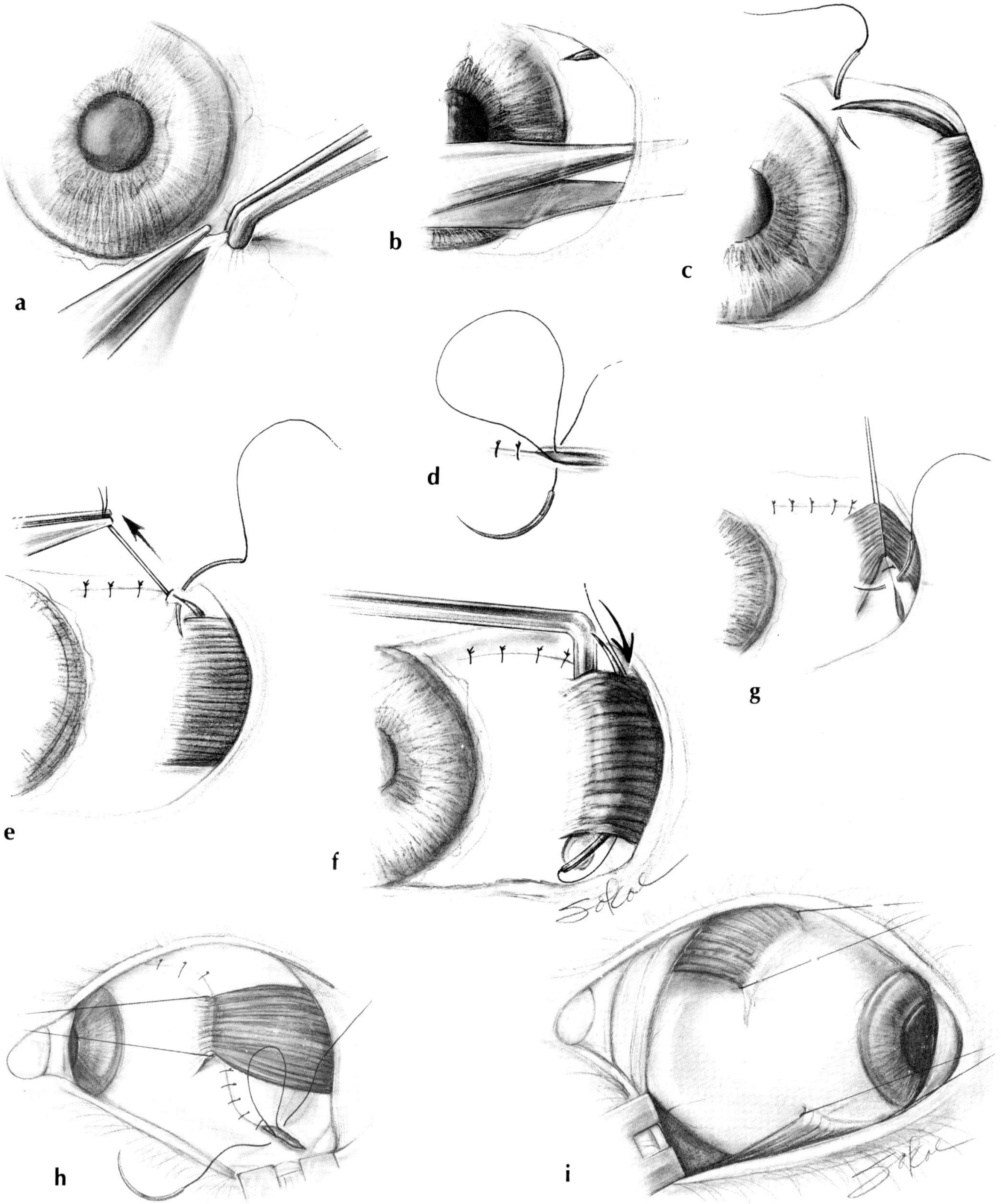

Figure 13.18 *Closure of a scleral wound extending posterior to an extraocular muscle insertion.* **(a,b)** *Conjunctival peritomy exposing the wound.* **(c,d)** *Suturing the anterior wound with interrupted sutures.* **(e)** *Exposure for further suturing obtained by traction on a previously placed suture.* **(f)** *Placement of stay suture beneath rectus muscle.* **(g)** *Traction on stay suture provides further exposure.* **(h)** *Closure of posterior wound.* **(i)** *Examination of other quadrants for injury*

wound, cryotherapy and scleral buckling are best performed at the time of this operation. Usually, however, vitreous hemorrhage prevents visualization of the fundus, and complete repair of the injury requires both vitreous and retinal reattachment surgery, either at this time or at later surgery. If the operating surgeon performs vitreoretinal surgery, consideration can be given to proceeding immediately with definitive repair. The surgeon may instead choose to repair only the laceration and perform a reoperation later or refer the patient to a vitreoretinal surgeon for possible reoperation. Scleral buckling in these eyes is described later in this chapter.

The conjunctival incisions are closed with 6/0 catgut sutures and subconjunctival injections of antibiotic (such as gentamicin 20 mg) and corticosteroid (such as dexamethasone 2 mg) are given.

Management of other problems associated with posterior segment injury

Removal of cataract and hyphema

If an eye has a scleral laceration that extends posterior to the ora serrata and there is also a cataract, lens removal is justified to allow visualization and treatment of the retinal break and any retinal detachment. This surgery can be done at the time of the original repair of the traumatic wound or as a secondary operation. An eye with a hyphema and cataract can have removal of both. An eye with a hyphema, but in which the lens cannot be seen, should have surgery deferred if ultrasonography shows the retina is attached. After the hyphema clears, it may be possible to treat the retinal break in the attached retina without removing a clear lens. If a retinal detachment is present on ultrasonography, lensectomy, removal of the hyphema, vitrectomy and retinal reattachment surgery should be done.

For eyes with a cataract and a scleral laceration or rupture that does not extend posterior to the ora serrata, and in which no retinal detachment is present on ultrasonography, lens removal may be deferred until the eye recovers from the initial injury and is stable.

When an intraocular foreign body is present in the posterior segment, it should be removed unless it is known to be small and non-reactive. This requires lens removal if a cataract is present and possibly removal of a clear lens if significant hyphema is present, obscuring a view of the fundus.

The crystalline lens should be spared when possible, but with severe injuries removal of a clear lens may be justified if it makes vitreous surgery easier and more likely to succeed. When a lens must be removed in an eye with posterior segment trauma, a vitrectomy instrument or an ultrasonic fragmentation and aspirating instrument is used. A vitrectomy instrument is capable of removing only soft lenses, and an ultrasonic instrument is required for harder lenses.

A lens can be removed through the limbus or pars plana. A limbal approach is preferred in eyes: (*1*) in which the anterior chamber is filled with blood so that the lens cannot be seen; (*2*) when the retina is highly detached on ultrasonography and the lens is opaque; and (*3*) when there are large choroidal detachments. Lens removal is then performed as described earlier (see p. 417). When these conditions are not present, a pars plana entry site is preferred because it allows better access for lens removal and the same entry sites can be used for vitreous surgery. A pars plana approach also often allows better removal of incarcerated tissue from corneal wounds than is possible through limbal entry sites.

Pars plana lensectomy is described in Chapter 8. For eyes that have had trauma, it is performed in the same general fashion except that the longer 6 mm infusion cannula is used because it is safer than a 4 mm cannula when the Ocutome system is used and lens removal is performed. The longer 6 mm cannula has a better chance of fully penetrating through all pars plana tissue and into the vitreous cavity in an eye that might have choroidal detachment from trauma, and this lessens the risk of inadvertently infusing fluid into the choroid. The 6 mm cannula is placed through the inferotemporal pars plana 3.0 mm or 3.5 mm posterior to the limbus. Every attempt is made to visualize the tip of the infusion cannula to confirm that the tip has fully penetrated into the vitreous cavity. If it cannot be seen, a 20 gauge infusion needle or cannula can be temporarily inserted through the limbus into the anterior chamber. Infusion into the anterior chamber is used until enough lens is removed so that the pars plana cannula tip can be seen to confirm that it has penetrated all pars plana tissue. Once this has been confirmed, the pars plana cannula can be used for further infusion. To remove the lens, a 20 gauge ultrasonic fragmentation and aspiration needle is inserted through a pars plana sclerotomy site in one of the superior quadrants. The lens is removed by ultrasonic vibration and aspiration, first removing the nearest part of the lens nucleus and then progressively removing more of the lens nucleus as the instrument tip passes to the opposite side of the lens (*Figure 13.19a–d*). After the lens nucleus has been removed, lens cortex is fully removed. Lens capsule and any residual lens cortex is then removed with the vitrectomy instrument (*Figure 13.19e*), and any opacities or blood in the anterior chamber are also removed. If the anterior chamber has no opacities, the anterior lens capsule can be left intact to minimize damage to the corneal endothelium from the irrigating solution during vitrectomy. The anterior lens capsule is removed near the end of the vitrectomy.

Removal of vitreous hemorrhage in eyes with no retinal damage or intraocular foreign body

Eyes with blunt trauma or a lacerating injury anterior to the ora serrata can have vitreous hemorrhage without any retinal breaks or detachment. Such eyes can have surgery postponed to see if the hemorrhage will clear spontaneously. If hemorrhage does not clear, it can be removed as described in Chapter 8. The same techniques are used in eyes with posterior scleral wounds and intraocular foreign bodies, and these techniques will be described more fully below.

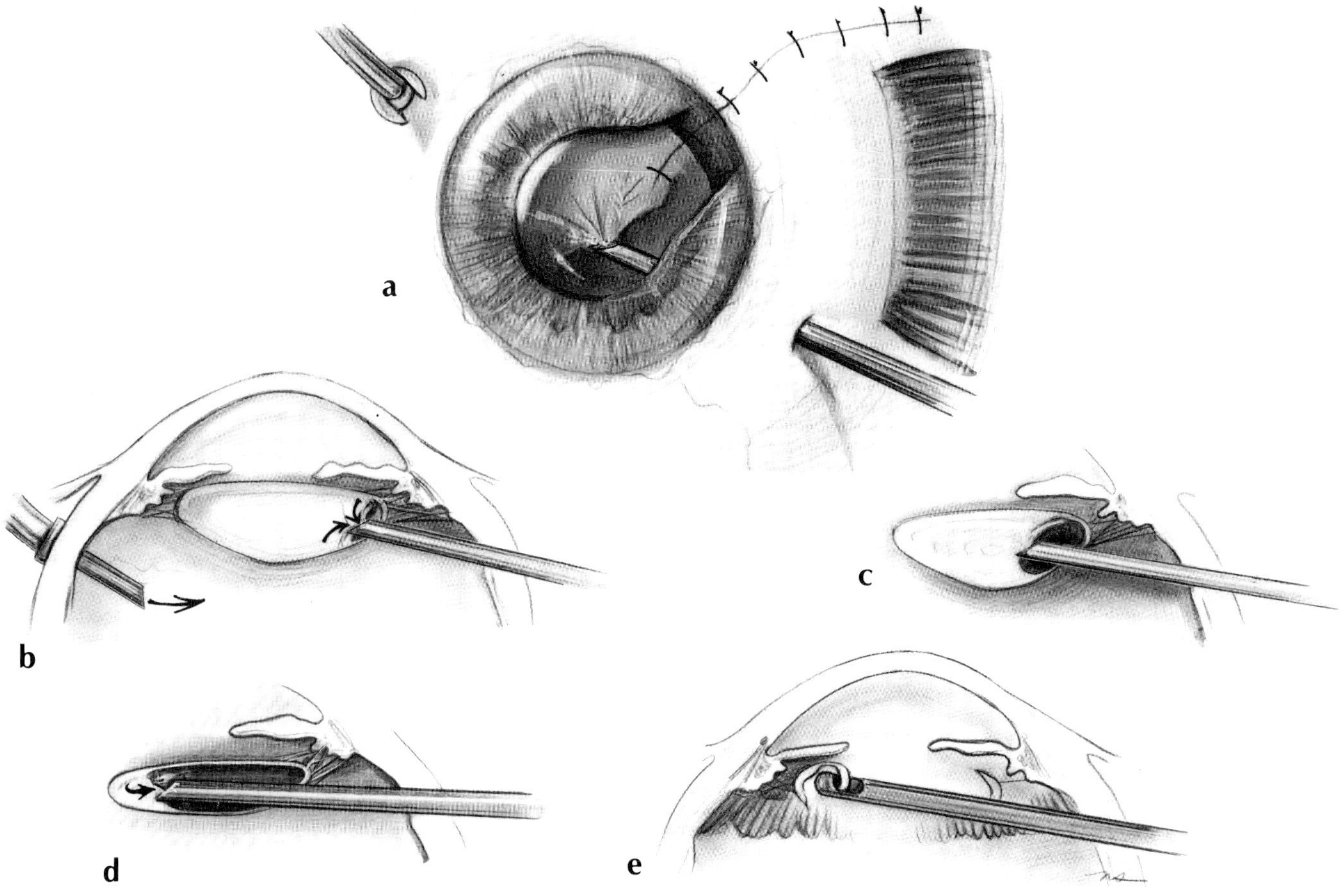

Figure 13.19 *Pars plana lensectomy.* **(a–d)** *After closing the wound and placing an infusion cannula, an ultrasonic fragmenting and aspirating instrument removes the lens nucleus and cortex.* **(e)** *Vitrectomy instrument removes residual lens cortex and lens capsule*

Eyes with vitreous hemorrhage and also posterior scleral laceration, intraocular foreign body or retinal detachment need vitrectomy to remove vitreous hemorrhage earlier, so that these coexisting conditions can be treated. The removal of vitreous hemorrhage as part of repair of these other conditions is described below.

Temporary keratoprosthesis for eyes needing vitreous surgery

In eyes with severe corneal damage and corneal opacity, from a corneoscleral laceration for example, a temporary keratoprosthesis may be used to permit vitreous surgery, perhaps needed to remove an intraocular foreign body or to repair a retinal detachment associated with scleral rupture or laceration. First, if possible, the corneal laceration is closed with interrupted 10/0 monofilament nylon sutures (*Figure 13.20a*). A 6 mm corneal trephine is used to remove a central corneal button (*Figure 13.20b*). The threaded, plastic, temporary keratoprosthesis is screwed into the cornea and sutured in place if necessary (*Figure 13.20c*). Vitrectomy is performed, the keratoprosthesis removed, and a 6.5 mm donor corneal button is sutured into place with 10/0 monofilament nylon sutures (*Figure 13.20d*).

Removal of intraocular foreign bodies

Vitreous surgery allows removal of many non-magnetic foreign bodies that previously could be removed only at considerable risk to the eye. Because the success rate of removal with vitreous surgery is good, and because vitreous surgery can be used to treat coexisting ocular damage, removal is now attempted in most eyes. On occasion, however, foreign materials can be tolerated in an eye without damage or inflammation, although any foreign body can potentially produce physical damage to the retina or other ocular tissues, or can cause endophthalmitis. If a small piece of glass is trapped in the vitreous gel, it can be left in place unless vitreous surgery is needed to treat other damage. If a non-reactive, non-magnetic foreign body lies in an inaccessible position on the pars plana in a phakic eye, removal is likely to damage the lens. Most other foreign bodies, however, should be removed.

Most intraocular foreign bodies are magnetic and many result from pounding with a hammer on another iron-containing metal. We prefer to attempt removal of magnetic foreign bodies with a hand-held electromagnet when they can be seen, unless they are large and embedded in the retina posterior to the equator in a phakic eye. For a phakic eye with a large posterior foreign body,

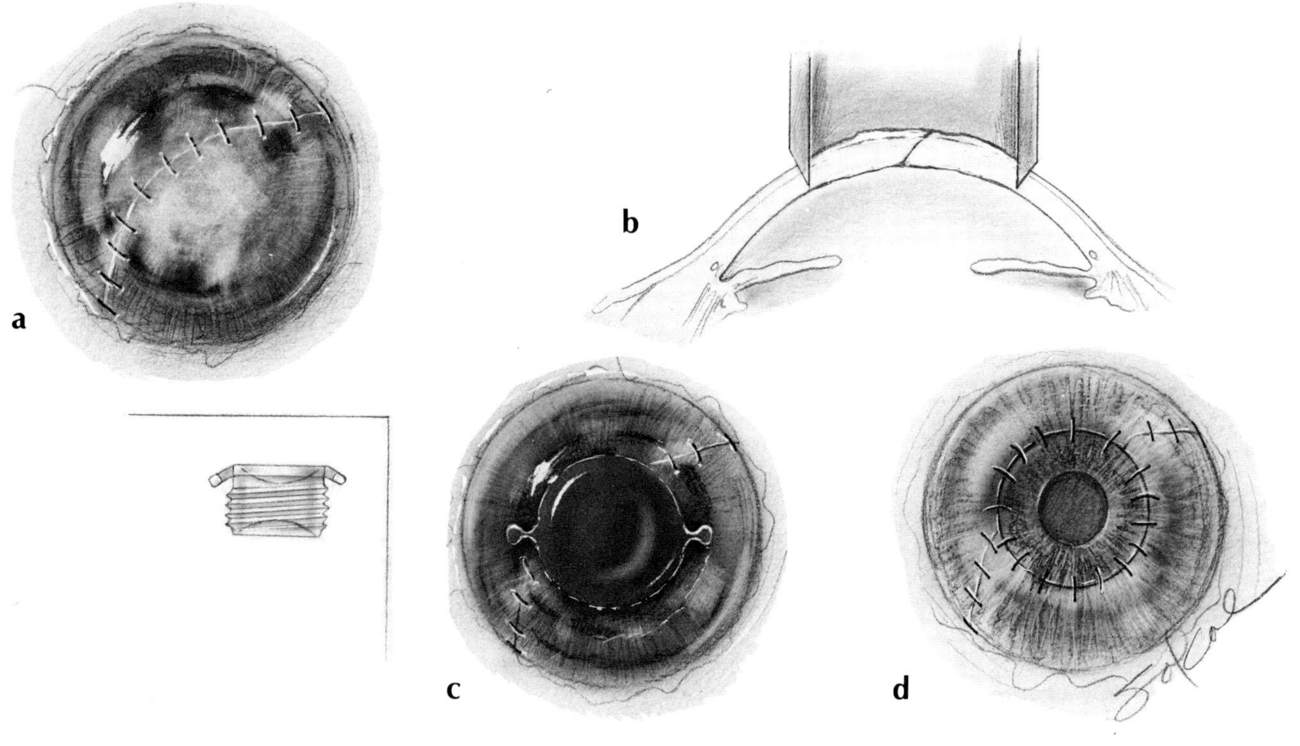

Figure 13.20 *Use of temporary keratoprosthesis to allow vitrectomy in eye with corneal opacity.* **(a)** *Opacified cornea with laceration closed.* **(b)** *Removal of a central 6 mm corneal button with a corneal trephine.* **(c)** *Placement of temporary keratoprosthesis.* **(d)** *6.5 mm corneal button sutured into place after removal of temporary keratoprosthesis*

removal through a pars plana incision with a magnet can be done, but there is a risk of the foreign body hitting and damaging the retina or lens. For this type of case or for non-magnetic foreign bodies in most positions, vitreous surgery and removal with foreign body forceps is preferred.

Prophylactic scleral buckling surgery is performed in most eyes that have foreign body removal. This is used to treat flat peripheral retinal holes produced by the foreign body if they are present, but also prophylactically to treat and buckle the peripheral retina to prevent later retinal detachment in eyes that have no holes. Vitreous traction often occurs after foreign body removal because vitreous gel is generally lost through the removal site. Traction extends from this site to the vitreous base, often later producing retinal holes and detachment.

Removal of magnetic foreign bodies with a magnet

Ophthalmoscopically visible, small or medium-sized magnetic foreign bodies in the vitreous gel, over the pars plana or embedded in the retina posterior to the equator can be removed with a magnet through a pars plana incision. A hand-held electromagnet is used, and the shortest and bluntest tip is chosen for the magnet to maximize the magnetic force. When there is difficulty pulling the foreign body from the eye, the magnet is repeatedly turned on and off to 'rock' the foreign body and to avoid overheating the magnet, which results in loss of magnetic flux.

For magnetic removal through the pars plana, any external corneal or scleral wound is first closed. A site is chosen on the pars plana such that when the foreign body is pulled to this site it does not strike the lens and is not dragged along the retina. A circumferentially oriented incision is made in the pars plana 4 mm behind the limbus, using a sharp stiletto or other similar sharp instrument (*Figure 13.21a*). Ciliary body bleeding is treated with bipolar diathermy. A 6/0 silk suture is passed through the scleral lips of the wound and is looped out and held on each side with non-magnetic forceps to draw the lips of the wound apart. The sterile, hand-held electromagnet tip is placed on the wound, activated and used to withdraw the foreign body (*Figure 13.21b*). If the wound is too small, it is enlarged and another attempt at removal is made. Sometimes the wound must be converted to a T-shaped incision, with a radial cut extending anteriorly. During removal every attempt is made to minimize loss of vitreous gel. Vitreous is cleaned from the pars plana wound, and the wound is closed with interrupted 7/0 polyglycolate or 8/0 monofilament nylon sutures. We usually apply prophylactic 360° cryotherapy to the peripheral retina and place a peripheral encircling band, as described below, to prevent later retinal detachment. The conjunctiva is closed, and subconjunctival antibiotic solution is injected.

A small or medium-sized magnetic foreign body embedded in the retina and choroid at or anterior to the equator, or sometimes even slightly posterior to the equator, is best removed through the eyewall with a magnet. The position of the foreign body is localized on the external

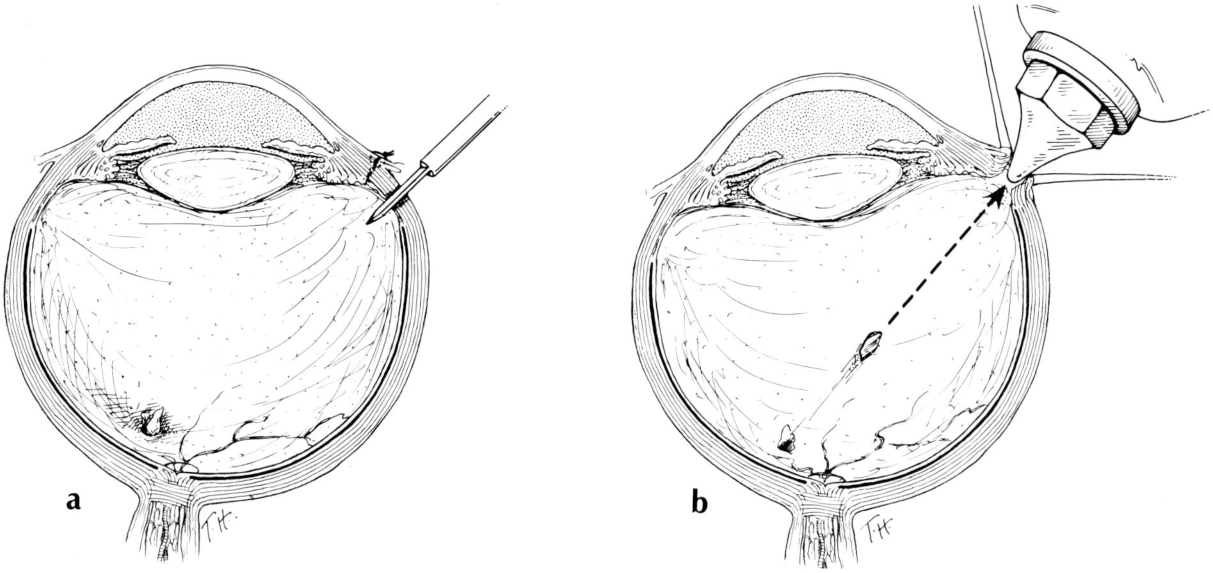

Figure 13.21 *Removal of intraocular magnetic foreign body through a pars plana incision with hand-held electromagnet.* **(a)** *After closure of the anterior entry site wound, a circumferentially oriented pars plana incision is made with a sharp knife.* **(b)** *A preplaced suture through the incision is looped out of the wound, and traction is applied to the sutures to open the wound. The hand-held electromagnet removes the magnetic foreign body. The wound is then closed*

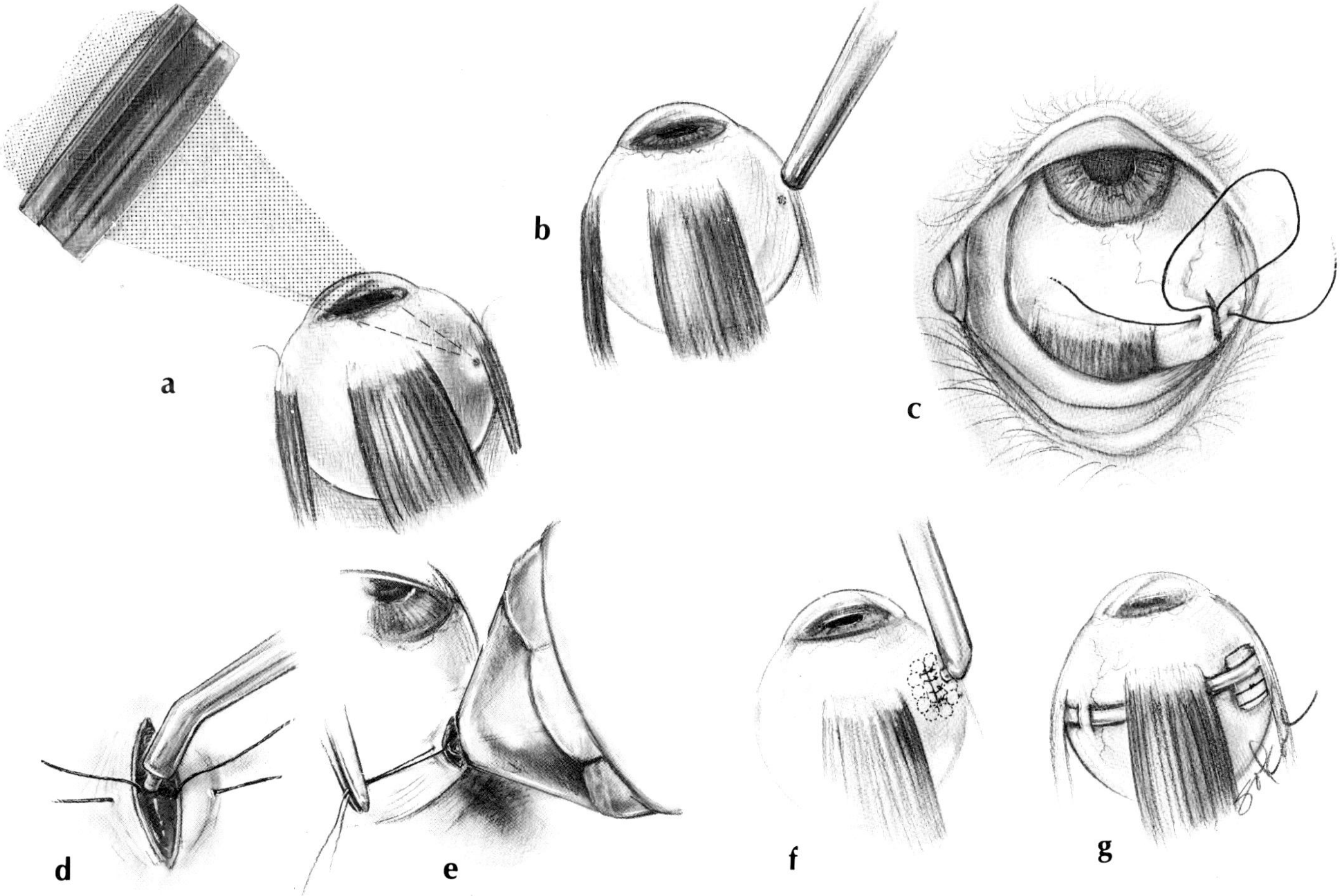

Figure 13.22 *Removal of a magnetic foreign body embedded in the midperipheral retina through the eyewall.* **(a)** *Foreign body is localized externally by transillumination .* **(b)** *Foreign body is localized externally with an electronic metal-localizing instrument.* **(c)** *Scleral incision over the foreign body with a preplaced suture.* **(d)** *Bare choroid is treated with diathermy.* **(e)** *Hand-held electromagnet pulls foreign body through choroid.* **(f)** *Wound is closed with interrupted sutures, and cryotherapy is applied around the retinal hole.* **(g)** *The retinal hole is buckled with a radial silicone sponge with an overlying encircling band*

sclera by transillumination (*Figure 13.22a*). Transillumination can be achieved by having the surgical assistant use an indirect ophthalmoscope and viewing lens to look at the foreign body in the eye. The foreign body casts a shadow visible on the sclera externally, and this position is marked. The foreign body can also be localized by indirect ophthalmoscopy with a scleral-depressor or a metal-localizing instrument (*Figure 13.22b*). If the foreign body is small, a small radial scleral incision is made external to the foreign body down to bare choroid, and a 6/0 silk suture is placed through the scleral lips (*Figure 13.22c*). The underlying choroid is treated with diathermy to close all choroidal vessels (*Figure 13.22d*). The suture in the incision is looped out and held with non-magnetic forceps on each side to draw the wound edges apart. The electromagnet tip is held against the choroid and the magnet is activated to pull the foreign body out through the choroid (*Figure 13.22e*). The wound is closed with multiple interrupted sutures after tying the preplaced suture. One row of external cryotherapy is applied around the retinal hole, monitoring the freezes internally with ophthalmoscopy (*Figure 13.22f*). One row of prophylactic cryotherapy is also usually applied for 360° to the peripheral retina just posterior to the ora serrata, and a prophylactic encircling band is placed around the eye with the anterior portion of this band 2.5–3.0 mm posterior to the ora serrata. An encircling band in this position buckles and supports the posterior vitreous base. A split-thickness, radially oriented silicone sponge is placed to buckle the retinal hole at the sclerotomy, with the anterior part of the sponge beneath the encircling band and the posterior part indented by a horizontal mattress suture (*Figure 13.22g*).

If the foreign body is medium-sized and to be removed through the sclera, it is better to make a rectangular or triangular half-thickness scleral trapdoor incision with preplaced sutures in it. In the bed of this scleral flap the sclera is incised, the choroid treated and the foreign body removed. Closure using a scleral flap after removal of a medium-sized foreign body usually is more secure than can be achieved with a simple full-thickness incision.

Removal of intraocular foreign bodies with vitreous surgery

Vitreous surgery is used to remove: (*1*) accessible non-magnetic foreign bodies; (*2*) some magnetic foreign bodies with severe vitreous hemorrhage; (*3*) magnetic foreign bodies embedded or encapsulated in the posterior retina that cannot be pulled free with a magnet; and (*4*) large magnetic foreign bodies in a phakic eye. Occasionally a non-magnetic foreign body embedded in the peripheral retina or pars plana that is inaccessible to removal by vitreous surgery can be removed through the eyewall. The technique used is similar to that described above for removing a magnetic foreign body through the eyewall except, of course, a magnet cannot be used to pull the foreign body from the eye. Instead, after cutting down to the choroid and treating the choroid with diathermy, a cut is made through the choroid, and pressure is applied to the globe to raise the intraocular pressure and express the foreign body through the incision.

Usually, however, vitreous surgery is used to remove non-magnetic foreign bodies and those magnetic foreign bodies described above. In an eye with clear media and no significant open wound, it is desirable to apply preoperative laser treatment to the retina and choroid around the foreign body. This eliminates the need for applying posterior transscleral cryotherapy or other intraoperative treatment to create a chorioretinal adhesion around the retinal hole. Laser treatment around the foreign body is applied as one or two confluent rows of moderate-intensity 500 μm burns.

To remove an intraocular foreign body using vitreous surgery, the corneal or anterior wound is closed watertight (*Figure 13.23a,b*). An infusion cannula is placed through the pars plana if using the Ocutome system. If a cataract is present, it is removed through the pars plana using the ultrasonic fragmenting and aspirating instrument (*Figure 13.23c*). The vitrectomy instrument is used to remove the vitreous gel which may contain blood (*Figure 13.23d*). In particular, the vitreous tract through which the foreign body passed is removed to prevent growth of fibrous tissue along this tract and resulting anterior-to-posterior traction. If the foreign body is encapsulated, a dissecting pick is used to open the capsule. Occasionally, if a magnetic foreign body has passed through the retina to a subretinal position adjacent to the retinal hole, a miniaturized intraocular magnet with a 20 gauge probe tip is inserted into the eye and used to 'tease' the foreign body back out of the hole. Once the foreign body is freed from its posterior attachments, a traction suture is placed through the incision to facilitate opening the lips of the wound, and the pars plana wound is enlarged circumferentially from its original 20 gauge size to a size large enough to allow extraction of the foreign body (*Figure 13.23e,f*). Intraocular forceps, chosen so that they are the correct size for grasping the foreign body, are introduced into the eye. The foreign body is grasped and removed (*Figure 13.23g,h*), and the pars plana wound is closed (*Figure 13.23i*). If the foreign body is very large, it may be necessary to remove it through a limbal incision after first removing the crystalline lens.

Although damage from the foreign body itself may produce enough irritation to cause a chorioretinal scar sealing the retinal hole, it is desirable to insure a good adhesion with some form of treatment. Preoperative laser treatment, as mentioned, can be used. Intraoperative endocryotherapy or endophotocoagulation can be used just before or after removing the foreign body with forceps. External (transscleral) cryopexy can be applied after the foreign body is removed, although this is dangerous for very posterior foreign bodies because it can result in accidental treatment of the macula or optic nerve.

If there is localized retinal detachment around the retinal hole, or any suggestion that it might occur, a fluid-air exchange is done, as described in Chapter 8, to place a large air bubble in the vitreous cavity. The patient is positioned face-down postoperatively to use the bubble to tamponade and flatten the retinal hole. It is also advisable to apply 360° prophylactic peripheral cryopexy and a peripheral encircling silicone band around the eye to prevent later peripheral retinal detachment.

A foreign body in the vitreous gel is usually easier to remove. The foreign body is grasped in the vitreous and extracted after removing overlying and adherent vitreous gel with a vitrectomy instrument.

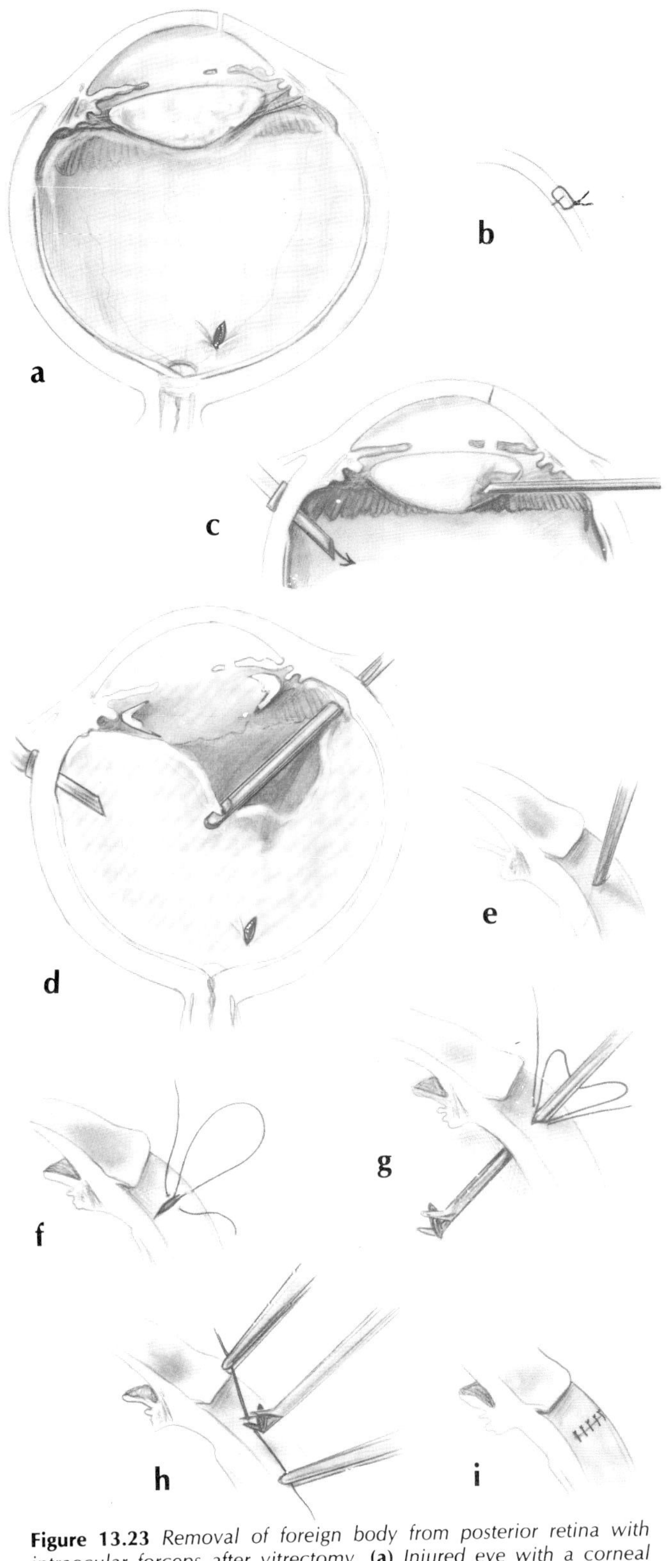

Figure 13.23 *Removal of foreign body from posterior retina with intraocular forceps after vitrectomy.* **(a)** *Injured eye with a corneal wound, cataract, and a foreign body embedded in the retina.* **(b)** *Corneal wound closed.* **(c)** *Cataract removed with ultrasonic fragmenting instrument.* **(d)** *Vitrectomy removes vitreous gel including the vitreous tract of foreign body.* **(e)** *Entry site enlarged with sharp knife.* **(f)** *Traction suture placed through pars plana entry site.* **(g)** *Foreign body grasped by intraocular forceps.* **(h)** *Foreign body removed.* **(i)** *Sclerotomy site closed*

Vitrectomy and retinal reattachment surgery for penetrating wounds through the retina

Penetrating injuries through the retina have a poor prognosis even with vitreous surgery. Less severe, smaller wounds, especially if they are in the anterior retina, can often be repaired and vision salvaged. The types of wounds that are seen and their associated injuries are variable. Wounds may result from a scleral rupture, a laceration that extends posteriorly or a double-penetrating injury with an anterior entry site and a posterior exit site. Most eyes have opaque media due to corneal opacity, cataract, vitreous hemorrhage, or a combination of these, but occasionally the media are clear. The retina can be attached despite a large retinal hole, especially if the patient is young and has non-liquefied vitreous gel. In other eyes the retina is detached. Most eyes with these wounds require vitreoretinal surgery if they are to be salvaged.

Prophylactic scleral buckling in eyes with penetrating injury

Prophylactic scleral buckling surgery is used for certain eyes that are at high risk of developing retinal detachment after injury. These include eyes with attached retina that have: (*1*) clear media and scleral laceration anterior to the ora serrata with massive vitreous loss and traction; (*2*) a scleral laceration posterior to the ora serrata; or (*3*) foreign bodies removed from the posterior segment.

If an eye has a corneoscleral laceration with vitreous loss, the wound is repaired, the lens is removed if a cataract is present, and an anterior vitrectomy is performed to remove vitreous if vitreous is incarcerated in the wound. Even with vitrectomy, some vitreous often remains incarcerated anteriorly and exerts traction on the vitreous base (*Figure 13.24a*). This traction can cause a peripheral traction retinal detachment or a peripheral retinal break and rhegmatogenous detachment. Such eyes are prophylactically treated with 360° of peripheral retinal cryopexy and an encircling silicone band or buckle at the time of the primary repair (*Figure 13.24b*). This treatment lessens the chance of later rhegmatogenous retinal detachment.

A prophylactic scleral buckle should be used in eyes in which there is scleral laceration involving the retina but in which no retinal detachment is present. In rare instances, an eye with a scleral laceration extending posterior to the ora serrata may have clear enough media after wound closure to allow ophthalmoscopic visualization of retinal and vitreous incarceration in the internal aspect of the wound (*Figure 13.25a*). One row of external cryotherapy is applied around the wound under direct visualization, and cryotherapy is applied in one or two contiguous rows just posterior to the ora serrata elsewhere (*Figure 13.25b*). A split-thickness, radially oriented silicone sponge is placed over the laceration with an encircling band around the eye. Mattress sutures indent the posterior portion of the sponge and the anterior portion is indented by the overlying encircling band (*Figure 13.25c,d*). The encircling band is held in position by scleral tunnels (belt-loops) or

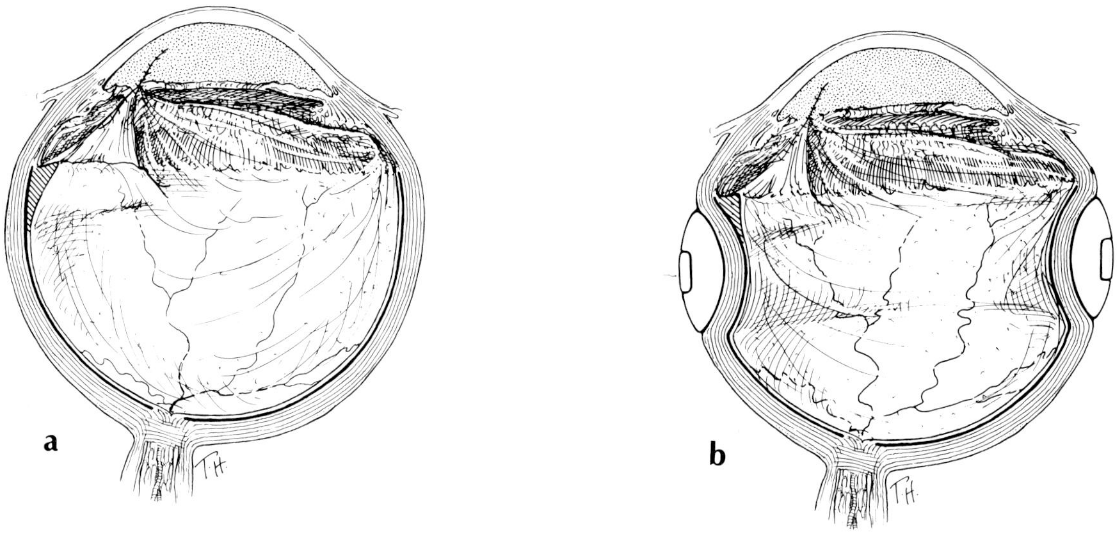

Figure 13.24 *Placement of prophylactic cryotherapy and encircling scleral buckle in an eye with vitreous traction.* **(a)** *Anterior corneoscleral wound not involving the retina is closed. Vitreous incarceration and vitreous traction on the peripheral retina remains.* **(b)** *Prophylactic encircling buckle placed, after 360° cryotherapy, to prevent rhegmatogenous retinal detachment*

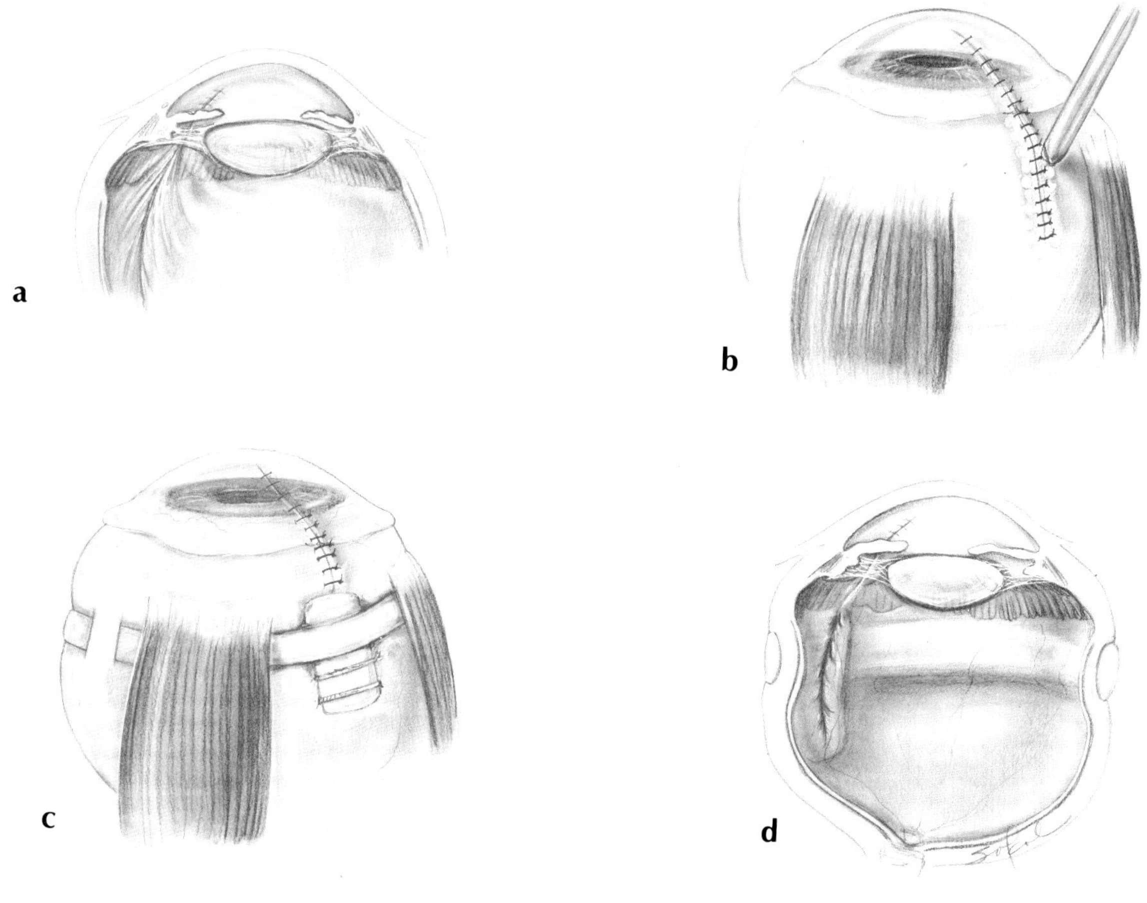

Figure 13.25 *Prophylactic buckling of scleral laceration involving the retina but without retinal detachment.* **(a)** *Corneoscleral laceration extending into the retina after external closure. Vitreous and retina are incarcerated in the wound.* **(b)** *Cryotherapy is applied around the wound posterior to the ora serrata and to the peripheral retina for 360°.* **(c)** *An encircling band is placed with a radially oriented, silicone sponge over the laceration.* **(d)** *Internal view of eye after scleral buckling*

sutures. Lacerations oriented differently are supported by other types of scleral buckles.

In an eye with a cataract or vitreous hemorrhage (as is usually the case), it is necessary to perform a lensectomy, vitrectomy or both before applying cryotherapy and a scleral buckle to treat the retinal break. For example, pars plana vitrectomy is used to remove vitreous hemorrhage (*Figure 13.26a*). If there is a posterior vitreous separation, cortical vitreous is removed where possible. Vitreous will remain incarcerated in the wound, however, and vitreous extending to this wound is cut with the vitrectomy instrument to lessen vitreous traction (*Figure 13.26b*). Tangential traction from vitreous running along the retinal surface and into the wound is gently isolated with a dissecting pick (*Figure 13.26c*) and cut with the vitrectomy instrument (*Figure 13.26d*). Not all such vitreous can be safely removed, but the goal is to eliminate as much traction as possible. Excessive pulling on the vitreous and the edge of the retinal wound is avoided to try to prevent opening the edge of the retinal laceration, which will cause rhegmatogenous retinal detachment. Cryotherapy is applied around the laceration (*Figure 13.26e*) and to the peripheral retina for 360°. An encircling buckle is placed around the eye to support the retinal break (*Figure 13.26f*).

In double-penetrating injuries it is not always necessary or advisable to close the posterior wound if the wound is small and self-sealing. Attempts to close the scleral wound externally can result in loss of intraocular tissue or bleeding. A posterior scleral wound in such eyes therefore is not closed externally. Laser treatment, transvitreal cryopexy or endophotocoagulation is used around the retinal hole internally, and an air bubble is placed in the eye. Vigorous attempts at peeling non-detached posterior cortical vitreous from the retinal surface are avoided to lessen the chance of causing retinal detachment, although as much vitreous gel as possible, including the tract of injury through the gel, is removed. Prophylactic cryotherapy and an encircling band are placed around the eye. If there is significant residual traction on the posterior retinal wound and the wound is accessible on the external sclera and can be closed first, a radial buckle of silicone sponge can be placed to support the retinal break after cryotherapy.

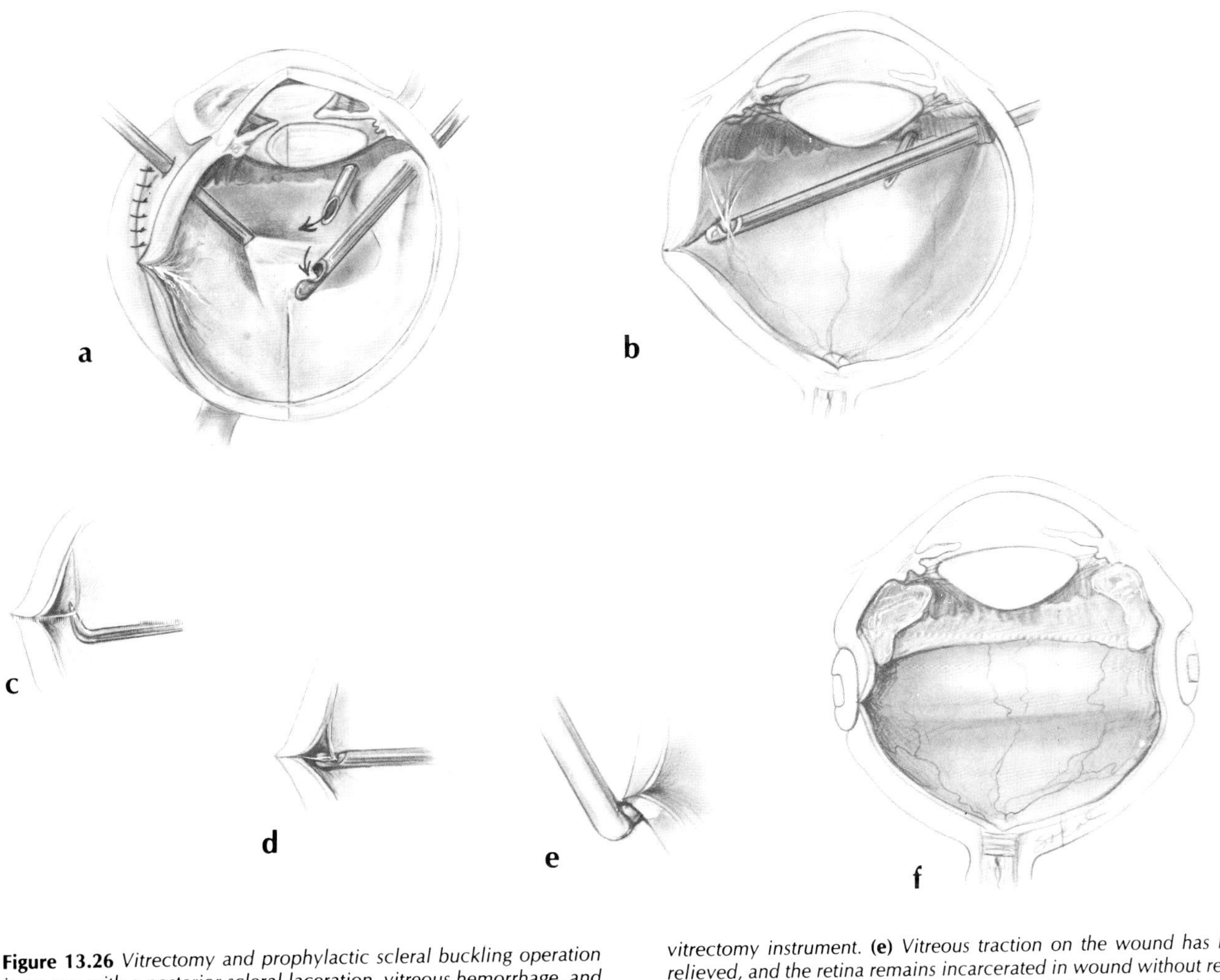

Figure 13.26 *Vitrectomy and prophylactic scleral buckling operation in an eye with a posterior scleral laceration, vitreous hemorrhage, and laceration involving the retina without a retinal detachment.* **(a)** *Vitrectomy removes opaque vitreous hemorrhage.* **(b)** *Vitreous strands extending to wound are cut.* **(c,d)** *Additional vitreous incarcerated in wound is gently elevated with a dissecting pick and removed with a vitrectomy instrument.* **(e)** *Vitreous traction on the wound has been relieved, and the retina remains incarcerated in wound without retinal detachment. Cryotherapy is applied around the wound and to the peripheral retina for 360°.* **(f)** *The wound and peripheral retina are supported on an encircling buckle*

Combined vitrectomy and retinal reattachment surgery for scleral laceration with retinal detachment

Vitrectomy is useful in the repair of eyes with retinal detachment resulting from a scleral laceration or rupture. It allows not only removal of opacities from the media but also the cutting of traction from vitreous or other tissue incarcerated in the wound. In addition, after vitrectomy, ancilliary techniques such as fluid-gas exchange increase the chance of reattaching the retina. Vitrectomy is useful in managing eyes with retinal detachment with anterior scleral wounds not extending posterior to the ora serrata or more posterior wounds involving the retina.

Figure 13.27a shows a posterior penetrating wound in which the scleral wound has been closed. Vitreous is incarcerated in the wound internally and exerts traction across the vitreous cavity. Retina is also incarcerated and an open retinal break near the wound causes a rhegmatogenous retinal detachment. A vitrectomy instrument is first used to remove hemorrhagic vitreous gel and vitreous strands extending to the wound (*Figure 13.27b*). If the posterior cortical vitreous is separated from the detached retina, it can be removed; but, if not, removal from detached retina is too hazardous and is not attempted because of the risk of cutting the adherent, detached retina. After removing the vitreous, transvitreal drainage of subretinal fluid is sometimes performed using a 'vacuum-cleaner' needle. The blunt needle tip is passed through the retinal break, and subretinal fluid is removed. This may be performed simultaneously with fluid-air exchange, which removes vitreous fluid and replaces it with air that is injected through the infusion cannula (*Figure 13.27c* and see *Figure 8.38*). The injected air flattens the retinal break against the choroid. Cryotherapy is applied externally around the retinal break and treatment is also applied to the peripheral retina for 360° (*Figure 13.27d*). The posterior laceration is buckled with a split-thickness, radially oriented silicone sponge, and the peripheral retina is buckled with a silicone band for 360°. Postoperatively, the patient is positioned face-down to keep the air bubble up against the retinal break to tamponade and flatten it (*Figure 13.27e*).

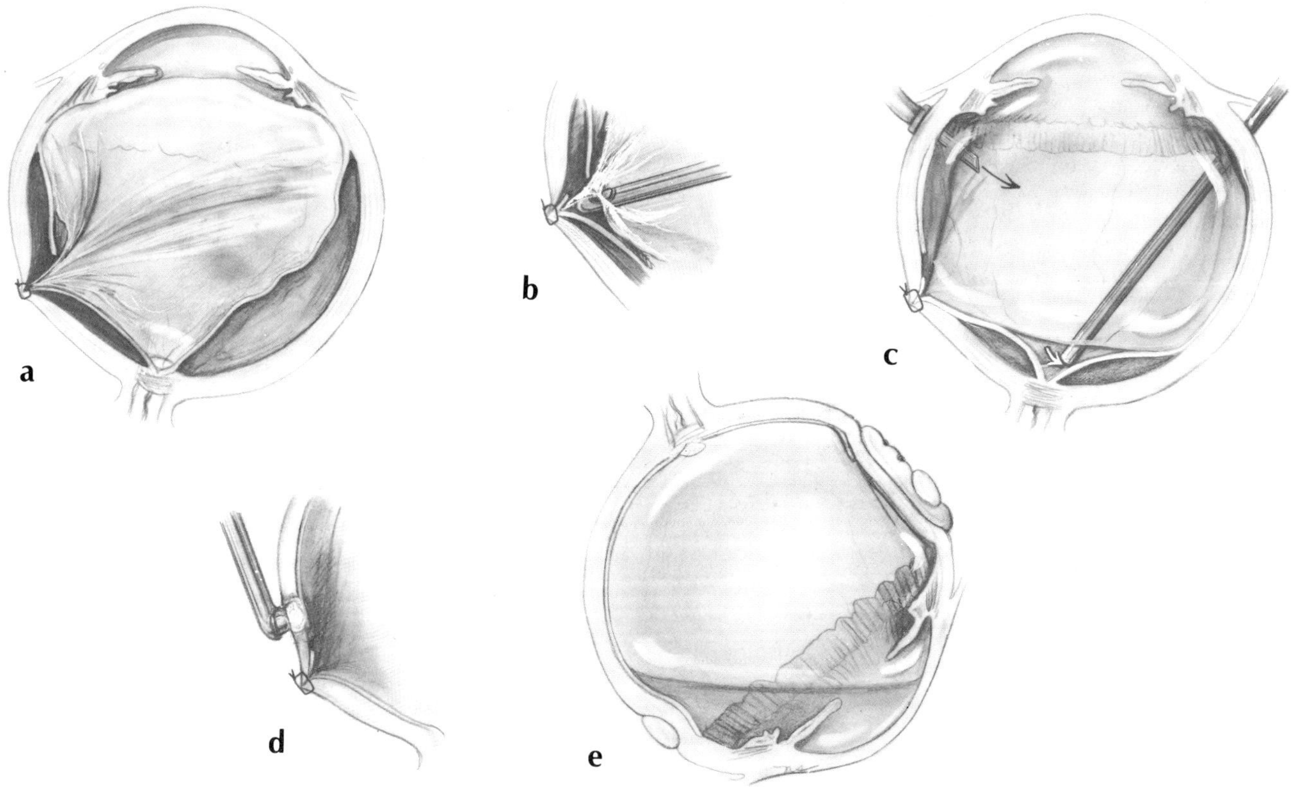

Figure 13.27 *Vitrectomy, intraocular gas and scleral buckling in an eye with a posterior scleral laceration and retinal detachment.* **(a)** *Eye with lacerated, detached retina after external closure of a scleral laceration. Vitreous and the posterior edge of the retinal laceration are incarcerated in the wound.* **(b)** *Vitrectomy removes vitreous gel and vitreous extending to wound.* **(c)** *Fluid-gas exchange performed, filling vitreous cavity with air and flattening the retinal break against the choroid.* **(d)** *Cryotherapy applied around flattened retinal break. Cryotherapy is also applied to the peripheral retina for 360°.* **(e)** *Laceration is buckled with a radially oriented, silicone sponge, and the peripheral retina is buckled with an encircling band. Patient is positioned face-down postoperatively to use bubble to flatten and tamponade the retinal break*

Postoperative care

Postoperative care after surgery for traumatic injury is similar to that used after intraocular or retinal reattachment surgery. The operated eye is protected with an eye shield from accidental postoperative trauma that might rupture a sutured wound. In an eye with a penetrating wound, the intravenous broad-spectrum antibiotics that were administered prophylactically before surgery are continued postoperatively to complete at least a 5-day course of treatment. Topical steroid and antibiotic drops are administered and topical cycloplegic drops may also be used if appropriate.

The patient's vision is checked daily after surgery to detect worsening; and in eyes with poor vision, light perception and light projection are checked. In eyes that have had trauma involving the posterior segment, the fundus is examined to make certain the retina remains attached. When the fundus cannot be seen because of vitreous hemorrhage or other opacity, ultrasonography is performed to detect retinal detachment.

Reoperations may be necessary. For example, if an eye that had simple closure of a scleral laceration with no preoperative retinal detachment later develops retinal detachment, vitrectomy and retinal reattachment surgery may be necessary. Other types of reoperations may also be necessary for other postoperative problems or complications.

Enucleation is indicated before 2 weeks after severe injury if there is no light perception or there is bare light perception and no chance of salvaging the eye. This lessens the chance of sympathetic ophthalmia[17]. Sometimes a severely injured eye with poor light perception and a retinal detachment on ultrasonography can have an 'exploratory' vitrectomy to determine the extent of intraocular damage, and enucleation can be performed at the same operation if the eye cannot be repaired.

Complications

In eyes with extensive traumatic injuries, it is often difficult to differentiate a preoperative or postoperative complication from damage produced by the original injury itself. Definite complications occur, however, and some are preventable. An eye with an open wound can have extrusion of intraocular contents as a result of external pressure or choroidal hemorrhage. To prevent this, open wounds should be closed promptly, with re-establishment of a normal intraocular pressure. Lacerations or tears of the extraocular muscles or periocular scarring from injury or surgery can cause strabismus, and damage to an extraocular muscle should be repaired. Corneal bloodstaining, usually associated with glaucoma, results from blood in the anterior chamber. If early corneal bloodstaining is detected, surgery should be done to remove the anterior chamber blood and reduce the intraocular pressure. Secondary glaucoma can develop from a variety of causes and should be treated medically, or surgically, if indicated. Phthisis bulbi is a frequent result of severe ocular trauma and usually occurs in an irreparably damaged eye with ciliary body injury, cyclitic membranes or retinal detachment. Successful retinal reattachment in some eyes may prevent phthisis bulbi.

Later retinal detachment is a frequent complication in traumatically injured eyes. Detachment results from unrecognized retinal breaks, posterior vitreous separation with production of new retinal breaks, vitreous traction, fibrous traction bands that pull on the retina, traumatic macular holes, and other causes. Retinal detachment can be prevented in some eyes by vitrectomy to remove or prevent vitreous traction, prophylactic scleral buckling, or both. If a retinal detachment occurs, surgery can successfully reattach the retina in some eyes.

A retained intraocular foreign body can be the source of endophthalmitis or can cause progressive physical damage. If a reactive foreign body is not removed from the eye, it may also produce metalosis or severe inflammation. Because of these potential dangers, we attempt to remove most intraocular foreign bodies. Removal may be more difficult if delayed for several weeks if the foreign body becomes encapsulated. For this reason earlier removal is preferred.

Sympathetic ophthalmia is a feared complication in patients that have had a penetrating eye injury or a ruptured globe. Because vitreous surgery allows some badly damaged eyes to be saved so that enucleation is unnecessary, there is a risk of sympathetic ophthalmia in these patients. The risk is low enough, so that a severely injured eye with potential for visual recovery should not be removed[20]. Nevertheless every attempt should be made to determine if such eyes cannot be saved so that if not, they can be removed within 2 weeks of the injury.

Endophthalmitis can occur in any eye with a penetrating injury or rupture. Prompt removal of necrotic tissue and foreign bodies, and closure of wounds reduces the risk of infection. If there is any suspicion of infection at the time of primary repair, aqueous and vitreous samples should be taken for culture and microscopic examination[21]. Prophylactic intravenous broad-spectrum antibiotics are given as previously described. If signs of endophthalmitis develop postoperatively, prompt vitreous and aqueous aspirations are performed to obtain specimens, and the type of antibiotic treatment is reassessed. Vitrectomy and intravitreal antibiotics[22] may be used in the management of overt endophthalmitis.

Results

The prognosis for recovery of vision after injury depends on both the severity of the injury and the surgical management of the injury. Many eyes with severe trauma have no chance of recovering vision; however, microsurgical techniques have improved the repair of anterior segment injuries, and vitreous surgery has improved the management of both anterior and posterior segment injuries.

Comparison of surgical results from different published studies has limited validity because of the diversity of injuries treated and the variation in their surgical management in the different studies. It is clear that injuries involving only the anterior segment have a better prognosis than those involving the vitreous and retina. In one series, 87 per cent of eyes with penetrating injury confined to the cornea and lens achieved 20/40 visual acuity[23]. For eyes with posterior segment penetrating injuries managed without vitreous surgery, only 13 per cent achieved 20/40 visual acuity[23,24]. By using vitreous surgery when indicated for posterior segment injuries, the percentage of eyes recovering 20/40 or better vision increased from 28 per cent[25] in one study to 44 per cent[19] in another study. The percentage of such eyes recovering a lower but 'functional' level of vision in various studies ranged from 49 per cent to 78 per cent[9,18,25,26].

Summary

Management of ocular trauma requires a thorough preoperative evaluation, meticulous surgery performed in a logical stepwise fashion, management of postoperative complications, and often one or more reoperations. Microsurgical techniques together with vitreous surgery allow a high proportion of eyes with anterior segment injury to be salvaged. The chance of achieving functional vision in eyes with posterior segment injuries is not as good but has improved with the use of vitreous surgery.

References

1. Cleary, P. E., Ryan, S. J. Method of production and natural history of experimental posterior penetrating eye injury in the rhesus monkey. American Journal of Ophthalmology 1979; 88:212–220
2. Cleary, P. E., Ryan, S. J. Vitrectomy in penetrating eye injury: results of a controlled trial of vitrectomy in an experimental posterior penetrating eye injury in the rhesus monkey. Archives of Ophthalmology 1981; 99:287–292
3. Topping, T. M., Abrams, G. W., Machemer, R. Experimental double-perforating injury of the posterior segment in rabbit eyes: the natural history of intraocular proliferation. Archives of Ophthalmology 1979; 97:735–742
4. Abrams, G. W., Topping, T. M., Machemer, R. Vitrectomy for injury: The effect on intraocular proliferation following perforation of the posterior segment of the rabbit eye. Archives of Ophthalmology 1979; 97:743–748
5. Cox, M. S., Freeman, H. M. Retinal detachment due to ocular penetration. I. Clinical characteristics and surgical results. Archives of Ophthalmology 1978; 96:1354–1361
6. Hughes, W. E. Alkali burns of the eye. I. Review of the literature and summary of present knowledge. Archives of Ophthalmology 1946; 35:423–449
7. Hirst, L. W., Stark, W. J., Jensen, A. D. Tissue adhesives: new perspectives in corneal perforations. Ophthalmic Surgery 1979; 10:58–64
8. Keeney, A. H. Intralenticular foreign bodies. Archives of Ophthalmology 1971; 86:499–501
9. Goldberg, M. F. Sickled erythrocytes, hyphema, and secondary glaucoma. I. The diagnosis and treatment of sickled erythrocytes in human hyphemas. Ophthalmic Surgery 1979; 10:17–31
10. McCuen, B. W., Fung, W. E. The role of vitrectomy instrumentation in the treatment of severe traumatic hyphema. American Journal of Ophthalmology 1979; 88:930–934
11. Diddie, K. R., Ernest, J. T. Rotoextractor evacuation of total hyphema. Ophthalmic Surgery 1976; 7:49–51
12. Stern, W. H., Mondal, K. M. Vitrectomy instrumentation for surgical evacuation of total anterior chamber hyphema and control of recurrent anterior chamber hemorrhage. Ophthalmic Surgery 1979; 10:34–37
13. Radius, R. L., Finkelstein, D. Central retinal artery occlusion (reversible) in sickle trait with glaucoma. British Journal of Ophthalmology 1976; 60:428–430
14. Paterson, C. A., Pfister, R. R., Levinson, R. A. Aqueous humor pH changes after experimental alkali burns. American Journal of Ophthalmology 1975; 79:414–419
15. Pfister, R. R., Paterson, C. A. Additional clinical and morphological observations on the favorable effect of ascorbate in experimental ocular alkali burns. Investigative Ophthalmology and Visual Science 1977; 16:478–487
16. Pfister, R. R., Paterson, C. A., Hayes, S. A. Topical ascorbate decreases the incidence of corneal ulceration after experimental alkali burns. Investigative Ophthalmology and Visual Science 1978; 17:1019–1024
17. Joy, H. H. A survey of cases of sympathetic ophthalmia occurring in New York State. Archives of Ophthalmology 1935; 14: 733–741
18. Ryan, S. J., Allen, A. W. Pars plana vitrectomy in ocular trauma. American Journal of Ophthalmology 1979; 88:483–491
19. Coleman, D. J. Early vitrectomy in the management of the severely traumatized eye. American Journal of Ophthalmology 1982; 93:543–551
20. Allen, J. C. Sympathetic ophthalmia: A disappearing disease. Journal of the American Medical Association 1969; 209:1090
21. Forster, R. K., Zachary, I. G., Cottingham, A. J., Norton, E. W. D. Further observations on the diagnosis, cause and treatment of endophthalmitis. American Journal of Ophthalmology 1976; 81:52–56
22. Forster, R. K., Abbot, R. I., Gelender, H. Management of infectious endophthalmitis. Ophthalmology 1980; 87:313
23. Eagling, E. M. Perforating injuries of the eye. British Journal of Ophthalmology 1976; 60:732–736
24. Adhikary, H. P., Taylor, P., Fitzmaurice, D. J. Prognosis of perforating eye injury. British Journal of Ophthalmology 1976; 60:737–739
25. Brinton, G. S., Aaberg, T. M., Reeser, F. H., Topping, T. M., Abrams, G. W. Surgical results in ocular trauma involving the posterior segment. American Journal of Ophthalmology 1982; 93:271–278
26. Hutton, W. L., Snyder, W. B., Vaiser, A. Vitrectomy in the treatment of ocular perforating injuries. American Journal of Ophthalmology 1976; 81:733–739

Index